WHO Classification of Tum

Haematolymphoid Tumours

Part B

WHO Classification of Tumours Editorial Board

International Agency for Research on Cancer

World Health Organization

Suggested citation
WHO Classification of Tumours Editorial Board. Haematolymphoid tumours.
Lyon (France): International Agency for Research on Cancer; 2024.
(WHO classification of tumours series, 5th ed.; vol. 11).
https://publications.iarc.who.int/637.

Sales, rights, and permissions
Print copies are distributed by WHO Press, World Health Organization, 20 Avenue Appia, 1211 Geneva 27, Switzerland
Tel.: +41 22 791 3264; Fax: +41 22 791 4857; email: bookorders@who.int; website: https://whobluebooks.iarc.who.int/

To purchase IARC publications in electronic format, see the IARC Publications website (https://publications.iarc.who.int).

Requests for permission to reproduce or translate IARC publications – whether for sale or for non-commercial distribution – should be submitted through the IARC Publications website (https://publications.iarc.who.int/Rights-And-Permissions).

First print run (12 500 copies)

Updated corrigenda can be found at https://publications.iarc.who.int

IARC Library Cataloguing-in-Publication Data
Names: WHO Classification of Tumours Editorial Board.
Title: Haematolymphoid tumours / edited by WHO Classification of Tumours Editorial Board.
Description: Fifth edition. | Lyon: International Agency for Research on Cancer, 2024. | Series: World Health Organization classification of tumours. | Includes bibliographical references and index.
Identifiers: ISBN 9789283245209 (pbk.) | ISBN 9789283245216 (ebook)
Subjects: MESH: Hematologic Neoplasms – classification. | Lymphoma – classification.
Classification: NLM WH 490

The WHO classification of haematolymphoid tumours presented in this book reflects the views of the WHO Classification of Tumours Editorial Board that convened via video conference from 30 March to 1 April 2022, as well as subsequent consultation.

The WHO Classification of Tumours Editorial Board

The molecular data presented in this volume was provided with support from the
Compendium of Cancer Genome Aberrations (CCGA)

www.ccga.io

For the complete list of all contributors and their affiliations, see pages 815–833.

The WHO Classification of Tumours Editorial Board (continued)

Standing members

For the complete list of all contributors and their affiliations, see pages 815–833.

WHO Classification of Tumours

Haematolymphoid Tumours

Edited by	The WHO Classification of Tumours Editorial Board
IARC Editors	Faiq Ahmed Ian A. Cree Daphne de Jong Anil Felix Angelo Fonseca Gabrielle Goldman-Lévy Dilani Lokuhetty
Project Assistant	Asiedua Asante
Assistant	Anne-Sophie Bres
Production Editor Editorial Consultancy	Jessica Cox Julia Slone-Murphy
Principal Information Assistant Information Assistant	Alberto Machado Catarina Marques
Layout	Meaghan Fortune Catarina Marques
Printed by	Omnibook 74370 Argonay, France
Publisher	International Agency for Research on Cancer (IARC) 25 Av. Tony Garnier, CS 90627 69366 Lyon, CEDEX 07, France

Contents

Please note that the contents of this volume have been split into two parts for publication in print: Part A (in the accompanying book) and Part B (in this book).

List of abbreviations

3D	three-dimensional
ATP	adenosine triphosphate
BL-IPI	Burkitt Lymphoma International Prognostic Index
bp	base pair
CI	confidence interval
CMV	cytomegalovirus
CNS	central nervous system
CT	computed tomography
CXR	chest X-ray
DNA	deoxyribonucleic acid
EBV	Epstein–Barr virus
ELN	European LeukemiaNet
ESR	erythrocyte sedimentation rate
EUS-FNAB	endoscopic ultrasound–guided fine-needle aspiration biopsy
EWOG-MDS	European Working Group of Myelodysplastic Syndrome
FDG	18F-fluorodeoxyglucose
FISH	fluorescence in situ hybridization
FNA	fine-needle aspiration
FNAB	fine-needle aspiration biopsy
FNAC	fine-needle aspiration cytology
GHSG	German Hodgkin Study Group
H&E	haematoxylin and eosin stain
HBV	hepatitis B virus
HCV	hepatitis C virus
HIV	human immunodeficiency virus
HPF	high-power field
HPV	human papillomavirus
HRS cell	Hodgkin/Reed–Sternberg cell
HRS-like cell	Hodgkin/Reed–Sternberg–like cell
HTLV-1	human T-lymphotropic virus type 1
IARC	International Agency for Research on Cancer
ICD-11	International Classification of Diseases, 11th revision
ICD-O	International Classification of Diseases for Oncology
IMWG	International Myeloma Working Group
kb	kilobase
kDa	kilodalton
KSHV/HHV8	Kaposi sarcoma–associated herpesvirus / human herpesvirus 8
M:F ratio	male-to-female ratio
MIM number	Mendelian Inheritance in Man number
MRI	magnetic resonance imaging
mRNA	messenger ribonucleic acid
N:C ratio	nuclear-to-cytoplasmic ratio
NCI	Untied States National Cancer Institute
NK cell	natural killer cell
NOS	not otherwise specified
NSAID	non-steroidal anti-inflammatory drug
Pap	Papanicolaou stain
PAS staining	periodic acid–Schiff staining
PCR	polymerase chain reaction
PET	positron emission tomography
PET-CT	positron emission tomography–computed tomography
RNA	ribonucleic acid
RT-PCR	reverse transcription polymerase chain reaction
SEER Program	Surveillance, Epidemiology, and End Results Program
SNP	single-nucleotide polymorphism
SNV	single-nucleotide variant
TNM	tumour, node, metastasis
TNMB	tumour, node, metastasis, blood

Foreword

The WHO Classification of Tumours is a taxonomy of cancer, published as a series of books (also known as the WHO Blue Books) and now as a website (https://tumourclassification.iarc.who.int). It is an essential tool for standardizing diagnostic practice worldwide. It also serves as a vehicle for the translation of cancer research into practice. The diagnostic criteria and standards that make up the classification are underpinned by evidence evaluated and debated by experts in the field. More than 400 authors and editors participated in the production of this volume, and they gave their time freely to this task. We are very grateful for their help; it is a remarkable international team effort of great significance to both patients and their doctors.

This volume of the fifth edition of the WHO Blue Books has been a considerable challenge for all involved. It has been completely rewritten and reorganized, so it has taken more than 18 months to produce. Along the way we have had many excellent scientific discussions, and we hope that the final product meets with your approval. Classifications evolve over time, and there will be an opportunity in the next edition to make changes on the basis of new evidence. This volume has been coordinated as much as possible with other later fifth-edition WHO Classification of Tumours volumes, although there may still be some differences between volumes.

This volume, like the rest of the fifth edition, has been led by the WHO Classification of Tumours Editorial Board, composed of standing and expert members. The standing members, who have been nominated by pathology organizations, are the equivalent of the series editors of previous editions. The expert members for each volume, equivalent to the volume editors of previous editions, are selected on the basis of informed bibliometric analysis and advice from the standing members. The diagnostic process is increasingly multidisciplinary, and we are delighted that several radiology and clinical experts have joined us to address specific needs.

The most conspicuous change to the format of the books in the fifth edition is that tumour types common to multiple systems are dealt with together. There is also a chapter on genetic tumour syndromes associated with haematolymphoid tumours.

We have attempted to take a more systematic approach to the multifaceted nature of tumour classification; each tumour type is described on the basis of its localization, clinical features, epidemiology, etiology, pathogenesis, histopathology, diagnostic molecular pathology, staging, and prognosis and prediction. We have also included information on macroscopic appearance and cytology, as well as essential and desirable diagnostic criteria. This standardized, modular approach makes it easier for the books to be accessible online, and it also enables us to call attention to areas in which there is little information, and where serious gaps in our knowledge remain to be addressed. Genetic disorders are of increasing importance to diagnosis in individual patients, and the study of these disorders has undoubtedly informed our understanding of tumour biology and behaviour over the past decade.

The organization of the WHO Blue Books content now follows the normal progression from benign to malignant – a break with the fourth edition, but one we hope will be welcome.

Table A Approximate number of fields per 1 mm^2 based on the field diameter and its corresponding area

Field diameter (mm)	Field area (mm^2)	Approximate number of fields per 1 mm^2
0.40	0.126	8
0.41	0.132	8
0.42	0.138	7
0.43	0.145	7
0.44	0.152	7
0.45	0.159	6
0.46	0.166	6
0.47	0.173	6
0.48	0.181	6
0.49	0.188	5
0.50	0.196	5
0.51	0.204	5
0.52	0.212	5
0.53	0.221	5
0.54	0.229	4
0.55	0.237	4
0.56	0.246	4
0.57	0.255	4
0.58	0.264	4
0.59	0.273	4
0.60	0.283	4
0.61	0.292	3
0.62	0.302	3
0.63	0.312	3
0.64	0.322	3
0.65	0.332	3
0.66	0.342	3
0.67	0.352	3
0.68	0.363	3
0.69	0.374	3

Most volumes are still organized by anatomical site (digestive system, breast, soft tissue and bone, etc.), and each tumour type is listed within a taxonomic classification that follows the format below, which helps to structure the books in a systematic manner:

Site: e.g. lung

Category: e.g. tumours

Family (class): e.g. papillomas

Type: e.g. bronchial papillomas

Subtype: e.g. glandular papilloma

For this volume, however, we have replaced sites by lineages (e.g. myeloid, lymphoid), and these serve as the headings for the chapters, within which the categories are further defined on the basis of differentiation (e.g. precursor B-cell neoplasms, mature B-cell neoplasms). Within each category, families are defined (e.g. marginal zone lymphoma), and finally tumour types (e.g. primary cutaneous marginal zone lymphoma, nodal marginal zone lymphoma).

The issue of whether a given tumour type represents a distinct entity rather than a subtype continues to exercise pathologists, and it is the topic of many publications in the literature. We continue to deal with this issue on a case-by-case basis, but we believe there are inherent rules that can be applied. For example, tumours in which multiple histological patterns contain shared truncal mutations are clearly of the same type, despite the differences in their appearance. Equally, genetic heterogeneity within the same tumour type may have implications for treatment. A small shift in terminology in the fifth edition is that the term "variant" in reference to a specific kind of tumour has been wholly superseded by "subtype", in an effort to more clearly differentiate this meaning from that of "variant" in reference to a genetic alteration. Genetic tumour syndromes associated with haematolymphoid tumours are addressed in a dedicated chapter at the end of the volume.

Another important change in this edition of the WHO Classification of Tumours series is the conversion of mitotic count from the traditional denominator of 10 HPF to a defined area expressed in mm^2 {836}. This serves to standardize the true area over which mitoses are enumerated, because different microscopes have high-power fields of different sizes. This change will also be helpful for anyone reporting using digital systems. The approximate number of fields per 1 mm^2 based on the field diameter and its corresponding area is presented in Table A.

We are continually working to improve the consistency and standards within the classification. In addition to having moved to the International System of Units (SI) for all mitotic counts, we have standardized genomic nomenclature by using Human Genome Variation Society (HGVS) notation. This includes the recent move in fusion gene notation to the separation of involved genes by a double colon (e.g. *BCR*::*ABL1*) {474}. We have also standardized our use of units of length, adopting the convention used by the International Collaboration on Cancer Reporting (https://www.iccr-cancer.org/) and the UK Royal College of Pathologists (https://www.rcpath.org/), so that the size of tumours is now given exclusively in millimetres (mm) rather than centimetres (cm). This is clearer, in our view, and avoids the use of decimal points – a common source of medical errors.

The WHO Blue Books are much appreciated by pathologists of all types, and they are of increasing importance to practitioners of other clinical disciplines involved in cancer management, as well as to researchers. We, along with the entire editorial board, certainly hope that the series will continue to meet the need for standards in diagnosis and to facilitate the translation of diagnostic research into practice worldwide. It is particularly important that cancers continue to be classified and diagnosed according to the same standards internationally so that patients can benefit from multicentre clinical trials, as well as from the results of local trials conducted on different continents.

Dr Ian A. Cree

Former Head, WHO Classification of Tumours Programme
International Agency for Research on Cancer

Dr Dilani Lokuhetty

Head, WHO Classification of Tumours Programme
International Agency for Research on Cancer

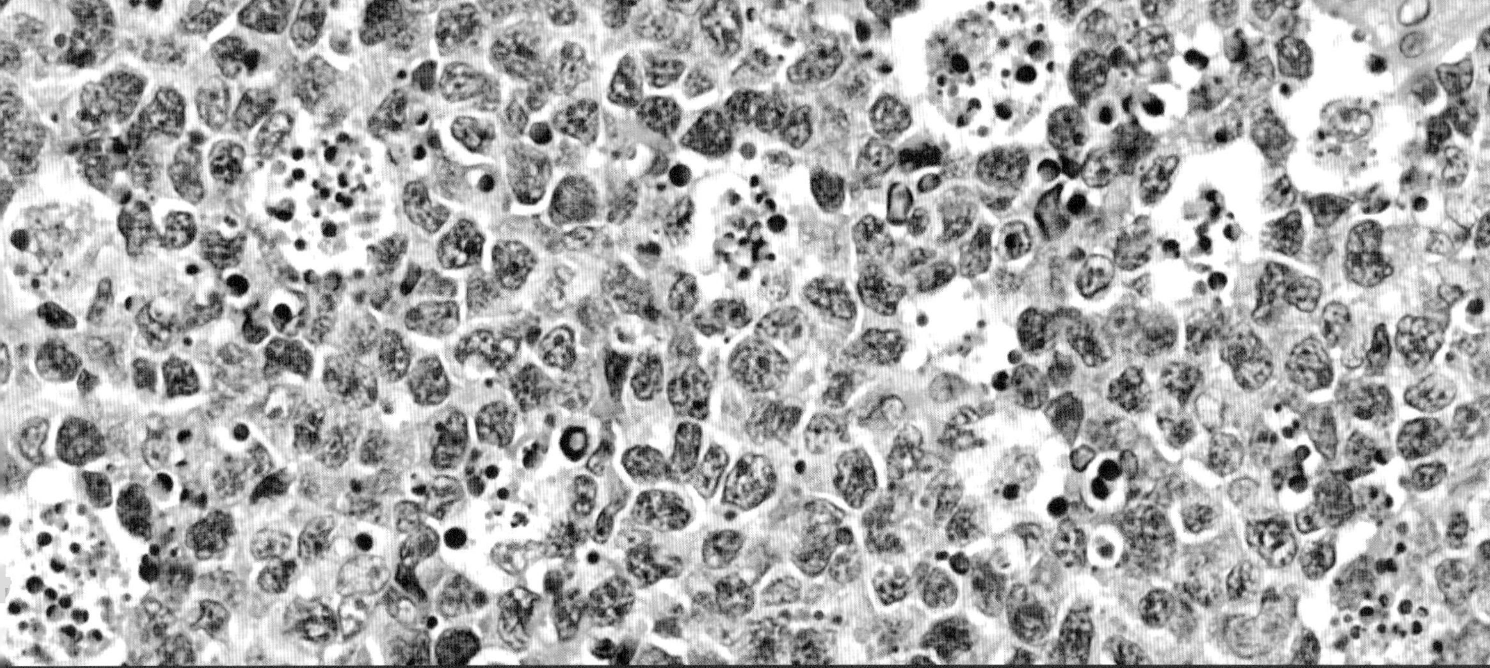

4

B-cell lymphoid proliferations and lymphomas

Edited by: Akkari Y, Alaggio R, Chan JKC, Chng WJ, Coupland SE, Dave SS, de Jong D, Du MQ, Ferry JA, Gujral S, Khoury JD, Lazar AJ, Moch H, Nagai H, Naresh KN, Ott G, Sayed S, Schuh A, Sewell WA, Siebert R, Thompson LDR, Washington MK, Wood BL

(Continued on next page)

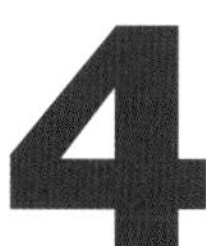

B-cell lymphoid proliferations and lymphomas (continued)

- Follicular lymphoma
  - Paediatric-type follicular lymphoma
  - Duodenal-type follicular lymphoma
- Cutaneous follicle centre lymphoma
  - Primary cutaneous follicle centre lymphoma
- Mantle cell lymphoma
  - In situ mantle cell neoplasm
  - Mantle cell lymphoma
  - Leukaemic non-nodal mantle cell lymphoma
- Transformations of indolent B-cell lymphomas
  - Transformations of indolent B-cell lymphomas
- Large B-cell lymphomas
  - Diffuse large B-cell lymphoma NOS
  - T-cell/histiocyte–rich large B-cell lymphoma
  - Diffuse large B-cell lymphoma / high-grade B-cell lymphoma with *MYC* and *BCL2* rearrangements
  - ALK-positive large B-cell lymphoma
  - Large B-cell lymphoma with *IRF4* rearrangement
  - High-grade B-cell lymphoma with 11q aberration
  - Lymphomatoid granulomatosis
  - EBV-positive diffuse large B-cell lymphoma
  - Diffuse large B-cell lymphoma associated with chronic inflammation
  - Fibrin-associated large B-cell lymphoma
  - Fluid overload–associated large B-cell lymphoma
  - Plasmablastic lymphoma
  - Primary large B-cell lymphoma of immune-privileged sites
  - Primary cutaneous diffuse large B-cell lymphoma, leg type
  - Intravascular large B-cell lymphoma
  - Primary mediastinal large B-cell lymphoma
  - Mediastinal grey zone lymphoma
  - High-grade B-cell lymphoma NOS
- Burkitt lymphoma
  - Burkitt lymphoma
- KSHV/HHV8-associated B-cell lymphoid proliferations and lymphomas
  - Primary effusion lymphoma
  - KSHV/HHV8-positive diffuse large B-cell lymphoma
  - KSHV/HHV8-positive germinotropic lymphoproliferative disorder
- Lymphoid proliferations and lymphomas associated with immune deficiency and dysregulation
  - Hyperplasias arising in immune deficiency/dysregulation
  - Polymorphic lymphoproliferative disorders arising in immune deficiency/dysregulation
  - EBV-positive mucocutaneous ulcer
  - Lymphomas arising in immune deficiency/dysregulation
  - Inborn error of immunity–associated lymphoid proliferations and lymphomas

Hodgkin lymphoma
- Classic Hodgkin lymphoma
- Nodular lymphocyte-predominant Hodgkin lymphoma

Plasma cell neoplasms and other diseases with paraproteins
- Monoclonal gammopathies
  - Cold agglutinin disease
  - IgM monoclonal gammopathy of undetermined significance
  - Non-IgM monoclonal gammopathy of undetermined significance
  - Monoclonal gammopathy of renal significance
- Diseases with monoclonal immunoglobulin deposition
  - Immunoglobulin-related amyloidosis (AL amyloidosis)
  - Monoclonal immunoglobulin deposition disease
- Heavy chain diseases
  - Mu heavy chain disease
  - Gamma heavy chain disease
  - Alpha heavy chain disease
- Plasma cell neoplasms
  - Plasmacytoma
  - Plasma cell myeloma / multiple myeloma
  - Plasma cell neoplasms with associated paraneoplastic syndrome

Introduction to B-cell lymphoproliferative disorders and neoplasms

Naresh KN
Du MQ
Ferry JA

The term "B-cell lymphoproliferative disorder" is used to describe both non-clonal and clonal expansions of B cells. Many non-clonal expansions occurring in response to infections or antigenic challenges can mimic neoplasms. In contrast, B-cell lymphomas are clonal tumours of mature and immature B cells. B-cell lymphomas have a highly variable clinical presentation – nodal or extranodal, localized or systemic, and indolent or aggressive. Although some B-cell lymphomas recapitulate the stages of normal B-cell differentiation and can be classified according to their corresponding normal stage, certain other B-cell lymphomas do not have a clearcut normal cell counterpart. The relatedness of B-cell lymphomas to their normal B-cell counterparts is a key aspect of the nomenclature in their classification. Many are also classified according to distinct genetic/genomic changes, association with specific infectious agents, or distinctive clinical presentation. Changes from the revised fourth edition of the WHO classification of haematolymphoid tumours are captured in Table 4.01, Table 4.02 (p. 298), and Table 4.03 (p. 298).

Normal B-cell maturation

Normal B-cell development begins in the bone marrow, with a haematopoietic stem cell (HSC) giving rise to a pro-B cell, which later develops into an immature B cell via a pre-B-cell stage. These B-cell precursors, also known as B lymphoblasts, undergo immunoglobulin (IG) V(D)J gene rearrangement and

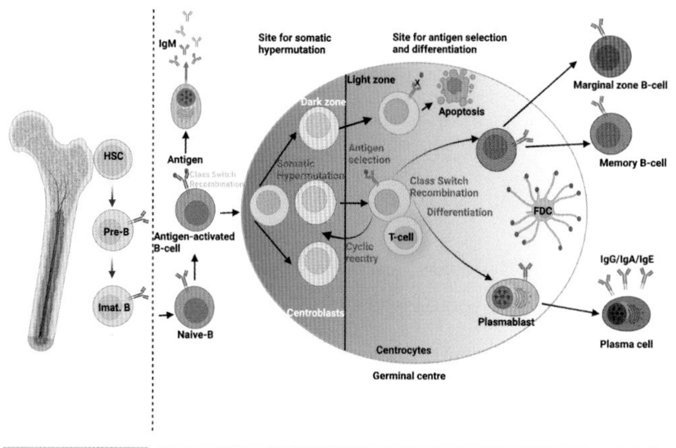

Fig. 4.01 Normal B-cell development and maturation. Normal B-cell development begins in the bone marrow, with a haematopoietic stem cell (HSC) giving rise to a pro-B cell, which later develops into an immature B-cell via a pre-B-cell stage. Immunoglobulin V(D)J gene rearrangement occurs in the bone marrow at the pre-B-cell stage, finally resulting in IgM+/IgD+ naïve B cells. Upon encountering an antigen, naïve B cells can differentiate into IgM-producing plasma cells or enter a germinal centre and undergo affinity maturation, ultimately differentiating into antibody-secreting plasma cells and memory B cells. Centroblasts within the dark zone of the germinal centre undergo somatic hypermutation of the rearranged IG genes to improve their binding to antigen. These cells enter the light zone as centrocytes, where germinal-centre B cells expressing the highest-affinity B-cell receptors undergo class-switch recombination, which makes them switch from IgM production to IgG, IgA, or IgE production {1197,264,2043}. FDC, follicular dendritic cell. Figure created with BioRender.com.

Table 4.01 B-cell lymphoproliferative disorders and neoplasms introduced in the fifth-edition WHO classification of haematolymphoid tumours

Entity	Comment
Tumour-like lesions with B-cell predominance	Reactive B-cell–rich lymphoid proliferations that can mimic lymphoma; IgG4-related disease; different types of Castleman disease
B-lymphoblastic leukaemia/lymphoma with *ETV6::RUNX1*-like features	
B-lymphoblastic leukaemia/lymphoma with *TCF3::HLF* fusion	
Splenic B-cell lymphoma/leukaemia with prominent nucleoli	Encompasses hairy cell leukaemia variant and some cases of B-cell prolymphocytic leukaemia
Primary cutaneous marginal zone lymphoma	Previously included under extranodal marginal zone lymphoma of mucosa-associated lymphoid tissue
Transformations of indolent B-cell lymphomas	
Fibrin-associated large B-cell lymphoma	Previously considered a subtype of diffuse large B-cell lymphoma associated with chronic inflammation
Fluid overload–associated large B-cell lymphoma	
Primary large B-cell lymphoma of immune-privileged sites	Encompasses primary diffuse large B-cell lymphoma of the CNS, primary large B-cell lymphoma of the vitreoretinal areas, and primary large B-cell lymphoma of the testis
Lymphoid proliferations and lymphomas associated with immune deficiency and dysregulation	Encompasses the full range of lymphoid proliferations occurring in the settings of post–haematopoietic stem cell transplantation, post–solid organ transplantation, HIV infection, other iatrogenic immunodeficiency-associated settings, and primary immune disorders, among others.
Cold agglutinin disease	
Monoclonal gammopathy of renal significance	

Table 4.02 Significant changes to nomenclature in the fifth-edition WHO classification of haematolymphoid tumours

Fifth edition	Revised fourth edition
B-lymphoblastic leukaemia/lymphoma with high hyperdiploidy	B-lymphoblastic leukaemia/lymphoma with hyperdiploidy
B-lymphoblastic leukaemia/lymphoma with *BCR::ABL1* fusion	B-lymphoblastic leukaemia/lymphoma with t(9;22)(q34.1;q11.2); *BCR-ABL1*
B-lymphoblastic leukaemia/lymphoma with *BCR::ABL1*-like features	B-lymphoblastic leukaemia/lymphoma, *BCR-ABL1*–like
B-lymphoblastic leukaemia/lymphoma with *KMT2A* rearrangement	B-lymphoblastic leukaemia/lymphoma with t(v;11q23.3); *KMT2A*-rearranged
B-lymphoblastic leukaemia/lymphoma with *ETV6::RUNX1* fusion	B-lymphoblastic leukaemia/lymphoma with t(12;21)(p13.2;q22.1); *ETV6-RUNX1*
B-lymphoblastic leukaemia/lymphoma with *TCF3::PBX1* fusion	B-lymphoblastic leukaemia/lymphoma with t(1;19)(q23;p13.3); *TCF3-PBX1*
B-lymphoblastic leukaemia/lymphoma with IGH::*IL3* fusion	B-lymphoblastic leukaemia/lymphoma with t(5;14)(q31.1;q32.1); IGH/*IL3*
In situ follicular B-cell neoplasm	In situ follicular neoplasia
Diffuse large B-cell lymphoma / high-grade B-cell lymphoma with *MYC* and *BCL2* rearrangements	High-grade B-cell lymphoma with *MYC* and *BCL2* and/or *BCL6* rearrangements
High-grade B-cell lymphoma with 11q aberration	Burkitt-like lymphoma with 11q aberration
EBV-positive diffuse large B-cell lymphoma	EBV-positive diffuse large B-cell lymphoma NOS
Mediastinal grey zone lymphoma	B-cell lymphoma, unclassifiable, with features intermediate between diffuse large B-cell lymphoma and classic Hodgkin lymphoma
KSHV/HHV8-positive diffuse large B-cell lymphoma	HHV8-positive diffuse large B-cell lymphoma NOS
KSHV/HHV8-positive germinotropic lymphoproliferative disorder	HHV8-positive germinotropic lymphoproliferative disorder
Immunoglobulin-related amyloidosis	Primary amyloidosis
Monoclonal immunoglobulin deposition disease	Light chain and heavy chain deposition diseases

differentiate into mature but antigen-naïve B cells expressing surface immunoglobulin (IgM+, IgD+) {1197}. Naïve B cells are small resting lymphocytes that circulate in the peripheral blood and occupy primary lymphoid follicles and mantle zones of secondary follicles of peripheral lymphoid tissues {1721, 2033}. Upon encountering an antigen that fits their surface immunoglobulin receptors, naïve B cells are activated, and they proliferate and ultimately differentiate into memory B cells and antibody-secreting plasma cells. Activated B cells derived from naïve B cells that have encountered antigen may mature directly into plasma cells that produce the early IgM antibody response to antigen. This T-cell–independent maturation can take place outside the germinal centre (GC) {714}. Alternatively, antigen-exposed B cells migrate into the centre of a primary follicle, differentiate into centroblasts, and rapidly proliferate, forming a GC or secondary follicle {2389,2463}. GC centroblasts that mainly occupy the dark zone of the GC express low levels of surface immunoglobulin and lack expression of BCL2; they are highly susceptible to apoptosis {3388}. Two key events occur in the GC B cells: somatic hypermutation (SHM) of the rearranged IG genes, and class-switch recombination (CSR). The SHM process introduces mostly somatic point mutations in the rearranged IG gene to improve antibody affinity, although it can also result in deleterious changes due to nonsense or frameshift mutations. Centroblasts differentiate into centrocytes that are predominantly seen in the light zone of the GC, and they can undergo multiple rounds of the SHM process by transiting between the dark and light zones. Centrocytes expressing high-affinity surface immunoglobulin receive pro-survival signals from B-cell receptor (BCR) signalling and T-cell help and are rescued from apoptosis and allowed to exit the GC to further differentiate into memory B cells or plasma cells {2463,264, 2043}. By CSR, B cells switch from IgM production to IgG, IgA, or IgE production. Through SHM and CSR mechanisms, GC B cells express higher-affinity class-switched antibodies {2464}. Post-GC memory B cells circulate in the peripheral blood and populate the marginal zones of B-cell follicles in lymph nodes, spleen, and mucosa-associated lymphoid tissue. Plasma cells produced in the GC enter the peripheral blood and home to the bone marrow. They express predominantly cytoplasmic IgG, IgA, or IgE, and they lack surface immunoglobulin. This is a simplified concept of GC biology, and novel single-cell RNA sequencing studies are likely to provide a more detailed understanding of the GC structure, with the identification of a larger number of subpopulations.

Table 4.03 Entities excluded from the fifth edition of the WHO classification of haematolymphoid tumours and their equivalents in the previous version

Fifth edition	Revised fourth edition
Prolymphocytic progression of chronic lymphocytic leukaemia / small lymphocytic lymphoma or splenic B-cell lymphoma/leukaemia with prominent nucleoli	B-cell prolymphocytic leukaemia
Splenic B-cell lymphoma/leukaemia with prominent nucleoli	Hairy cell leukaemia variant

Transcriptional regulation of B-cell maturation

During early B-cell development, HSCs give rise to lymphoid-primed multipotent progenitors with lymphoid and limited myeloid potential that further differentiate into common lymphoid progenitors, then into pro-B and pre-B cells. PU.1 (a purine-rich sequence binding factor), Ikaros (IKZF1), RAG1, and E2A are key transcription factors during the transition from HSC to lymphoid-primed multipotent progenitor; during this transition, RAG1 is essential for V(D)J recombination. Furthermore, E2A, EBF1, and PAX5

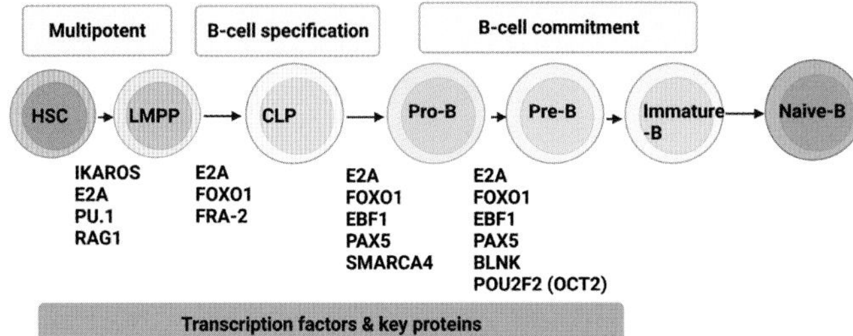

Fig. 4.02 Transcription factors and key proteins during early B-cell development. During early B-cell development, haematopoietic stem cells (HSCs) give rise to lymphoid-primed multipotent progenitors with lymphoid and limited myeloid potential (LMPPs) that further differentiate into common lymphoid progenitors (CLPs), then giving rise to pro-B and pre-B cells. Multiple transcriptional factors (as shown) are key for this transition. E2A, EBF1, and PAX5 are essential for the commitment of cells to the B lineage {1197}. Figure created with BioRender.com.

are essential for the commitment of cells to the B lineage {1197, 2360,3745}. PU.1 and Ikaros (IKZF1) are key factors for controlling lymphoid versus myeloid cell fate. E2A initiates the B-lineage transcriptional programme by activating the gene *FOXO1*. FOXO1 activates EBF1 in a feed-forward loop, and EBF1 then activates PAX5. EBF1 and PAX5 activate the B-cell programme while repressing the myeloid programme genes.

Several transcription factors are key regulators of the initiation and maintenance of the GC stage. A concerted action of sequentially expressed and repressed transcription factors drives the differentiation of an antigen-engaged naïve B cell into a proliferating B cell in the dark zone of the GC. NF-κB and IRF4 are expressed and active at the initiation of the GC, while their expression and/or activation is downmodulated in dark-zone cells. Similarly, MYC is expressed at GC initiation, after which it is repressed by BCL6, the master regulator of the GC, and thus most of the dark-zone GC cells do not express MYC. The proliferative activity in the dark-zone cells is governed by cyclin D3 (encoded by *CCND3*). MYC is transiently expressed in a very small subset of light-zone B cells and may help these cells to re-enter the dark zone to undergo further steps of proliferation and SHM. Along with BCL6, BACH2 maintains the GC programme and also represses the expression of Blimp1 (PRDM1), a transcription factor essential for plasma cell differentiation. Components of NF-κB complexes are active in the light-zone cells and are essential for B-cell maturation. Simultaneous stimulation of BCR through engagement with the antigen and costimulatory interaction with T follicular helper (TFH) cells via CD40 / CD154 (CD40L) result in activation of the transcription factor NF-κB. NF-κB transactivates IRF4, which represses BCL6. The repression of BCL6 leads to the expression of Blimp1 (PRDM1), which triggers plasma cell differentiation. Apart from maturing into plasma cells, an alternative fate of the selected light-zone cells is to exit the GC as memory B cells or marginal zone B cells. The molecular mechanisms underlying the differentiation of memory B cells from centrocytes are not yet fully understood {3360,2198,3098,265,4450,1660,3786,519,988, 2044,1549,936}. The plasma cell programme depends on two opposing sets of transcription factors: the suppression of PAX5, EBF1, and BCL6, and the expression of Blimp1, IRF4, and XBP1. Thereby, Blimp1 is a master regulator for plasma cell differentiation as it suppresses PAX5 and BCL6 {1048,2590,4030,3700}.

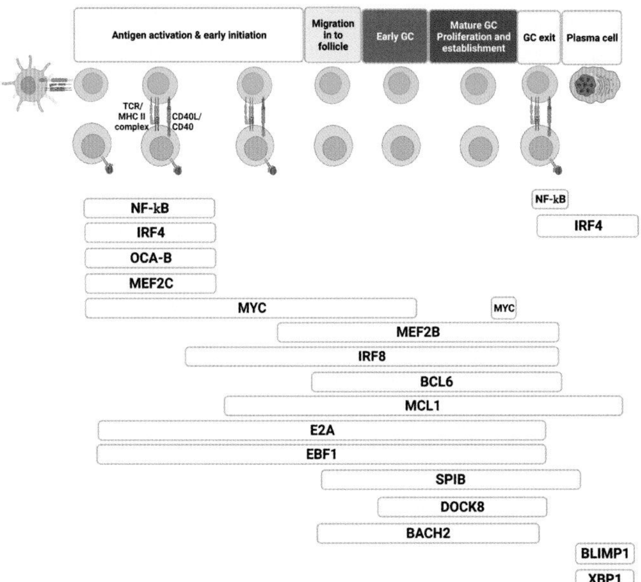

Fig. 4.03 Transcription factors and key proteins during B-cell maturation in peripheral lymphoid tissues. Several transcription factors are key for the initiation and maintenance of the germinal centre (GC). Initiation of the GC after antigen activation of T and B cells requires NF-κB, IRF4, BOB1 (OCA-B), MEF2C, and MYC. Formation of an early germinal centre further requires interactions of MEF2B, BCL6, IRF8, MCL1, and E2A. EBF1, SPIB, DOCK8, and BACH2 are essential for the proliferation and maintenance of the GC {936}. TCR, T-cell receptor. Figure created with BioRender.com.

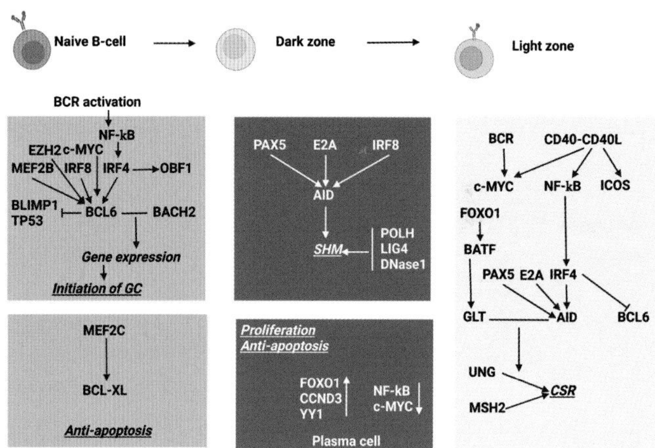

Fig. 4.04 Interactions of transcription factors and key proteins in germinal-centre B cells. Several transcription factors and key proteins are responsible for the initiation and maintenance of the germinal centre (GC). Initiation of GC formation starts after antigen activation of a naïve B cell. BCL6 is essential for the initiation of germinal centre; MEF2B, IRF8, IRF4, Blimp1, EZH2, MYC (c-MYC), and p53 (TP53) are involved in regulating the expression of BCL6. BCL6 and BACH2 cooperatively allow the establishment of the GC B-cell programme. MEF2C is required for B-cell survival after antigen stimulation by upregulating BCL-XL. In the dark zone, activation-induced cytidine deaminase (AID) is a key enzyme regulating somatic hypermutation (SHM), and the expression of AID is controlled by PAX5, E2A, and IRF8. POLH, LIG4, and DNase I are also required for SHM and are highly expressed in dark zone B cells. FOXO1, cyclin D3 (CCND3), and YY1 are key proteins required for maintaining the GC dark zone B-cell programme. In the GC light zone, B-cell receptor (BCR) binding by antigen and CD40 stimulation by T follicular helper (TFH) cells trigger activation of NF-κB, which transactivates IRF4 expression. IRF4 suppresses BCL6 but enhances Blimp1 expression, hence initiating plasma cell differentiation. PAX5, E2A, and IRF4 are key factors in regulating AID expression in the light zone. BATF, downstream of FOXO1, regulates germline transcripts (GLTs) in centrocytes. GLT and AID in turn regulate class-switch recombination (CSR) in centrocytes {3786}.

Impact of the microenvironment on B-cell maturation

In the bone marrow, B-cell development from the HSCs is dependent on its interactions with bone marrow stromal cells that provide the necessary growth factors and cytokines essential for survival and differentiation. The B-cell developmental niches in the bone marrow include mesenchymal cells, osteoblasts, endothelial cells, and HSCs {1048}. In the lymph node and other peripheral lymphoid organs, B-cell entry into the GC, migration between the dark and light zones, and maturation to memory B cells and plasma cells all depend on interactions with stromal cells, follicular dendritic cells, T cells, and macrophages. Antigen-primed naïve B cells upregulate the chemokine receptor CCR7, which facilitates the migration of B cells towards the CCR7 ligands CCL19 and CCL21, expressed in the T-cell zone. B cells present antigen on MHC class II to CD4+ helper T cells, triggering costimulatory signals via an interaction between CD40 and CD154 (CD40L). B cells proliferate and will either initiate the GC response or differentiate into short-lived extrafollicular plasma cells. Centroblasts in the dark zone express the chemokine receptor CXCR4, and the stromal cells in the dark zone express CXCL12, which functions as the ligand for CXCR4. Once centroblasts have undergone SHM in the dark zone, they downregulate CXCR4, migrate to the light zone, and transform as centrocytes that express CXCR5 {3821,3223,3035,1944,232}. Centrocytes interact with follicular dendritic cells in the light zone, where B cells are exposed to immune complexes presented by those cells. B cells with antigen receptors that have the highest affinity to the antigen can capture the greatest amounts of antigen, thus providing them with an advantage in the interaction with TFH cells that deliver the required pro-survival signals to the B cells, ultimately leading to positive selection {1048}. The mutual survival/costimulatory signals between B cells and TFH cells delivered via CD40 / CD154 (CD40L), CD80/CD28, and CD86/CD28 interactions are balanced by co-inhibitory signals between B cells and T follicular regulatory cells delivered via PDL1/PD1 and TNFRSF14 (HVEM) / BTLA interactions modulating B-cell competition and affinity maturation {1962,4423}.

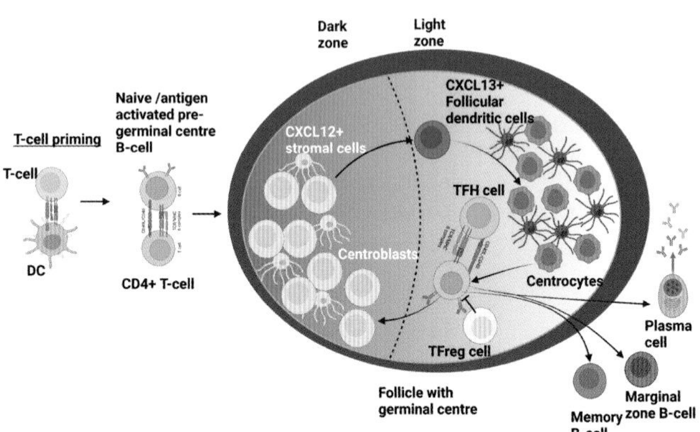

Fig. 4.05 The role of the microenvironment in B-cell maturation in peripheral lymphoid tissues. The initial interaction of an antigen-activated naïve B cell with a primed T cell is facilitated by CCR7, after which the formation of the germinal centre (GC) is initiated. The GC dynamics are further facilitated by a specialized microenvironment. The GC has two distinct compartments. The dark zone has a network of CXCL12-producing reticular cells; GC B-cell proliferation and somatic hypermutation occur in the dark zone. Centroblast traffic follows a CXCL13 gradient to enter the light zone as centrocytes. In the light zone, centrocytes capture antigen presented on follicular dendritic cells (FDCs) and internalize, process, and subsequently present it to T follicular helper (TFH) cells in order to undergo selection. This process is regulated by T follicular regulatory (TFreg) cells. The mutual survival/costimulatory signals between B cells and TFH cells delivered via CD40 / CD154 (CD40L), CD80/CD28, and CD86/CD28 interactions are balanced by co-inhibitory signals between B cells and TFreg cells involving PDL1/PD1 and TNFRSF14 (HVEM) / BTLA interactions modulating B-cell competition and affinity maturation. Such positively selected centrocytes re-enter the dark zone for further rounds of proliferation and somatic hypermutation, after which they exit the GC as memory B cells or high-affinity antibody-secreting plasma cells. Figure adapted from {3821}.

Impact of ontogeny on the classification of B-cell lymphomas

Most B-cell lymphomas have a certain resemblance to the characteristic morphological, immunophenotypic, epigenetic, and gene-expression features of different stages in B-cell development. These features are also impacted and altered by lymphoma-associated genomic changes. This resemblance and variation are extremely useful in the diagnosis and classification of B-cell lymphomas. For example, B-lymphoblastic leukaemia/lymphoma (B-ALL/LBL) has many features of normal B-cell precursors; however, normal B-cell precursors are spread across discrete stages of maturation, each with a defined immunophenotype. Although the cells of B-ALL/LBL have morphological and immunophenotypic features of precursor B cells, they do not fully align with the maturation pathway of maturing B-cell precursors, and they may also show aberrant antigen expression {3664,647,3988,3986}. Follicular lymphoma cells express phenotypic features of GC B cells; however, unlike normal GC B cells, they express BCL2, which is a result of the IGH::*BCL2* translocation {3493,2267}. On similar principles, lymphoma cells of entities such as mantle cell lymphoma, Burkitt lymphoma, diffuse large B-cell lymphoma NOS, and plasma cell neoplasms resemble their normal cell counterparts: mantle zone B cells, dark-zone centroblasts, light-zone centroblasts or post-GC immunoblasts, and plasma cells, respectively, with certain alterations as modulated by their underlying genomic changes. Other lymphomas have a relation to more heterogeneous normal counterparts. As an example, some cases of chronic lymphocytic leukaemia / small lymphocytic lymphoma (CLL/SLL) resemble pre-GC or naïve-like B cells, whereas others resemble post-GC or memory-like B cells. There are also several B-cell lymphomas in which assigning B-cell ontogeny is difficult. It should also be noted that even the B-cell lymphomas that resemble their normal ontogenic counterparts are not strictly frozen to that morphology or immunophenotype. Their attributes can be altered by the microenvironment and additional genetic changes. Examples of this include plasmacytic differentiation occurring in several small B-cell lymphomas such as marginal zone lymphoma (MZL) and follicular lymphoma, and colonization of residual follicles by MZL.

Characteristic genetic/genomic changes in B-cell lymphomas or their subtypes

Several B-cell neoplasms have characteristic genetic or genomic abnormalities that are important in determining their biological features and thereby lend support for classification (see Table 4.04) {1269,3232,193,1771,887,1882,2289}. Furthermore, characteristic epigenetic changes or methylome signatures are also noted in B-cell malignancies such as CLL/SLL and other lymphomas. Many of the genetic abnormalities are not restricted to a single lymphoma entity. In translocations

Table 4.04 Examples of characteristic genomic/genetic changes in B-cell lymphomas

Type of abnormality	Specific lesion	B-cell lymphoma
Chromosomal translocations		
	BCR::ABL1 *ETV6::RUNX1* *KMT2A* rearrangement	B-lymphoblastic leukaemia/lymphoma
	IGH::*CCND1*	Mantle cell lymphoma Plasma cell myeloma
	IGH::*BCL2*	Follicular lymphoma Diffuse large B-cell lymphoma NOS
	IGH::*MYC*	Burkitt lymphoma Diffuse large B-cell lymphoma NOS Plasmablastic lymphoma
	IG::*IRF4*	Large B-cell lymphoma with *IRF4* rearrangement
	BIRC3::MALT1 IGH::*BCL10* IGH::*MALT1* IGH::*FOXP1*	Extranodal marginal zone lymphoma of mucosa-associated lymphoid tissue
	BCL6 rearrangement	Diffuse large B-cell lymphoma NOS
	CLTC::ALK	ALK-positive large B-cell lymphoma
Point mutations		
	BRAF p.V600E	Hairy cell leukaemia Langerhans cell histiocytosis and other histiocytic neoplasms
	MYD88 p.L265P	Lymphoplasmacytic lymphoma Diffuse large B-cell lymphoma, activated B-cell-like subtype
	EZH2 *TNFRSF14* *STAT6* *RRAGC*	Follicular lymphoma
Chromosomal copy-number alterations		
	iAMP21	B-lymphoblastic leukaemia/lymphoma
	7q31-32 deletion	Splenic marginal zone lymphoma
	1p36 deletion	Follicular lymphoma
	11q gain/loss	High-grade B-cell lymphoma with 11q aberration
Gene expression		
	ETV6::RUNX1-like *BCR::ABL1*-like	B-lymphoblastic leukaemia/lymphoma
	GCB and ABC	Diffuse large B-cell lymphoma NOS
Combination of chromosomal translocations and mutations		
	MCD, BN2, N1, EZB, A53, and ST2	Diffuse large B-cell lymphoma NOS

A53, aneuploidy with *TP53* inactivation; ABC, activated B cell; BN2, *BCL6* translocations and *NOTCH2* mutations; EZB, *EZH2* mutations and *BCL2* translocations; GCB, germinal-centre B cell; iAMP21, intrachromosomal amplification of chromosome 21; MCD, *MYD88* p.L265P and *CD79B* mutations; N1, *NOTCH1* mutations; ST2, *SGK1* and *TET2* mutations.

involving an IG gene, an oncogene comes under the influence of the IG enhancer, and the product of the oncogene is either overexpressed or inappropriately expressed; examples of this include BCL2 in follicular lymphoma, cyclin D1 in mantle cell lymphoma, and MYC in Burkitt lymphoma. These events have significant consequences. For example, in follicular lymphoma, the overexpression of BCL2 blocks apoptosis and mediates preferential expansion within the follicle centre. Translocations involving some of the other genes, such as *BCL6* in follicular lymphoma and diffuse large B-cell lymphoma (DLBCL), can involve an IG or a non-IG gene; such abnormalities nevertheless deregulate *BCL6*, leading to BCL6 overexpression {2127, 244}. Some of the other translocations result in fusion genes, leading to the expression of chimeric proteins. Examples of such gene fusions include *BIRC3::MALT1* in extranodal MZL, where N-terminal *BIRC3* is fused to the C-terminal sequences of *MALT1*; and the fusion of *ALK* with *CLTC* or various other genes in ALK-positive large B-cell lymphoma {3849,1739}.

Characteristic mutations are seen in several mature B-cell lymphomas {4016,2949,2895}. Like translocations, these mutations are not specific to a particular B-cell malignancy, and they can be seen in other lymphoid or other haematological malignancies. Mutation in *BRAF*, commonly seen in hairy cell leukaemia, is also seen in Langerhans cell histiocytosis and other histiocytic neoplasms, whereas *MYD88* mutation, commonly seen in lymphoplasmacytic lymphoma, is also seen in a subset of DLBCL. Changes in copy numbers of genes or chromosomal loci, including amplifications and deletions, are characteristic of several B-cell malignancies, such as B-ALL/LBL with intrachromosomal amplification of chromosome 21 (iAMP21), splenic MZL with 7q32 deletion, a subset of follicular lymphoma with 1p36 deletion, and high-grade B-cell lymphoma with 11q aberration {1509,1234,193,2895}. Hyperdiploidy is the defining feature of B-ALL/LBL with high hyperdiploidy (comprising 51–65 chromosomes) and a subset of plasma cell neoplasm

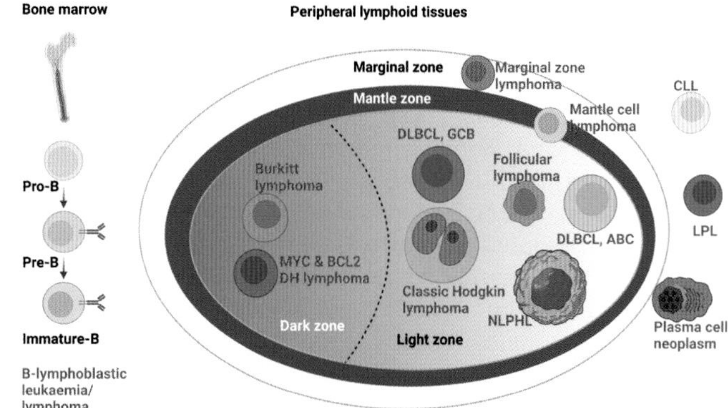

Fig. 4.06 Ontogeny of B-cell lymphomas. Different B-cell malignancies show features characteristic or reminiscent of B cells at specific points during their differentiation/ maturation. Please note that the image represents ontogenic relationships, not the morphological patterns of the lymphoma entities. CLL, chronic lymphocytic leukaemia; DLBCL, ABC, diffuse large B-cell lymphoma, activated B-cell–like subtype; DLBCL, GCB, diffuse large B-cell lymphoma, germinal-centre B-cell–like subtype; LPL, lymphoplasmacytic lymphoma; MYC & BCL2 DH lymphoma, double-hit lymphoma, diffuse large B-cell lymphoma / high-grade B-cell lymphoma with *MYC* and *BCL2* rearrangements; NLPHL, nodular lymphocyte-predominant Hodgkin lymphoma. Figure created with BioRender.com.

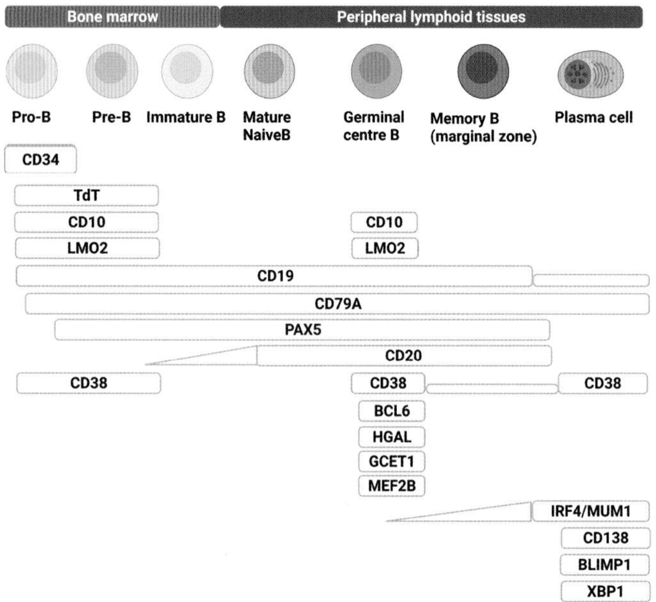

Fig. 4.07 B-cell lymphoproliferative disorders and neoplasms. Key antigens and proteins expressed at different stages of B-cell maturation and used in diagnostic practice. Figure created with BioRender.com.

with hyperdiploidy (multiple trisomies of the odd-numbered chromosomes) {3171,2153}.

Characteristic gene expression profiles define some B-cell neoplasms such as B-ALL/LBL with *ETV6*::*RUNX1*-like features and B-ALL/LBL with *BCR*::*ABL1*-like features {3102,1705}. Gene expression profiling was initially used to distinguish two major molecular subtypes of DLBCL, the germinal-centre and activated B-cell types {73}. More recent approaches towards the genomic classification of DLBCL have used a combination of gene expression and genetic abnormalities {4417,3629,644, 3386}. Using such strategies, six genetic subtypes of DLBCL have been identified: MCD (*MYD88* p.L265P and *CD79B* mutations), BN2 (*BCL6* translocations and *NOTCH2* mutations), N1 (*NOTCH1* mutations), EZB (*EZH2* mutations and *BCL2* translocations), A53 (aneuploidy with *TP53* inactivation), and ST2 (*SGK1* and *TET2* mutations) {4417}. Some of the small B-cell lymphomas, such as CLL/SLL, splenic MZL, and splenic diffuse red pulp small B-cell lymphoma, show skewed IG gene usage resulting in BCR stereotypy or the presence of (quasi-) identical BCRs shared by unrelated patients, supporting the selection and expansion of clonal B cells bearing BCRs specific for discrete antigens {33,3816,1780,4446}. The gene IGHV1-2*04 is employed by about 30% of all cases of splenic MZL {4446}. Splenic diffuse red pulp small B-cell lymphoma cases show biased usage of the genes IGHV3-23 and IGHV4-34 {364, 1780}. It is important to note that none of the presumed driver genetic abnormalities are sufficient on their own for the development of a lymphoma. For example, IGH::*BCL2*-positive B-cell clones can be detected in the peripheral blood at very low levels (~1–100 cells per 1 million B cells) in > 70% of healthy adults, the vast majority of whom will never develop follicular lymphoma {3488,2351,986}. Furthermore, most people with in situ follicular B-cell neoplasm, which can be noted in the lymph nodes of about 2% of the population, do not develop an overt follicular lymphoma {1793,3953,3029}. A complex interplay of the primary genetic abnormality with secondary genetic abnormalities and a supportive microenvironment is necessary for lymphomagenesis.

Key etiopathogenetic factors in B-cell lymphomas

Infectious agents, other environmental factors, immune deficiency/dysregulation, and autoimmunity are some of the factors implicated in the etiopathogenesis of B-cell lymphomas (see Table 4.05). Viruses such as EBV, KSHV/HHV8, and HCV have been associated with various lymphomas {1480,3295, 2632, 4055, 1695, 3929, 3300, 904, 2390, 2408, 1850, 595, 3042, 436, 4543}. EBV and KSHV/HHV8 infect B cells and are present within the neoplastic cells. In contrast, other infectious agents do not infect B cells. EBV is present in nearly 100% of endemic Burkitt lymphoma cases. Furthermore, the presence of EBV in the neoplastic B cells is the defining feature of EBV-positive DLBCL, lymphomatoid granulomatosis, DLBCL associated with chronic inflammation, and EBV-positive mucocutaneous ulcer. In contrast, only a proportion of several other lymphomas, such as classic Hodgkin lymphoma, show association with EBV. KSHV/HHV8 is found in primary effusion lymphoma, KSHV/HHV8-positive multicentric Castleman disease, KSHV/HHV8-positive DLBCL, and KSHV/HHV8-positive germinotropic lymphoproliferative disorder. Lymphoid cells in primary effusion lymphoma and KSHV/HHV8-positive germinotropic lymphoproliferative disorder are infected with KSHV/HHV8 and very often coinfected with EBV. Bacteria and immune responses to bacterial antigens have also been implicated in the pathogenesis of MALT lymphomas at various sites {1693,2932, 4410,4411,593,23,635,3501,3299,3363}. Genetic and familial associations have been identified in several B-cell lymphomas through epidemiological studies {3867}. It should be noted that familial clustering does not necessarily imply genetic predisposition; it can also imply common exposures to infectious agents or chemicals.

Epidemiological studies have implicated environmental exposures to herbicide and pesticide use, as well as the use of hair dyes, in the development of follicular lymphoma and DLBCL {785,1512,4572}. Disruption in T-cell immunosurveillance is thought to play a major role in the development of B-cell lymphomas arising in the background of immune deficiencies and immune dysregulation. Most typical clinical scenarios include posttransplantation (both solid-organ and haematopoietic stem cell), iatrogenic / therapy-related, and HIV infection settings. Inborn errors of immunity, autoimmune diseases, and various forms of immunotherapy also increase the risk of developing lymphomas and lymphoproliferative disorders. These lymphomas and lymphoproliferative disorders are frequently associated with EBV and/or KSHV/HHV8, and, in comparison with similar types of lymphoma in patients without immune defects, these lymphomas carry fewer genetic alterations, and some may regress upon restoration of the immune response {2845, 2652,3296,2340,4007,3399}.

A large proportion of B-cell lymphomas have characteristic chromosomal translocations where an oncogene comes under the transcriptional regulation of an IG gene. Such chromosomal translocations are considered to occur because of an erroneous IG gene recombination during B-cell development. For translocations involving genes such as *CCND1*, *BCL2*, and *MALT1*, breaks at the IG gene are usually directly adjacent to D or J segments. In some of the other translocations involving genes such as *BCL6* or *MYC*, breaks in the IG gene can also involve the IGH class-switch regions during an erroneous CSR event {2338}.

Table 4.05 Examples of factors involved in the etiology and pathogenesis of B-cell lymphomas

Etiopathogenic factors	Lymphoma entities
Infectious agents and chronic autoimmune disorders	
Helicobacter pylori (gastric) *Borrelia burgdorferi* (cutaneous) *Chlamydia psittaci* (ocular adnexa) *Campylobacter jejuni* (intestinal) *Achromobacter xylosoxidans* (pulmonary) Sjögren syndrome (salivary gland) Hashimoto thyroiditis (thyroid)	Extranodal marginal zone lymphoma of mucosa-associated lymphoid tissue
HCV	Lymphoplasmacytic lymphoma associated with type II cryoglobulinaemia Splenic marginal zone lymphoma Nodal marginal zone lymphoma Diffuse large B-cell lymphoma
EBV	EBV-positive diffuse large B-cell lymphoma Lymphomatoid granulomatosis DLBCL associated with chronic inflammation EBV-positive mucocutaneous ulcer Fibrin-associated diffuse large B-cell lymphoma Immune deficiency/dysregulation–associated lymphoproliferative disorders Plasmablastic lymphoma
EBV	Burkitt lymphoma
KSHV/HHV8	Multicentric Castleman disease KSHV/HHV8-positive diffuse large B-cell lymphoma Primary effusion lymphoma
KSHV/HHV8 and EBV	Primary effusion lymphoma KSHV/HHV8-positive germinotropic lymphoproliferative disorder
Environmental exposures	
Herbicides and pesticides	Follicular lymphoma
Hair dyes	Diffuse large B-cell lymphoma
Immune deficiency/dysregulation	
Solid organ transplantation Haematopoietic stem cell transplantation Iatrogenic/therapy-related immunodeficiency HIV infection Inborn errors of immunity Autoimmune diseases Various forms of multichemotherapy and immunotherapy	Lymphoproliferative disorders Lymphomas

Principles of classification, subtyping, and workup

Classification of lymphoid neoplasms is based on multiple parameters: clinical presentation, clinical/imaging investigations, and a multitude of laboratory investigations. It is not based on any single investigation, although morphology remains the key component of diagnostic decision-making. In addition to morphology, immunohistochemistry or immunophenotyping plays a major role in disease classification. B-cell lymphomas have immunophenotypic similarities to their ontogenic normal counterparts. Over the past two to three decades, we have noticed the immense impact of genetic/genomic investigations (performed using many different technologies) on lymphoma classification and subtyping. These have led to the discovery of distinct lymphomas and improved lymphoma subtyping. Such an approach has also impacted disease classification and stratification in a clinically meaningful manner.

In lymphoma diagnosis and classification, general consideration needs to be given to the following aspects:

FNA alone is generally insufficient for the diagnosis and classification of lymphomas, and it is not the recommended procedure for primary lymphoma diagnosis unless an extraordinary situation demands such an approach {608,2622}. FNA can be a good screening tool to exclude non-haematological diseases. In low- and middle-income (LMIC) settings, FNA can be an effective alternative diagnostic procedure, when limited financial and/or technical resources preclude complete histology-based lymphoma classification. In most instances, it is needed to revert the diagnosis to a higher hierarchical level in the classification (family, category) in such cases.

Given the multiparametric approach necessary to make an optimal diagnosis, having sufficient tissue is critical. Core needle biopsies are often not optimal for primary diagnosis, and every attempt should be made either for an excisional biopsy in patients with peripheral lymphadenopathy or for a larger biopsy in other situations. If these are not feasible because of the patient's clinical condition or the location of the lesion, performing (multiple) core needle biopsies should be considered.

Although immunohistochemistry is the preferred mode of investigating antigen/protein expression in the workup of lymphomas, immunophenotyping (flow cytometry) can be complementary and provide useful information in many situations. In the bone marrow, peripheral blood, or other fluid-based lymphomas, flow cytometry has distinct advantages.

Morphology and immunophenotype are sufficient for the diagnosis of most lymphoid neoplasms. However, no single immunophenotypic marker is specific for any neoplasm, and a combination of morphological features and a panel of immunophenotypic markers is necessary for correct diagnosis. Most B-cell lymphomas have characteristic immunophenotypic profiles that are very helpful for their diagnosis. Many lymphomas are defined by genetic abnormalities or by association with infectious agents. Appropriate genetic studies addressing chromosomal translocations, gains, and deletions, as well as molecular studies addressing clonality, chromosomal translocations, copy-number alterations, mutations, and gene expression, would be essential for precise disease classification in these situations. Performing investigations on platforms that can undertake a large and standardized panel of tests may impact precision diagnosis and help shape future versions of the WHO classification.

Multidisciplinary tumour board discussions remain key for optimal lymphoma diagnosis and management.

The practice of lymphoma classification in the setting of limited resources or limited sample (available material for investigation)

Limitations posed by resources and/or technology are a major stumbling block for the practice of high-quality lymphoma diagnosis. If availability of resources is the main limiting factor, establishing minimal panels of immunohistochemistry that can be used in a staged algorithmic manner can be a strategy to adopt for arriving at a precise diagnosis of B-cell lymphoma, albeit at the cost of additional time and effort. Previous studies have shown that a correct diagnosis is achievable in as many as 70% of B-cell lymphomas with the application of a limited set of antibodies (three to five) in such a setting {965,2901}. The lack of infrastructure to perform FISH studies can be a major limitation for the diagnosis of Burkitt lymphoma in parts of the world such as sub-Saharan Africa, where the incidence of Burkitt lymphoma is high. In the WHO classification, Burkitt lymphoma is defined by the presence of *MYC* translocation. In an appropriate clinical and histological context, the presence of MYC protein expression in > 80% of the lymphoma cells correlates very highly with the presence of *MYC* translocation, thereby serving as a surrogate for FISH studies. In places with infrastructural constraints, an algorithmic approach can be used to diagnose Burkitt lymphoma in most cases, even in the absence of FISH studies {2903}.

The structure of the fifth edition of the WHO classification also assists the practice of lymphoma diagnosis in the setting of resource or sample limitations. Diagnostic entities are ordered in increasing levels of specification: category (e.g. mature B-cell), family/class (e.g. large B-cell lymphomas), entity/type (e.g. diffuse large B-cell lymphoma NOS), and subtype (e.g. diffuse large B-cell lymphoma NOS, germinal-centre B-cell–like subtype). Furthermore, the criteria for diagnosis are grouped under essential and desirable diagnostic criteria for each entity. In most instances, the essential criteria can be met in many parts of the world. In circumstances where these essential criteria, including molecular parameters if listed, are not achievable, a diagnostic label based on the family name of that entity can be applied, with the clarification "not further classified".

Conclusion

The multiparameter approach adopted for the fifth edition of the WHO classification is essential for achieving reproducibility of diagnosis and optimal management. The reliability of the results of clinical and translational research studies is dependent on precise and reproducible diagnoses.

Tumour-like lesions with B-cell predominance: Introduction

Ferry JA

These sections discuss a group of diseases that are rich in B cells, and that could be considered in the differential diagnosis of lymphoma, but that do not represent lymphoid neoplasms. They are included for the first time in the WHO classification of haematolymphoid tumours. Reactive B-cell–rich proliferations that can mimic lymphoma include lymph nodal proliferations characterized by distortion of the normal architecture and/or the presence of atypical cells, as well as unusually dense, extensive extranodal lymphoid infiltrates showing cytological atypia.

IgG4-related disease is characterized by extranodal lymphoplasmacytic infiltrates rich in IgG4+ plasma cells, accompanied by sclerosis; some patients also have lymphadenopathy. The clinical and pathological differential

Table 4.06 Diagnostic criteria and helpful features for the subtypes of Castleman disease (continued on next page)

	Hyaline-vascular unicentric Castleman disease[a]	Mixed/plasmacytic unicentric Castleman disease
Major criteria (all three required)		
Enlarged lymph nodes	One enlarged lymph node (> 10 mm in the short axis diameter) or multiple enlarged lymph nodes in one lymph node station	One enlarged lymph node or multiple enlarged lymph nodes in one lymph node station
Morphological features consistent with Castleman disease spectrum	Including grade 2–3 regressed follicles / hyaline-vascular follicles[b] and: • Prominent stroma • Prominent high endothelial vessels • Relatively few plasma cells	Including grade 2–3 plasmacytosis; regressed follicles / hyaline-vascular follicles can be seen
KSHV/HHV8 LANA IHC	Negative	Negative
Additional supportive histopathological features (not required)		
	Variably prominent interfollicular stroma Compressed sinuses Plasmacytoid dendritic cell clusters No grade 2–3 plasmacytosis Indolent T-lymphoblastic proliferation	Usually includes a mix of atrophic and hyperplastic follicle features, but usually at least one regressed hyaline-vascular follicle is present
Other supportive features (not required)		
	Mass lesion Lack of symptoms (in most cases) Co-occurring autoimmune diseases (in ~5%; paraneoplastic pemphigus, myasthenia gravis, bronchiolitis obliterans, etc.)	Mass lesion Lack of symptoms (in most cases) Inflammatory syndrome (in a subset) Constitutional symptoms Laboratory abnormalities including cytopenias, hypoalbuminaemia, polyclonal hypergammaglobulinaemia, elevated CRP and/or IL-6, etc.
Exclusion criteria[c]		
Infection	HIV[d], KSHV/HHV8, CMV, etc.	HIV, KSHV/HHV8, COVID-19, syphilis, etc.
Autoimmune, inflammatory, or immunodeficiency disorders	SLE, rheumatoid arthritis, etc.	SLE, rheumatoid arthritis, adult-onset Still disease, juvenile idiopathic arthritis, IgG4-related disease, etc.
Malignancy	Non-Hodgkin lymphoma, Hodgkin lymphoma, thymoma	Non-Hodgkin lymphoma, Hodgkin lymphoma, plasma cell myeloma / plasmacytoma, POEMS syndrome, etc.

ALPS, autoimmune lymphoproliferative syndrome; CRP, C-reactive protein; DAT, direct antiglobulin test; eGFR, estimated glomerular filtration rate; IHC, immunohistochemistry; iMCD, idiopathic multicentric Castleman disease; LANA, latency-associated nuclear antigen; POEMS, polyneuropathy, organomegaly, endocrinopathy, myeloma protein, and skin changes; SLE, systemic lupus erythematosus; TAFRO, thrombocytopenia, anasarca, fever / inflammatory symptoms, renal dysfunction / bone marrow reticulin fibrosis, organomegaly.
[a]The follicular and interfollicular changes in hyaline-vascular unicentric Castleman disease are usually better developed and more characteristic than in the other forms of Castleman disease. [b]Hyaline-vascular follicles are regressed follicles with hyalinization and lymphoid depletion, a concentric onion-skin appearance to the rings of the mantle zone cells, and penetrating vessels (lollipop). [c]Some patients with Castleman disease may also have some of these processes in addition to Castleman disease; careful clinical evaluation is needed. [d]HIV-positive patients can have hyaline-vascular unicentric Castleman disease. [e]See {1110}. [f]Patients with KSHV/HHV8+ multicentric Castleman disease should be carefully evaluated for other KSHV/HHV8-associated diseases (Kaposi sarcoma, primary effusion lymphoma / extracavitary primary effusion lymphoma, etc.). [g]Conditions combined from {4120} and {1321}. References: {1110,4308,2967,4120,1321}.

Table 4.06 Diagnostic criteria and helpful features for the subtypes of Castleman disease (continued from previous page, continued on next page)

	iMCD-NOS	iMCD-TAFRO
Major criteria (all three required)		
Enlarged lymph nodes	Enlarged lymph nodes in at least two lymph node stations	Enlarged lymph nodes in at least two lymph node stations
Morphological features consistent with Castleman disease spectrum	Including: Grade 2–3 regressed follicles **OR** grade 2–3 plasmacytosis	Including: Grade 2–3 regressed follicles **OR** grade 2–3 plasmacytosis
KSHV/HHV8 LANA IHC	Negative	Negative
Major criteria for further subclassification of iMCD-TAFRO (all five required)		
	Does not demonstrate all five required features of iMCD-TAFRO	Anasarca (includes pleural effusions, ascites, subcutaneous oedema) Thrombocytopenia (< 10 × 10^4/μL) Systemic inflammation: Fever > 37.5 °C **AND/OR** CRP ≥ 2 mg/dL Organomegaly (CT): Small-volume lymphadenopathy (often < 10 mm in greatest diameter) in more than two lymph node stations **AND/OR** hepatomegaly **AND/OR** splenomegaly At least one of the following: Bone marrow with reticulin fibrosis and/or megakaryocytic hyperplasia without another cause **OR** renal insufficiency (pretreatment; eGFR < 60 mL/min/1.73 m^2; creatinine > 1.3 mg/dL in male patients, > 1.1 mg/dL in female patients) or renal failure (dialysis)
Minor criteria	Need at least two of the criteria below, with at least one laboratory criterion	
Laboratory criteria	Anaemia (< 12.5 g/dL in male patients, < 11.5 g/dL in female patients) Thrombocytopenia (platelet count < 15 × 10^4/μL) or thrombocytosis (platelet count > 40 × 10^4/μL) CRP > 1 mg/dL Renal dysfunction or proteinuria Polyclonal hypergammaglobulinaemia	If the above major criteria are met, then the criteria for iMCD-TAFRO are fulfilled
Clinical criteria	Constitutional symptoms Large spleen and/or liver Fluid accumulation (oedema, effusions, anasarca) Eruptive cherry haemangiomatosis or violaceous papules Lymphocytic interstitial pneumonitis	If the above major criteria are met, then the criteria for iMCD-TAFRO are fulfilled
Additional supportive histopathological features (not required)		
	Grade 2–3 vascularity often present (hypervascular > hyaline-vascular) Lymph nodes borderline enlarged (often ≤ 10 mm)	Grade 2–3 hyperplastic germinal centres often present (mixed/plasmacytic histopathological features) At least one lymph node measuring > 10 mm on the short axis
Other supportive features (not required)		
	Elevated levels of IL-6, sIL-2R, VEGF, and/or B2M Elevated alkaline phosphatase without elevation in bilirubin or transaminases	Elevated levels of IL-6, sIL-2R, VEGF, IgA, IgE, LDH, and/or B2M Reticulin marrow fibrosis Typically associated with thrombocytosis and hypergammaglobulinaemia Disorders associated with iMCD[e]
Exclusion criteria[c]		
Infection	EBV, COVID-19, HIV, KSHV/HHV8, tuberculosis, etc.	EBV, COVID-19, HIV, KSHV/HHV8, tuberculosis, etc.
Autoimmune, inflammatory, or immunodeficiency disorders	SLE, rheumatoid arthritis, adult-onset Still disease, juvenile idiopathic arthritis, Sjögren syndrome, ALPS, haemophagocytic lymphohistiocytosis, IgG4-related disease, etc.	SLE, rheumatoid arthritis, adult-onset Still disease, juvenile idiopathic arthritis, Sjögren syndrome, ALPS, IgG4-related disease, etc.
Malignancy	Non-Hodgkin lymphoma, plasma cell myeloma / plasmacytoma, metastatic cancer, POEMS syndrome, etc.	Non-Hodgkin lymphoma, Hodgkin lymphoma, plasma cell myeloma / plasmacytoma, follicular dendritic cell sarcoma, POEMS syndrome, etc.

ALPS, autoimmune lymphoproliferative syndrome; CRP, C-reactive protein; DAT, direct antiglobulin test; eGFR, estimated glomerular filtration rate; IHC, immunohistochemistry; iMCD, idiopathic multicentric Castleman disease; LANA, latency-associated nuclear antigen; POEMS, polyneuropathy, organomegaly, endocrinopathy, myeloma protein, and skin changes; SLE, systemic lupus erythematosus; TAFRO, thrombocytopenia, anasarca, fever / inflammatory symptoms, renal dysfunction / bone marrow reticulin fibrosis, organomegaly.
[a]The follicular and interfollicular changes in hyaline-vascular unicentric Castleman disease are usually better developed and more characteristic than in the other forms of Castleman disease. [b]Hyaline-vascular follicles are regressed follicles with hyalinization and lymphoid depletion, a concentric onion-skin appearance to the rings of the mantle zone cells, and penetrating vessels (lollipop). [c]Some patients with Castleman disease may also have some of these processes in addition to Castleman disease; careful clinical evaluation is needed. [d]HIV-positive patients can have hyaline-vascular unicentric Castleman disease. [e]See {1110}. [f]Patients with KSHV/HHV8+ multicentric Castleman disease should be carefully evaluated for other KSHV/HHV8-associated diseases (Kaposi sarcoma, primary effusion lymphoma / extracavitary primary effusion lymphoma, etc.). [g]Conditions combined from {4120} and {1321}.
References: {1110,4308,2967,4120,1321}.

Table 4.06 Diagnostic criteria and helpful features for the subtypes of Castleman disease (continued)

	KSHV/HHV8-MCD[f]
Major criteria (all three required)	
Enlarged lymph nodes	Enlarged lymph nodes in at least two lymph node stations
Morphological features consistent with Castleman disease spectrum	Including: • Grade 2–3 regressed follicles **AND/OR** • Grade 2–3 plasmacytosis; plasmablasts
KSHV/HHV8 LANA IHC	Positive plasmablasts
Minor criteria	Need fever and CRP > 2 mg/dL and at least three laboratory/clinical criteria that are not related to other HIV infection complications[g]
Laboratory criteria	Hyponatraemia Hypoalbuminaemia Thrombocytopenia Anaemia (including autoimmune haemolytic anaemia) *For flares (after original diagnosis):* Elevated KSHV/HHV8 viral load
Clinical criteria	Splenomegaly Fatigue Weight loss Respiratory symptoms Gastrointestinal symptoms Neuropathy Headache Oedema Rash Myalgia Fluid accumulation (oedema, effusions)
Additional supportive histopathological features (not required)	
	Plasmablasts express monotypic lambda light chain Very prominent vascularity may be seen (hypervascular > hyaline-vascular) Kaposi sarcoma is often also present
Other supportive features (not required)	
	Elevated KSHV/HHV8 viral load Positive DAT Elevated levels of vIL-6, IL-6, IL-10 Haemophagocytic lymphohistiocytosis Other KSHV/HHV8-associated disease(s)
Exclusion criteria[c]	
Infection	EBV, COVID-19, tuberculosis, etc.
Autoimmune, inflammatory, or immunodeficiency disorders	SLE, rheumatoid arthritis, etc.
Malignancy	KSHV/HHV8-negative non-Hodgkin lymphoma, Hodgkin lymphoma, plasma cell myeloma / plasmacytoma, metastatic cancer, etc.

ALPS, autoimmune lymphoproliferative syndrome; CRP, C-reactive protein; DAT, direct antiglobulin test; eGFR, estimated glomerular filtration rate; IHC, immunohistochemistry; iMCD, idiopathic multicentric Castleman disease; LANA, latency-associated nuclear antigen; POEMS, polyneuropathy, organomegaly, endocrinopathy, myeloma protein, and skin changes; SLE, systemic lupus erythematosus; TAFRO, thrombocytopenia, anasarca, fever / inflammatory symptoms, renal dysfunction / bone marrow reticulin fibrosis, organomegaly.
[a]The follicular and interfollicular changes in hyaline-vascular unicentric Castleman disease are usually better developed and more characteristic than in the other forms of Castleman disease. [b]Hyaline-vascular follicles are regressed follicles with hyalinization and lymphoid depletion, a concentric onion-skin appearance to the rings of the mantle zone cells, and penetrating vessels (lollipop). [c]Some patients with Castleman disease may also have some of these processes in addition to Castleman disease; careful clinical evaluation is needed. [d]HIV-positive patients can have hyaline-vascular unicentric Castleman disease. [e]See {1110}. [f]Patients with KSHV/HHV8+ multicentric Castleman disease should be carefully evaluated for other KSHV/HHV8-associated diseases (Kaposi sarcoma, primary effusion lymphoma / extracavitary primary effusion lymphoma, etc.). [g]Conditions combined from {4120} and {1321}. References: {1110,4308,2967,4120,1321}.

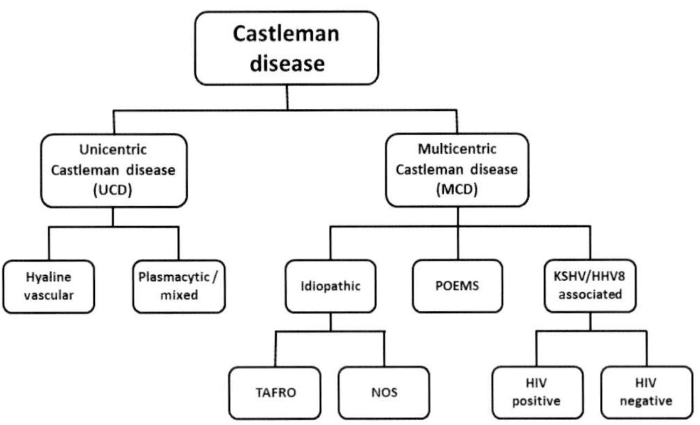

Fig. 4.08 Classification of Castleman disease. Structure of the classification of Castleman disease. POEMS, polyneuropathy, organomegaly, endocrinopathy, myeloma protein, and skin changes (see *Plasma cell neoplasms with associated paraneoplastic syndrome*, p. 631); TAFRO, thrombocytopenia, anasarca, fever / inflammatory symptoms, renal dysfunction / bone marrow reticulin fibrosis, organomegaly.

diagnosis of IgG4-related disease is broad and includes malignancy, antineutrophil cytoplasmic antibody (ANCA) vasculitides, nonspecific chronic inflammatory changes, and others; establishing a diagnosis requires a multidisciplinary approach, incorporating clinical, pathological, radiographic, and serological findings.

Castleman disease is not a single disorder, but rather several different, etiologically unrelated diseases (see Table 4.06, p. 305). Nearly all cases of unicentric Castleman disease are of hyaline-vascular type; hyaline-vascular Castleman disease has well-defined pathological features and probably represents a neoplasm of stromal origin with abundant associated reactive lymphoid tissue. Multicentric Castleman disease (MCD) includes cases related to KSHV/HHV8 infection (KSHV/HHV8-MCD) and cases of uncertain etiology (idiopathic MCD). In a patient known to have multifocal lymphadenopathy, a diagnosis of KSHV/HHV8-MCD can be readily established on the basis of histological features and immunohistochemistry for KSHV/HHV8. Establishing a diagnosis of idiopathic MCD can be an elusive enterprise; it requires careful clinicopathological correlation, with integration of laboratory findings. A subset of cases of idiopathic MCD fulfil criteria for TAFRO (thrombocytopenia, anasarca, fever / inflammatory symptoms, renal dysfunction / bone marrow reticulin fibrosis, organomegaly). Recognition of this MCD type is important because of its differing prognosis and expected response to therapy.

Reactive B-cell–rich lymphoid proliferations that can mimic lymphoma

Louissaint A Jr
Ferry JA
Natkunam Y

Definition

These are non-neoplastic proliferations of lymphoid tissue in nodal or extranodal sites that may occasionally or frequently resemble B-cell lymphoma.

ICD-O coding

None

ICD-11 coding

4B07 Acquired lymphocytosis

Related terminology

Acceptable: lymphadenitis.

Subtype(s)

None

Localization

See Table 4.07 (p. 310).

Clinical features

Patients present with lymphadenopathy, enlarged tonsils or salivary glands, and/or mucosal ulceration. Symptoms vary by cause and organs involved. Manifestations may be more severe in immunodeficient patients.

Epidemiology

See Table 4.07 (p. 310).

Etiology

See Table 4.07 (p. 310).

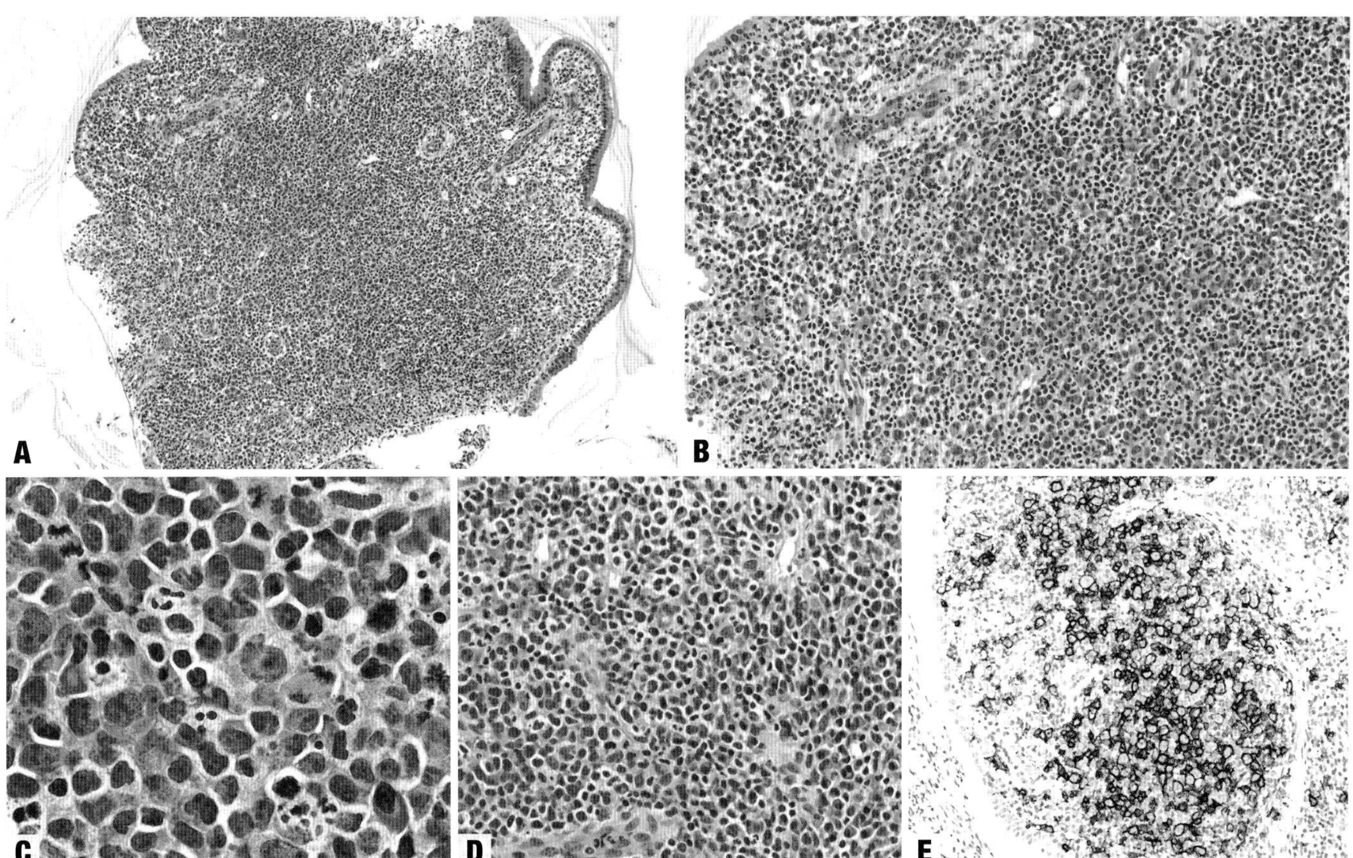

Fig. 4.09 Florid reactive lymphoid hyperplasia (lymphoma-like lesion) of the cervix. **A** Low-power view shows endocervix with a dense lymphoid infiltrate that fills the stroma and involves the surface epithelium. **B** Higher-magnification view shows a mixture small and large lymphoid cells, plasma cells, and neutrophils, with surface epithelial involvement. Large cells are present in a vaguely nodular pattern. **C** The infiltrate includes small and frequent large lymphoid cells, a few plasma cells, and frequent mitoses. **D** A focus with many large cells blends with an area with marked chronic cervicitis with many small lymphocytes and plasma cells. **E** The large cells are positive for CD20; they expressed CD30 (subset) and had a high proliferation index. Plasma cells were polytypic.

Pathogenesis

Infectious agents, drugs/toxins, or autoimmune phenomena

Macroscopic appearance

Patients may present with enlarged lymph nodes, expanded extranodal lymphoid tissue, or ulceration, sometimes associated with necrosis.

Histopathology

Reactive conditions mimicking lymphoma show one of several patterns. Key examples are described below.

Nodal follicular / nodular proliferations

Florid follicular hyperplasia

Florid follicular hyperplasia may be associated with a variety of reactive or inflammatory conditions, or conditions of infectious etiology, and can pose problems in its distinction from follicular lymphoma. Patients with autoimmune diseases such as rheumatoid arthritis and systemic lupus erythematosus, as well as those with HIV infection (particularly before HIV-specific treatment), sometimes present with florid follicular hyperplasia. Generally, follicles are widely spaced, are of uneven size and shape, and contain prominent germinal centres (GCs) with polarization and tingible-body macrophages. GC cells are negative for BCL2 expression, and the Ki-67 proliferation index is high.

Table 4.07 Reactive B-cell–rich lymphoid proliferations that can mimic lymphoma[a] (continued on next page)

Etiology	Entity	Patient characteristics	Clinical features and location	Histopathology	Differential diagnosis and differentiating features
Nodal follicular / nodular proliferation					
Unknown/ multiple	Florid follicular hyperplasia	Children / young adults; can be seen at all ages	Adenotonsillar hypertrophy; cervical or axillary lymphadenopathy Location: Lymph nodes, tonsils, adenoids	Follicles are widely spaced and of uneven size and shape, and they contain prominent germinal centres with polarization and tingible-body macrophages; varying degrees of paracortical and sinusoidal hyperplasia may be present	Follicular lymphoma: CD20 and germinal-centre B-cell markers highlight a preserved architecture; no aberrant BCL2 expression within follicles
Unknown/ multiple	Progressive transformation of germinal centres	Young/middle-aged adults; M > F	No or minor localized lymph node enlargement Location: Lymph nodes	Enlarged follicles with involution of mantle zone B cells with resulting disruption of germinal centres	NLPHL: In progressive transformation of germinal centres there is a lack of CD20+ LP cells and of PD1+ T-cell rosettes; mantle zone B cells are best highlighted by stains for IgD and BCL2
Autoimmune	Systemic lupus erythematosus	Young/middle-aged adults; F > M; more common in people of African American, Hispanic, and Asian descent	Variable symptoms with periodic flares; treated with NSAIDs, corticosteroids, immunosuppressants, and biologicals; end-organ damage in kidney, brain, lung, heart, and blood vessels Location: Lymph nodes	Paracortical expansion by immunoblasts, histiocytes, apoptotic and amorphous debris; neutrophils and granulomas are absent; prominent plasma cells	MZL: Immunohistochemistry for CD20, MNDA, CD43, kappa, and lambda helps rule out MZL; absence of IG rearrangements
Extranodal follicular / nodular proliferation					
Autoimmune	Sjögren syndrome	Adults aged > 40 years; F > M	Dry eyes and dry mouth; some patients also have rheumatoid arthritis or SLE; increased risk of EMZL or DLBCL Location: Salivary glands	Lymphoepithelial sialadenitis: follicular hyperplasia and prominent lymphoepithelial lesions	EMZL
Unknown/ multiple	Lymphoma-like lesions of the female genital tract	Women of reproductive age	Variable Location: Cervix, uterus, vulva	Lymphoid hyperplasia, atypical variably sized B cells in polymorphous background	DLBCL
Unknown/ multiple	Rectal tonsil	Middle-aged adults	Localized, raised mass lesion Location: Rectum, lamina propria and submucosa	Discrete nodule of organized lymphoid tissue with follicular hyperplasia	Follicular lymphoma, MZL: Rectal tonsil shows hyperplastic germinal centres without excess extrafollicular B cells or clonal plasma cells; lacks clonal IGH rearrangements

CHL, classic Hodgkin lymphoma; DLBCL, diffuse large B-cell lymphoma; EMZL, extranodal marginal zone lymphoma; LP, lymphocyte-predominant; MZL, marginal zone lymphoma; NLPHL, nodular lymphocyte-predominant Hodgkin lymphoma; NMZL, nodal marginal zone lymphoma SLE, systemic lupus erythematosus.
[a]Histiocytic necrotizing lymphadenitis (Kikuchi–Fujimoto disease) can have an immunoblastic proliferation that mimics lymphoma, but it is composed of T-lineage immunoblasts and so is not included in this table. [b]See separate sections on IgG4-related disease and mucocutaneous ulcer.

Table 4.07 Reactive B-cell–rich lymphoid proliferations that can mimic lymphoma[a] (continued)

Etiology	Entity	Patient characteristics	Clinical features and location	Histopathology	Differential diagnosis and differentiating features
Unknown/ multiple	IgG4-related disease[b]	Middle-aged and older adults; M > F	Variable symptoms with periodic flares; treated with NSAIDs, corticosteroids, immunosuppressants, and biologicals; end-organ damage in kidney, brain, lung, heart, and blood vessels; good response to steroids and/or rituximab in most cases Location: Enlargement of salivary glands (submandibular > parotid) and/or lacrimal gland, and/or orbital soft tissue masses +/− lymphadenopathy +/− lesions beyond head and neck	Extranodal sites: follicular hyperplasia, mixed infiltrate of eosinophils and many plasma cells; obliterative phlebitis; storiform fibrosis; increased number and percentage of IgG4+ plasma cells Lymph nodes: follicular and/or paracortical hyperplasia, some with progressively transformed germinal centres, some with sclerosis; some cases reminiscent of Castleman disease; increased number and percentage of IgG4+ plasma cells	Very broad (see main text)
Unknown/ multiple	Marginal zone hyperplasia	Unilateral or bilateral tonsillar enlargement or pharyngeal mass +/− dyspnoea or apnoea; other patients have involvement of appendix	Patients alive and well after excision of lesion	Expanded marginal zones with numerous B cells invading crypt epithelium +/− invasion of germinal centres, composed of CD20+ B cells that are usually CD43+, CD21+, IgM+, IgD+, monotypic lambda light chain +, IRF4 (MUM1)−, IRTA1+, high proliferation index	NMZL: Absent clonal IGH or immunoglobulin light chain by gene rearrangement studies
Nodal immunoblastic proliferation (interfollicular, paracortical, or diffuse pattern)					
Iatrogenic	Postvaccination lymphadenitis	Variable	Variable Location: Lymph nodes	Variable pattern, commonly mononucleosis-like	DLBCL and CHL: Immunohistochemistry: immunoblasts show polytypic kappa/ lambda light chain expression in reactive proliferations, and monotypic expression in lymphoma; CD15 is positive in CHL Hodgkin variants, whereas reactive immunoblasts are CD15-negative; immunohistochemistry for CMV can help identify CMV lymphadenitis Serology: serological testing for EBV may be helpful Molecular: gene rearrangement studies
Iatrogenic	Drug sensitivity, e.g. to phenytoin	Variable	Variable Location: Lymph nodes	Variable pattern, commonly mononucleosis-like	
Infection	Infectious mononucleosis	Mainly adolescents and young adults	Fever, fatigue, sore throat, cervical lymphadenopathy, atypical lymphocytosis in peripheral blood; usually self-limited Location: Lymph nodes	Tonsils and/or lymph nodes: interfollicular/paracortical expansion by B-lineage immunoblasts, small and medium-sized lymphoid cells, plasma cells +/− Reed–Sternberg–like B cells, frequent mitoses and necrosis	
Infection	CMV	Immunocompetent and immunodeficient patients over a broad age range	Localized or generalized lymphadenopathy, +/− symptoms similar to those of infectious mononucleosis; usually self-limited in immunocompetent patients Location: Lymph nodes	Lymph nodes with florid follicular and monocytoid B-cell hyperplasia; rarely, there may be an immunoblastic proliferation	
Extranodal immunoblastic proliferation					
Infection	EBV+ mucocutaneous ulcer[b]	Immunosuppressed patients (elderly, iatrogenic, posttransplant)	Single, shallow, often painful ulcer; most cases regress spontaneously; respond to withdrawal of immunosuppression (if possible) or localized treatment Location: Ulcerated lesion of skin, oral mucosa, tonsils, palate, gastrointestinal tract	Well-circumscribed ulcer with small and medium-sized lymphoid cells, plasma cells, and immunoblasts, +/− HRS-like cells and necrosis	DLBCL, Hodgkin lymphoma
Other proliferations					
Unknown/ multiple	Indolent B-lymphoblastic proliferation (haematogone hyperplasia)	Children	Nonspecific lymphadenopathy or tonsillar hypertrophy Location: Lymph nodes, tonsils	Paracortical or sinusoidal proliferation of TdT-positive B cells	B-lymphoblastic lymphoma: Lack of uniform expression of TdT and B-lineage markers

CHL, classic Hodgkin lymphoma; DLBCL, diffuse large B-cell lymphoma; EMZL, extranodal marginal zone lymphoma; LP, lymphocyte-predominant; MZL, marginal zone lymphoma; NLPHL, nodular lymphocyte-predominant Hodgkin lymphoma; NMZL, nodal marginal zone lymphoma SLE, systemic lupus erythematosus.
[a]Histiocytic necrotizing lymphadenitis (Kikuchi–Fujimoto disease) can have an immunoblastic proliferation that mimics lymphoma, but it is composed of T-lineage immunoblasts and so is not included in this table. [b]See separate sections on IgG4-related disease and mucocutaneous ulcer.

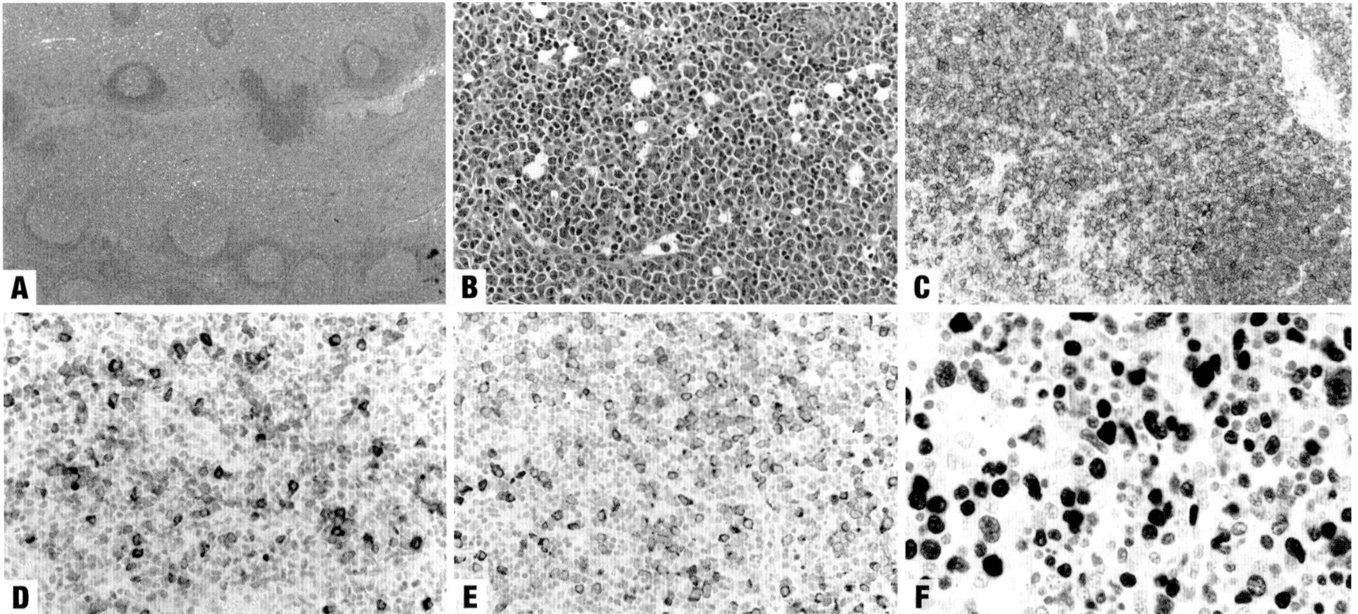

Fig. 4.10 Infectious mononucleosis. **A** Tonsil with polymorphous diffuse interfollicular expansion. **B** Higher-magnification view shows interfollicular expansion by a predominance of immunoblasts, with admixed small and medium-sized lymphocytes and plasma cells. **C** Immunohistochemistry for CD20 shows that the infiltrate contains sheets of B-lineage immunoblasts. A reactive follicle present in the lower-right corner. **D,E** Immunohistochemistry for immunoglobulin light chain shows polytypic expression of kappa (**D**) and lambda (**E**) light chain. **F** In situ hybridization for EBV-encoded small RNA (EBER) shows staining of cells of a wide range of sizes.

Progressive transformation of germinal centres

Progressive transformation of GCs has an unknown etiology and most frequently affects the cervical lymph nodes of children and young adults, in a background of reactive follicular hyperplasia {1491,1188,450}. The nodules are large and well-circumscribed, and they show infiltration of GCs by mantle zone B cells with gradual dismantling of GCs {1822,1526}. Rarely, progressive transformation of GCs may mimic nodular lymphocyte-predominant Hodgkin lymphoma, and may precede, co-occur with, or follow it.

Immunohistochemistry shows CD20+ GCs lacking lymphocyte-predominant cells and PD1+ rosettes; they are composed of IgD/BCL2+ mantle zone B cells admixed with varying proportions of GC B cells. Progressive transformation of GCs may also rarely resemble floral variant of follicular lymphoma or mantle cell lymphoma, which can be excluded by immunohistochemistry.

Extranodal follicular / nodular proliferations

Florid reactive lymphoid hyperplasia / lymphoma-like lesion of female genital tract

The cervix and (less often) the endometrium and vulva are rarely involved by florid reactive lymphoid hyperplasia mimicking lymphoma (lymphoma-like lesions) {1462,4517}. Patients are usually of reproductive age. Lymphoma-like lesions can cause abnormal vaginal bleeding or may be an incidental finding. They may be associated with EBV, *Chlamydia trachomatis*, HIV, and HPV infection, or with intrauterine devices, or they may occur after surgery {1462,1327,3356}. They are typically superficially located, associated with erosion of overlying epithelium, lacking a mass lesion, and composed of a polymorphous infiltrate of small and large lymphoid cells, often with polytypic plasma cells and neutrophils. Large cells are mostly B cells. Sclerosis is absent {1462,4517}. Clonal IGH rearrangement is not

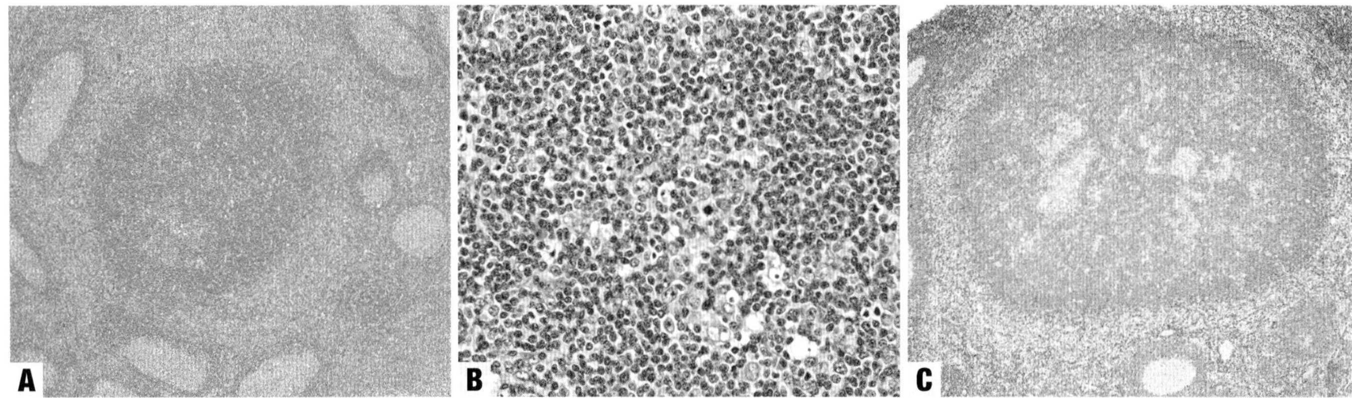

Fig. 4.11 Reactive lymphoid hyperplasia with progressive transformation of germinal centres. **A** Low-power view shows an enlarged, dark, progressively transformed germinal centre with adjacent small, typical reactive follicles. **B** High-power view shows a predominance of small lymphocytes and remnants of a germinal centre (large lymphoid cells, mitotic figure, and apoptotic debris). **C** An immunostain for BCL2 shows staining of most cells in a large follicle with a progressively transformed germinal centre; remnants of the germinal centre are negative for BCL2.

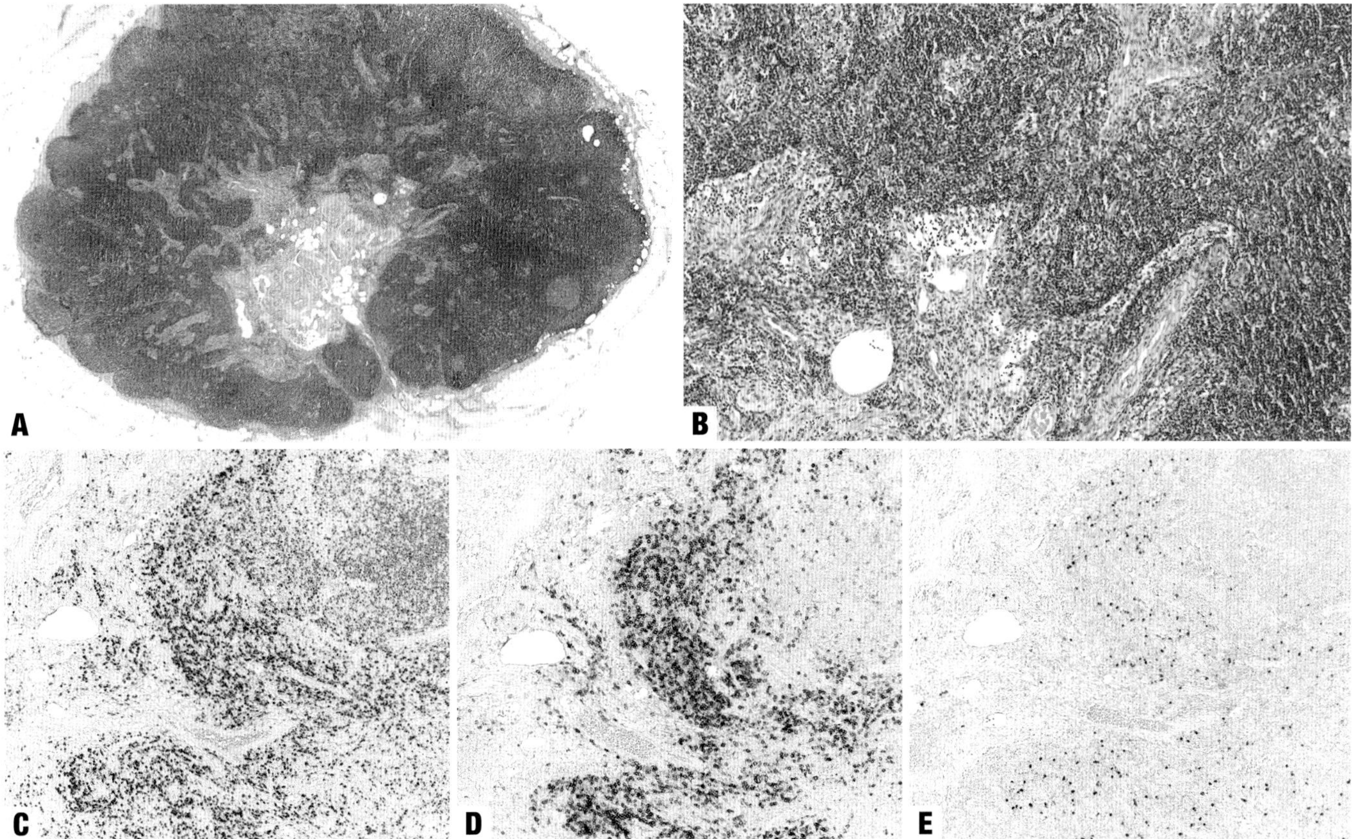

Fig. 4.12 Indolent B-lymphoblastic proliferation. **A** The lymph node has preservation of the normal architecture. **B** In areas with immature B cells, there is no significant cytological atypia. **C** In the medulla, close to the hilus, are frequent B cells expressing PAX5 more strongly than other B cells. **D** CD10+ cells are present in a distribution similar to that of the strongly PAX5+ cells. T cells were sparse in areas with CD10+ cells. **E** A subset of the CD10+ cells are TdT+.

uncommon, although patients are free of lymphoma on follow-up {4517,1327,3356}.

Nodal/extranodal immunoblastic proliferations

Infectious mononucleosis (IM)

IM is caused by EBV in adolescents and young adults who present with lymphadenopathy and tonsillar enlargement. Later stages may show architectural distortion with paracortical expansion and increased numbers of large immunoblasts in a background of small lymphocytes and plasma cells. Occasionally, a diffuse proliferation of immunoblasts, including some resembling HRS cells, may mimic a large B-cell lymphoma or classic Hodgkin lymphoma (CHL), respectively. IM often shows incomplete architectural effacement and a mixed cellular infiltrate, with a predominance of CD8+ T cells, whereas the CHL microenvironment has an elevated CD4:CD8 ratio. IM immunoblasts usually have a post–germinal-centre phenotype (IRF4 [MUM1]+, CD10−, BCL6−) and show polytypic light chain expression. HRS-like cells in IM usually express both CD30 and CD45, but lack CD15, and include both B and T immunoblasts, in contrast to CHL. In CHL, EBV is positive in the HRS cells, whereas in IM, EBV is positive in a range of cells including large immunoblasts and background small lymphocytes.

Extranodal immunoblastic proliferation

See *EBV-positive mucocutaneous ulcer* (p. 565).

Other proliferations

Indolent B-lymphoblastic proliferations (haematogone hyperplasia)

Expansions of TdT-positive B-lymphoblastic proliferations in reactive lymph nodes and tonsils may be mistaken for involvement by lymphoblastic lymphoma. These cells are typically small and involve the paracortex and/or medulla of the lymph node, and they occur most frequently in reactive lymph nodes in children. In contrast, B-lymphoblastic lymphoma is characterized by larger blasts with a uniform expression of TdT and B-cell markers {3065}. The clinical context further helps in distinguishing indolent proliferations.

Cytology

The distinction between reactive B-cell–rich lymphoid proliferations and B-cell lymphoma is challenging on FNA specimens. Flow cytometric analysis to assess for evidence of B-cell light chain monotypia may be supportive in this setting {3618}.

Diagnostic molecular pathology

Occasional cases may show such distortion of the normal architecture or cytological atypia as to raise the question of lymphoma. In such cases, gene rearrangement studies are useful to show the absence of a clonal B- or T-cell population. Genetic techniques can assist with the identification of certain infectious agents {3303}.

Essential and desirable diagnostic criteria

Essential: identification of appropriate histological features along with documentation of the nature of the proliferation through supporting ancillary studies (see Table 4.07, p. 310), with no diagnostic evidence of lymphoma or another neoplasm.

Desirable: where appropriate, identification of an infectious agent by immunohistochemistry, special stains, microbiology culture, or molecular techniques; recognition of an underlying autoimmune disease, immunodeficiency, or other disease by clinical or laboratory criteria.

Staging

Not applicable

Prognosis and prediction

The outcome is dependent on the underlying disease and available therapy. Most cases due to infection resolve spontaneously or respond to antibiotics. The outcome in patients with autoimmune diseases or immunodeficiency is variable.

IgG4-related disease

Cheuk W
Bledsoe JR
Deshpande V
Ferry JA
Flanagan M
Sato Y
Yamamoto H
Zen Y

Definition

Immunoglobulin G4–related disease (IgG4-RD) is an immune-mediated disease characterized by mass-forming lesions with a lymphoplasmacytic infiltrate rich in IgG4+ plasma cells and storiform fibrosis, usually with an elevated serum IgG4 titre.

ICD-O coding

9760/1 IgG4-related disease

ICD-11 coding

4A43.0 IgG4-related disease

Related terminology

Not recommended: IgG4-related autoimmune disease; IgG4-related sclerosing disease.

Subtype(s)

None

Localization

IgG4-RD can affect almost any organ, with the pancreas, salivary glands, and orbit being the most common {463}. Multiorgan involvement, synchronously or metachronously, is typical, with three organs being affected on average {4283,4122}. Four distinctive patterns of involvement have been described: pancreas/liver/biliary, retroperitoneum/aorta, head and neck, and systemic phenotypes {4283}. About 30–60% of patients show lymphadenopathy (> 10 mm) {2482,4282,4467}, most often involving the mediastinal, intra-abdominal, axillary, and cervical nodes {699}. Lymphadenopathy attributable to IgG4-RD has been termed IgG4-related lymphadenopathy, which commonly occurs concurrently with IgG4-RD, but may precede extranodal involvement, and typically involves lymph nodes regional to the extranodal site but may be more extensive and sometimes diffuse {3585,373}. Bone marrow involvement is rare {1858,1710, 2000,1696,4147}.

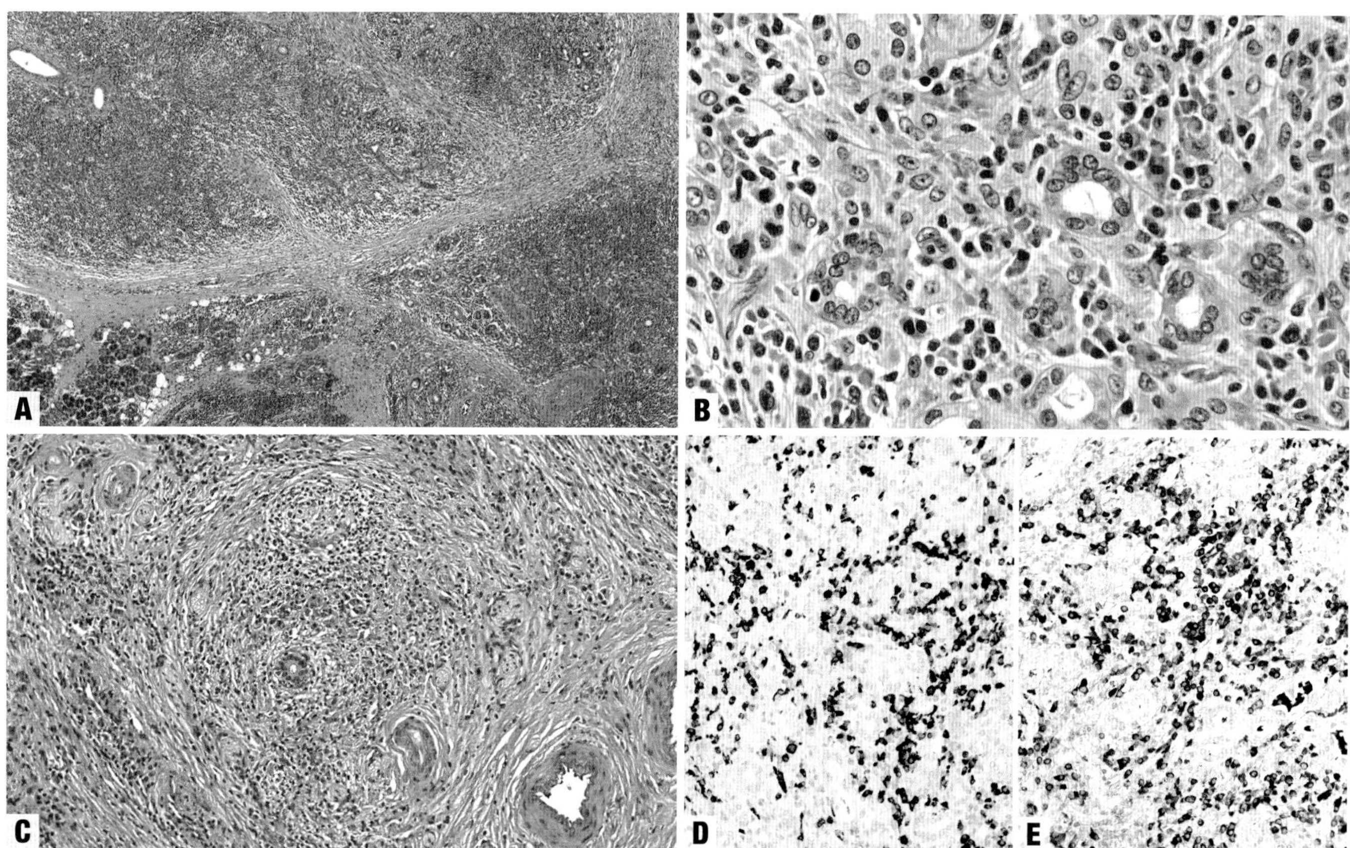

Fig. 4.13 IgG4-related sialadenitis. **A** Low-power magnification shows variable degrees of inflammation, glandular atrophy, and fibrosis in different areas of the submandibular gland. Note the accentuated lobular architecture. **B** Periductal lymphocytic and plasma cell infiltrate is present, and lymphoepithelial lesions are typically absent. **C** There is an atrophic area with storiform fibrosis and a few residual ducts. **D,E** IgG immunostaining shows IgG4+ plasma cells (**D**) constituting > 60% of all IgG+ plasma cells (**E**).

Clinical features

The patients, usually in good general condition, present with symptoms attributable to mass lesions or their localized effects, frequently mimicking malignancies clinically (see Table 4.08). Lymph nodes are usually non-tender and only moderately enlarged (< 30 mm), lacking necrosis and perinodal infiltration on imaging {699,1931}.

Elevated serum IgG4 generally correlates with disease activity, although it is not specific for IgG4-RD {2222}. Elevated eosinophil count, serum IgE, ESR, antinuclear antibodies, and rheumatoid factor are common, as are low complement levels, but serum LDH, IgA, and IgM are normal, and autoantibodies specific for other diseases are negative. C-reactive protein and IL-6 are typically normal {3585,3587,2966}, except in IgG4-related aortitis/periaortitis {1903}. IgG4-RD is FDG-avid on PET, which may reflect disease activity {290}.

Epidemiology

IgG4-RD is an uncommon condition affecting adults, with a median age in the fifth or sixth decade of life, and a male predilection. Pancreatic/hepatic/biliary and retroperitoneal/aortic involvement is more common in White people and men, whereas head and neck involvement appears to be more common in people of Asian descent and women {4283}. Paediatric cases are rare {1889,2222}.

Etiology

The etiology is unknown. IgG4-RD may be associated with chronic antigenic stimulation by self (ANXA11, laminin-511, galectin-3, prohibitin) or unidentified antigens in genetically susceptible individuals with impaired immunological tolerance {1003,1672,3203,2564,3729,1746}.

Pathogenesis

Studies suggest that chronic antigenic stimulation and a breach of immune tolerance lead to oligoclonal expansion of circulating plasmablasts and CD4+ cytotoxic T cells. Meanwhile, increased follicular T helper cell subsets promote plasmablastic differentiation, IgG4 isotype switching, and germinal-centre formation in affected sites {2593,2592,56}. CD4+ cytotoxic T cells, IgG4+ plasmablasts, and locally recruited M2 macrophages in affected sites express profibrotic cytokines, leading to fibroblast activation and collagen production {3204}. IgG4 probably plays an anti-inflammatory role in an unsuccessful attempt to dampen the aberrant immune response.

Macroscopic appearance

The lymph nodes are rubbery to firm or fibrotic, with tan-white cut surfaces. The extranodal lesions are non-circumscribed and firm; fibrosis can extend into the surrounding tissues.

Table 4.08 Common sites involved by IgG4-related disease, and corresponding clinical features

Site	Clinical presentation	IgG4+/mm²
Pancreas	Parenchymal mass lesion mimicking pancreatic carcinoma (painless obstructive jaundice, pancreatic mass, abdominal pain) and/or pancreatic insufficiency (new-onset diabetes mellitus, steatorrhoea)	> 40 (biopsy) > 200 (excision)
Hepatobiliary system	Biliary obstruction mimicking cholangiocarcinoma (obstructive jaundice, abnormal liver function tests) or sclerosing cholangitis exhibiting dramatic response to steroids {1859} Gallbladder mass mimicking cancer (right upper quadrant pain, jaundice) {1152} Hepatic mass mimicking cancer (right upper quadrant pain, jaundice) or abnormal liver function tests {2252}	> 40 (biopsy) > 200 (excision)
Orbit	Unilateral or bilateral painless orbital swelling, proptosis, and diplopia; rarely, eye pain and visual impairment {698,2005}	> 400
Salivary glands	Unilateral or bilateral painless swelling; occasionally simultaneous bilateral lacrimal, parotid, and submandibular gland involvement (Mikulicz disease); xerostomia is usually mild and responds well to steroids {2318}	> 400
Retroperitoneum	Asymptomatic or nonspecific constitutional symptoms (fatigue, anorexia, fever, weight loss), low back or flank pain, leg oedema, abnormal renal function test, hydronephrosis on imaging {2705,731}	> 120
Mediastinum	Asymptomatic or dyspnoea, haemoptysis, dysphagia, and chest pain {3933}	> 120
Aorta	Asymptomatic or low back pain; some patients may present with aortic aneurysm or dissection {2963,2705}	> 200
Lymph node	Asymptomatic or local mass effects (hydronephrosis or lower limb swelling for pelvic lymph nodes) {4561}	> 400
Kidney	Incidental finding on imaging (nodular or wedge-shaped lesions, diffuse involvement, thickening of the renal pelvis) or abnormal renal function tests / urinalysis, hypocomplementaemia or elevated serum IgE {3519}	> 40 (biopsy) > 120 (excision)
Dura	Headache, cranial nerve palsies, visual impairment, motor weakness, numbness, seizures, cognitive decline, and gait instability {8,2629}	> 40
Pituitary	Headache, visual field defect, hyperprolactinaemia (galactorrhoea), hypopituitarism (diabetes insipidus, fatigue, amenorrhoea) {2323}	> 40
Skin and soft tissue	Plaques or indurated nodules frequently in the head and neck region; local neurological symptoms (numbness and shoulder drop) due to associated nerve involvement are common {696}	> 800
Lung and pleura	Incidental finding of abnormal chest imaging; or cough, chest pain, dyspnoea, haemoptysis Nodules, ground-glass opacities, bronchial wall / bronchovascular bundle thickening, interlobular septal wall thickening, infiltrative shadow, pleural thickening or effusion {2587,2775}	> 80 (biopsy) > 200 (excision)
Thyroid	Goitre and/or hypothyroidism {3942}	> 80

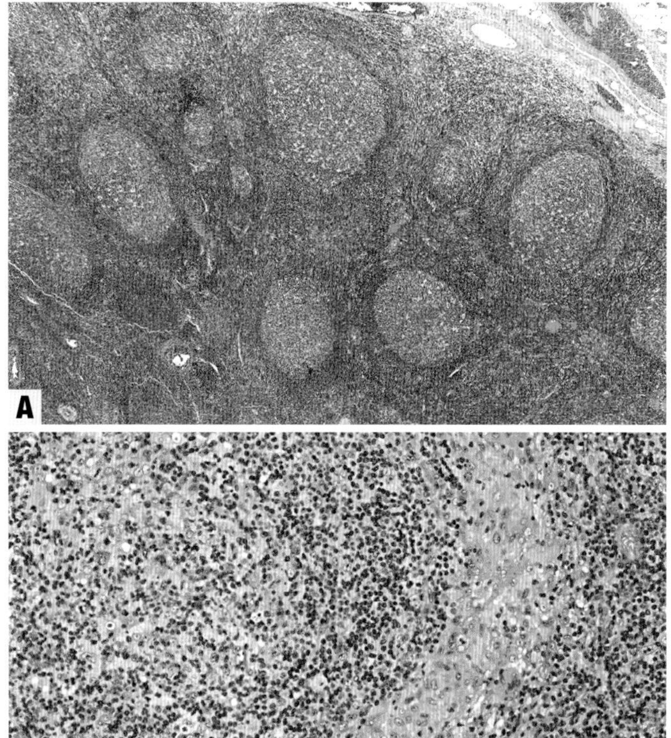

Fig. 4.14 IgG4-related lymphadenopathy, follicular hyperplasia pattern. The follicular hyperplasia pattern is marked by many reactive lymphoid follicles (**A**) with perifollicular ring-like granulomas (**B**).

Histopathology

The unifying morphological features of IgG4-RD are an IgG4+ plasma cell–rich lymphoplasmacytic and eosinophilic infiltrate, and storiform fibrosis, the former predominating in the early (inflammatory) phase and the latter in the late (fibrotic) phase. Because superficially located lesions (e.g. in the orbit, salivary gland, or skin) often present earlier than deep-seated counterparts (e.g. in the pancreas, retroperitoneum, or meninges), the diagnostic IgG4+ plasma cell count differs according to the site. Nevertheless, elevation of both the absolute IgG4+ cell count and the IgG4+:IgG+ ratio (> 40%) is required for the diagnosis {935}.

Admixed reactive lymphoid follicles are common, particularly in head and neck lesions. Obliterative phlebitis, characterized by a transmural inflammatory infiltrate and fibrous occlusion of venous lumina, is common but is not always found {1184,4548}. Elastic stain is useful to demonstrate completely obliterated veins. Necrosis, abscess, neutrophilic infiltration, necrotizing vasculitis, and granulomas are not typical of IgG4-RD and should prompt consideration of alternative diagnoses.

Lymphadenopathy in patients with established IgG4-RD shows a spectrum of morphological patterns that are usually but not consistently associated with increased IgG4 count and IgG4+:IgG+ ratio (> 40%) {3585,373}. In the multicentric Castleman disease–like pattern (type I), hyperplastic and regressed follicles are accompanied by immature to mature plasma cells, small lymphocytes, and eosinophils, with abundant IgG4+ plasma cells {3587,2966}.

Similar features can be seen in patients with hyper–IL-6 syndrome (e.g. multicentric Castleman disease, rheumatoid arthritis), but the sheet-like proliferation of mature plasma cells and frequent haemosiderin deposition in this syndrome are not seen in IgG4-related lymphadenopathy {2966,3587}, and patients typically have prominent constitutional symptoms and elevated IL-6, C-reactive protein, IgA, and IgM {3585,3587,2966}. The follicular hyperplasia pattern (type II) features reactive follicular hyperplasia with many IgG4+ plasma cells in germinal centres or the interfollicular zone. The interfollicular expansion pattern (type III) shows a markedly expanded interfollicular zone with many high endothelial venules, small lymphocytes, immunoblasts, plasmablasts, plasma cells, and eosinophils. This pattern can be distinguished from angioimmunoblastic T-cell lymphoma by the absence of atypical T cells and irregularly expanded follicular dendritic cell meshworks. The progressive transformation of germinal centres pattern (type IV) shows transformed follicles that are two to four times as large as normal follicles, with markedly thickened mantle zones with inward extension breaking up the germinal centres, and many IgG4+ plasma cells in the germinal centres. The inflammatory pseudotumour–like pattern (type V) is the least common, featuring focal to extensive fibrosclerosis of the nodal parenchyma and infiltration of IgG4+ plasma cells and eosinophils.

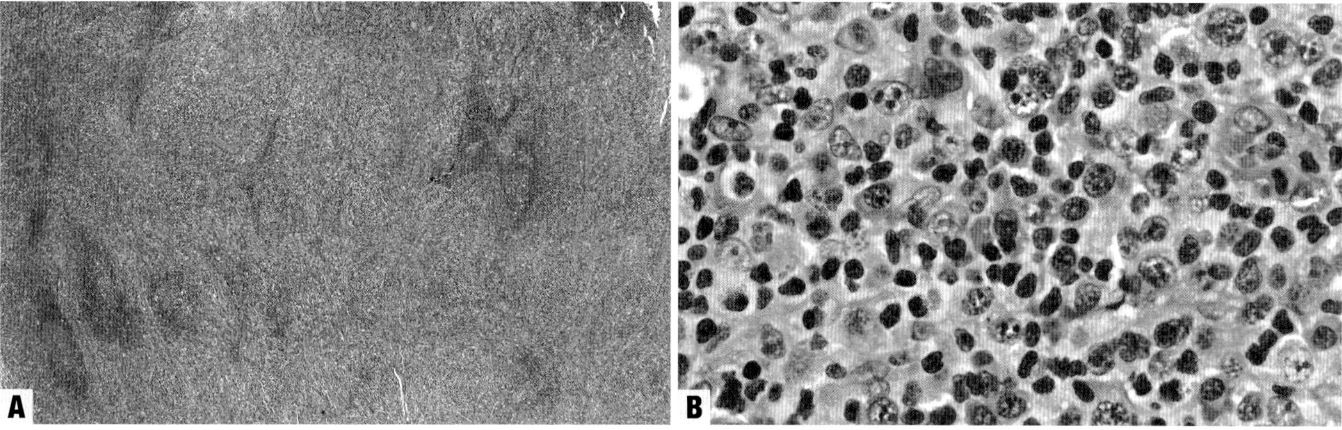

Fig. 4.15 IgG4-related lymphadenopathy, interfollicular expansion pattern. The interfollicular expansion pattern is characterized by a markedly expanded interfollicular region with a few follicles (**A**) and activated large cells, immature plasma cells, eosinophils, and some lymphocytes in the interfollicular region (**B**).

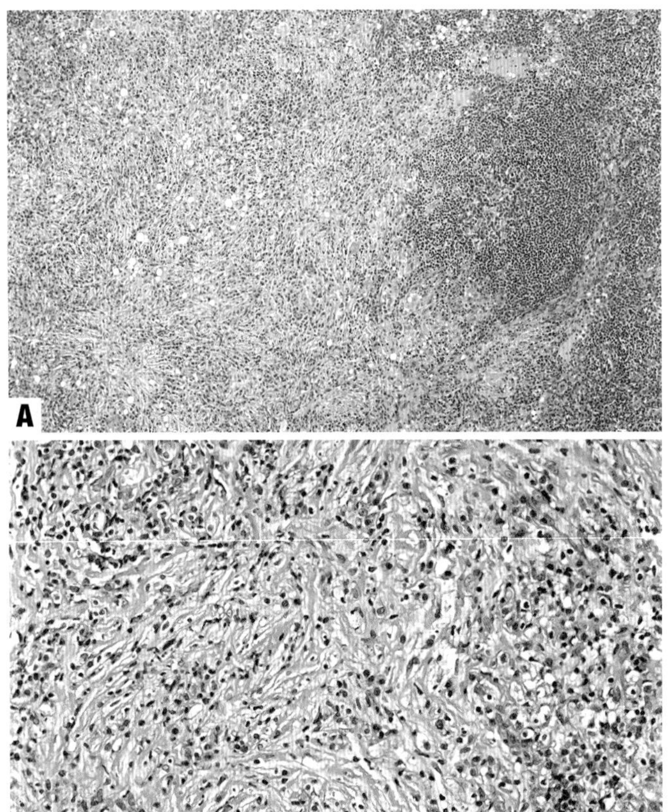

Fig. 4.16 IgG4-related lymphadenopathy, inflammatory pseudotumour–like pattern. The inflammatory pseudotumour–like pattern shows partial effacement of nodal parenchyma by fibrosis and lymphoplasmacytic infiltrate (**A**) and storiform fibrosis with lymphocytes, plasma cells, and eosinophils (**B**).

A lymph node may show a combination of patterns, and different patterns can be found in different nodes. An inflammatory pseudotumour–like pattern and the presence of increased IgG4+ plasma cells and IgG4+:IgG+ ratio, with eosinophils in the fibrotic and/or interfollicular zones, are relatively specific features for IgG4-related lymphadenopathy {4114,373}. The presence of an isolated increase in intrafollicular IgG4+ plasma cells, Castleman disease–like features, follicular hyperplasia patterns, and progressive transformation of germinal centres patterns are less specific {373}. Perifollicular ring-like granulomas and phlebitis are useful but nonspecific morphological features that should prompt consideration of IgG4-RD, particularly in lymph nodes with plasmacytosis {271,373}. Obliterative phlebitis is rarely encountered in lymph nodes. However, none of these patterns are entirely specific for IgG4-RD {2550}. Hence, IgG4-related lymphadenopathy can only be confidently diagnosed in the context of IgG4-RD, sometimes retrospectively in patients who subsequently develop IgG4-RD. The biological nature of isolated lymphadenopathy with increased IgG4+ plasma cells is not certain. Lymph nodes from patients with established IgG4-RD may not demonstrate increased IgG4+ plasma cells or any specific pathological change.

IgG4+ plasma cells in IgG4-RD are polyclonal. Immunostaining or in situ hybridization for kappa and lambda light chains is recommended in all potential cases of IgG4-RD to demonstrate polyclonality and exclude an IgG4-expressing lymphoma with plasmacytic differentiation or plasma cell neoplasm {376,1329, 4210}. Rarely, oligoclonal expansions of IgG4+ plasma cells may be encountered in nodal or extranodal sites, which may raise the possibility of lymphoma or a plasma cell neoplasm {375}.

Cytology

In extranodal sites, the aspirate is low in cellularity, comprising fibrous stromal fragments associated with a lymphoplasmacytic infiltrate. Scattered ductal structures enveloped by collagen bundles can be seen in aspirates from exocrine glands {693,1928}.

Diagnostic molecular pathology

Not applicable

Essential and desirable diagnostic criteria

Extranodal presentation

Essential: a lymphoplasmacytic infiltrate with increased IgG4+ plasma cells and an IgG4+:IgG+ plasma cell ratio of > 40%; storiform fibrosis; exclusion of well-defined entities that mimic IgG4-RD (e.g. antineutrophil cytoplasmic antibody [ANCA]-associated vasculitis, rheumatoid arthritis, multicentric Castleman disease, Rosai–Dorfman disease, inflammatory myofibroblastic tumour, chronic infection, lymphoma, plasma cell neoplasia).

Desirable: obliterative phlebitis; clinically compatible features: IgG4-RD in other body sites, elevated serum IgG4, and response to steroids/rituximab.

Nodal presentation

Essential: presence of extranodal IgG4-RD (prior, synchronous, or subsequent development); polytypic IgG4+ plasma cells > 400/mm^2, and an IgG4+:IgG+ plasma cell ratio of > 40%; exclusion of well-defined entities that mimic IgG4-RD (as listed above), hyper–IL-6 syndrome, and syphilis.

Desirable: IgG4+ plasma cells and eosinophils in the fibrotic and/or interfollicular zones of lymph nodes.

Staging

Not applicable

Prognosis and prediction

Although highly responsive to steroids, IgG4-RD follows a remitting and relapsing course and can lead to organ dysfunction and even death if not properly diagnosed and treated {698, 1682,243}. Multiorgan disease and high baseline IgG4, IgE, and peripheral eosinophilia are risk factors for relapse. Maintenance therapy with steroids, immunomodulators, and biological agents like rituximab have been used with variable success {2221}. An increased incidence of malignancy, including carcinoma and lymphoma, has been suggested in patients with IgG4-RD {1682,2570,158,3965,52}, but a causal relationship is still unclear {1593,1724,2403}.

Unicentric Castleman disease

Chadburn A
Bower M
Cesarman E
Elenitoba-Johnson KSJ
Fajgenbaum DC
Iwaki N
Medeiros LJ
Meignin V
Natkunam Y
van Rhee F

Definition

Unicentric Castleman disease (UCD) is a benign lymphoproliferative disorder with distinctive morphological features that involves a single lymph node or group of lymph nodes in one lymph node station.

ICD-O coding

None

ICD-11 coding

4B2Y Other specified disorders involving the immune system

Related terminology

None

Subtype(s)

Hyaline-vascular unicentric Castleman disease (HV-UCD); mixed/plasmacytic unicentric Castleman disease

Localization

UCD usually involves a single lymph node, or occasionally, one group of lymph nodes. The most common nodal stations are the mediastinum, neck, abdomen, and retroperitoneum {3949}. Rarely, extranodal sites are involved {3949,2476}.

Clinical features

Individuals of any age can develop UCD (median age: fourth decade of life) {4569,433,4308,4165}. There is a slight female predominance {4569,433}. Most patients are asymptomatic, and lesions are detected incidentally on physical examination or (more commonly) by imaging studies performed for unrelated reasons {4165,3884}. Depending on the size and location of UCD, patients may have symptoms related to compression. Autoimmune or paraneoplastic diseases are present in approximately 5% of patients with the hyaline-vascular subtype (HV-UCD) {3878}. A subset of patients with UCD, usually those with the mixed/plasmacytic subtype and uncommonly those with the HV-UCD subtype, have an inflammatory syndrome similar to that in patients with multicentric Castleman disease, including constitutional symptoms, hepatosplenomegaly, effusions, oedema, and laboratory abnormalities {4165,4564,3043,4524}. Secondary amyloid deposition of serum amyloid AA (AA amyloidosis) can occur in patients with the mixed/plasmacytic subtype {1146}. Approximately 15–20% of patients with UCD may have complicating disorders such as paraneoplastic pemphigus, bronchiolitis obliterans, follicular dendritic cell sarcoma, or lymphoma {433,4165}.

Epidemiology

UCD represents 50–70% of all Castleman disease cases {2842, 4569}. The incidence of UCD is 16–19 cases per 1 million person-years, with 5000–6000 new patients per year in the USA {2842, 4165}. Approximately 70–80% of UCD cases are of the HV-UCD subtype {4569,4165}.

Etiology

Unknown

Pathogenesis

Evidence suggests that HV-UCD is a benign clonal neoplasm derived from lymph node stromal cells, possibly follicular dendritic cells (FDCs). The evidence includes the detection of clonal karyotypes, the results of human androgen receptor alpha (HUMARA) testing {630,507}, and the results of mutation analyses showing gene mutations (most commonly *PDGFRB*) in a subset of cases {2328}. Evidence suggesting an FDC origin is the observation of FDC dysplasia in occasional cases, rare FDC sarcomas that have arisen in UCD, and the absence of IG and TR gene rearrangements {630}.

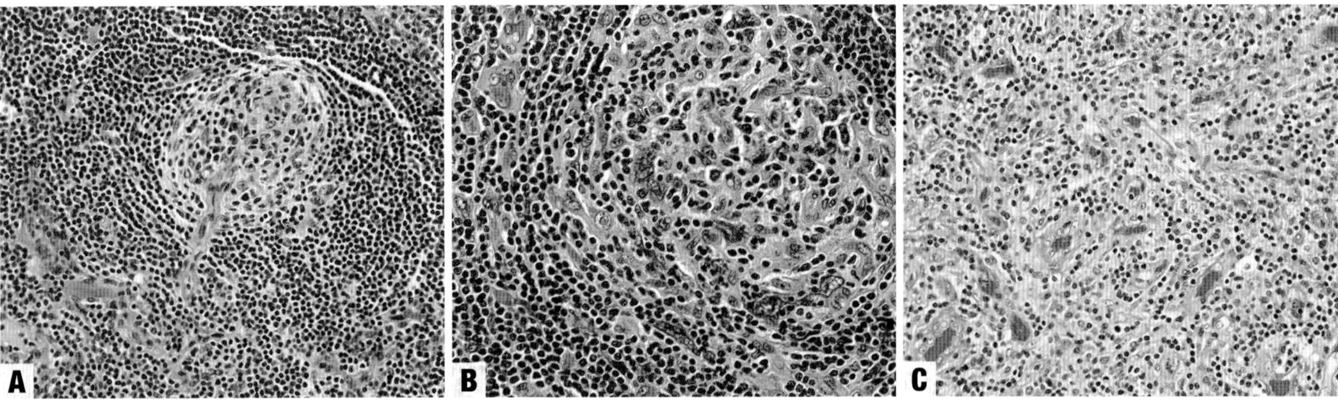

Fig. 4.17 Unicentric Castleman disease, hyaline-vascular subtype. **A** A follicle showing a hyaline-vascular lesion, also known as a lollipop lesion, with a regressed germinal centre and a prominent radial blood vessel with sclerosis. **B** The involuted follicle is relatively depleted of lymphocytes and contains multiple dysplastic, cytologically atypical follicular dendritic cells, including multinucleated forms. **C** The interfollicular (stromal) region is occupied by many small lymphocytes and a proliferation of many high endothelial blood vessels and other spindle-shape cells.

The pathogenesis of mixed/plasmacytic UCD is unknown. Cytokine dysregulation is involved, particularly IL-6, which is probably the cause of systemic inflammatory-type symptoms and/or laboratory abnormalities.

Macroscopic appearance

Lymph nodes vary in size, ranging from 20 to 200 mm {866}. HV-UCD lymph nodes tend to be large, with a firm, white, nodular cut surface. Dystrophic calcifications may be present. Lymph nodes involved by the mixed/plasmacytic UCD tend to be smaller and less firm.

Histopathology

The overall lymph node architecture is distorted, with variable prominence of the follicular and interfollicular/stromal components (see Table 4.06, p. 305, in *Tumour-like lesions with B-cell predominance: Introduction*) {866,4308}.

HV-UCD subtype

Follicles are increased in number and size throughout the lesion. Germinal centres are lymphocyte-depleted and enriched in FDCs that may occasionally show dysplasia. Radially oriented hyalinized or sclerotic blood vessels penetrate into germinal centres, forming hyaline-vascular (lollipop) lesions. Mantle zones are expanded with lymphocytes arranged in concentric (onion-skin) rings around germinal centres. Follicles may contain two or more small germinal centres surrounded by a single mantle (twinning). Interfollicular areas, which can predominate, are populated predominantly by small lymphocytes, with few or no activated large lymphoid cells, and contain many (often sclerotic) high endothelial venules, clusters of plasmacytoid dendritic cells and increased fibrosis. Sinuses are compressed and usually obliterated. The lymph node capsule is fibrotic and thickened, and sclerotic bands may be present.

Mixed/plasmacytic subtype

Unlike in the HV-UCD subtype, the lymph node architecture is usually well preserved. Interfollicular areas are expanded by numerous mature plasma cells in groups and sheets associated with variably prominent blood vessels {4308}. Follicles range from large and hyperplastic to small with regressive changes. Characteristic hyaline-vascular follicles may be present but are usually less well formed than in HV-UCD {4165}.

Immunohistochemistry

Immunohistochemistry shows numerous concentric rings of CD21+, CD23+, CD35+, and (usually) CD106 (VCAM1)+ FDCs. Germinal centres are variably lymphocyte-depleted, with the remaining B lymphocytes being CD10+, BCL6+, and BCL2−. Expanded mantle zones are composed of IgD+, BCL2+ B cells that may exhibit dim CD5 expression. Interfollicular blood vessels express vascular-associated markers such as CD31. Plasmacytoid dendritic cells are CD68+, CD123+, and TCL1+. The interfollicular plasma cells are usually polytypic, but there are reports of very rare cases describing the presence of monotypic plasma cells. TdT-positive cells can be present and rarely are numerous, consistent with a concomitant indolent T-lymphoblastic proliferation. CD3+ T cells show no evidence of an aberrant immunophenotype. In some cases, interfollicular regions may contain FDC hyperplasia (CD21+, CD35+) or smooth actin-positive spindle cells (angiomyoid areas) {2356}. KSHV/HHV8 latency-associated nuclear antigen (LANA) is negative. In situ hybridization for EBV-encoded small RNA (EBER) is negative or highlights rare bystander lymphocytes {4308}.

Differential diagnosis

The differential diagnosis of the HV-UCD subtype includes follicular hyperplasia and lymphomas with a nodular component (particularly follicular, mantle cell, or nodal marginal zone lymphoma). The differential diagnosis of the mixed/plasmacytic subtype includes autoimmune diseases (particularly rheumatoid arthritis, infectious disorders, lymphadenopathy of IgG4-related disease) and various neoplastic processes (particularly Hodgkin lymphomas and plasmacytoma). For the cases with monotypic plasma cells, POEMS syndrome (polyneuropathy, organomegaly, endocrinopathy, M protein, and skin changes), lymphoplasmacytic lymphoma, marginal zone lymphoma, and plasmacytoma should be excluded. Evaluation of histological and immunophenotypic features and correlation with clinical and laboratory findings is necessary to distinguish UCD from other disorders (see Table 4.06, p. 305, in *Tumour-like lesions with B-cell predominance: Introduction*).

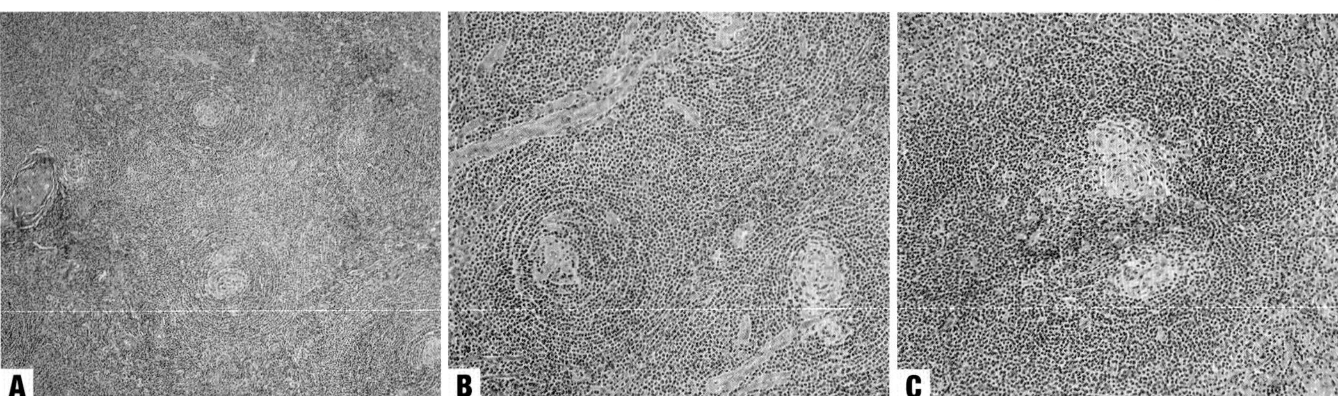

Fig. 4.18 Unicentric Castleman disease, hyaline-vascular subtype. **A** Low-power magnification showing large follicles composed of small, regressed germinal centres and expanded mantle zones with an onion-skin appearance. **B** Two follicles are shown, both with small, regressed germinal centres. One follicle has a prominent blood vessel penetrating the follicle, consistent with a hyaline-vascular lesion. **C** A large follicle contains two small, lymphocyte-depleted germinal centres, known as twinning.

Cytology

Cytological examination of HV-UCD (as well as other types of Castleman disease) shows characteristic features {2854}; however, the findings are often not sufficiently specific to establish a definitive diagnosis {1807,3756}.

Diagnostic molecular pathology

Molecular genetic testing is typically not required to establish a diagnosis.

Essential and desirable diagnostic criteria

HV-UCD subtype

Essential: involvement of a single lymph node or multiple lymph nodes in a single lymph node station, requiring clinical/radiographic correlation; hyaline-vascular follicles; fibrotic and hypervascular stroma with sinus compression.

Mixed/plasmacytic subtype

Essential: involvement of a single lymph node or multiple lymph nodes in a single lymph node station, requiring clinical/radiographic correlation; dense, interfollicular sheets of plasma cells, extending to the cortex; polytypic, or rarely monotypic, plasmacytosis; variably sized lymphoid follicles, including some with regressive changes.

Staging

Not applicable

Prognosis and prediction

Complete surgical excision is adequate in most cases, regardless of subtype; recurrence is rare {4165,3297}. Patients with asymptomatic unresectable disease may be followed. For patients with compression symptoms and unresectable disease, radiation therapy, immunochemotherapy, or embolization may be used {4569,286}. For patients with inflammatory symptoms and unresectable disease, anti–IL-6 therapy (e.g. siltuximab or tocilizumab), or alternatively, immunotherapy with or without steroids, is considered the most appropriate initial treatment {4165}. UCD patients with paraneoplastic pemphigus, bronchiolitis obliterans, follicular dendritic cell sarcoma, or lymphoma have a less favourable prognosis {433,4165}.

Idiopathic multicentric Castleman disease

Chadburn A
Bower M
Cesarman E
Elenitoba-Johnson KSJ
Fajgenbaum DC
Iwaki N
Medeiros LJ
Meignin V
Natkunam Y
van Rhee F

Definition

Idiopathic multicentric Castleman disease (iMCD) is a lymphoproliferative disorder involving two or more lymph node sites, associated with systemic inflammatory symptoms and organ dysfunction related to hypercytokinaemia. The diagnosis requires fulfilment of morphological, clinical, and laboratory criteria, and exclusion of other diseases, including HIV infection, KSHV/HHV8 infection, and other forms of Castleman disease.

ICD-O coding

None

ICD-11 coding

4B2Y Other specified disorders involving the immune system

Related terminology

Not recommended: angiofollicular lymph node hyperplasia (obsolete).

Subtype(s)

iMCD-TAFRO (thrombocytopenia, anasarca, fever / inflammatory symptoms, renal dysfunction / bone marrow reticulin fibrosis, organomegaly); iMCD-NOS

Localization

iMCD occurs in lymph nodes in any site, most frequently the neck, mediastinum, axilla, and abdomen, and in the spleen.

Clinical features

More than 80% of patients present with systemic symptoms {4524,2831,4304}. The major clinical and laboratory findings are listed in the introduction (see Table 4.06, p. 305, in *Tumour-like lesions with B-cell predominance: Introduction*). Patients with iMCD often have fever, renal dysfunction, and abnormal laboratory values (including elevated C-reactive protein, elevations in cytokines, anaemia, and hypoalbuminaemia) {2831,4304,1110, 1256,3043,2371,2486,2967}. Whereas thrombocytopenia and significant fluid overload, including localized oedema, generalized oedema (anasarca), and body cavity effusions, are more frequent in iMCD-TAFRO, thrombocytosis and polyclonal hypergammaglobulinaemia are often present in iMCD-NOS {1256, 2486,2967,1753}. Many patients have a remitting and relapsing course, even on therapy, whereas others have severe and progressive disease, which may be fatal. In general, patients with iMCD-TAFRO are more likely to have multiorgan dysfunction, more aggressive disease, and shorter survival than patients with iMCD-NOS {4524,1256,2371,2486,968,1108,1238}.

Epidemiology

iMCD can occur in individuals at any age (median age: ~50 years), with an M:F ratio close to 1:1 {4524,1256,2831,4304, 1753,2371,2486,284,1711,2569,3043,4523}. It can occur in a variety of ethnicities {4524,1753,2486,3043,4523}. The incidence of iMCD in the USA is estimated to be 3–3.5 cases per 1 million person-years {2831}, whereas in Japan it is 2.4–5.8 cases per 1 million person-years. TAFRO may be more common in Japan, with an incidence rate of 0.9–4.9 cases per 1 million person-years. Although TAFRO is found throughout the world, data from Europe and the USA are limited {2831,2371, 2486,2567}.

Etiology

The underlying cause of hypercytokinaemia is unknown but may be inflammatory, neoplastic, or viral in origin, although molecular studies have not identified an associated virus or any significant recurring underlying genomic alterations {968,1108,1111,2861, 2875,507,1376}. Serum proteomic studies show heterogeneous iMCD profiles, suggesting multiple etiologies {3231}.

Pathogenesis

The pathogenesis of iMCD is complex and incompletely understood, but many of the disease manifestations appear related to elevations in cytokines, such as IL-6, IL-2R, and VEGF {1108}. In many cases, the disease is probably driven by IL-6, given the correlation between serum IL-6 levels and disease flares, as well as the clinical effectiveness of IL-6 inhibitors {285,4167}. Limited in vivo, in vitro, serum proteomics, gene-set enrichment, sequencing, and genome-wide association studies have shown a variety of abnormalities, including increased T-cell activation, elevated serum VEGF levels, IG rearrangements, mutations in chromatin-remodelling genes, and alterations in pathways such as PIK3/AKT/mTOR, MAPK, JAK/STAT, and interleukin signalling {284,3231,146,1109,1376,507,2875}. However, the causative basis of iMCD has not been definitively determined.

Macroscopic appearance

The lymph nodes in iMCD, by definition, must be ≥ 10 mm in short-axis diameter in at least two lymph node stations. The lymph nodes in iMCD-NOS tend to be larger than those in iMCD-TAFRO {1110,2568}.

Histopathology

The histopathological findings in iMCD are variable and nonspecific. iMCD is evaluated according to five morphological features in lymph node biopsies (tissues from other sites cannot be used for grading): degree and number of regressed germinal centres, follicular dendritic cell prominence, vascularity, number of hyperplastic follicles, and degree of plasmacytosis, each graded on a scale of 0–3 {1110}. Grade 2 or 3 regressed germinal centres or plasmacytosis is required for diagnosis. In both clinicopathological subtypes, the morphological findings are a spectrum ranging from hypervascular to mixed to plasmacytic, and they overlap with those seen in unicentric Castleman disease, MCD associated with POEMS syndrome (polyneuropathy,

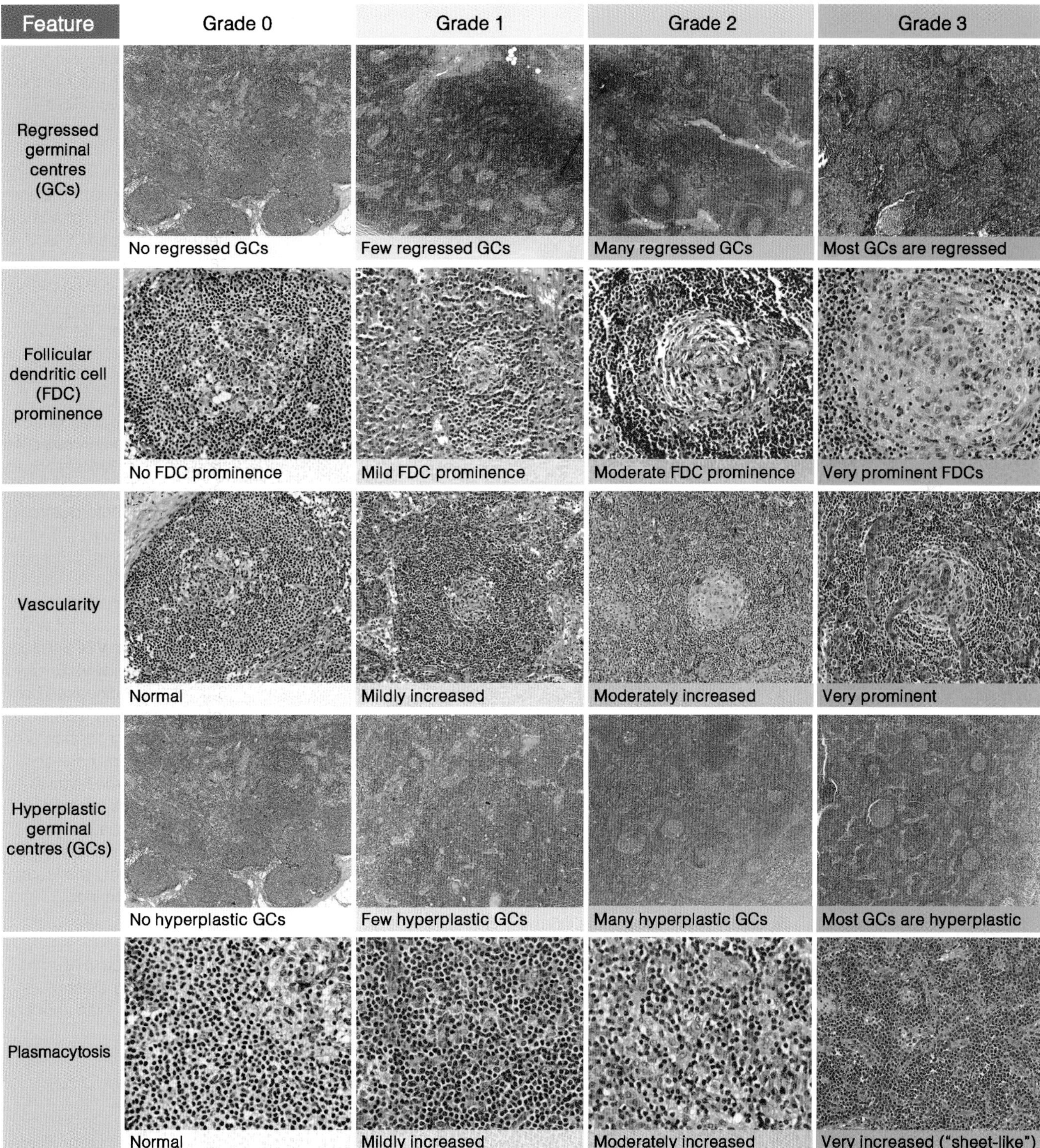

Fig. 4.19 Idiopathic multicentric Castleman disease. Grading of idiopathic multicentric Castleman disease in lymph node biopsies in four grade levels (0–3) (depicted in the columns) on the basis of five morphological features (depicted in the rows).

organomegaly, endocrinopathy, myeloma protein, and skin changes), and KSHV/HHV8-associated MCD. However, iMCD-TAFRO cases tend to have more atrophic follicles, more high endothelial venules, and fewer interfollicular plasma cells, whereas iMCD-NOS cases tend to have more interfollicular plasma cells and fewer atrophic follicles. In comparison to unicentric Castleman disease, in iMCD dysplastic follicular dendritic cells are uncommon, sinuses are usually patent, and penetrating blood vessels are less sclerotic {1110,2967,1753,1238, 2568,4308,4420}. Initial studies employing these diagnostic criteria have correlated well with historical diagnosis and clinical impression and are currently undergoing prospective validation by the Castleman Disease Collaborative Network {3043,2486}. Bone marrow in iMCD-NOS often shows plasmacytosis and increased megakaryocytes {4524,1238,2121}, whereas bone marrow in iMCD-TAFRO is often hypercellular, with megakaryocytic hyperplasia and clustering and increased reticulin fibres {2486,2967,1753,4420}.

Immunohistochemistry

Immunohistochemistry shows CD20+ B cells and CD3+ T cells in appropriate locations, although the atrophic germinal centres are depleted of B cells. The interfollicular plasma cells are polytypic. Increased numbers of cells positive for phosphorylated ribosomal protein S6 and phosphorylated 4EBP1, consistent with mTOR pathway activation, have been seen in the interfollicular area. No KSHV/HHV8 latency-associated nuclear antigen (LANA)-positive cells should be present {1753,146,1109,4308,4420}.

Differential diagnosis

The differential diagnosis includes KSHV/HHV8-associated MCD, MCD associated with POEMS syndrome, HIV-related lymphadenopathy, lymphadenopathy associated with autoimmune disorders, IgG4-related disease, Hodgkin lymphoma, and non-Hodgkin lymphomas. Immunostaining for LANA, immunoglobulin light chains, IgG/IgG4, CD30, and other pertinent markers, as well as IG and TR gene rearrangement studies and careful evaluation of the clinical history, are all helpful in separating these lesions {4308,4420,3084}.

Cytology

The presence of branching or fragmented small vessels with a heterogeneous population of predominately small lymphocytes, variable numbers of plasma cells, and follicular dendritic cells may be helpful clues, but establishing a definitive diagnosis based on cytology is not possible {1334,932,3756,2854}.

Diagnostic molecular pathology

There is typically no evidence of monoclonal antigen receptor gene rearrangements.

Essential and desirable diagnostic criteria

Essential: enlarged lymph nodes in at least two sites; lymph node morphology showing grade 2 or 3 regressed germinal centres or plasmacytosis; clinical, laboratory, and exclusion criteria fulfilled (see Table 4.06, p. 305, in *Tumour-like lesions with B-cell predominance: Introduction*).

Staging

Not relevant

Prognosis and prediction

Because the etiology is unclear, identifying appropriate treatments for iMCD has been difficult {4182}. Anti–IL-6 therapy (siltuximab or tocilizumab) is recommended as the first-line treatment for all patients; very ill patients may require chemotherapy upon progression {1255,4166}. Approximately one third of patients will respond to anti–IL-6 therapy {4167}. For nonresponders, treatment with steroids, chemotherapy, other monoclonal antibodies (including rituximab), immunomodulators, intravenous immunoglobulin, and thalidomide, alone or in various combinations, may reduce or eliminate symptoms {2831,1753,968,1108,1111,4182}. New data, such as the identification of elevated numbers of cells positive for phosphorylated S6 and phosphorylated 4EBP1 in lymph nodes from patients with iMCD, may support the use of mTOR inhibitors. However, additional targeted therapies are needed. The clinical course of iMCD-TAFRO is more aggressive, with significantly worse survival than that of iMCD-NOS {1256,968,1109}. The risk for both haematolymphoid and solid malignancies is suggested to be increased in patients with iMCD {2371}.

KSHV/HHV8-associated multicentric Castleman disease

Chadburn A
Bower M
Cesarman E
Elenitoba-Johnson KSJ
Fajgenbaum DC
Iwaki N
Meignin V
Natkunam Y
van Rhee F

Definition

Kaposi sarcoma–associated herpesvirus / human herpesvirus 8 (KSHV/HHV8)-associated multicentric Castleman disease (KSHV/HHV8-MCD) is a lymphoproliferative disorder featuring characteristic KSHV/HHV8-infected plasmablasts, idiopathic multicentric Castleman disease (iMCD)-like morphology, and systemic inflammatory symptoms due to proinflammatory hypercytokinaemia.

ICD-O coding

None

ICD-11 coding

4B2Y Other specified disorders involving the immune system

Related terminology

Acceptable: HHV8-positive multicentric Castleman disease.
Not recommended: plasmablastic multicentric Castleman disease.

Subtype(s)

None

Localization

KSHV/HHV8-MCD involves lymph nodes (most frequently axillary, abdominal, pelvic, mediastinal, and cervical) and the spleen {436, 1024}. Bone marrow involvement has been reported {204,1706}.

Clinical features

Patients present with fever and other systemic symptoms, including fatigue, weight loss, and myalgias. They exhibit many laboratory abnormalities, including elevated C-reactive protein, anaemia, and hypoalbuminaemia. Nearly all have diffuse lymphadenopathy, and many have hepatosplenomegaly, effusions, and oedema. Some patients have pulmonary and/or gastrointestinal symptoms, autoimmune haemolytic anaemia, or haemophagocytic lymphohistiocytosis. Most patients, even with treatment, experience recurrent episodes of systemic inflammatory symptoms (flares), which correlate with elevations in KSHV/HHV8 viral load and cytokine levels, particularly human interleukin-6 (huIL-6), IL-10, and KSHV/HHV8-associated vIL-6 {436,1610, 3272,3145,3043,3358,4043,2860,3044,3271}. The majority have Kaposi sarcoma, and 10–20% have a concurrent or subsequent diagnosis of lymphoma, which is often KSHV/HHV8-related {436, 1024,1610,3145,3043,3358,4043,2860,3801,1369,3042}.

Epidemiology

The majority (~80%) of patients with KSHV/HHV8-MCD are HIV-positive {3450}. In HIV-positive patients, the M:F ratio is 8:1, the median age is about 40–45 years, the HIV viral load is low or undetectable, and the median CD4+ cell count is usually 150–300/mL {436,1610,3272,3043,3358,4043,3801,3450,1322}. HIV-negative patients are older (median age is about 65 years) with a lower M:F ratio (2.4:1) {3145,3043,3801}. Most reported cases are in White people; however, KSHV/HHV8-MCD is likely to be underreported in sub-Saharan Africa {3043,3358,4043,2860}. The incidence of KSHV/HHV8-MCD is increasing in HIV-positive patients and is most recently at 8.3 cases per 10 000 patient-years {3289}.

Etiology

KSHV/HHV8 is the etiological agent, although immunosuppression (e.g. related to HIV infection or immune senescence) and genetic characteristics are additional contributing factors {3043,3801,381,3602}.

Pathogenesis

The pathogenesis of KSHV/HHV8-MCD is complex and incompletely understood. Many of the manifestations are secondary

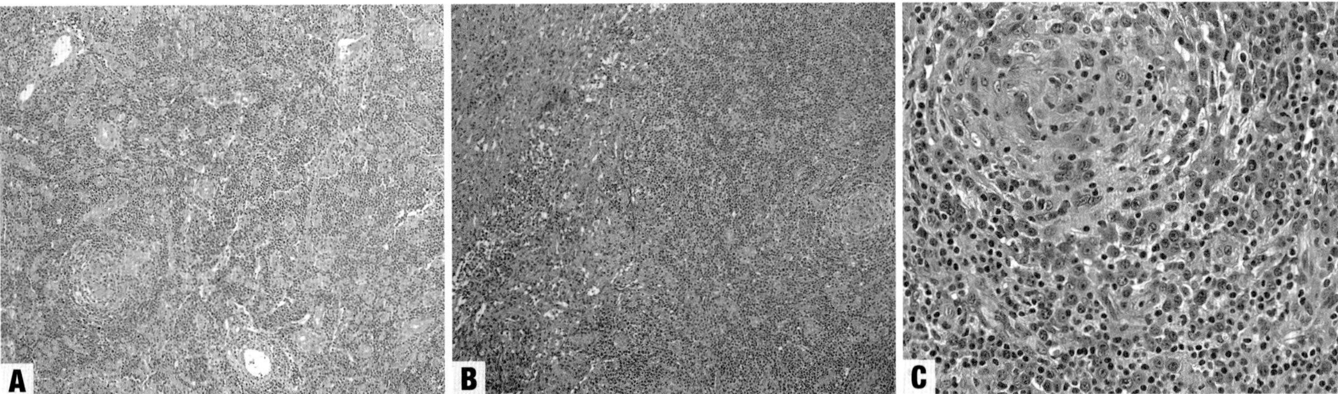

Fig. 4.20 KSHV/HHV8-associated multicentric Castleman disease. **A** The lymph node shows an involuted follicle and a hypervascular interfollicular compartment and interfollicular plasmacytosis. **B** Cases can be associated with Kaposi sarcoma (left side of image). **C** High magnification showing plasmablasts at the periphery of an involuted germinal centre.

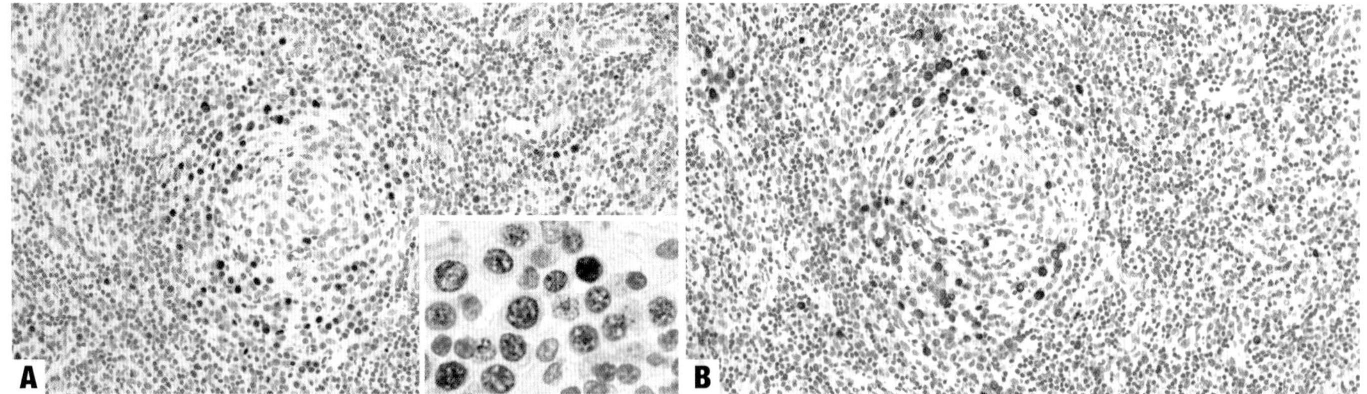

Fig. 4.21 KSHV/HHV8-associated multicentric Castleman disease. **A** The plasmablasts, based on immunostaining for latency-associated nuclear antigen (LANA; ORF73), are infected with KSHV/HHV8. This KSHV/HHV8 gene product tethers the virus to the human DNA. **Inset:** At higher magnification, immunostaining for LANA in the KSHV/HHV8-infected cells shows a characteristic nuclear-dot pattern. **B** A significant number of the LANA-positive plasmablasts also express vIL-6.

to hypercytokinaemia and B-cell proliferation. A key role of B cells is demonstrated by the effectiveness of B-cell depleting therapies, such as rituximab {1610,1322,594}. The KSHV/HHV8-encoded vIL-6 is a key cytokine expressed in the infected cells, promoting cell proliferation, differentiation, and survival, as well as angiogenesis and huIL-6 secretion {2860,649,129,465}. Other KSHV/HHV8 gene products, including vFLIP, vIRF3/LANA2, and viral microRNAs, impact KSHV/HHV8-infected cell survival, the host immune response, and cytokine production {594,465,226,1691}. Expression of other lytic viral genes, in addition to vIL-6, has been reported in KSHV/HHV8-MCD {1907}. Furthermore, infected B cells may represent a source of viraemia, contributing to the clinical manifestations {3271}. Cellular proteins (such as XBP1, which activates vIL-6 directly) and suboptimal invariant natural killer T-cell response may also play a role in disease development {3602,4306}.

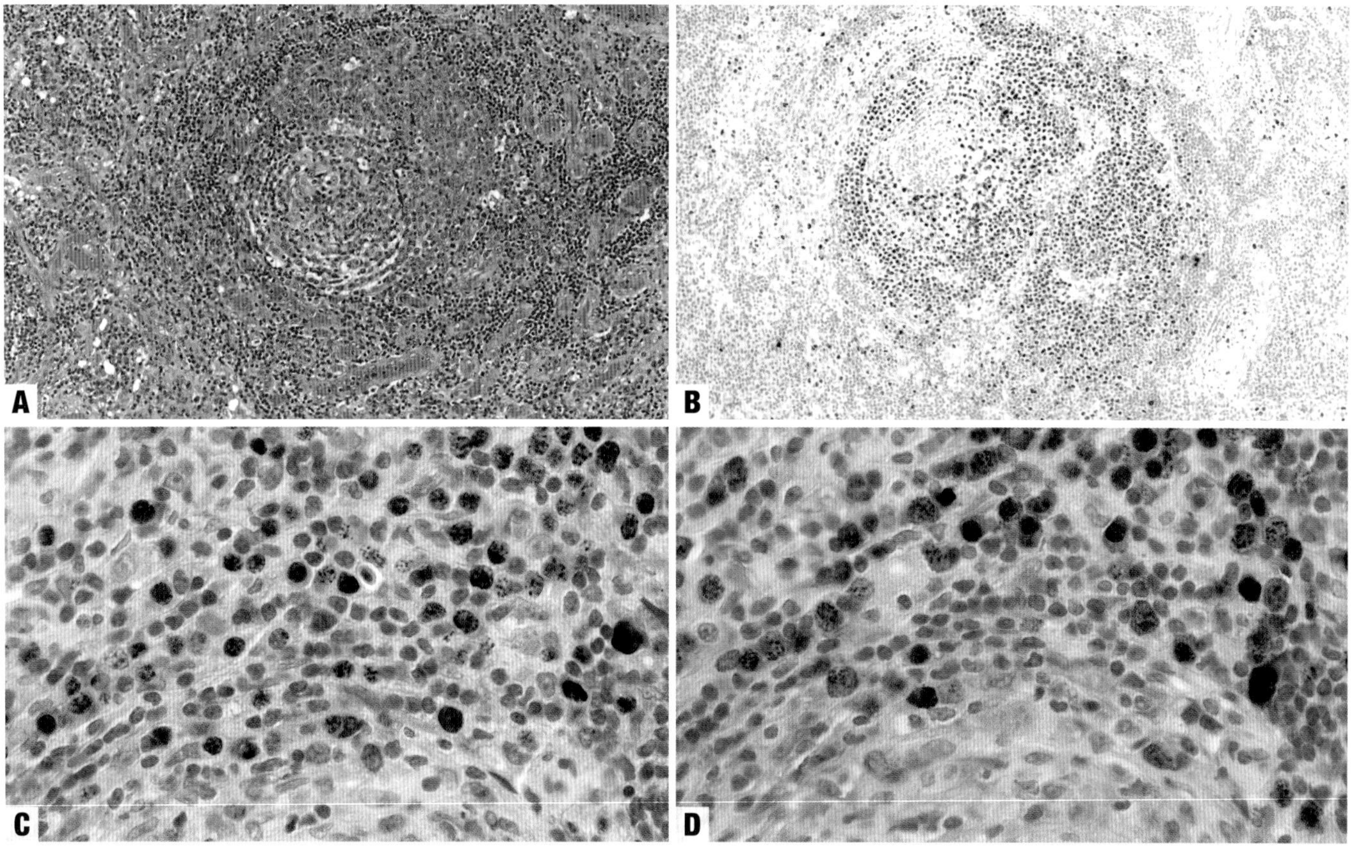

Fig. 4.22 KSHV/HHV8-associated multicentric Castleman disease. **A** Large groups of plasmablasts can be seen in KSHV/HHV8-associated multicentric Castleman disease. **B** The plasmablast aggregates are composed of KSHV/HHV8-positive cells, as demonstrated by immunostaining for latency-associated nuclear antigen (LANA) (immunoperoxidase staining). **C,D** Plasmablasts are polyclonal according to IG gene rearrangement studies, but at the protein level are lambda immunoglobulin light chain monotypic, as demonstrated by double immunostaining for LANA (brown) and kappa or lambda immunoglobulin light chain (red), in which the KSHV/HHV8-positive cells are kappa light chain–negative (immunoperoxidase staining, LANA, and streptavidin, kappa light chain) (**C**) but lambda light chain–positive (immunoperoxidase staining, LANA, and streptavidin, lambda light chain) (**D**).

Macroscopic appearance

The macroscopic appearance is similar to that of iMCD.

Histopathology

Lymph nodes and splenic white pulp show histological features similar to those seen in iMCD, with most cases exhibiting plasmacytic or mixed patterns (see Table 4.06, p. 305, in *Tumour-like lesions with B-cell predominance: Introduction*). KSHV/HHV8-MCD, in contrast to iMCD, contains a variable number of plasmablasts, which are medium-sized to large cells with one to two nucleoli and a moderate amount of amphophilic cytoplasm. The plasmablasts are located primarily in the mantle zone but may be seen in intrafollicular and perifollicular areas. Plasmablasts may be scattered individually, or occasionally form small clusters or larger aggregates (plasmablastic aggregates, formerly called microlymphomas). Foci of Kaposi sarcoma are often present {1024,3145,2860,1110,604,3045}.

The plasmablasts are immunopositive for latency-associated nuclear antigen (LANA), a product of the KSHV/HHV8 gene *ORF73* {1024,3145,604,1011}. A proportion of plasmablasts are positive for vIL-6; expression of other KSHV/HHV8-related proteins, such as vIRF1, has been documented. The plasmablasts are positive for IRF4 (MUM1) and Blimp1 and express monotypic cytoplasmic IgM lambda. They are dim to negative for CD20 and other B-cell markers, negative for T-cell antigens, and they lack CD138 expression {1024,3145,604,1011,3144}. Although there is monotypic lambda light chain expression, the plasmablasts are polyclonal B cells according to molecular studies {1011}. In general, the KSHV/HHV8-infected plasmablasts are negative for EBV {1024,3145,604,1011}. Interfollicular KSHV/HHV8-negative polytypic plasma cells are numerous and usually IgM-negative {1024}.

The differential diagnosis includes iMCD, HIV-associated lymphadenopathy (particularly mixed follicular hyperplasia/involution and follicular involution), MCD associated with POEMS syndrome (polyneuropathy, organomegaly, endocrinopathy, myeloma protein, and skin changes), lymphadenopathy associated with autoimmune disorders, classic Hodgkin lymphoma, and non-Hodgkin lymphomas such as follicular lymphoma with small hypocellular follicles {605,4308,3247}. Clinical correlation, IG and TR gene rearrangement studies, and immunostaining for immunoglobulin light chains, IgM, IgG, IgG4, CD30, and LANA are helpful in separating these lesions.

Cytology

KSHV/HHV8-MCD cannot be diagnosed by FNA with certainty. FNAs can show changes associated with reactive lymph nodes, and there are reports documenting a heterogeneous lymphoid cell population with branching capillaries often closely associated with groups of germinal centre cells {932}.

Diagnostic molecular pathology

Molecular studies are not necessary for the diagnosis.

Essential and desirable diagnostic criteria

Essential: lymph node showing the histological features of iMCD with KSHV/HHV8-positive plasmablasts (LANA-positive by immunostaining) in a patient with clinical and laboratory findings as outlined in Table 4.06 (p. 305) in *Tumour-like lesions with B-cell predominance: Introduction*.

Staging

Not relevant

Prognosis and prediction

KSHV/HHV8-MCD is a relapsing and remitting disease punctuated by flares, with systemic symptoms, elevated cytokine levels, elevated KSHV/HHV8 viral load, and lymphadenopathy. Patients with KSHV/HHV8-MCD have an increased risk of developing lymphoma; many have other KSHV/HHV8-associated diseases {436,3043,3358,3042,594}. In the past, overall survival was ≤ 2 years {2860,3045}. However, with better treatments, particularly rituximab (with liposomal doxorubicin for those with concurrent Kaposi sarcoma) and, in HIV-positive patients, antiretroviral therapy (ART), survival is much improved. Treatment with rituximab (and ART in HIV-positive patients) is also associated with a decreased risk of lymphoma development {1610,1322,594,4121}.

B-lymphoblastic leukaemias/lymphomas: Introduction

Wood BL
Akkari Y
Gujral S

B-lymphoblastic leukaemia/lymphoma (B-ALL/LBL) is diagnosed by a combination of morphology and immunophenotyping, whereas further classification is now largely by defined cytogenetic and/or molecular abnormalities. These genetic types form the basis of the present classification, and they may be associated with characteristic morphological, immunophenotypic, or clinical features with prognostic and/or therapeutic implications {3102,2023,1794}. The type/entity of "B-ALL/LBL-NOS" should only be used for cases lacking defined genetic abnormalities after comprehensive testing. In the absence of complete testing for genetic abnormalities, definitive diagnosis may not be possible {2708,1777} and the category "B-ALL/LBL not further classified" should be used. "B-ALL/LBL" should not be used for mature B-cell neoplasms (e.g. leukaemic Burkitt lymphoma). The general features of B-ALL/LBL and the overall classification structure are summarized in the next section, and the sections on each B-ALL/LBL type defined by genetics highlight the respective characterizing features. B-ALL/LBL subtypes with newly described or uncommon genetic drivers that may (or may not) become defined types in future editions of the classification are grouped under B-ALL/LBL with other defined genetic alterations.

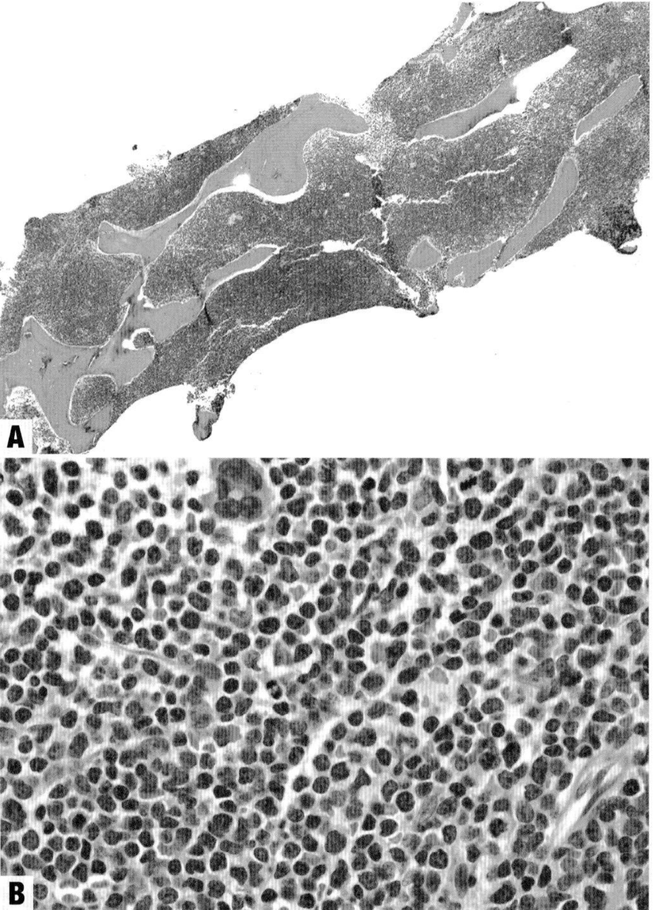

Fig. 4.23 B-lymphoblastic leukaemia/lymphoma. Histopathology at diagnosis. **A** Bone marrow trephine core biopsy showing that the maturing haematopoiesis is largely replaced by sheets of lymphoblasts. **B** The lymphoblasts are relatively monomorphic and show mitotic activity; some megakaryopoiesis is preserved.

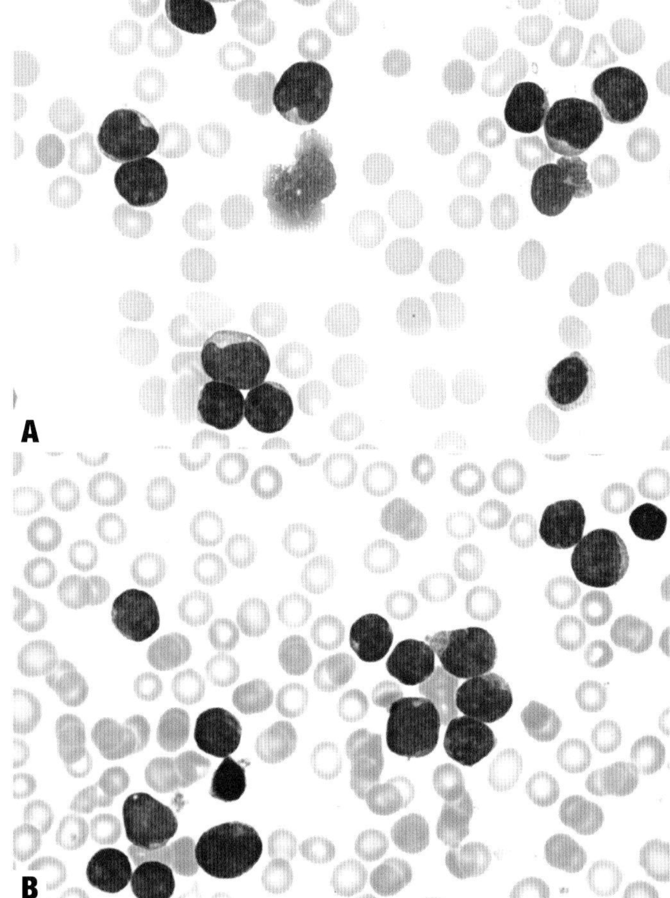

Fig. 4.24 B-lymphoblastic leukaemia/lymphoma. Bone marrow aspirate smears (Wright–Giemsa). The blasts are variably larger than red blood cells. The nuclei show irregular nuclear contours and finely dispersed chromatin. Nucleoli are typically indistinct. Pale vacuoles (**A**) and fine granules (**B**) are noted.

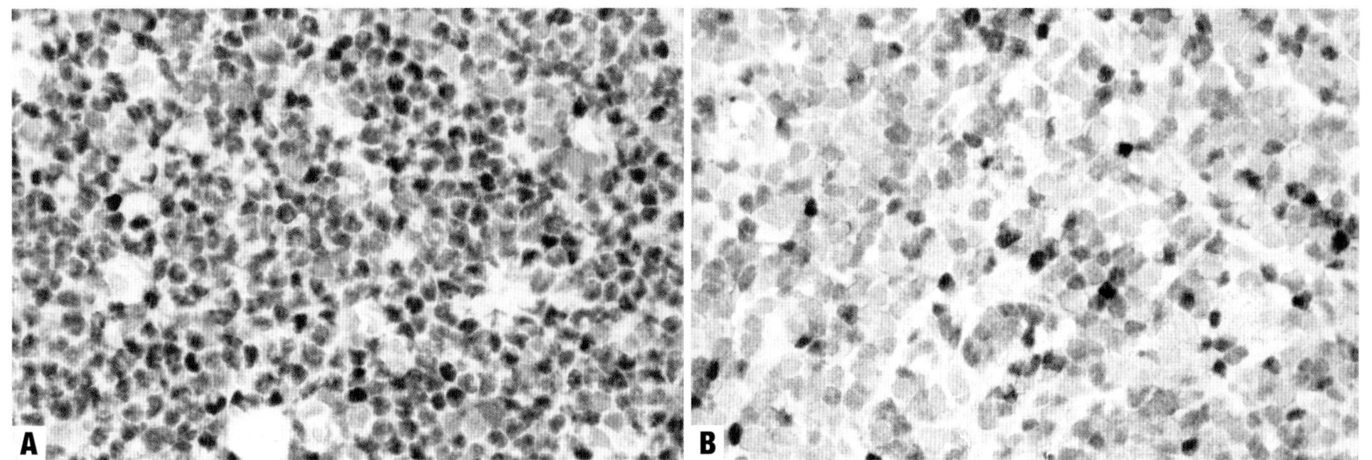

Fig. 4.25 Extramedullary B-lymphoblastic lymphoma presenting as a paraspinal mass. Neoplastic cells are positive for PAX5 (**A**) and TdT (**B**).

B-lymphoblastic leukaemia/lymphoma

Wood BL
Gujral S

Definition

B-lymphoblastic leukaemia/lymphoma (B-ALL/LBL) is a neoplasm of precursor lymphoid cells committed to the B-cell lineage, involving bone marrow and usually peripheral blood (B-lymphoblastic leukaemia [B-ALL]) and often involving nodal or extranodal sites, which by definition are the primary sites of involvement in B-lymphoblastic lymphoma (B-LBL).

ICD-O coding

9811/3 B-lymphoblastic leukaemia/lymphoma

ICD-11 coding

2A70.0 B-lymphoblastic leukaemia or lymphoma, not elsewhere classified

Related terminology

Acceptable: B-cell acute lymphoblastic leukaemia (B-ALL); precursor B-cell acute lymphoblastic leukaemia; B precursor or B-lymphoblastic leukaemia of defined precursor maturational stage (pro-B, pre-pre-B, pre-B, common, etc.).

Subtype(s)

None

Localization

B-ALL always involves the bone marrow and usually also involves the peripheral blood. Extramedullary involvement is common and is by definition the primary site of involvement in B-LBL, with frequent sites being the CNS, testes, lymph nodes, liver, spleen, skin, and soft tissues {330,2357,2487}. Involvement of the CNS and testes is of special clinical importance, affecting treatment decisions for optimal disease control. Unlike in T-lymphoblastic leukaemia/lymphoma, mediastinal masses are uncommon {330,2487,3563}.

By convention, the term "leukaemia" (B-ALL) is used when peripheral blood and bone marrow are the primary site of involvement, and the term "lymphoma" (B-LBL) when the primary involvement is of lymph nodes or extranodal sites. The distinction becomes arbitrary when both bone marrow and non–bone marrow sites are involved. Unlike for myeloid neoplasms, a defined number of blasts in the blood or marrow is not a prerequisite for the diagnosis of B-ALL/LBL, although in practice the diagnosis should be made with caution when blasts are < 20%. Of note, there is no convincing evidence to suggest outcome is adversely affected by deferring therapy until blasts reach 20%.

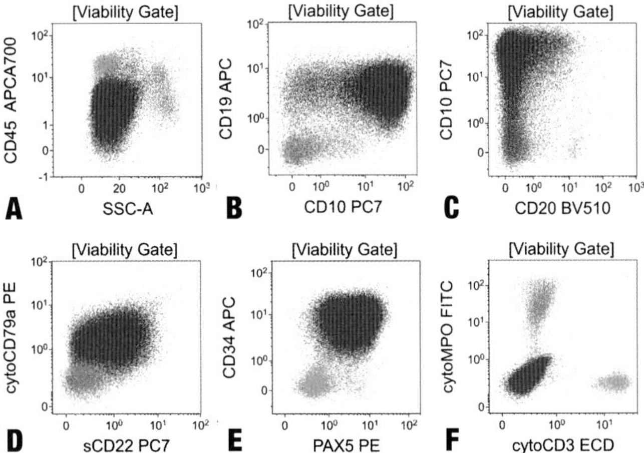

Fig. 4.26 B-precursor lymphoblastic leukaemia. Flow cytometry dot plots. B-lymphoblastic leukaemia blasts (red dots) show low side scatter and dim to negative CD45 (**A**), moderate CD19 and bright CD10 (**B**), dim to negative CD20 expression (**C**), moderate to dim sCD22 and cCD79a (**D**), and moderate CD34 and cytoplasmic PAX5 expression (**E**), but negative expression of cytoplasmic myeloperoxidase and cCD3 (**F**).

Clinical features

Patients with B-ALL commonly present with bone marrow failure evidenced by thrombocytopenia, anaemia, and/or neutropenia. The leukocyte count is often elevated, sometimes markedly, but it may be normal or decreased. Lymphadenopathy and hepatosplenomegaly are frequent, and bone pain and arthralgias may be prominent symptoms. B-LBL is usually asymptomatic at presentation, with limited-stage disease including < 25% blasts in blood and marrow by definition {2357,2487}. Head and neck presentations of B-LBL are common, especially in children.

Most cases of B-ALL/LBL are now characterized by defined cytogenetic and/or molecular abnormalities, which form the basis for subclassification. These may be associated with characteristic morphological, immunophenotypic, or clinical features and may have prognostic and/or therapeutic implications. The category "B-ALL/LBL-NOS" should be used only for cases lacking defined genetic abnormalities after comprehensive testing. In the absence of complete testing for genetic abnormalities, definitive subclassification may not be possible {2708}, and the category "B-ALL/LBL not further classified" should be used.

Epidemiology

B-ALL occurs predominantly in children, with 75% of all patients aged < 6 years, and is the most common leukaemia in the paediatric age group {1449}. However, the incidence is bimodal, with a second, smaller peak in the fifth decade of life {3166}. The estimated incidence worldwide is 1–4.75 cases per 100 000 person-years {3385}. B-LBL represents about 10% of lymphoblastic lymphoma cases, the remainder being of T lineage, and the majority of cases occur in patients aged < 18 years {417,2487}.

Etiology

The etiology of B-ALL/LBL is unknown. Children with Down syndrome and other constitutional genetic disorders have an increased risk of B-ALL {4588}. Genome-wide association studies have shown an association of B-ALL with SNPs in a number of genes (*GATA3*, *ARID5B*, *IKZF1*, *CEBPE*, *CDKN2A*, and *CDKN2B*) {3131,3189}. However, true familial B-ALL is rare, with some kindreds described having mutations in *PAX5* {3690}, *ETV6*, and *TP53* {3288}. Translocations associated with B-ALL have been identified in neonatal specimens long before the development of leukaemia, and monozygotic twins with leukaemia often share the same genetic abnormalities that are thought to be acquired mutations {1400,2784}.

Pathogenesis

The postulated normal counterpart is a haematopoietic precursor cell committed to B lineage. Multiple molecular pathways seem to be affected for leukaemogenesis.

Macroscopic appearance

Not relevant

Histopathology

On smears and touch preparations, B-ALL/LBL lymphoblasts vary from small cells with scant cytoplasm, condensed chromatin, and indistinct nucleoli to larger cells with moderate pale blue-grey cytoplasm with occasional vacuolation, dispersed chromatin, and multiple variably prominent nucleoli. Nuclei may be round or show convolutions. Coarse, cytoplasmic azurophilic granules may be seen in roughly 10% of cases, and cytoplasmic pseudopods may be present (hand-mirror cells). Normal B-cell precursors (haematogones) have a similar appearance, but with a higher N:C ratio, more uniform dispersed chromatin, and no discernible nucleoli. Morphological discrimination between B-ALL and normal B-cell precursors is challenging, and specialized techniques such as immunophenotyping are required for definitive assessment.

In marrow biopsies, blasts form mid-marrow sheets or loose collections that displace or admix with normal marrow elements. The lymphoblasts have a relatively uniform appearance, with scant cytoplasm, round to oval to indented or convoluted nuclei, fine chromatin, and variably distinct nucleoli. Mitotic figures vary in number. Lymph nodes show a diffuse or (less commonly) paracortical infiltrate, often with numerous mitotic figures and, in some cases, interspersed macrophages (starry-sky pattern). No morphological features reliably distinguish B- and T-lineage lymphoblastic neoplasms.

Cytochemical stains are still often performed for the subtyping of acute leukaemia, particularly in resource-limited settings, but immunophenotyping is required for definitive lineage assignment. Lymphoblasts are invariably negative for myeloperoxidase but may stain light-grey and weakly with Sudan Black B when granules are present. Nonspecific esterase may show multifocal punctate or Golgi staining that is variably inhibited by sodium fluoride. PAS shows coarse, chunky cytoplasmic staining in some cases.

Immunophenotype

The lymphoblasts in B-ALL/LBL essentially always express the B lineage–associated antigens CD19, cytoplasmic CD79a, and cytoplasmic and surface CD22, best demonstrated by flow cytometry. PAX5 is the most sensitive and specific B-lineage antigen demonstrated in tissue sections by immunohistochemistry, and cCD79a is also often used {4049}. However, CD19, cCD79a, and PAX5 may each be seen in acute myeloid leukaemia (AML) with t(8;21)(q22;q22.1), and cCD79a is commonly expressed at a variably low level in T-lymphoblastic leukaemia/lymphoma {1530}. Thus, although not entirely specific for B lineage individually, their presence in combination, or at an intensity approaching that seen in their normal B counterparts, indicates B lineage. CD13, CD33, and CD66c may be expressed individually or in combination, particularly in cases with t(9;22), but are not indicative of myeloid lineage {2036}. Myeloperoxidase may be seen infrequently by either immunohistochemistry or flow cytometry, but it does not suggest myeloid lineage unless at moderate to high intensity or with the variable intensity characteristic of normal early myeloid maturation, in which case either AML or B/myeloid mixed-phenotype acute leukaemia should be considered {137,1145}. Intriguingly, *ZNF384*-rearranged, *DUX4*-rearranged, and *PAX5* p.P80R B-ALL may show monocytic differentiation after therapy or even at diagnosis {2982,3613}, having implications for residual disease monitoring after therapy.

Patterns of antigen expression associated with B-cell immaturity are commonly present and imperfectly recapitulate stages of early B-cell maturation. These include CD45 expression (invariably lower than in mature lymphocytes), CD10 (often of moderate to high intensity), variably low to absent CD20, CD34

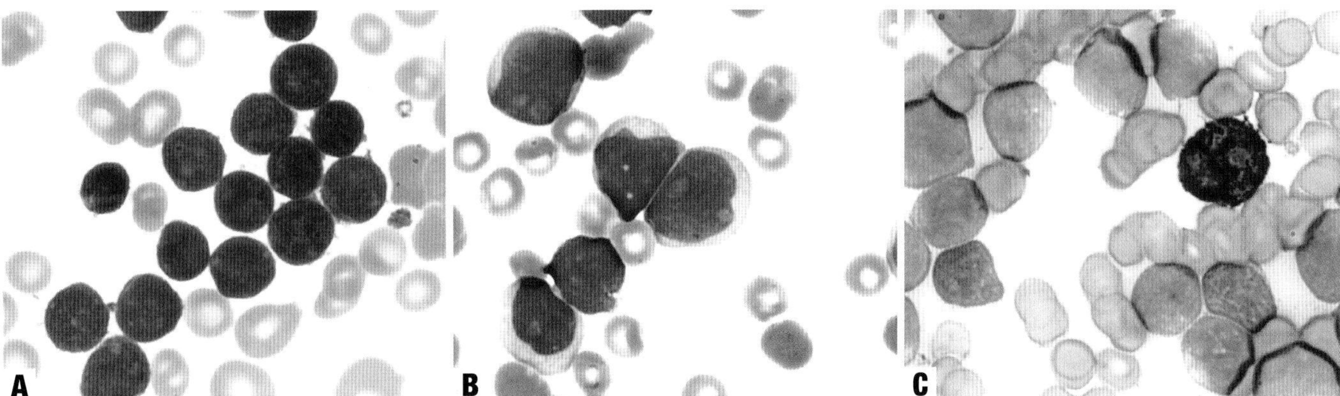

Fig. 4.27 B-lymphoblastic leukaemia/lymphoma. Bone marrow smears show small, monomorphic-looking blasts with scant blue cytoplasm, condensed nuclear chromatin, and indistinct nucleoli (Giemsa) (**A**); or larger blasts with moderate pale or blue-grey cytoplasm with occasional vacuolation, dispersed chromatin, multiple variably prominent nucleoli, and nuclei that may be round or show convolutions (Giemsa) (**B**). Cytochemical stain for myeloperoxidase is negative in blasts; internal control neutrophil is positive (**C**).

(in many cases), and TdT (in the majority of cases). Historically, immunophenotypic similarity to stages of normal B-cell development were recognized, i.e. pro-B (CD19, cCD79, cCD22, TdT), common-B (CD10), pre-B (cytoplasmic mu), and transitional pre-B (heavy chain without light chains). Clonal surface light chains are typically absent but may be seen in up to 4% of cases, often associated with a more mature immunophenotype {2925}. Recognition of these immunophenotypic maturational stages is of limited clinical utility, in contrast to genetic classification. Nevertheless, there are immunophenotypic correlates to some genetic lesions, as described when relevant in the sections that follow, and these may be used as imperfect surrogates in resource-limited settings.

Immunophenotypic differences from normal B-cell precursors (haematogones) are invariably present and are very useful for the identification of residual leukaemia after therapy. Normal B-cell maturation proceeds through a series of relatively discrete stages with defined immunophenotypes, and comparing leukaemic cells with their closest normal counterpart is required for sensitive recognition of aberrant antigen expression. Common aberrancies include decreased expression of CD45 (below that of even the most immature normal B progenitors); increased or decreased expression of CD10; increased CD19; decreased expression of CD38 and CD81 {3664}; increased and uniform CD58; and increased CD66c, CD73, CD86, CD123, and CD304 {530,666,647,3988,3986}. These immunophenotypic differences may change after therapy, so reliance on the persistence of any single immunophenotypic abnormality is ill-advised.

Cytology

See *Histopathology*, above.

Diagnostic molecular pathology

Genetic abnormalities are now the fundamental basis of the classification of B-ALL/LBL. Although some entities can be defined by traditional karyotype or FISH analysis, many of the newer entities require next-generation sequencing or transcriptomics to identify defining (often cryptic) abnormalities. Thus, the comprehensive subclassification and risk stratification of B-ALL/LBL relies on a combination of genetic techniques (see Table 4.09).

Table 4.09 Overview of defined genetic abnormalities associated with B-lymphoblastic leukaemia/lymphoma types and subtypes (continued on next page)

Genetic entity	Additional genetic changes	Frequency	Genetic testing	Immunophenotypic correlates	Prognosis
Aneuploidy: hypodiploidy (24–43 chromosomes)	In near hypodiploidy: RTK/RAS pathway mutations (*NF1*), *IKZF3* deletion In low hypodiploidy: *RB1*, *CDKN2A/B*, *IKZF2* deletions; *TP53* mutations (as many as 50% of *TP53* mutations are germline variants) {786}	~2% of childhood cases are near-hypodiploid ~1% of childhood cases and 10% of adult cases are low-hypodiploid	Karyotyping/FISH	Flow cytometry DNA index can be used to estimate ploidy in situations where cytogenetics has failed or not been performed; it is especially useful to detect masked hypodiploidy characterized by duplication of the hypodiploid genome {563}	Unfavourable {786} for near and low hypodiploidy
Aneuploidy: high hyperdiploidy (> 50 chromosomes)	RAS pathway (*KRAS*, *NRAS*, *FLT3*, *PTPN11*) and *CREBBP* mutations	As many as 30% of childhood cases	Karyotyping/FISH		Favourable {3172, 3171}
BCR::ABL1 fusion {1206}	*IKZF1* deletions (in 80%) co-occurring with deletions of *PAX5* and *CDKN2A/B* {2834}; *EBF1* mutations (in 14%)	2–5% in children, 6% in adolescents and young adults, and > 25% in adults	Karyotyping/FISH, PCR, or RNA sequencing for detection of *BCR::ABL1* fusion; RT-PCR and/or ddPCR for monitoring responses	CD19+, CD10+; often aberrant CD13/CD33 expression {2887,3090,3101,1269,812}; IL2RA (CD25) overexpression is frequent {2887,3090}	Unfavourable, but incorporation of TKI targeted therapy has improved outcomes {2834}; unfavourable for *IKZF1*-rearranged
KMT2A rearrangement {4388, 3162,2673}	> 90 partners of *KMT2A* described, of which *AFF1* (*AF4*), *MLLT3*, *MLLT1*, *MLLT10*, and *MLLT6* are common	70–85% in infants, 2% in children and adults	Karyotyping/FISH; whole-genome or targeted RNA sequencing	Dim/absent CD10 and CD24; frequent positivity for CD15, CD65, and CSPG4 (NG2) {1648,3143,415,4545}	Unfavourable
TCF3 fusion {1728}	*PBX1* is the most common partner; others include *ZNF384*, *NOP2* (*NOL1*), *TFPT*, and *HLF1*	*TCF3::PBX1* in 4–6%	Karyotyping/FISH for *TCF3::PBX1*; whole-genome or targeted RNA sequencing for uncommon partners	*TCF3::PBX1*-rearranged cases frequently express bright CD9 and negative CD34 {418,1033}	*TCF3::PBX1* has better outcomes with contemporary therapeutic regimens; *TCF3::HLF* has a universally dismal prognosis
IGH::*IL3* fusion {1224}	Frequent *IKZF1* deletion	Rare	Karyotyping/FISH	Marked eosinophilia	Intermediate
IG::*MYC* rearrangement {4265,1433}	Frequent mutations in genes involving RAS pathway, 1q gain	Rare in children, ~2% of adults	Karyotyping/FISH; genetic and epigenetic profile distinct from Burkitt lymphoma	MYC overexpression	Unfavourable

B-ALL, B-lymphoblastic leukaemia; ddPCR, droplet digital PCR; iAMP21, intrachromosomal amplification of chromosome 21; LOH, loss of heterozygosity; MPAL, mixed-phenotype acute leukaemia; MRD, measurable residual disease; Ph, Philadelphia chromosome; RTK, receptor tyrosine kinase; TKI, tyrosine kinase inhibitor.

Table 4.09 Overview of defined genetic abnormalities associated with B-lymphoblastic leukaemia/lymphoma types and subtypes (continued from previous page, continued on next page)

Genetic entity	Additional genetic changes	Frequency	Genetic testing	Immunophenotypic correlates	Prognosis
ETV6::RUNX1 fusion {496,2620}		Nearly 25% of patients aged 2–10 years; < 3% of adults	FISH/PCR/RNA sequencing for detection of *ETV6::RUNX1*; RT-PCR and/or ddPCR for monitoring responses	Absent or partial expression of CD9, CD20, and CD66c; moderate to bright CD27 and dim to negative CD44 {419, 909,1648}	Favourable
iAMP21 {3431, 2769}	Defined by ≥ 5 copies of *RUNX1* per cell, with ≥ 3 copies on a single abnormal chromosome 21 {1505}	1–2%	FISH for *ETV6::RUNX1* used to identify iAMP21	None	Unfavourable; outcomes may improve with intensive chemotherapy
BCR::ABL1-like features {3962, 3504,1571,1774, 3426,3162,4352, 558,3962}	ABL-class fusions, involving *ABL1, ABL2, CSF1R, LYN, PDGFRA, PDGFRB* JAK/STAT abnormalities, including enhancer-hijacking of promoter regions (IGH::*CRLF2*, *P2RY8::CRLF2*), fusions and mutations (e.g. *JAK2* p.R683G or *JAK1* p.V658F) in *JAK1*/*JAK2*/*JAK3* genes, and fusions / truncating deletions of *EPOR* (e.g. *EPOR*::IGH) Miscellaneous fusions involving *FGFR1, NTRK3*, etc. Frequently associated with *IKZF1* deletions and copy-number alterations in B-lymphoid transcription factors Activating mutations involving cytokine receptors (e.g. IL7R and CRLF2) also constitute an underlying genetic abnormality	Frequency increases with age; 10–15% of children, 20–25% of adults	Whole-transcriptome or targeted RNA sequencing is the most reliable method for diagnosis; when unavailable, derivative methods like TaqMan low-density arrays, multiplex PCR, and FISH panels using break-apart probes may be used	CRLF2 overexpression by flow cytometry is a useful rapid screen for *CRLF2* aberrations and JAK/STAT pathway activation {2101, 487}	Unfavourable, associated with high MRD positivity rates; targeting the underlying genetic abnormality may improve survival rates
ETV6::RUNX1-like features {2342, 4530,2965}	Fusions or copy-number alterations involving *ETV6, ERG, FLI1, IKZF*, or *TCF3* are common	3% of children	Whole-transcriptome or targeted RNA sequencing; increased frequency of *ETV6*-like B-ALL may be seen in patients with germline *ETV6* variants	Moderate to bright CD27 and dim to absent CD44 {4530}	Unfavourable
DUX4 rearrangement {4489, 4531}	Fusions involving IGH are common, resulting in *DUX4* overexpression and *ERG* deletions	4–7% of children; slightly higher frequency in the adolescent and young adult population	Difficult to identify using FISH and PCR, because of repetitive genome; whole-transcriptome or targeted RNA sequencing is more reliable	Aberrant CD2 and CD371 expression; monocytic differentiation may be seen, particularly after therapy	Favourable
MEF2D rearrangement {3892}	*BCL9* is the most common translocation partner; others include *HNRNPUL1, DAZAP1, CSF1R, SS18*, and *FOXJ2*	4% of children, 10% of adults	*MEF2D::BCL9* is difficult to detect using FISH; whole-transcriptome or targeted RNA sequencing is more reliable	Dim/absent CD10, positivity for CD38 and PKCμ; aberrant CD5 expression variable {3013,1432}	Unfavourable
ZNF384 rearrangement {3316, 1590,2982}	Numerous partners reported (*EP300, EWSR1, TAF15, TCF3*), either transcription partners or chromatin modifiers; *FLT3* overexpression also described	5% of children and 10% of adults with B-ALL; 48% of patients with B/myeloid MPAL	FISH; whole-transcriptome or targeted RNA sequencing	Dim CD10 and aberrant CD13/CD33; lineage may change during disease progression	Favourable for *EP300::ZNF384*; unfavourable for *TCF3::ZNF384*

B-ALL, B-lymphoblastic leukaemia; ddPCR, droplet digital PCR; iAMP21, intrachromosomal amplification of chromosome 21; LOH, loss of heterozygosity; MPAL, mixed-phenotype acute leukaemia; MRD, measurable residual disease; Ph, Philadelphia chromosome; RTK, receptor tyrosine kinase; TKI, tyrosine kinase inhibitor.

Table 4.09 Overview of defined genetic abnormalities associated with B-lymphoblastic leukaemia/lymphoma types and subtypes (continued)

Genetic entity	Additional genetic changes	Frequency	Genetic testing	Immunophenotypic correlates	Prognosis
PAX5[alt]/*PAX5* p.P80R {2982}	Numerous fusion partners; copy-number alterations are common; *PAX5* p.P80R is an inactivating mutation with a distinct expression profile and is commonly associated with deletion of alternate allele or copy-neutral LOH	*PAX5*[alt] in 7% and *PAX5* p.P80R in 3%	FISH; whole-transcriptome or targeted RNA sequencing	None	Intermediate for *PAX5*[alt] in children and unfavourable in adults; *PAX5* p.P80R may be unfavourable in children
NUTM1 rearrangement {3835,387}	Numerous partners reported, either transcription partners or epigenetic regulators	< 2%	Whole-transcriptome or targeted RNA sequencing	NUT protein overexpression	Favourable

B-ALL, B-lymphoblastic leukaemia; ddPCR, droplet digital PCR; iAMP21, intrachromosomal amplification of chromosome 21; LOH, loss of heterozygosity; MPAL, mixed-phenotype acute leukaemia; MRD, measurable residual disease; Ph, Philadelphia chromosome; RTK, receptor tyrosine kinase; TKI, tyrosine kinase inhibitor.

Genetic abnormalities in B-ALL/LBL can be broadly classified according to the techniques that can define them most readily.

Genetic abnormalities evident with conventional cytogenetic techniques

Aneuploidy

The gain or loss of chromosome numbers (aneuploidy) is a defining feature in nearly 30% of B-ALL/LBL cases. This is commonly detected through conventional karyotyping, FISH, or flow cytometry. The prognostic significance depends upon the type of abnormality detected (see Table 4.09, p. 332).

Recurrent rearrangements

B-ALL/LBL with *BCR*::*ABL1* fusion is often identified by conventional karyotyping, although FISH or PCR may be required for more cryptic or unusual rearrangements. *KMT2A* gene rearrangements involving > 90 partners have been described and can often be detected using conventional karyotyping, FISH (using break-apart probes), and global or targeted RNA sequencing {4388,3162,2673}. B-ALL/LBL with *TCF3*::*PBX1* fusion and other *TCF3* partners can be identified by conventional karyotype analysis and FISH, including B-ALL/LBL with *TCF3*::*HLF* fusion (now recognized as a distinct entity). B-ALL/LBL with IGH::*IL3* fusion is a morphologically distinct entity that may be confused with a myeloproliferative process and can be identified by FISH.

Genetic abnormalities not evident by conventional karyotyping but diagnosed by FISH

B-ALL with *ETV6*::*RUNX1* fusion is one of the most common subtypes of paediatric B-ALL/LBL and has a favourable prognosis. Intrachromosomal amplification of chromosome 21 (iAMP21) is a rare type of B-ALL/LBL with a poor prognosis that can show grossly abnormal chromosome 21 on karyotype analysis but is often observed by FISH while screening for *ETV6*::*RUNX1*.

Genetic abnormalities defined by transcriptomic analysis and largely driven by chimeric gene fusions

B-ALL/LBL with *BCR*::*ABL1*-like features and B-ALL/LBL with *ETV6*::*RUNX1*-like features are phenocopies of their established types, harbouring diverse underlying alterations identified by gene expression profiling (see Table 4.09, p. 332). This underlying heterogeneity makes screening for these disorders challenging. Where genomic methods are not available, other approaches can sometimes be used; for example, CRLF2 expression by flow cytometry may be used to identify a major subset of B-ALL/LBL with *BCR*::*ABL1*-like features {2101,487}. This edition recognizes a number of recently identified entities with distinct clinical, phenotypic, and/or prognostic features, described together under B-ALL/LBL with other defined genetic alterations. These include B-ALLs with *DUX4* {4489, 2342}, *MEF2D* {1432}, *ZNF384* {1590}, *NUTM1* {1629}, and *MYC* {4265,1700} rearrangements, as well as with *PAX5* alterations (*PAX5*[alt]) {1433} and *PAX5* p.P80R {3153} alterations.

In cases of familial B-ALL/LBL, germline testing for monogenic predisposition (e.g. linked to mutations in *PAX5* {3690}, *ETV6*, and *TP53* {3288}) and probable multigenic risk variants (e.g. in *GATA3*, *ARID5B*, *IKZF1*, *CEBPE*, *CDKN2A*, or *CDKN2B*) {3131,3189} should be considered. Suspicion should be raised by a strong family history.

Essential and desirable diagnostic criteria

Essential: for B-ALL: predominantly peripheral blood and/or bone marrow presentation with demonstration of increased immunophenotypically abnormal lymphoblasts by flow cytometry; for B-LBL: predominantly lymph node or extranodal presentation and/or diffuse organ infiltration with effacement of the architecture by abnormal lymphoblasts; B-cell lineage supported by expression of CD19, CD22, cCD79a, and/or PAX5 by flow cytometry or immunohistochemistry; immature phenotype supported by TdT and CD34 (although CD34 and TdT expression may be absent in rare cases), and/or bright CD10, low CD45, low/absent CD20, and absent surface immunoglobulin light chain expression by flow cytometry or immunohistochemistry.

Desirable: demonstration of specific recurrent genetic abnormalities; demonstration of immunophenotypic profiles associated with specific recurrent genetic abnormalities.

Staging

Not relevant

Prognosis and prediction

Risk-stratified treatment approaches have led to significant improvements in the outcomes of B-ALL in children, with long-term remission rates of > 90% {1718}. However, the benefit in adult B-ALL/LBL has been more modest, because of the adverse biology and treatment toxicity in adult patients. Novel approaches based on disease biology have shown promise in recent years. The use of tyrosine kinase inhibitors in B-ALL/LBL with *BCR*::*ABL1* fusion, monoclonal antibodies (rituximab), antibody–drug conjugates (inotuzumab ozogamicin), bispecific antibodies (blinatumomab), and chimeric antigen receptor (CAR) T cells have demonstrated potential to improve outcomes {3557}.

The benefits of high cure rates in children, however, do not extend uniformly across the globe, and where a child is born is still the most important predictor of survival. It is estimated that the global 5-year net survival rate for B-ALL is currently 56.1%, varying from 22.4% in Africa to 52.6% in Asia and 82.8% in North America {1306}. Of the estimated 74 500 global cases of childhood B-ALL in 2015, approximately three quarters occurred in Asia and Africa {4320}, indicating that most children with B-ALL in the world are still not cured, and highlighting the importance of therapeutic implementation along with biological insights to improve survival.

Adverse prognostic factors include age (< 1 year or > 10 years), an elevated white blood cell count (> 50 000/μL), slow blast clearance with initial therapy, certain genomic entities (e.g. hypodiploidy), and the presence of residual disease at defined time points early after therapy (end of induction or consolidation) {827,3648,3748,4155}. The presence of CNS disease at diagnosis is associated with an adverse outcome and requires specific therapy. The prognosis of B-LBL is relatively favourable, more so in children than adults, similarly to for B-ALL {2487}. Genomic abnormalities are important prognostic factors and are discussed in the following sections.

B-lymphoblastic leukaemia/lymphoma with high hyperdiploidy

Harrison CJ
Ketterling RP
Parihar M
Rabin KR
Yasuda T

Definition

B-lymphoblastic leukaemia/lymphoma (B-ALL/LBL) with high hyperdiploidy is a neoplasm of lymphoblasts of B-cell lineage defined by a karyotype comprising 51–65 chromosomes, characterized by recurrent, non-random gains of one or more copies of entire chromosomes (usually the X chromosome and chromosomes 4, 6, 10, 14, 17, 18 and 21) in the absence of type-defining gene fusions and rearrangements.

ICD-O coding

9815/3 B-lymphoblastic leukaemia/lymphoma with high hyperdiploidy

ICD-11 coding

2A70.Y & XH24C7 Other B-lymphoblastic leukaemia/lymphoma with recurrent genetic abnormalities & B-lymphoblastic leukaemia/lymphoma with hyperdiploidy

Related terminology

None

Subtype(s)

None

Localization

B-ALL and B-LBL represent the same disease. B-ALL always involves the bone marrow and usually also involves the peripheral blood. Extramedullary involvement is common and is by definition the primary site of involvement in B-LBL. For details, see *B-lymphoblastic leukaemia/lymphoma* (p. 330).

Clinical features

The clinical features of B-ALL/LBL with high hyperdiploidy are similar to those of other subtypes, except that B-ALL/LBL with high hyperdiploidy generally has low white blood cell counts {1460}.

Epidemiology

Although rare in infants, high-hyperdiploid B-ALL/LBL is most frequent in children (25–35% of all B-ALL/LBL cases) and less common in adults (7–8% of all B-ALL/LBL cases) {2822}.

Etiology

No unique features

Pathogenesis

Although pathogenetic mechanisms are poorly understood, chromosomal gains are early events in the pathogenesis of B-ALL/LBL with high hyperdiploidy and are the main driver. Mutations in the receptor tyrosine kinase / RAS signalling pathway (*FLT3*, *NRAS*, *KRAS*, and *PTPN11* genes) are reported in about 51% of cases, suggesting that the receptor tyrosine kinase / RAS pathway and histone modifiers are involved in the pathogenesis {3172}.

Macroscopic appearance

No unique features

Histopathology

No unique features

Cytology

No unique features

Diagnostic molecular pathology

B-ALL/LBL with high hyperdiploidy is identified by chromosomal analysis, FISH, flow cytometric DNA index, or SNP array analysis. Karyotyping identifies clones with 51–65 chromosomes with non-random trisomies (most frequently of the X chromosome and chromosomes 4, 6, 10, 14, 17, and 18) and trisomy/tetrasomy 21. FISH studies can complement cytogenetic analysis to identify the common chromosomal gains

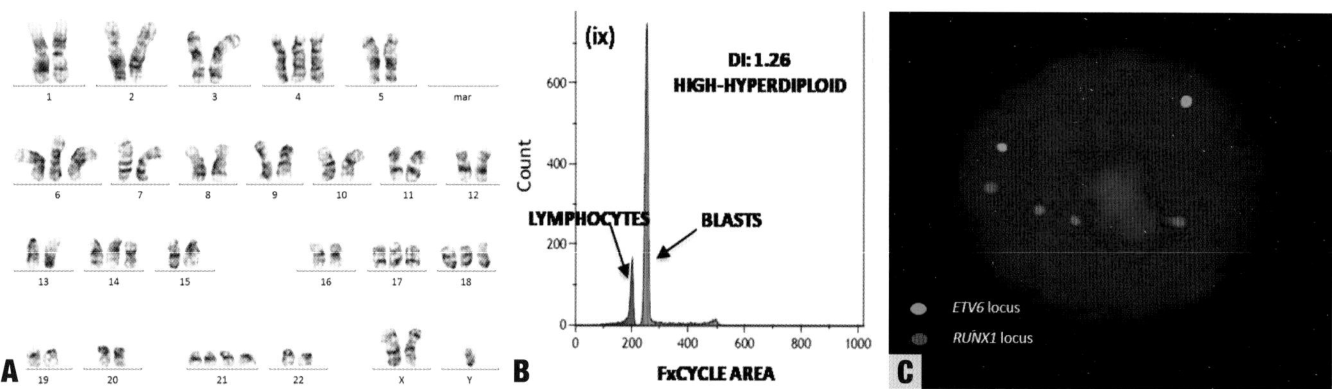

Fig. 4.28 B-lymphoblastic leukaemia/lymphoma with high hyperdiploidy. **A** Karyotype showing 54 chromosomes with trisomies of the X chromosome and chromosomes 4, 6, 14, 17, and 18, and tetrasomy 21. **B** A flow cytometry–based DNA index showing a peak of 1.2, consistent with a diagnosis of B-lymphoblastic leukaemia/lymphoma with high hyperdiploidy. **C** Interphase FISH analysis using dual-colour/dual-fusion *ETV6::RUNX1* probes indicates four discrete copies of *RUNX1*, consistent with gain of chromosome 21.

(chromosomes 4, 10, 17, and 21) {3170} or as a surrogate for the detection of high hyperdiploidy hidden within a normal or failed karyotype {2768,1507,3171,3133}. Chromosomal microarrays are also useful to characterize high hyperdiploidy, particularly in distinguishing possible pseudohyperdiploidy due to a doubled-up hypodiploid clone. Such cases may also be identified by flow cytometry–based DNA index analysis, which may show two peaks, corresponding to the hypodiploid and pseudohyperdiploid clones (see *B-lymphoblastic leukaemia/lymphoma with hypodiploidy*, p. 338).

Because chromosome 21 is universally gained in high-hyperdiploid B-ALL/LBL, the presence of multiple (three to five) discrete *RUNX1* signals seen when using *ETV6*::*RUNX1* FISH probes suggests the presence of high hyperdiploidy {1506}. This status can be confirmed using centromeric probes targeting chromosomes 4, 10, and 17 in patients with a normal karyotype or failed cytogenetic result {3170}.

Essential and desirable diagnostic criteria

Essential: meets the diagnostic criteria for B-ALL/LBL (see *B-lymphoblastic leukaemia/lymphoma*, p. 330); demonstration of high-hyperdiploidy status (comprising 51–65 chromosomes) by karyotyping and/or FISH; exclusion of pseudohyperdiploidy by flow cytometry DNA index and/or SNP array analysis; absence of other subtype-defining translocations.

Staging

Not relevant

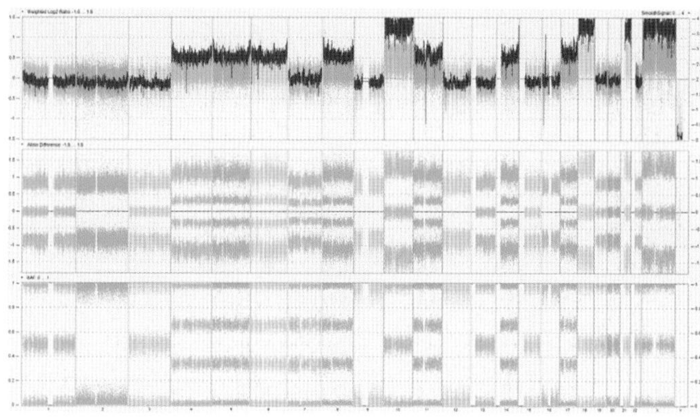

Fig. 4.29 B-lymphoblastic leukaemia/lymphoma with high hyperdiploidy. The SNP array profile shows evidence of one-copy gain of chromosomes 4, 5, 6, 8, 11, 14, and 17, as well as two- to three-copy gain of chromosomes 10, 18, 21, and X.

Prognosis and prediction

B-ALL/LBL with high-hyperdiploidy has a very favourable prognosis, with long-term overall survival in > 90% of children, especially among children with a favourable US National Cancer Institute (NCI) risk profile and low measurable residual disease. Outcome has been shown to be linked to the specific chromosomal gains {2768,1085}. Associated structural abnormalities, including translocations, usually have no impact on the good outcome {2768}. Adverse risk factors such as advanced patient age and a high white blood cell count may adversely affect prognosis, but these patients may not fare as badly as others without this favourable genetic abnormality {712}.

B-lymphoblastic leukaemia/lymphoma with hypodiploidy

Harrison CJ
Locatelli F
Parihar M
Rabin KR
Yasuda T

Definition

B-lymphoblastic leukaemia/lymphoma (B-ALL/LBL) with hypodiploidy is a neoplasm of lymphoblasts of B-cell lineage defined by the presence of ≤ 43 chromosomes.

ICD-O coding

9816/3 B-lymphoblastic leukaemia/lymphoma with hypodiploidy
9816/3 B-lymphoblastic leukaemia/lymphoma with hypodiploidy, near-haploid
9816/3 B-lymphoblastic leukaemia/lymphoma with hypodiploidy, low hypodiploid
9816/3 B-lymphoblastic leukaemia/lymphoma with hypodiploidy, high hypodiploid

ICD-11 coding

2A70.Y & XH2MD9 Other B-lymphoblastic leukaemia/lymphoma with recurrent genetic abnormalities & B-lymphoblastic leukaemia/lymphoma with hypodiploidy (hypodiploid ALL)

Related terminology

None

Subtype(s)

Near-haploid B-ALL/LBL with hypodiploidy (24–31 chromosomes); low-hypodiploid B-ALL/LBL with hypodiploidy (32–39 chromosomes); high-hypodiploid B-ALL/LBL with hypodiploidy (40–43 chromosomes)

Localization

B-ALL and B-LBL represent the same disease. B-ALL always involves the bone marrow and usually also involves the peripheral blood. Extramedullary involvement is common and is by definition the primary site of involvement in B-LBL. For details, see *B-lymphoblastic leukaemia/lymphoma* (p. 330).

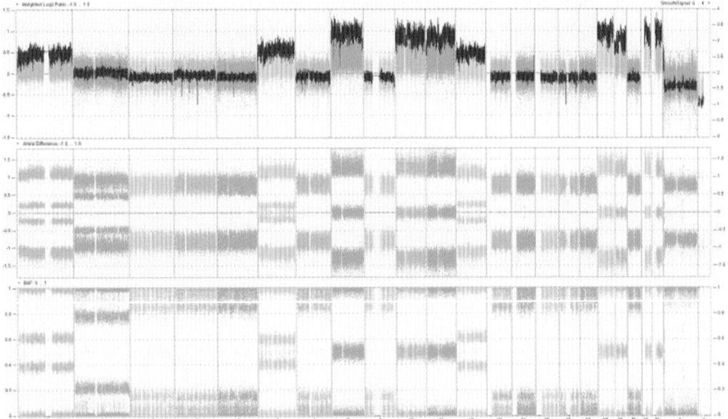

Fig. 4.30 B-lymphoblastic leukaemia/lymphoma with hypodiploidy. SNP array profile shows evidence of a doubled near-haploid/low-hypodiploid clone. Copy-neutral loss of heterozygosity is apparent for chromosomes 2–5, 7, 9, 13–17, 20, and X, indicating that the disomic state for these chromosomes was achieved through endoreduplication.

Clinical features

No unique features

Epidemiology

Although low-hypodiploid B-ALL/LBL is rare in children (< 1%), the frequency increases with age, accounting for 5% of B-ALL/LBL cases in adolescents and young adults, and > 10% of cases in adults. The near-haploid subtype accounts for < 2% of paediatric B-ALL/LBL cases and is rare in adults.

Etiology

Approximately 50% of children with low-hypodiploid B-ALL/LBL have germline *TP53* variants (Li–Fraumeni syndrome, an autosomal dominant inherited disorder associated with mutations of *TP53*) {2830,1620}.

Pathogenesis

p53 is one of the most prominent tumour suppressors. Its activation as a transcription factor stimulates downstream pathways leading to protective cellular processes, including cell-cycle arrest, apoptosis, and senescence, to prevent the propagation of genetically altered cells {4246}. Evidence indicates that p53 also regulates other important processes, such as cell oxidative metabolism (the cellular response to nutrient deprivation), fertility, ferroptosis, and stem cell maintenance. The extent and consequences of the biological response elicited by p53 vary according to the stress and cell type {1905}. The functions of p53 rely mainly on its transcriptional activity, but it can also act via interactions with various proteins {2531, 2111}. Cells from individuals with Li–Fraumeni syndrome exhibit genomic instability, telomere dysfunction, and spontaneous immortalization {3128}.

Macroscopic appearance

No unique features

Histopathology

No unique features

Cytology

No unique features

Diagnostic molecular pathology

Karyotype, flow cytometry DNA index, FISH, and SNP arrays are all useful in establishing the diagnosis. Several genetic alterations are associated with specific hypodiploid subtypes {1620}. Near-haploid B-ALL/LBL frequently exhibits alterations in receptor tyrosine kinase and RAS pathway signalling, *IKZF3* deletions, and focal deletions of a histone gene cluster at 6p22. Low-hypodiploid B-ALL/LBL harbours *TP53* alterations in > 90% of cases; approximately half are somatic mutations and half are germline variants, the latter of which are associated with Li–Fraumeni syndrome {2830,1620}. *IKZF2* deletions and *RB1* mutations are also frequent in low-hypodiploid B-ALL/LBL.

Differential diagnosis

Near-haploid and low-hypodiploid B-ALL/LBL may undergo doubling, resulting in a pseudohyperdiploid or near-triploid clone containing up to 78 chromosomes. If the original hypodiploid clone is not present, the hypodiploidy is regarded as masked, and the case may be mistaken for high-hyperdiploid B-ALL/LBL, resulting in an inappropriate prognostication {563, 835}. The two subtypes may be differentiated by SNP array analysis, demonstrating copy-neutral loss of heterozygosity for doubled monosomic chromosomes. The DNA index assessed by flow cytometry may also be helpful if distinct peaks representing the hypodiploid and doubled clones are both detectable {4519}. FISH and karyotype analysis demonstrating characteristic patterns of chromosomal gain and loss may also aid in differentiation.

Essential and desirable diagnostic criteria

Essential: meets the diagnostic criteria for B-ALL/LBL (see *B-lymphoblastic leukaemia/lymphoma*, p. 330); demonstration of hypodiploidy (≤ 43 chromosomes) by karyotyping and/or FISH analysis; flow cytometry DNA index analysis and/or SNP array analysis to identify masked hypodiploidy.

Staging

Not relevant

Prognosis and prediction

Both near-haploid and low/high-hypodiploid B-ALL/LBL have a poor prognosis. Near-diploid cases (44–45 chromosomes) are not included in the hypodiploid category in clinical therapy–directed classification schemes because they do not share the poor prognosis observed {3310} in cases with ≤ 43 chromosomes. Lower modal chromosome numbers are associated with increasingly poor outcomes, and allogeneic haematopoietic stem cell transplantation does not appear to provide a significant outcome benefit {3310,2623,2862}.

B-lymphoblastic leukaemia/lymphoma with iAMP21

Harrison CJ
Parihar M
Rabin KR

Definition

B-lymphoblastic leukaemia/lymphoma (B-ALL/LBL) with intrachromosomal amplification of chromosome 21 (iAMP21) is a neoplasm of lymphoblasts of B lineage, defined by the presence of gains and gross rearrangements involving the long arm of chromosome 21.

ICD-O coding

9811/3 B-lymphoblastic leukaemia/lymphoma with iAMP21

ICD-11 coding

2A70.Y & XH0KD4 Other B-lymphoblastic leukaemia/lymphoma with recurrent genetic abnormalities & B-lymphoblastic leukaemia/lymphoma with iAMP21

Related terminology

None

Subtype(s)

None

Localization

B-ALL and B-LBL represent the same disease. B-ALL always involves the bone marrow and usually also involves the peripheral blood. Extramedullary involvement is common and is by definition the primary site of involvement in B-LBL. For details, see *B-lymphoblastic leukaemia/lymphoma* (p. 330).

Clinical features

No unique features

Epidemiology

Patients are usually older children (median age: 9 years) with low white blood cell counts. B-ALL/LBL with iAMP21 accounts for approximately 2% of paediatric B-ALL/LBL cases and is rare in adults {417,2487}.

Etiology

Individuals with the rare constitutional Robertsonian translocation between chromosomes 15 and 21, rob(15;21)(q10;q10)c, have a > 2700-fold increased risk of developing B-ALL/LBL with iAMP21. Carriers of constitutional ring chromosome 21, r(21)c, also have an increased risk {1509,2326}.

Pathogenesis

Macroscopic appearance

No unique features

Histopathology

No unique features

Cytology

No unique features

Diagnostic molecular pathology

B-ALL/LBL with iAMP21 is defined by the identification of a grossly abnormal chromosome 21 in the karyotype, supported by FISH using a probe for *RUNX1*, which detects additional copies of the *RUNX1* signal. To date, the FISH definition of B-ALL/LBL with iAMP21 is ≥ 5 copies of *RUNX1* per cell, with ≥ 3 copies on a single abnormal chromosome 21 {1505}. Care must be taken not to misinterpret the FISH result when ≥ 5 copies of *RUNX1* per cell are seen in interphase cells, because high-hyperdiploid B-ALL harbours additional copies of whole chromosome 21 and can produce the same FISH signal pattern. More recently, for a definitive diagnosis of B-ALL/LBL with iAMP21, the distinctive SNP array profile of chromosome 21 seen in these patients has been used to

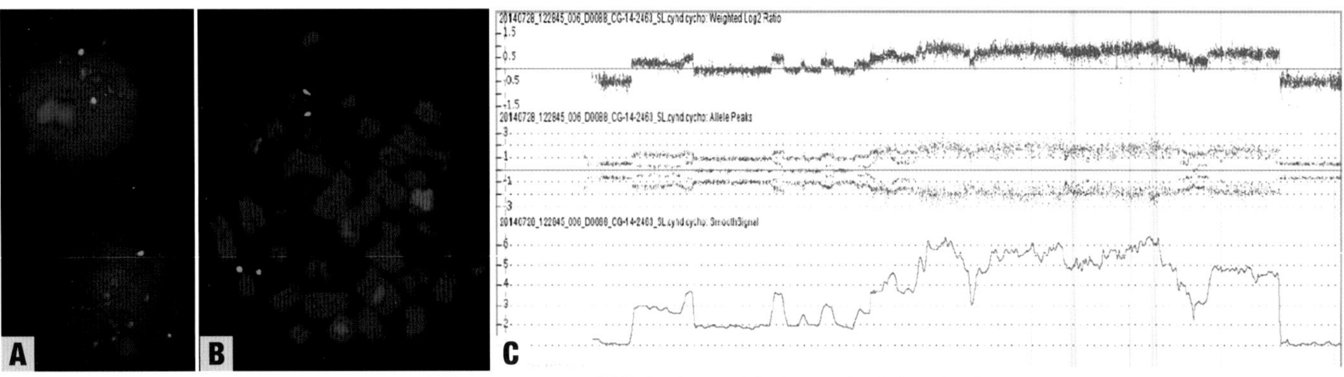

Fig. 4.31 B-lymphoblastic leukaemia/lymphoma with iAMP21. **A** Interphase FISH showing multiple *RUNX1* signals in red and two *ETV6* signals in green. **B** Metaphase cell showing the expected (two) *RUNX1* signals on each chromatid of the normal chromosome 21 (upper-left red signals) and the remaining *RUNX1* signals clustered together on the iAMP21 chromosome (lower-right red signals). **C** Typical SNP array profile of chromosome 21 showing evidence of iAMP21 as illustrated by the alternating copy-number changes across the entire chromosome, in addition to amplification across the *RUNX1* locus and terminal copy-number loss.

validate the FISH result {1025,1505,1508}. This is of particular importance when the *RUNX1* signal pattern differs from the expected result, for example < 5 signals per cell or involving other chromosomes in addition to chromosome 21 {1814}. Although these situations rarely occur, the region of highest gain on chromosome 21 may not always include *RUNX1*; other chromosomes may be involved in rearrangements with the iAMP21 chromosome, or it may be duplicated. Common associated secondary chromosomal abnormalities include gain of the X chromosome, abnormalities of chromosomes 7 and 11, and deletions of *RB1* and *ETV6*. *P2RY8*::*CRLF2* fusion occurs at a higher frequency than in other B-ALL subtypes. The co-occurrence of iAMP21 with additional driver abnormalities like *BCR*::*ABL1*-like features is rare. In such cases, iAMP21 should take precedence, because additional fusions are regarded as secondary events {2255}.

Essential and desirable diagnostic criteria

Essential: meets the diagnostic criteria for B-ALL/LBL (see *B-lymphoblastic leukaemia/lymphoma*, p. 330); demonstration of a grossly abnormal chromosome 21 by karyotyping; demonstration of ≥ 5 copies of *RUNX1* per cell, with ≥ 3 copies on a single abnormal chromosome 21 by karyotyping and FISH analysis.

Desirable: confirmation of FISH findings by SNP array analysis.

Staging

No unique features

Prognosis and prediction

It was previously reported that B-ALL/LBL with iAMP21 is associated with a high relapse risk on standard therapy. Treatment with more intensive therapy overcomes this adverse risk {1546, 2770}.

B-lymphoblastic leukaemia/lymphoma with *BCR::ABL1* fusion

Nardi V
Cassaday RD
Cazzaniga G
Harris MH
Hu S
Leventaki V
Weinstock DM

Definition

B-lymphoblastic leukaemia/lymphoma (B-ALL/LBL) with *BCR::ABL1* fusion is a neoplasm of lymphoblasts of B lineage defined by the presence of a rearrangement between *BCR* on chromosome 22q11.2 and the oncogene *ABL1* on chromosome 9q34.1.

ICD-O coding

9812/3 B-lymphoblastic leukaemia/lymphoma with *BCR::ABL1* fusion

ICD-11 coding

2A70.1 B-lymphoblastic leukaemia or lymphoma with t(9:22)(q34;q11.2); *BCR-ABL1*

Related terminology

Not recommended: Philadelphia chromosome–positive (Ph+) B-ALL/LBL.

Subtype(s)

None

Localization

B-ALL and B-LBL represent the same disease. B-ALL always involves the bone marrow and usually also involves the peripheral blood. Extramedullary involvement is common and is by definition the primary site of involvement in B-LBL. For details, see *B-lymphoblastic leukaemia/lymphoma* (p. 330).

Clinical features

The clinical features of B-ALL/LBL with *BCR::ABL1* fusion are similar to those of other subtypes, and there tends to be a high white blood cell count.

Epidemiology

The proportion of patients with B-ALL/LBL who harbour *BCR::ABL1* increases with age: 2–4% of B-ALL cases in children aged < 15 years, 10% in patients aged 15–39 years, 25% in patients aged 40–49 years, and 20–40% in patients aged > 50 years {2766,3311,3668,497}.

Etiology

No unique features

Pathogenesis

The chimeric BCR::ABL1 protein has a constitutively active tyrosine kinase. The majority (80–90%) of B-ALL/LBL cases with *BCR::ABL1* harbour a 190 kDa fusion protein (p190; transcript e1a2). Fewer *BCR::ABL1*-positive B-ALL/LBL cases harbour a 210 kDa fusion protein (p210; transcripts e13a2 or e14a2), which is more commonly found in chronic myeloid leukaemia (CML) (see Table 4.10). It should be noted that *BCR::ABL1* is not unique to the entity B-ALL/LBL with *BCR::ABL1* and can be acquired as a secondary event during treatment or follow-up in cases of various other types/entities of the B-ALL/LBL family.

Macroscopic appearance

No unique features

Histopathology

In addition to B-lineage markers, blasts frequently express the myeloid-associated antigens CD13 and CD33. CD25 is also frequently expressed {3101,1269}.

Cytology

No unique features

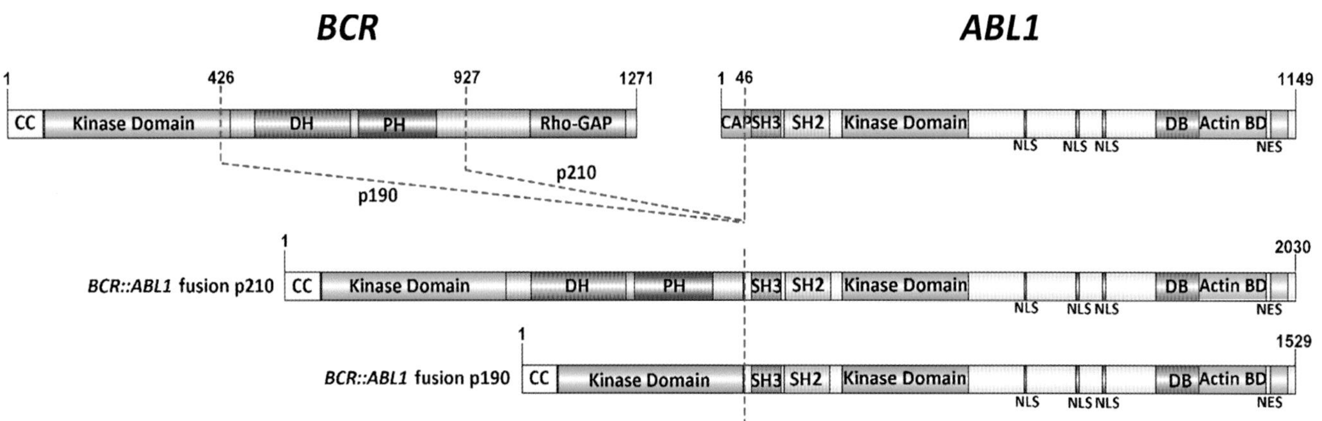

Fig. 4.32 B-lymphoblastic leukaemia/lymphoma with *BCR::ABL1* fusion. Schematic illustration of *BCR::ABL1* fusion, and the functional domains and breakpoints. The dotted red line indicates the breakpoint, and the number denotes amino acids {2095,3384}. Actin BD, F-actin binding domain; CAP, N-terminal cap; CC, coiled-coil; DB, DNA-binding site; DH, double homology; NES, nuclear export signal; NLS, nuclear localization signal; PH, pleckstrin homology; Rho-GAP, Rho GTPase–activating protein.

Table 4.10 Typical and atypical/variant *BCR::ABL1* transcripts

BCR exon	*ABL1* exon	*BCR::ABL1* transcript type	Protein size (kDa)	Typical and atypical breakpoints and transcripts {927,2218}	Frequency in CML (overall and among the non-atypical major breakpoint cluster region[a]) {3318,198}	Frequency in *BCR::ABL1*+ B-ALL {498,934,199,1364}
e13 (b2)	a2	e13a2 (b2a2)	p210	Major breakpoint cluster region	~37.9%	17.50%[b]
e14 (b3)	a2	e14a2 (b3a2)	p210	Major breakpoint cluster region	~62.1%	12.5%[b]
e1	a2	e1a2	p190	Minor breakpoint cluster region	< 1%, 16.9%	~70%
e19	a2	e19a2	p230	Micro breakpoint cluster region	< 1%, 39.8%	Not available
e1	a3	e1a3	p190	Atypical/variant transcript	< 1%, 1.2%	< 1%
e13	a3	e13a3 (b2a3)	p203	Atypical/variant transcript	< 1%, 7.2%	< 1%
e14	a3	e14a3 (b3a3)	p203	Atypical/variant transcript	< 1%, 13.3%	< 1%
e6	a2	e6a2	p195	Atypical/variant transcript	< 1%, 3.6%	< 1%
e8	a2	e8a2	p200	Atypical/variant transcript	< 1%, 8.4%	Not available
e12	a2	e12a2	Not available	Atypical/variant transcript	< 1%, 1.2%	Not available
e1	a8	e1a8	p200	Atypical/variant transcript	Not available	< 1%

CML, chronic myeloid leukaemia.
[a]This category includes also unusual *BCR::ABL1* e13a2 transcripts (7.2%) and unusual *BCR::ABL1* e14a2 transcripts (1.2%), with insertions or inversions at the junction sites. [b]Calculated on the basis of a total p210-positive rate of about 30% and referring to the 58.5% frequency of *BCR::ABL1* e13a2 versus *BCR::ABL1* e14a2 (+/− *BCR::ABL1* e13a2) {199}.

Diagnostic molecular pathology

Detection of the *BCR::ABL1* fusion via karyotyping, FISH, PCR, DNA, or RNA sequencing is required for the diagnosis of B-ALL/LBL with *BCR::ABL1*. Identification of the specific *BCR::ABL1* fusion transcripts (see Table 4.10) is useful for quantifying disease burden and monitoring therapeutic response. In patients who relapse or are refractory to initial *ABL1* tyrosine kinase inhibitor (TKI) therapy, mutation analysis of the *ABL1* kinase domain is recommended to guide the selection of TKIs {2767,4362}. Gain of a Ph chromosome, monosomy 7, +8, +X, +21, and del(9p) are among the commonly associated secondary abnormalities {2767,4362}. In the rare case when an additional subtype-defining cytogenetic finding is noted along with *BCR::ABL1* fusion, the presence of *BCR::ABL1* (as long as not subclonal) appears to govern the clinical features of the disease, and the disease should be subclassified as B-ALL/LBL with *BCR::ABL1* fusion {3803}. More than 80% of patients with B-ALL/LBL with *BCR::ABL1* fusion have deletion or splicing abnormalities of *IKZF1*. As many as 50% of patients have deletions, mutations, or rearrangements of *PAX5* {1127,1703}, and deletions of *CDKN2A* and/or *CDKN2B* {2836}.

B-ALL/LBL with *BCR::ABL1* fusion should be differentiated from the B-lymphoid blast phase of CML showing *BCR::ABL1* with a p210 fusion protein {679}. *BCR::ABL1* can also be present in rare cases of T-lymphoblastic leukaemia and mixed-phenotype acute leukaemia {3345,3340,1363,3928,67}.

Essential and desirable diagnostic criteria

Essential: meets the diagnostic criteria for B-ALL/LBL (see *B-lymphoblastic leukaemia/lymphoma*, p. 330);

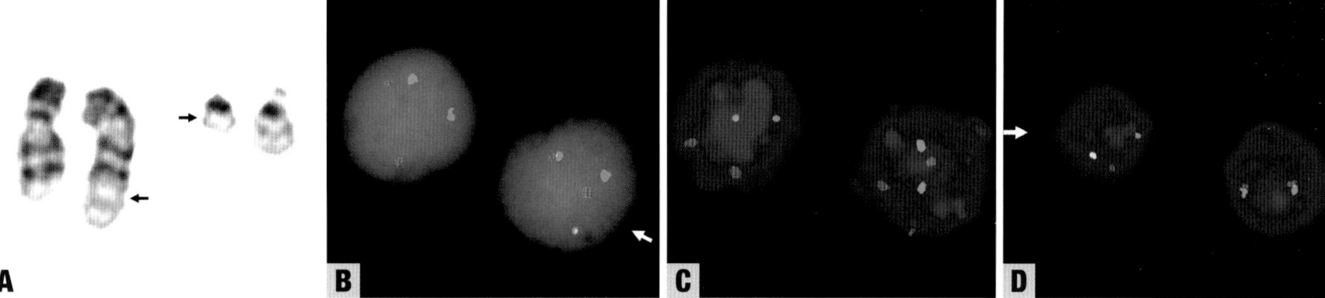

Fig. 4.33 B-lymphoblastic leukaemia/lymphoma with *BCR::ABL1* fusion. **A** The translocation results from the breakage and rejoining of bands 9q34 and 22q11.2. G-banded normal chromosomes 9 and 22 are shown on the outside of each pair of homologues, and the points of rearrangement on the derivative chromosomes 9 and 22 from the translocation are indicated by black arrows. **B** Dual-colour, dual-fusion FISH strategy with probes for *ABL1* (9q34) and *BCR* (22q11.2). Representative interphase nucleus with abnormal *BCR::ABL1* dual-fusion signal pattern (white arrow) (one red normal *ABL1*, one green normal *BCR*, and two *BCR::ABL1* fusion signals indicating the 9;22 translocation). A normal nucleus is also present (two red signals for normal *ABL1* and two green signals for normal *BCR*). **C** Dual-colour, dual-fusion FISH strategy with probes for *ABL1* (9q34) and *BCR* (22q11.2). Representative interphase nuclei with three *ABL1* signals and no *BCR::ABL1* rearrangement (white arrow) (three red *ABL1* and two normal *BCR*, which may indicate gain of *ABL1* at 9q34 or rearrangement of one *ABL1* locus with a partner other than *BCR*). A normal nucleus is also present (two red signals for normal *ABL1* and two green signals for normal *BCR*). **D** Break-apart probe strategy for *ABL1* (9q34). Representative interphase nucleus with abnormal *ABL1* rearrangement signal pattern (white arrow) (one normal intact fusion signal, and one separated green 5′ *ABL1* and red 3′ *ABL1*; this confirms that the pattern of three *ABL1* signals shown in **C** represents one normal *ABL1* signal and *ABL1* rearrangement with a partner other than *BCR* for consideration as a separate subtype). A normal nucleus is also present (two intact fusion signals).

demonstration of the *BCR::ABL1* fusion; exclusion of cases of B-ALL in which *BCR::ABL1* is acquired as a secondary event during treatment or follow-up; exclusion of B-lymphoid blast crisis of CML.

Staging

Not relevant

Prognosis and prediction

Historically, B-ALL/LBL with *BCR::ABL1* fusion had a relatively poor prognosis, even with more liberal use of haematopoietic stem cell transplantation in first remission {1359}. Incorporation of TKIs in the treatment of B-ALL/LBL with *BCR::ABL1* fusion has significantly improved the long-term survival rates for this leukaemia, which are now surpassing those of *BCR::ABL1*-negative acute lymphoblastic leukaemia in several studies in adults. Measurable residual disease is a strong predictor of disease relapse and overall survival {3734,583,4567}. The goal of therapy now is to achieve undetectable *BCR::ABL1* transcript, with a sensitivity of 0.01%, which, if achieved, identifies patients with a favourable prognosis {3734,583,4567}. *IKZF1* alterations are associated with a poor response to TKIs and worse overall survival {2834, 1702,4151,3762}. Discrepancies in measurable residual disease monitoring may reflect different subgroup involvement {1644,2873}.

B-lymphoblastic leukaemia/lymphoma with *BCR::ABL1*-like features

Nardi V
Cassaday RD
Harris MH
Ketterling RP
Weinstock DM

Definition

BCR::ABL1-like B-lymphoblastic leukaemia/lymphoma (B-ALL/LBL) is a neoplasm of lymphoblasts of B-cell lineage defined by DNA alterations that induce a phenotype similar to that of *BCR::ABL1*-positive B-ALL but lack the pathognomonic *BCR::ABL1* rearrangement.

ICD-O coding

9819/3 B-lymphoblastic leukaemia/lymphoma with *BCR::ABL1*-like features

ICD-11 coding

2A70.Y & XH1D04 Other B-lymphoblastic leukaemia/lymphoma with recurrent genetic abnormalities & B-lymphoblastic leukaemia/lymphoma, *BCR-ABL1*-like

Related terminology

Acceptable: Philadelphia-like (Ph-like) B-ALL; *BCR::ABL1*-like B-ALL/LBL.

Subtype(s)

None

Localization

B-ALL and B-LBL represent the same disease. B-ALL always involves the bone marrow and usually also involves the peripheral blood. Extramedullary involvement is common and is by definition the primary site of involvement in B-LBL. For details, see *B-lymphoblastic leukaemia/lymphoma* (p. 330).

Clinical features

B-ALL/LBL with *BCR::ABL1*-like features has clinical features similar to those of other subtypes, but it more often has a high white blood cell count {3427}.

Epidemiology

The fraction of B-ALL cases that have *BCR::ABL1*-like features ranges from 10–15% in children to 25–30% in adolescents and young adults and 20–25% in older adults. In patients with Down syndrome, the fraction of all B-ALL cases that are B-ALL/LBL with *BCR::ABL1*-like features is 50–60% {2833,1574,3426,3397}. The M:F ratio for this subtype is about 2:1 {1705}.

Etiology

No unique features

Pathogenesis

B-ALL/LBL with *BCR::ABL1*-like features harbours mutations or rearrangements that constitutively activate JAK/STAT, ABL-class, or other kinase signalling pathways {3428,3427}. Approximately 50% of cases have rearrangements of *CRLF2* with IGH (t(X/Y;14)) or *P2RY8* (intrachromosomal deletion in the pseudoautosomal region of the X or Y chromosome) that lead to aberrant expression of CRLF2 {2833,1574,4500}. In these cases, additional mutations lead to constitutive JAK/STAT activation downstream of *CRLF2* and include CRLF2 p.F232C or activating mutations of *JAK1* (most commonly p.V658F), *JAK2* (most commonly codon R683) or *IL7R*. *JAK2* gene fusions occur in about 7% of cases of B-ALL with *BCR::ABL1* features, and *EPOR* rearrangements occur in about 5% {1701}. Alterations in *SH2B3*, *IL2RB*, and *TYK2* genes occur in about 7% of patients and also activate JAK/STAT. Distinct from these leukaemias are cases with rearrangements of ABL-class kinase genes (*ABL1*, *ABL2*, *CSF1R*, *PDGFRA*, *PDGFRB*, and *LYN*), RAS pathway activating mutations (in *KRAS*, *NF1*, and *PTPN11*), or uncommon fusions involving *NTRK3*, *PTK2B*, *FLT3*, and *FGFR1*. *IKZF1* deletions occur in about 70–80% of adult patients and about 40–60% of paediatric patients {4150,929}, particularly in fusion-positive cases. Copy-number aberrations in cell-cycle regulators (*CDKN2A/B*, *TP53*, *RB1*) and in genes involved in B-cell development (*ETV6*, *PAX5*, *EBF1*), as well as extra copies of chromosome 21 (or intrachromosomal amplification of chromosome 21 [iAMP21]) {386} are also recurrent. Cases with *CRLF2* rearrangements commonly harbour additional copies of the X or Y chromosome. Of note, some of these genetic alterations (e.g. *P2RY8::CRLF2*) can be subclonal and not the main driving force of the acute lymphoblastic leukaemia {1086,2774,4228}.

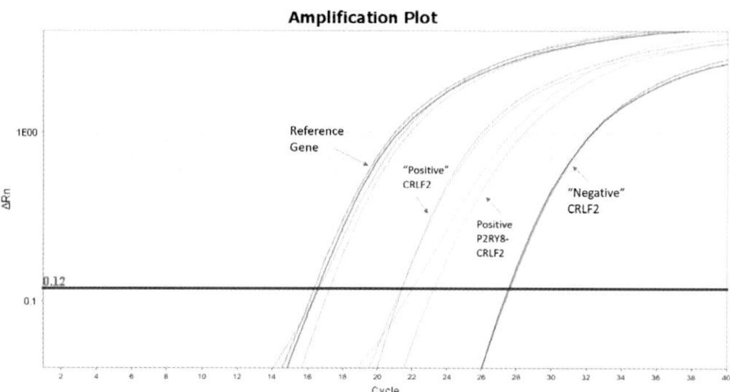

Fig. 4.34 B-lymphoblastic leukaemia/lymphoma (B-ALL/LBL) with *BCR::ABL1*-like features detected with a quantitative RT-PCR–based low-density array assay. Quantitative RT-PCR–based low-density array evaluates the expression levels of 15 previously described genes (and a control gene) shown to be associated with the diagnosis of B-ALL/LBL with *BCR::ABL1*-like features {1527}. A score based on a composite of the individual amplification curves is generated to determine whether the case shows expression levels at or above the validated threshold of positivity. The assay also screens for multiple fusions that would preclude the diagnosis of B-ALL/LBL with *BCR::ABL1*-like features and fusions that are commonly associated with B-ALL/LBL with *BCR::ABL1*-like features, such as *P2RY8::CRLF2*. In this example, there is increased expression of *CRLF2* and *P2RY8::CRLF2* compared with a negative control, consistent with a positive result in a patient with B-ALL/LBL with *BCR::ABL1*-like features due to del(X)(p22.33;p22.33) causing *P2RY8::CRLF2* rearrangement.

Macroscopic appearance

No unique features

Histopathology

Immunophenotype

TSLPR (encoded by *CRLF2*) overexpression by flow cytometric analysis is a useful surrogate for *CRLF2* rearrangement {3975, 487}.

Cytology

No unique features

Diagnostic molecular pathology

Whole-transcriptome analysis was traditionally used to define B-ALL/LBL with *BCR::ABL1*-like features, but it is not routinely available as a clinical assay. Quantitative RT-PCR of selected gene sets may be a valid alternative for identifying a *BCR::ABL1*-like signature {1872}. Whether or not this initial screening is performed,

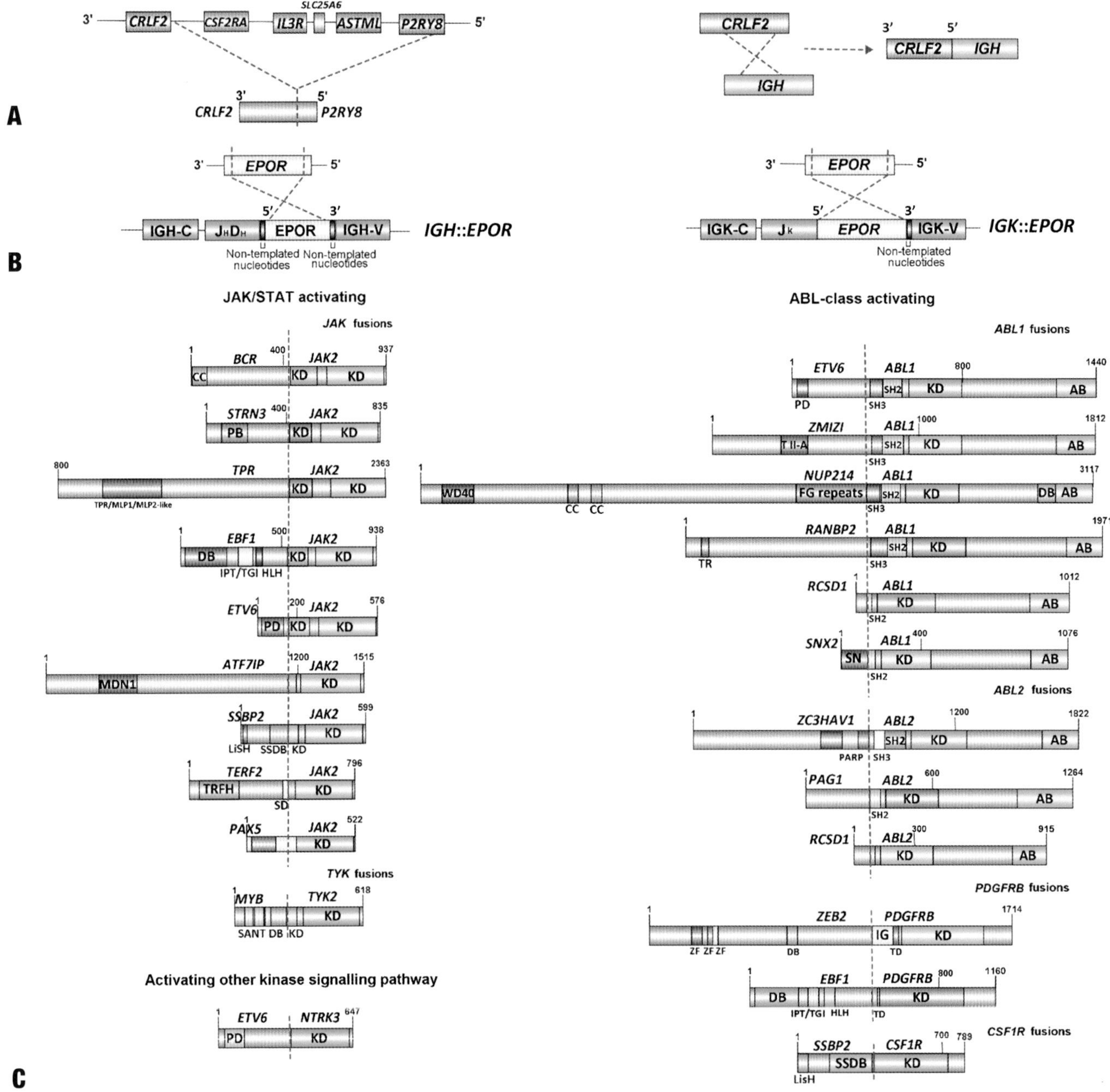

Fig. 4.35 B-lymphoblastic leukaemia/lymphoma with *BCR::ABL1*-like features. Schematic illustration of representative fusions with *BCR::ABL1*-like features, and their functional domains and breakpoints. Dotted red lines indicate the breakpoints, and numbers denote amino acids (**A** {1034,3976}; **B** {1701}; **C** {3427,3428}). AB, actin-binding domain; CC, coiled-coil oligomerization domain; DB, DNA-binding domain; FG, phenylalanine glycine; HLH, helix-loop-helix; IG, immunoglobulin-like domain; IPT/TIG, immunoglobulin-like fold, plexins, transcription factors / transcription factor immunoglobulin; KD, kinase domain; LisH, Lis homology; PARP, PARP catalytic domain; PB, paired-box domain; PD, pointed domain; SD, SANT DNA binding domains; SH, SRC homology domain; SN, sorting nexin, N-terminal; SSDB, single-stranded DNA-binding domain; T II-A, topoisomerase II–associated protein; TD, transmembrane domain; TR, tetratricopeptide repeat; TRFH, telomeric repeat binding factor; ZF, zinc finger domain.

the specific genetic alteration driving *BCR*::*ABL1*-like B-ALL/LBL should be identified because it could have therapeutic implications. In most cases of B-ALL/LBL with *BCR*::*ABL1*-like features, rearrangements are cytogenetically cryptic. However, cytogenetics and FISH can be used to rule out known molecular subgroups, which are usually mutually exclusive. Break-apart FISH probes are available for identifying the major rearrangements (involving *ABL1*, *ABL2*, *CRLF2*, *JAK2*, and *PDGFRB* as 3′ partners). Similarly, multiplex RT-PCR can be used to rapidly detect the most common gene fusions. DNA and RNA sequencing can provide additional information on JAK/STAT and RAS pathway mutations, as well as detecting rarer rearrangements (e.g. *ETV6*::*NTRK3*, *FLT3* rearrangements). Co-occurrence of iAMP21 with additional driver abnormalities including *BCR*::*ABL1*-like features is rare. In such cases iAMP21 should take precedence, because additional fusions are regarded as secondary events {2255}.

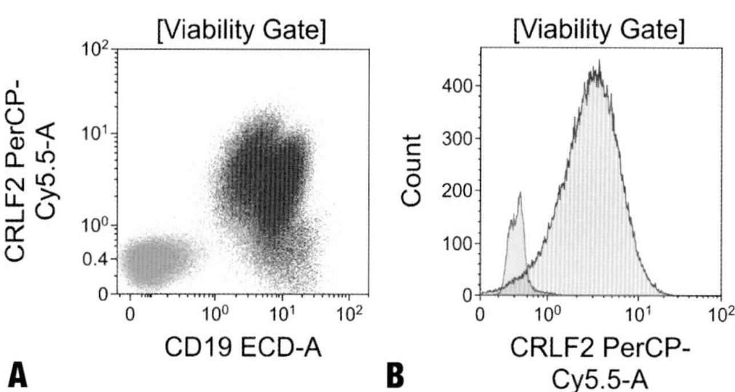

Fig. 4.36 B-lymphoblastic leukaemia/lymphoma with *BCR*::*ABL1*-like features. B-lymphoblastic leukaemia with CRLF2 expression: flow cytometry dot plot and histogram. **A** B-lymphoblastic leukaemia blasts show moderate expression of TSLPR (CRLF2). **B** An overlay histogram shows TSLPR (CRLF2)-positive B-lymphoblastic leukaemia blasts (red peak) and negative lymphocytes (blue peak).

Essential and desirable diagnostic criteria

Essential: meets the diagnostic criteria for B-ALL/LBL (see *B-lymphoblastic leukaemia/lymphoma*, p. 330); demonstration of a *BCR*::*ABL1*-like gene expression signature and/or demonstration of major *BCR*::*ABL1*-like B-ALL/LBL-associated rearrangements.

Staging

No unique features

Prognosis and prediction

B-ALL/LBL with *BCR*::*ABL1*-like features is associated with high-risk clinical features, such as an elevated leukocyte count at diagnosis and a poor treatment response. B-ALL/LBL with *BCR*::*ABL1*-like features has a worse 5-year and overall survival, a higher likelihood of measurable residual disease at the end of induction therapy, and a higher likelihood of relapse than other B-ALL/LBL types {1774,3426,1571,558}. Cases lacking *IKZF1* alterations may have a better prognosis than those with *IKZF1* alterations {3427}. Measurable residual disease–directed treatment has been shown to improve outcomes in patents with B-ALL/LBL with *BCR*::*ABL1*-like features. Recent studies have shown promising outcomes for B-ALL/LBL with *BCR*::*ABL1*-like features with the addition of tyrosine kinase inhibitors directed against specific genomic lesions {4352,558,3962}.

B-lymphoblastic leukaemia/lymphoma with *KMT2A* rearrangement

Harris MH
Cassaday RD
Ketterling RP
Weinstock DM

Definition

B-lymphoblastic leukaemia/lymphoma (B-ALL/LBL) with *KMT2A* rearrangement is a neoplasm of lymphoblasts of B-cell lineage defined by the presence of a rearrangement between *KMT2A* and one of the numerous fusion partners.

ICD-O coding

9813/3 B-lymphoblastic leukaemia/lymphoma with *KMT2A* rearrangement

ICD-11 coding

2A70.Y & XH8GG0 Other B-lymphoblastic leukaemia/lymphoma with recurrent genetic abnormalities & B-lymphoblastic leukaemia/lymphoma with t(v;11q23); *MLL*-rearranged

Related terminology

Not recommended: B-lymphoblastic leukaemia/lymphoma with t(v;11q23), *MLL*-rearranged.

Subtype(s)

None

Localization

B-ALL and B-LBL represent the same disease. B-ALL always involves the bone marrow and usually also involves the peripheral blood. Extramedullary involvement is common and is by definition the primary site of involvement in B-LBL. For details, see *B-lymphoblastic leukaemia/lymphoma* (p. 330).

Clinical features

B-ALL/LBL with *KMT2A* rearrangement has clinical features similar to those of other clinical subtypes, but it more often has a high white blood cell count. CNS involvement is also common at presentation.

Epidemiology

B-ALL with *KMT2A* rearrangement accounts for 70–80% of leukaemia cases in infants aged < 1 year {3232}. It is less common in older children and then becomes increasingly common with age into adulthood.

Etiology

The etiology is unknown. In infants and young children, the *KMT2A* rearrangement is typically acquired in utero {1275,1141}. *KMT2A* breakpoints predominantly occur within an 8.3 kb region that includes multiple repeat sequences, DNase hypersensitivity sites, and targets for topoisomerase II cleavage, although the specific factors that affect breakage remain undefined {131}.

Pathogenesis

KMT2A (also known as MLL) is a histone H3 lysine 4 (H3K4) methyltransferase. Rearrangements typically delete the methyltransferase domain and fuse *KMT2A* to a gene involved in transcription elongation {2540}. This dysregulates both H3K4 and H3K79 methylation, resulting in upregulation of HOXA genes {3036}. *KMT2A* rearrangement may be sufficient to drive leukaemogenesis, although leukaemias may harbour alterations of epigenetic modifiers or MAPK genes, including *FLT3* {117}.

Macroscopic appearance

No unique features

Histopathology

There are no unique morphological features.

Immunophenotype

Cases of B-ALL/LBL with *KMT2A* rearrangements, especially t(4;11), typically have a CD19+, CD10−, CD24− immunophenotype and are often positive for the myeloid markers CD15 and

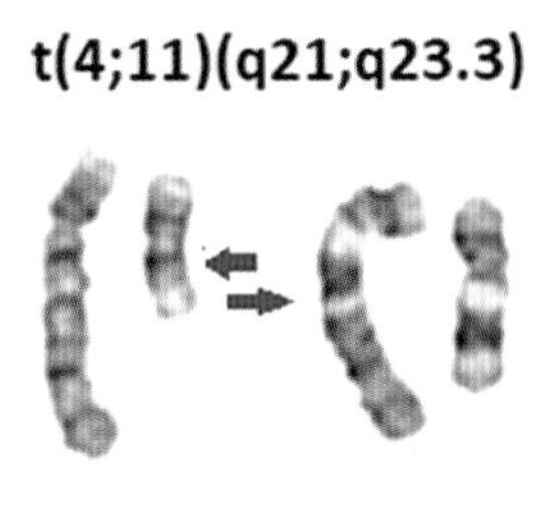

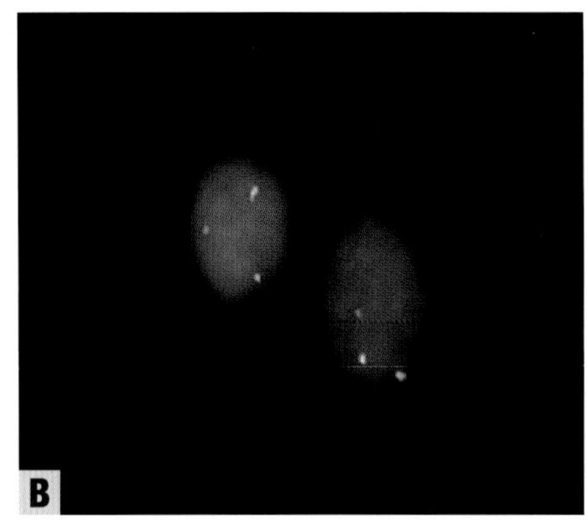

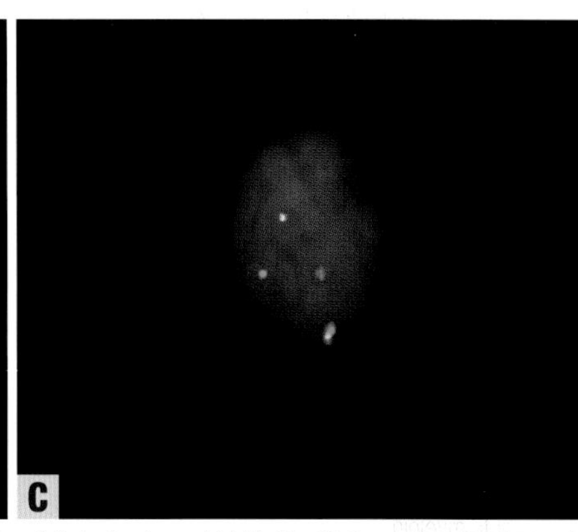

Fig. 4.37 B-lymphoblastic leukaemia/lymphoma with *KMT2A* rearrangement. **A** Partial karyotype of chromosomes 4 and 11, indicating a t(4;11)(q21;q23.3) translocation (arrows). **B** Interphase nuclei with an abnormal *KMT2A* rearrangement signal pattern (one intact fusion signal, one red signal separated from one green signal indicating a break) using a *KMT2A* break-apart probe. **C** Interphase nucleus with an abnormal *KMT2A::AFF1* fusion signal pattern (one red signal for the normal *AFF1* gene, one green signal for the normal *KMT2A* gene, and two *KMT2A::AFF1* fusion signals indicating a translocation) using a *KMT2A::AFF1* dual-colour, dual-fusion probe.

CD65s, as well as the neural/glial antigen CSPG4 (NG2) {1648, 3143,415,4545}. TdT negativity, which is uncommon in B-ALL/LBL overall, is also relatively frequent in B-ALL/LB with *KMT2A* rearrangement {2037}.

Differential diagnosis

In some cases, it may be possible to recognize distinct lymphoblastic and monoblastic populations, a finding that can be confirmed by immunophenotyping; at diagnosis, such cases should be considered B/myeloid mixed-phenotype acute leukaemia. B-ALL/LBL with *KMT2A* rearrangement may undergo a lineage switch after either conventional therapy or anti-CD19–directed therapy {3484,1004}.

Cytology

No unique features

Diagnostic molecular pathology

More than 90 different gene partners for *KMT2A* have been identified across all leukaemia types {2672}. The seven most common fusion partners account for > 90% of cases (see Table 4.11).

B-ALL/LBL with *KMT2A* rearrangement is suspected by translocations/inversions at 11q23 in chromosome studies but requires verification by FISH, RT-PCR, or next-generation sequencing evaluation. *KMT2A* rearrangements can be cryptic by karyotype and/or FISH studies and require next-generation sequencing evaluation, which exemplifies the variable and complex genomics that can occur with *KMT2A*, particularly in infant/paediatric leukaemia {2940,370}.

Essential and desirable diagnostic criteria

Essential: meets the diagnostic criteria for B-ALL/LBL (see *B-lymphoblastic leukaemia/lymphoma*, p. 330); immunophenotyping by FACS and/or immunohistochemistry to explore a frequently present immunophenotype (negative for CD10, CD24, and TdT; positive for myeloid markers CD15, CD65s, and NG2); demonstration of *KMT2A* rearrangement by FISH and/or RT-PCR and/or next-generation sequencing analysis.

Desirable: identification of *KMT2A* rearrangement partner.

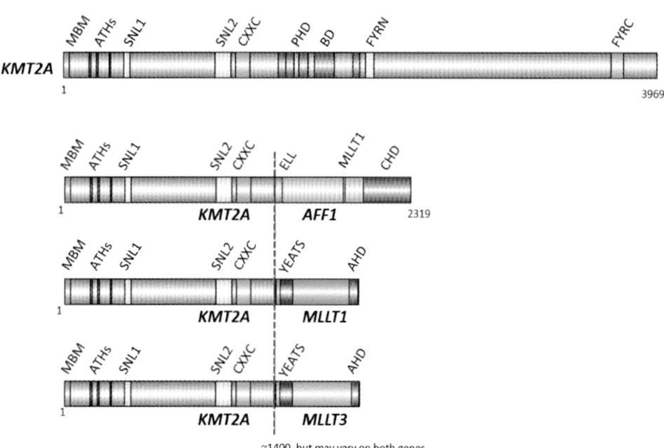

Fig. 4.38 B-lymphoblastic leukaemia/lymphoma with *KMT2A* rearrangement. Schematic illustration of *KMT2A*-involved fusions, and their functional domains and breakpoints. The dotted red line indicates the breakpoint and the number denotes amino acids {464,1275,3761}. AHD, Anc1 homology domain; ATHs, N-terminal AT hooks region; BD, bromodomain; CHD, chromodomain helicase DNA-binding domain; CXXC, DNA-binding CXXC region; ELL, ELL binding domain; FYRC, FY-rich C-terminal domains; FYRN, FY-rich N-terminal domains; MBM, menin binding motif; MLLT1, MLLT1 binding domain; PHD, plant homeodomain fingers; SNL, subnuclear localization domains; YEATS, YEATS domain.

Staging

No unique features

Prognosis and prediction

B-ALL/LBL with *KMT2A* rearrangement generally has a poor prognosis compared with other genetic types across age groups. The relative risk associated with different *KMT2A* partners continues to be a topic of investigation {3403,3232, 3309}.

Table 4.11 Common fusion partners in *KMT2A*-rearranged B-lymphoblastic leukaemia/lymphoma (B-ALL/LBL) {2672,3208}

Fusion partner	Previous names	Cytogenetic band	Infant ALL/LBL	Paediatric ALL/LBL	Adult ALL/LBL	Karyotype	Other considerations
AFF1	*AF4, MLLT2*	4q21.3-q22.1	49%	44%	80%	t(4;11)(q21;q23)	Most common partner in ALL/LBL across age groups
MLLT3	*AF9*	9p21.3	16%	18%	2%	t(9;11)(p21;q23) or t(9;11)(p22;q23)	Also common in AML, particularly in paediatric and adult cases
MLLT1	*ENL*	19p13.3	22%	18%	12%	t(11;19)(q23;p13.3)	Easy to miss by karyotype banding; common partner in T-ALL
MLLT10	*AF10*	10p12.31	6%	4%	0%	t(10;11)(p12;q23)	Typically complex; genes in cis orientation
AFDN	*AF6, MLLT4*	6q27	0%	5%	2%	t(6;11)(q27;q23)	Easy to miss by karyotype banding; common partner in T-ALL
EPS15	*MLLT5, AF-1P*	1p32.3	2%	2%	1%	t(1;11)(p32;q23)	None
AFF3	*LAF4, MLLT2*-like	2q11.2	0%	2%	0%	t(2;11)(q11;q23)	None
Total			**95%**	**93%**	**97%**		

AML, acute myeloid leukaemia; T-ALL, T-lymphoblastic leukaemia.

B-lymphoblastic leukaemia/lymphoma with *ETV6::RUNX1* fusion

Kovach AE
Buldini B
Cazzaniga G
Inaba H
Ketterling RP
Locatelli F

Definition
B-lymphoblastic leukaemia/lymphoma (B-ALL/LBL) with *ETV6::RUNX1* fusion is a neoplasm of lymphoblasts of B-cell lineage defined by the presence of rearrangement between *ETV6* on chromosome 12p13.2 and *RUNX1* on chromosome 21q22.1.

ICD-O coding
9814/3 B-lymphoblastic leukaemia/lymphoma with *ETV6::RUNX1* fusion

ICD-11 coding
2A70.Y & XH4KA2 Other B-lymphoblastic leukaemia/lymphoma with recurrent genetic abnormalities & B-lymphoblastic leukaemia/lymphoma with t(12;21)(p13;q22); *TEL-AML1* (*ETV6-RUNX1*)

Related terminology
Not recommended: B-lymphoblastic leukaemia/lymphoma with t(12;21)(p13;q22); *TEL-AML1* (*ETV6-RUNX1*).

Subtype(s)
None

Localization
B-ALL and B-LBL represent the same disease. B-ALL always involves the bone marrow and usually also involves the peripheral blood. Extramedullary involvement is common and is by definition the primary site of involvement in B-LBL. For details, see *B-lymphoblastic leukaemia/lymphoma* (p. 330).

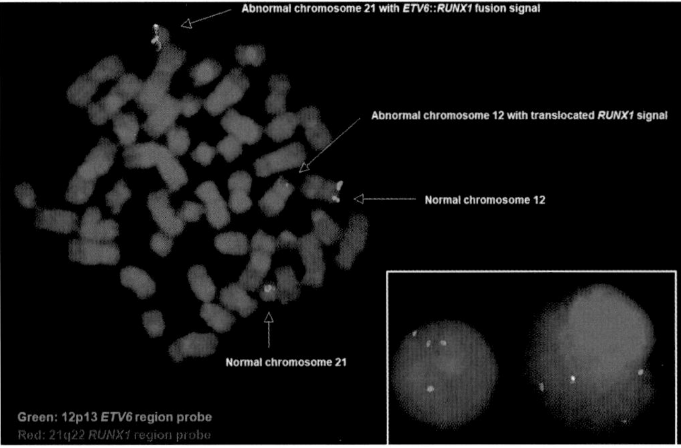

Fig. 4.39 B-lymphoblastic leukaemia/lymphoma with *ETV6::RUNX1* fusion. Abnormal FISH pattern with the *RUNX1* (21q22) (red) and *ETV6* (12p13) (green) probes in a metaphase cell and interphase nuclei (**inset**) in B-lymphoblastic leukaemia/lymphoma with t(12;21)(p13.2;q22.1)/*ETV6::RUNX1*. The probe set utilizes the extra-signal (ES)-FISH strategy, producing the two red, one green, and one fusion signal pattern (2R1G1F) in abnormal cells. In the metaphase cell, the fusion signal indicative of an *ETV6::RUNX1* translocation is shown on derivative chromosome 21 (top, yellow signal). In interphase nuclei, the normal cell (**inset**, left) shows two red and two green signals corresponding to normal copies of the *RUNX1* and *ETV6* genes, respectively, and the abnormal cell (**inset**, right) shows the 2R1G1F pattern, consistent with an *ETV6::RUNX1* rearrangement.

Clinical features
No unique features

Epidemiology
ETV6::RUNX1 is the most common recurrent translocation in childhood B-ALL/LBL, representing approximately 25% of B-ALL/LBL cases diagnosed in patients aged 2–10 years {2538,3735,2620,1282}. It is extremely rare in adults and infants {2708,1771}.

Etiology
The *ETV6::RUNX1* fusion has been identified in archival blood spots of neonates who go on to develop this leukaemia in childhood, and in as many as 5% of healthy newborns, suggesting that it is an early event necessary but not sufficient for leukaemogenesis {4369,3607}. There is no known specific environmental or immunological trigger {1399}.

Pathogenesis
B-ALL/LBL with *ETV6::RUNX1* fusion appears to derive from a B-cell progenitor rather than a haematopoietic stem cell {574, 4153}. The *ETV6::RUNX1* fusion results in the production of a fusion protein that probably acts in a dominant negative fashion to interfere with the normal function of the transcription factor RUNX1 and other proteins {2801}. This leukaemia appears to have a unique gene expression signature {4495}, including a characteristic high RAG1 expression signature {659} and high levels of expression of IGF2BP3 {2491}; abnormalities of the intact *ETV6* allele {578}; and *PAX5*, JAK/STAT pathway, *EPOR*, and DNA methylation abnormalities {4152,4403,4153,1271}.

Macroscopic appearance
No unique features

Histopathology
There are no unique features.

Immunophenotyping
Negative or partially positive CD9, CD20, and CD66c appear relatively specific for this subtype {419,909,1648}. A CD27-positive, CD44-low-to-negative immunophenotype is seen in B-ALL/LBL with *ETV6::RUNX1* fusion, as well as in B-ALL/LBL with *ETV6::RUNX1*-like features {4188,4081}. Myeloid-associated antigens, especially CD13 and CD33, are frequently expressed {257,3014,1033}.

Cytology
Not relevant

Diagnostic molecular pathology

The *ETV6::RUNX1* fusion is identifiable by FISH, RT-PCR, and RNA sequencing methods {468} and not readily identifiable by standard cytogenetics. Derivative chromosomes and other non-prognostic karyotypic changes may be present {171}. Co-occurrence of other recurrent genetic abnormalities in B-ALL/LBL is rare {1430,218,1019}.

Essential and desirable diagnostic criteria

Essential: meets the diagnostic criteria for B-ALL/LBL (see *B-lymphoblastic leukaemia/lymphoma*, p. 330); demonstration of *ETV6::RUNX1* fusion.

Staging

Not relevant

Prognosis and prediction

B-ALL/LBL with *ETV6::RUNX1* fusion has a very favourable prognosis, in part due to chemosensitivity {1244}. Age, presenting white blood cell count, and measurable residual disease after induction chemotherapy are important prognostic factors, but this entity may still have better outcomes than other B-ALL/LBL types with these adverse factors {2589,1794}. Relapses often occur later than do those of other types of B-ALL/LBL. It has been suggested that some late relapses derive from persistent preleukaemic clones that harbour the translocation and undergo additional genetic events after the first leukaemic clone has been eliminated {1218}. Derivative chromosomes by karyotype do not appear to alter the prognosis. Patients with relapsed B-ALL/LBL with *ETV6::RUNX1* fusion have a considerable chance of rescue.

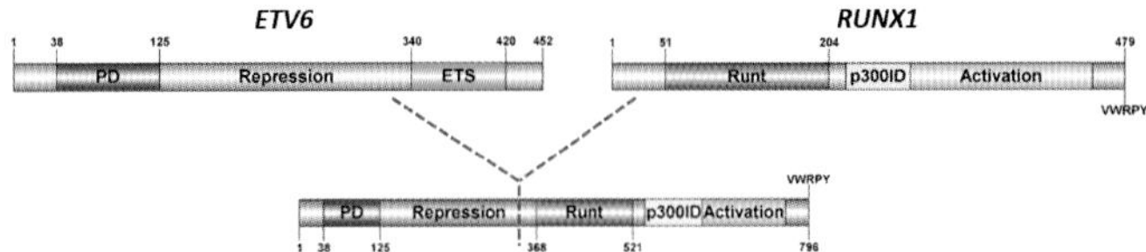

Fig. 4.40 B-lymphoblastic leukaemia/lymphoma with *ETV6::RUNX1* fusion. Schematic illustration of *ETV6::RUNX1* fusion and the functional domains and breakpoints. The dotted red line indicates the breakpoint, and the numbers denote amino acids {4547}. ETS, erythroblast transformation specific domain; p300ID, p300 HAT interacting domain; PD, pointed domain.

Chapter 4

B-lymphoblastic leukaemia/lymphoma with *ETV6::RUNX1*-like features

Kovach AE
Buldini B
Cazzaniga G
Inaba H
Ketterling RP
Locatelli F

Definition

B-lymphoblastic leukaemia/lymphoma (B-ALL/LBL) with *ETV6::RUNX1*-like features is a neoplasm of lymphoblasts of B-cell lineage characterized by a gene expression profile similar to that of B-ALL with *ETV6::RUNX1*, in the absence of the *ETV6::RUNX1* translocation.

ICD-O coding

9814/3 B-lymphoblastic leukaemia/lymphoma with *ETV6::RUNX1*-like features

ICD-11 coding

2A70.Y Other B-lymphoblastic leukaemia/lymphoma with recurrent genetic abnormalities

Related terminology

Acceptable: B-ALL, *ETV6::RUNX1*-like.

Subtype(s)

None

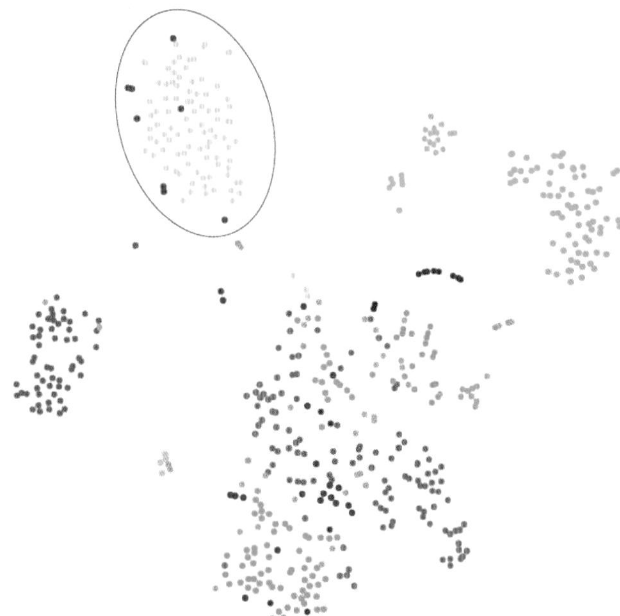

Fig. 4.41 B-lymphoblastic leukaemia/lymphoma (B-ALL/LBL) with *ETV6::RUNX1*-like features. Relationship of RNA sequencing gene expression signatures of B-ALL/LBL with *ETV6::RUNX1* and B-ALL/LBL with *ETV6::RUNX1*-like features. Compared with other B-ALL subtypes, B-ALL/LBL with *ETV6::RUNX1* rearrangement (yellow, *n* = 84) shares a unique distribution with B-ALL/LBL with *ETV6::RUNX1*-like features (red, *n* = 9) by t-distributed stochastic neighbour embedding (t-SNE) plot (*N* = 519).

Localization

B-ALL and B-LBL represent the same disease. B-ALL always involves the bone marrow and usually also involves the peripheral blood. Extramedullary involvement is common and is by definition the primary site of involvement in B-LBL. For details, see *B-lymphoblastic leukaemia/lymphoma* (p. 330).

Clinical features

No unique features

Epidemiology

Like B-ALL/LBL with *ETV6::RUNX1* fusion, B-ALL/LBL with *ETV6::RUNX1*-like features is more frequent in childhood, representing 1–3% of B-ALL/LBL cases in this population {2342}, and uncommon in adults {3102}.

Etiology

Unknown

Pathogenesis

Combined *ETV6* and *IKZF1* rearrangements or deletions appear common and specific to this entity, and they may underlie an alternative mechanism for *RUNX1* disruption in place of an *ETV6::RUNX1* fusion {2835,3055,2342}. *ETV6* rearrangement partners in this category identified to date include *BCL2L14*, *BORCS5*, *CREBBP*, *MSH6*, *NID1*, and *PMEL* {2342}. *ARPP21* deletion may be a secondary genetic event {4530}.

Macroscopic appearance

Not relevant

Histopathology

Immunophenotype

Like B-ALL/LBL with *ETV6::RUNX1* fusion, this type also demonstrates a CD27-positive, CD44-low-to-negative immunophenotype {4530}.

Cytology

Not relevant

Diagnostic molecular pathology

The optimal clinical methods for the identification of this entity have not yet been established {2298}. Like in B-ALL/LBL with *ETV6::RUNX1* fusion, a high *RAG1* signature {659} and *IGF2BP3* {2491} expression and a CD27-positive, CD44-low-to-negative immunophenotype {4530} are suggestive but not fully specific {1779}.

Essential and desirable diagnostic criteria

Essential: meets the diagnostic criteria for B-ALL/LBL (see *B-lymphoblastic leukaemia/lymphoma*, p. 330); lack of *ETV6::RUNX1* translocation and other defined recurrent genetic abnormalities in B-ALL/LBL; gene expression profile similar to that of B-ALL/LBL with *ETV6::RUNX1*.

Desirable: demonstration of a recognized *ETV6* fusion partner, with or without associated *IKZF1* alterations; demonstration of CD27-positive / CD44-low-to-negative immunophenotype.

Staging

Not relevant

Prognosis and prediction

Because the number of patients identified as having B-ALL with *ETV6::RUNX1*-like features is small, the outcome of patients with this subtype is still undefined. However, several relapses have been reported {1794}. *IKZF1* deletions and other alterations may not confer an unfavourable prognosis in this context like they do in others {2835}. Further studies are needed to determine the outcome of patients affected by B-ALL/LBL with *ETV6::RUNX1*-like features.

B-lymphoblastic leukaemia/lymphoma with *TCF3::PBX1* fusion

Kovach AE
Buldini B
Cazzaniga G
Harris MH
Inaba H
Ketterling RP
Locatelli F
Rabin KR

Definition

B-lymphoblastic leukaemia/lymphoma (B-ALL/LBL) with *TCF3::PBX1* fusion is a neoplasm of lymphoblasts of B-cell lineage defined by the presence of rearrangement between *TCF3* on chromosome 19 and *PBX1* on chromosome 1.

ICD-O coding

9818/3 B-lymphoblastic leukaemia/lymphoma with *TCF3::PBX1* fusion

ICD-11 coding

2A70.Y & XH3GU8 Other B-lymphoblastic leukaemia/lymphoma with recurrent genetic abnormalities & B-lymphoblastic leukaemia/lymphoma with t(1;19)(q23;p13.3); *E2A-PBX1* (*TCF3-PBX1*)

Related terminology

Not recommended: B-lymphoblastic leukaemia/lymphoma with *E2A::PBX1*.

Subtype(s)

None

Localization

B-ALL and B-LBL represent the same disease. B-ALL always involves the bone marrow and usually also involves the peripheral blood. Extramedullary involvement is common and is by definition the primary site of involvement in B-LBL. For details, see *B-lymphoblastic leukaemia/lymphoma* (p. 330).

Clinical features

There are no unique features (see *B-lymphoblastic leukaemias/lymphomas: Introduction*, p. 328).

Epidemiology

B-ALL/LBL with *TCF3::PBX1* fusion is relatively common in children, accounting for approximately 5% of paediatric B-ALL/LBL cases, and it is rare in adults {496}.

Etiology

Unknown

Pathogenesis

The *TCF3::PBX1* fusion, usually resulting from t(1;19)(q23;q13.3), has been identified in 0.6% of healthy newborns {1548},

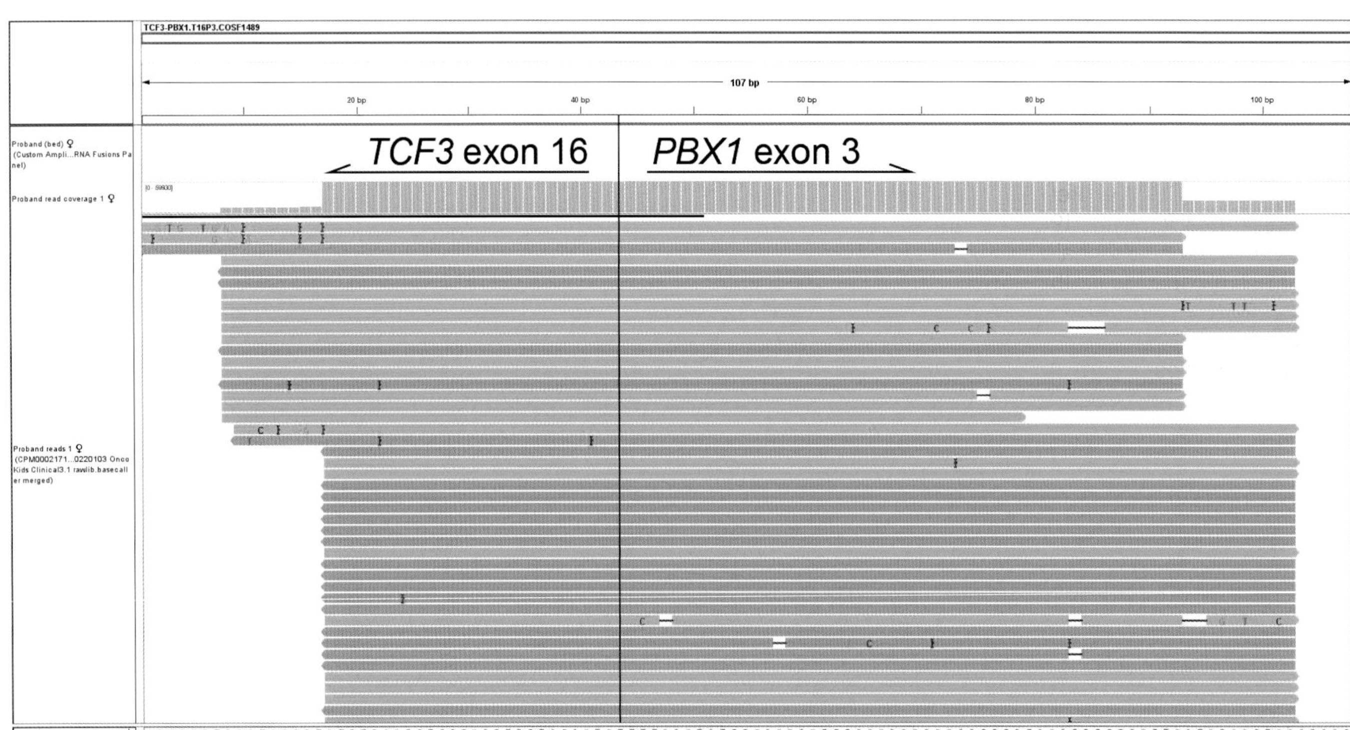

Fig. 4.42 B-lymphoblastic leukaemia/lymphoma with *TCF3::PBX1* fusion. Sequencing reads obtained after PCR amplification and next-generation sequencing of the *TCF3::PBX1* fusion junction using cDNA obtained from leukaemia cells. The presence of chimeric reads with sequence from *TCF3* exon 16 and *PBX1* exon 3 confirms the presence of the abnormal *TCF3::PBX1* fusion in the leukaemic clone.

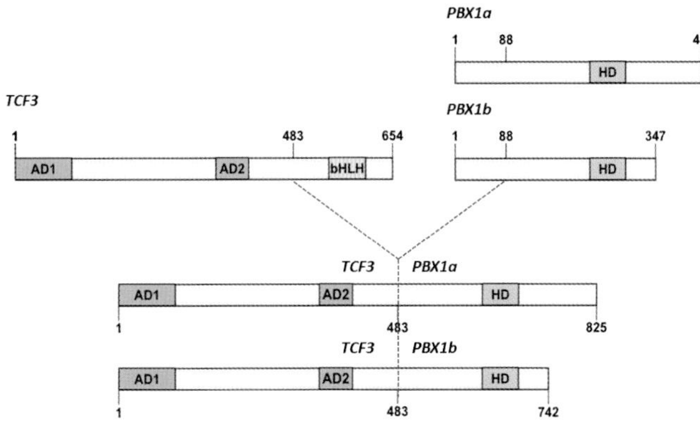

Fig. 4.43 B-lymphoblastic leukaemia/lymphoma with *TCF3::PBX1* fusion. Schematic illustration of *TCF3::PBX1* fusion, and the functional domains and breakpoints. The dotted red line indicates the breakpoint, and the numbers denote amino acids {2246}. AD, activation domain; bHLH, basic helix-loop-helix domain; HD, homeodomain.

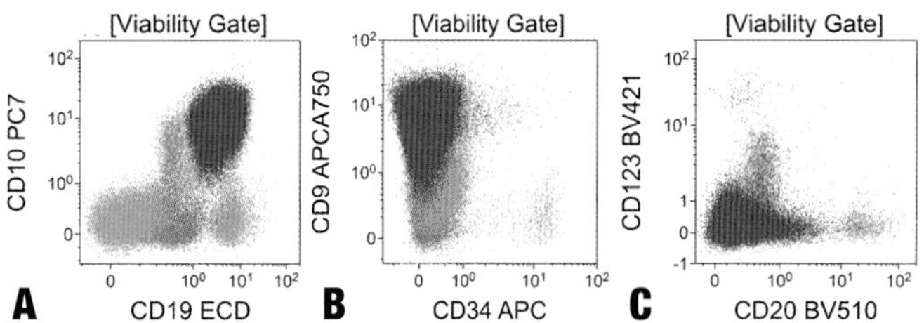

Fig. 4.44 B-lymphoblastic leukaemia/lymphoma (B-ALL/LBL) with *TCF3::PBX1* fusion. Flow cytometry dot plots. B-ALL/LBL tumour cells (in red) show moderate CD19 and moderate CD10 expression (**A**), moderate CD9 but negative CD34 expression (**B**), and negative CD123 and negative CD20 expression (**C**).

suggesting that like *ETV6::RUNX1*, *TCF3::PBX1* is an early lesion necessary but not sufficient for leukaemogenesis. The *TCF3::PBX1* fusion results in the production of a fusion protein that has an oncogenic role as a transcriptional activator; it also probably interferes with the normal function of the transcription factors encoded by *TCF3* and *PBX1* {2246}. Gene expression profiling studies have identified a signature unique to this lesion {4495}, and *PHF6* mutations have been described {4116}. Downstream WNT signalling and PI3K abnormalities have been implicated in pathogenesis {1059,1901}.

Macroscopic appearance

Not relevant

Histopathology

There are no unique morphological features.

Immunophenotype

The abnormal B lymphoblasts show strong CD9 expression, dim to negative CD34 expression, and at least partial absence of CD20, in addition to CD19 and CD10 expression {418,1033}. Cytoplasmic mu heavy chain expression is frequently present but not entirely specific for this entity {1033}.

Cytology

No unique features

Diagnostic molecular pathology

The *TCF3::PBX1* fusion is detectable by karyotype, FISH, and molecular methods {238,468}. The functional fusion gene resides on chromosome 19, and there may be loss of the derivative chromosome 1 in a majority of cases, resulting in an unbalanced translocation on karyotype analysis. Molecular methods may help identify cryptic translocations {3550} as well as alternate fusion partners {3494}.

Importantly, B-ALL/LBL with *TCF3* partners other than *PBX1* are not included in this entity. *TCF3* break-apart FISH is not sufficient, as this will not distinguish between *TCF3::PBX1* and *TCF3::HLF*. B-ALL/LBL with *TCF3::HLF* rearrangement carries a poor prognosis and is classified separately. In addition, cases of B-ALL/LBL, commonly with hyperdiploidy, have a karyotypically identical t(1;19) that involves neither *TCF3* nor *PBX1* and should not be classified as B-ALL/LBL with *TCF3::PBX1* fusion.

Essential and desirable diagnostic criteria

Essential: meets the diagnostic criteria for B-ALL/LBL (see *B-lymphoblastic leukaemia/lymphoma*, p. 330); demonstration of *TCF3::PBX1* rearrangement.

Staging

Not relevant

Prognosis and prediction

With modern intensive therapy, B-ALL/LBL with *TCF3::PBX1* fusion is associated with intermediate to relatively favourable clinical outcomes {496,1158,2352,4499,4315,3102,1794,4579, 3401}. However, there may be an increased relative risk of CNS relapse in these patients {1795}. Relapsed patients appear to have a dismal prognosis.

B-lymphoblastic leukaemia/lymphoma with IGH::*IL3* fusion

Leventaki V
Cassaday RD
Harris MH
Ketterling RP
Weinstock DM

Definition

B-lymphoblastic leukaemia/lymphoma (B-ALL/LBL) with IGH::*IL3* fusion is a neoplasm of lymphoblasts of B lineage defined by the juxtaposition of the IGH enhancer and the *IL3* promoter, with characteristic peripheral blood and bone marrow eosinophilia.

ICD-O coding

9817/3 B-lymphoblastic leukaemia/lymphoma with IGH::*IL3* fusion

ICD-11 coding

2A70.Y & XH4ZL2 Other B-lymphoblastic leukaemia/lymphoma with recurrent genetic abnormalities & B-lymphoblastic leukaemia/lymphoma with t(5;14)(q31;q32); *IL3*-IGH

Related terminology

None

Subtype(s)

None

Localization

B-ALL and B-LBL represent the same disease. B-ALL with IGH::*IL3* fusion always involves the bone marrow and usually also involves the peripheral blood. Extramedullary involvement is common and is by definition the primary site of involvement in B-LBL. For details, see *B-lymphoblastic leukaemia/lymphoma* (p. 330). Eosinophilic infiltrates can involve solid organs, including the lungs, heart (Loeffler endocarditis), and CNS, even without infiltration by leukaemic blasts {397,2069,1224}.

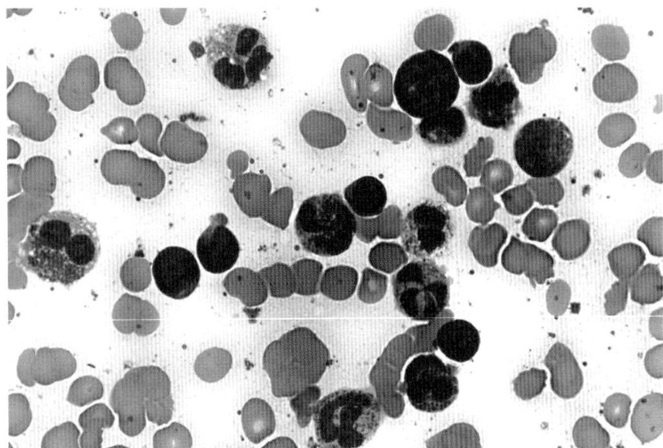

Fig. 4.45 B-lymphoblastic leukaemia/lymphoma with IGH::*IL3* fusion. Bone marrow aspirate with increased eosinophils and eosinophilic precursors and a smaller population of lymphoblasts.

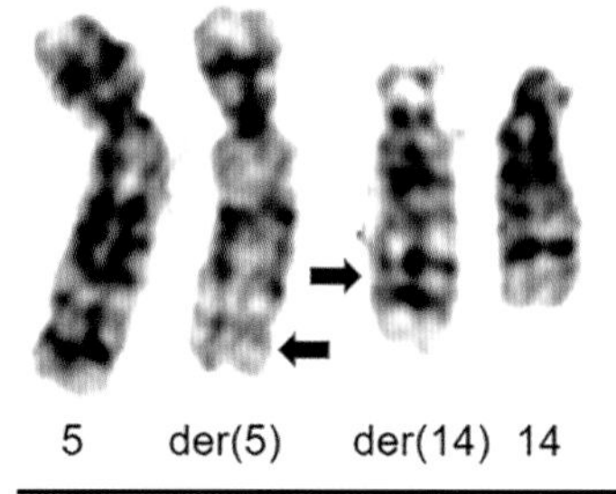

Fig. 4.46 B-lymphoblastic leukaemia/lymphoma with IGH::*IL3* fusion. A partial karyotype showing t(5;14)(q31.1;q32) (arrows).

Clinical features

The clinical presentation can be quite variable, including a typical presentation of B-ALL/LBL with increased blasts; asymptomatic eosinophilia with low or absent peripheral blood blasts; or clinical manifestations of hypereosinophilic syndrome with organomegaly, dyspnoea, skin involvement, neurological symptoms, thromboembolic events, and eosinophilic cardiomyopathy {4044,1224,4029}.

Epidemiology

This is a very rare type (< 1%) of B-ALL/LBL, with only case reports or small case series described in the literature. Most reported cases are in children and young adults (median age: 14.3 years), with a male predominance {1224}.

Etiology

Unknown

Pathogenesis

The IGH::*IL3* fusion is most commonly due to a balanced t(5;14)(q31.1;q32) that joins the IGH enhancer (14q32) to the *IL3* gene promoter (5q31.1) {2627,1418}. This results in IL-3 overexpression that drives the leukaemic clone in an autocrine manner and induces eosinophil maturation in the bone marrow and reactive eosinophilia in the peripheral blood {2064,2069}.

Macroscopic appearance

Not relevant

Histopathology

The bone marrow may show partial infiltration by lymphoblasts in a background of increased eosinophils. Peripheral blood blasts may be low, with a normal or slightly decreased haemoglobin and platelet count {1224,4521}.

Immunophenotype

The lymphoblasts show typical expression of CD19 and CD10. A subset of cases shows expression of myeloid markers, CD33 and/or CD13 {1348,1224}. Both lymphoblasts and eosinophils express the IL-3 receptor, CD123 {2069}.

Cytology

Peripheral blood and bone marrow aspirate smears commonly show increased eosinophils and variable numbers of lymphoblasts.

Diagnostic molecular pathology

The t(5;14)(q31.1;q32) translocation can be detected by karyotyping or FISH, but detection can be challenging in cases with a low blast count or a cytogenetically cryptic rearrangement. FISH for IGH rearrangement can be applied, but it is not diagnostic. Next-generation sequencing assays may identify IGH::*IL3* fusion with greater sensitivity {1435,1224}.

Essential and desirable diagnostic criteria

Essential: meets the diagnostic criteria for B-ALL/LBL (see *B-lymphoblastic leukaemia/lymphoma*, p. 330); demonstration of IGH::*IL3* fusion.

Staging

Not relevant

Prognosis and prediction

There are too few cases to be certain about the prognosis. A small case series suggested an intermediate prognosis, with a poor response to treatment and high levels of measurable residual disease at the end of induction {1224}. Blast percentage at diagnosis is not considered to be a prognostic factor. An increase in eosinophils during and after treatment may suggest relapsed disease.

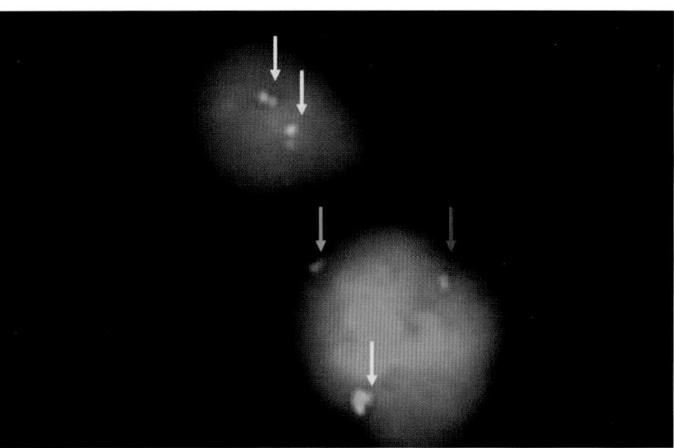

Fig. 4.47 B-lymphoblastic leukaemia/lymphoma with IGH::*IL3* fusion. Dual-colour FISH. Representative interphase nucleus with abnormal IGH rearrangement signal pattern (one intact fusion signal [yellow arrow], and separated red and green signals indicating a disruption [red and green arrows]), using an IGH break-apart probe. A normal nucleus is also present with a normal IGH signal pattern (two intact IGH fusion signals [yellow arrows]).

Chapter 4

B-lymphoblastic leukaemia/lymphoma with *TCF3::HLF* fusion

Harris MH
Buldini B
Cazzaniga G
Kovach AE
Locatelli F
Rabin KR

Definition

B-lymphoblastic leukaemia/lymphoma (B-ALL/LBL) with *TCF3::HLF* fusion is a neoplasm of lymphoblasts of B-cell lineage defined by the presence of rearrangement between *TCF3* at 19p13.3 and *HLF* at 17q22.

ICD-O coding

9818/3 B-lymphoblastic leukaemia/lymphoma with *TCF3::HLF* fusion

ICD-11 coding

2A70.Y Other B-lymphoblastic leukaemia/lymphoma with recurrent genetic abnormalities

Related terminology

Not recommended: B-lymphoblastic leukaemia/lymphoma with *E2A::HLF* fusion.

Subtype(s)

B-ALL/LBL with *TCF3::HLF* has a distinct transcriptional profile. Rare cases of B-ALL/LBL with *TCF4::HLF* cluster with B-ALL/LBL with *TCF3::HLF* {2301,1433}.

Localization

B-ALL and B-LBL represent the same disease. B-ALL always involves the bone marrow and usually also involves the peripheral blood. Extramedullary involvement is common and is by definition the primary site of involvement in B-LBL. For details, see *B-lymphoblastic leukaemia/lymphoma* (p. 330).

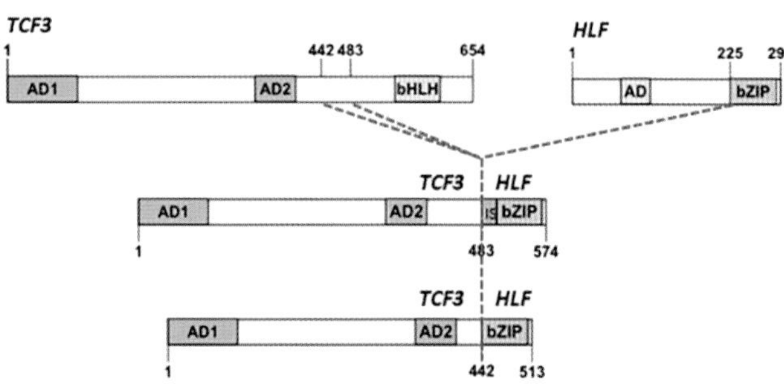

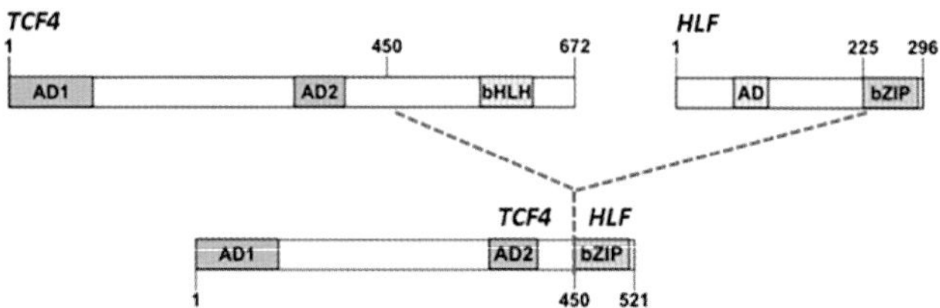

Fig. 4.48 B-lymphoblastic leukaemia with *TCF3::HLF* rearrangement. Schematic illustration of *TCF3::HLF* and *TCF4::HLF* fusion, and their functional domains and breakpoints. The dotted red lines indicates the breakpoint, and the numbers denote amino acids {1684,2246,1196,2301}. AD, activation domain; bHLH, basic helix-loop-helix domain; IS, intronic sequence.

Clinical features

Patients often present with hypercalcaemia and coagulopathy {1728}. PTHrP plays a major role in the development of hypercalcaemia, resulting in impairment of renal function {1728}.

Epidemiology

B-ALL/LBL with *TCF3::HLF* fusion is rare across age groups (< 1% of childhood B-ALL cases) {1433}. Most reported cases have been in children; rare cases have been described in adults {3940,3102}.

Etiology

Unknown

Pathogenesis

The *TCF3::HLF* fusion couples the transactivation domains (TADs) of *TCF3* fused to the DNA-binding and dimerization domains of *HLF*. Expression of *TCF3::HLF* leads to transcriptional reprogramming towards an immature state. Accompanying genetic lesions, including deletion of B-cell differentiation genes (*PAX5*, *VPREB1*, or *BTG1*), deletions of *CDKN2A/B*, and mutations in signalling pathways driving proliferation, are frequently observed {1196}.

Macroscopic appearance

Not relevant

Histopathology

There are no unique morphological features.

Immunophenotype

CD19 expression is typically high {2817}, but this feature is not specific.

Cytology

Not relevant

Diagnostic molecular pathology

Karyotype, FISH, and molecular methods are useful in establishing the diagnosis. *TCF3* break-apart FISH is not sufficient, because it cannot distinguish between *TCF3::HLF* and *TCF3::PBX1*. RT-PCR requires multiple primers to cover alternative fusion variants {1684,3123,2270}. Next-generation sequencing of RNA, either of targeted panels or of the whole transcriptome, can identify all transcript variants.

Essential and desirable diagnostic criteria

Essential: meets the diagnostic criteria for B-ALL/LBL (see *B-lymphoblastic leukaemia/lymphoma*, p. 330); demonstration of *TCF3::HLF* fusion.

Staging

Not relevant

Prognosis and prediction

B-ALL/LBL with *TCF3::HLF* fusion is characterized by dismal outcomes and until recently was considered incurable despite treatment intensification and allogeneic haematopoietic stem cell transplantation {1196}. Relapse usually occurs early. In view of the high and homogeneous expression of CD19 on blasts of this leukaemia subtype, these patients may benefit from CD19-directed immunotherapy, including bispecific T-cell engager (BiTE) molecules and chimeric antigen receptor (CAR) T cells {2817,2394}. The BCL2 inhibitor venetoclax has shown promising results in preclinical models {1196,1236}.

B-lymphoblastic leukaemia/lymphoma with other defined genetic alterations

Choi JK
Fisher KE
Greipp PT
Hodge JC
Hunger SP
Mejstrikova E
Yasuda T

Definition

B-lymphoblastic leukaemia/lymphoma (B-ALL/LBL) with other defined genetic abnormalities includes neoplasms of lymphoblasts of B-cell lineage defined by the presence of specific newly described or uncommon genetic drivers.

ICD-O coding

9811/3 B-lymphoblastic leukaemia/lymphoma with other defined genetic alterations
9811/3 B-lymphoblastic leukaemia with *DUX4* rearrangement
9811/3 B-lymphoblastic leukaemia with *MEF2D* rearrangement
9811/3 B-lymphoblastic leukaemia with *ZNF384* rearrangement
9811/3 B-lymphoblastic leukaemia with *PAX5*alt
9811/3 B-lymphoblastic leukaemia with *PAX5* p.P80R
9811/3 B-lymphoblastic leukaemia with *NUTM1* rearrangement
9811/3 B-lymphoblastic leukaemia with *MYC* rearrangement

ICD-11 coding

2A70.Y Other B-lymphoblastic leukaemia/lymphoma with recurrent genetic abnormalities

Related terminology

Acceptable: B-cell lymphoblastic leukaemia/lymphoma NOS.
Not recommended: precursor B-lymphoblastic leukaemia/lymphoma; B-cell acute lymphoid leukaemia; B-lymphoblastic lymphoma.

Subtype(s)

B-lymphoblastic leukaemia with *DUX4* rearrangement; B-lymphoblastic leukaemia with *MEF2D* rearrangement; B-lymphoblastic leukaemia with *ZNF384* rearrangement; B-lymphoblastic leukaemia with *PAX5*^{alt}; B-lymphoblastic leukaemia with *PAX5* p.P80R; B-lymphoblastic leukaemia with *NUTM1* rearrangement; B-lymphoblastic leukaemia with *MYC* rearrangement

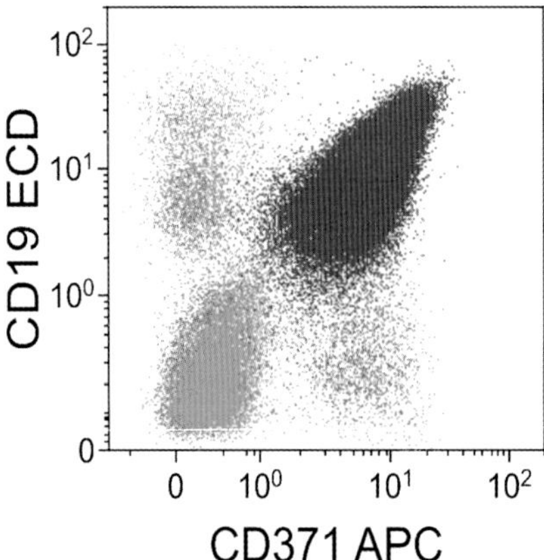

Fig. 4.49 B-lymphoblastic leukaemia/lymphoma with other defined genetic alterations. Flow cytometric scatterplot of B-lymphoblastic leukaemia with *DUX4* rearrangement. CD371 is expressed by leukaemic blasts (red) and normal granulocytes (brown), but not normal B cells or mature lymphocytes (blue).

Localization

B-ALL and B-LBL represent the same disease. B-ALL always involves the bone marrow and usually also involves the peripheral blood. Extramedullary involvement is common and is by definition the primary site of involvement in B-LBL. For details, see *B-lymphoblastic leukaemia/lymphoma* (p. 330).

Clinical features

The presenting features are similar to those seen in other B-ALLs (see *B-lymphoblastic leukaemias/lymphomas: Introduction*, p. 328).

Epidemiology

These represent approximately 10–15% of paediatric B-ALL/LBL cases and 20–35% of adult B-ALL/LBL cases {3102,1794}; the individual subtypes are detailed in Table 4.12.

Etiology

Like for other types, the initiating causes of these B-ALL/LBLs are unknown. For some B-ALL/LBL with other defined genetic alterations, a genetic predisposition is suggestive. Susceptibility to B-ALL/LBL has been described in patients with germline variants in the haematopoietic transcription factor gene *PAX5* {3690,186,1026}.

Pathogenesis

The development of B-ALL/LBL, like other cancers, occurs secondary to cumulative disruptions of key cell regulatory pathways {1485,437,1662}. In particular, most dysregulations involve genes for self-renewal, cell proliferation, apoptosis, differentiation, or their signalling pathways {2406,4595,2714,1501,2501}.

DUX4 activates the cleavage-specific transcriptional programme during embryogenesis, but it is normally repressed in adult tissue except for testis {1552}. *DUX4* rearrangement induces ectopic DUX4 expression in immature B cells and promotes leukaemogenesis in murine experimental models {4489}. DUX4 overexpression results in loss of function of ERG, either by depletion or induced expression of a novel isoform, showing the interplay between DUX4 and ERG deregulation in leukaemogenesis in this subtype {4559}.

MEF2D encodes a transcription factor expressed throughout B-cell differentiation and involved in early B-cell development {1553,1561}. Chimeric proteins created by *MEF2D* fusion genes gain aberrant function mediated by the MEF2D transcriptional activation domain and confer haematopoietic self-renewal {1432}. Mouse transplantation assays show that MEF2D fusion proteins have leukaemogenic activity in murine pro-B cells {4489}. MEF2D fusion proteins alter the transcription of downstream genes, resulting in upregulation of pre-B-cell receptor

Table 4.12 B-lymphoblastic leukaemia/lymphoma (B-ALL/LBL) with other defined genetic alterations: clinical and immunophenotypic features

Subtype: B-ALL/LBL with...	Frequency at different ages			Prognosis[a], children	Prognosis[a], adults	Immunophenotype
	≤ 15 years	16–39 years	≥ 40 years			
DUX4 **rearrangement** {4489,2342,4559,3014,3613}	4–5%	8%	3%	Good, high early MRD	Good	CD2+ (70%), CD13++, CD34++, CD38++, CD371+
MEF2D **rearrangement** {3013}	1–4%	3%	1%	Intermediate to poor	Intermediate to poor	CD10−, CD5, CD38+, cMu+
ZNF384 **rearrangement** {1589,1590}	1–4%	4%	3%	Intermediate; dependent on partner	Intermediate	CD10− (73%), CD13+, CD33+, CD65−, CD15−, CD25+ (25%), myeloperoxidase− (+ in MPAL)
PAX5 **alteration** {3690}	3–9%	9%	3%	Intermediate	Poor	No association reported
PAX5 **p.P80R** {3690}	1–2%	3%	4%	Intermediate	Good	CD2+, CD33+, CD65−, CD15−
NUTM1 **rearrangement** {3613,1629,387}	1–2%; 3–5% in infants	0%	0%	Good to intermediate	Not applicable	No association reported
MYC **rearrangement**[b] {2925,3844}	< 1%	1–2%	2–3%	Intermediate	Poor	No association reported

MPAL, mixed-phenotype acute leukaemia; MRD, measurable residual disease.
[a]The designations of poor, intermediate, and good are relative measures within each age group; for example, for B-ALL/LBL with *DUX4* rearrangement, the "good" prognosis reflects a 5-year event-free survival rate of 95% in children but only 80% in adults. Children ≤ 15 years, adolescents and young adults 16–39 years, adults ≥ 40 years. [b]B-ALL/LBL with *MYC* rearrangement in children is treated as Burkitt lymphoma at many institutions. In adults, diffuse large B-cell lymphoma / high-grade B-cell lymphoma with *MYC* and *BCL2* rearrangements needs to be excluded.
Additional references, pertaining to multiple subtypes: {4116,3102,1794,1700,4116,1433,2388}.

components that contributes to B-cell proliferation and survival {3518,4563}.

ZNF384 (*CIZ*) at 12p13.31 encodes a zinc finger transcription factor important for regulation of extracellular matrix genes {2882}. *ZNF384* rearrangements are understood to occur in a subset of haematopoietic stem cells {67,484}. More than 10 *ZNF384* translocation partners exist, including *EP300*, *TCF3*, *CREBBP*, *SMARCA2*, *TAF15*, and *ARID1B* {1433,2301,4532,1589,3687}. These cryptic translocations that fuse the *ZNF384* coding region in-frame to the partner gene forming the 3′ part of the fusion gene {4533} can be observed in both B-ALL and B/myeloid mixed-phenotype acute leukaemia with the same transcriptional profile, and both leukaemias demonstrate lineage plasticity at diagnosis and relapse {67}.

PAX5 encodes a transcription factor that regulates numerous signalling, adhesion, migration, differentiation, and proliferation genes important for normal B-cell development {3608,3800}. *PAX5* mutations are frequently detected in the *TCF3::PBX1*, *BCR::ABL1*, and *BCR::ABL1*-like subtypes {3051,1127} and can be seen rarely in mature B-cell lymphomas {3283}. Current models propose that *PAX5* functions overall as a tumour suppressor gene and that its mutations, including p.P80R, reduce or abolish its normal function, thereby promoting B-cell leukaemogenesis {3690,1433}. The *PAX5*[alt] subtype accounts for about 7.5% of B-ALL cases and differs from B-ALL with *PAX5* p.P80R in its expression profile, immunophenotype, and prognosis in adults {1433,3102}. Most of the *PAX5*[alt] leukaemias have a diverse variety of *PAX5* alterations, including rearrangements, point mutations other than p.P80R, and intragenic amplifications {1433}. More than two dozen translocation partner genes have been reported, all of which create in-frame fusion proteins, with *PAX5::ETV6* being the most common. *PAX5* p.P80R mutations impair B-lymphoid development, and B-cell leukaemogenesis occurs when a second *PAX5* alteration is acquired {3690,1433}. Mutations of the second *PAX5* allele, via loss of heterozygosity or an additional *PAX5* mutation, are present in nearly all cases {1700}. Signalling pathway mutations (RAS and JAK/STAT pathway genes, *FLT3*, *BRAF*, and *PIK3CA*) are present in almost all *PAX5* p.P80R cases {1433}.

NUTM1 normally functions as a chromatin modifier by increasing histone acetylation in postmeiotic spermatogenic cells {3730}. *NUTM1* rearrangements occur in as many as one third of infant B-ALL cases that have germline *KMT2A* variants, and are associated with a favourable prognosis {1148}. The majority of the *NUTM1* coding sequence fuses in-frame to the 5′ portion of multiple different transcription factor or epigenetic regulator partner genes including *ACIN1*, *AFF1*, *ATAD5*, *BRD9*, *CHD4*, *CUX1*, *IKZF1*, *RUNX1*, *SLC12A6*, and *ZNF618* {117,1432,2301,1433,1629,4116,1148,1794,387}. These fusions result in aberrant NUTM1 overexpression that may potentially alter global chromatin acetylation {1629,2301}, conferring sensitivity to histone deacetylase inhibitors, and possibly to bromodomain inhibitors in *NUTM1::BRD9* fusion cases.

MYC encodes a transcription factor that regulates many genes important for proliferation, differentiation, apoptosis, and immune regulation in many cell types {48}. *MYC* is overexpressed or dysregulated in > 70% of human cancers and is actively studied as a target of precision therapy {3799,2468}. Within B-cell neoplasms, *MYC* overexpression, because of its translocation to the IGH, IGK, and IGL loci, occurs in Burkitt lymphoma, diffuse large B-cell lymphoma, and plasmablastic lymphoma {3906}. IGH::*MYC*, IGK::*MYC*, or IGL::*MYC* is detected in 0.1% and 4.3% of paediatric and adult B-ALL, respectively {2925,3102}.

Macroscopic appearance

Not relevant

Histopathology

There are no unique morphological features.

Immunophenotype

DUX4 rearrangement

Expression of CD371 is seen in almost all cases and CD2 in a major subset {3014,3613}. Monocytic differentiation with expression of CD14, gain of CD45 and CD33, and loss of B-cell antigens is often seen early after induction therapy but may also be present at diagnosis.

ZNF384 rearrangement

Concurrent monocytic differentiation may be seen at diagnosis or early after induction therapy, and the distinction between B-ALL and mixed-phenotype acute leukaemia for this entity is unclear {67,4533}. It may be reasonable to consider cases where monocytic differentiation is seen on < 5% of the leukaemic cell population as B-ALL until more data emerge. See also *Acute leukaemia of ambiguous lineage with other defined genetic alterations* (p. 210).

Cytology

There are no unique cytological features.

Diagnostic molecular pathology

These subtypes are defined by their genetic abnormalities as detected by genomic sequencing (DNA or RNA) and/or expression profiling (see the sections on individual subtypes, and Table 4.13). Many cases have additional mutations, but these do not alter the subclassification or diagnosis. Criteria for definitive B-ALL types must not be met, because these frequently have similar mutations {1127,4116}.

DUX4 rearrangement

Next-generation sequencing (RNA and/or DNA) is needed to detect *DUX4* rearrangement, mostly with IGH or *ERG* {4559, 4489,2342}. Detection of *DUX4* rearrangement by conventional cytogenetic approaches is challenging because of the repetitive nature of *DUX4* and the insertion of *DUX4* into the IGH locus {4559}.

MEF2D rearrangement

RNA sequencing or RT-PCR is needed to detect the various *MEF2D* rearrangements, mostly with *BCL9* or *HNRNPUL1* {4489,1432}. These rearrangements are often cryptic on conventional karyotype analysis {1432}.

ZNF384 rearrangement

Break-apart FISH or next-generation sequencing (RNA and/or DNA) is necessary to detect the classically cryptic *ZNF384* translocations {3687,1590}.

PAX5 p.P80R and PAX5^{alt}

Next-generation sequencing (RNA and/or DNA) is needed to detect the various *PAX5* mutations, consisting of sequence mutations, intragenic amplifications, and rearrangement with > 20 different partners {1433,4116}.

B-ALL with *PAX5* p.P80R is defined by acquired *PAX5* (NM_016734.3) missense mutations that result in a proline-to-arginine replacement at amino acid 80 (p.P80R) within the *PAX5* DNA-binding domain (DBD). Detection of *PAX5* p.P80R requires DNA sequencing methods. Structural rearrangements of chromosome arm 9p and/or 7p, as well as secondary mutations in signalling pathway genes (Table 4.13), are often observed {3153,1433}. *PAX5* p.P80R mutations appear mutually exclusive and are not reported in other B-ALL subtypes {4532}. Other *PAX5* alterations, including gene rearrangements, non-p.P80R sequence mutations, or focal intragenic amplifications, should be classified as B-ALL/LBL with *PAX5*^{alt}, with the exception of *PAX5::JAK2* (Philadelphia [Ph] chromosome–like B-ALL) and *PAX5::ZCCHC7*, which occurs in cases with other class-defining alterations {1433}.

NUTM1 rearrangement

Although karyotype analysis can identify a subset of *NUTM1* rearrangements with aberrations at 15q14, the exact band is often difficult to discern {117,387} and requires break-apart FISH with a *NUTM1* probe or RNA and/or DNA sequencing {1629, 1794,387}. Of note, *NUTM1* break-apart FISH was negative in a *SLC12A6::NUTM1* fusion case, probably because of a small inversion limiting signal separation {1629}.

MYC rearrangement

Karyotype or FISH analysis can detect IGH::*MYC*, IGK::*MYC*, or IGL::*MYC*. Gene expression profiling of this B-ALL/LBL type

Table 4.13 B-lymphoblastic leukaemia/lymphoma (B-ALL/LBL) with other defined genetic alterations: genetics

Subtype: B-ALL/LBL with...	Diagnostic genetics	Gene function	Additional mutations	References
DUX4 **rearrangement**	*DUX4* rearrangement, overexpression, gene expression profile	Transcription factor	*ERG, IKZF1, KMT2D, TP53, ZEB2, TBL1XR1*	{3102,1794}
MEF2D **rearrangement**	*MEF2D* rearrangement, gene expression profile	Transcription factor	*PHF6, CDKN2A/B*	{3102,1794}
ZNF384 **rearrangement**	*ZNF384* rearrangement, gene expression profile	Transcription factor	*NRAS, KRAS, PTPN11, EZH2,* KMT2 (*MLL2*), *ASH1L*	{3102,1794}
PAX5 **alteration**	Expression profile cluster enriched with *PAX5* alterations	Transcription factor	*CDKN2A, RB1, BTG1, KDM6A, KMT2A, ATRX*	{1433,3102,1794}
PAX5 p.P80R	*PAX5* p.P80R, gene expression profile	Transcription factor	*NRAS, KRAS, IL7R, CDKN2A/B, IKZF1*	{3153,1433}
NUTM1 **rearrangement**	*NUTM1* rearrangement, expression profile	Histone acetylation	*TP53, KRAS, CREBBP, KMT2D, SETD1B*	{2301,1433,387}
MYC **rearrangement**	*MYC* rearrangement, expression profile	Transcription factor	*BCL2, BCL6, NRAS, KRAS*	{4265,1700}

is distinct from other B-ALL/LBL types {1433} and from Burkitt lymphoma {4265}.

Essential and desirable diagnostic criteria

Essential: meets the general criteria for B-ALL/LBL (see *B-lymphoblastic leukaemia/lymphoma*, p. 330); demonstration of a specific genetic abnormality as defined in this section; absence of genetic mutations of other B-ALL/LBL types.

Desirable: in B-ALL/LBL with *DUX4* rearrangement, increased *DUX4* gene expression and/or demonstration of CD371 expression; in adult B-ALL/LBL with *MYC* rearrangement, exclusion of diffuse large B-cell lymphoma / high-grade B-cell lymphoma with *MYC* and *BCL2* rearrangements.

Staging

Not relevant

Prognosis and prediction

As with other B-ALL/LBL types, the prognosis is influenced in part by the genetic mutations (see Table 4.12, p. 361), but other criteria such as age, white blood cell count, CNS status, early response to therapy, and additional mutations contribute. Of the types listed, *DUX4*-rearranged B-ALL/LBL has the best outcome, equating to a 5-year event-free survival rate of 95% in children versus 80% in adults {1433,3102,1794}, despite a poor measurable residual disease (MRD) response {2982, 2329}. The presence of *TP53* mutations in this subtype is associated with a poor prognosis {4116}. *MEF2D* rearrangement has an intermediate to poor outcome, with a 5-year overall survival rate of about 70% for children and about 30% for adults {1432, 3102}. Some cases with *DUX4* rearrangement, *PAX5* p.P80R, and *ZNF384* rearrangement may switch to monocytic lineage during therapy {2982}. In adults, *MYC*-rearranged B-ALL/LBL has an inferior outcome, with a 5-year overall survival rate of < 20% for adults {3844,3102}; it has been suggested that Burkitt lymphoma therapy may improve outcome {2325}. In children, *MYC*-rearranged B-ALL/LBL is usually treated with Burkitt lymphoma therapy and has a better outcome than the adult counterpart {2925,2675,4554}. The prognosis is likely to continue to change as new therapies are introduced and treatments are altered based on minimal/measurable residual disease detection {4002}.

B-lymphoblastic leukaemia/lymphoma NOS

Choi JK
Cassaday RD
Chandy M
Harrison CJ
Kovach AE
Leventaki V
Nardi V
Saha V
Tembhare PR

Definition

B-lymphoblastic leukaemia/lymphoma (B-ALL/LBL) NOS is a neoplasm of lymphoblasts of B-cell lineage that includes B-ALL/LBL cases that do not meet the criteria for any B-ALL/LBL types that are defined by defined genetic abnormalities.

ICD-O coding

9811/3 B-lymphoblastic leukaemia/lymphoma, NOS

ICD-11 coding

2A70.0 B-lymphoblastic leukaemia or lymphoma, not elsewhere classified

Related terminology

Acceptable: B-cell lymphoblastic leukaemia/lymphoma NOS; pro-B lymphoblastic leukaemia; pre-B-lymphoblastic leukaemia; pro-/pre-B-lymphoblastic leukaemia; B-cell acute lymphoblastic leukaemia.

Not recommended: precursor B-lymphoblastic leukaemia/lymphoma; B-cell acute lymphoid leukaemia; B-lymphoblastic lymphoma; common precursor B-lymphoblastic leukaemia/lymphoma; common lymphoblastic leukaemia.

Subtype(s)

None

Localization

B-ALL and B-LBL represent the same disease. B-ALL always involves the bone marrow and usually also involves the peripheral blood. Extramedullary involvement is common and is by definition the primary site of involvement in B-LBL. For details, see *B-lymphoblastic leukaemia/lymphoma* (p. 330).

Clinical features

No unique features

Epidemiology

Currently, B-ALL/LBL-NOS represents approximately 5–10% of all B-ALL/LBLs, excluding definitive and provisional entities {3102,1794,2301,1433}. This proportion will likely decrease with the identification of additional genetic drivers.

Etiology

Unknown

Pathogenesis

B-ALL/LBL development probably involves cumulative dysregulations of key regulatory pathways of self-renewal, cell proliferation, apoptosis, differentiation, and/or their signalling pathways, many of which are in common among all B-ALL/LBL subtypes, including B-ALL/LBL-NOS {4595,2406,2714,1501,2501}.

Macroscopic appearance

Not relevant

Histopathology

No unique features

Cytology

No unique features

Diagnostic molecular pathology

Other definitive and provisional subtypes must be excluded through cytogenetic analysis (karyotype, FISH, chromosomal microarray), genetic sequencing (RNA, DNA), and/or gene expression profiling. Molecular profiling has identified rare but recurrent genetic alterations in cases currently classified as B-ALL/LBL-NOS {3102,2301,1433}.

Essential and desirable diagnostic criteria

Essential: meets the diagnostic criteria for B-ALL/LBL (see *B-lymphoblastic leukaemia/lymphoma*, p. 330); does not meet criteria for any defined B-ALL/LBL types after comprehensive testing.

Staging

No unique features

Prognosis and prediction

In children, the prognosis of this group is intermediate, with a 5-year event-free survival rate of 86%, and probably encompasses B-ALLs with heterogeneous clinical behaviour {1794}.

Preneoplastic and neoplastic small lymphocytic proliferations: Introduction

Naresh KN

The following sections cover chronic lymphocytic leukaemia / small lymphocytic lymphoma (CLL/SLL) and the broad group monoclonal B-cell lymphocytosis (MBL). The diagnosis of MBL (and its distinction from CLL/SLL) requires documentation of < 5 × 10^9/L peripheral blood B cells in the absence of lymphadenopathy, organomegaly, and any feature diagnostic of another B-cell lymphoproliferative disorder or a lymphoma. MBL is further subtyped as low-count MBL or clonal B-cell expansion when the clonal B-cell count is < 0.5 × 10^9/L and the B cells have a CLL/SLL phenotype; CLL/SLL-type MBL when the clonal B-cell count is ≥ 0.5 × 10^9/L, the total B-cell count is < 5 × 10^9/L, and the B cells have a CLL/SLL phenotype; and non–CLL/SLL-type MBL when the phenotype of the clonal B cells is not that of CLL/SLL. Most cases of non–CLL/SLL-type MBL have phenotypic features akin to marginal zone B cells {3694,3380,4448}. A tissue equivalent of CLL/SLL-type MBL is also recognizable in normal-sized lymph nodes with preserved architecture. Approximately 0.5–2% of individuals with CLL/SLL-type MBL progress to CLL/SLL each year.

A diagnosis of CLL/SLL can be made on a peripheral blood sample or on a biopsy of a lymph node or other tissues. Cytomorphological and immunophenotypic features are characteristic. Investigating patients for appropriate prognostic/predictive genomic biomarkers plays a major role in disease management. An accelerated form of CLL/SLL is recognized. In the peripheral blood, the accelerated form is recognized by the presence of > 15% prolymphocytes among all lymphocytes, and the disease is termed prolymphocytic progression; the presence of *TP53* alteration should be considered and a blastoid variant of mantle cell lymphoma excluded {1471,1083}. In lymph nodes and other tissues, the accelerated form is recognized by very large, prominent/confluent proliferation centres (broader than a 20× field) or high proliferation indexes (> 2.4 mitoses per proliferation centre or > 40% Ki-67+ cells in proliferation centres) and is termed histologically aggressive CLL/SLL; this should be distinguished from Richter transformation (RT) {1345}. RT can be clonally related or unrelated. Clonally unrelated RT has a favourable prognosis and is managed differently from clonally related RT. Comparative IG rearrangement studies on CLL/SLL-phase and RT samples are therefore recommended {2052, 790A,1102}.

Monoclonal B-cell lymphocytosis

Rawstron AC
Eichhorst B
Rai K
Rosenquist R
Rossi D
Shanafelt TD
Stamatopoulos KE
Stilgenbauer S
Wu CJ

Definition

Monoclonal B-cell lymphocytosis (MBL) is an asymptomatic condition characterized by the presence of a monoclonal B-cell population in the absence of lymphadenopathy, organomegaly, and any features diagnostic of another B-cell lymphoproliferative disorder (B-LPD).

ICD-O coding

9823/1 Monoclonal B-cell lymphocytosis, chronic lymphocytic leukaemia type

9591/1 Monoclonal B-cell lymphocytosis, non–chronic lymphocytic leukaemia type

ICD-11 coding

4B0Y & XH73D5 Other specified immune system disorders involving white cell lineages & Monoclonal B-cell lymphocytosis, NOS

4B0Y & XH5M35 Other specified immune system disorders involving white cell lineages & Monoclonal B-cell lymphocytosis, non-CLL type

Related terminology

None

Subtype(s)

MBL, chronic lymphocytic leukaemia / small lymphocytic lymphoma (CLL/SLL) type; MBL, low count or clonal B-cell expansion (CLL/SLL type); MBL, non-CLL/SLL type

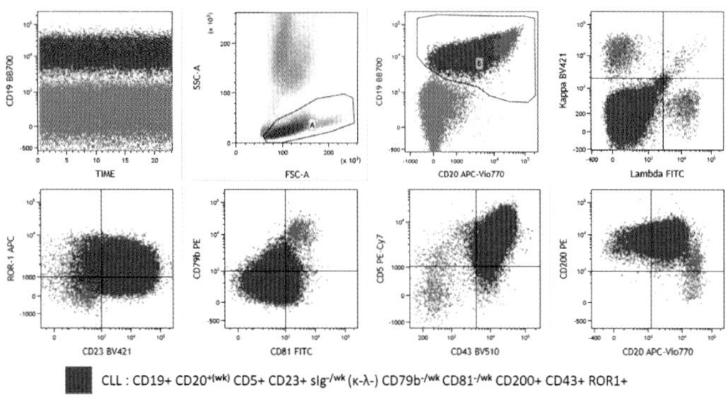

Fig. 4.50 Monoclonal B-cell lymphocytosis (MBL). Peripheral blood sample from an 81-year-old man with an absolute lymphocyte count of 3.2 × 10^9/L, haemoglobin 157 g/L, platelet count 144, no palpable lymphadenopathy, and B cells 0.37 × 10^9/L: the chronic lymphocytic leukaemia / small lymphocytic lymphoma (CLL/SLL)-type MBL cells are coloured red, and normal polyclonal mature B cells are green; the CLL/SLL-type MBL cells are CD19+, CD20weak/+, light chain−/weak, CD5+, CD23+, CD200+, CD43+, CD79b−/weak, ROR1+, CD81−/weak, CD22+/weak, and CD25+.

Localization

MBL is present in the peripheral blood and may be detectable in bone marrow and secondary lymphoid tissue.

Clinical features

MBL is an asymptomatic condition and frequently found incidentally to other investigations. Symptoms of tiredness/fatigue, unplanned weight loss, night sweats, and an increased frequency of infections may be an initial reason for investigations. Their presence does not necessarily exclude a diagnosis of MBL if there are no other features of a haematological malignancy.

There is immune impairment to a varying degree in all subtypes of MBL, with suboptimal responses to vaccination and an increased risk of infection {2778,838,3693,4363,2827}.

Epidemiology

The incidence and prevalence of MBL vary according to the sensitivity of diagnostic tests applied. High-sensitivity flow cytometry assays can detect CLL/SLL-type clonal B-cell expansion in as many as 5% of people aged 40–50 years, 5–25% of people aged 65–80 years, and 50–75% of people aged > 90 years {3378,1331, 2960}. The reported incidence of CLL/SLL-type MBL may be up to half that of CLL/SLL, with a similar age distribution and a median age at diagnosis of 70–75 years {522,2203}. The geographical distribution of MBL appears to reflect the incidence of associated clinical disease types, with relatively low proportions of CLL/SLL-type monoclonal B-cell expansions reported in African, Eastern Mediterranean, and Western Pacific regions {75,3381,4451}.

Etiology

The etiology is unknown. Genetic predisposition to CLL/SLL and CLL/SLL-type MBL is evident from family studies, with multiple SNPs associated with an increased risk of developing both {845,2046}.

Pathogenesis

Highly similar stereotyped B-cell receptors are found in both CLL/SLL-type MBL and CLL/SLL but very rarely in low-count MBL, indicating that B-cell receptor signalling is likely to play a central role in the development of CLL/SLL-type MBL {4185,34}. Genomic aberrations and gene mutations prevalent in CLL/SLL can be found in CLL/SLL-type MBL, albeit at a lower frequency {3377,1147,2773,249,36}. Similarly, abnormalities central to post-germinal-centre B-LPD, such as *MYD88* mutations, are common in non–CLL/SLL-type MBL {1855}.

Macroscopic appearance

Not relevant

Histopathology

The cytomorphology of MBL is typically similar to that of CLL/SLL for CLL/SLL-type MBL, or centrocyte-like cells for non–CLL/

SLL-type MBL. Cells with irregular nuclei, nucleoli, and larger cells (other than lymphoplasmacytic forms) should not be evident.

Bone marrow and lymph node investigations are not indicated for MBL. However, if a biopsy is taken for other reasons, then an infiltrate corresponding to MBL is likely to be detectable. By definition, lymph nodes are < 15 mm with preserved architecture and residual normal follicles. The CLL/SLL-type infiltrate can form diffuse, interfollicular, intrasinusoidal, perifollicular, or follicular-colonizing patterns, but proliferation centres are absent. The focal abnormal B-cell infiltrates are highlighted with CD5 expression and confirmed by other immunophenotypic features of CLL/SLL {742,1540,1340,1461}. Lymph node appearance in non–CLL/SLL-type MBL is not well characterized. In the bone marrow, lymphoid cells with a CLL/SLL phenotype may be visible as focal or interstitial aggregates {3365} and represent a median 20% of bone marrow cells (with a large range, reportedly to as high as 65%) {3479}. Patients with MBL typically have bone marrow involvement of < 30%, but even in cases with bone marrow involvement of > 30%, a primary diagnosis of CLL/SLL is not fulfilled unless peripheral blood B cell counts are ≥ 5 × 10^9/L or there is presence of lymph node enlargement {1472}.

Flow cytometry

B-cell clonality is defined by an immunoglobulin light chain kappa-to-lambda ratio of > 3:1 or < 0.3:1, or by > 25% of mature B cells lacking surface immunoglobulin {2543}. The CLL/SLL phenotype is defined as coexpression of CD5 and CD23 on > 20% of the clonal CD19+ B cells, with weak expression of CD20 and immunoglobulin light chain (with "weak" defined as a median fluorescence intensity at least 20% lower than the median expression level by normal CD20+ peripheral blood B cells stained under the same conditions) and no CD10 expression. In addition, CD43, CD200, and ROR1 would typically be expressed on > 20% of clonal B cells, with weak or absent CD79b and CD81 coexpression {3379}. The immunophenotype of the abnormal B cells in non–CLL/SLL-type MBL is similar to that in marginal zone lymphoma or lymphoplasmacytic lymphoma, and the abnormal B cells are admixed with normal B cells. The abnormal B cells negative for CD5 and CD10 are usually identified by the different intensity in the expression of B-cell markers or light chains.

Differential diagnosis

The main differential diagnosis is with CLL/SLL. The presence of monoclonal B cells without a CLL/SLL immunophenotype in the peripheral blood should trigger comprehensive clinical, imaging, and pathological lymphoma investigations.

The three subtypes are defined:

Low-count MBL or clonal B-cell expansion: Clonal CLL/SLL-phenotype B-cell count < 0.5 × 10^9/L with no other features diagnostic of B-LPD. The arbitrary threshold is based on the distribution of clonal B-cell counts in population studies compared with clinical cohorts {3380}.

CLL/SLL-type MBL: Monoclonal CLL/SLL-phenotype cell count ≥ 0.5 × 10^9/L and total B-cell count < 5 × 10^9/L with no other features diagnostic of CLL/SLL {2543}. The threshold of < 5 × 10^9/L is arbitrary but identifies a group with a very low likelihood of requiring treatment compared with individuals with B-cell counts of 5–10 × 10^9/L {3694}.

Non–CLL/SLL-type MBL: Any monoclonal non–CLL/SLL-phenotype B-cell expansion with no symptoms or features diagnostic of another mature B-cell neoplasm. The majority of cases have features consistent with a marginal zone origin {4448}. Thresholds have yet to be formally defined.

Cytology

Not applicable

Diagnostic molecular pathology

There are no molecular abnormalities diagnostic of MBL. The spectrum of molecular abnormalities overlaps with related conditions, with 13q14 deletions being common in CLL/SLL-type MBL and *MYD88* mutation in non–CLL/SLL-type MBL. *TP53* mutation/deletion may be detectable in a small proportion of cases but does not necessarily confer an increased risk of progression {249,36,3377,2773,1147}.

Essential and desirable diagnostic criteria

Essential: demonstration of a monoclonal B-cell population (light chain restriction or lack of surface light chain expression by flow cytometry, or monoclonal IG gene rearrangement with a peripheral B-cell count of < 5 × 10^9/L); absence of lymphadenopathy, organomegaly, and any features diagnostic of another B-LPD; for low-count MBL / clonal B-cell expansion: clonal B-cell count < 0.5 × 10^9/L and typical CLL/SLL phenotype; for CLL/SLL-type MBL: clonal B-cell count ≥ 0.5 × 10^9/L and typical CLL/SLL phenotype; for non–CLL/SLL-type MBL: any clonal B-cell expansion without the typical CLL/SLL phenotype.

Desirable: expression patterns that would be atypical for CLL/SLL (e.g. strong CD20 / CD79b / CD81 / surface immunoglobulin, or weak/undetectable CD43/CD200/ROR1 expression) may also warrant further investigation to exclude other B-LPDs.

Staging

Not relevant

Prognosis and prediction

Progression to CLL/SLL occurs in approximately 0.5–2% of individuals with CLL/SLL-type MBL per year. The risk of progression to CLL/SLL is higher if the clonal B-cell count is > 3 × 10^9/L, but very low if it is < 1–1.5 × 10^9/L {3377,3694}. In addition to the absolute B-cell count, unmutated IGHV genes and serum B2M > 3.5 g/L are associated with more rapid time to first treatment and shorter overall survival {3377,3479,3136}. Low-count MBL / clonal B-cell expansion is associated with a negligible risk of developing CLL/SLL in general, but it can occur in familial CLL/SLL {838,3760}. If disease progression is suspected (e.g. there is new lymphadenopathy with stable clonal B-cell counts), a full evaluation is required in order to investigate the possibility of an unrelated lymphoma or other disease.

Chronic lymphocytic leukaemia / small lymphocytic lymphoma

Naresh KN
Akinola NO
Burger JA
Chiattone C
Chiorazzi N
Eichhorst B
Ferry JA
Geddie WR
Rai K
Rawstron AC
Rosenquist R
Rossi D
Slager SL
Stamatopoulos KE
Stilgenbauer S
Varghese AM
Wu CJ
Yang SM

Definition

Chronic lymphocytic leukaemia / small lymphocytic lymphoma (CLL/SLL) is a B-cell lymphoma comprising monomorphic small mature B cells that frequently coexpress CD5 and CD23. A peripheral blood diagnosis of chronic lymphocytic leukaemia (CLL) requires a B-cell count of ≥ 5 × 10^9/L, with the characteristic morphology and immunophenotype. A tissue-based diagnosis of small lymphocytic lymphoma (SLL) requires organ enlargement (e.g. lymphadenopathy > 15 mm) and its infiltration by the above neoplastic B cells. Although CLL and SLL represent the same disease, the latter term is used for cases with < 5 × 10^9/L circulating B cells and nodal, splenic, or other extramedullary involvement.

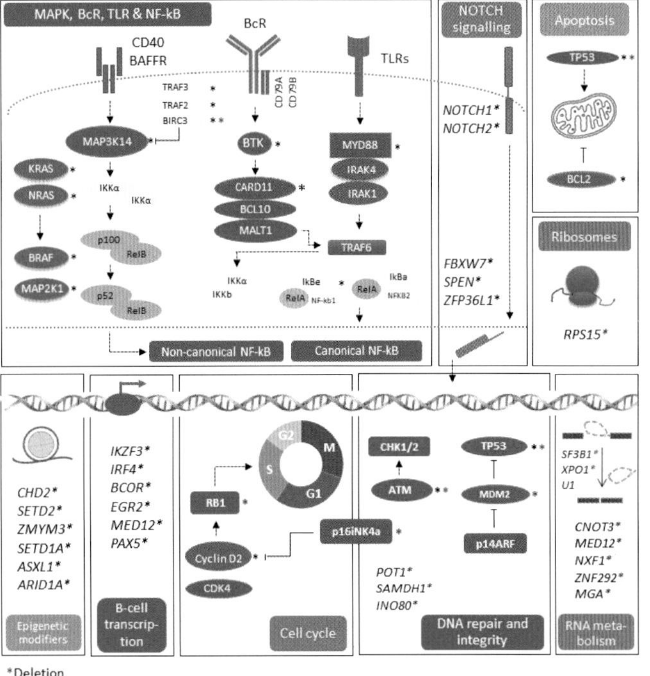

Fig. 4.51 Chronic lymphocytic leukaemia / small lymphocytic lymphoma genetics. Affected pathways and cellular processes in chronic lymphocytic leukaemia include DNA damage response (*ATM*, *TP53*, *SAMHD1*, *POT1*), cell cycle (*CCND2*, *CDKN2A*), RNA splicing and metabolism (*SF3B1*, *U1*, *DDX3X*, *XPO1*, *RPS15*, *ZNF292*, *NXF1*, *MED12*, *CNOT3*), B-cell transcription (*MGA*, *IKZF3*, *IRF4*, *BCOR*, *EGR2*, *PAX5*), and chromatin modifiers (*CHD2*, *SETD2*, *ZMYM3*, *SETD1A*, *ASXL1*, *ARID1A*). Mutations also cluster around microenvironment-dependent signalling pathways, such as those involving NOTCH1 (*NOTCH1*, *FBXW7*, *SPEN*), BcR (*KLHL6*), toll-like receptors (*MYD88*), the MAPK/ERK pathway (*KRAS*, *NRAS*, *BRAF*, *MAP2K1*, *PTPN11*), and NF-κB (*TRAF2*, *TRAF3*, *BIRC3*, *NFKBIE*, *NFKB2*) {2210,501,3307}. Black asterisks denote recurrent single nucleotide variants (SNVs) and indels, and red asterisks deletions. BcR, B-cell receptor; TLR, toll-like receptor.

ICD-O coding

9823/3 Chronic lymphocytic leukaemia / small lymphocytic lymphoma

ICD-11 coding

2A82.0Z Chronic lymphocytic leukaemia or small lymphocytic lymphoma

Related terminology

Acceptable: B-cell chronic lymphocytic leukaemia / small lymphocytic lymphoma.

Subtype(s)

None

Localization

CLL/SLL involves the peripheral blood, bone marrow, and lymphoid tissues such as lymph nodes, spleen, and tonsils. Less frequently, extranodal sites such as the liver, skin, CNS, kidney, pleura, and bones may be involved {3371}. In rare cases, CLL/SLL may be detected in the parotid gland, lacrimal glands, tongue, ocular structures, prostate, lung, pericardium, or intestinal mucosa, and it may accompany other pathologies at these sites {3572}.

Clinical features

Patients may be asymptomatic initially, with the diagnosis only being established with a demonstration of lymphocytosis, lymphadenopathy, or splenomegaly. Symptoms related to cytopenia (anaemia, thrombocytopenia, and rarely neutropenia, due to bone marrow infiltration or autoimmune mechanisms), recurrent infections (due to hypogammaglobulinaemia but also defective cellular immunity), lymphadenopathy, and/or splenomegaly may occur at presentation or subsequently. Constitutional B symptoms (chronic fatigue, unplanned weight loss of > 10% of body weight over a period of 6 months, fever of unknown origin, and/or night sweats) may occur at any disease stage and can indicate progressive disease or Richter transformation (RT) {1605,3572}. Rapid and asymmetrical growth of lymph nodes or one or more extranodal masses is also suggestive of transformation {3481}. About 15% of patients have low-level IgM or IgG paraproteinaemia at diagnosis {803}, and 25% of patients who have normal IgG levels will develop hypogammaglobulinaemia during long-term follow-up {3135}.

Epidemiology

CLL/SLL is most common in fair-skinned populations, with an age-adjusted incidence of 4.9 cases per 100 000 person-years. It is much less common in Asian and Latin American populations, with age-adjusted incidence rates of 0.1–0.5 and 0.5–1.4 cases per 100 000 person-years, respectively. The incidence among African people is unknown {3685,708,2263, 2694,704,2065,263}. The median age at diagnosis in fair-skinned populations (≥ 70 years) is higher than in Asian and African people (58–62 years). There is a male predominance in Europe and the USA (M:F ratio: 1.5–2.1:1), whereas in Asian and African populations, the ratio is variable {4486}.

Etiology

The etiology is unknown. A family history of CLL is a risk factor for developing CLL and monoclonal B-cell lymphocytosis {2046,466}. Cancer registry data suggest that family members of patients with CLL or related lymphomas, such as lymphoplasmacytic lymphoma and mantle cell lymphoma {3867}, have a 5- to 8-fold increased risk of CLL. These studies support an inherited genetic contribution to CLL etiology. To date, large genome-wide association studies among individuals of European ancestry have identified > 40 SNPs associated with the risk of CLL {941,844,2047,2046}. The effect of each individual SNP on CLL risk is small (1.1- to 1.8-fold risk). However, when combining them into a polygenic risk score, individuals in the top quintile have a 2.5-fold increased risk of CLL compared with individuals in the middle quintile {2046,2047}.

Pathogenesis

The cellular origin of CLL/SLL remains unclear; however, transcriptomic and epigenetic analyses suggest that CLL/SLL cells most closely resemble antigen-experienced, memory-like B cells {2126,2992}. CLL/SLL could derive from normal B cells differentiating via follicular or extrafollicular maturation pathways, reflected by the presence or absence of somatic hypermutation (SHM), respectively {2941,1072}.

Microenvironment

The centrality of CLL/SLL microenvironment interactions in the development of CLL/SLL is highlighted by the therapeutic efficacy of kinase inhibitors targeting the B-cell receptor (BCR)-related kinases (i.e. Syk, BTK, and PI3K). Of these, BTK has emerged as the most effective therapeutic target {491,493}.

CLL/SLL cell growth occurs in proliferation centres (PCs) within lymph nodes, where they interact with T helper cells, mesenchymal stromal cells, and macrophages called nurse-like cells, leading to BCR signalling {1570,1562,494}. The BCR and its downstream signalling molecules are central drivers of CLL/SLL cell growth.

Untreated CLL/SLL lacks activating BCR pathway mutations. Instead, BCR activation follows the principles of normal B lymphocytes, with dependence upon the BCR's interactions with antigens. The BCRs bind microbial antigens and autoantigens or engage each other in homotypic interactions, leading to cell-autonomous BCR signalling {741,1575,2217,1017,2689}. Skewed IG gene usage in CLL/SLL culminates in BCR stereotypy, which is the presence of (quasi-)identical BCRs in unrelated patients {1107,2667,3816}. Different BCR stereotypes are found in as many as 41% of patients with CLL/SLL, supporting the notion that CLL/SLL cells bearing BCRs specific for discrete antigens have a significant selection benefit {33}.

The relevance of BCR signalling for CLL/SLL cell proliferation is also underscored by associations between the SHM status of the rearranged IGHV gene utilized in clonotypic BCRs and clinical outcomes. CLL/SLL patients with IGHV genes bearing few or no SHMs (IGHV-unmutated CLL/SLL) typically experience more aggressive disease than those with IGHV genes bearing significant SHM loads (IGHV-mutated CLL/SLL) {861, 1478,713}.

Genetics

The genomic landscape of CLL/SLL is very heterogeneous, lacking a unifying genetic lesion. The most frequent chromosomal aberrations are del(13q), del(11q), (del(17p), and trisomy 12. Occurring in 50–60% of patients, del(13q) removes the *DLEU2*-miR-15-16 cluster, which regulates the expression of antiapoptotic and cell-cycle regulatory proteins {2045, 749}. Del(11q), detected in 10–20% of patients, removes *ATM*, whereas del(17p) (in 5–10% of patients) results in loss of *TP53*. Trisomy 12 occurs in 15–20% of patients, although the genes involved remain unknown {2210,501,3307}. The most frequently mutated genes in CLL/SLL at the time of first treatment are

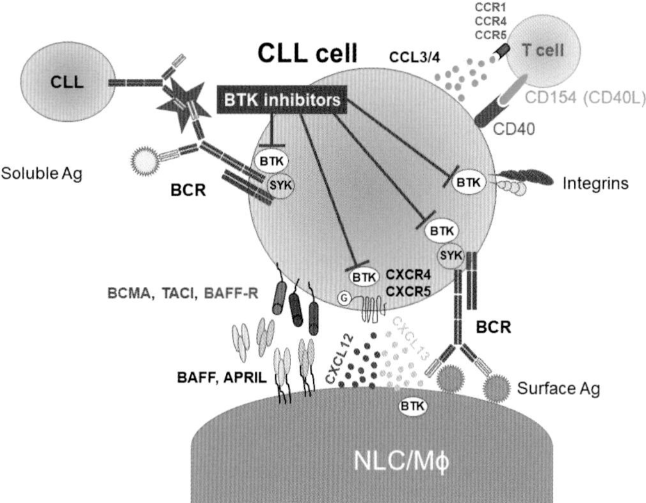

Fig. 4.52 Chronic lymphocytic leukaemia (CLL) microenvironment. The tissue microenvironment activates multiple signalling pathways in CLL. CLL cells proliferate in the microenvironment of secondary lymphatic organs (i.e. lymph nodes, spleen). CLL cells engage in crosstalk with non-malignant cells that constitute the microenvironment. Nurse-like cells (NLCs), which are CLL-associated macrophages (Mϕ), and T lymphocytes are important elements of the microenvironment. B-cell receptor (BCR) activation and downstream signalling promote the proliferation and survival of CLL cells. BCR signalling is activated in secondary lymphatic organs after engagement of the BCR with soluble or surface bound antigens (Ag). An alternative mechanism of BCR activation is through homotypic interactions between two BCR molecules (red star, upper-left corner). Other molecules that contribute to survival and proliferation are BAFF and APRIL (also known as also known as TNFSF13), which are expressed by NLCs and activate corresponding receptors on CLL cells (BAFFR), (BCMA), and TACI (TNFRSF13B). Activated T helper cells express CD154 (CD40L), which can promote the growth of CLL cells via CD40 engagement. NLCs and other stromal cells secrete chemotactic factors (chemokines, e.g. CXCL12 and CXCL13), which attract and retain CLL cells within the tissue compartment by engaging corresponding chemokine receptors (CXCR4, CXCR5) on CLL cells. The primary target of the BTK inhibitors is BCR signalling. However, BTK also plays a role in the signalling of other surface receptors, such as chemokine receptors and adhesion molecules (integrins). Furthermore, BTK is expressed not only by B cells but also by bystander cells in the microenvironment, such as in NLCs. Thus, BTK inhibitors disrupt several CLL–microenvironment interactions. Disrupted signalling of chemokine receptors and adhesion molecules explains the redistribution lymphocytosis that is characteristically seen in patients with CLL treated with BTK inhibitors.

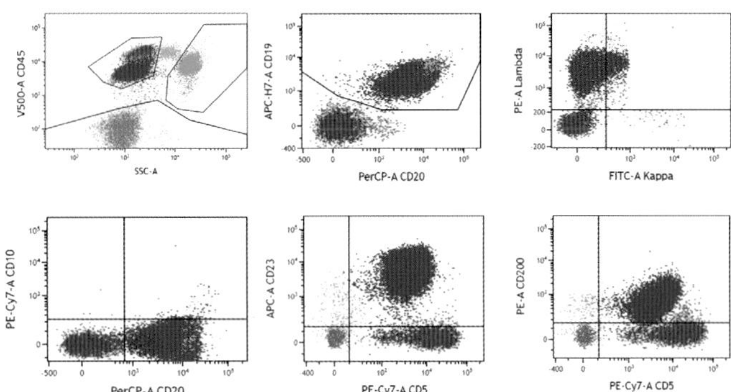

Fig. 4.53 Chronic lymphocytic leukaemia in peripheral blood in a patient with asymptomatic lymphocytosis. Total B-cell count = 5.8 × 10^9/L. The upper-left scatter plot shows CD45 expression against side scatter (SSC-A) of all leukocytes with chronic lymphocytic leukaemia cells (blue), T cells (red), monocytes (light blue), and granulocytes (light green). The other scatter plots show antigen expression on the gated T-cell and B-cell lymphocyte populations and also include NK cells (green) and normal polyclonal B cells (orange). Note the characteristically low CD5 mean fluorescence intensity typical of chronic lymphocytic leukaemia (lower-right scatter plot).

NOTCH1 (10–15%), *ATM* (10–15%), *SF3B1* (10%), *TP53* (5–10%), and *BIRC3* (5%) {2210,3307}.

Collectively, gene mutations impact diverse pathways and cellular programmes. The frequencies and patterns of chromosomal abnormalities and mutations differ according to IGHV gene SHM status and among different subsets of patients with distinct stereotyped BCR (see Table 4.14) {3307,3890}. Cases presenting as SLL have trisomy 12 more frequently than do those presenting as CLL (37% vs 15–20%), but they show the same distribution of driver gene mutations {2556}.

Progressing cases rarely acquire new genetic lesions after watch-and-wait management, but large clonal shifts in CLL/SLL can occur after treatment {1428,1438,3646}. Chemoimmunotherapy leads to frequent *TP53* aberrations (20–30%), *MYC* gain (15%), and *CDKN2A* loss (10%) in CLL/SLL cells, and these are often seen at relapse {1042,2210,3632}.

The genetics of histologically aggressive CLL/SLL is poorly understood. Trisomy 12 and del(17p) are more frequent in cases with enlarged PCs {1345,748}. Diffuse large B-cell lymphoma (DLBCL) transformed from CLL/SLL (i.e. clonally related RT) shows greater molecular heterogeneity and complexity than CLL/SLL, a mutation profile different from that of de novo DLBCL, a lack of specific recurrent genetic alterations causing transformation, and either linear or branching evolution {1103,706,3480,2052}. Genetic aberrations commonly involve *TP53* mutations and/or del(17p) (60–70% of cases), *NOTCH1* mutations (30%), activation of *MYC* by translocation, amplification or mutation (30%), and 9p21 deletion affecting *CDKN2A* (20%). One or more of these abnormalities is present in 90% of RT cases, typically acquired at transformation {1103,3478,3480,706}.

Epigenetics

Although the CLL/SLL DNA methylome reflects the cell of origin, it is also characterized by disease-specific changes. Distinct CLL/SLL subtypes bearing distinct DNA methylation signatures have been identified: one similar to germinal centre–experienced B cells, termed memory-like CLL (m-like CLL); and another resembling germinal centre–inexperienced B cells, termed naïve-like CLL (n-like CLL) {2146,2992,2145,3323,514}. The m-CLL and n-CLL subsets have prognoses that correspond largely to IGHV-mutated CLL/SLL and IGHV-unmutated CLL/SLL, respectively {2992,2523}. A third group with an intermediate DNA methylation profile has an intermediate prognosis {2145,2992}. Recent studies show that CLL with an intermediate DNA methylation profile is enriched for stereotyped subset #2 (IGHV3-21/IGLV3-21) and IGLV3-21R110, which are associated with a more aggressive clinical course; the remaining cases of CLL with an intermediate DNA methylation profile mostly belong to IGHV-mutated CLL/SLL and follow a more indolent disease course {2865,348}. Although the DNA methylation profiles remain relatively stable in patients with untreated CLL/SLL, those with progressive/relapsing disease display a higher degree of epigenetic changes and evolution, parallel to the genetic evolution {514,4082,2991}.

Macroscopic appearance

Not relevant

Histopathology

Peripheral blood and bone marrow aspirate

Bone marrow and peripheral blood smears typically show small lymphoid cells with clumped chromatin; indistinct or absent nucleoli; and scant, pale to lightly basophilic cytoplasm. Nuclear chromatin can have a cracked-mud or soccer-ball patch-like pattern. Smudge cells are common in blood smears.

Table 4.14 Genetic and clinical features according to IGHV gene somatic hypermutation status and B-cell receptor IG stereotypy

Feature	M-CLL	U-CLL	B-cell receptor stereotyped subset			
			#1	#2	#4	#8
Frequency	50–60%	30–40%	2.2%	2.5%	0.9%	0.5%
Immunogenetic features	< 98% identity to germline	> 98% identity to germline	IGHV1/5/7 / IGKV1(D)-39 (U-CLL)	IGHV3-21 / IGLV3-21 (M-CLL and U-CLL)	IGHV4-34 / IGKV2-30 (M-CLL)	IGHV4-39 / IGKV1(D)-39 (U-CLL)
Chromosomal alterations	del(13q), trisomy 12	del(11q), del(17p), trisomy 12	del(11q), del(17p)	del(13q), del(11q)	del(13q) or none	Trisomy 12
Gene mutations	*MYD88*, *CDH2*	*TP53*, *ATM*, *SF3B1*, *NOTCH1*, *EGR2*, etc.	*TP53*, *NFKBIE*, *NOTCH1*	*SF3B1*, *ATM*	None	*NOTCH1*
Clinical features	Long TTFT/OS	Short TTFT/OS	Short TTFT/OS	Short TTFT/OS	Long TTFT/OS	Short TTFT/OS High risk of RT

M-CLL, chronic lymphocytic leukaemia with mutated IGHV status; OS, overall survival; RT, Richter transformation; TTFT, time to first treatment; U-CLL, chronic lymphocytic leukaemia with unmutated IGHV status.

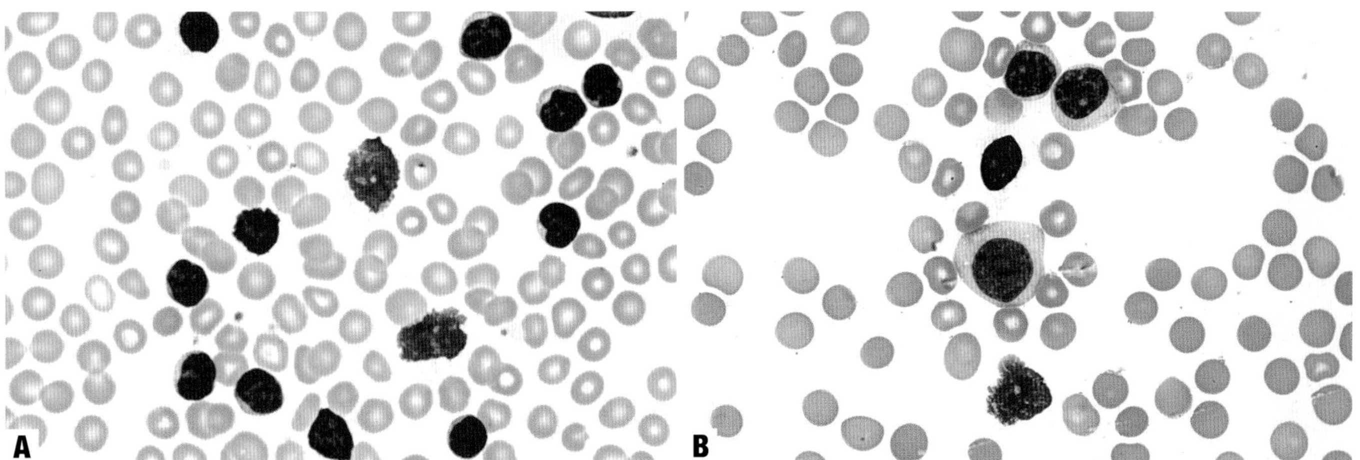

Fig. 4.54 Chronic lymphocytic leukaemia / small lymphocytic lymphoma, peripheral blood. **A** Peripheral blood film in chronic lymphocytic leukaemia showing small lymphoid cells with scant cytoplasm and nuclei with coarsely clumped chromatin. Smudge cells are seen in the background. **B** Prolymphocytes are larger and have more abundant cytoplasm, larger nuclei, and a single central prominent nucleolus.

Bone marrow core biopsy

Marrow involvement may be nodular, interstitial, diffuse, or a combination of the three. Paratrabecular and intrasinusoidal aggregates are not typical; there is usually a spared paratrabecular zone where normal marrow remains, even in heavily involved marrow. Infiltration patterns correlate with prognosis: nodular and interstitial patterns are seen mainly in early CLL/SLL, whereas a diffuse pattern is seen in advanced disease and is associated with bone marrow failure {2716,2760,222}. PCs are less common in bone marrow than in lymph nodes but are reported in about 10% of cases {1291}. Immune-related cytopenia is associated with a normal or increased proportion

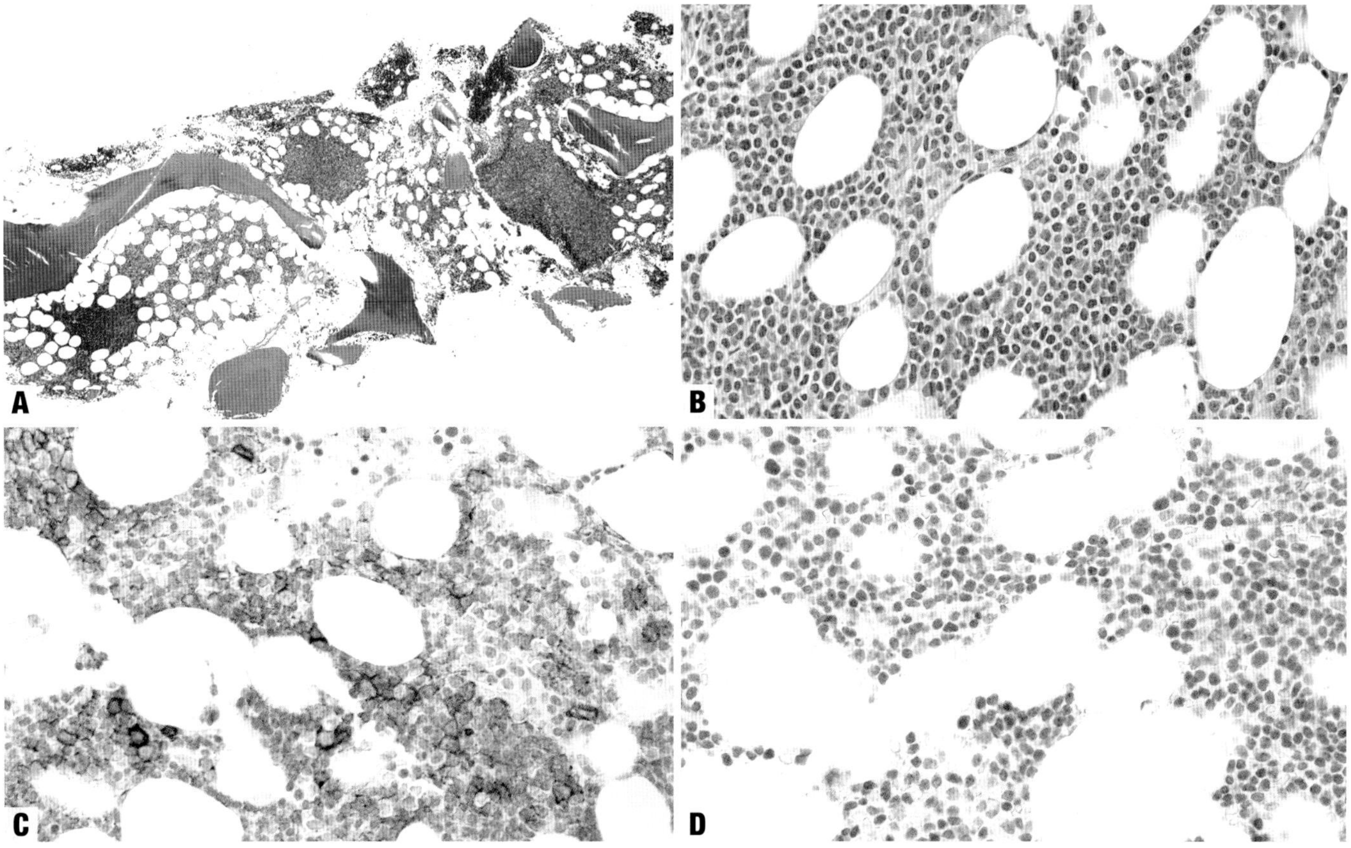

Fig. 4.55 Chronic lymphocytic leukaemia / small lymphocytic lymphoma involving bone marrow. **A** Bone marrow core biopsy in chronic lymphocytic leukaemia showing intertrabecular nodular aggregates of small lymphoid cells. **B** There is a predominance of small cells with oval to irregular dark nuclei and scant cytoplasm. A few medium-sized prolymphocytes with open chromatin and distinct nucleoli are intermixed. **C** The neoplastic cells are weakly CD20+ by immunohistochemistry. **D** Neoplastic B cells are weakly to moderately LEF1+ by immunohistochemistry.

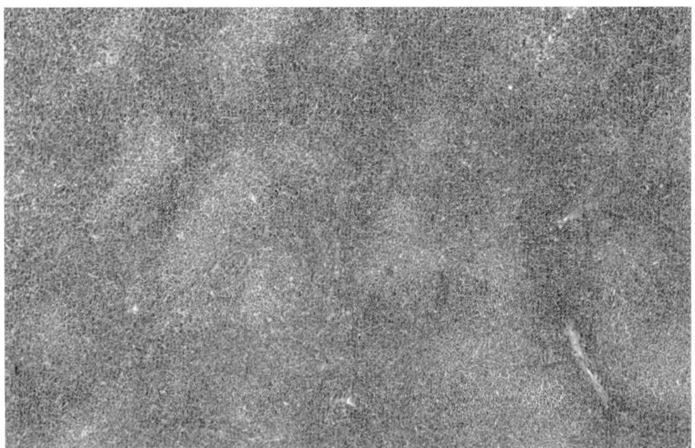

Fig. 4.56 Chronic lymphocytic leukaemia / small lymphocytic lymphoma. Lymph node involved by chronic lymphocytic leukaemia, showing prominent proliferation centres.

of the affected lineage's cells without dysplastic features {4085, 2782,4240}. Pure red cell aplasia (either immune-related or viral infection–related) is characterized by a near-complete absence of erythroid precursors {4085}.

Lymph node

Lymph nodes are enlarged with diffuse infiltration of small lymphoid cells, often with variably prominent pale-staining PCs containing larger cells (either prolymphocytes or paraimmunoblasts, which are larger cells with round to oval nuclei, dispersed chromatin, central nucleoli, and pale cytoplasm), and may be entirely or partially effaced. Neoplastic B cells are slightly larger than normal mature B cells and have clumped chromatin within round, occasionally irregular nuclei. Mitoses are infrequent. PCs contain a spectrum of small lymphoid cells, medium-sized prolymphocytes, and paraimmunoblasts {399,2274}. Plasmacytic differentiation can be seen, but it is rare {3907}.

Spleen

White pulp involvement is usually prominent, but the red pulp can be infiltrated. Diffuse infiltration leads to loss of distinction between the red and white pulp.

Immunophenotype by flow cytometry

By flow cytometry, neoplastic cells are typically monotypic surface IgM dim+, IgD+/– (IgG+ in ~10% of cases), CD19+, CD5+, CD23+, CD43+, CD200+, CD20 dim+, CD11c variable, CD10–, CD79b–, FMC7–, CD25–, and CD103–, along with showing light chain restriction (dim expression). Atypical immunophenotypes (e.g. CD5–, CD23–, FMC7+, CD79b+, or strongly expressed surface immunoglobulin) are known {839, 2599,2119}. In such cases, other small B-cell lymphomas must be carefully excluded. Strong expression of CD200 and ROR1

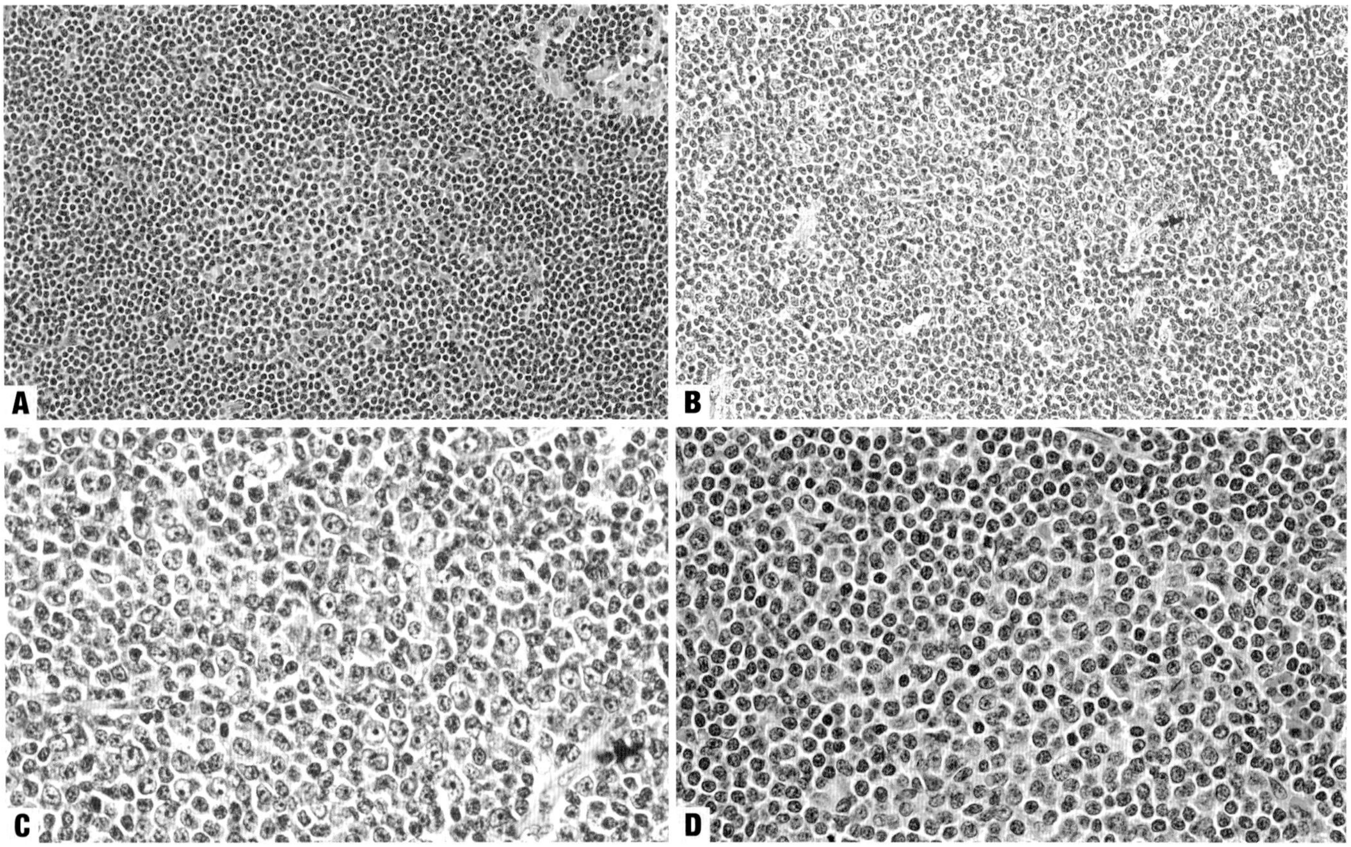

Fig. 4.57 Chronic lymphocytic leukaemia / small lymphocytic lymphoma. **A** Low magnification shows a proliferation centre and a background of small lymphocytes. **B** Giemsa staining in this case more clearly highlights the presence of prolymphocytes. **C,D** At higher magnification, the cellular detail of small lymphocytes, slightly larger prolymphocytes, and interspersed larger paraimmunoblasts with light chromatin and a single nucleolus is appreciated (**C**), as well as small lymphocytes and slightly larger cells within the proliferation centre (**D**).

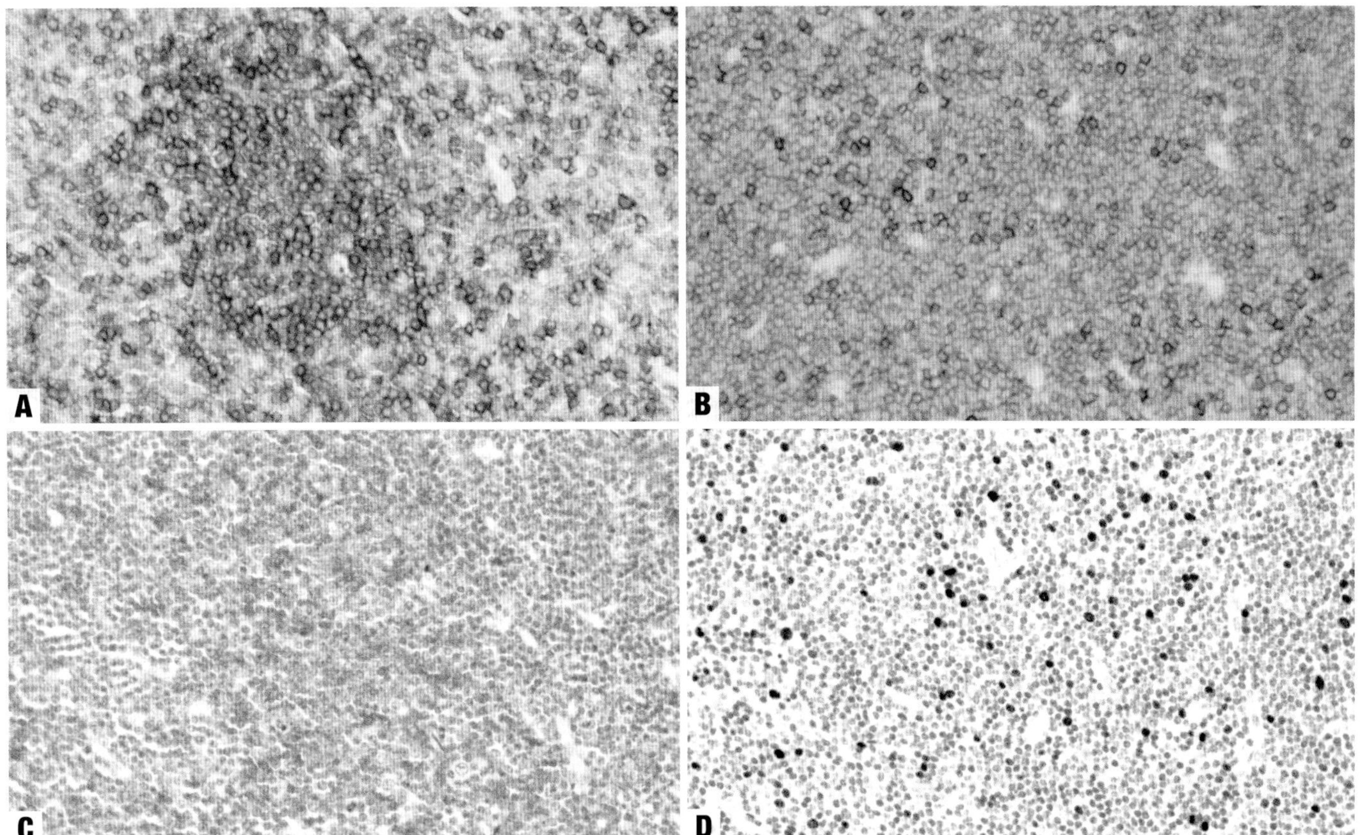

Fig. 4.58 Chronic lymphocytic leukaemia / small lymphocytic lymphoma. Immunophenotype. **A** Lymphoid cells show variable expression of CD20, with cells in the proliferation centres showing stronger expression. **B** Aberrant expression of CD5. **C** Weak expression of CD23; it is often stronger in cells within the proliferation centres. **D** About 10–15% of cells express Ki-67.

{4117,1139} and an absence of CD81 expression {30} characterize CLL. Expression of CD38 and CD49d is associated with a worse prognosis {920}. A major consensus effort identified CD19, CD5, CD20, CD23, kappa, and lambda as markers essential to be tested for a diagnosis of CLL, and CD43, CD79b, CD81, CD200, CD10, and ROR1 as additional markers useful in the differential diagnosis from other small B-cell lymphomas/leukaemias {3379}.

Immunohistochemistry

CLL/SLL cells express pan–B-cell markers (CD19, CD20, CD79a, and PAX5), CD5, and CD23, and are negative for CD10 and other germinal-centre markers. As many as 95% of cases express LEF1, which is rarely expressed in other small B-cell lymphomas {2654,2649,3964}. Usually, cyclin D1 and SOX11 are negative. In rare cases, scattered cells in PCs are cyclin D1+, but diffuse expression of cyclin D1 excludes CLL/SLL {5,1386}. The cells in the PCs may variably express MYC {3906}. IRF4 (MUM1), CD20, and CD23 expression is usually stronger in PCs than in diffuse areas {3778,2900,2205}. The proliferation index is low overall but elevated in PCs. Minimal antibody panels for the diagnosis of B-cell lymphomas have been described {965}.

Accelerated CLL/SLL

Histologically aggressive CLL/SLL

The size of PCs and the numbers of prolymphocytes or paraimmunoblasts vary between cases. Those with very large, prominent/confluent PCs (traditionally spanning the diameter of a visual field using a 20× objective lens and a 10× ocular lens) or with high proliferation indexes (> 2.4 mitoses per PC or > 40% Ki-67+ cells in PCs, whereby traditionally PC size is not defined) are arbitrarily designated as histologically aggressive CLL/SLL.

Prolymphocytic progression

If the total proportion of prolymphocytes (medium-sized cells with basophilic cytoplasm and a prominent nucleolus) is > 15% in peripheral blood, prolymphocytic progression is established {1083,2637,316,1471}. It should be noted that cases with > 55% prolymphocytes, that have otherwise immunophenotypic features of CLL and that were classified as B-prolymphocytic leukaemia in the previous edition of the WHO classification of haematolymphoid tumours, are now classified as prolymphocytic progression of CLL/SLL (not as B-prolymphocytic leukaemia). A blastoid variant of mantle cell lymphoma should be excluded in these cases.

Histologically aggressive CLL/SLL or prolymphocytic progression are seen in approximately 5% of cases of CLL/SLL. Such cases often show *TP53* disruption and have a clinical outcome between that of typical CLL/SLL and RT {1345}, the latter occurring in about 5% of cases of CLL/SLL {1342}.

Richter transformation

The diagnosis of RT is optimally based on lymph node excisional biopsy; on needle biopsy, it may be difficult to distinguish prominent PCs from DLBCL {3481}. DLBCL-type RT (DLBCL-RT) is characterized by sheets of large atypical B cells, which almost always have a non–germinal centre B immunophenotype, whereas background histiocytes express PDL1 {288, 4313}. CD5 is occasionally expressed, CD23 is typically negative, and EBV is usually absent {3481}. Rare cases of CLL/SLL with progression to lymphoma resembling classic Hodgkin lymphoma (CHL) (classic Hodgkin lymphoma–type RT [CHL-RT]) also occur (< 1%). These cases show both the typical neoplastic cells and the characteristic milieu of CHL, with mixed-cellularity CHL being the most common subtype {382}. Reed–Sternberg cells and variants are usually EBV-positive. Survival of patients with CHL-RT is generally better than that of DLBCL-RT, possibly because most cases of CHL-RT are clonally unrelated to the original CLL/SLL {3481}. The presence of scattered Reed–Sternberg cells or Reed–Sternberg–like cells (EBV+/–), without the milieu of CHL, can also be seen in cases of CLL/SLL without transformation {382, 2028}. Some RT cases, of both CHL and DLBCL type, are due to underlying immune deficiency/dysregulation, mostly occurring after (poly)chemotherapy for CLL/SLL. These are generally clonally unrelated and EBV+, and they should be interpreted as immune deficiency/dysregulation–associated B-lymphoproliferations and lymphomas in an iatrogenic setting (see respective sections).

In very rare cases, patients with CLL/SLL develop histiocytic/dendritic cell neoplasms, probably representing clonal evolution and transdifferentiation of the original CLL/SLL clone, with loss of characteristic morphology and B-antigen expression {1230,3696}. Extremely rare cases of mature T-cell lymphoma have arisen in association with CLL/SLL {2547,439, 4149,4076}.

Cytology

See above.

Diagnostic molecular pathology

In > 80% of patients with CLL/SLL, at least one of four recurrent chromosomal alterations can be seen when using FISH: del(11q), del(13q), del(17p), and trisomy 12 {982}. Of those with *TP53* disruption, about 60% of cases carry both del(17p) and *TP53* mutation, and roughly 30% display *TP53* mutations without del(17p) {533}. Therefore, before therapy, comprehensive assessment of *TP53* requires investigation of both deletion of the *TP53* locus and mutations of *TP53* by a sufficiently sensitive sequencing method {2503,1472}. Because *TP53* aberrations can emerge during the disease, in particular at the time of progression after chemoimmunotherapy, the *TP53* status should be reassessed at progression in previously *TP53*-wildtype cases. Unlike other B-cell malignancies, translocations involving the IG gene loci are uncommon in CLL/SLL. Exceptions include t(14;18)(q32;q21)/IGH::*BCL2* and its light chain variants (2% of cases) {816,3134} and the rare t(14;19)(q32;q13)/IGH::*BCL3* {816,3391,2563}. Unlike

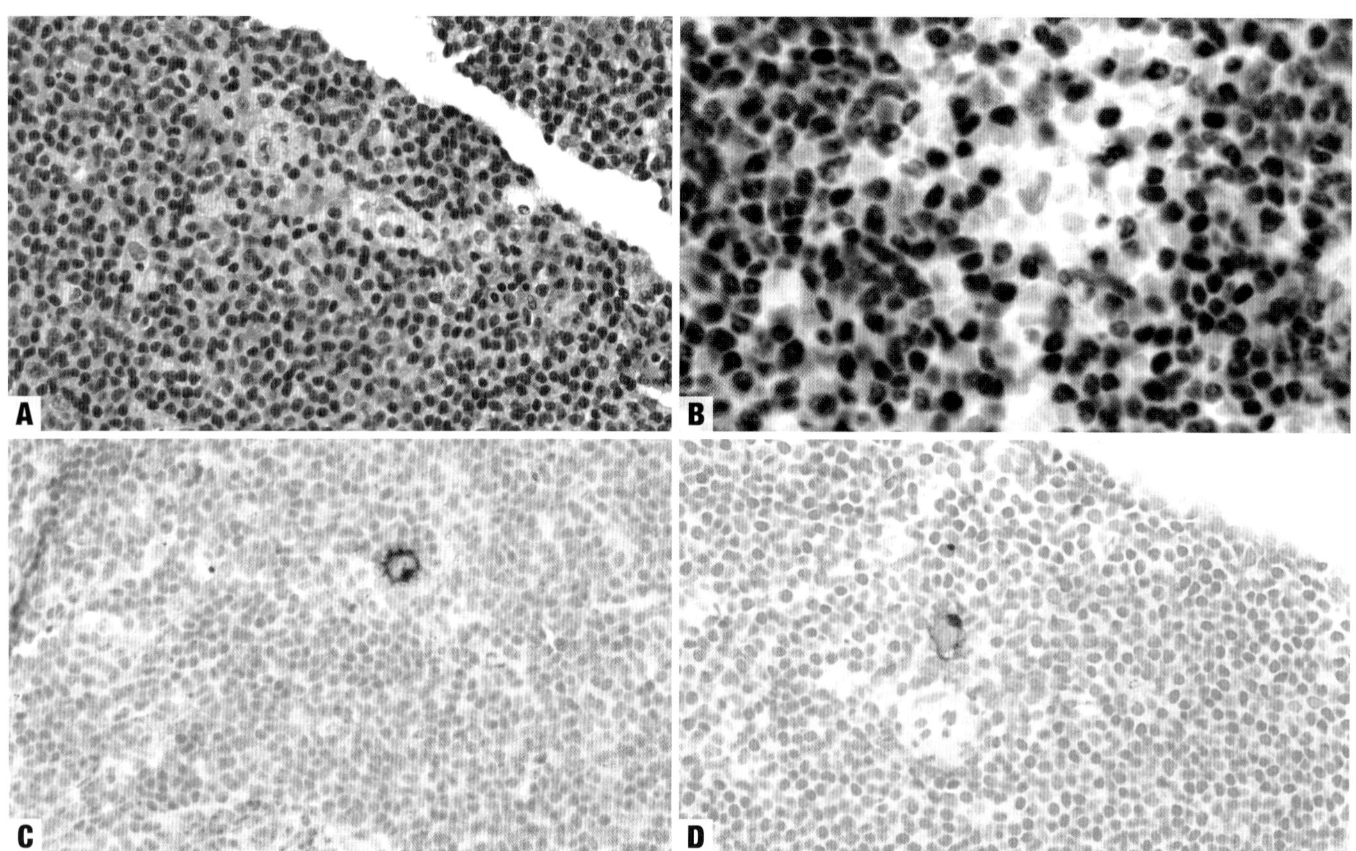

Fig. 4.59 Chronic lymphocytic leukaemia / small lymphocytic lymphoma. **A** The presence of scattered Hodgkin/Reed–Sternberg (HRS)-like cells does not qualify for transformation. **B** Chronic lymphocytic leukaemia cells show strong expression of PAX5, whereas the HRS-like cells weakly express PAX5. **C,D** HRS-like cells are positive for CD30 (**C**) and often express CD15 (**D**).

Table 4.15 Essential and desirable diagnostic criteria for chronic lymphocytic leukaemia / small lymphocytic lymphoma (CLL/SLL)

	Positive	Negative/weak
Essential diagnostic criteria		
For peripheral blood	Classic morphology of CLL cells Absolute monoclonal B-cell count ≥ 5 × 10^9/L	
Immunophenotyping	CD19, CD5, CD20, CD23 (variable), and light chain (weak)	
For tissue	Lymphadenopathy/organomegaly or altered architecture on microscopy; classic morphology of SLL[a]	
Immunohistochemistry	CD20 (positive/weak), CD5 (positive/weak), CD23 (variable)	Cyclin D1 (weak positivity in subset of cells in proliferation centres is allowed) {965}
Desirable diagnostic criteria		
Immunophenotyping	CD200, ROR1, CD43	FMC7, CD79b (weak/negative), CD10, CD81
Immunohistochemistry	CD23, LEF1, CD43, IRF4 (MUM1) (proliferation centres)	CD10, SOX11

CLL, chronic lymphocytic leukaemia; SLL, small lymphocytic lymphoma.
[a]The majority of cases of CLL/SLL present with a leukaemic phase and diagnosis can be established on peripheral blood without the need for either bone marrow or lymph node examination. These are only required to confirm the diagnosis of small lymphocytic lymphoma {1472}.

mantle cell lymphoma, CLL/SLL does not harbour t(11;14)(q13;q32) {816}.

The assessment of the SHM status of the clonotypic rearranged IGHV gene is recommended for all patients with CLL/SLL before therapy commencement {3469,1472}. If the germline identity of the rearranged IGHV gene is < 98%, the patient is considered to have IGHV-mutated CLL/SLL, whereas patients classified as having IGHV-unmutated CLL/SLL show a germline identity ≥ 98% {1478,861}. As for all cut-off values, there exist borderline-mutated cases, with a germline identity of 97–97.9%, and these may have diverse clinical outcomes. Caution is warranted in such cases regarding the prognosis {3469}. The subset #2 configuration (IGHV3-21/IGLV3-21) of the IG gene rearrangement, mostly classified as IGHV-mutated CLL/SLL, heralds a poorer prognosis, similar to that of IGHV-unmutated CLL/SLL {220,1786}. Because the IG gene rearrangement and IGHV gene SHM status do not change over time, the test only needs to be performed once for each patient.

In familial cases, germline determination of polygenic risk scores might be considered {2046,2047}.

Essential and desirable diagnostic criteria

See Table 4.15.

Recommended investigations for prognosis/prediction

See Table 4.16 (p. 376).

Essential: evaluation of del(11q), del(13q), del(17p), and trisomy 12; *TP53* mutation analysis; IGHV gene SHM analysis and subset #2 configuration.
Desirable: demonstration of complex karyotype; *BTK*, *PLCG2*, and *BCL2* mutation analysis.

Staging

The Rai and Binet systems are used; they are based on blood cell counts and physical examination (see Table 4.17, p. 377). Stage of SLL is determined with the Lugano modifications to the Ann Arbor system, which is based on CT and bone marrow biopsy {688}. PET-CT may help differentiate progressive CLL/SLL from RT, and in cases with a high maximum standardized uptake value of > 10, a diagnostic biopsy should be undertaken.

Prognosis and prediction

Despite significant improvements in clinical outcome since the introduction of targeted therapies, CLL/SLL remains largely incurable. Clinical staging is relevant for prognostication and decision on therapy initiation. Although del(13q), presenting as the sole aberration, is associated with indolent disease, *TP53*

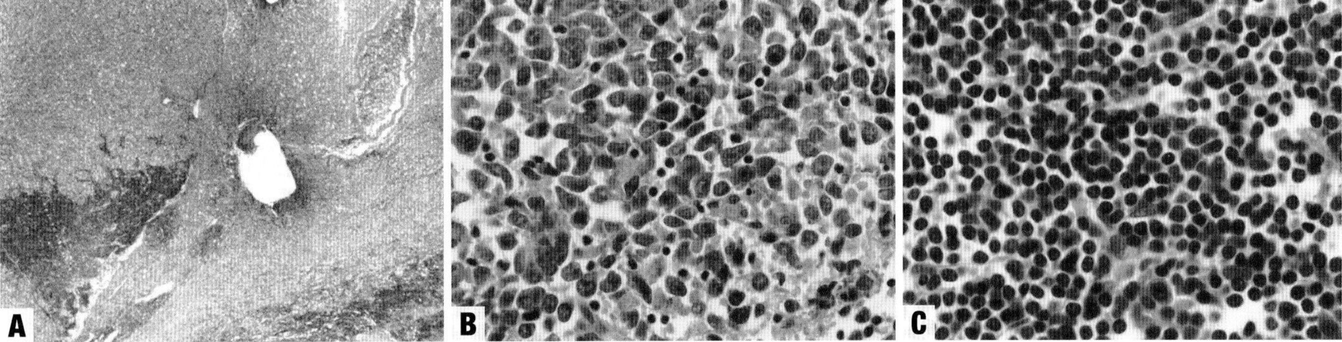

Fig. 4.60 Diffuse large B-cell lymphoma–type Richter transformation. **A** Most of the lymph node shows diffuse large B-cell lymphoma with areas of residual chronic lymphocytic leukaemia. **B,C** At higher magnification, diffuse large B-cell lymphoma areas are composed of monomorphic large cells with centroblastic and immunoblastic features (**B**) intermingled with sheets of residual chronic lymphocytic leukaemia (**C**).

Table 4.16 Overview of the most relevant prognostic and predictive markers in chronic lymphocytic leukaemia (CLL)

Parameter	Frequency	Prognostic impact	Predictive impact	Comment
del(17p) and/or *TP53* mutation (~60% of cases carry both del(17p) and TP53 mutation) {533}	del(17p) 4–8% and *TP53* mutation 5–12% in early-stage CLL {533} del(17p) 5–8% and *TP53* mutation 8–12% at start of first-line therapy {4549,3838,1194,4414} 40–50% in relapsed and refractory CLL {533}	Strong negative prognostic impact on PFS and OS without therapy and with CIT, less adverse impact with targeted therapy (BTK and BCL2 inhibitors) {3838,533}	Predictive for poor response and shorter response duration, PFS, and OS with CIT, as compared with longer response duration, PFS, and OS with BTK and BCL2 inhibitors {533}	Repeated testing at relapse is recommended Associated with a higher risk of RT
Complex karyotype: defined as ≥ 3 or ≥ 5 aberrations	15% detectable by chromosome banding analysis {221}	Independent negative prognostic impact in most studies, particularly for ≥ 5 aberrations in *TP53*-wildtype cases {221,2266}	Not clear, because the predictive impact is also dependent on involved chromosomal and genetic abnormalities; limited evidence from prospective trials	Strong correlation with *TP53* aberrations, but still an independent prognostic factor The optimal definition with respect to defining a number of chromosomal aberrations is unclear The role of involved chromosomal and genetic abnormalities beyond *TP53* is to be evaluated {221}
IGHV status: U-CLL with ≥ 98% identity vs M-CLL with < 98% identity	~30% U-IGHV in early-stage CLL {792} 50–75% U-IGHV in advanced stages {861,1478,3838}	U-IGHV: negative prognostic impact on PFS and OS without therapy and with CIT, less adverse impact with targeted therapy (BTK and BCL2 inhibitors) {1726,1195, 492,87}	U-IGHV: predictive for shorter response duration, PFS, and OS with CIT, as compared with longer response duration, PFS, and OS with BTK and BCL2 inhibitors	No repeated testing, because IGHV gene somatic hypermutation status does not change over time
***BTK* mutation**	None in BTK-inhibitor treatment–naïve patients {1126,2209}; 23–57% of relapsed CLLs on ibrutinib had *BTK* mutations after a median of 3 years {1824,3329}; 60–80% of ibrutinib-resistant CLLs had *BTK* mutations, which were retrospectively detectable at a median of 8–9 months (range: 3–18 months) before clinical progression {50,4413,2209}	Not tested as an independent parameter	Predictive for progression on therapy with covalent BTK inhibitors within the next 3–18 months {4413}	No routine testing so far
***PLCG2* mutation**	13% of relapsed CLLs after 3 years on ibrutinib had *PLCG2* mutations in addition to *BTK* mutations {3329} 6% of ibrutinib-resistant CLLs had sole *PLCG2* mutation, and 13% had *PLCG2* and *BTK* mutation {4413}	Not tested as an independent parameter	Predictive for progression on therapy with (covalent and non-covalent) BTK inhibitors {4413}	No routine testing so far
***BCL2* mutation**	45–47% of patients with venetoclax-resistant CLL have detectable *BCL2* mutations {377,2440}	Not tested as an independent parameter	Predictive for progression on venetoclax monotherapy {377,2440}	No routine testing so far
Serum B2M	Elevated in 34% of patients with CLL {1726,533}	Independent negative prognostic factor {1726}	None	
≥ 15% prolymphocytes in peripheral blood	Unclear, possibly as high as 33% {2637}	Not tested	Not tested	
Bone marrow infiltration pattern with proliferation centres	Unclear	Not tested	Not tested	Some correlation with *TP53* aberration and complex karyotype {1291}
Large confluent proliferation centres in lymph node	As high as 23% in advanced CLL {1345}	Not tested	Not tested	Expanded proliferation centres (broader than a 20× field) and high proliferation (either > 2.4 mitoses/ proliferation centre or Ki-67 > 40%/ proliferation centre) are associated with poor prognosis and defined as accelerated CLL {1345}

CIT, chemoimmunotherapy; CT, chemotherapy; M-CLL, CLL with mutated IGHV status; OS, overall survival; PFS, progression-free survival; RT, Richter transformation; U-CLL, CLL with unmutated IGHV status.

Table 4.17 Rai and Binet staging systems for chronic lymphocytic leukaemia

Stage according to Rai	Definition by Rai	Stage according to Binet	Definition by Binet
Rai 0	Lymphocytosis > 5 × 10^9/L	**Binet A**	Haemoglobin ≥ 100 g/L (6.21 mmol/L), platelets ≥ 100 × 10^9/L, fewer than three involved lymphoid sites
Rai I	Lymphocytosis and lymphadenopathy		
Rai II	Lymphocytosis and hepatomegaly and/or splenomegaly with/without lymphadenopathy	**Binet B**	Haemoglobin ≥ 100 g/L (6.21 mmol/L), platelets ≥ 100 × 10^9/L, at least three involved lymphoid sites
Rai III	Lymphocytosis and haemoglobin < 110 g/L (6.83 mmol/L) with/without lymphadenopathy/organomegaly	**Binet C**	Haemoglobin < 100 g/L and/or platelets < 100 × 10^9/L
Rai IV	Lymphocytosis and platelets < 100 × 10^9/L with/without lymphadenopathy/organomegaly		

deletion and/or mutation is a biomarker that predicts resistance to chemoimmunotherapy {533,2503,1472}. An unmutated IGHV gene is predictive of shorter progression-free survival if patients are treated with chemoimmunotherapy {1195,492,3979}.

Prognostic markers with the highest impact on outcome should be evaluated at the time of therapy, to aid therapeutic strategy decision-making. Markers that may develop later during the disease, due to clonal evolution, should be tested repeatedly {2210}. Among the chromosomal and molecular genetic aberrations, del(17p) and/or *TP53* mutation have the strongest impact on the prognosis and the prediction of therapeutic outcome (see Table 4.16), even with the use of targeted agents {4549,49}. Furthermore, IGHV-mutated and unmutated CLL/SLL show different kinetics with respect to proliferation and therefore have different time to therapy and time to relapse with time-limited chemotherapy-based regimens {861,1478}. Stereotyped subset #2, independent of its IGHV gene SHM status, is associated with poor responses to chemoimmunotherapy {1786}.

IGHV mutation status and presence of *TP53* aberrations are both included in the CLL International Prognostic Index (CLL-IPI) {1726}, along with age, stage, and B2M level. The International Prognostic Score for Early-Stage CLL/SLL (IPS-E) includes IGHV mutation status, an absolute lymphocyte count of > 15 × 10^9/L, and the presence of palpable lymph nodes {792}.

Cases progressing under treatment with BTK inhibitors often (60–80% of cases) show mutations of *BTK* (mostly in the kinase domain), *PLCG2*, and others. Furthermore, *BTK* and *PLCG2* mutations may occur in patients with RT on BTK inhibitor therapy. Genetic aberrations associated with RT after novel agents are like those observed after chemoimmunotherapy {4412,684, 3329,50,4413,1824,2209,1847,2469,1861,1563,116}. In about 50% of cases progressing on treatment with BCL2 inhibitors, the CLL/SLL cells acquire mutations in *BCL2* (disrupting the drug-binding site) or amplification of 1q (involving *MCL1*) {377, 3978,2440,380,1437}.

Complex karyotype and genomic complexity can be identified by a variety of different methods, including chromosome banding analysis, microarrays, or whole-genome sequencing {221,2266,2053}. The precise definition of complex karyotype depends on the technology used and is predictive of resistance to chemoimmunotherapy in *TP53*-wildtype cases {221,1820, 2035,2266}.

Overexpression of ZAP70 (intracellular), CD38, and CD49d (membrane-associated) reflects activation and proliferation of CLL/SLL and tends to correlate with unfavourable genetic markers, such as unmutated IGHV genes {2502,310}. Similarly, the presence of PCs in marrow biopsies is often associated with *TP53* abnormalities and complex karyotype {1291}. The presence of either > 15% prolymphocytes in the peripheral blood (prolymphocytic progression) or of large confluent PCs in lymph nodes (histologically aggressive CLL/SLL) is associated with disease evolution and with poorer outcomes (i.e. accelerated CLL/SLL) {1083,2637,316,1471,1345}.

Among the serum parameters, B2M is an independent prognostic marker in early and advanced CLL/SLL. Elevated LDH appears to reflect an inferior prognosis in relapsed CLL/SLL {1726,49,2715}.

Splenic B-cell lymphomas and leukaemias: Introduction

Naresh KN

The sections on splenic B-cell lymphomas/leukaemias in this fifth edition of the WHO classification of haematolymphoid tumours include hairy cell leukaemia (HCL), splenic marginal zone lymphoma (SMZL), splenic diffuse red pulp small B-cell lymphoma (SDRPL), and splenic B-cell lymphoma/leukaemia with prominent nucleoli (SBLPN) (see Table 4.18 and Table 4.19). The term "hairy cell leukaemia variant" has been removed as a diagnostic entity, in recognition that the biology of this disease is unrelated to HCL.

HCL is a well-recognized mature B-cell neoplasm with a clinicopathological definition that includes characteristic cytomorphology, immunophenotype, and clinical features. These defining parameters have not changed since the first inclusion of HCL in the 2001 WHO classification. The presence of *BRAF* p.V600E (NP_004324.2) in ≥ 95% of cases has further established HCL as a distinct entity {4016}. A diagnosis of HCL can be made reliably on peripheral blood, bone marrow aspirate, and/or bone marrow trephine samples.

SMZL and SDRPL share, to a large extent, overlapping clinical, morphological, and immunophenotypic features, often precluding a definite diagnosis on peripheral blood or bone marrow samples in the absence of a splenectomy specimen (or possibly a splenic biopsy sample). Of these, SMZL is the better defined. In the spleen, the infiltrate typically involves both white and red pulp. The white pulp is expanded, and the infiltrate in the red pulp involves both sinuses and cords. Also in the bone marrow trephine, the growth pattern often has a nodular component in addition to interstitial and intrasinusoidal infiltrates. Plasmacytoid differentiation may be observed. Lymphoid cells with relatively abundant cytoplasm and villous projections reminiscent of

Table 4.18 Summary of the main histopathological and immunophenotypic features of splenic diffuse red pulp small B-cell lymphoma (SDRPL), splenic marginal zone lymphoma (SMZL), splenic B-cell lymphoma/leukaemia with prominent nucleoli (SBLPN), and hairy cell leukaemia (HCL) {1780,850,3549,4067,4061,364}

Feature	SDRPL	SMZL	SBLPN	HCL
Histopathology				
Spleen pattern	Diffuse	Predominantly macronodular; less frequently diffuse	Diffuse	Diffuse
Bone marrow pattern	Predominantly intrasinusoidal Interstitial Nodular Mixed	Interstitial Intrasinusoidal Nodular Mixed	Intrasinusoidal	Interstitial
Morphology/cytology	Monomorphic	Small cells Marginal-zone cells Isolated large cells	Monomorphic with visible nucleoli	Monomorphic
Peripheral blood cytology				
	Monomorphic: villous lymphocytes (round and regular nucleus; clumped chromatin; small or not visible nucleolus; basophilic cytoplasm with polar, well-visible projections)	Polymorphous: small lymphocytes (round nucleus, condensed chromatin in small irregular clumps) admixed with lymphoplasmacytic cells	Monomorphic: intermediate between prolymphocytes and hairy cells, and distinguished from villous lymphocytes by prominent nucleolus	Monomorphic: hairy cells (oval and indented nucleus, dispersed chromatin, abundant and pale cytoplasm with circumference projections)
Immunophenotype by immunohistochemistry				
Cyclin D1	–	–	–	+
Cyclin D3	+	–	–	–
ANXA1	–	–	–	+
Immunophenotype by flow cytometry				
CD11c	Bright in ~67% of cases	Moderate in ~70% of cases	Bright in ~25% of cases	Bright in 100% of cases
CD180	Strong in 100% of cases	Moderate in 93% of cases	Not described	Strong in 100% of cases
CD200	Dim in 40% of cases	Moderate 93% of cases	Not described	Strong in 100% of cases
CD103	Positive in ~20% of cases	Negative	Positive in 65–100% of cases	Bright in 100% of cases
CD123	Positive in 3% of cases	Negative	Positive in 9% of cases	Bright in 100% of cases

hairy cells can be seen on smears, whereas nucleolated cells reminiscent of prolymphocytes are sparse. The immunophenotype is mostly characterized by the absence of markers that are diagnostic for other B-cell lymphomas such as HCL, chronic lymphocytic leukaemia, and mantle cell lymphoma. No positive defining immunophenotypic markers are available. The cytological and immunophenotypic features of the neoplastic cells in SDRPL are similar to those of SMZL in peripheral blood and bone marrow specimens, although nodular infiltrates in the bone marrow are rare. The distinction of SDRPL from SMZL is best made in the spleen, where SDRPL shows atrophic white pulp and diffuse involvement of the red pulp {4063}.

In this edition, the new term "splenic B-cell lymphoma/leukaemia with prominent nucleoli" (SBLPN) has been introduced for those primary splenic lymphomas that, based on currently available biological and clinical data, cannot be separated into biologically meaningful entities. These cases share the cytomorphological features of medium-sized to large atypical lymphoid cells with a large prominent single nucleolus reminiscent of prolymphocytes, have poorly defined cytoplasmic projections reminiscent of hairy cells {3528,2597}, and lack class-defining immunohistochemical markers. In splenic specimens, diffuse red pulp involvement is usually prominent; and in bone marrow biopsies, the intrasinusoidal infiltrates are generally present. SBLPN therefore has a morphological definition and is introduced to accommodate cases previously diagnosed as "hairy cell leukaemia variant" in recognition that the biology of this disease is unrelated to HCL and its quality as a separate entity is unproven {126,2489}. Moreover, the class also absorbs cases previously termed CD5-negative B-prolymphocytic leukaemia (B-PLL).

The entity B-PLL has, therefore, been omitted from the new edition. Since its introduction into the WHO Classification of Tumours in 2001, its heterogeneous nature had always been debated {1065}. As previously indicated in the revised fourth edition, the large majority of so-called B-PLLs represent either blastoid subtypes of mantle cell lymphoma with a prominent leukaemic component, or progression of underlying chronic lymphocytic leukaemia / small lymphocytic lymphoma (CLL/SLL), which can both be recognized using appropriate immunohistochemical and molecular markers. The remaining cases with morphological features defining SBLPN can be classified as such. It should be noted that SBLPN is not intended as a definite defined entity but should be regarded as a placeholder for those morphologically defined cases of primary splenic B-cell lymphoma that cannot be classified into biologically distinct entities on the basis of current evidence-based knowledge, awaiting further data to better define or refute SBLPN as representing one or more distinct lymphoma entities.

Table 4.19 Summary of the main molecular features of splenic diffuse red pulp small B-cell lymphoma (SDRPL), splenic marginal zone lymphoma (SMZL), splenic B-cell lymphoma/leukaemia with prominent nucleoli (SBLPN), and hairy cell leukaemia (HCL) {1780,850,3549,4067,4061,364,4016,3264,1030,3264,958,2488,4328,2488,2548}

Genetic lesion	SDRPL	SMZL	SBLPN	HCL
***BRAF* p.V600E mutations**	–	–	–	+ (> 95%)
7q deletions	+ (18%)	+ (~30%)	+ (~20%)	+ (up to 20%)
***CDKN1B* mutations**	Rare	–	–	+ (16%)
***KMT2C* mutations**	–	–	+ (25%)	+ (16%)
***KLF2* mutations**	Rare	+ (~20–40%)	–	+ (16%)
***KLF2* deletions**	–	+ (11%)	–	–
***TP53* deletions and/or mutations**	Rare	+ (~15–20%)	+ (33%)	Rare
***MAP2K1* mutations**	+ (10%)	Rare	+ (38–42%)	–
***NOTCH2* mutations**	Rare	+ (~15–25%)	–	–
***CCND3* mutations**	+ (~25%)	Rare	+ (21–24%)	–
***U2AF1* mutations**	Rare	–	+ (13%)	–
***BCOR* mutations/ deletions**	+ (16–24%)	+ (< 10%)	–	–
NF-κB pathway gene alterations[a]	–	+ (~35%)	–	–

+, genetic lesion present (in the indicated percentage of cases); –, genetic lesion absent.
[a]Including *IKBKB, TNFAIP3, TRAF3, MAP3K14, TRAF2, BIRC3*, and *MYD88*.

Hairy cell leukaemia

Lim MS
Molina TJ
Montes-Moreno S
Siebert R
Stamatopoulos KE
Tiacci E

Definition

Hairy cell leukaemia (HCL) is an indolent mature B-cell neoplasm composed of neoplastic cells with abundant cytoplasm and characteristic hairy projections that usually involve the bone marrow, peripheral blood, and spleen and bear the *BRAF* p.V600E somatic mutation in ≥ 95% of cases.

ICD-O coding

9940/3 Hairy cell leukaemia

ICD-11 coding

2A82.2 Hairy cell leukaemia

Related terminology

None

Subtype(s)

None

Localization

HCL involves the bone marrow, spleen, and peripheral blood. Significant lymphocytosis is infrequent. Lymphadenopathy and infiltration of extranodal sites, such as the liver, bone, skin, breast, and brain, occur rarely {3465,784,3525,3240,4501,3199,1142}.

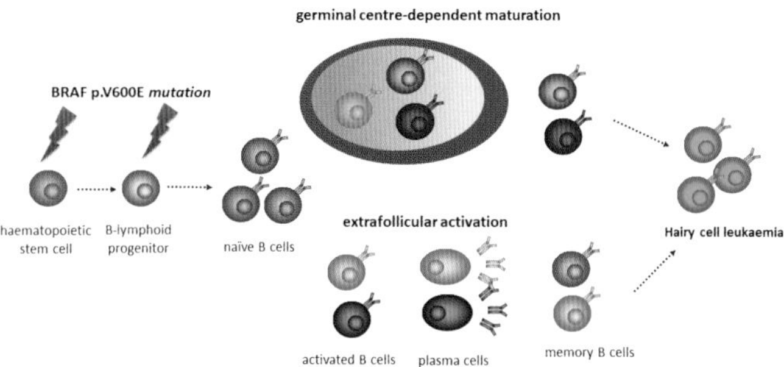

Fig. 4.61 Putative cellular origin of hairy cell leukaemia (HCL). Pinning down with certainty the exact cell of origin of HCL is currently not possible, because of several distinctive features of the malignant cells, including frequent coexpression in the same cell of multiple switched and unswitched immunoglobulin transcripts with a dominance in the IgG3 subclass {2057,1216,1217}; AID (AICDA) expression {1603,1079}; lack of allelic exclusion of immunoglobulin light chains, which occurs at a higher frequency (3–4% of HCL cases) {3804} than in the normal human peripheral repertoire (< 0.5%) {1336}; and a lack of CD27 expression {1215,1214}. Together, this constellation of features renders the quest for the normal counterpart of HCL cells particularly challenging, with possibilities abounding, including cells that could follow follicular or extrafollicular maturation pathways. It is unclear whether neoplastic transformation of one such cell requires additional genetic lesions developing after *BRAF* p.V600E occurrence in the stem/B-progenitor compartment, and/or whether neoplastic transformation is licensed by a permissive epigenetic landscape that is exclusive of a particular mature B-cell differentiation stage in a particular microenvironment with its specific cues (e.g. antigenic stimulation). The latter hypothesis may be favoured by the fact that genetic lesions other than in *BRAF* recur in a small minority of HCL cases (see Table 4.19, p. 379), whereas BRAF inhibition in the full-blown leukaemic clone appears sufficient to consistently repress several key tumour traits of HCL {3216,4015}.

Clinical features

Patients usually present with pancytopenia (including monocytopenia), low-level circulating leukaemic cells, and splenomegaly. The presence of related signs and symptoms (fatigue, fever, opportunistic infections, bleeding, discomfort or pain in the upper-left quadrant, night sweats) is variable and correlates with the extent of disease, disease duration, and degree of cytopenias {1413,3328}. Hepatomegaly can occur, whereas lymphadenopathy is uncommon at disease onset. Rarely, HCL can be associated with paraneoplastic/autoimmune vasculitis, arthritis, dermatitis, or neuropathy {3922}.

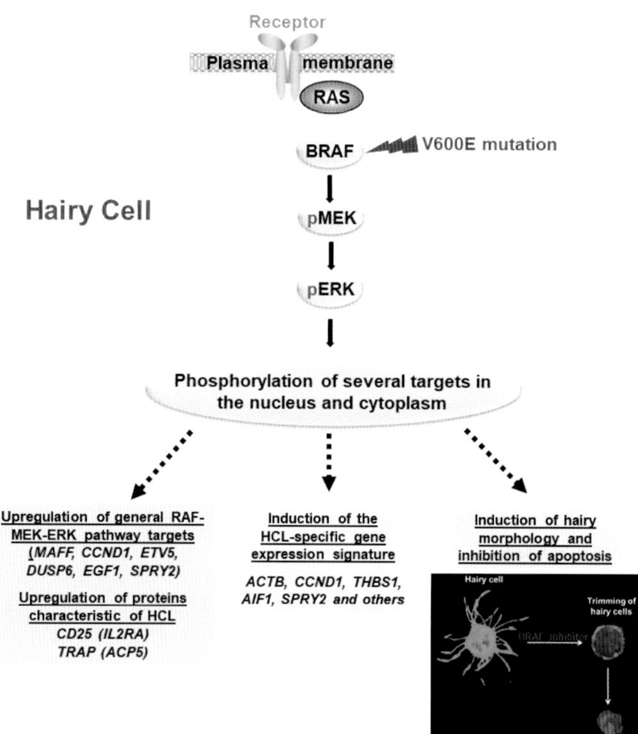

Fig. 4.62 Hairy cell leukaemia (HCL). Pathogenetic role of *BRAF* p.V600E mutations in HCL. The p.V600E missense mutation in the cytosolic serine-threonine kinase BRAF leads to its constitutive activation (independent from upstream regulation by RAS at the plasma membrane) and hence to downstream phosphorylation of the kinases MAP2K1 (MEK1) and MAP2K2 (MEK2) (pMEK) that in turn phosphorylate the kinase ERK1/2 (pERK). Subsequent phosphorylated ERK–mediated phosphorylation of numerous targets in the nucleus and the cytoplasm promotes, in general, survival, proliferation, growth, and motility; in the specific context of the HCL cell, among the genes transcriptionally upregulated by the RAF/MEK/ERK signalling pathway, there are not only those common to most cell types but also some characteristic markers of this leukaemia (i.e. CD25 and TRAP) and the whole expression signature distinguishing HCL from normal mature B-cell subsets and mature B-cell neoplasms. Finally, aberrant pathway activity induces the typical hairy morphology and inhibits apoptosis, as shown in the confocal immunofluorescence image of a primary HCL cell exposed in vitro to the BRAF inhibitor vemurafenib, which first trims the hairy projections (rich in F-actin and thus labelled in green by the cytoskeleton marker phalloidin) and then induces apoptosis (red, ANXA5; blue, nuclear dye DRAQ5).

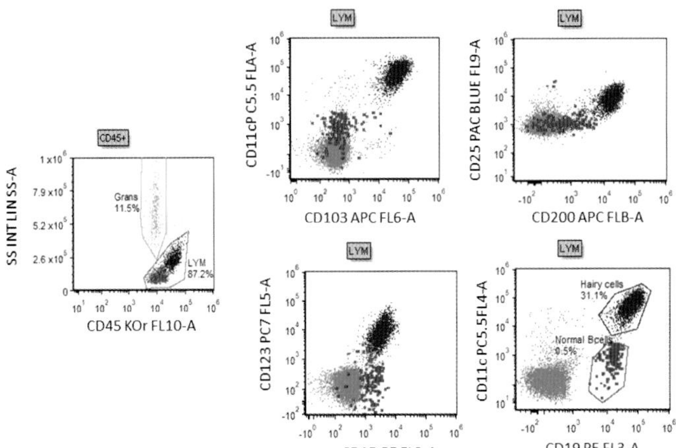

Fig. 4.63 Hairy cell leukaemia. Flow cytometric analysis of hairy cell leukaemia demonstrates CD19-positive B cells with coexpression of CD11c, CD103, CD25, CD200, CD123, and CD1d.

Epidemiology

HCL is a rare disease, accounting for 2% of all leukaemias, and its incidence is 0.28–0.3 cases per 100 000 person-years in Europe and the USA {3993,1302}. HCL is less frequent in individuals of Asian, African, and Arab descent than in individuals of European descent {3921}. There is a male predominance (M:F ratio: ~4:1) and the median age at diagnosis is about 60 years {628,1834}. It is extremely rare in children and young adults.

Etiology

The precise etiology is unknown. Inherited susceptibility to HCL is suggested by the overrepresentation of the HLA-DRB*11 allele in patients of European descent compared with a matched healthy control population {150} and, potentially, by the rare occurrence of familial cases {4429,4234,3503,2772, 3184}. Farming and exposure to pesticides have been associated with an increased risk of HCL {757,756,2731,1498}. High exposure to benzene may also be a risk factor {3364}.

Pathogenesis

The somatic genetic lesion underlying almost all HCL cases (> 95%) is the activating *BRAF* p.V600E (NP_004324.2) mutation, a founding clonal event stable throughout the disease course {4016}. The mutation results in constitutive activation of the kinase BRAF and aberrant downstream signalling through the MEK/ERK pathway {4018}. *BRAF* p.V600E (NP_004324.2) mutation is the key driver genetic event and profoundly contributes to the unique morphological, immunophenotypic, and transcriptional identity of HCL, while sustaining leukaemic growth {3216,4015}. Rare cases carrying alternative *BRAF* mutations {4092} or *BRAF* translocation to the IGH locus {4005} have also been described. The *BRAF* p.V600E (NP_004324.2) mutation arises and expands in haematopoietic stem and B-lymphoid progenitor cells {745}. However, because HCL invariably carries clonal IG gene rearrangements, it originates from the neoplastic transformation of a single *BRAF*-mutant mature B cell. Indeed, HCL has a transcriptional signature most similar to that of post–germinal-centre memory B cells {266}; this finding, combined with the substantial load of somatic hypermutation in the clonotypic immunoglobulin heavy chain and/or light chain variable genes in > 90% of cases {4009,2559, 1217}, implicates derivation from an antigen-experienced B cell. However, the corresponding normal cell counterpart of HCL is uncertain. Additional genetic lesions are present in HCL at relatively low frequencies (see Table 4.19, p. 379, in *Splenic B-cell lymphomas and leukaemias: Introduction*), including heterozygous deletion of 7q with loss of the wildtype *BRAF* allele at 7q34 (thus resulting in hemizygosity for the mutant *BRAF* allele) as well as mutations of the transcription factor *KLF2* (involved in marginal zone B-cell differentiation) {765,3264,4016}, the cyclin-dependent kinase inhibitor *CDKN1B*, and the histone methyltransferase *KMT2C* {1030,3264,958,2488}.

Macroscopic appearance

The spleen is markedly enlarged; cut sections show diffuse expansion of the red pulp with scattered blood lakes. Splenic infarction can be present {430}.

Histopathology

Peripheral blood

In the peripheral blood or marrow smear, neoplastic cells are small to intermediate in size with oval to indented kidney-shaped nuclei with bland ground-glass chromatin that is less clumped than that of normal lymphocytes. Nucleoli are inconspicuous or absent. The cytoplasm is variably abundant and pale blue with prominent and fine villous (hairy) projections circumferentially located, and it may have small vacuoles {341,3705}.

Bone marrow

The diagnosis of HCL is usually made on a bone marrow biopsy. The neoplastic cells primarily involve the marrow, with a patchy or interstitial pattern and variable preservation of background haematopoietic elements. Infiltration is usually diffuse when the disease burden is high; in exceptional cases, isolated intrasinusoidal involvement can be observed {3260,2676,2561}. The low-power appearance of the neoplastic cells often exhibits a characteristic fried-egg appearance attributable to the abundant cytoplasm widely spacing the oval or indented nuclei and prominent cell-to-cell borders. The infiltration pattern of HCL differs from that of other indolent B-cell neoplasms, which usually feature discrete aggregates with more densely packed nuclei. Mitotic figures are virtually never seen. Because of the small size of neoplastic cells with minimal cytological atypia, low-level

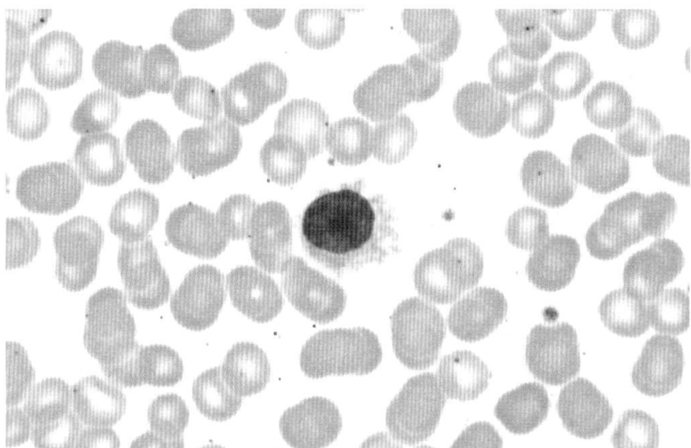

Fig. 4.64 Hairy cell leukaemia. Peripheral blood smear demonstrates neoplastic cells that are small to intermediate-sized lymphocytes with bland ground-glass chromatin. The cytoplasm is variably abundant with fine villous projections.

involvement may be difficult to identify by histological examination alone. Extravasated erythrocytes, sometimes surrounded by neoplastic cells, are often observed in infiltrated areas. The extent of involvement is variable and, in some cases, associated with a hypocellular marrow, mimicking aplastic anaemia. Reticulin fibrosis is induced by the HCL infiltrate and frequently leads to a dry tap or a haemodiluted marrow aspirate.

Spleen, liver, and other tissues

HCL typically diffusely involves the red pulp of the spleen, accompanied by atrophy of the white pulp. The blood lakes recognized on macroscopic examination are composed of pools of red blood cells that may be surrounded by aggregates of HCL cells thought to result from disrupted blood flow in the red pulp {341,3705}. The liver may also show sinusoidal infiltrates. The lymph node may be involved in advanced disease and typically shows infiltration of the interfollicular and paracortical areas.

Immunophenotype

The characteristic immunophenotype of HCL is expression of bright surface immunoglobulin, CD20, CD22, CD11c, CD103, CD25, CD123, TBX21 (T-bet), ANXA1, FMC7, CD200, and cyclin D1 (usually weak, sometimes focal) {2691,1117,1818,3712, 1299,4409}. CD5 or CD10 can rarely be expressed in HCL {675,1770}. Immunohistochemical staining for BRAF p.V600E (NP_004324.2) mutant protein using the mutation-specific VE1 antibody clone is helpful to identify HCL cells {4105}.

Differential diagnosis

Patients with HCL are sometimes initially referred for the suspicion of other conditions with a partially overlapping clinical picture, including myelodysplastic neoplasms and megaloblastic or aplastic anaemia. Cases with partial HCL infiltration can show some dyserythropoiesis in the form of hyperplastic pro-erythroblasts and basophilic erythroblasts, which may further confound the differential diagnoses above. The major differential diagnoses are other small B-cell lymphomas with splenomegaly but little or no lymphadenopathy and the presence of circulating lymphoid cells with or without villous projections, including splenic B-cell lymphoma/leukaemia with prominent nucleoli, splenic diffuse red pulp small B-cell lymphoma, and splenic marginal zone lymphoma (see Table 4.18, p. 378, in *Splenic B-cell lymphomas and leukaemias: Introduction*, for a summary of the morphological, immunophenotypic, and molecular differential features of these entities). Thereby, ANXA1 expression is a highly specific marker of HCL {1117}, and molecular features including mutation status of MAPK pathway genes (*BRAF*, *MAP2K1*), NOTCH pathway genes (*NOTCH1*, *NOTCH2*), BCOR alterations, and IGHV gene usage can be supportive {152,151,4328,2488,2122}.

Cytology

See above.

Diagnostic molecular pathology

A clonal *BRAF* p.V600E (NP_004324.2) mutation is the genetic hallmark of HCL and is useful for confirming the diagnosis and

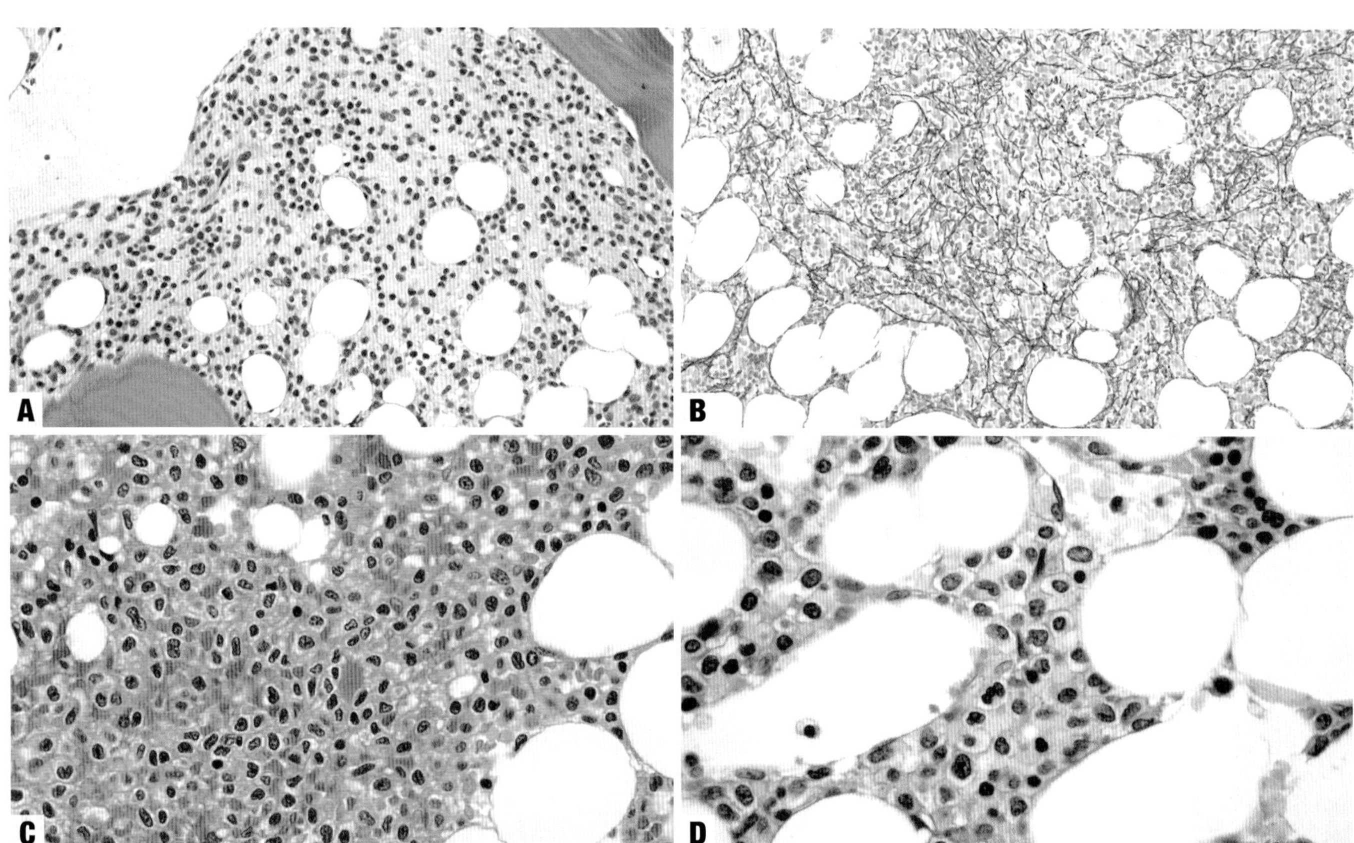

Fig. 4.65 Hairy cell leukaemia, bone marrow involvement. **A** Bone marrow core biopsy with interstitial infiltration of small lymphocytes with abundant cytoplasm and variable preservation of background haematopoietic elements. **B** Higher magnification demonstrates characteristic fried-egg appearance with abundant cytoplasm widely spacing the cells with prominent cell-to-cell borders. **C** Extravasated erythrocytes and small blood lakes are present. **D** Note the diffuse increase in reticulin fibrosis.

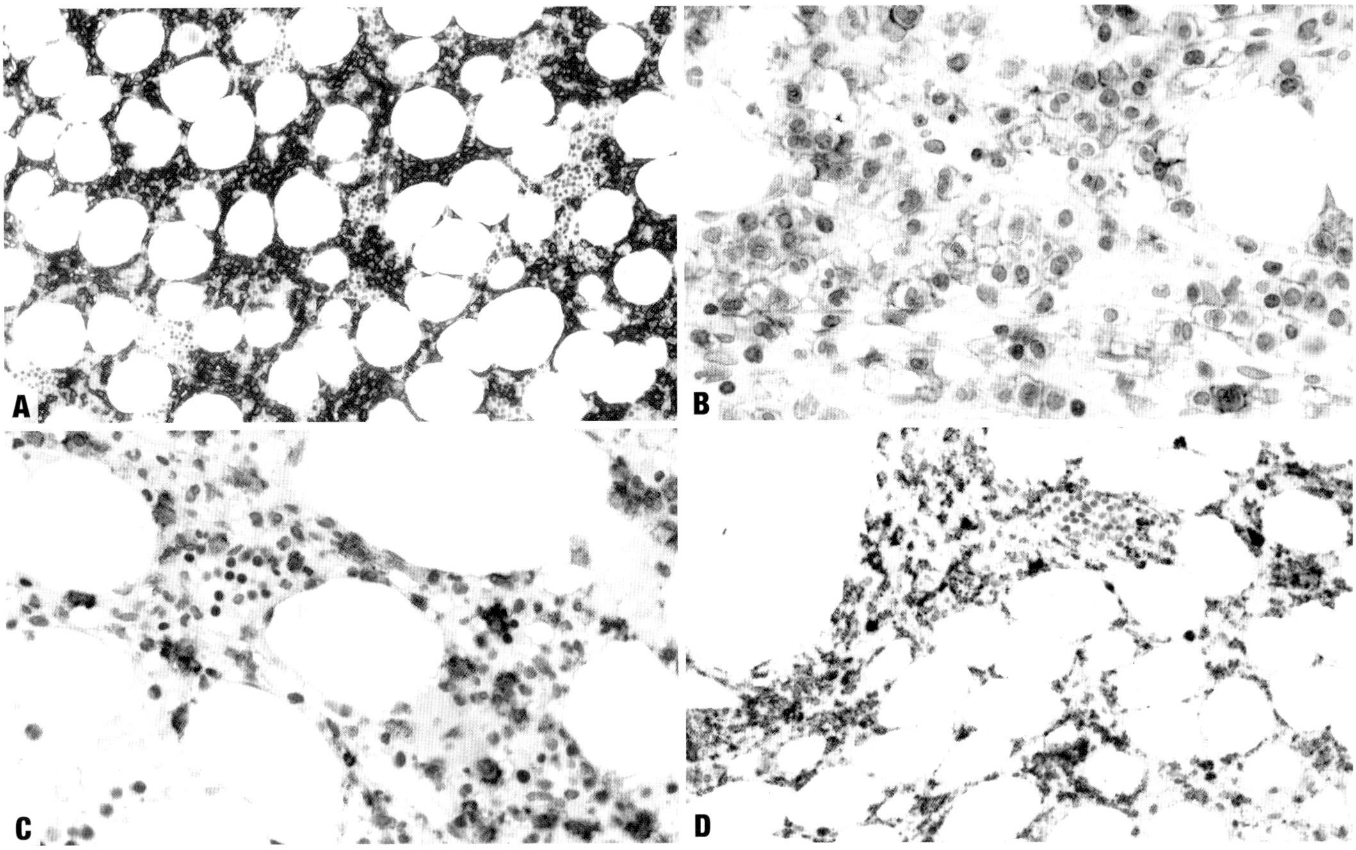

Fig. 4.66 Hairy cell leukaemia. Immunophenotype. **A** CD20 highlights an interstitial pattern of bone marrow infiltration. The neoplastic cells are highlighted by CD103 (**B**) and show partial expression of DBA44 (**C**). **D** Immunohistochemistry using a BRAF p.V600E antibody is positive.

for distinguishing HCL from the other splenic small B-cell neoplasms, particularly splenic B-cell lymphoma/leukaemia with prominent nucleoli and splenic diffuse red pulp small B-cell lymphoma, which lack this genetic lesion {4016}. However, the clinicopathological context appropriate for HCL should also be present, as anecdotal cases of *BRAF* p.V600E (NP_004324.2)-positive splenic marginal zone lymphoma or chronic lymphocytic leukaemia have been reported {4105,1344}. *BRAF* p.V600E (NP_004324.2) can be detected by allele-specific PCR (conventional or digital) {4017,143,3633,1436}, targeted deep sequencing {1030,2488} or, when DNA is not available {1414}, immunohistochemistry with the mutation-specific VE1 antibody clone {122,469,4127}.

Essential and desirable diagnostic criteria

Essential: characteristic morphology in a blood or marrow smear (small to intermediate-sized cells with oval to indented nuclei with bland ground-glass chromatin, absent or inconspicuous nucleoli, and variably abundant pale-staining cytoplasm with circumferential fine villous cytoplasmic projections) and/or in a marrow biopsy (characteristic fried-egg appearance, with cells having oval or indented nuclei, abundant cytoplasm,

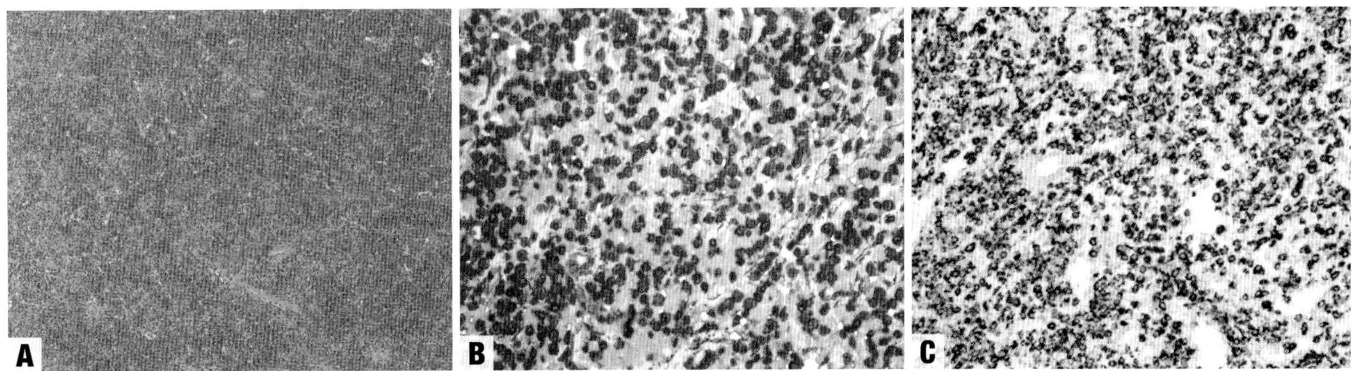

Fig. 4.67 Hairy cell leukaemia. **A** Characteristic infiltrates involving the splenic red pulp and atrophy of the white pulp. Pools of red blood cells surround aggregates of hairy cell leukaemia cells. **B** The neoplastic cells involving the spleen are highlighted by ANXA1. **C** Immunohistochemistry using BRAF p.V600E antibody demonstrates infiltration of the splenic red pulp by neoplastic cells.

and prominent cell-to-cell borders); strong positivity for CD20 and ANXA1 by immunohistochemistry or coexpression of CD20/CD11c/CD103/CD25 by flow cytometry and/or immunohistochemistry.

Desirable: clonal *BRAF* p.V600E (NP_004324.2) mutation; positivity for CD123, CD22 (bright), CD200 (bright), surface immunoglobulins (bright), cyclin D1, and TBX21 (T-bet) by flow cytometry and/or immunohistochemistry.

Staging

No staging system is routinely used in the management of HCL. Treatment initiation is guided by the degree of cytopenia and disease-related symptoms {3423,1414}.

Prognosis and prediction

Chemotherapy with purine analogues (cladribine and pentostatin) is highly effective as a first-line treatment for HCL, but there are no validated clinical or molecular prognostic factors to identify the minority of patients with a suboptimal response. Clonal *BRAF* p.V600E (NP_004324.2) mutation and bright CD22 expression may explain the high effectiveness respectively shown by BRAF inhibitors (either alone or, even more, with rituximab) and anti-CD22 immunotoxin therapy in patients who relapse after or are refractory to chemotherapy {3603,2339,4013,2123,3422}. Persistence of minimal/measurable residual disease after response to chemotherapy or targeted drugs correlates with a shorter time to relapse {707, 2123,3422}.

Splenic marginal zone lymphoma

Lim MS
Arcaini L
Naresh KN
Rossi D
Traverse-Glehen A

Definition
Splenic marginal zone lymphoma (SMZL) is an indolent mature B-cell neoplasm primarily presenting in the spleen, preferentially involving the white pulp, often with villous lymphocytes in the peripheral blood, with or without involvement of splenic hilar lymph nodes.

ICD-O coding
9689/3 Splenic marginal zone lymphoma

ICD-11 coding
2A82.Y & XH0MV1 Other specified mature B-cell neoplasm with leukaemic behaviour & Splenic marginal zone B-cell lymphoma

Related terminology
Not recommended: splenic lymphoma with villous lymphocytes.

Subtype(s)
None

Localization
SMZL typically presents with splenomegaly and involvement of the splenic hilar lymph nodes, bone marrow, and peripheral blood, and occasionally with microscopic hepatic involvement. Lymph nodes other than splenic hilar nodes are typically uninvolved {1481,434}.

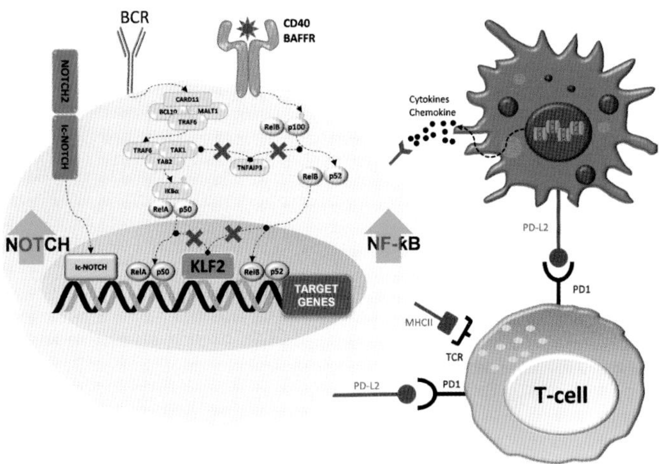

Fig. 4.68 Key molecular alterations and microenvironmental interactions of splenic marginal zone lymphoma. Main genes and pathways that are molecularly deregulated are schematically represented. The most frequently mutated genes are colour-coded on the basis of the consequences of the mutations: in purple are genes that lose function, and in red are genes whose function is upregulated. The interactions between macrophages (at the top) and T cells (at the bottom) with the splenic marginal zone lymphoma tumour cells are shown, with the key factors involved in the interaction. BCR, B-cell receptor.

Clinical features
SMZL is often diagnosed after the incidental finding of lymphocytosis or splenomegaly. Other patients present with symptoms related to cytopenias or massive splenomegaly (e.g. early satiety and left upper abdominal discomfort). Such symptoms may also develop with progression {2732}. Systemic symptoms (e.g. fever and night sweats) are rare and suggest transformation to an aggressive lymphoma {790,64}. Approximately 30% of patients have a low-level paraprotein without significant hyperviscosity {2732}. Twenty per cent of patients present with autoimmune manifestations {3751} (acquired angio-oedema due to C1 esterase inhibitor deficiency {570}, cold agglutinin disease {321,3910}, warm antibody autoimmune haemolytic anaemia {3551}, and mixed cryoglobulinaemia {2757}).

Epidemiology
Patients are mostly middle-aged and older adults, with a median age in the seventh decade of life. The age-standardized incidence rate of SMZL is 1.7 cases per 1 million person-years. Incidence increases exponentially with age and is slightly higher among men and non-Hispanic White people {587}. The relative frequency of SMZL is similar in high-income countries and low- and middle-income countries {3198}.

Etiology
The etiology is unknown in most cases. A family history of lymphoma and a personal medical history of autoimmune conditions are associated with SMZL {442}. Genetic variations in the MHC influence SMZL susceptibility {4232}. Epidemiological and clinical evidence supports the role of HCV in the pathogenesis of a subset of SMZL, particularly in areas with a high seroprevalence of HCV. HCV infection is a predisposing condition for SMZL, and the risk increases when complicated by cryoglobulinaemia. Furthermore, successful treatment of HCV may reduce the risk of lymphoma in patients who achieve a sustained virological response, particularly those treated with interferon, and it may lead to regression of lymphoma in patients with SMZL {142}.

Pathogenesis
Immunoglobulin heavy and light chain genes are clonally rearranged. Somatic mutations of the rearranged IG genes with ongoing diversification occur in most cases. IGHV gene usage is significantly skewed in SMZL; IGHV1-2*04 is employed by about 30% of all cases {4446}. The immunogenetic features highlight (auto)antigen selection pressure as a driver of lymphomagenesis and point towards a marginal zone B-cell as the cell of origin. At the cytogenetic level, about 30% of SMZLs show hemizygous deletion of 7q31-32, which is otherwise virtually absent in B-cell lymphoproliferative disorders; the specific genes targeted by this deletion remain unknown

{2582,3502,4196,4330,1234,4329}. Co-occurrence of trisomies of chromosomes 3 and 18 is observed in about 25% of cases {3414}, shared among the three marginal zone lymphoma entities, but it is infrequent in other B-cell neoplasms. Rarely, SMZL harbours a recurrent translocation juxtaposing the oncogene *CDK6* to transcriptionally active IG gene loci {804,1270}, whereas it lacks the translocations of *MALT1* (and others), *BCL2*, and *CCND1* that are recurrent in extranodal marginal zone lymphoma, follicular lymphoma, and mantle cell lymphoma, respectively.

Two prominent genetic clusters have been defined in SMZL, termed NNK (4-[N-methyl-N-nitrosamino]-1-[3-pyridyl]-1-butanone), occurring in about ~60% of cases, and DMT (differentially methylated targets), occurring in about 30% of cases. NNK-SMZLs are dominated by mutations affecting NF-κB (e.g. *TNFAIP3*), including non-canonical pathway genes (e.g. *TRAF3*, *BIRC3*), NOTCH (e.g. *NOTCH2*, *NOTCH1*, *SPEN*), and *KLF2*, a master transcriptional regulator of both NOTCH and NF-κB signalling. DMT-SMZLs are characterized by mutations in DNA damage response genes (e.g. *TP53*, *ATM*), MAPK (e.g. *BRAF*), and toll-like receptor signalling genes (e.g. *MYD88*) {401}. NNK-SMZLs are enriched in IGHV1-2*04 usage and 7q31-32 deletion, whereas DMT-SMZL lack both of these features {401}. SMZL is characterized by two distinct types of immune microenvironment, of which one is dominantly immunosuppressive (50% of cases, associated with inflammatory cells and immune checkpoint activation) and the other is immune-silent (50% of cases, associated with an immune-excluded phenotype) {401} (see Table 4.19, p. 379, in *Splenic B-cell lymphomas and leukaemias: Introduction*).

Macroscopic appearance

Splenectomy specimens show parenchymal abnormalities, with variably sized, pale white-yellow nodules consistent with expanded white pulp.

Histopathology

In most cases the diagnosis of SMZL rests on peripheral blood and bone marrow findings. A diagnosis of SMZL is made on splenectomy specimens in only a minority of cases.

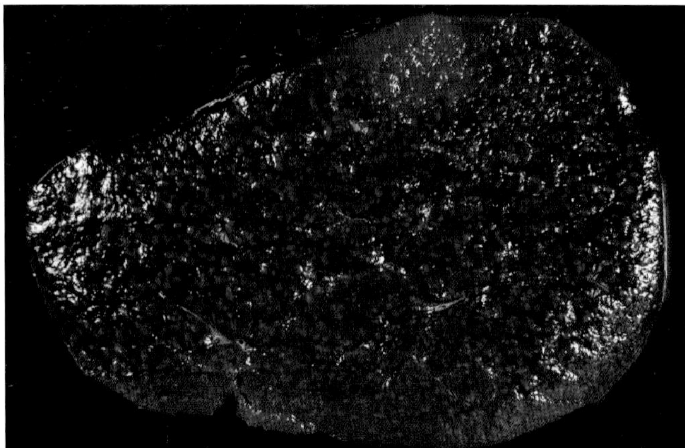

Fig. 4.69 Splenic marginal zone lymphoma. This markedly enlarged spleen, weighing 3300 g and measuring 340 mm in greatest dimension, shows prominent white pulp.

Spleen

The spleen typically shows involvement of both the white pulp and the red pulp. There is typically prominent white pulp, characterized by a variably expanded population of small lymphoid cells that surround reactive germinal centres, with a peripheral zone of cells with moderately abundant pale cytoplasm. Neoplastic lymphocytes also infiltrate the red pulp, forming small clusters and typically involving both sinuses and cords. Lymphoid cells have round to oval nuclei that are frequently minimally indented/cleaved. Scattered larger cells with nucleoli usually account for a small minority of neoplastic cells. Germinal centres may show follicular colonization. Small aggregates of epithelioid histiocytes may be seen both within and outside the white pulp. Some cases show plasmacytoid differentiation {2719,1738,1481,2600}.

Splenic hilar lymph nodes

Lymph nodes show variable involvement by neoplastic cells. Sinuses are typically dilated. Neoplastic lymphocytes populate marginal zones surrounding follicles but also may form irregular clusters.

Bone marrow

The extent of marrow involvement is variable. The biopsy commonly shows intertrabecular nodules along with interstitial and focally intrasinusoidal infiltrates of small lymphoid cells with a scant to moderate amount of pale cytoplasm. Occasionally, neoplastic cells diffusely infiltrate the marrow. Rare cases show marginal zone expansion surrounding reactive follicles. CD20 immunostaining is often helpful in identifying intrasinusoidal infiltrates {1228,185,2600}. Normal haematopoietic elements may be increased, particularly in cases with hypersplenism.

Peripheral blood

Peripheral blood shows mild to moderate lymphocytosis. Neoplastic cells are mature small to medium-sized lymphoid cells with round nuclei, condensed chromatin, and basophilic cytoplasm with short villi, which may be unevenly distributed or concentrated at one or two poles of the cell. There is often morphological heterogeneity, featuring small lymphoid cells without specific features, lymphoplasmacytoid cells, lymphocytes with nuclear clefts, and/or medium-sized lymphoid cells with relatively abundant pale cytoplasm {2638}.

Immunophenotype

The neoplastic cells express CD20, CD79a, PAX5, FMC7, CD27, CD38 (dim), IgM, and IgD and are negative for BCL6, ANXA1, CD103, cyclin D1, SOX11, and LEF1. A small subset of cases expresses CD11c, CD123, CD5 (usually weak), or CD43. Rare cases are positive for CD10. About one third to half of cases express CD25 and DBA44. CD200 expression is usually dim {2598,3595,2600,260,2092,4207,609}. When SMZL forms nodules, CD21 often identifies associated FDC meshworks. Cases with plasmacytic or plasmacytoid differentiation may show light chain restriction on paraffin sections. Residual reactive germinal centres in splenic white pulp are CD10+ and BCL2–, with a high Ki-67 proliferation index. Ki-67 is elevated in peripherally located proliferating marginal zone cells, highlighting a targetoid pattern. BCL2 is positive in the neoplastic cells.

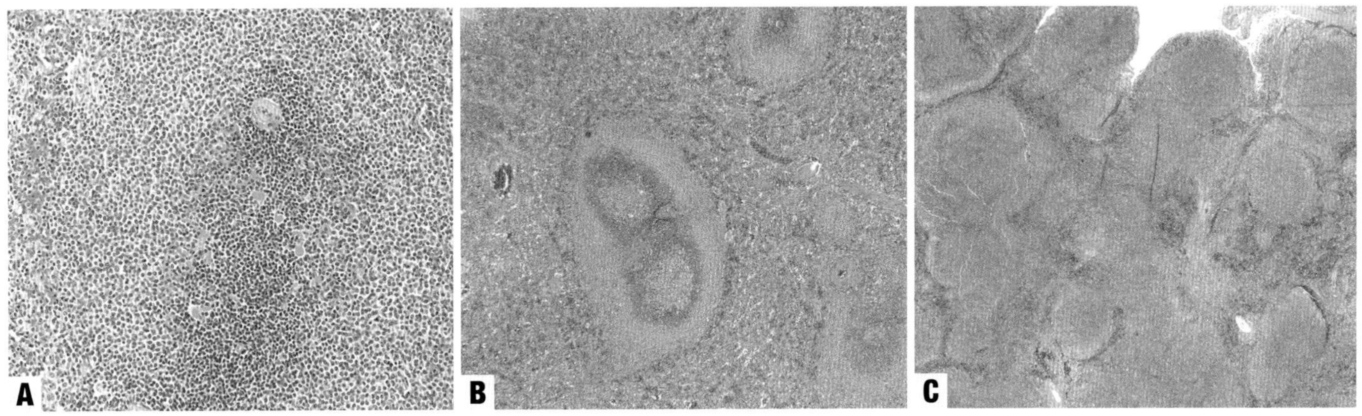

Fig. 4.70 Splenic marginal zone lymphoma. **A** An atypical population of small to medium-sized lymphocytes with variably abundant cytoplasm and plasmacytoid differentiation involves the splenic white and red pulp. **B** A striking targetoid pattern in the white pulp can be present. **C** Perihilar lymph node involvement with expansion of the marginal zones by monocytoid B cells.

Comprehensive immunophenotypic characterization is helpful in distinguishing SMZL from other small B-cell lymphomas that may involve the spleen.

Differential diagnosis

SMZL may be difficult to distinguish from other B-cell lymphomas, especially on bone marrow and peripheral blood evaluation. In some instances, a definitive diagnosis of SMZL can be established only after extensive clinical, radiographic, and pathology workup, including the integration of cytogenetic and molecular findings. Other small B-cell lymphomas, such as follicular lymphoma, chronic lymphocytic leukaemia / small lymphocytic lymphoma (CLL/SLL), hairy cell leukaemia, and mantle cell lymphoma, should be excluded using immunophenotypic and genetic studies. Other splenic lymphomas, including hairy cell leukaemia, splenic B-cell lymphoma/leukaemia with prominent nucleoli (encompassing cases previously called hairy cell leukaemia variant, a subset of those previously called B-prolymphocytic leukaemia, and a few others), and splenic diffuse red pulp small B-cell lymphoma, predominantly involve the red pulp and may all be associated with circulating lymphoma cells with variably abundant cytoplasm with or without villous projections. Splenic diffuse red pulp lymphoma shows a monomorphic diffuse infiltration of red pulp with atrophic white pulp and may rarely be difficult to distinguish from massive white and red pulp infiltration by SMZL (see Table 4.18, p. 378, in *Splenic B-cell lymphomas and leukaemias: Introduction*).

Cytology

Touch preparations of spleen show small to medium-sized lymphoid cells with a relative abundance of pale cytoplasm.

Diagnostic molecular pathology

Immunoglobulin heavy and light chain genes are clonally rearranged. Deletion of 7q31-32 is the sole molecular biomarker that specifically associates with SMZL. *NOTCH2* and *KLF2* mutations occur in both SMZL and nodal marginal zone lymphoma, although they are rare in other small B-cell lymphomas. Translocations that are characteristic of other small B-cell lymphomas are not observed in SMZL and may help in the distinction.

Essential and desirable diagnostic criteria

Essential: small B-cell lymphoma involving bone marrow and/or peripheral blood, composed of small lymphoid cells with villous processes; positive expression of pan–B-cell markers, IgM, and IgD, and negative for BCL6, ANXA1, CD103, cyclin D1, SOX11, and LEF1; exclusion of other splenic and nodal B-cell lymphomas; clinical or imaging studies that show splenomegaly.

Desirable: neoplastic cells that are negative for CD5 and CD10.

Staging

Staging uses the Lugano modifications of the Ann Arbor system {688}. Imaging studies help assess splenomegaly and involvement of hilar and extrahilar lymph nodes. Peripheral blood and bone marrow biopsies are useful to identify and quantify leukaemic disease. PET-CT may assist in directing biopsies in cases of suspected large-cell transformation.

Prognosis and prediction

The clinical course of SMZL is generally indolent, with a median survival time of > 10 years {1204}. Like in other indolent lymphomas, early progression after treatment, which occurs in about 20% of patients, is the strongest prognostic biomarker

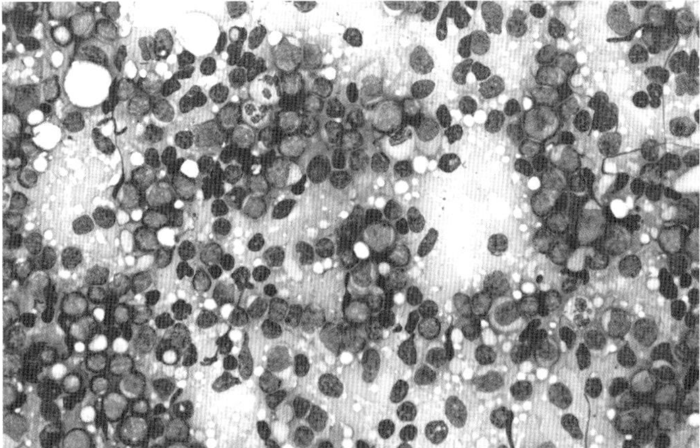

Fig. 4.71 Splenic marginal zone lymphoma. Giemsa-stained touch preparation of splenic marginal zone lymphoma demonstrates a spectrum of atypical medium-sized lymphocytes with variably abundant cytoplasm.

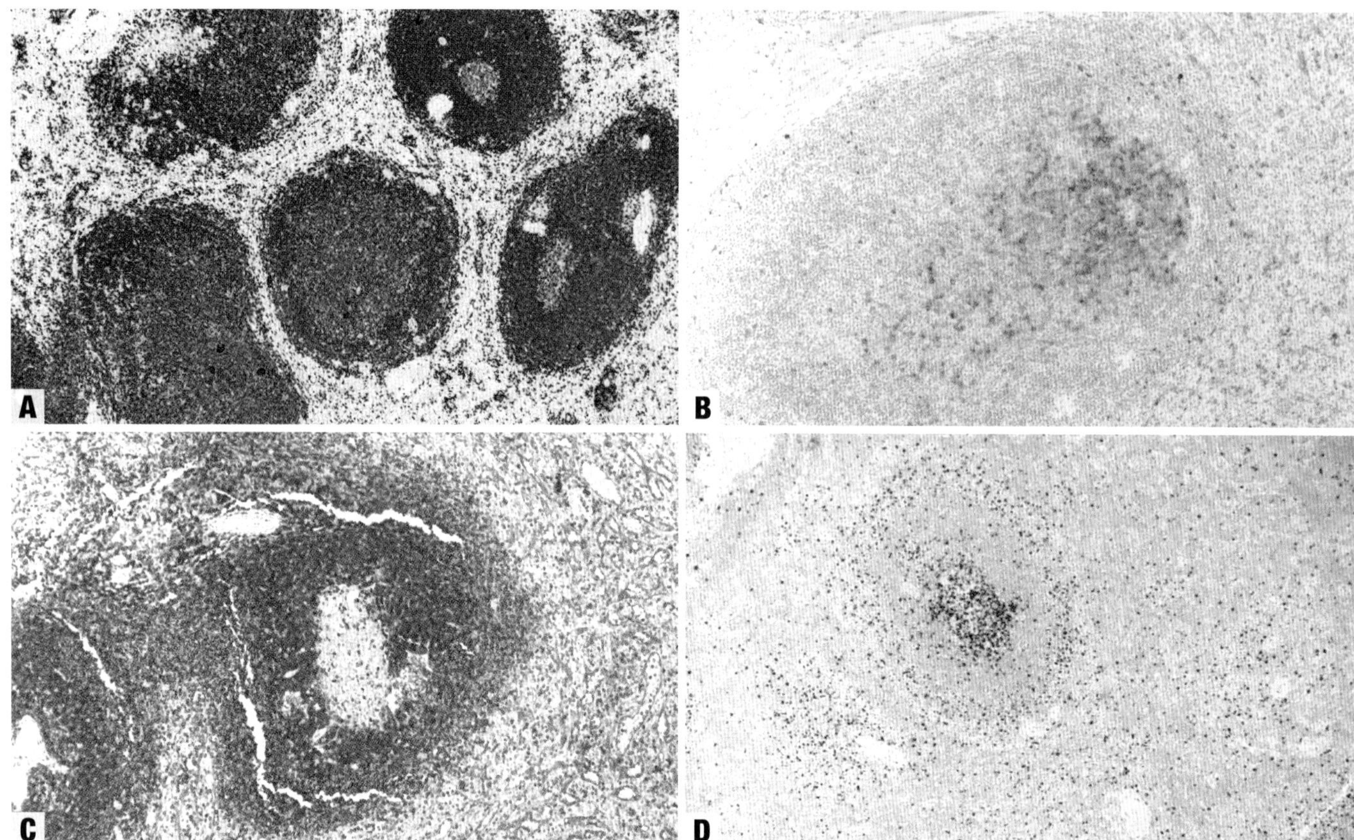

Fig. 4.72 Splenic marginal zone lymphoma. **A** CD20-positive neoplastic cells with a nodular and marginal zone growth pattern. **B** CD10 highlights mildly disrupted germinal centres, which are surrounded by the neoplastic cells. **C** BCL2 highlights the expanded marginal zones by neoplastic cells, whereas the naked reactive germinal centres are negative. **D** Reactive germinal centres show high proliferation, and proliferating neoplastic cells within the expanded marginal zone are accentuated by Ki-67 staining against the low proliferation of non-malignant mantle and marginal zones.

affecting survival: patients with early progression of disease (< 24 months) have a median survival time of only 3–5 years, whereas patients without early progression of disease have a survival time similar to that of the matched general population {2447}. Transformation into an aggressive lymphoma is a poor prognostic biomarker {2671,790,64}. The HPLL score, based on specific clinical biomarkers (i.e. low haemoglobin, low platelet count, high LDH level, and occurrence of extrahilar lymphadenopathy), is validated and may be used for the prognostic stratification of SMZL {2732}. Patients with SMZL harbouring *NOTCH2* mutations, *KLF2* mutations, and the NNK molecular genotype have inferior outcomes {401}.

Splenic diffuse red pulp small B-cell lymphoma

Traverse-Glehen A
Lim MS
Molina TJ
Mollejo M
Montes-Moreno S
Siebert R
Stamatopoulos KE

Definition

Splenic diffuse red pulp small B-cell lymphoma (SDRPL) is a small B-cell lymphoma involving the spleen, bone marrow, and peripheral blood, characterized by diffuse infiltration of the splenic red pulp by a monomorphic lymphoid population associated with circulating tumour cells bearing cytoplasmic projections.

ICD-O coding

9591/3 Splenic diffuse red pulp small B-cell lymphoma

ICD-11 coding

2A82.Y & XH99V9 Other specified mature B-cell neoplasm with leukaemic behaviour & Splenic diffuse red pulp small B-cell lymphoma

Related terminology

Not recommended: splenic B-cell lymphoma/leukaemia, unclassifiable; splenic red pulp lymphoma with numerous basophilic villous lymphocytes; splenic marginal zone B-cell lymphoma with villous lymphocytes; splenic lymphoma with villous lymphocytes; splenic marginal zone lymphoma, diffuse variant; prolymphocytic variant of hairy cell leukaemia.

Subtype(s)

None

Localization

The neoplastic cells involve the spleen, bone marrow, and peripheral blood {2718,3130,4062,1869,4063,4067}. The splenic hilar lymph nodes are usually involved, and the involvement of other lymph nodes is extremely rare. Liver involvement is infrequent.

Clinical features

Most patients present with pronounced splenomegaly and lymphocytosis; pancytopenia is infrequent, mostly seen in cases with hypersplenism. Serum M component of IgM, IgG, or both has been reported, and B symptoms are infrequent {2718,3130,1869,4063,4067}.

Epidemiology

SDRPL is a rare neoplasm, accounting for < 1% of all non-Hodgkin lymphomas. It accounts for about 10% of lymphomas diagnosed in spleen specimens and 0.5% of all chronic lymphoid malignancies with peripheral blood involvement {4067}. Most patients are male, with a median age of < 75 years. Precise information on incidence rates is not available.

Etiology

Unknown

Pathogenesis

Most cases express B-cell receptor immunoglobulin with somatically hypermutated IGHV genes. The IGHV gene repertoire is biased, with a predominance of IGHV3-23 and IGHV4-34 {4062,364,1780}. These findings may suggest an antigen drive in the pathogenesis of SDRPL. Recurrent mutations and copy-number variations have been reported with variable frequency in *NOTCH1*, *NOTCH2*, *MYD88*, *TP53*, *MAP2K1*, *CCND3*, *BCOR*, *ARID1A*, and *SYK*, among others {3549,364,4061,4067,850,1780} (see Table 4.19, p. 379, in *Splenic B-cell lymphomas and leukaemias: Introduction*).

Macroscopic appearance

The spleen is enlarged and shows a diffuse congested pattern without a micronodular appearance {2718,3130,4062,1869,4063,4067}.

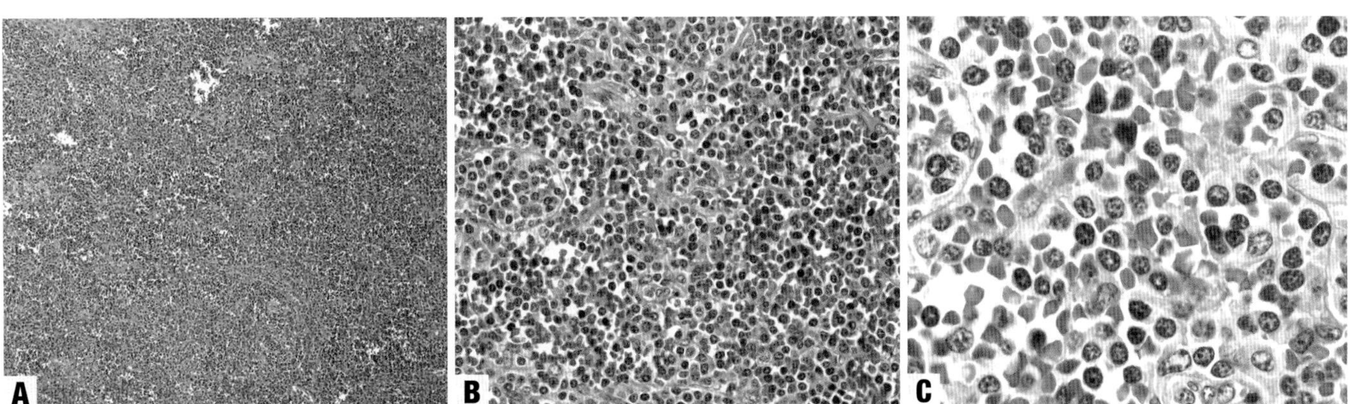

Fig. 4.73 Splenic diffuse red pulp small B-cell lymphoma. **A** The spleen shows a monomorphic diffuse red pulp infiltration in cords and sinuses, with architectural destruction of the red pulp. The white pulp is atrophic. **B** At higher magnification, the spleen shows the formation of pseudosinuses filled with neoplastic cells. **C** The cells have a relatively round hyperchromatic nucleus with clumped chromatin and basophilic cytoplasm, giving them a plasmacytoid appearance.

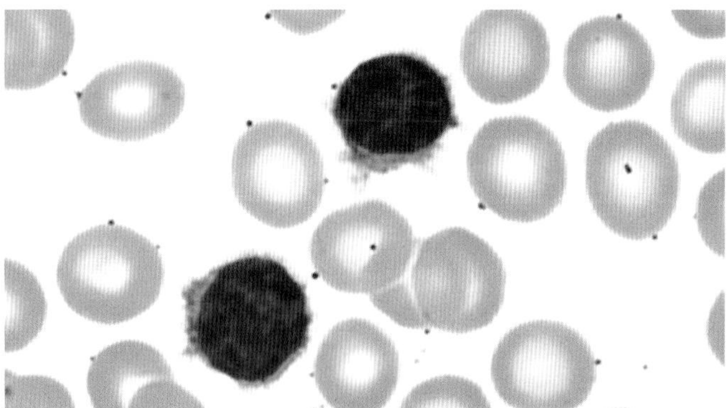

Fig. 4.74 Splenic diffuse red pulp small B-cell lymphoma. Cytology in peripheral blood. The cells have round or oval nuclei with moderately basophilic cytoplasm. Cytoplasmic or villous projections are visible, broad-based, and unevenly distributed around the cells with a polar distribution (one to four poles).

Histopathology

Peripheral blood

Peripheral blood smears show a homogeneous infiltrate of small to medium-sized cells with round or oval nuclei and clumped chromatin. The cytoplasm is variable in amount and moderately basophilic. Cytoplasmic or villous projections are well visible, broad-based, and unevenly distributed around the cells with a polar distribution (1–4 poles). The nucleolus is small or not visible in the large majority of the cells and is rarely prominent {1869,4063,4067}.

Bone marrow

Bone marrow biopsy shows variable cellularity, with sufficient residual haematopoiesis present and mild fibrosis. The most frequent patterns of infiltration are intrasinusoidal and/or interstitial, with a predominance of the former; nodular infiltrates are rare {4062,1869}.

Spleen

The spleen shows a monomorphic diffuse red pulp infiltration in cords and sinuses. Blood lakes with architectural destruction of the red pulp are frequently present, with neoplastic cells lining the resulting pseudosinuses. The white pulp is atrophic and not discernible. The cells usually have a relatively round, hyperchromatic nucleus with clumped chromatin and basophilic cytoplasm, giving them a plasmacytoid appearance {2718,1869,4063,4067}.

Immunophenotype

SDRPL is positive for B-cell markers (CD20, CD19, CD79a), DBA44, and IgG, but negative for CD5, CD23, CD43, cyclin D1, CD21, CD10, CD25, CD38, and ANXA1 {3130,1869,4063,4067}, although rare exceptions (for markers other than cyclin D1 and ANXA1) have been described {3130}. Cyclin D3 is expressed in 70% of cases {850}. Expression of IgD, CD11c, CD123, and CD103 has been reported in very few cases. The proliferation index (Ki-67) is usually low. p53 seems to be more frequently expressed than in splenic marginal zone lymphoma (SMZL).

By flow cytometry, CD180 {2683} is a very useful marker for distinguishing SDRPL from hairy cell leukaemia (HCL) and SMZL, and the sensitivity and specificity of SDRPL diagnosis are improved if CD180 is associated with CD200 and expressed as a median fluorescence intensity (MFI) ratio: a CD200 MFI to CD180 MFI ratio of < 0.5 favours a diagnosis of SDRPL rather than HCL or SMZL {1144}. On peripheral blood immunophenotyping, the identification of isolated monoclonal B-cell lymphocytosis with an immunophenotype consistent with marginal zone derivation may constitute an early stage of SDRPL or SMZL {4447}.

Differential diagnosis

This includes other splenic small B-cell lymphomas such as SMZL, HCL, and splenic B-cell lymphoma/leukaemia with prominent nucleoli (SBLPN). It can be difficult to distinguish these entities because of their similar clinical presentation and absence of specific immunophenotypic features, especially for SMZL, SDRPL, and SBLPN. Lymphocytosis is moderate and many cells lack prominent nucleoli, in contrast to splenic B-cell lymphoma/leukaemia with prominent nucleoli. Monocytopenia typically seen in HCL is not characteristic of SDRPL. As outlined in Table 4.18 (p. 378) in *Splenic B-cell lymphomas and leukaemias: Introduction*, macroscopic and microscopic patterns of involvement of the spleen, and (to some extent) the pattern of bone marrow infiltration, are helpful. Immunophenotypically, CD25, cyclin D1, and ANXA1, typically expressed in HCL, are absent in SDRPL. The CD200MFI:CD180MFI ratio by flow cytometry can help in the differential diagnosis {1144}.

When it is not possible to establish a definitive classification, which is often the case when no splenectomy specimen is available, the descriptive term "splenic B-cell leukaemia/lymphoma, not further classified (NFC)" should be used. In cases where cells display prominent nucleoli, the term "splenic B-cell lymphoma/leukaemia with prominent nucleoli" may be more appropriate.

Cytology

See above.

Diagnostic molecular pathology

No molecular test is pathognomonic of SDRPL. Molecular studies may also contribute to its distinction from HCL. *BRAF* p.V600E (NP_004324.2) mutation, observed in > 95% of HCL cases, is not present in SDRPL {4067}. Mutations in *NOTCH2* and *KLF2*, which are frequent in SMZL, are only rarely observed in SDRPL {4067}. The IGHV1-2*04 allele, which predominates by far in the repertoire of SMZL (relative frequency: ~30%), is underrepresented in SDRPL (< 5%) and HCL (< 1%) {4062,364,1780}.

Essential and desirable diagnostic criteria

Essential: diffuse infiltration of the spleen by monomorphic small B cells, accompanied by atrophic white pulp; peripheral blood with circulating small cells with abundant cytoplasm, well-visible broad-based and unevenly distributed cytoplasmic villous projections, and an inconspicuous nucleolus; immunophenotype compatible with SDRPL.

Desirable: absence of *BRAF* p.V600E (NP_004324.2) mutation; absence of lymphadenopathy other than splenic hilar lymph node involvement.

Staging

No staging system is routinely used.

Prognosis and prediction

The information available is limited. Aggressive behaviour has been noted in cases associated with mutations in *NOTCH1*, *TP53*, or *MAP2K1* in one study {2548}.

Splenic B-cell lymphoma/leukaemia with prominent nucleoli

Traverse-Glehen A
Lim MS
Molina TJ
Mollejo M
Montes-Moreno S
Siebert R
Stamatopoulos KE

Definition

Splenic B-cell lymphoma/leukaemia with prominent nucleoli (SBLPN) is a splenic B-cell neoplasm with some but not all of the cytomorphological and immunophenotypic features of cells of hairy cell leukaemia (HCL); it lacks *BRAF* mutation and is resistant to conventional HCL therapy. Characteristically, the cells have a single large nucleolus.

ICD-O coding

9591/3 Splenic B-cell lymphoma/leukaemia with prominent nucleoli

ICD-11 coding

2A82.3 Splenic B-cell lymphoma or leukaemia, unclassifiable

Related terminology

Acceptable: splenic B-cell lymphoma/leukaemia, unclassifiable.
Not recommended: hairy cell leukaemia variant; B-prolymphocytic leukaemia.

Subtype(s)

None

Localization

The spleen, bone marrow, and peripheral blood are involved. Peripheral lymphadenopathy is uncommon. Hepatomegaly is observed in less than one third of patients {126}.

Clinical features

The main clinical features are splenomegaly, high lymphocytosis, and cytopenia without monocytopenia. Autoimmune phenomena are rare {126}.

Epidemiology

SBLPN is rare and accounts for approximately 0.4% of chronic lymphoid malignancies {2603,3420,3421}, with an incidence of approximately 0.03 cases per 100 000 person-years {581, 540}. The disease mostly affects elderly patients (median age: 71 years), with a slight male predominance (M:F ratio: 1.6:1), which is much less marked than that of HCL (M:F ratio: 4:1). Because the definition of SBLPN is evolving, the incidence figures are likely to be imprecise.

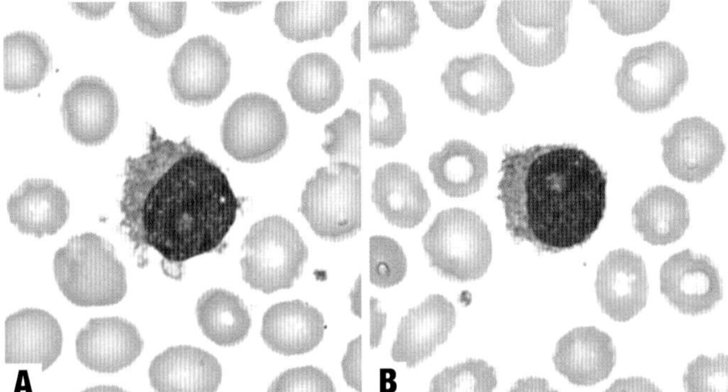

Fig. 4.75 Splenic B-cell lymphoma/leukaemia with prominent nucleoli. **A** Atypical medium-sized to large lymphocytes with abundant basophilic to pale cytoplasm and fine or poorly defined projections. **B** A prominent single nucleolus is seen.

Etiology

The etiology is unknown. There is no evidence suggesting that genetic or environmental factors play a role in its pathogenesis {2603}.

Pathogenesis

Because SBLPN is a newly introduced entity absorbing cases previously classified as HCL variant and cases of CD5-negative B-prolymphocytic leukaemia, aspects of pathogenesis need to be revised as the definition evolves. Based on limited data from series on HCL variant and B-prolymphocytic leukaemia, cases are probably biased for their IG gene repertoire, with a predominance of IGHV4-34 gene usage, and most cases carry a relatively low load of somatic hypermutation within the clonotypic rearranged IGHV genes {1602}. Complex karyotypes involving 14q32 as well as 8q24, 7p deletion, and trisomy 12 have been reported {462,4140}. *BRAF* p.V600E (NP_004324.2) mutation is absent, but *MAP2K1* mutations are present probably in 38–42% of cases {919,4434,1601,4328,2573}. Other genetic events include *KMT2C* mutations, *U2AF1* and *CCND3* mutations (~21–24%), and 7q deletions. *TP53* mutations and/or 17p deletions and *MYC* alterations seem to be associated with a high risk {3421,2594}. Molecular evidence supports the biological distinction from HCL and splenic marginal zone lymphoma (SMZL) {2594,1065,126,401} (see Table 4.19, p. 379, in *Splenic B-cell lymphomas and leukaemias: Introduction*).

Macroscopic appearance

The spleen is enlarged and shows a diffuse homogeneous appearance without presence of a micronodular aspect.

Histopathology

Peripheral blood

In the peripheral blood, the proportion of atypical lymphoid cells ranges from 20% to 95% {3528,2601,597}. These cells are medium-sized to large and have abundant basophilic or pale cytoplasm with variably defined projections. They typically have a large, prominent single nucleolus, but the nucleolus may be smaller and less conspicuous in some cases. The cells are smaller than those of HCL, but occasionally large cells with a bilobed nucleus can be identified. In contrast to HCL, the cells typically do not have circumferential villous processes.

Bone marrow

The bone marrow shows normal or increased cellularity, with a variable (often mild) degree of lymphoid infiltration and mild

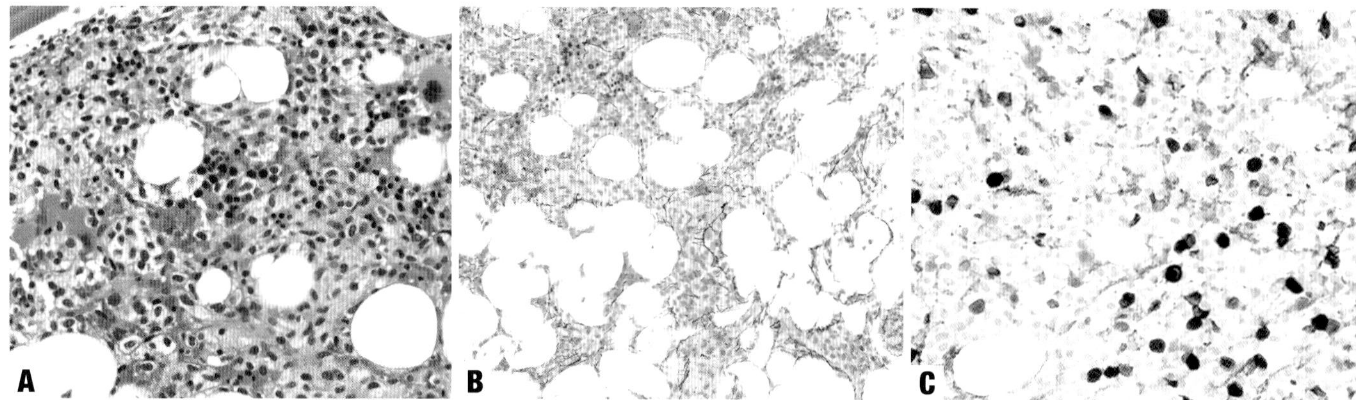

Fig. 4.76 Splenic B-cell lymphoma/leukaemia with prominent nucleoli. **A** Bone marrow core biopsy with interstitial lymphoid infiltrates. **B** Reticulin stain of bone marrow shows mild fibrosis. **C** Bone marrow biopsy involved by splenic B-cell lymphoma/leukaemia with prominent nucleoli demonstrating an absence of ANXA1 expression. Note the ANXA1 expression in background granulocytes, which serves as a positive internal control.

fibrosis. On the trephine biopsy, the most common pattern of infiltration is interstitial and intrasinusoidal. Cases with a mixed nodular and interstitial pattern occur; a diffuse pattern may be seen in the later stages of the disease. The key diagnostic feature is the cytomorphology of the cells: medium-sized atypical lymphoid cells with relatively abundant cytoplasm, a round nucleus, and a generally prominent nucleolus {2601,2597}.

Spleen

The spleen shows diffuse involvement of the red pulp with atrophic white pulp. There is prominent intrasinusoidal involvement in the red pulp. Blood lakes may be seen occasionally but are not typical as in HCL or splenic diffuse red pulp small B-cell lymphoma (SDRPL) {2595,2597}. The neoplastic cells are medium-sized atypical lymphoid cells with abundant cytoplasm, a round nucleus, and a generally prominent nucleolus.

Immunophenotype

The neoplastic cells express monotypic surface immunoglobulin (most frequently IgG, either alone or with another isotype), pan–B-cell antigens (CD19, CD20, and CD22), DBA44, CD11c, CD103, and FMC7, but not HCL markers (CD25, ANXA1, TRAP, and CD123) {2601,918,597,2595}.

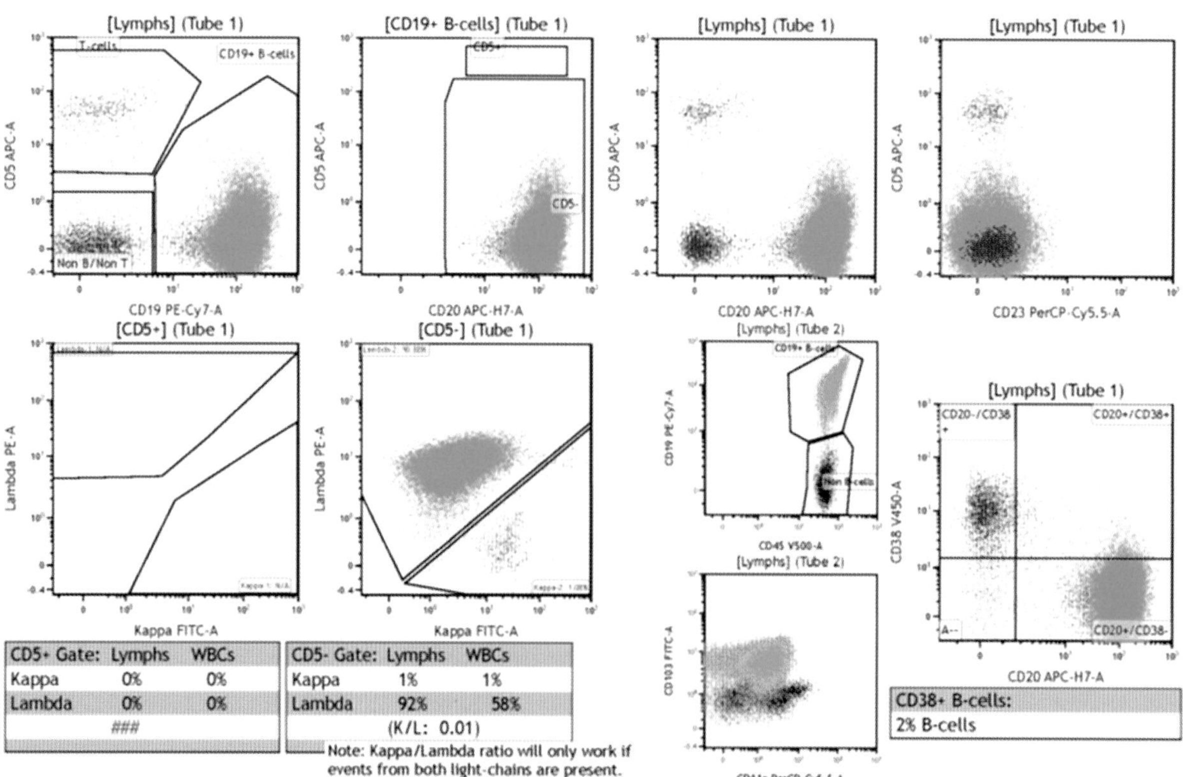

Fig. 4.77 Splenic B-cell lymphoma/leukaemia with prominent nucleoli. Flow cytometry demonstrates expression of bright CD19, CD20, CD11c, and CD103, but not CD5, CD23, or CD38, in immunoglobulin lambda light chain–positive splenic B-cell lymphoma/leukaemia with prominent nucleoli.

Differential diagnosis

SBLPN should be distinguished from other splenic B-cell lymphomas/leukaemias (HCL, SMZL, and SDRPL). SBLPN characteristically differs from other splenic B-cell lymphomas/leukaemias by its cytological atypia and a generally prominent, single nucleolus. SBLPN can be distinguished from HCL by the immunophenotype and the lack of *BRAF* mutation. Like patients with SBLPN, patients with SMZL and SDRPL may show intrasinusoidal infiltrates in bone marrow core biopsies; however, intrasinusoidal infiltrates are mixed with other patterns, and in SMZL, an intrasinusoidal pattern is less prominent. Furthermore, the lymphoid cells in SMZL and SDRPL lack the atypia and prominent nucleoli seen in SBLPN (see Table 4.18, p. 378, in *Splenic B-cell lymphomas and leukaemias: Introduction*).

Cytology

See above.

Diagnostic molecular pathology

No molecular test is pathognomonic of SBLPN, because its genetics remain to be characterized.

Essential and desirable diagnostic criteria

Essential: circulating medium-sized lymphoid cells with prominent nucleoli or convoluted nuclei – rare cells in the peripheral blood may show poorly defined cytoplasmic projections, but circumferential fine villous (hairy) projections are absent; presence of B-cell antigens (CD19, CD20, CD79a, or PAX5); absence of the characteristic phenotype of HCL, including expression of CD25, ANXA1, cyclin D1, and TRAP.

Desirable: diffuse involvement of the splenic red pulp with atrophic white pulp, but most cases are diagnosed without a spleen specimen; absence of *BRAF* mutation.

Staging

No staging system is routinely used.

Prognosis and prediction

The clinical course is variable, with half of the patients dying from unrelated causes. The evolution seems to be more aggressive than that of classic HCL. The median survival time is approximately 9 years, with only 15% of patients surviving for longer than 15 years {2601,2603,2602}. There is limited information on therapy, and treatment responses to a variety of agents have been disappointing. In contrast to classic HCL, patients with splenic B-cell lymphoma/leukaemia with hairy cell features do not usually respond to interferon alfa, and only half of them achieve transient partial responses to the purine analogues pentostatin (2′-deoxycoformycin) and cladribine (2′-chlorodeoxyadenosine) {3528, 2601, 3421, 2597, 2594}. Splenic B-cell lymphoma/leukaemia with hairy cell features may undergo transformation (reported in 6% of cases), which appears to be more frequent in cases harbouring 17p deletion {4140}.

Lymphoplasmacytic lymphoma

Montes-Moreno S
Geddie WR
Kersten MJ
Lin P
Maruyama D
Siebert R
Treon SP

Definition

Lymphoplasmacytic lymphoma (LPL) is a neoplasm comprising small B lymphocytes, plasmacytoid lymphocytes, and plasma cells, usually involving the bone marrow and sometimes involving the lymph nodes and spleen. Waldenström macroglobulinaemia (WM) is defined by the combination of LPL in the bone marrow and an IgM monoclonal component in the blood.

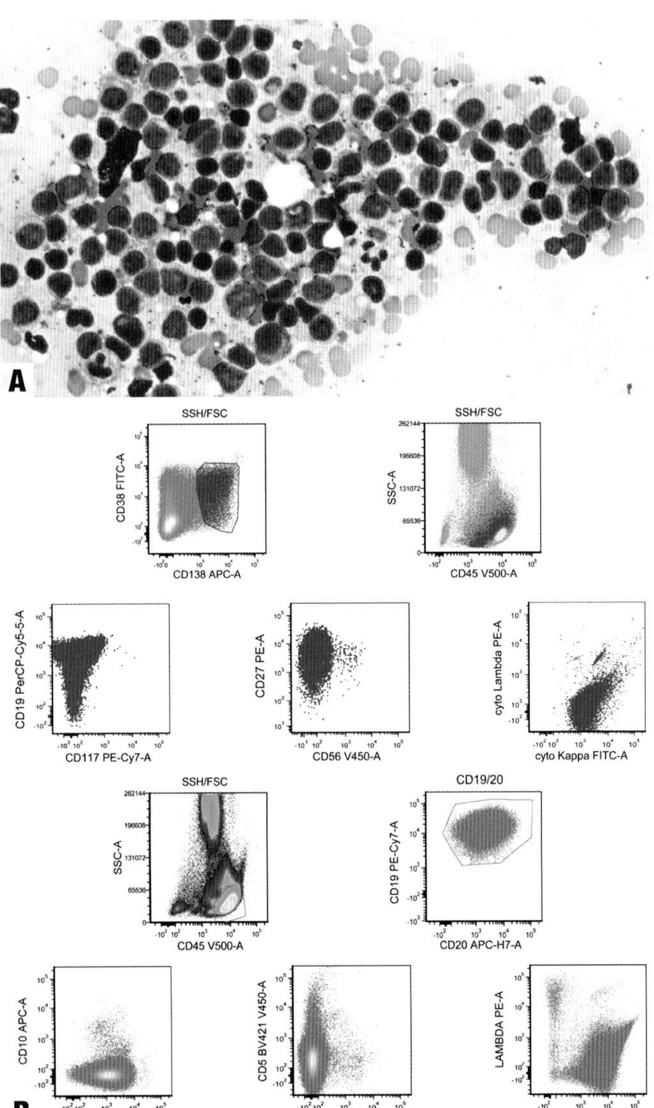

Fig. 4.78 Lymphoplasmacytic lymphoma. **A** Bone marrow aspirate smear from a patient with lymphoplasmacytic lymphoma showing a polymorphic population of small lymphocytes, plasmacytoid lymphocytes, plasma cells, and mast cells (Giemsa). **B** The corresponding flow cytometry immunophenotyping shows both monotypic cytoplasmic kappa restricted plasma cells (blue) and monotypic surface kappa light chain–restricted B cells (pink) expressing CD19, CD20, and CD22, and lacking CD5 and CD10. The plasma cells are positive for CD19 and negative for CD56, which is typical for lymphoplasmacytic lymphoma and different from plasma cells in plasma cell myeloma, which are nearly always negative for CD19 and usually positive for CD56.

ICD-O coding

9671/3 Lymphoplasmacytic lymphoma
9761/3 IgM-type lymphoplasmacytic lymphoma / Waldenström macroglobulinaemia
9761/3 Non–IgM-type lymphoplasmacytic lymphoma / Waldenström macroglobulinaemia

ICD-11 coding

2A85.4 Lymphoplasmacytic lymphoma

Related terminology

None

Subtype(s)

IgM-type lymphoplasmacytic lymphoma / Waldenström macroglobulinaemia (IgM-type LPL/WM); non–IgM-type lymphoplasmacytic lymphoma / Waldenström macroglobulinaemia (non–IgM-type LPL/WM)

Localization

LPL typically involves the bone marrow and less frequently the lymph nodes and spleen. LPL cells may infrequently involve other extranodal sites, including the CNS (Bing–Neel syndrome), skin, pleural cavities (resulting in malignant effusions), or other sites usually involved by extranodal marginal zone lymphoma.

Clinical features

Many patients with an IgM paraprotein are asymptomatic at diagnosis. The most common presenting symptoms in WM are fatigue and constitutional symptoms. The anaemia can be caused by LPL infiltration in the bone marrow and/or by increased hepcidin levels, interfering with iron uptake in the gut. Thrombocytopenia and leukopenia are less common. Fewer than 25% of patients present with lymphadenopathy and/or hepatosplenomegaly at diagnosis, but this percentage increases to 50–60% at relapse. Other common symptoms are directly related to the IgM paraprotein. As many as 30% of patients present with hyperviscosity syndrome, with blurred vision, headache, epistaxis, and shortness of breath {1298}. The syndrome is more likely to occur when IgM levels are > 6 g/dL {1456}. Bleeding tendency can occur, due to acquired von Willebrand disease and/or thrombocytopenia. The IgM paraprotein can also have autoantibody or cryoglobulin activity, resulting in autoimmune phenomena or type II cryoglobulinaemia (leading to vasculitis, skin lesions, renal complications, and neuropathy). IgM-related neuropathy is seen in approximately 20% of cases; this may result from reactivity of the IgM paraprotein with myelin sheath antigens (anti–myelin-associated glycoprotein [MAG] antibodies) and has a typical clinical picture of gradually worsening distal sensory loss, ataxic gait, and tremor, as well as a demyelinating pattern on electromyography. Other types of neuropathy more rarely observed in WM include amyloid peripheral neuropathy and CANOMAD syndrome (chronic ataxic neuropathy with ophthalmoplegia, M protein, cold agglutinins, and disialosyl ganglioside antibodies) {1000}, cryoglobulin-associated neuropathy, and small fibre neuropathy.

Non–IgM-type LPL/WM represents about 5% of LPL cases. This category includes cases with IgG or IgA monoclonal proteins and those with non-secretory LPL (the IgG type is more common than the IgA or non-secretory types), as well as cases of IgM-type LPL without bone marrow involvement {4186,2026, 543,1873,573,4109}. Compared with patients with IgM-type LPL/WM, these patients may show clinical heterogeneity, with less frequent hyperviscosity syndrome and neuropathy {573}; more frequent lymph node, extranodal, and spleen involvement; and less frequent serum paraprotein and bone marrow involvement {4186}. Data regarding overall survival in comparison with IgM-type LPL are conflicting among retrospective series, with similar {4186,573} or worse {543,1873} outcomes reported. Time to treatment requirement is usually shorter in cases with non–IgM-type LPL {4186,573}.

Epidemiology

LPL has an incidence of 3–7 cases per 1 million person-years in the USA and Europe and represents approximately 2% of all haematological malignancies. Most patients are diagnosed at ≥ 65 years of age, and LPL is more common in men and in White people {3670,856,3813}.

Etiology

The etiology is unknown. Acquired risk factors for LPL are a pre-existing IgM monoclonal gammopathy of undetermined significance (MGUS) and a history of HCV infection in specific geographical areas {4187,579,2635,2271}. Familial predisposition has been described in nearly 20% of cases with WM-type LPL {89,4072,3433,4073}.

Pathogenesis

In 93–97% of LPL/WM cases, the driver mutation is *MYD88* p.L265P (NP_002459.2) {2949}. Other mutations have also been identified in 1–2% of all patients with LPL/WM. These mutations result in gain of function of MYD88 and constitutive activation of the NF-κB pathway. *MYD88* mutations are also detectable in as many as 80% of IgM MGUS cases but not in IgG or IgA MGUS. Patients with IgM MGUS with mutated *MYD88*, and those with a higher mutated allele burden, are at higher risk of progression to WM.

The next most common somatic mutations are nonsense and frameshift mutations of *CXCR4* that affect its C-terminal region. CXCR4 is essential for the homing and migration of WM cells. These *CXCR4* mutations are seen in as many as 40% of patients with LPL/WM, mostly concurrently with *MYD88* mutations {1687,1685}. *CXCR4* mutations are essentially unique to WM, with only a few cases of marginal zone lymphoma (MZL) and activated B-cell diffuse large B-cell lymphoma reported so far. *CXCR4* mutations are associated with high serum IgM, symptomatic hyperviscosity, von Willebrand factor deficiency, and earlier time to treatment. These *CXCR4* activating mutations also confer resistance to ibrutinib therapy. The subclonal nature of *CXCR4* mutations, and their paucity in IgM MGUS suggest that they are acquired after *MYD88* mutation.

Clonal deletions of chromosome 6, targeting regions 6q21-q25, are found in 40–50% of patients with WM and appear to be exclusively associated with *CXCR4* mutations in treatment-naïve patients. Such deletions in 6q increase in frequency from IgM MGUS through asymptomatic WM and to symptomatic WM, suggesting that loss of genes within this region may facilitate disease progression.

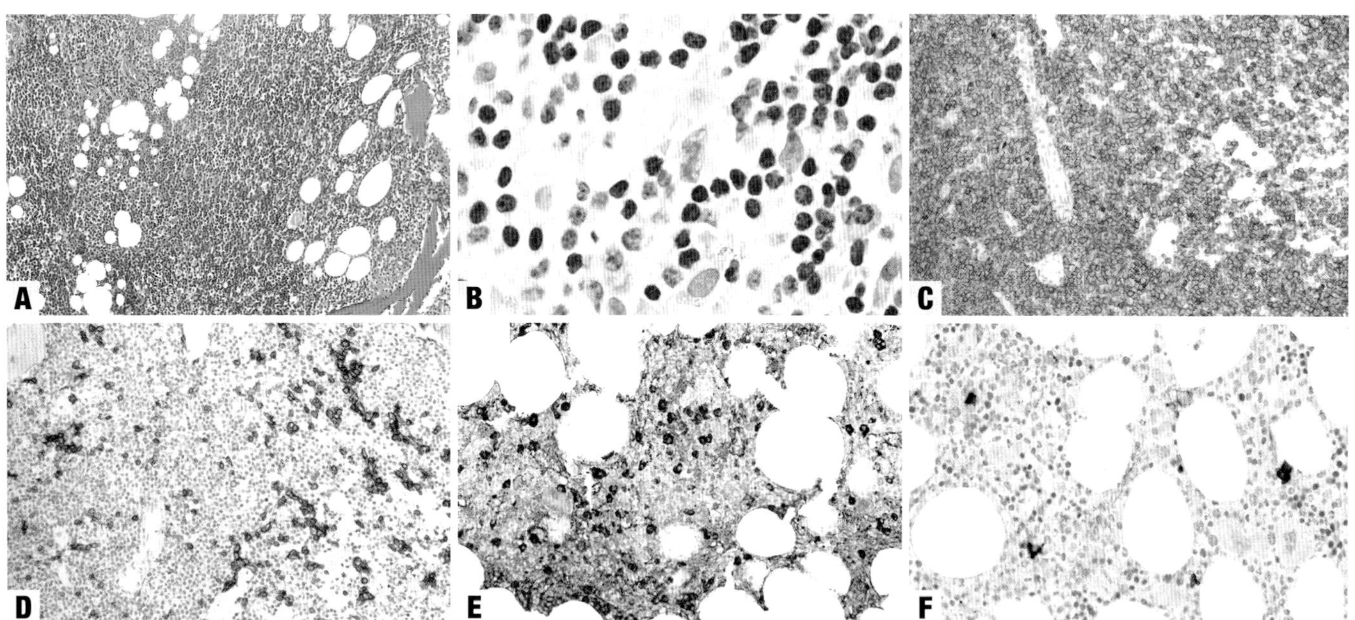

Fig. 4.79 Lymphoplasmacytic lymphoma. **A** Predominantly interstitial infiltrates are found in a case with significant bone marrow infiltration. **B** The infiltrate is composed of lymphocytes, plasmacytoid lymphocytes, and scattered plasma cells. Haemosiderin-laden histiocytes are noted. **C** CD20 immunohistochemistry highlights the B cells. **D** CD138 immunohistochemistry highlights the scattered plasma cells. **E** Kappa light chain restriction is noted. **F** The tumour cells are negative for lambda light chain.

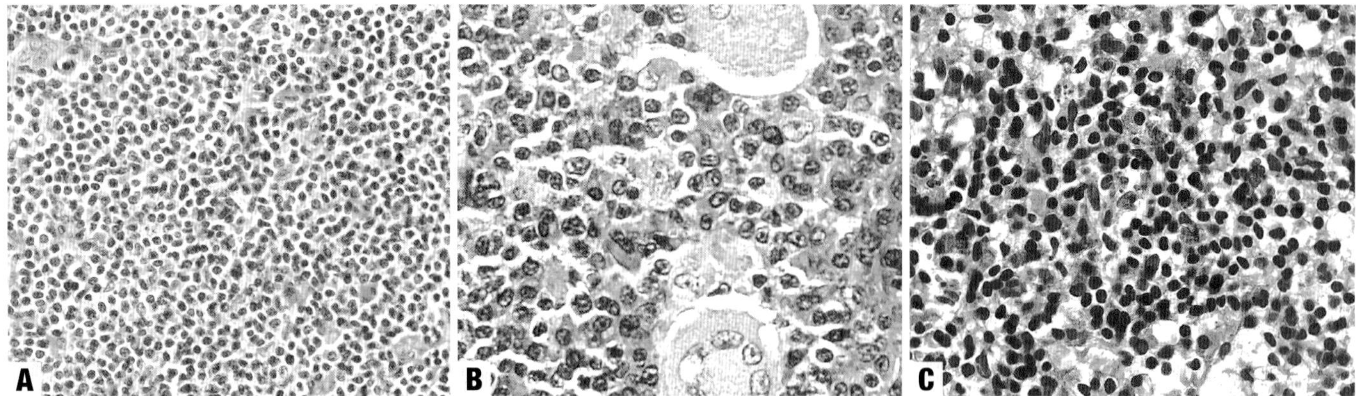

Fig. 4.80 Lymphoplasmacytic lymphoma. **A** The most common lymph node presentation is characterized by a diffuse infiltrate with architectural sparing. Follicular colonization may be present. **B** The crystal-storing histiocytosis pattern shows a prominent histiocytic reaction, with clusters of macrophages with foreign body–type reaction and crystalline inclusions in the cytoplasm. **C** Lymphocytes and plasmacytoid lymphocytes are present. Note the presence of immunoglobulin nuclear inclusions (Dutcher bodies).

Macroscopic appearance

Rare cases show enlarged lymph nodes and spleen.

Histopathology

Bone marrow

The bone marrow is infiltrated by small B lymphocytes, plasmacytoid cells, and plasma cells. Plasmacytoid differentiation with Dutcher bodies is useful in the differential diagnosis with MZL {262}. Another helpful feature is the increase in reactive mast cells as well as haemosiderin-laden histiocytes. Most cases show a combined paratrabecular and interstitial infiltration pattern {2026, 262,1296,1132}. In contrast, MZL and chronic lymphocytic leukaemia cases show predominantly interstitial growth patterns, combined with intrasinusoidal growth in the case of MZL. Uncommonly, nodular interstitial infiltrates may show a population of follicular dendritic cells {262}. Light chain amyloid deposition can be found in association with LPL infiltrates. In some cases, particularly after treatment, absence of the lymphoid component and pure monotypic plasma cell infiltrates with or without granulomatous reactions can be found. The differential diagnosis based on morphology includes MZL and lymphocyte-like morphological variants of multiple myeloma. Cases with patchy interstitial infiltrates characterized by minute interstitial cell clusters positive for B-cell markers are IgM MGUS rather than LPL. In cases with more advanced disease, large cells may be increased in number and the neoplastic infiltrate may appear more polymorphic, possibly heralding a transformation to large cell lymphoma. Rouleaux formation and plasmacytoid lymphocytes can be found in the peripheral blood.

Lymph node

The classic pattern is characterized by a relatively monomorphic, predominantly lymphoid, lymphoplasmacytoid, and plasmacytic infiltrate with a diffuse growth pattern, intact or dilated sinuses, follicular preservation, and scattered haemosiderin-laden macrophages. Rarely, morphological patterns comprising almost exclusively small lymphocytes or exclusively plasma cells may be present {1477,3907}. There is an absence of pseudofollicles. Follicular colonization can be found. Some cases may show a frank histiocytic infiltrate with cytoplasmic immunoglobulin (crystal-storing histiocytosis pattern).

Differential diagnosis with MZL

The differentiation from MZL may be difficult in some cases (see Table 4.20). The demonstration of *MYD88* p.L265P mutation favours LPL {2359,1477}.

Spleen

The spleen usually shows involvement of both the white pulp and the red pulp; in the former, the neoplastic cells are often localized to the mantle and marginal zones. Both lymphoplasmacytoid-predominant and plasmacytic types have been recorded. Such a degree of plasmacytic differentiation is unusual in splenic MZL {2554}.

Other extranodal sites

Lymphoma infiltrates in the skin and other mucosal sites can be difficult to distinguish from MZL and may require mutation testing for *MYD88* p.L265P. In the case of suspected CNS infiltration, the

Table 4.20 Differential diagnosis for Waldenström macroglobulinaemia–type lymphoplasmacytic lymphoma (LPL-WM), IgM monoclonal gammopathy of undetermined significance (IgM MGUS), and IgM-related disorders

Entity	IgM monoclonal protein	Bone marrow infiltration	IgM-related symptoms	Tumour-related symptoms (i.e. anaemia/adenopathy)
LPL-WM (symptomatic)	+	+	+/–	+
Asymptomatic LPL-WM	+	+	–	–
IgM MGUS	+	–	–	–
IgM-related disorders[a]	+	+/–	+	–

[a]Cold agglutinin haemolytic anaemia, type II cryoglobulinaemia, neuropathy, amyloidosis.

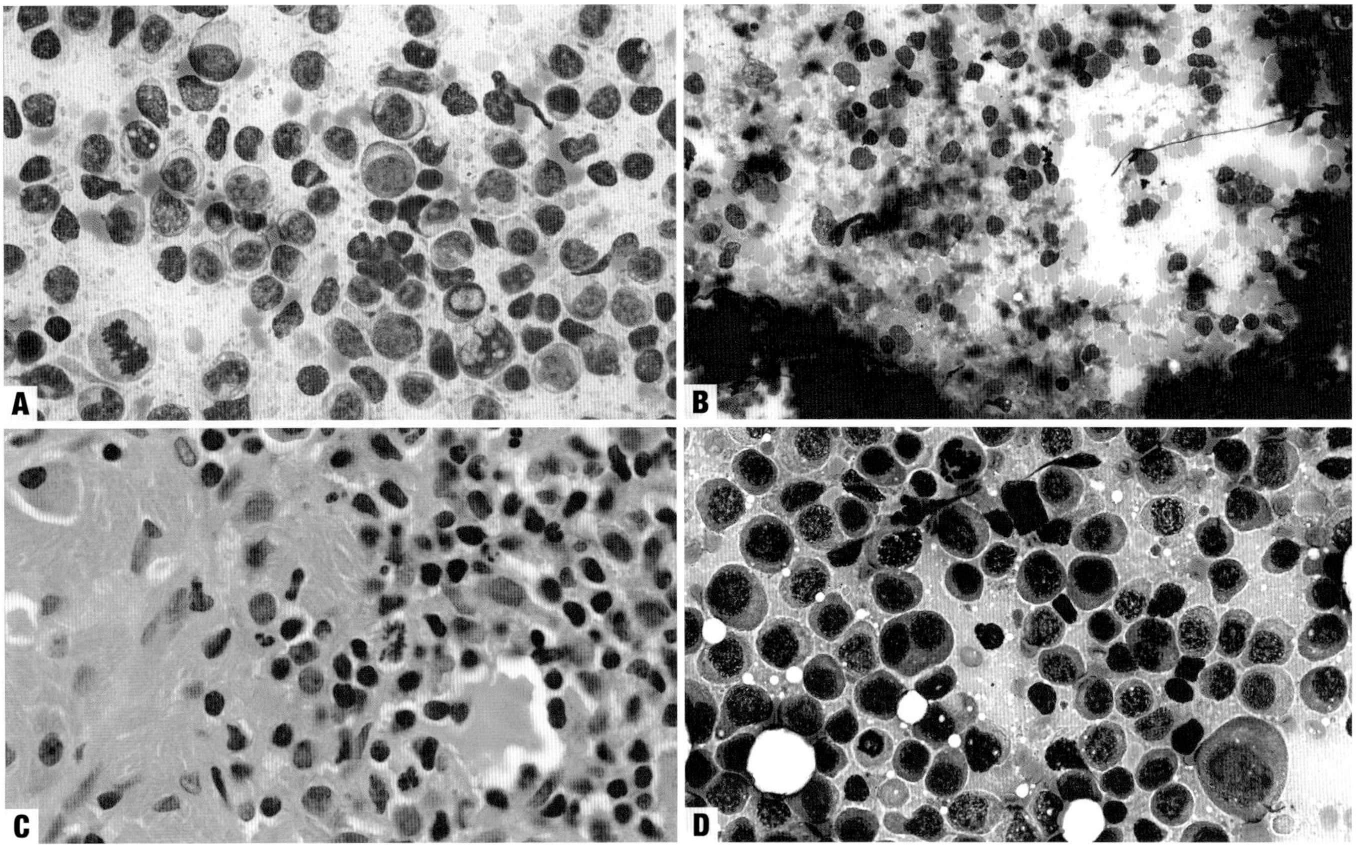

Fig. 4.81 Lymphoplasmacytic lymphoma cytology. **A** Fine-needle aspirate of an orbital mass, direct smear, showing plasmacytoid lymphocytes and scattered large cells. Dutcher bodies are noted. The differential diagnosis includes lymphoplasmacytic lymphoma and extranodal marginal zone lymphoma (Giemsa). **B** Fine-needle aspirate of lymph node (para-aortic), direct smear, showing pink amorphous material consistent with amyloid in the background of neoplastic lymphocytes (Giemsa). **C** Endobronchial ultrasound (EBUS)-guided transbronchial needle fine-aspirate of a mediastinal lymph node: cell block section showing crystal-storing histiocytosis characterized by plasmacytoid small lymphocytes and histiocytes distended with eosinophilic immunoglobulin crystals. **D** Fine-needle aspirate of an axillary lymph node, direct smear, showing numerous large immunoblasts and only occasional plasma cells, consistent with transformation to diffuse large B-cell lymphoma (Giemsa).

detection of a clonal B-cell population, possibly with the *MYD88* mutation, is of value in securing the diagnosis {2690}.

Immunophenotype

LPL cells express B-cell antigens such as CD20, CD19, CD22, CD79a, and PAX5 {1646,3558}. Other markers, such as CD45, CD25, and CD38, are usually positive. Light chain restriction can be demonstrated by both immunohistochemistry and flow cytometry. Most cases show IgM expression by immunohistochemistry, rarely IgG or IgA. IgD is usually negative. LPL cells are typically negative for CD10, CD5, CD23, CD103, and DBA44, but variable expression of CD5, CD23, and/or CD10 has been reported. Plasma cells express IRF4 (MUM1) and CD138, and these populations may predominate in posttreatment samples. Flow cytometry and immunohistochemistry show similar results regarding the cellular phenotype {1646}, but flow cytometry may underestimate the number of clonal B cells, compared with tissue-based immunohistochemistry against CD20 {1296}. Some LPLs are biclonal for IgM and IgG. Cases of IgG or IgA type usually show similar phenotypic features but may show more prominent plasmacytic differentiation.

Cytology

Cytological findings from fine core needle biopsies of lymph nodes or extranodal sites are sometimes the first demonstration of a lymphoproliferative disorder in patients being investigated for possible LPL/WM, and they may also document amyloid or crystal-storing histiocytosis {347,1743,4031,1863}. Fine core needle biopsy may also be useful to collect tissues for immunophenotyping and molecular testing {3573}. In patients with an

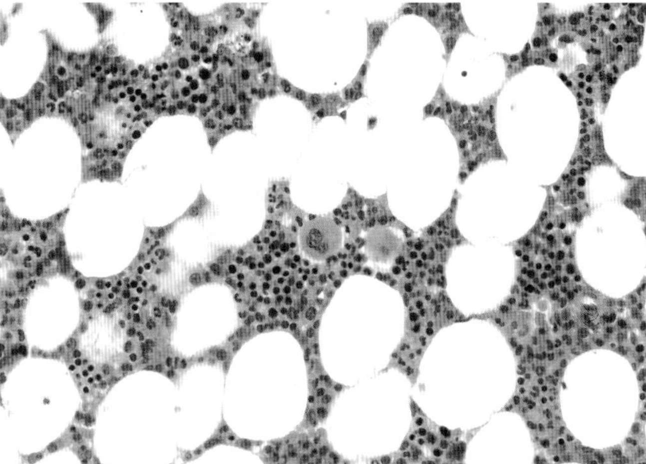

Fig. 4.82 IgM monoclonal gammopathy of undetermined significance. Bone marrow core biopsy. Scattered lymphocytes and plasmacytoid cells are found but are difficult to identify without immunohistochemistry.

Table 4.21 Summary of genetic features in lymphoplasmacytic lymphoma (LPL)

Gene	Frequency of genetic lesion	Type of genetic lesion
MYD88	> 90% in WM-type LPL 60–90% in non-WM–type LPL 80% in IgM MGUS	Missense somatic mutation (p.L265P >> other)
CXCR4	40% in WM-type LPL	Nonsense and frameshift mutations in C-terminus
del(6q)	40%	Deletion
KMT2D[a]	25%	Somatic mutation
ARID1A	10%	Somatic mutation
CD79B	< 10%	Somatic mutation
TBL1XR1[a]	< 10%	Somatic mutation
PTPN13[a]	< 10%	Somatic mutation
TP53[a]	< 10%	Somatic mutation

MGUS, monoclonal gammopathy of undetermined significance; WM, Waldenström macroglobulinaemia.
[a]Prevalent mutations in *MYD88* p.L265P–wildtype cases {1685,4075,1686,1687,4186}.

established diagnosis of LPL, fine core needle biopsy may be used to look for evidence of large-cell transformation and guide site selection for excisional or core biopsy.

Diagnostic molecular pathology

MYD88 p.L265P (NP_002459.2) change can be identified in 93–97% of patients with LPL/WM, and other rare *MYD88* mutations have also been identified in 1–2% of all patients with LPL/WM {4074} (see Table 4.21). Genetic testing may yield false negative results, largely due to low tumour cell content in bone marrow {2079}; negative results should therefore be interpreted with caution. The *MYD88* mutation can also be detected in peripheral blood samples, skin lesions, cerebrospinal fluid, pleural effusions, and cell-free DNA from the peripheral blood of patients with LPL/WM.

Essential and desirable diagnostic criteria

Essential: significant bone marrow infiltration by clonal small lymphocytes with plasmacytoid and/or plasma cell differentiation; immunophenotype of LPL cells: IgM+ (rarely IgG+ or IgA+), CD19+, CD20+, CD22+, CD25+, CD10−, CD23−, CD103−, CD138+/−.

Desirable: detection of *MYD88* p.L265P (NP_002459.2); detection of *CXCR4* somatic sequence variant; serum electrophoresis and immunofixation showing presence of monoclonal IgM (rarely IgG or IgA).

Staging

The modified Lugano staging system for underlying lymphoma applies.

Prognosis and prediction

The WM International Prognostic Scoring System (WM IPSS) incorporates five adverse covariates: advanced age (> 65 years), haemoglobin ≤ 11.5 g/dL, platelet count ≤ 100 × 10^9/L, B2M > 3 mg/L, and serum monoclonal protein concentration > 7.0 g/dL. It retains its prognostic significance independent of age and in patients treated with alkylating agents as well as with nucleoside analogues {2779}. *MYD88* mutation status may also impact survival; those with wildtype *MYD88* tend to harbour NF-κB pathway activating mutations that are also seen in diffuse large B-cell lymphoma {1685}. These patients have a higher risk of transformation to diffuse large B-cell lymphoma, and thereby a shorter overall survival. The presence of *CXCR4* mutations does not appear to impact overall survival {4071}.

Marginal zone lymphoma: Introduction

Ferry JA
Du MQ

Extranodal marginal zone lymphoma of mucosa-associated lymphoid tissue (EMZL), nodal marginal zone lymphoma, and splenic marginal zone lymphoma (SMZL) appeared as distinct entities in the fourth edition of the *WHO classification of tumours of haematopoietic and lymphoid tissues* and are retained in the fifth edition. Primary cutaneous marginal zone lymphoma appears as an entity in the fifth edition for the first time, as it has clinical and pathological features that distinguish it from other EMZLs. Similarly, paediatric nodal marginal zone lymphoma is recognized as a distinct type of lymphoma and is discussed separately.

These lymphomas have overlapping histological and immunophenotypic features: the neoplastic cells are small mature B cells typically negative for CD5 and CD10, and the lymphomas variably show plasmacytic differentiation. Associated reactive follicles are often present.

However, their clinical features differ significantly (see Table 4.22). Their differential diagnosis includes other types of small B-cell lymphomas and, in some instances, reactive processes. SMZL is discussed under splenic B-cell neoplasms but is included in this table to highlight features that distinguish it from other MZLs.

Despite having shared histological and immunophenotypic features, nodal marginal zone lymphoma, EMZL, and SMZL have differing etiologies. Since the previous edition, the most important advances have been in the refinement of their somatic genetic features, which differ among these three entities {4145,3808,3243,4200,401}. In addition, there are significant differences in the mutation landscapes among EMZLs arising in different anatomical sites, such as the ocular adnexa {1626,2761}, salivary glands {2762,2107}, thyroid {4423}, skin {2608}, and others. Better definition of the underlying genetic changes of these lymphomas opens the door to improved treatment options.

Table 4.22 Summary of clinicopathological and molecular features of extranodal marginal zone lymphoma (EMZL), nodal marginal zone lymphoma (NMZL), and splenic marginal zone lymphoma (SMZL) (continued on next page)

Features	EMZL	NMZL	SMZL
Etiology	Site-dependent and variable in different geographical regions: chronic infection by *Helicobacter pylori* (stomach), *Chlamydia psittaci* (ocular adnexa), Sjögren syndrome (salivary glands), Hashimoto thyroiditis (thyroid)	Unknown	HCV infection, subset Unknown, most cases
Clinical features	Symptoms vary according to sites and underlying inflammatory disorders May be asymptomatic	May be asymptomatic and show painless non-bulky peripheral adenopathy, or rarely lymphocytosis	Symptoms related to cytopenias, splenomegaly, or autoimmunity May be asymptomatic
Sites involved	Almost any anatomical site, but most frequently involving stomach, ocular adnexa, lung, and salivary glands	Peripheral lymph nodes, often in head and neck	Spleen, splenic hilar lymph nodes, blood, and bone marrow
Peripheral blood	Usually not involved	Cytopenias uncommon and may develop during disease progression	Mild to moderate lymphocytosis; mature small to medium-sized lymphoid cells with short polar villi
Bone marrow	Infrequent and subtle	Typically involved; interstitial or intertrabecular lymphoid aggregates	Variably involved; typically intertrabecular nodular and/or intrasinusoidal infiltrate of small lymphoid cells with scant to moderate amount of pale cytoplasm
Histology	Proliferation of small to medium-sized lymphoid cells (centrocyte-like, monocytoid, small lymphocytes) with admixed centroblasts/immunoblasts and frequent plasmacytic differentiation in a marginal zone and/or diffuse pattern Lymphoma cells may form lymphoepithelial lesions and colonize B-cell follicles	Small lymphoid cells with minimal atypia in nodular, interfollicular, or diffuse distribution with partial or complete effacement of nodal architecture; monocytoid and plasmacytoid differentiation may be seen	White pulp: variably expanded population of small lymphoid cells surrounding reactive germinal centres and a peripheral zone of medium-sized cells with abundant pale cytoplasm Red pulp: small clusters of neoplastic cells, involving both sinuses and cords
Usual immunophenotype	Positive for CD20, CD79a, PAX5, and IgM, occasionally other immunoglobulin classes Negative for CD5, germinal-centre markers, CD23, cyclin D1, and SOX11	Positive for CD20, CD19, CD79a, and PAX5; coexpression of CD43, MNDA, and IRTA1; majority express IgM Negative for germinal-centre markers, cyclin D1, and LEF1	Positive for CD20, CD79a, PAX5, FMC7, CD27, CD38 (dim), IgM, and IgD Negative for germinal-centre markers, ANXA1, CD103, cyclin D1, SOX11, and LEF1

DMT, differentially methylated targets; GPCR, G protein–coupled receptor; NNK, 4-(N-methyl-N-nitrosamino)-1-(3-pyridyl)-1-butanone.

Table 4.22 Summary of clinicopathological and molecular features of extranodal marginal zone lymphoma (EMZL), nodal marginal zone lymphoma (NMZL), and splenic marginal zone lymphoma (SMZL) (continued)

Features	EMZL	NMZL	SMZL
IG gene mutation and usage	Clonal IG rearrangements with somatic hypermutation and frequent intraclonal variations; frequently biased usage of IGHV genes that confer reactivity to autoantigens	Clonal IG rearrangements with somatic hypermutations and frequently biased usage of *IGHV4-34* and *IGHV1-69*	Clonal IG rearrangements with somatic hypermutation in most cases, and biased usage of *IGHV1-2*04* in ~30%
Cytogenetic changes	Frequent trisomies 3 and 18	Gains of chromosome 2p and 6p and loss of 1p and 6q; frequent trisomies 3, 12, and 18; no 7q31-32 deletion	7q31-32 deletion in 30% Frequent trisomies 3 and 18
	Variable and site-dependent chromosome translocation: • Stomach: t(11;18) (*BIRC3*::*MALT1*) (24%) • Lung: t(11;18) (*BIRC3*::*MALT1*) (40%) The following are infrequent: • t(1;14) (IGH::*BCL10*), t(14:18) (IGH::*MALT1*), t(3;14) (IGH::*FOXP1*), t(X;14) (IGH::*GPR34*)	No recurrent translocations	No recurrent translocations
Somatic variants	Variable and site-dependent frequent changes: • Ocular adnexa: *TNFAIP3* (35%) • Salivary glands: *GPR34* (19%) • Skin: *FAS* (63%) • Thyroid: *CD274* (68%), *TNFRSF14* (53%), and *TET2* (86%)	Frequent in *KMT2D* (34%), *PTPRD* (~20%), *NOTCH2* (20%), *KLF2* (17%); recurrent in *CARD11*, *FAS*, *TNFAIP3*, *CREBBP*, *TET2*, and *TBL1XR1* Rare in *BRAF*, *MYD88*, and *CXCR4*	Frequent in *KLF2* (20–40%) and *NOTCH2* (~22%) Recurrent in a number of genes involved in NOTCH and NF-κB pathways, epigenetic regulation, and DNA damage responses
Molecular pathogenesis	Enhanced NF-κB activation through B-cell receptor stimulation, T-cell help, and genetic changes in these pathways Enhanced GPCR signalling due to crosstalk between inflamed epithelium and lymphoma cells and related genetic changes	Enhanced *NOTCH2* and NF-κB activations by genetic changes	Two genetic clusters: NNK cluster, dominated by mutations enhancing NOTCH and NF-κB activation; and DMT cluster, characterized by mutations impairing DNA damage responses
Prognosis	Indolent, with median survival > 10 years in majority; early progression is unfavourable; transformation occurs in 2–3% of patients	Indolent, with median survival > 10 years; transformation occurs in 5% of patients	Indolent, with median survival > 10 years; early progression and high-grade transformation associated with inferior survival

DMT, differentially methylated targets; GPCR, G protein–coupled receptor; NNK, 4-(N-methyl-N-nitrosamino)-1-(3-pyridyl)-1-butanone.

Extranodal marginal zone lymphoma of mucosa-associated lymphoid tissue

Cheuk W
Cheng CL
Cooper WA
Delabie J
Du MQ
Geddie WR
Inagaki H
Kakkar A
Kempf W
Ott G
Raderer M
Tallini G

Definition

Extranodal marginal zone lymphoma of mucosa-associated lymphoid tissue (EMZL) is an indolent primary extranodal B-cell lymphoma with cytological and architectural features reminiscent of Peyer patch lymphoid tissue, the prototypical mucosa-associated lymphoid tissue (MALT). EMZL typically arises from marginal zone B cells of acquired MALT and is often associated with an underlying chronic inflammatory disorder.

ICD-O coding

9699/3 Extranodal marginal zone lymphoma of mucosa-associated lymphoid tissue
9762/3 Immunoproliferative small intestinal disease (alpha heavy chain disease)

ICD-11 coding

2A85.3 & XH1V99 Extranodal marginal zone B-cell lymphoma, primary site excluding stomach or skin & Extranodal marginal zone lymphoma of mucosa-associated lymphoid tissue

Related terminology

Acceptable: mucosa-associated lymphoid tissue (MALT) lymphoma; extranodal marginal zone lymphoma of MALT.
Not recommended: MALToma.

Subtype(s)

Immunoproliferative small intestinal disease (alpha heavy chain disease; see also *Alpha heavy chain disease*, p. 619)

Localization

Almost any anatomical site can be affected, including sites lacking mucosa. The most commonly affected sites are the stomach, ocular adnexa, salivary gland, skin, lung, breast, thyroid, and thymus. Others include the upper aerodigestive tract, small and large intestines, hepatobiliary system, pancreas, dura and brain, urogenital tract, female genital tract, and soft tissues {1801, 1293, 2088, 3872, 1967, 3225, 4206, 315, 223, 1812, 2187}. Synchronous involvement of two or more sites can occur at presentation, with a propensity to involve other extranodal sites during the course of disease {980,3343}.

Distribution of EMZL at a tertiary care centre in Vienna (1999-2018) (n=415)

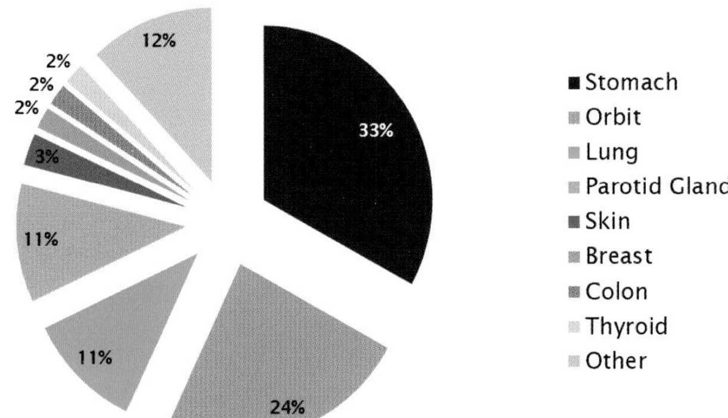

Fig. 4.83 Extranodal marginal zone lymphoma. Relative frequency of primary-presenting extranodal sites in patients with extranodal marginal zone lymphoma.

EMZL at various sites

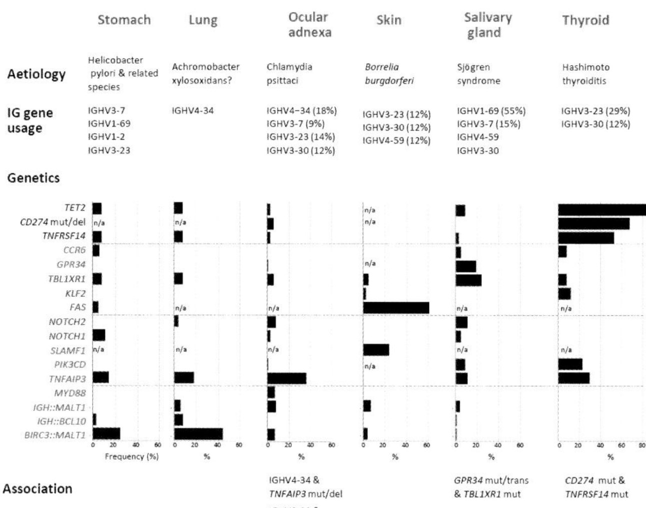

Fig. 4.84 Extranodal marginal zone lymphoma (EMZL). Etiology, IG gene usage, and recurrent genetic abnormalities in EMZL of various sites. Many of the EMZL-derived immunoglobulins are autoreactive, and where possible the estimated frequency of their usage is provided. As many of the genes involved in EMZL have not been uniformly investigated across different sites, only the recurrent genetic changes fundamental to the understanding of EMZL pathogenesis are presented {4423,4200}. The genes are grouped in different colour schemes according to their function. Known association among immunoglobulin usage and genetic changes is indicated. del, deletion; mut, mutation; n/a, data not available; trans, translocation.

Clinical features

Patients with EMZL present with symptoms related to a mass lesion, or they are asymptomatic, with the lymphoma being incidentally discovered. B symptoms are rare (see Table 4.23, p. 403). The lymphoma is often diagnosed while the disease is localized, with a low tumour burden {3342}. Regional lymph node involvement or disseminated disease may be found upon thorough staging in 25–50% of patients {3343,4594}, being significantly more common in extragastric EMZL (40–50%) than in gastric EMZL (25%) {3342}. Bone marrow involvement is found in 2–5% {2080,336}. The serum LDH and B2M levels are usually normal. Monoclonal gammopathy, usually of IgG or IgM type, can be detected in as many as one third of patients at diagnosis; the titre may correlate with therapeutic response {4398, 4054}.

Epidemiology

EMZL constitutes 5–8% of B-cell lymphomas, with an incidence rate of 0.5–2.6 cases per 100 000 person-years {3811,2730}. It is slightly more common in Asian people, and it represents the most common low-grade B-cell lymphoma in China and the Republic of Korea {3880,853}. The overall incidence of EMZL, with the exception of gastric EMZL, has increased over the years {2446,587}. EMZL occurs over a wide age range, mostly in adults (median age: 61 years) {2976}. A female predilection is observed in EMZL of the salivary gland, thyroid, and thymus, due to the higher prevalence of the associated autoimmune disorders in female patients. EMZL is rare in the paediatric population but is the most common primary cutaneous B-cell lymphoma in children and adolescents {1949,3995,398}.

Etiology

EMZL usually arises in acquired MALT at extranodal sites, which results from a chronic inflammatory process caused by infection, autoimmunity, or unknown factors. The development of gastric EMZL has been linked to chronic *Helicobacter pylori* infection by epidemiological and in vivo studies {3147,4411}. A causative relationship is supported by observations that *H. pylori* is capable of stimulating lymphoma cell proliferation in vitro {1693}, and its eradication by antibiotics leads to lymphoma remissions in about 80% of patients {4410,1009,3506,4594}. Since the introduction of antibiotic therapy for *H. pylori*–associated gastritis, the incidence of gastric EMZL has declined. Conversely, the incidence of *H. pylori*–negative gastric EMZL has increased, accounting for 10–30% of cases, partially due to other *Helicobacter* species {2883,3947,1984}. A similar role has been suggested for *Campylobacter jejuni* infection in the development of immunoproliferative small intestine disease (alpha heavy chain disease, see *Alpha heavy chain disease*, p. 619) {2248,86}, a disease that is disappearing with the worldwide availability of antibiotics {86}.

There is also a link between *Borrelia burgdorferi* and *Chlamydia psittaci* infection and primary cutaneous and ocular adnexal EMZL, respectively, and evidence of lymphoma response to antibiotic treatment in a proportion of cases {1289, 2166,1181,1182,1006,3280}. However, these associations vary greatly according to geographical regions.

EMZL of the salivary gland and thyroid are commonly preceded by Sjögren syndrome and Hashimoto thyroiditis, respectively, whose histological features are almost invariably identifiable in the involved sites. Patients with Sjögren syndrome or Hashimoto thyroiditis have a 14- to 19-fold or 9- to 17-fold increased risk, respectively, of developing lymphoma, particularly EMZL {2335,2968,3396,1913}. EMZL of the thymus also shows a strong association with Sjögren syndrome {1719}. Rare EMZL arises in patients with immune deficiency/dysregulation. An etiological association to the immune deficiency/dysregulation setting can only be substantiated in those cases that are EBV-associated (see *Lymphomas arising in immune deficiency/dysregulation*, p. 568) {1362}.

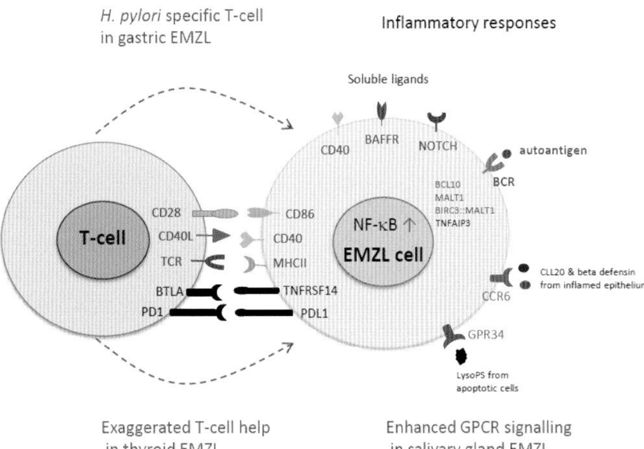

Fig. 4.85 Extranodal marginal zone lymphoma (EMZL). The proposed model of molecular pathogenesis of EMZL. The development of EMZL is the result of oncogenic cooperation among dysregulated immune responses and somatic genetic changes. The genetic changes vary considerably among EMZL of various sites but commonly affect the molecular pathways important for marginal B cells, particularly those leading to NF-κB activation. In general, the canonical NF-κB pathway is activated by chronic B-cell receptor (BCR) signalling triggered by autoantigens and genetic changes such as IGH::*BCL10*, IGH::*MALT1*, *BIRC3*::*MALT1*, and *TNFAIP3* mutation/deletion, whereas the noncanonical NF-κB pathway is activated by helper T cells, soluble ligands (CD40, BAFF), and *BIRC3*::*MALT1* fusion. In gastric EMZL, helper T cells are triggered by *Helicobacter pylori*–mediated immune responses, whereas in thyroid EMZL, these may result indirectly from genetic inactivation of *CD274* (*PDL1*) and *TNFRSF14*. In salivary gland EMZL, *GPR34* activation is triggered by mutation, rarely translocation, but more commonly by ligands produced by lymphoepithelial lesions. Similarly, CCR6 is activated by mutation and ligands from the inflamed epithelium in lesions of the salivary glands and stomach. Negative regulators are in black text; positive regulators are in different colour themes. GPCR, G protein–coupled receptor; TCR, T-cell receptor.

Pathogenesis

The genesis of EMZL is the result of oncogenic cooperation among dysregulated immune responses and somatic genetic changes {1007,1008}. The clonally rearranged IG genes in EMZL show somatic hypermutations {1012,4000} and frequent intraclonal variations {1012,4000}, suggesting that the lymphoma cells remain responsive to T-cell–dependent immune responses, consistent with their frequent involvement of existing B-cell follicles (follicular colonization). EMZLs, particularly those of the ocular adnexa and salivary glands, show a biased usage of IG genes, expressing autoreactive antigen B-cell receptor {855,4585,4163, 307,2762,306}. B-cell receptor engagement by autoantigens triggers its chronic activation, with extensive downstream molecular signalling including the canonical NF-κB pathway.

Studies of gastric EMZL show that the lymphoma cell growth critically depends on *H. pylori*–mediated T-cell help, involving both cognate interactions and stimulation by soluble ligands such as CD154 (CD40L) and BAFF {1693,925,1409,831,2156}, which activate the non-canonical NF-κB pathway. T-cell help may also operate in EMZL of other sites.

Apart from trisomy of chromosomes 3 and 18, all other genetic changes occur at highly variable frequencies in EMZL of different sites, with the majority affecting common molecular pathways important for marginal zone B cells.

A t(11;18)(q21;q21)/*BIRC3*::*MALT1* fusion is frequently seen in EMZL of the stomach (24%) and lung (40%), but rarely in other sites, and it is not recurrent in other B-cell lymphomas {4492, 3851}. The *BIRC3*::*MALT1* fusion is capable of activating both canonical and non-canonical NF-κB pathways {3464,1007}. The t(1;14)(p22;q32)/IGH::*BCL10*, t(14;18)(q32;q21)/IGH::*MALT1*, and t(3;14)(p14;q32)/IGH::*FOXP1* are infrequent and cause overexpression of the involved oncogenes {4490,4491,1355}. BCL10 and MALT1 connect B-cell receptor signalling to the

Table 4.23 Clinicopathological features and site-specific differential diagnosis of extranodal marginal zone lymphoma of mucosa-associated lymphoid tissue (EMZL) in common sites (continued on next page)

Site	Clinical features	Endoscopic/radiological/ macroscopic findings	Site-specific pathological features	Differential diagnosis
Stomach	Nonspecific symptoms (dyspepsia, weight loss, abdominal pain); less frequently, vomiting; asymptomatic in a small proportion of cases	Mass with ulceration (50%), hypertrophic mucosal folds or multinodular pattern (25%), normal or hyperaemic mucosa (12%), exophytic lesion (10%) {4598,2884}	LELs common and may show eosinophilic degeneration forming incomplete glands, short cords, or signet ring–like cells mimicking carcinoma The GELA scoring system can be used to assess post–*Helicobacter* eradication gastric biopsy (see Table 4.24, p. 408); however, clonal molecular analysis is not recommended because B-cell clones with no clinical impact can persist after complete histological remission {3129, 4293,4594,798,801,335}	Florid chronic gastritis / acquired MALT: Organized lymphoid infiltrate with reactive follicles surrounded by T cells; usually limited to lamina propria, LELs rare and not prominent Russell body gastritis: Plasma cells polytypic
Ocular adnexa	Conjunctiva: Slow-growing, painless, salmon-pink fleshy patch or swelling Lacrimal gland: Painless mass, exophthalmos, decreased eye motility, diplopia and ptosis Eyelid and orbital soft tissue: Painless mass Lacrimal sac: Epiphora, swelling, dacryocystitis and acquired nasolacrimal obstruction {1185,1287,4254}	CT/MRI shows an infiltrative mass that moulds along the eyeball	Polykaryocytes and perivascular hyalinization are common {1185,821, 1588}	IgG4-related disease: Preserved lymphoid architecture; storiform fibrosis with eosinophils and polytypic plasma cells
Salivary gland	Painless mass, sometimes bilateral; occasionally pain or facial nerve palsy {4059,376,4556}	Ultrasound shows hypoechoic solid nodules interspersed with linear echogenic septations (tortoiseshell pattern) Non-circumscribed, firm, tan-coloured tumours with interspersed cysts formed by dilated ducts	LEL with prominent monocytoid cells Presence of a pale zone (collar) of monocytoid cells around LELs is an early sign of EMZL Cystic changes in the interspersed ducts are common {4556,1698}	Lymphoepithelial sialadenitis: Preserved lobular architecture of salivary gland; lacks sheet-like B-cell proliferation and monotypic plasma cells IgG4-related sialadenitis: Preserved lymphoid architecture; storiform fibrosis with eosinophils and polytypic plasma cells, no LELs
Skin	Solitary, often multifocal red or violaceous plaques or nodules, preferentially on trunk and upper arm; waxing and waning course; spontaneous regression possible {1319,1608,3679,1043,1320,1360, 1608,3683,1171,3902}	Plaque or nodules usually covered by intact epidermis	Heavy chain class-switched form (more common): Dense multinodular infiltrate of small lymphocytes in dermis with a lymphoplasmacytoid appearance; aggregates of monotypic plasma cells; reactive follicles in the background; abundant reactive T cells; expression of IgG, IgA, or IgE; IgG4 found in 13–35% of cases but without IgG4-related disease; CXCR3 is negative Non–class-switched form (less common): Expression of IgM and CXCR3; large sheets of B cells dominating over T cells {1951,452,907,561,1043,4162, 560,219,1319,1360,3902}	Cutaneous lymphoid hyperplasia: Lacks monotypic plasma cells and clonal IG gene rearrangement Secondary cutaneous EMZL: Predominance of monocytoid cells and IgM expression; need clinical correlations {1043}
Lung	Often incidental findings or nonspecific respiratory symptoms (cough, dyspnoea, or chest pain)	One or several unilateral or bilateral solid masses on CT; air bronchogram common; some show ground-glass opacities or interstitial infiltrates Consolidated masses with a yellow to cream-coloured cut surface {3822,2163,555}	Alveoli effaced by dense sheets of neoplastic cells; LELs prominent; neoplastic cells often track along bronchovascular bundles at the periphery	Nodular lymphoid hyperplasia and lymphocytic interstitial pneumonia: Lack sheets of CD20+ B cells, monotypic plasma cells, and clonal IG gene rearrangement

LEL, lymphoepithelial lesion; MALT, mucosa-associated lymphoid tissue.

Table 4.23 Clinicopathological features and site-specific differential diagnosis of extranodal marginal zone lymphoma of mucosa-associated lymphoid tissue (EMZL) in common sites (continued)

Site	Clinical features	Endoscopic/radiological/ macroscopic findings	Site-specific pathological features	Differential diagnosis
Thymus	Higher incidence in Asian populations Asymptomatic or presenting with chest pain, dyspnoea, and haemoptysis {1719,4310}	CXR/CT/MR shows multiloculated or cystic mass Well-circumscribed masses comprising fleshy, tan-coloured tissue, commonly multiple variably sized cysts filled with proteinaceous material	Scattered epithelium-lined cysts, reactive lymphoid follicles surrounded by neoplastic cells with conspicuous monocytoid and plasmacytic differentiation; thymic epithelium, Hassall corpuscles and epithelial cyst lining are massively expanded by lymphoma cells (LELs) imparting a pale nodular appearance at low magnification; IgA expression is common {1719}	Multilocular thymic cyst and thymic follicular hyperplasia: Organized reactive lymphoid tissue, normal distribution of B and T cells; lacks monotypic plasma cells Hyaline-vascular Castleman disease: Usually involves mediastinal nodes; hyaline-vascular follicles; abundant high endothelial venules in the interfollicular region; B cells mostly confined to follicles while T cells are abundant in interfollicular zone
Thyroid	Asymptomatic or presenting as an enlarging thyroid mass {4326,93, 930}	Markedly hypoechoic mass, cold by scintigraphy {4484} Solid, non-circumscribed mass with a white cut surface	Thyroid follicles expanded by neoplastic cells forming the characteristic (although not pathognomonic) MALT balls; LELs; Hashimoto thyroiditis in the background {3178,3757,930,4326,203,930}	Hashimoto and lymphocytic thyroiditis: Lacks extensive destruction of thyroid parenchyma and clonal IG gene rearrangement {4326}
Breast	Mass lesion {2204,3951}	Mass lesion by mammography {2546}	Lymphoma cells in close proximity to mammary epithelium, LELs uncommon {3951,2591,987,322}	Lymphocytic mastopathy: Keloid-like stroma; epithelioid myofibroblasts; polytypic plasma cells usually IgG+ {322} IgG4-related mastitis: Reactive follicles; interfollicular lymphoplasmacytic and eosinophilic infiltrate; polytypic plasma cells

LEL, lymphoepithelial lesion; MALT, mucosa-associated lymphoid tissue.

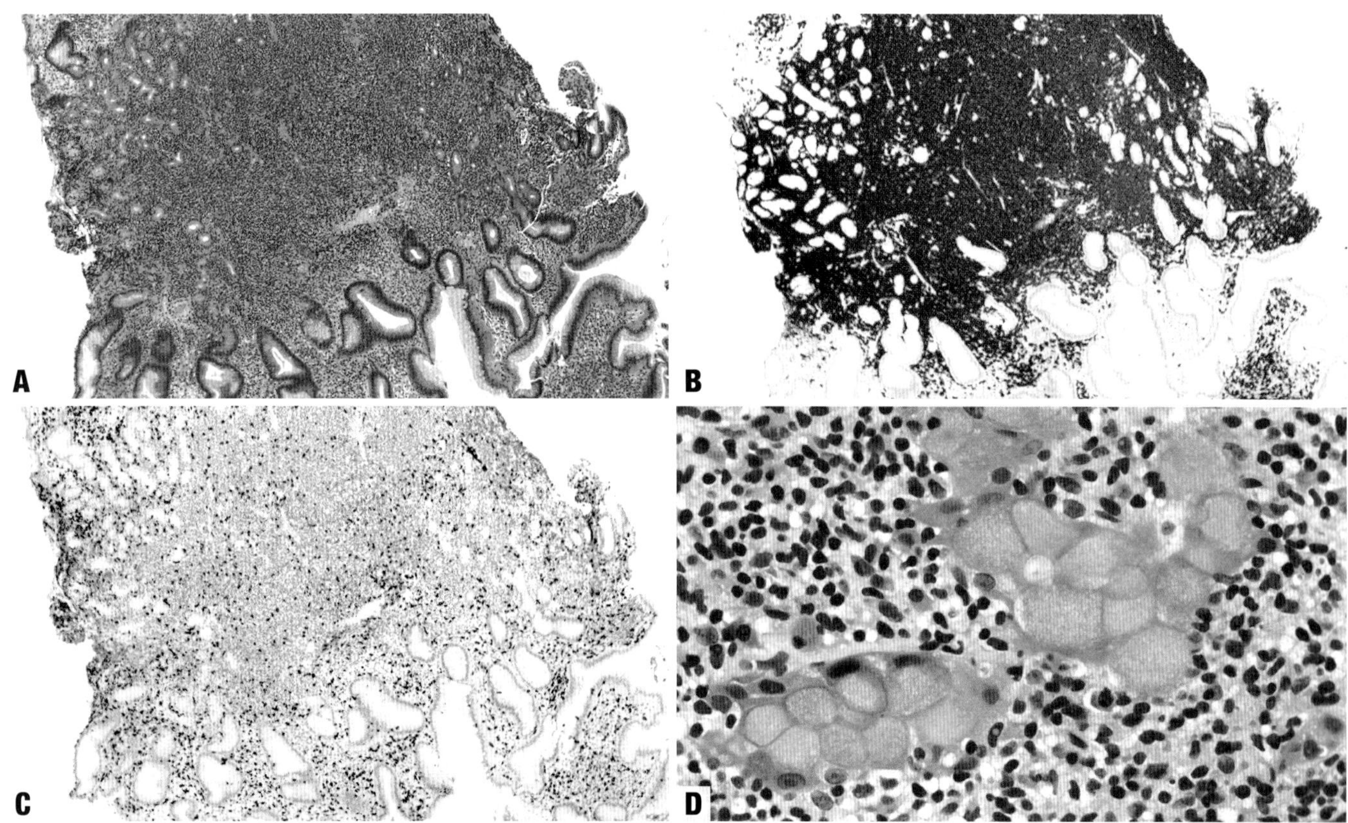

Fig. 4.86 Extranodal marginal zone lymphoma, gastric localization. The lamina propria is replaced by dense sheets of lymphoma cells (**A**). The infiltrate is positive for CD20 (**B**), with only scarce CD3-positive T cells (**C**). A signet ring–like appearance of the residual glandular cells may be seen (**D**).

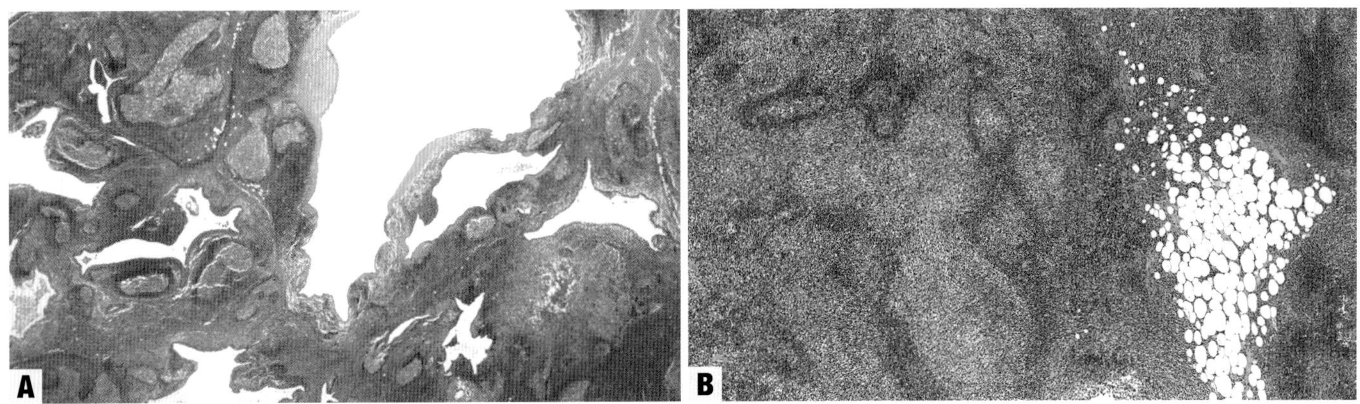

Fig. 4.87 Extranodal marginal zone lymphoma. **A** Parotid localization shows many cystically dilated ducts resulting from the compressive effects of the lymphoid proliferation. **B** Thymus involvement shows pale areas of monocytoid cells with scattered residual follicles.

canonical NF-κB pathway, and their overexpression causes constitutive NF-κB activation {1007}, while FOXP1 represses the expression of proapoptotic genes and cooperates with NF-κB to promote cell survival {4159}.

A number of genes are somatically mutated in EMZL. *TNFAIP3* (*A20*), a global negative regulator of the canonical NF-κB pathway, is frequently somatically inactivated by mutation and/or deletion in EMZL. In ocular adnexal EMZL, *TNFAIP3* mutations/deletions are the most frequent and are associated with IGHV4-34 usage, suggesting their potential cooperation in NF-κB activation {1626,634,2761}.

Several G protein–coupled receptors show recurrent activating mutations in EMZL, with *GPR34* mutation and rarely t(X;14)(p11;q32)/IGH::*GPR34* occurring exclusively in EMZL of the salivary glands (16%) {2762,4423}. Additionally, GPR34 signalling may be maintained by ligands produced by lymphoepithelial lesions (LELs) in salivary gland EMZL {2107}. Similarly, CCR6 signalling may also be triggered by ligands (CCL20, defensins) produced by the inflamed epithelium in EMZL of salivary glands and stomach {2106}. The stimulatory cross-talks between inflamed epithelium and B cells may explain the emergence of neoplastic B cells and their expansion surrounding LELs.

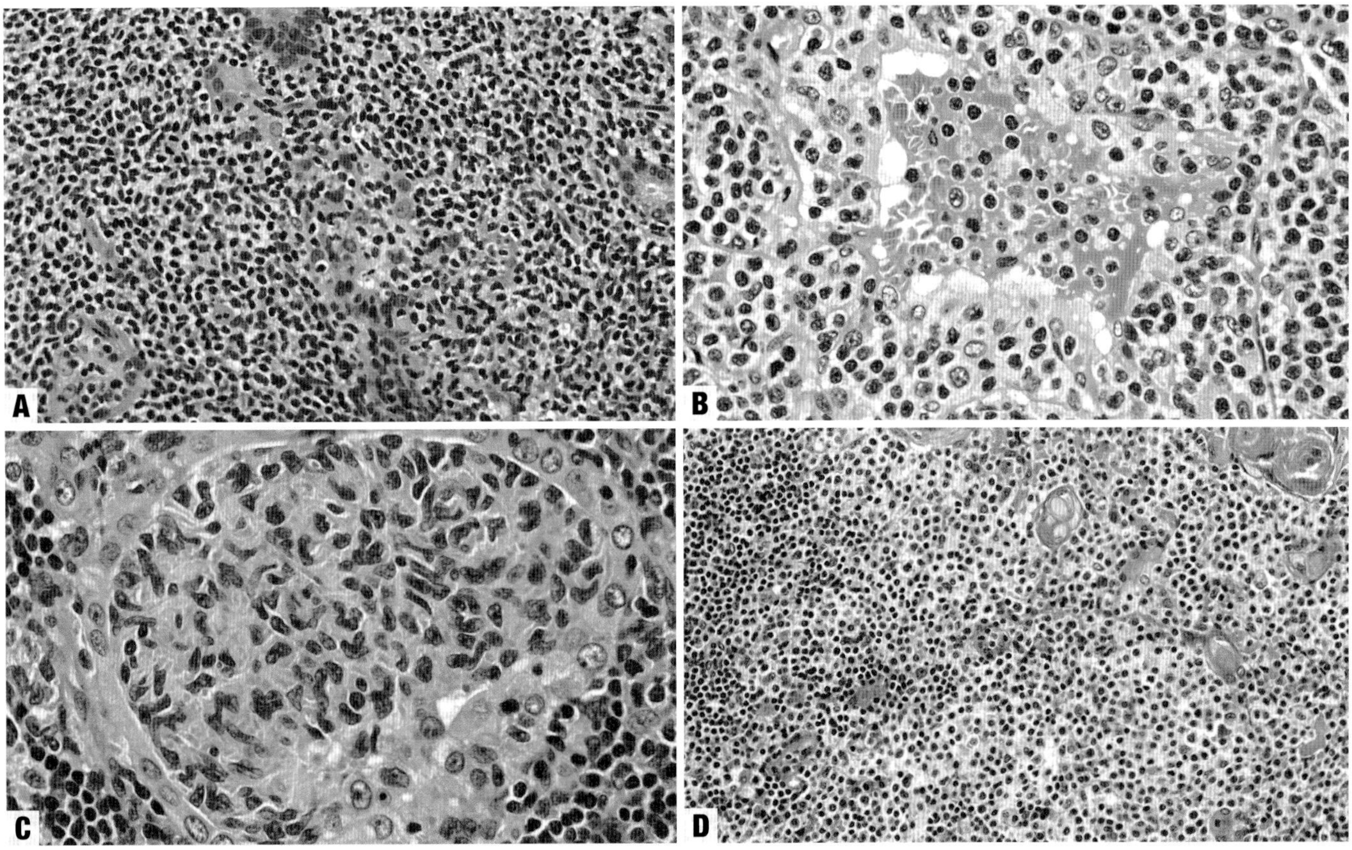

Fig. 4.88 Extranodal marginal zone lymphoma lymphoepithelial lesion (LEL). **A** In a LEL in the stomach, the glands are infiltrated, partially destroyed, and focally expanded by the lymphoma cells. **B** LEL appearance in the lung. **C** Mucosa-associated lymphoid tissue (MALT)-ball LEL in the thyroid. **D** LEL with residual Hassall corpuscles in the thymus.

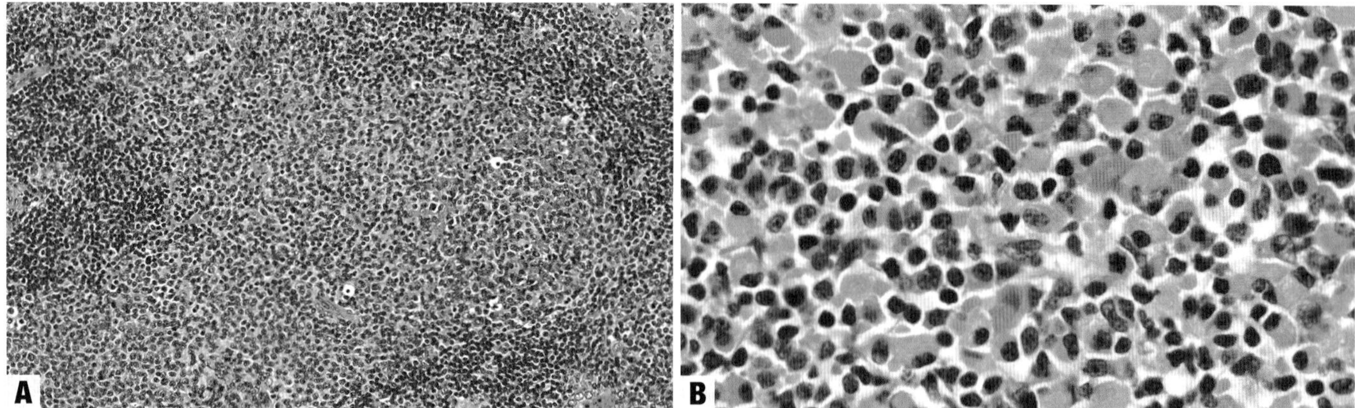

Fig. 4.89 Extranodal marginal zone lymphoma. **A** Extranodal marginal zone lymphoma tumour cells colonize the germinal centre of the follicle. Some residual germinal centre cells are noted. **B** In some cases, neoplastic plasmacytic cells are predominant and immunoglobulin-laden (submandibular localization).

In contrast, thyroid EMZLs are characterized by highly frequent and concurrent inactivating mutations in *TET2*, *CD274*, and *TNFRSF14* {4423}. *CD274* (*PDL1*) and *TNFRSF14* encode ligands for the co-inhibitory receptor PD1 and BTLA on T helper cells, respectively, and their inactivation may dysregulate their interaction with T cells, promoting costimulation and impairing peripheral tolerance {4423}, thus contributing to lymphomagenesis.

Macroscopic appearance

See Table 4.23 (p. 403).

Histopathology

The key microscopic feature of EMZL is a proliferation of atypical small to medium-sized lymphoid cells that efface the architecture of the affected sites, with or without site-specific LELs. The neoplastic cells comprise variable proportions of small lymphocytes with round nuclei and condensed chromatin; marginal zone cells (sometimes called centrocyte-like cells) with small to medium-sized slightly irregular nuclei, smooth chromatin, and pale cytoplasm {4594}; and monocytoid cells with abundant pale cytoplasm. Monocytoid cells are particularly prominent in EMZL of the salivary glands and thymus. There are often admixed plasma cells, shown to be monotypic in one third of cases, which can form large aggregates and may show Dutcher bodies, Russell bodies, or other immunoglobulin inclusions (crystals or globules) or be accompanied by crystal-storing histiocytosis or amyloid deposition {2088,3508}. Scattered centroblast- or immunoblast-like cells are common. Large-cell transformation is diagnosed when there are sheets of large cells unassociated with follicular dendritic cell meshworks {790,2473, 1985,4594}. Lymphoma cells display confluent growth, and they often surround remnants of reactive follicles in a marginal zone pattern. The germinal centres can be variably replaced by the lymphoma cells (follicular colonization), mimicking follicular lymphoma. The lymphoma cells infiltrate, expand, and distort the epithelial structures, forming LELs. When EMZL involves regional lymph nodes, it often shows interfollicular expansion, marginal zone, or perisinusoidal growth patterns {2885}.

Immunohistochemistry

Neoplastic cells express CD20, CD79a, and PAX5; usually IgM; occasionally IgG or IgA; and exceptionally IgD. IgA expression is overrepresented in thymic EMZL. IgG4 expression can be found in dural EMZL and primary cutaneous marginal zone lymphoma, without associated IgG4-related disease {1719, 4210,452,907}. EMZLs are typically negative for CD5, CD10, BCL6, CD23, cyclin D1, and SOX11 {1362}. A small subset (< 4%) of EMZL expresses CD5, which may be associated with more aggressive behaviour {4360,1185,1790}. IRTA1 (FCRLF4, CD307d), a marker of marginal zone cell differentiation, is expressed in 40–90% of EMZLs {1114,4316}. MNDA is frequently

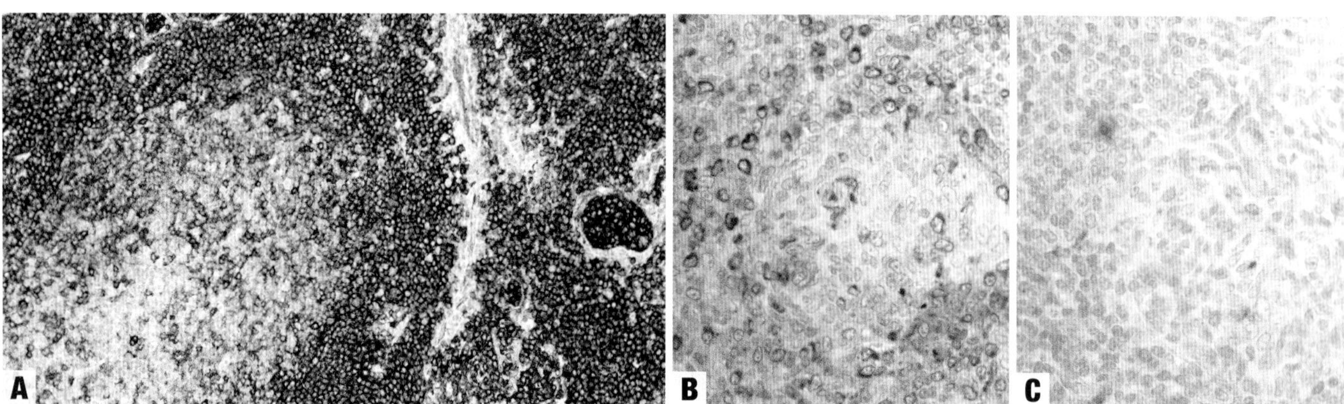

Fig. 4.90 Extranodal marginal zone lymphoma. **A** Strong IRTA1 immunostaining in the marginal zone surrounding germinal centres and lymphoepithelial lesions (thyroid localization). **B,C** The neoplastic cells express kappa (**B**) but not lambda (**C**).

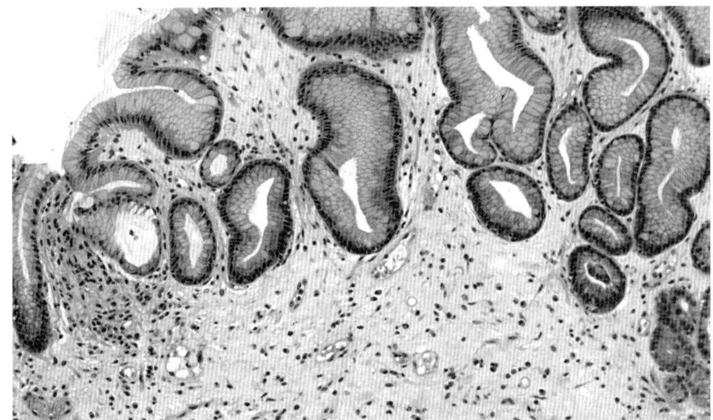

Fig. 4.91 Extranodal marginal zone lymphoma. Gastric extranodal marginal zone lymphoma with complete response after *Helicobacter*-eradication therapy, with an empty-looking lamina propria with glandular atrophy and rare lymphocytic infiltrate.

positive in EMZL, but it is also expressed in a subset of other types of B-cell lymphoma {1870,4316}. Aberrant expression of CD43 (in 20–40%) {2197} or TBX21 (T-bet) (in 40–89%) {2402} and immunoglobulin light chain restriction can aid in the distinction from reactive lymphoid proliferations. CD21 highlights expanded follicular dendritic cell meshworks in the background of the lymphoma, encompassing both reactive follicles and also colonized follicles. Cytokeratin can highlight subtle LELs.

In immunoproliferative small intestinal disease, the lymphocytes and plasma cells express cytoplasmic alpha heavy chain without associated light chains.

Differential diagnosis

EMZL can be distinguished from reactive hyperplasia by sheet-like or permeative infiltration of CD20+ B cells, effacement of architecture, monotypic plasma cells, and monoclonal IG gene rearrangements. Atypical marginal zone hyperplasia is a reactive lesion of children presenting with tonsillar enlargement, a pharyngeal mass, or appendicitis {180}. It shows reactive follicular hyperplasia, expanded marginal zones, and abundant B cells invading crypt epithelium or colonizing germinal centres. Lambda light chain restriction is often demonstrated, but no monoclonal IG gene rearrangement is found.

Other mature B-cell lymphomas (e.g. follicular lymphoma, mantle cell lymphoma, and chronic lymphocytic leukaemia / small lymphocytic lymphoma) can be excluded by a lack of CD10, BCL6, CD5, cyclin D1, and LEF1 protein expression. EMZL with prominent follicular colonization may mimic follicular lymphoma; the presence of an appreciable extrafollicular component of B cells, a lack of extensive expression of follicular-centre markers (particularly CD10) within and outside follicles {3287}, and an absence of *BCL2* gene translocation may support the former. Distinction between EMZL and lymphoplasmacytic lymphoma can be very difficult, especially in extranodal sites. Bone marrow and lymph node involvement at presentation, high-titre IgM paraproteinaemia, frequent Dutcher bodies, and *MYD88* p.L265P (NP_002459.2) mutation would favour the latter. Rare cases of EMZL show extensive plasma cell differentiation, mimicking plasmacytoma, but the presence of a component of CD20+ B cells, as well as presentation in a typical MALT site, would favour the former.

Cytology

The cytology is challenging, and it may be difficult to distinguish EMZL from reactive lymphoid hyperplasia. Smears are usually moderately to highly cellular, with a mixed cellular population. However, small to medium-sized cells may predominate. These cells have moderate amounts of pale cytoplasm, mild nuclear contour irregularities, and moderately dispersed and inconspicuous nucleoli (resembling centrocytes).

Diagnostic molecular pathology

Demonstration of monoclonal IG gene rearrangements may help establish a diagnosis when the histopathological and immunophenotypic findings are suspicious but not diagnostic. However, monoclonal IG gene rearrangements can be seen in some reactive conditions associated with EMZL {970, 2809,1832}. Where consecutive biopsies are available for initial diagnostic investigations, comparative clonality analyses should be performed to identify persistent and progressively expanding, hence potentially lymphoma-related, IG gene rearrangements, discriminating those from reactive B cells, which tend to be more variable although are occasionally recurrent. With the exception of t(11;18)/*BIRC3*::*MALT1*, which is frequently seen in EMZL of the stomach (in 24%) and lung (in 40%), other EMZL-associated genetic changes are at a low frequency or their diagnostic utility is unclear. Differentiating EMZL from other low-grade lymphomas is better approached by investigating the characteristic genetic changes in the latter.

Essential and desirable diagnostic criteria

Essential: primary lymphoma arising in an extranodal site; atypical small/medium-sized lymphoid cell proliferation mimicking reactive MALT and showing architectural distortion; expression of B-lineage markers; exclusion of other small B-cell neoplasms, e.g. follicular lymphoma, mantle cell lymphoma, small lymphocytic lymphoma, lymphoplasmacytic lymphoma, and plasmacytoma.

Desirable: demonstration of light chain restriction or clonal IG gene rearrangement; lymphoepithelial lesions; remnants of underlying inflammatory background (e.g. reactive lymphoid follicles, Hashimoto thyroiditis in the thyroid, or lymphoepithelial sialadenitis in the salivary gland).

Staging

The Lugano classification is used to stage EMZL. The Ann Arbor classification has often been used for non-gastric EMZL {4594,3343}.

Prognosis and prediction

EMZL is an indolent lymphoma. Local recurrences, relapses in other MALT sites, and nodal or distant metastasis may occur, but the 5- and 10-year overall survival rates reach 90% and 80%, respectively {3343}. A clinical prognostic index – the MALT Lymphoma International Prognostic Index (MALT-IPI) – has been developed for stratifying patients into three prognostic groups (low, intermediate, and high risk) according to the presence of 0, 1, and 2–3 of the following parameters: age > 70 years, stage III/IV, and elevated LDH {3999}, but further studies are needed to determine its value for tailoring treatment decisions. Among genetic changes, t(11;18)(q21;q21) is associated with

Table 4.24 GELA histological grading system for posttreatment evaluation of gastric extranodal marginal zone lymphoma of mucosa-associated lymphoid tissue (EMZL)

Score	Lymphoid infiltrate	Lymphoepithelial lesions	Stromal changes
Complete histological remission (CR)	Absent, or scattered plasma cells and small lymphoid cells in the lamina propria	Absent	Normal, or empty lamina propria and/or fibrosis
Probable minimal residual disease (pMRD)	Aggregates of lymphoid cells or lymphoid nodules in the lamina propria, muscularis mucosae, or submucosa	Absent	Empty lamina propria and/or fibrosis
Responding residual disease (rRD)	Dense, diffuse, or nodular, extending around glands in the lamina propria	Absent or present	Focal empty lamina propria and/or fibrosis
No change (NC)	Dense, diffuse, or nodular	Absent or present	No changes

more widespread disease and an impaired response of gastric EMZL to *H. pylori* eradication therapy, but high-grade transformation is extremely rare {2378,4428,3343,1985}. Large-cell transformation is associated with more aggressive behaviour {1986}. A grading system has been suggested for posttreatment histological evaluation (see Table 4.24).

Primary cutaneous marginal zone lymphoma

Geyer J
Willemze R

Definition

Primary cutaneous marginal zone lymphoma (PCMZL) is an indolent cutaneous B-cell lymphoma composed of neoplastic small B cells, plasma cells, and a variable number of reactive T cells.

ICD-O coding

9699/3 Primary cutaneous marginal zone lymphoma

ICD-11 coding

2A85.2 Extranodal marginal zone B-cell lymphoma, primary site skin

Related terminology

Acceptable: primary cutaneous marginal zone lymphoproliferative disorder.

Not recommended: primary cutaneous immunocytoma; primary cutaneous plasmacytoma.

Subtype(s)

Heavy chain class-switched form (IgG+, IgA+, or IgE+; ~90% of cases); non–class-switched form (IgM+; ~10% of cases)

Localization

The trunk and arms are the most common sites {1608,1319}.

Clinical features

Patients present with multifocal or (less frequently) solitary red or violaceous plaques or nodules.

Epidemiology

PCMZL accounts for 30–40% of all primary cutaneous B-cell lymphomas. PCMZL mostly affects adults in their fifth or sixth decade of life, with a male preponderance {3679}.

Etiology

The etiology of PCMZL is unknown in most cases. It may develop from chronic antigenic stimulation by intradermally applied antigens, such as tattoo pigments, vaccines, and tick-borne bacteria {454,1949}. An association with *Borrelia burgdorferi* infection is found in endemic areas in Europe, but not in the USA or Asia {593,1373,4406,3948}. Patients appear to have an increased frequency of various gastrointestinal disorders (reflux, gastric ulcers, positive *Helicobacter* serology, irritable bowel disease) and of various autoimmune diseases of uncertain significance {1443}.

Pathogenesis

Genetic sequencing studies identified deleterious somatic *FAS* mutations affecting the death domain of the apoptosis-regulating FAS (CD95) protein in > 60% of cases, suggesting that apoptosis defects underlie the pathogenesis of PCMZL {2608}. Somatic mutations have also recurrently been identified in *SLAMF1*, *SPEN*, and *NCOR2* {2608}.

Macroscopic appearance

Not relevant

Histopathology

PCMZL is characterized by a dense dermal infiltrate composed of small lymphocytes, plasma cells, and (in most cases) follicles with reactive germinal centres. The plasma cells are typically located at the periphery of the lymphoid infiltrates or in the subepidermal compartment.

The neoplastic B cells are positive for BCL2, and negative for CD5, CD10, BCL6, and cyclin D1. The reactive germinal centres contain BCL6-positive and BCL2-negative B cells and are highlighted by networks of follicular dendritic cells. Plasma cells show monotypic expression of immunoglobulin light

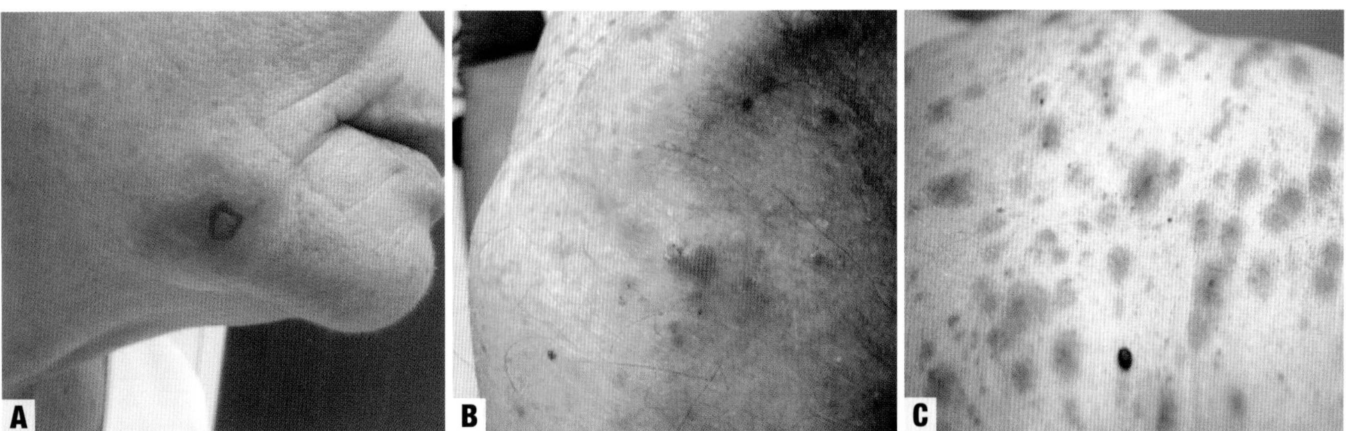

Fig. 4.92 Primary cutaneous marginal zone lymphoma. **A** Presentation with a solitary red nodule on the face. **B** A patient with multiple elevated plaques and nodules on the shoulder. **C** A rare presentation with extensive violaceous, rash-like plaques on the back that may typically be observed in epidermotropic primary cutaneous marginal zone lymphoma.

chains in most cases. The heavy chain class-switched form is characterized by the expression of IgG, IgA, or IgE, as well as a high number of T cells, and no expression of CXCR3. The non–class-switched form expresses IgM and CXCR3 and presents with large sheets of B cells and only a small number of T cells {4162,1043}. The class-switched cases more often have peripherally clustered monotypic plasma cells, in contrast to the scattered plasma cells in the non–class-switched cases {561}. Reactive T cells may be very prominent, occasionally obscuring the neoplastic B cells in the class-switched cases {1328}. Clusters of plasmacytoid dendritic cells (CD123+) are typically found in the periphery of the infiltrates {2167}. IgG4 is expressed by plasma cells in 13–35% of PCMZLs, but this finding is not associated with signs of IgG4-related disease {452,907}. Prominent monocytoid B cells and IgM expression should raise suspicion for a secondary cutaneous extranodal marginal zone lymphoma.

Cytology

Not applicable

Diagnostic molecular pathology

Heavy and light chain IG genes are clonally rearranged.

Essential and desirable diagnostic criteria

Essential: presence of CD5-negative, CD10-negative small B cells; demonstration of monotypic plasma cells, monotypic B cells, and/or clonal IG gene rearrangement; no evidence of

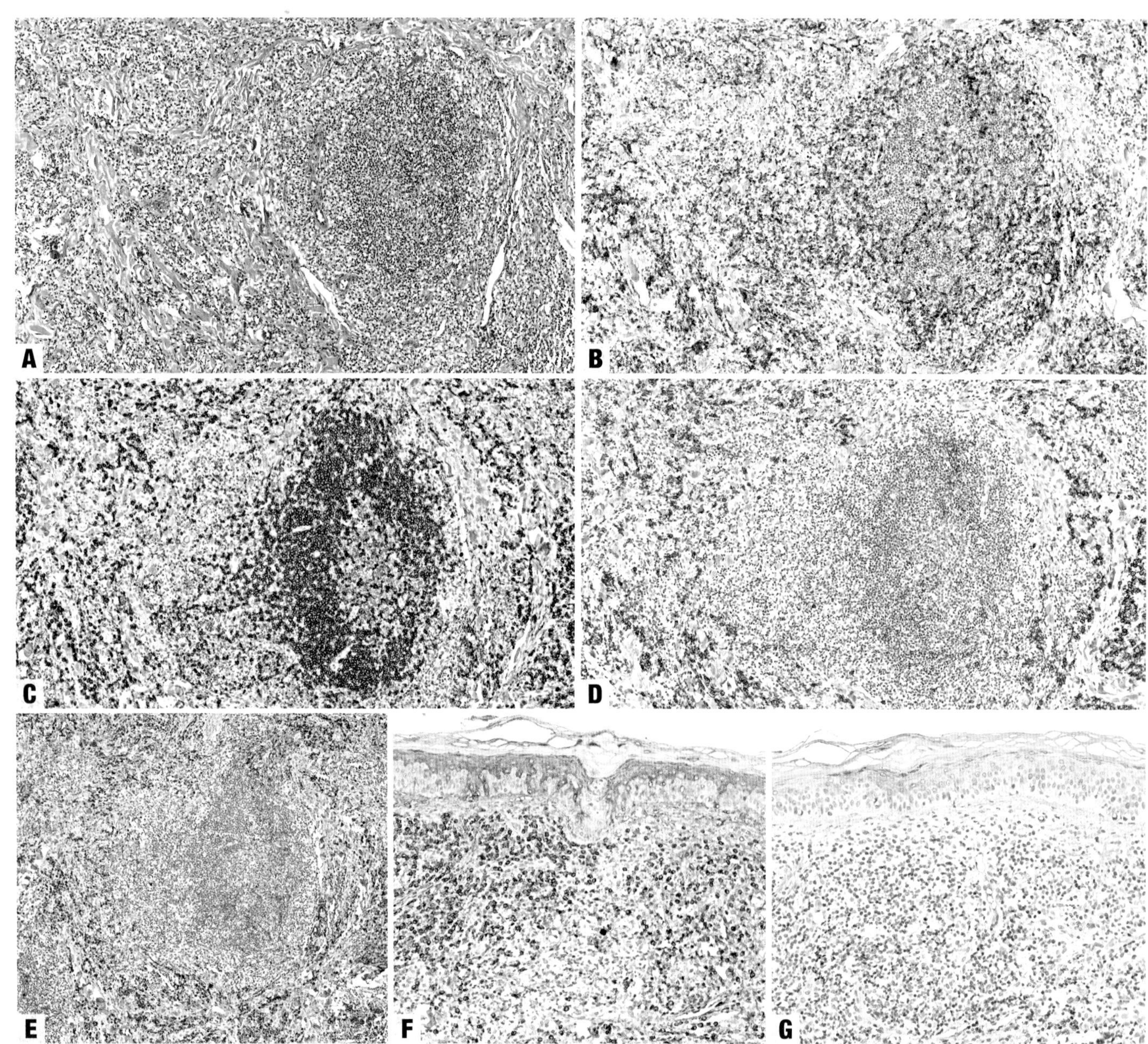

Fig. 4.93 Primary cutaneous marginal zone lymphoma. **A** Dense dermal lymphoid infiltrate that includes follicles with reactive germinal centres. **B** CD3 highlights numerous admixed T lymphocytes. **C** CD79a stains small B cells and plasma cells. **D** CD138 is positive in large aggregates of plasma cells at the periphery of the lymphoid infiltrate and in the subepidermal compartment. **E,F** The plasma cells express IgG (**E**) and monotypic kappa light chain (**F**). **G** Lambda light chain is negative.

extracutaneous disease at the time of diagnosis; exclusion of other cutaneous lymphomas.

Desirable: lesions on trunk or arms; reactive lymphoid follicles in lesion.

Staging

Cases are staged using the International Society for Cutaneous Lymphomas (ISCL) / European Organisation for Research and Treatment of Cancer (EORTC) TNM staging system for primary cutaneous lymphomas other than mycosis fungoides and Sézary syndrome {2015}.

Prognosis and prediction

The prognosis is favourable, with a 5-year disease-specific survival rate of > 98% {4378}. Recurrences are common. Extracutaneous spread rarely occurs (4% of all patients) and is more frequently observed in patients with longstanding multifocal disease, in the non–class-switched form and in PCMZL with transformation {1043,3683}. Some consider the class-switched cases as a clonal chronic cutaneous lymphoproliferative disorder rather than overt lymphoma {1043}.

Nodal marginal zone lymphoma

Natkunam Y
Attarbaschi A
Di Napoli A
Naresh KN
Ohgami RS
Rossi D

Definition

Nodal marginal zone lymphoma (NMZL) is a primary nodal lymphoma of small, mature B cells derived from marginal zone B cells, without involvement of extranodal sites or the spleen.

ICD-O coding

9699/3 Nodal marginal zone lymphoma

ICD-11 coding

2A85.0 Nodal marginal zone lymphoma

Related terminology

Not recommended: monocytoid B-cell lymphoma; parafollicular B-cell lymphoma.

Subtype(s)

None

Localization

NMZL involves single or multiple lymph nodes, most frequently in the head and neck, and often disseminates to the bone marrow. The peripheral blood may be involved, but lymphocytosis is uncommon {526,324,3004,4065}.

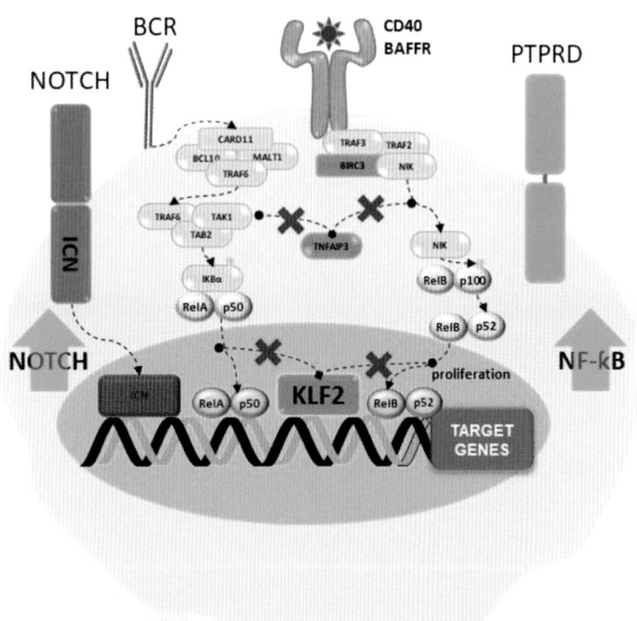

Fig. 4.94 Key molecular alterations in nodal marginal zone lymphoma. The main genes and pathways that are molecularly deregulated are schematically represented. The most frequently mutated genes are colour-coded on the basis of the consequences of the mutations: in purple are genes with loss of function, and in red are genes whose function is upregulated.

Clinical features

Patients may be asymptomatic at presentation and show painless, non-bulky peripheral adenopathy or (infrequently) lymphocytosis. An occult extranodal marginal zone lymphoma (EMZL) with spread to lymph nodes should be excluded in cases with localized lymphadenopathy {534}. Symptoms related to massive lymph node enlargement or cytopenias may occur at presentation in a minority of patients or arise during disease progression {526,141,2086,1547,4146,3437}. Systemic symptoms are rare and should raise suspicion of transformation to an aggressive lymphoma {790,4146}.

Paediatric nodal marginal zone lymphoma is discussed separately (see *Paediatric nodal marginal zone lymphoma*, p. 417).

Epidemiology

The age-adjusted incidence rate of NMZL is 6 cases per 1 million person-years. There is an exponential increase with age. The incidence is slightly higher among males and non-Hispanic White people {587}. Relative frequency is similar in high-, middle-, and low-resource countries {3198}. A family history of lymphoma, a history of autoimmune conditions, and HCV infection are risk factors {442}. Genetic variation in MHC loci influences susceptibility to NMZL {4232}.

Etiology

Unknown

Pathogenesis

NMZL shows clonal heavy and light chain IG gene rearrangements. More than 80% of cases show somatic IGHV mutations and biased usage towards IGHV4-34 and IGHV1-69 {789,4064, 3808,4446,1388}. Cytogenetic abnormalities and chromosomal copy-number changes (gains and losses) are common; in particular, gains of chromosomes 2p and 6p, and trisomy 3, 12, and 18. Losses of 1p and 6q are also seen. Recurrent translocations have not been identified {482,523,1,3414,4179,2130, 3243}. In marginal zone lymphomas, *PTPRD* mutation is skewed towards NMZL, although it occurs in only about 20% of cases. Translocations involving *BCL2* and *BCL6* (seen in follicular lymphoma and other B-cell lymphomas) and *MALT1*, *BIRC3*, *BCL10*, and *FOXP1* (seen in EMZL) are absent {3764,957,3392, 3850,3852,207,4179}.

Somatic mutation profiling of NMZL has demonstrated mutations recurrently affecting *KMT2D*, *PTPRD*, *KLF2*, *CARD11*, *FAS*, *TNFAIP3*, *CREBBP*, *TET2*, and *TBL1XR1*, although these mutations can be seen in other B-cell lymphomas {3907,4145, 3808,3243}. *NOTCH2* and *KLF2* mutations are common to both NMZL and splenic marginal zone lymphoma but are rare in other small B-cell lymphomas. *BRAF* mutations, including *BRAF* p.V600E (NP_004324.2), may occur in a small proportion of NMZLs {2238,3243}. *MYD88* and *CXCR4* mutations are

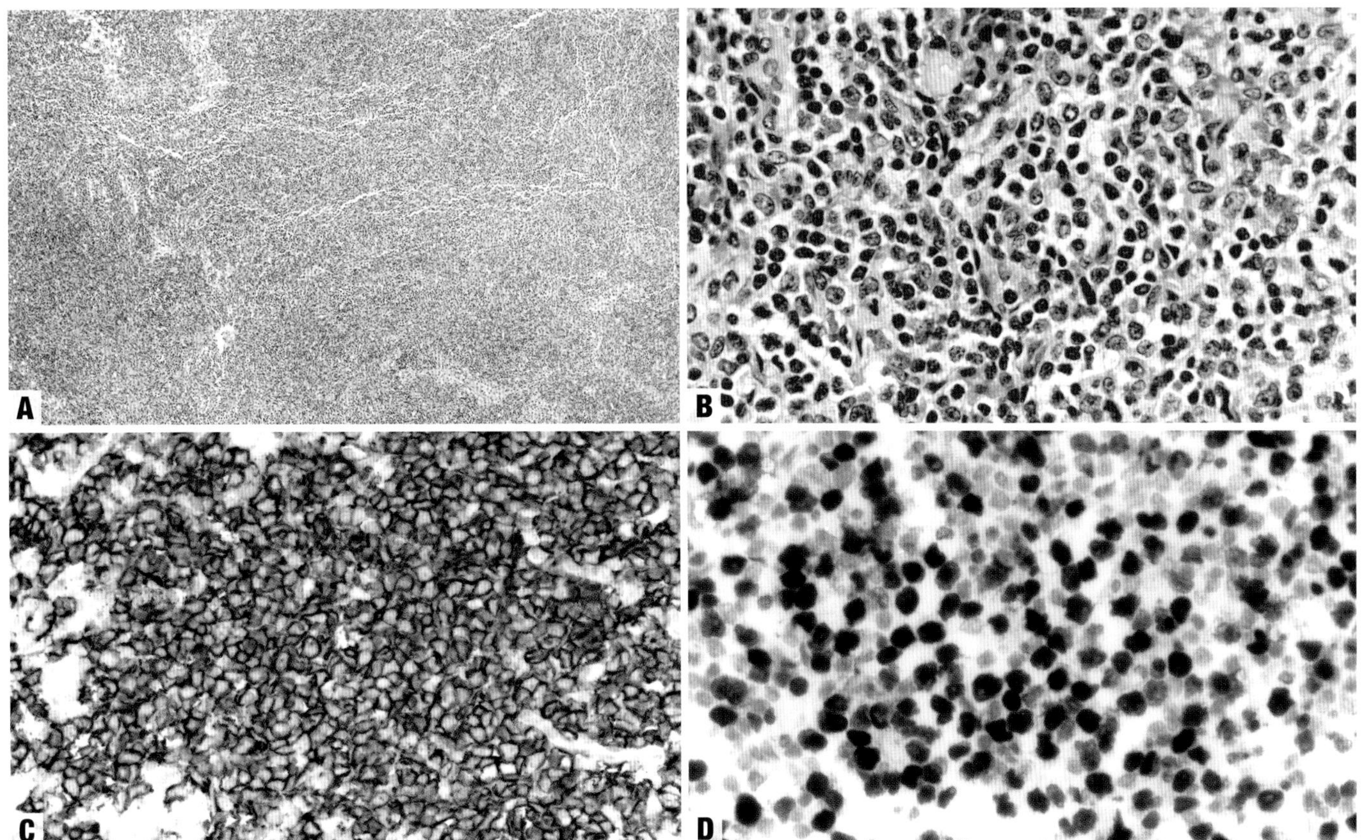

Fig. 4.95 Nodal marginal zone lymphoma, diffuse pattern. **A** Lymph node shows diffuse effacement of the architecture by a monotonous small lymphoid infiltrate. **B** The neoplastic cells are small lymphoid cells with minimally indented nuclei and moderate pale-staining cytoplasm. **C** Immunohistochemistry for CD20 shows sheets of small B cells effacing the lymph node architecture. **D** Immunohistochemistry for MNDA shows diffuse nuclear expression in the lymphoma cells.

common in lymphoplasmacytic lymphoma and rare in NMZL {1477,2554,3907,3808}.

Macroscopic appearance

Enlarged lymph nodes

Histopathology

Lymph nodes involved by NMZL demonstrate partial or complete effacement by a small lymphoid proliferation with a nodular/follicular, parafollicular, interfollicular, or diffuse growth pattern. There are varying degrees of follicular colonization {2914, 4065,2899,3538}. The neoplastic cells typically have minimally cleaved/indented nuclei, along with scant to moderate amount of cytoplasm; cells containing more abundant or pale-staining cytoplasm (monocytoid B cells), and plasmacytic differentiation may be seen. Scattered larger nucleolated cells, granulocytes, reactive plasma cells, and variable numbers of small, non-neoplastic lymphocytes may also be present {2914,526,4065, 2972}. Bone marrow involvement is variable and shows an interstitial or intertrabecular nodular distribution, sometimes with remnant germinal centres. An intrasinusoidal infiltration may be detected on immunostaining {1720,434}.

Immunohistochemistry

Most NMZLs express pan–B-cell markers (CD19, CD20, CD79a, or PAX5) and BCL2, and a variable proportion express CD43 {3538,4179}. A minority of NMZLs express CD5, CD23, or one of the germinal-centre B-cell markers {2899,4179,1035,1791}. Rare cases of NMZL express LEF1 {2654}, whereas cyclin D1 is absent {4179}. MNDA and IRTA1 are expressed in nearly 75% of cases {4179,2668}. The majority of NMZLs express IgM {526}, and a subset expresses IgD {534}. Light chain restriction may be documented by immunohistochemistry or in situ hybridization in plasma cells in cases with plasmacytic differentiation. Colonized follicles show at least partial replacement by neoplastic B cells that lack CD10 and BCL6 and have a low proliferation index, with associated follicular dendritic cell meshworks that may be disrupted {2899}. Remnant germinal-centre B cells that express CD10 and BCL6, with a high proliferation index, may be present.

Differential diagnosis

This includes other small B-cell lymphomas (particularly follicular lymphoma, mantle cell lymphoma, splenic marginal zone lymphoma, and lymphoplasmacytic lymphoma), plasma cell neoplasm, and reactive lymphoid hyperplasia {2914,4065,1035} (see Table 4.25, p. 414). Predominant splenomegaly suggests splenic marginal zone lymphoma. The minimal criteria required for recognizing transformation to diffuse large B-cell lymphoma are not well defined. However, the presence of unequivocal sheets of large B cells outside the confines of a germinal centre is consistent with transformation. An accelerated phase of NMZL has not been clearly defined. Composite lymphomas of NMZL and Hodgkin lymphoma have been reported {4552}.

Table 4.25 Differential diagnosis of nodal marginal zone lymphoma (NMZL)

Overlapping histological feature	Differential diagnostic considerations and recommended workup
Diffuse small B-cell proliferation	Other small B-cell lymphomas with a diffuse growth pattern: • Particularly challenging in superficial or core needle biopsies where architecture is limited • A panel of immunohistochemical markers may be necessary for definitive diagnosis and include LEF1 (positive in small lymphocytic lymphoma), BCL1 and SOX11 (positive in mantle cell lymphoma), diffuse follicular lymphoma (see follicular lymphoma below), and MNDA and CD43 (positive in NMZL)
Prominent follicular pattern	Follicular lymphoma: • Expression of one or more germinal-centre B-cell markers (CD10, BCL6, HGAL, LMO2, MEF2B) and FISH studies for *BCL2* and *BCL6* rearrangements support follicular lymphoma; MNDA and CD43 expression support NMZL • In a nodular proliferation of small B cells, coexpression of more than one germinal-centre B-cell marker, particularly in the interfollicular areas, is unusual and should raise suspicion for follicular lymphoma {1035}
Prominent plasma cell differentiation	Lymphoplasmacytic lymphoma: • The presence of typical clinicopathological features, IgM paraprotein, *MYD88* p.L265P and/or *CXCR4* mutations support lymphoplasmacytic lymphoma • Rarely, NMZL may show *MYD88* mutations, although mutations affecting p.L265P are less common in NMZL Plasma cell neoplasm: • Presence of small lymphoid cells or residual lymphoid follicles favours NMZL • Correlation with clinical features and imaging is required to exclude plasma cell myeloma
Frequent large nucleolated B cells	Colonized reactive follicles: • Immunohistochemistry for follicular dendritic cell markers (CD21 and CD23) and germinal-centre B-cell markers (CD10, BCL6, HGAL, LMO2, MEF2B) is helpful in highlighting remnant germinal centres

The absence of deletions of 7q31-32 and 13q14, of translocations involving *BCL2*, *BCL6*, *MALT1*, *BIRC3*, *BCL10*, *FOXP1*, and *CCND1*, and of mutations involving *MYD88* p.L265P and *CXCR4*, help to exclude other B-cell lymphomas (splenic marginal zone lymphoma, follicular lymphoma, EMZL, mantle cell lymphoma, and lymphoplasmacytic lymphoma) and establish a diagnosis of NMZL {3764,957,3392, 3850,3852,207,4179}.

Cytology

FNAC typically shows a population of small lymphoid cells with moderate amounts of pale cytoplasm with minimal nuclear irregularity, sometimes with admixed plasma cells and a few large cells. Flow cytometry typically shows a CD5−, CD10−, light chain–restricted B-cell population. However, establishing a specific diagnosis and excluding other types of B-cell lymphoma on a cytological specimen alone is challenging.

Diagnostic molecular pathology

Testing for clonal IG gene rearrangements may be necessary in some cases, to distinguish NMZL from reactive lymphoid hyperplasias. NMZL may be difficult to distinguish from other B-cell lymphomas and may require cytogenetic and molecular genetic studies to establish a diagnosis in some cases. Identification of *PTPRD* mutation may be helpful to support the diagnosis of NMZL.

Essential and desirable diagnostic criteria

Essential: proliferation predominantly of small, mature B cells with a scant to moderate amount of pale cytoplasm, with or without plasmacytic differentiation; architectural distortion

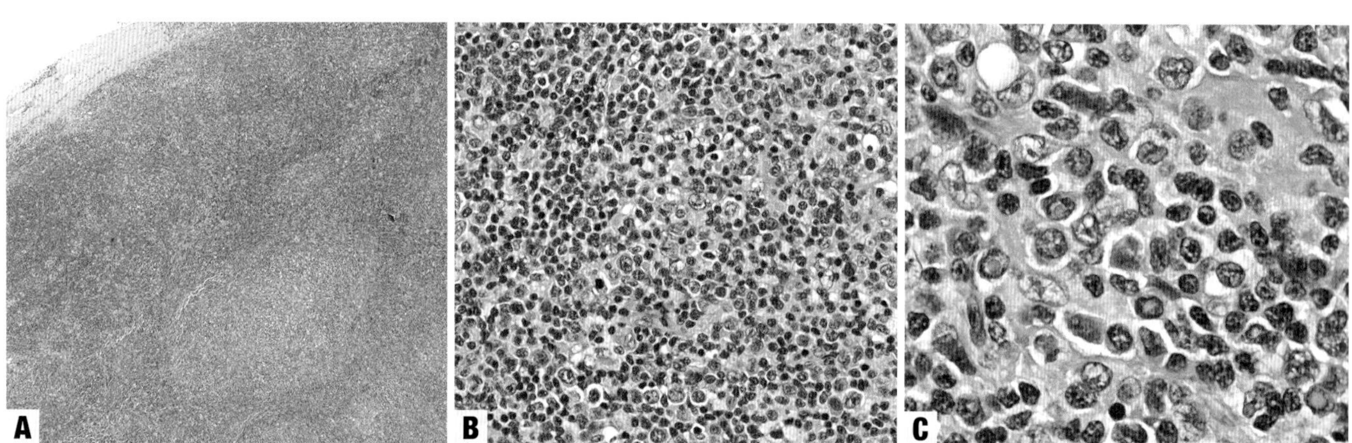

Fig. 4.96 Nodal marginal zone lymphoma, nodular pattern. **A** Low-power view shows architectural effacement by a vaguely nodular lymphoid proliferation. **B** Medium-power view of one nodule shows a range of cell types, including small lymphoid cells, plasmacytoid cells, and plasma cells. Occasional scattered larger cells are also present. **C** High-power view shows the presence of Dutcher bodies among the atypical cells by oil immersion.

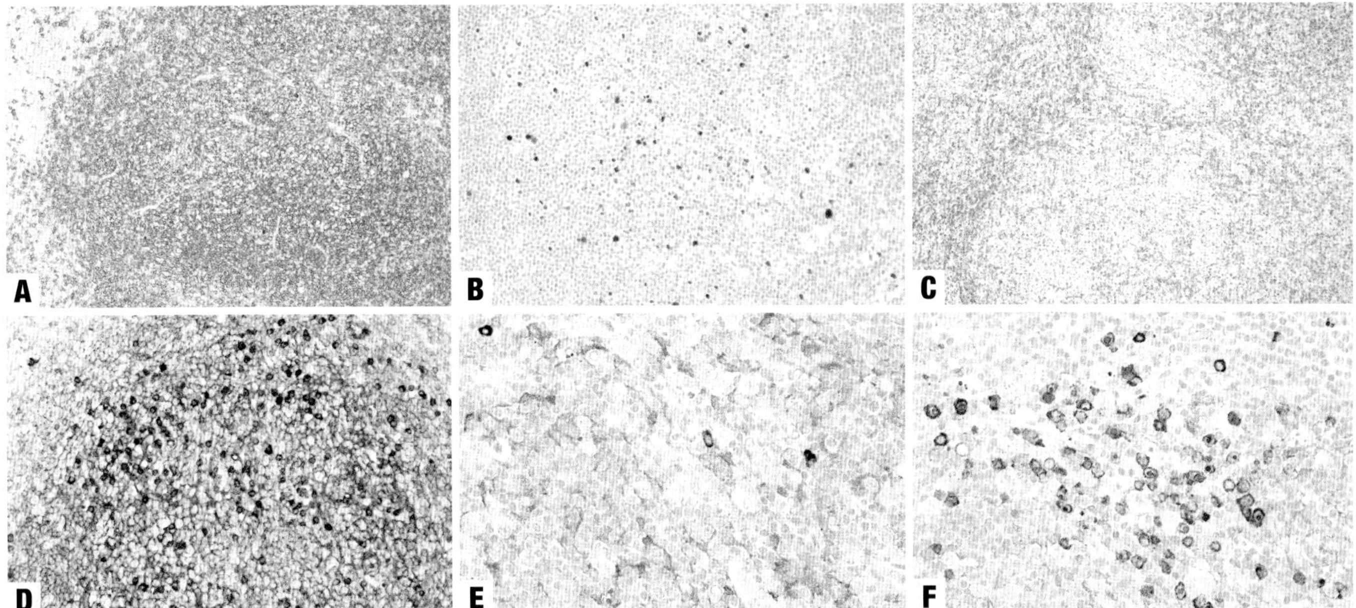

Fig. 4.97 Nodal marginal zone lymphoma, nodular pattern, immunohistochemistry. **A** There is a predominance of CD20-positive B cells, of a range of sizes, in nodules of neoplastic cells. **B** Only a few cells are BCL6-positive; these are probably residual germinal-centre cells in follicles colonized by neoplastic marginal zone cells (immunoperoxidase technique). Atypical cells were also negative for CD5 and CD10 (not shown). **C** B cells in colonized follicles are mostly negative for BCL2. **D** B cells and scattered plasmacytoid forms in nodules are IgM-positive. **E** Immunohistochemistry for kappa light chains shows a lack of staining in the lymphoma cells. **F** Immunohistochemistry for lambda light chains is positive in scattered plasmacytoid cells; note the presence of several lambda-positive Dutcher bodies.

in a nodular/follicular, parafollicular, interfollicular, or diffuse growth pattern; absence of markers supporting follicular lymphoma, mantle cell lymphoma, or other specific small B-cell lymphomas.

Desirable: presence of markers such as MNDA or IRTA1; residual follicles with follicular colonization; evidence of clonality by immunohistochemistry (light chain restriction in B cells and/or plasma cells) and/or by monoclonal IG rearrangements.

Staging

Stage of NMZL is determined by the Lugano modifications to the Ann Arbor system {688}. Imaging should evaluate the neck, chest, abdomen, and pelvis for lymphadenopathy and splenomegaly. Bone marrow and peripheral blood morphology and flow cytometry are also helpful in evaluating extent of disease. HCV serology testing has therapeutic consequences, because antiviral treatment results in haematological response and virological clearance {140}. Nodal spread of a clinically occult EMZL can be ruled out by carefully evaluating the extranodal tissues draining to the involved lymph nodes by imaging or endoscopy. PET-CT may be used to direct the diagnostic biopsy in cases of suspected large-cell transformation.

Prognosis and prediction

The clinical course of NMZL is generally indolent, with a median survival time exceeding 10 years, although it affects the overall

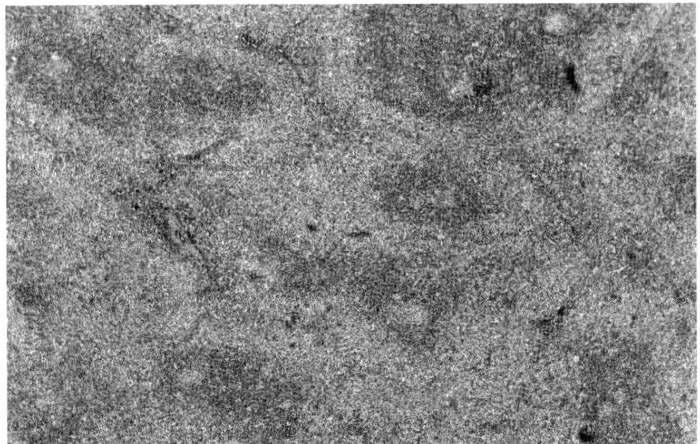

Fig. 4.98 Nodal marginal zone lymphoma, interfollicular pattern. The interfollicular pattern is characterized by neoplastic cells predominantly confined to the interfollicular areas, with relative sparing of secondary follicles containing intact germinal centres and mantle zones.

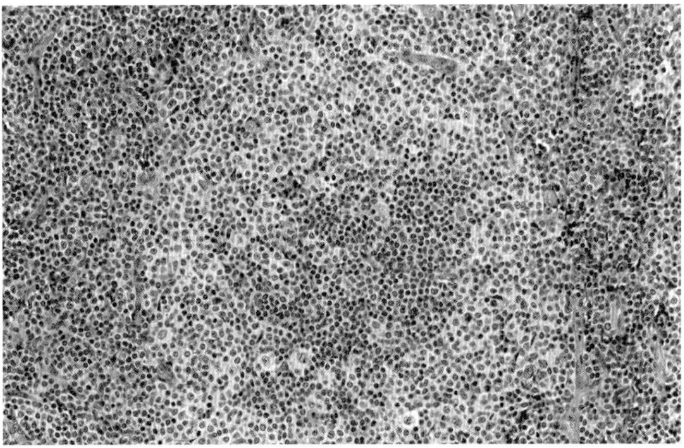

Fig. 4.99 Nodal marginal zone lymphoma, perifollicular pattern. Higher magnification of a single follicle shows an annular distribution of neoplastic cells with moderate amounts of pale cytoplasm surrounding a relatively well preserved secondary follicle. Tingible-body macrophages are present within the germinal centre.

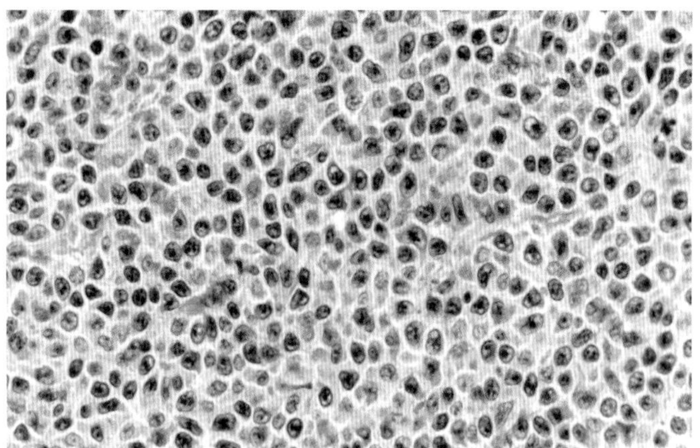

Fig. 4.100 Nodal marginal zone lymphoma with monocytoid features. The neoplastic cells show moderate to abundant pale-staining cytoplasm.

life expectancy {2612,3819,587}. Early progression after treatment (≤ 24 months; seen in ~20% of patients) is associated with a median survival time of 3–5 years and is the strongest predictor of prognosis {2447}. Histological transformation to an aggressive lymphoma occurs in 5% of patients and heralds a poor prognosis {2671,790,64}. Younger patients have a better prognosis {3920}. In HCV-seropositive cases, antiviral treatment results in haematological response, virological clearance, and improved overall survival {140}.

Paediatric nodal marginal zone lymphoma

Di Napoli A
Attarbaschi A
Oschlies I

Definition

Paediatric nodal marginal zone lymphoma (PNMZL) is a primary nodal mature B-cell neoplasm, mostly occurring in the head and neck region of adolescent boys. PNMZL shares the interfollicular expansion of clonal marginal zone B cells with usual nodal marginal zone lymphoma (NMZL). Nevertheless, the specific clinical and histomorphological features differ from those of the adult counterpart.

ICD-O coding

9699/3 Paediatric nodal marginal zone lymphoma

ICD-11 coding

2A85.Y Further specified mature B-cell neoplasms or lymphoma

Related terminology

Not recommended: monocytoid B-cell lymphoma; parafollicular B-cell lymphoma.

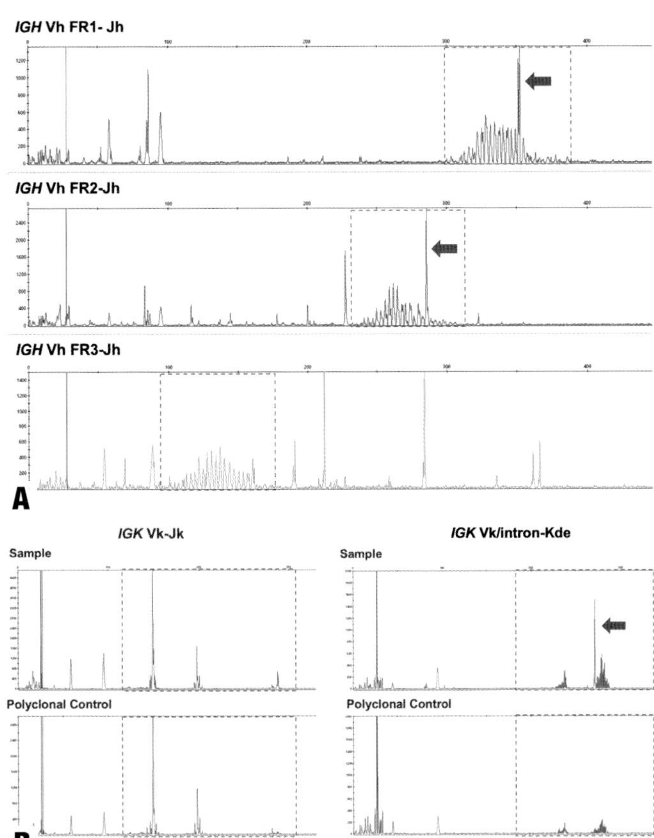

Fig. 4.101 Paediatric nodal marginal zone lymphoma. IGH and IGK gene rearrangement analysis by PCR and gene scan. A dominant peak (red arrow) of PCR products of identical size indicating a clonal expansion within a polyclonal background is evident in the IGH-FR1 and IGH-FR2 reactions (**A**) as well as in the IGK-DE amplification (**B**).

Subtype(s)

None

Localization

PNMZL often involves the lymph nodes of the head and neck region (i.e. cervical, submandibular, and supraclavicular lymph nodes) {2490,3457,212,4396,169}.

Clinical features

Patients with PNMZL usually present with peripheral lymphadenopathy without clinical symptoms, localized stage I/II disease {169}, and normal serum LDH levels {3920,2490,3457,4396,169}. However, stage III/IV disease has been reported, emphasizing the need for complete staging {3083,2490,3457,4396,169}. Splenic and extranodal marginal zone lymphomas are very rare in the paediatric age range and should not be included in this category.

Epidemiology

The overall incidence of PNMZL among patients with childhood non-Hodgkin lymphoma is < 2%. It is most commonly diagnosed in otherwise healthy adolescent boys (median age: 16 years) {3920,3419,3093,2490,3457,169} and rarely in adults {1895,1349}.

Etiology

In contrast to extranodal marginal zone lymphoma, PNMZL extremely rarely occurs in patients with pre-existing immunodeficiencies or autoimmune disorders, or in association with an infectious stimulus {1062,3920,758,39,3862,3194,2490,3457,269,3995,1698,1697,169}.

Pathogenesis

The pathogenetic mechanisms underlying the development of PNMZL are currently unknown, mainly because of the hitherto very limited molecular studies. In adult NMZL, studies on IGHV gene mutation status suggest that the lymphoma may originate from different subsets of marginal zone B cells: the naïve B cells expressing unmutated IGHV (VH) genes and the somatically hypermutated antigen-experienced B cells {2692,789,4064,3809,1388}. No evidence of EBV or bacterial infections has been documented in PNMZL {1062,3920,134,2055}.

Like in NMZL, trisomy 18 has been found in 21% of PNMZL cases, with 1 case showing concomitant trisomy 3 {3419}. Trisomy 13, monosomy 20, and translocation of IGH with an unknown partner gene have also been reported in single cases {1062,3419,134}. PNMZL lacks the t(14;18) IGH::*MALT1* rearrangement as well as *BCL10* and *FOXP1* translocations {3419}. A whole-exome sequencing study performed on four PNMZL cases reported isolated point mutations in genes of unknown pathogenetic potential, involved in cellular adhesion, cytokine regulatory elements, and cellular proliferation {3093}.

Macroscopic appearance

Enlarged and encapsulated lymph nodes without sclerosis or necrosis

Histopathology

The lymph node architecture is at least partly effaced by an interfollicular proliferation, with markedly expanded pale marginal zones and attenuated sinuses.

Immunophenotype

Characteristically, the follicles are often enlarged, with a disrupted CD23+ follicular dendritic cell meshwork and IgD+ mantle cells extending into the germinal centres, resembling progressively transformed germinal centres (PTGCs). However, in contrast to PTGCs, the peripheral rim of IgD+ mantle is irregular, owing to the infiltration of marginal zone cells. Widely spaced hyperplastic follicles partially colonized by IgD− cells but still containing residual typical germinal-centre cells (centrocytes and centroblasts) can also be present. Complete effacement of the lymph node architecture by a diffuse infiltration, as seen in adult NMZL, is rarely observed. The neoplastic population is represented by a polymorphic B-cell infiltrate composed of small to medium-sized B cells with monocytoid features (round nuclei, pale-staining cytoplasm) and centrocyte-like features (irregular nuclei, scant cytoplasm). Plasmacytoid cells and scattered immunoblasts and centroblast-like cells may be present {3920,3903,3419,134,3338,2103}. Sheets of large cells should not be present and would favour the diagnosis of a diffuse large B-cell lymphoma. The infiltrating cells may express BCL2 and in most cases are CD43+. BCL6 and CD10 are typically negative, although rare CD10+ exceptions have been reported {3338}. The proliferation index is low to moderate. Cytoplasmic light chain restriction consistent with plasmacytoid differentiation can be observed {3419,3338,2103}.

Differential diagnosis

Cases with overlapping features between paediatric-type follicular lymphoma and PNMZL have been reported, especially in PNMZL with extensive follicular colonization and paediatric-type follicular lymphoma with marginal zone differentiation {3338}. Differential diagnostic features in PNMZL are the expanded interfollicular areas of CD43+ marginal zone B cells, the presence of PTGC-like features, and the higher content in PD1+ T cells in the remaining germinal centres {2380,3338}.

Various forms of marginal zone hyperplasia should be excluded. Polyclonal expansions of IgD+ marginal zones with cytoplasmic light chain restriction and aberrant expression of CD43 can be observed in atypical marginal zone hyperplasia, a reactive condition mainly reported in the tonsils or in the gastrointestinal tract {180,524}. In lymph nodes, a similar condition with variable marginal zone hyperplasia, PTGC-like nodules, skewed light chain expression, and faint IgD positivity has been reported in association with *Haemophilus influenzae* infection {2055}. Flow cytometry may reveal surface light chain–restricted, CD19+, CD20+, CD10− B cells in both PNMZL and atypical marginal zone hyperplasia. Molecular testing for heavy and/or light chain rearrangements is therefore mandatory for the differential diagnosis {3920,1349,3419,134,2055,3338}.

Children affected by activated phosphatidylinositol-3-OH kinase δ syndrome (APDS) frequently present with lymphadenopathy with marked polyclonal marginal zone hyperplasia; the germinal centres, however, are commonly infiltrated by PD1+ T cells, and sometimes a few cells infected by EBV and CMV are detected {818,3755}.

Cytology

A cytology-based approach for the diagnosis of PNMZL is not recommended, because marginal zone lymphomas are composed of a polymorphic lymphoid population of centrocyte-like, monocytoid, and plasmacytoid cells that can be extremely difficult to distinguish from reactive cells on FNA specimens {833, 3654}.

Diagnostic molecular pathology

Monoclonal rearrangements of the immunoglobulin heavy and/or light chain genes (IGH, IGK) are detected in almost all cases of PNMZL. In contrast, atypical marginal zone hyperplasia can show monotypic light chain immunoglobulin expression by both immunohistochemistry and flow cytometry but an absence of clonality by molecular analyses {1062,3920,3419, 134,2055,3338,3554}. Combining morphological and immunophenotypic findings with molecular clonality assessments is therefore strongly recommended to support the diagnosis of PNMZL {3554}.

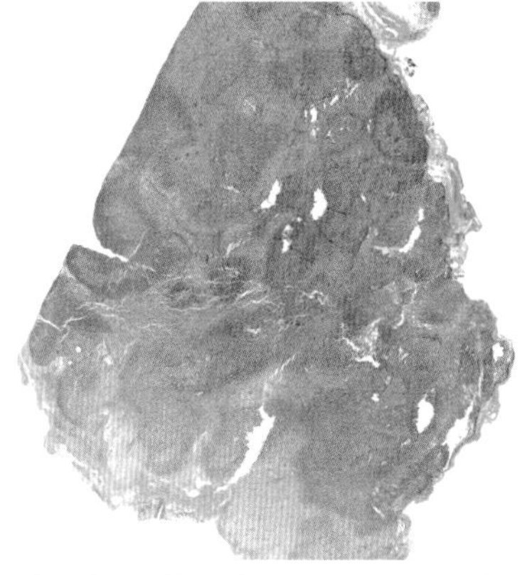

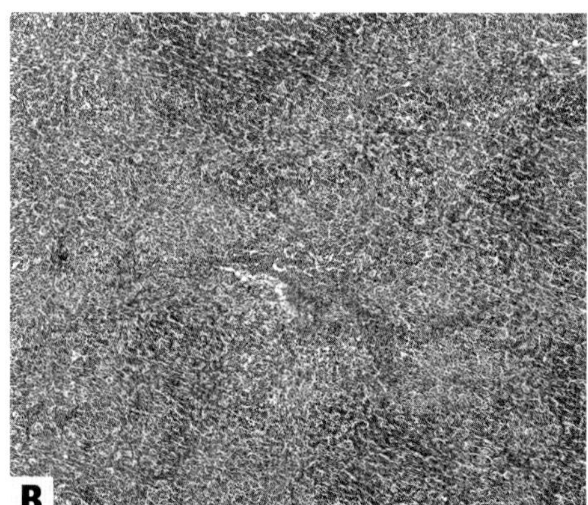

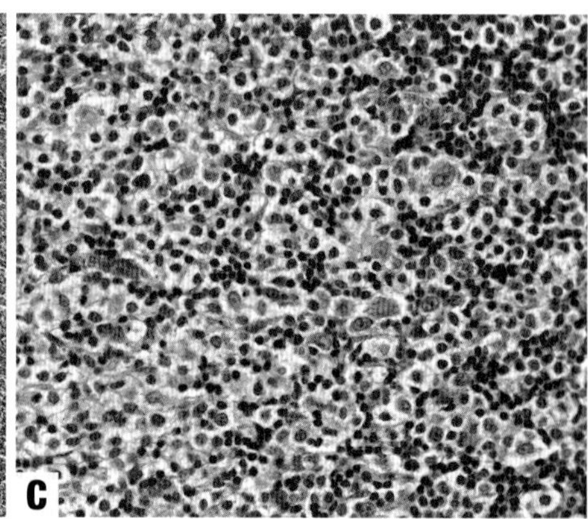

Fig. 4.102 Paediatric nodal marginal zone lymphoma. **A** At low magnification, an organoid architecture with follicles and pale, markedly expanded interfollicular areas is seen. **B** The paler marginal zone cells in part disrupt follicle mantles with follicular colonization. **C** There is a spectrum of small to medium-sized cells with clear cytoplasm and some intermingled large cells.

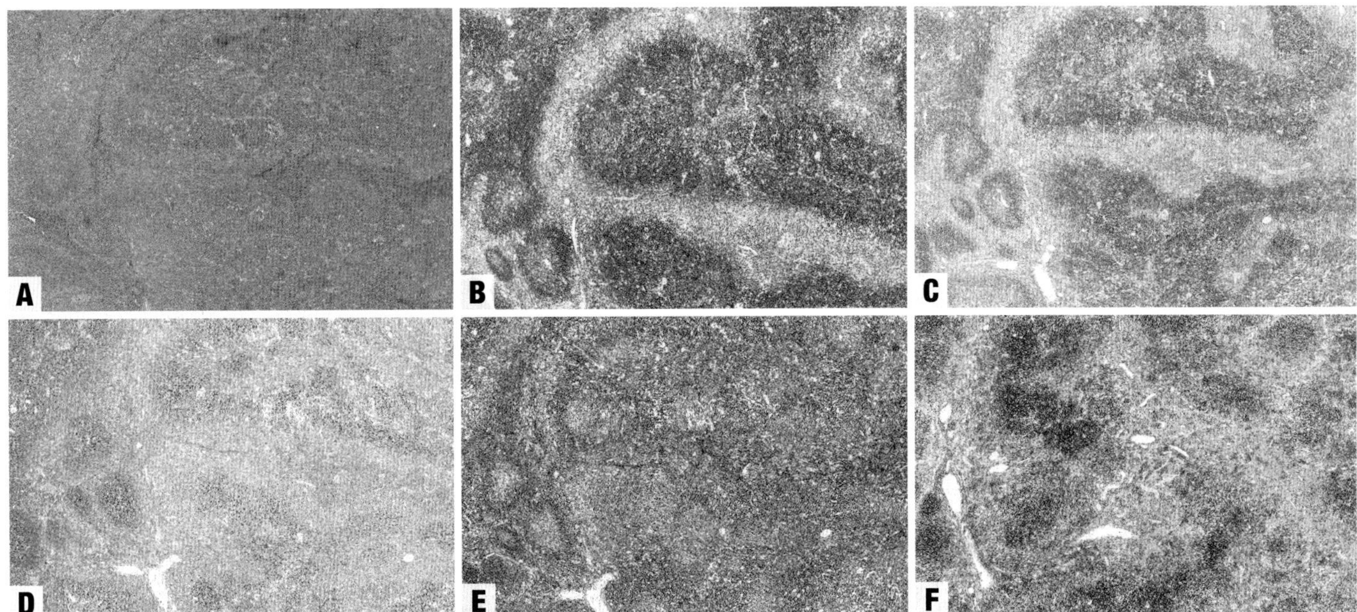

Fig. 4.103 Paediatric nodal marginal zone lymphoma. **A** Hyperplastic follicles resembling progressive transformation of germinal centres with expanded paler marginal zones. Some reactive germinal centres are also still present. **B** CD20 stains follicles and perifollicular and interfollicular B cells. **C** IgD-positive mantle cells penetrate the germinal centres that are infiltrated at the periphery by marginal zone cells. Remnants of reactive germinal centres are highlighted by the presence of CD10-positive B cells (**D**) and BCL2-negative B cells (**E**). **F** Residual germinal centres contain abundant PD1+ T cells.

Essential and desirable diagnostic criteria

Essential: partial effacement of lymph node architecture by an interfollicular proliferation of marginal zone cells with monocytoid and centrocyte-like morphology; evidence of clonality by monoclonal IG rearrangement; immunophenotype compatible with marginal zone B cells (BCL6−, CD43+/−).

Desirable: residual follicles with PTGC-like features; follicular colonization; light chain restriction in B cells and/or plasma cells; increased PD1+ cells in reactive germinal centres.

Staging

Although most patients with PNMZL present with localized disease of the head and neck region and lack B symptoms, complete staging should be performed according to the revised International Pediatric Non-Hodgkin Lymphoma Staging System (IPNHLSS) {3476,169}. Whether analysis of the bone marrow and cerebrospinal fluid is necessary is a matter of current debate, but it might be waived in a histologically and clinically typical situation of PNMZL {169}.

Prognosis and prediction

According to the literature available, most patients with limited-stage PNMZL underwent watchful waiting after complete resection {3920,2490,3457,4396,169}. Fewer than 5% of them relapsed but were cured with second-line therapy. Survival rates thus approach 100% {3920,2490,3457,4396,169}. Primary systemic therapy might be reserved for the very rare patients with advanced or relapsed/progressive disease. Observations of a few patients suggest that a period of delay before considering systemic therapy might be appropriate for incompletely resected localized PNMZL {2490,169}. Only a few patients with PNMZL have been primarily treated by local radiotherapy or systemic polychemotherapy; none of them relapsed {4396}. However, in view of the high cure rates, local irradiation is not indicated.

Follicular lymphoma: Introduction

Ott G
Dave SS
de Jong D

Follicular lymphoma (FL) is one of the more common lymphomas. In the fifth edition of the WHO classification of haematolymphoid tumours, we have adopted a new way of subtyping FL. The vast majority of FLs have a follicular growth pattern at least in part, are composed of centrocytes and centroblasts, and harbour the t(14;18)(q32;q21) translocation in about 85% of cases. These lymphomas are now termed classic FL and are set apart from less frequent subtypes.

The grading of FL has been a matter of discussion through successive editions of the WHO classification. Various studies have shown poor reproducibility of grading using the conventional method of counting centroblasts, limiting the practical value of the grading system {2670,3413,2133}. Poor reproducibility may be caused by various issues related to inadequate sampling (core needle vs excision biopsy), definition and morphological recognition of centroblasts, and methods of enumeration. The traditional method of grading FL is by assessing the density of centroblasts as the number of cells per high-power-field (HPF) using a 40× objective. Over the years, microscopes have evolved, and the sizes of microscopic fields have changed, even at the same magnification of 400× {836}. In recognition of these issues, this edition proposes that grading of FL be optional. This recommendation is also supported by the lack of a statistically significant difference in clinical outcomes between FL grades 1, 2, and 3A in the majority of the reported clinical trials using modern treatment protocols {2534,1578,3413,2802, 202}. In many parts of the world, it is accepted practice to treat these patients with similar protocols, both in clinical trials and in daily practice. Attempts have been made to improve the reproducibility of grading, such as through digital applications or by using a mitotic marker such as phosphohistone H3 and/or by expressing the centroblast count as cells/mm^2 {1975,2133}. The impact of these alternative methods, however, has not been validated on patient outcomes and requires prospective studies.

Rare cases of classic follicular lymphoma with cytological features of FL grade 3A can present with a prominent diffuse pattern. In the previous edition, such cases were defined as diffuse large B-cell lymphoma. Currently, it is uncertain whether such cases should be classified as FL or diffuse large B-cell lymphoma; and in such cases, individual treatment choices should be made in multidisciplinary conference settings taking into consideration clinical, laboratory, and imaging parameters. The presence of diffuse areas composed entirely or predominantly of large cells, however, warrants a diagnosis of diffuse large B-cell lymphoma.

Follicular large B-cell lymphoma largely corresponds to FL grade 3B in the previous edition. Two additional FL subtypes are now separately described: FL with a predominantly diffuse growth pattern, and FL with unusual cytological features, the latter defined by having particular cytomorphological features of either blastoid cells or large centrocytes {3619,1055,2231}. These two groups of FL tend to harbour the t(14;18)(q32;q21)/ IGH::*BCL2* fusion only rarely. The different genetic constitution further supports a rationale to separate these subtypes, whereas their FL nature is still supported by an FL-like mutation landscape, including mutations in genes such as *CREBBP*, *STAT6*, *TNFRSF14*, and others {3740,2895,2231}. Of note, testicular FL was not considered as a subtype in the present edition because of its extreme rarity, in addition to its immunophenotypic and genetic similarities with paediatric-type FL {3238,205,2405}.

In situ follicular B-cell neoplasm

Xerri L
Ardeshna KM
de Jong D
Herfarth K
Klapper W
Marafioti T
Nadel B

Definition

In situ follicular B-cell neoplasm (ISFN) is defined as partial or complete colonization of some reactive germinal centres by follicular B cells with IGH::*BCL2* fusion and strong BCL2 expression in otherwise normal reactive lymph nodes or lymphoid tissues at extranodal sites.

ICD-O coding

9695/1 In situ follicular B-cell neoplasm

ICD-11 coding

2A80.5 Follicular lymphoma in situ

Related terminology

Acceptable: in situ follicular neoplasia.
Not recommended: follicular lymphoma in situ.

Subtype(s)

None

Localization

ISFN can be seen in any lymph node or at an extranodal site harbouring reactive lymphoid tissue, including the intestine, spleen, tonsils, thyroid, and salivary glands {3953}.

Clinical features

Individuals with isolated ISFN are asymptomatic. ISFN may be detected concurrently with or subsequent to follicular lymphoma (FL) at another site {3242,1555}. It can also be diagnosed before, concurrently with, or after the diagnosis of any type of lymphoma. It can be incidentally found in specimens with non-haematological cancers {3953,976}. In some cases of ISFN with subsequent, clonally related diffuse large B-cell lymphoma, no clinically overt FL phase may be present {4245}.

Epidemiology

Because ISFN is an incidental finding in biopsy samples taken for other medical conditions, no reliable incidence data are available. The reported prevalence rates of ISFN in two large studies were 2.1% and 2.3% in the general population {1555,3029}. In one of these studies, the median age was 67 years {3029}.

Etiology

Unknown

Pathogenesis

ISFN shows genetic alterations seen in the early steps of FL pathogenesis, but it does not show or rarely shows other genetic features of classic FL. Like FL, ISFN demonstrates t(14;18)(q32;q21)/IGH::*BCL2* and shows imprints of activation-induced cytidine deaminase (AID)-mediated genomic instability. It also shows a restricted repertoire of genetic alterations recurrently seen in FL, including *BCL2*, *CREBBP*, *KMT2D*, and *TNFRSF14* mutations and acquisition of N-glycosylation sites in their rearranged IGH genes {1793,3622,2513,2512,2109, 3620}. Deletions at 1p36 encompassing *TNFRSF14* have also been detected {3622,2513}. ISFN may be regarded as the earliest histologically recognizable tissue involvement by the circulating t(14;18)(q32;q21)/IGH::*BCL2*-positive B cells. Clonally related ISFN and circulating IGH::*BCL2*-positive cells have been observed in the same patient {702,3886}, further suggesting that both are components of the same premalignant clonal dynamics {2511}. In cases with concurrent, clonally related ISFN and FL, there are secondary genetic events in FL that are not present in ISFN {407,3622}, such as *EZH2* mutation and further pathogenic mutations in *CREBBP* and *BCL2* in the FL component {1793,407,4245,976}. Rare patients have been reported with concurrent, clonally linked ISFN and duodenal-type FL {702,2511,3886,2894}.

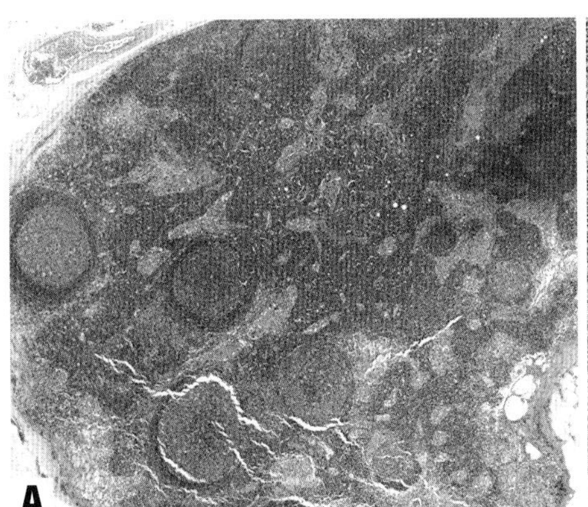

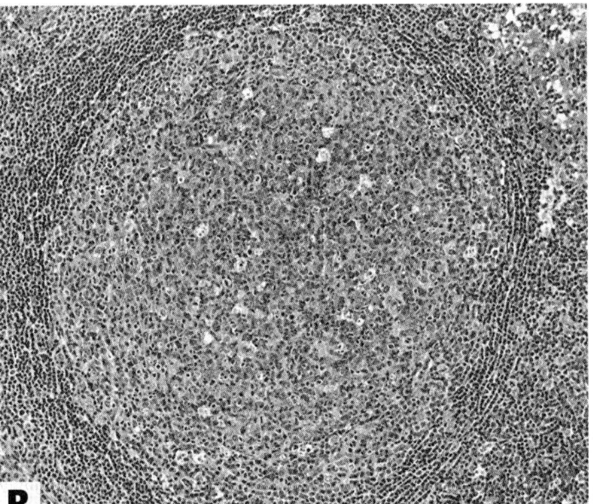

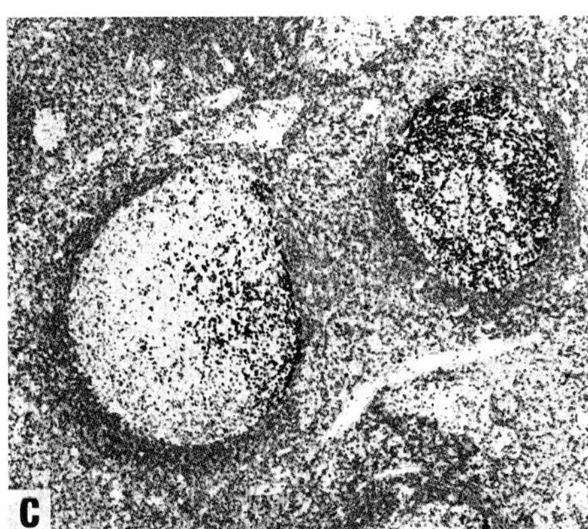

Fig. 4.104 In situ follicular B-cell neoplasm. **A** Lymph node with retained architecture along with secondary follicles without any obvious abnormality. **B** A secondary follicle composed of centrocytes, centroblasts, small lymphocytes, and tingible-body macrophages; no obvious abnormality is identifiable. **C** Two of the secondary follicles with germinal centres show partial colonization by cells strongly positive for BCL2.

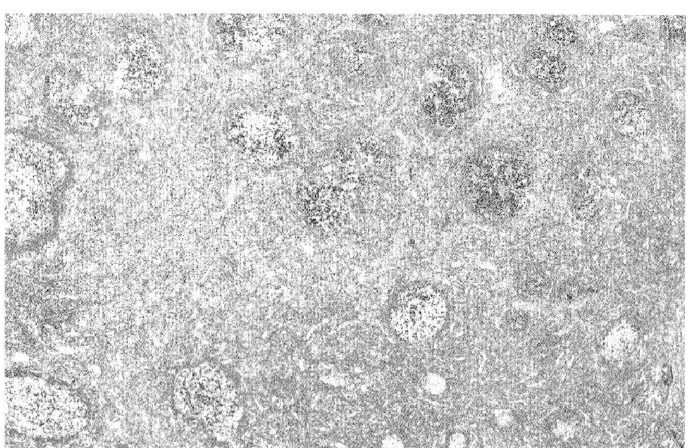

Fig. 4.105 In situ follicular neoplasia. BCL2 immunohistochemistry shows varying infiltration of pre-existing germinal centres by neoplastic in situ follicular B-cell neoplasm, ranging from very sparse to dense infiltrates.

Macroscopic appearance

The lymphatic tissue involved by ISFN may be enlarged due to lymphoid hyperplasia, a coexisting related or unrelated lymphoma, or another unrelated malignant or non-malignant disorder.

Histopathology

ISFN is usually not detectable on routine histological sections. The lymph node or extranodal tissue shows usual-appearing lymphoid hyperplasia with scattered reactive lymphoid follicles. Involved germinal centres resemble reactive follicles in their size, shape, and distribution {793}. ISFN may sometimes be suspected if there is a loss of polarization or focal abundance of closely packed centrocytes.

Immunohistochemistry

ISFN can be readily identified by immunostaining for BCL2 and CD10. The strong staining intensity of the t(14;18)-positive cells for BCL2 contrasts with that of the surrounding mantle zone B cells and T cells. CD10 expression is also strong in the ISFN cells. The abnormal B cells with strong expression of BCL2 and CD10 are limited to germinal centres and do not transgress the mantle zones or extend outside the follicles. The extent of involvement of the follicles is variable. Typically only a proportion of the follicles are involved, and colonization of individual follicles is also frequently partial. Immunoglobulin light chain restriction of CD10+/BCL2+ cells may be demonstrated by flow cytometry. Germinal centres colonized by ISFN are BCL6+ and show low Ki-67 proliferation indexes. ISFN can coexist in the same anatomical site with overt FL or other lymphomas, such as chronic lymphocytic leukaemia / small lymphocytic lymphoma, marginal zone lymphoma, mantle cell lymphoma, and classic Hodgkin lymphoma {2751,1793,3242,3000,4245}. ISFN may also co-occur with in situ mantle cell neoplasm {3489,3866}.

Differential diagnosis

ISFN should be distinguished from partial involvement by FL, which shows a partially effaced architecture with closely packed atypical follicles or blurred mantle cuffs {24}. BCL2 staining intensity in partial involvement by FL is not particularly strong; some centroblasts can be apparent, and CD10+/BCL2+ tumour cells can be observed outside the germinal centres, infiltrating mantle zones and perifollicular tissues. The number of secondary genetic alterations is higher than in ISFN {2513,3622}. Duodenal-type follicular lymphoma should not be regarded as a form of ISFN, because the neoplastic cells are not confined to the follicles but extend into the lamina propria outside the follicles.

Cytology

This diagnosis cannot be made by cytology alone, because it requires immunohistochemistry of germinal centres.

Diagnostic molecular pathology

Not relevant

Essential and desirable diagnostic criteria

Essential: variable numbers of B cells within germinal centres staining intensely for BCL2; maintained lymph node or extranodal lymphoid tissue architecture, and lacking features of classic FL.

Desirable: strong CD10 expression in the BCL2-positive B cells within the follicles.

Staging

Staging is not relevant for ISFN. However, if ISFN is diagnosed, there should be a search for overt lymphoma, and any other suspicious lymph node should be examined. Partial involvement by FL is commonly associated with low-stage disease {24, 2513}, but its detection cannot substitute clinical staging.

Prognosis and prediction

The precise risk of progression to overt FL cannot be reliably assessed, because the studies addressing progression involve relatively small cohorts of individuals. In such studies, progression to overt FL has been demonstrated in 5–10% of healthy individuals diagnosed with ISFN with up to 12 years of follow-up, and the time to subsequent FL diagnosis ranged from 2 to 10 years {1793,3953}. The predictive value of the number/proportion of follicles with ISFN features and its relationship to progression to FL remains controversial {1793,3242,3953}.

Follicular lymphoma

Xerri L
Ardeshna KM
Davies AJ
Fitzgibbon J
Karube K
Klapper W
Kridel R
Louissaint A Jr
Marafioti T
Medeiros LJ
Nadel B
Watanabe T

Definition

Follicular lymphoma (FL) is a neoplasm of germinal-centre (GC) B cells with varying proportions of centrocytes and centroblasts or large transformed cells and at least a partially follicular growth pattern. In rare cases with an entirely diffuse growth pattern, the neoplastic cells should still show GC B-cell morphology and immunophenotype.

ICD-O coding

9690/3 Follicular lymphoma
9698/3 Follicular large B-cell lymphoma
9690/3 Follicular lymphoma with uncommon features

ICD-11 coding

2A80.Z Follicular lymphoma, unspecified

Related terminology

Acceptable: FL grades 1, 2, 3A, and 3B; *BCL2*-R–negative CD23-positive follicle centre lymphoma (for some cases of FL with dominant diffuse growth pattern only).

Subtype(s)

Classic FL (cFL); FL with unusual cytological features (uFL); FL with a predominantly diffuse growth pattern (dFL); follicular large B-cell lymphoma (FLBCL)

Localization

FL predominantly affects lymph nodes. Involvement of the spleen and bone marrow is frequent. Rarely, the Waldeyer ring and peripheral blood are involved. More commonly affected sites include the gastrointestinal tract (often with mesenteric lymph node involvement), soft tissue, thoracic vertebrae, breast, and ocular adnexa. Primary testicular FL is very rare and has also been reported in children, in addition to adults {3238,205, 2405}.

Clinical features

Most patients have widespread disease at diagnosis, including peripheral and central (abdominal and thoracic) lymphadenopathy and splenomegaly. Most patients present with peripheral lymphadenopathy, but any nodal group can be involved. A pure extranodal presentation is uncommon but can occur in almost any extranodal site {4345,3706,120}. The bone marrow is involved in 40–70% of cases. Only 10–15% of patients present in stages I or II {998}. Patients are often asymptomatic, and B symptoms (e.g. fever and weight loss) are uncommon. Waxing and waning of involved sites without therapy may occur. The most common clinical course follows a chronic relapsing pattern. Early treatment does not appear to prolong survival {145,2912,144,998}.

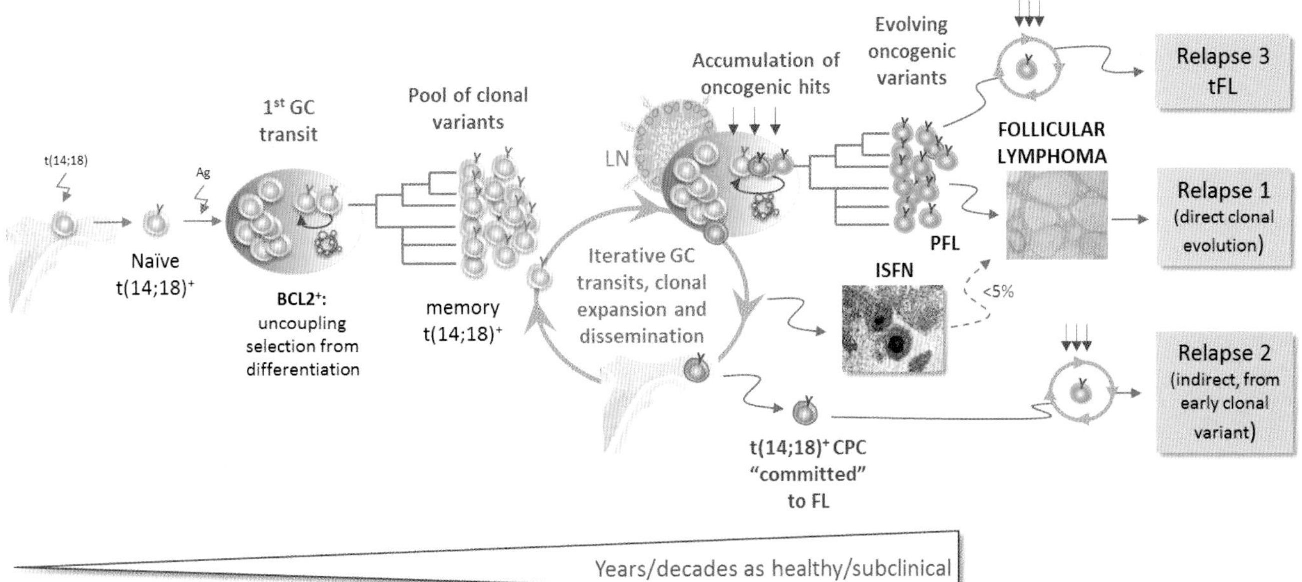

Fig. 4.106 The current model of follicular lymphoma (FL) development. Overt FL is preceded by an insidious phase of asymptomatic growth, probably emerging from widely disseminated precursor clones, evolving over years if not decades. Several premalignant intermediates have been identified or inferred as precursors (in situ follicular B-cell neoplasm [ISFN], partial involvement by FL [PFL]) or committed precursor clones (CPC), each of which could be at the origin of relapses. The major part of the transformation process is indolent. It includes illegitimate immunological stimulation, iterative cycles of germinal centre (GC) re-entry and reactions, increasing genomic instability, epigenetic switch, decommissioning from the GC B-cell programme, and escape from / adaptation to / instructive modification of the microenvironment. LN, lymph node; tFL, transformed follicular lymphoma.

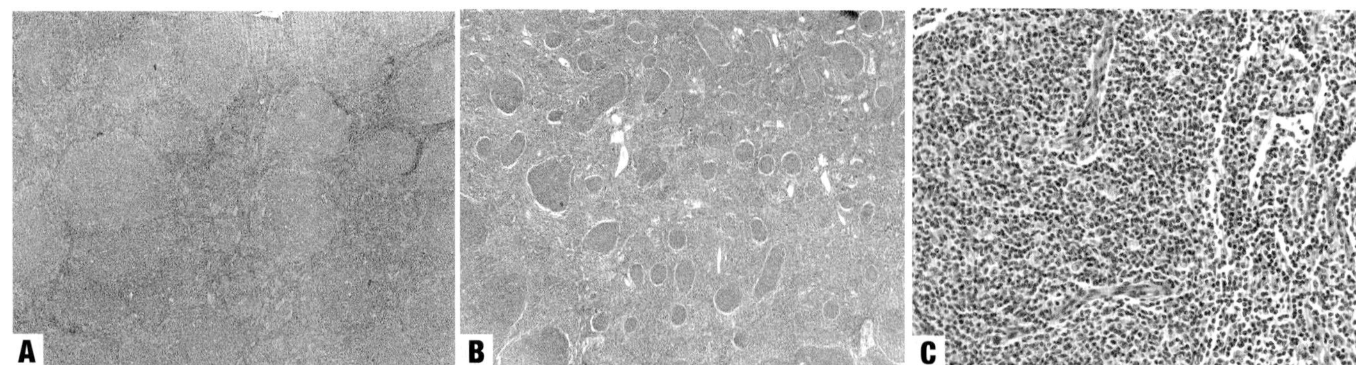

Fig. 4.107 Follicular lymphoma, cytomorphological spectrum. **A** The classic follicular lymphoma pattern shows effacement of the lymph node architecture by an accumulation of follicles of homogeneous size and cellular content. The mantle zones and macrophages (starry-sky pattern) are no longer visible. In rare classic follicular lymphoma cases, the architecture may be preserved or only slightly distorted (**B**), but the follicles harbour an obviously abnormal monomorphic cell population and the mantle zone is lacking (**C**).

In situ follicular B-cell neoplasm, paediatric-type FL, and duodenal-type FL are considered to be distinct entities, separate from FL.

Epidemiology

FL accounts for 10–20% of all lymphomas {3993}, with the highest proportions reported in the USA and western Europe, and the lowest in eastern Europe and Asia {115}. During the period 1993–2008, the incidence significantly increased in certain parts of the world, such as Japan {708}. Furthermore, studies have shown differences in regional distribution/incidence. In Canada, a higher incidence of FL was noted within cities or regions with high herbicide use, primary mining, and a strong manufacturing presence, supporting a possible role of environmental factors {2242}. The latter is also suggested by a higher incidence in cities and near industrial regions {903,2242}. The incidence is lower in low- and middle-income countries than in high-income countries {3198}. FL is two to three times as frequent in White populations as it is in Black populations in the USA {585}. FL predominantly affects adults (median age: 65 years) {1837}. There is no sex predilection {3993}, although a slight male predominance has been observed {585}.

Etiology

The etiology is unknown. Agricultural exposure to malathion {2117} and dichlorodiphenyltrichloroethane (DDT) {3612} (but none of other pesticide chemical groups {2279}), as well as cigarette smoking in women {2363}, occupational spray painting {2363}, HCV infection {860,2461}, and Sjögren syndrome {1054,2363} have been associated with an increased risk. For younger patients, obesity {721,2363} and having a first-degree relative with FL {1358,1123}, non-Hodgkin lymphoma {2363}, or haematological malignancies {3867} have been reported as risk factors {721,2363}.

Pathogenesis

FL with BCL2 rearrangement

Lymphomagenesis is a multi-hit process (see Table 4.26) escalating over many years {2687}. The t(14;18)(q32;q21) rearrangement involving IGH and *BCL2*, and leading to constitutive expression of *BCL2*, is considered the initiating event in FL and is found in 85–90% of cFL cases {2267,3493}. It arises from a V(D)J recombination error in a bone marrow pre-B cell. Rare translocation variants involve IGL instead of IGH. Whereas pre-B or naïve B cells harbouring t(14;18) have not been documented to date, differentiated t(14;18)+ memory-like B-cell clones can be detected in the peripheral blood at very low levels (~1–100 cells per 1 million B cells) in > 70% of healthy adults. Among them, the vast majority will never develop FL {3488,2351,986}. The frequency of detection of t(14;18)+ cells in peripheral blood increases with age, and t(14;18)+ cells have been detected at higher levels in individuals with environmental

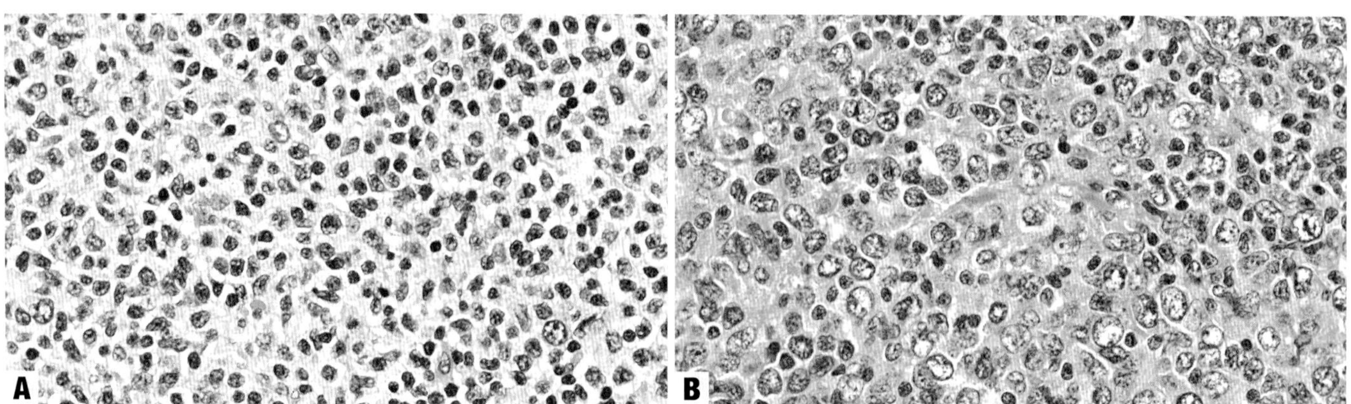

Fig. 4.108 Follicular lymphoma (FL), cytomorphological spectrum. Classic FL includes tumours composed of a majority of centrocytes (**A**) or with a substantial component of centroblasts mixed with centrocytes (**B**). Such tumours can be graded optionally as grade 1–2 FL (FL1–2) and grade 3A FL (FL3A), respectively. In contrast, follicular large B-cell lymphoma (grade 3B FL [FL3B]) is totally devoid of centrocytes.

Table 4.26 Most frequent gene alterations in *BCL2*-rearranged follicular lymphoma at diagnosis

Gene	Frequency of alterations[a]	Predominant type(s) of alteration
KMT2D (*MLL2*)	50–70%	Mutation
CREBBP	50–70%	Mutation (~60%), deletion
EPHA7	70%	Deletion, methylation
TNFRSF14	45–65%	Deletion, mutation (~30%)
BCL2	~50%	Mutation
SESN1	30–40%	Deletion
CDK4	~30%	Gain
EZH2	20–40%	Mutation (~20%), gain
H1-2 to *H1-5* (*HIST1H1B–E*)	15–30%	Mutation
CTSS	15–20%	Mutation (~5%), amplification
BCL6	~15%	Translocation, mutation (~5%)
FOXO1	10–15%	Mutation
STAT6	10–15%	Mutation
ARID1A	10–15%	Mutation
EP300	10–15%	Mutation
CARD11	10–15%	Mutation
MEF2B	10–15%	Mutation
ATP6V1B2	~10%	Mutation
ATP6AP1	~10%	Mutation
GNA13	~10%	Mutation
RB1	~10%	Deletion, mutation (< 5%)
SOCS1	~10%	Mutation
RRAGC	5–15%	Mutation
IRF8	5–15%	Mutation
POU2F2	5–10%	Mutation
SGK1	5–10%	Mutation
CDKN2A/B	5–10%	Deletion
TNFAIP3	5–10%	Deletion, mutation (< 5%)
HVCN1	5–10%	Mutation
EBF1	5–10%	Mutation
TP53	~5%	Mutation, deletion
CD79B	~5%	Mutation
FAS	< 5%	Mutation

[a]Approximate frequency of alterations; some alterations may be subclonal.

exposures such as pesticides {720,41}. These cells may also be found in the bone marrow, spleen, and lymph nodes of the same healthy individuals {41,3886}. In reactive lymph nodes, t(14;18)-positive B cells accumulate within GCs as centrocytes with a very low proliferation rate {3984,3886} and a high propensity to re-enter the GC and undergo iterative cycles of GC reaction, increasing the risk of accumulation of genomic instability {3886}. Circulating and resident clones usually carry IgM, whereas the translocated allele is often class-switched to IgG (known as the allelic paradox) {3488}. Significant somatic hypermutation is also observed on the translocated allele, with an evolution pattern suggesting that activation-induced cytidine deaminase (AID) expression is maintained or reactivated {41, 3886}. N-glycosylation sites are introduced within the V regions, an event not commonly encountered in normal B cells {2995}.

The dominant t(14;18)+ clone detected in healthy individuals may rarely develop into overt FL as long as a decade later, especially if the clonal cell frequency is > 10^{-4}; such individuals have a 23-fold higher risk of subsequent FL {1594,559,453, 4342,2513,3487}. These clones have been demonstrated to carry some mutations commonly found in established FL, such as *CREBBP* {3040,1403,2128,135,2995,975}. In situ follicular B-cell neoplasm and partial involvement of lymph nodes by FL may constitute intermediate steps of morphological progression in tissues.

Phylogenetic trees suggest divergent subclonal evolution from a common precursor cell driving FL at diagnosis and relapses. Although linear clonal evolution has been described, most FL cases follow a branching evolution. Multiple subclones can readily be identified in early disease phases {1402} and provide the substrate for progression and transformation {1401,2512,2493}. The sequences of events driving progression are largely unknown. Copy-number alterations are found in > 90% of FLs. They encompass chromosomal gains of 18, X, 1q, 2p, and 7, and less commonly of 17q, 6p, 8q, and 12q {4021,2999,1613,3321}. Deletions mainly include 6q and 1p, and less frequently 10q and 9p {3321}. The 1p36 region, containing *TNFRSF14*, is frequently deleted {2895}. Copy-neutral loss of heterozygosity of *TNFRSF14* is also observed. The evolution of FL is accompanied by gene mutations that occur over time {3040,2127,394}. The most frequent mutations are found in *KMT2D* and *CREBBP*; these represent early driver events and induce loss-of-function of chromatin modifiers {4558}. Epigenetic dysregulation comprises gain-of-function mutations of *EZH2*, encoding an H3K27 methyltransferase and (less frequently) mutations affecting *ARID1A*, *MEF2B*, and *KMT2C* {1678}. Loss-of-function mutations and deletions of *TNFRSF14* foster an FL-supporting milieu {394}. *BCL2* mutations are frequent, owing to AID activity {1679}. Other, less common, gene mutations are found in *STAT6*, *CARD11*, *FOXO1*, *BTK*, *TNFAIP3*, *NOTCH1*, *NOTCH2*, and *RRAGC*, all leading to perturbed intracellular signalling. Some recurrent mutations in genes such as *RRAGC* and *CTSS* are uncommon in lymphoma types other than FL {3040,939}. A number of genetic alterations are more often seen in transformed lymphoma than in preceding FL, such as inactivation of *TP53* and *CDKN2A*, as well as *MYC* translocations {3255,1060, 2426,2128,2127,848}.

FL with BCL6 rearrangement

Rearrangements affecting chromosomal band 3q27, resulting in structural *BCL6* alterations, can be found in any type of FL. Their frequency is 15–20% in FL with *BCL2* rearrangement (FL-*BCL2*-R) {4432,2127} and is higher (~35%) in FLs lacking *BCL2* rearrangement {2128,2127}. In FLBCL, structural alterations involving BCL6 can be found in about 40% of cases, reflecting their closer biological relationship to diffuse large B-cell lymphoma (DLBCL) {1923,244}.

FL lacking BCL2 and BCL6 rearrangements
The pathogenesis of FL lacking *BCL2* rearrangement is less well known and probably follows different pathways. These cases account for 10–15% of cFL cases {4432}; they are more common in FLBCL {3087,244}, dFL {3740}, primary testicular FL {205}, and paediatric-type FL {4396}. FLs lacking *BCL2* and *BCL6* rearrangements show evidence of somatic hypermutation, similarly to cells having transited through the GC. However, in contrast to FL-*BCL2*-R, which expresses GC B-cell signatures, the gene expression profile of FLs lacking *BCL2* rearrangement is reminiscent of late/post-GC cells {2268}. Thus, the postulated normal counterpart is a late GC B-cell that has not yet exited the GC stage of differentiation. Overall, FLs lacking *BCL2* rearrangement display copy-number alterations and mutations similar to those in FL-*BCL2*-R, but with different frequencies {4539,2895}. The most frequently mutated gene is *STAT6* (> 50%), which may play a pivotal role in some tumours {2656}, especially in localized stages {2425}. *KMT2D* is less often mutated (< 50%) {2895}. FL with a predominantly diffuse growth pattern lacking *BCL2* rearrangement frequently presents as limited-stage disease, often involving the inguinal lymph nodes, showing frequent coexpression of CD23 (correlated with *STAT6* mutation), 1p36 deletion, and *TNFRSF14* mutation {3740,2560,2895}.

Tumour microenvironment
The tumour microenvironment plays a crucial role in FL pathogenesis. FL cells reside within specific niches with a spatial architecture formed by follicular dendritic cells (FDCs), T follicular helper (TFH) cells, and different subsets of tumour-associated macrophages {878,2149}. Compared with normal lymph nodes, the GCs of FL contain increased numbers of CD4+ T-cell subsets, such as TFH cells and T regulatory (Treg) cells. Immune signalling pathways are skewed towards T-cell exhaustion and tolerance, leading to tumour immune evasion {2149}.

Some tumour microenvironment components such as TFH cells can directly stimulate the growth and survival of the neoplastic cells {106}. Non-immune components, such as endothelial cells, fibroblasts, and mesenchymal stromal cells, are also involved in the aberrant ecosystem {1440}.

Macroscopic appearance
The cut surface of lymph nodes involved by FL may display a vaguely nodular pattern. Splenic involvement by FL shows a uniform expansion of the white pulp, usually without obvious involvement of the red pulp.

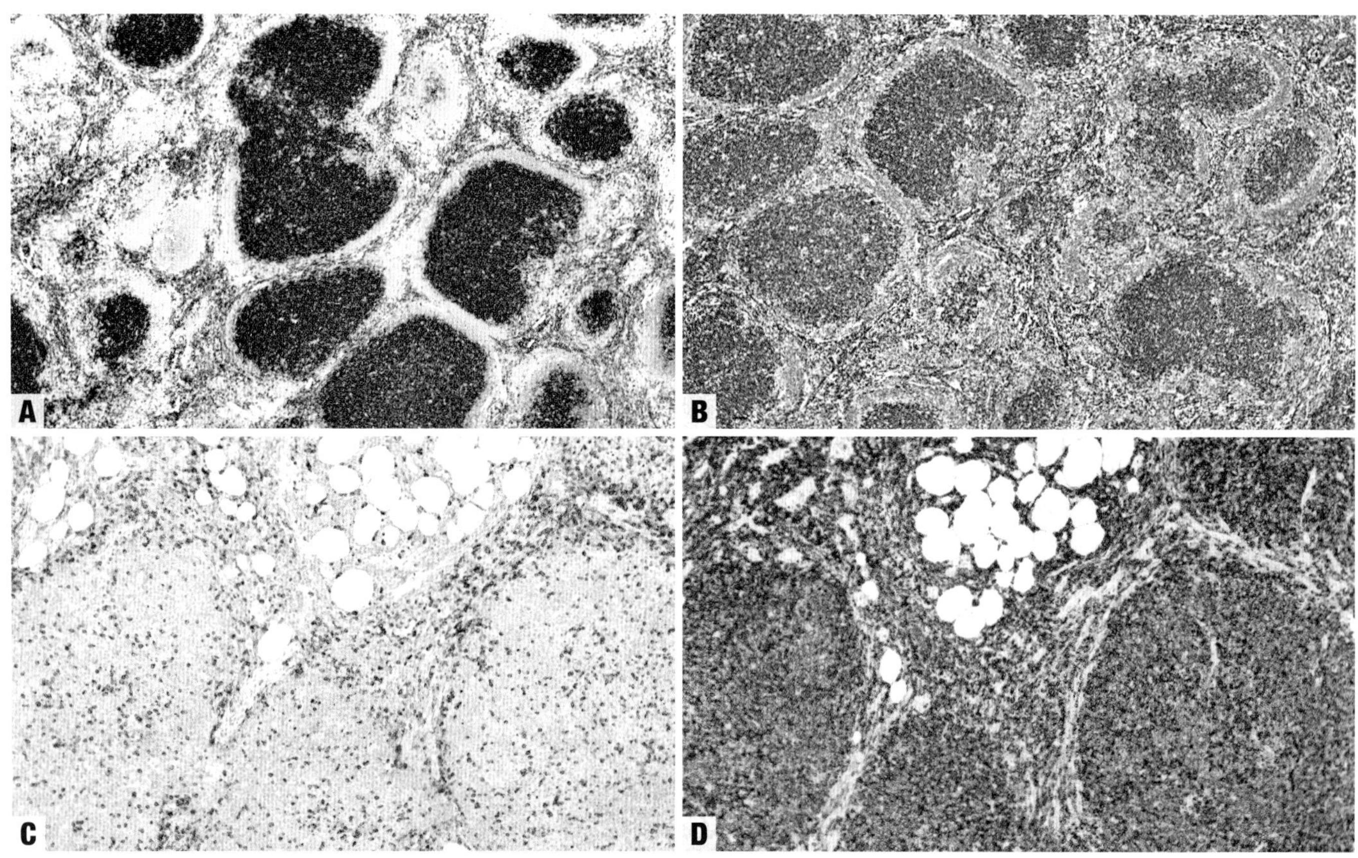

Fig. 4.109 Follicular lymphoma, immunophenotype. **A** Neoplastic follicles are usually positive for CD10, and there may also be CD10+ cells between follicles, indicating the presence of interfollicular invasion (and supporting the diagnosis of lymphoma). **B** Neoplastic follicles are usually positive for BCL2, and the intensity of staining may be stronger than in the non-neoplastic B cells and T cells. In a minority of cases, neoplastic cells appear to be negative for BCL2 when tested with monoclonal antibody BCL2 clone 124 (**C**), because of minor amino acid variations at the antibody binding site caused by mutations in *BCL2*. BCL2 expression may be demonstrable in these cases using the monoclonal antibody BCL2 clone SP66 (**D**).

Histopathology

Classic follicular lymphoma

Cellular composition

Follicles are organoid structures comprising neoplastic cells placed in a specific microenvironment composed of T cells, macrophages, and FDCs. cFL resembles GCs in its cellular composition, with a mixture of centrocytes and centroblasts / large transformed cells. Centrocytes and centroblasts are located mostly within the neoplastic follicles but are often found between and outside the follicles as well. Centrocytes are slightly larger than small lymphocytes and have angulated, elongated, twisted, or cleaved nuclei. The chromatin is less dense than in small lymphocytes, and the nucleoli are inconspicuous. The cytoplasm is scant, pale, and barely discernible in routinely stained sections. Centroblasts are large cells (usually at least three times the size of normal lymphocytes) but may sometimes be smaller (termed small centroblasts), depending in part on the staining/fixation. Their cytoplasm is usually fairly visible and lightly amphophilic (basophilic with Giemsa). The nuclei appear round or oval with vesicular chromatin and multiple peripherally located nucleoli. Transformed/blastic cells with similar chromatin and a single large nucleolus are immunoblasts and may be found as a minority of blasts. Rare cases harbour intrafollicular giant or multinucleated cells resembling HRS cells {4432}.

Patterns

Most cases present with at least a focal follicular pattern identifiable by morphology, but recognition may be facilitated by immunohistochemistry. Spread beyond the nodal capsule is often associated with sclerosis or diffuse areas.

The size and shape of the follicles vary substantially between cases. There is also variability in the extent and distribution of the follicles, which are commonly distributed over the whole lymph node, leading to effacement of the architecture (including a lack of sinuses). The follicles are often crowded, with a back-to-back arrangement. Most neoplastic follicles display attenuated or absent mantle zones, with poorly defined borders. They usually lack polarization of the GCs, i.e. the physiological demarcation between a centroblast-rich (dark) and a centrocyte-rich (light) zone is absent. The starry-sky pattern imparted by tingible-body macrophages, characteristic of the dark zone of reactive GCs, is usually not seen. Some cases show irregular or serpiginous follicles, which may resemble progressively transformed GCs and create a floral pattern. Involvement of the interfollicular regions is a frequent finding and should not be confused with a diffuse growth pattern. Interfollicular FL cells may be smaller, have less irregular nuclei, and show phenotypic differences (CD10/BCL6 downregulation, CD23 upregulation) as compared with the intrafollicular FL cells. Their detection can be facilitated by immunohistochemistry.

Marginal zone differentiation of FL presents with pale, marginal zone–like areas, mostly found at the outer borders of the follicles and containing lymphoma cells with a monocytoid appearance. Plasmacytic differentiation, characterized by the presence of light chain–restricted plasmacytoid cells mainly seen in interfollicular areas, is uncommon {1385,639}. Rarely, the neoplastic cells may assume a signet-ring cell appearance, in the form of either a clear cytoplasmic vacuole or a homogeneous eosinophilic globule (Russell-body type) compressing the nucleus {4566}. Occasional cases, frequently with

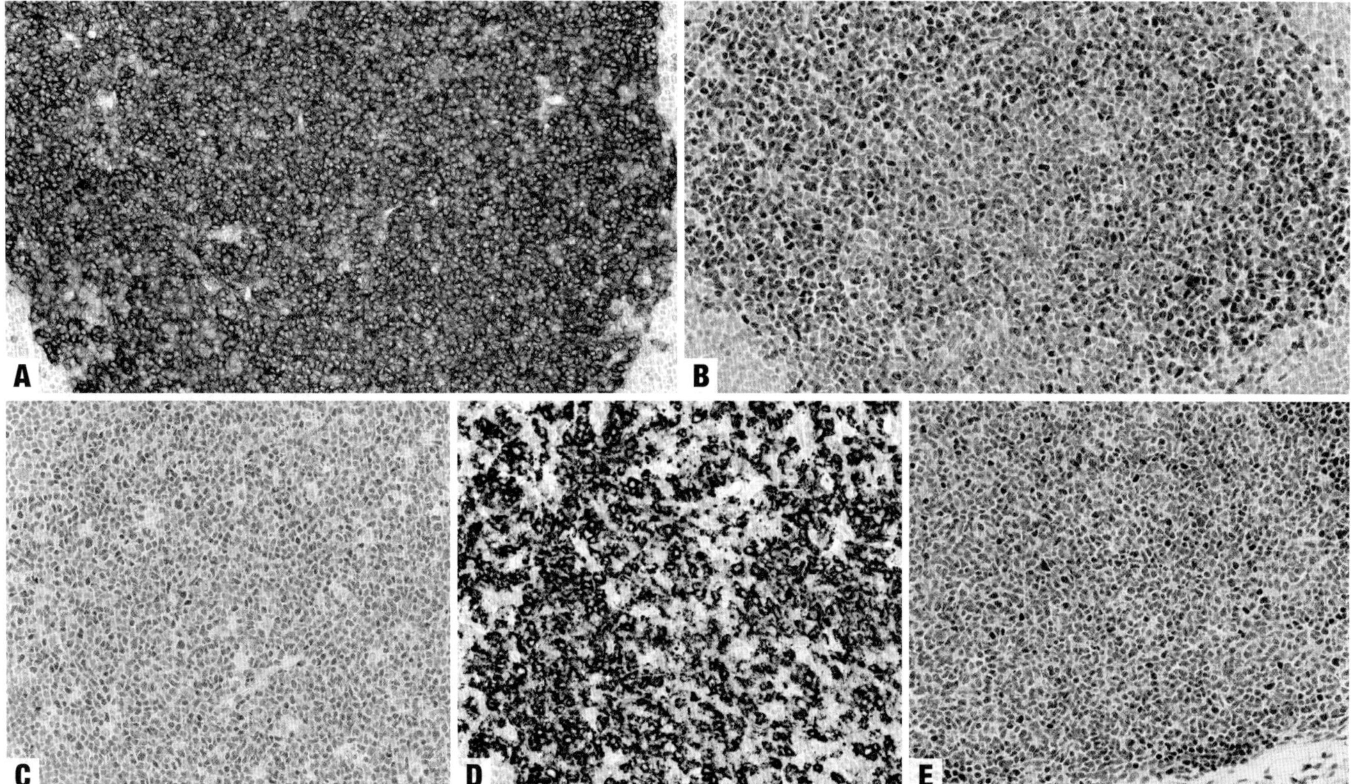

Fig. 4.110 Follicular lymphoma, immunophenotype. Follicular lymphoma cases express a variety of germinal-centre markers including CD10 (**A**), BCL6 (**B**), LMO2 (**C**), and stathmin (**D**). FOXP1 is often expressed at variable levels (**E**).

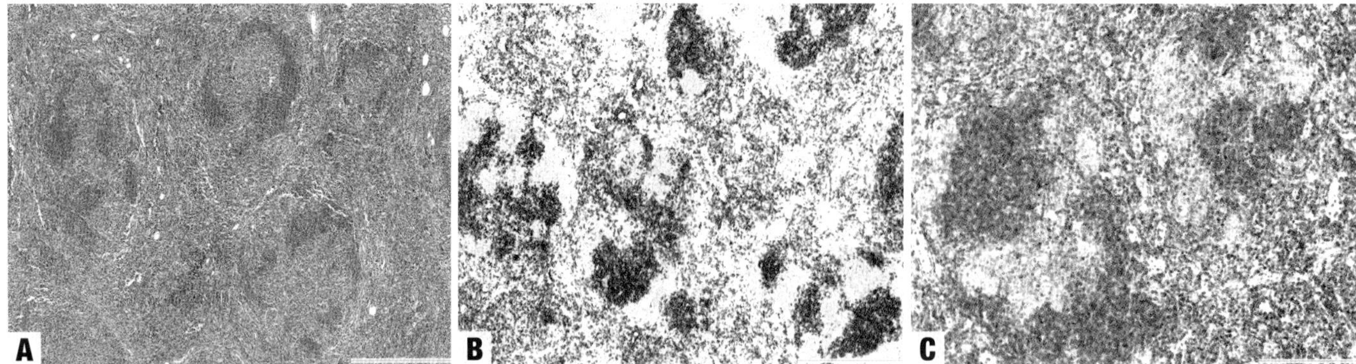

Fig. 4.111 Follicular lymphoma with prominent colonization of neoplastic follicles. In floral-pattern follicular lymphoma, neoplastic follicles are partly colonized by mantle zone cells, resulting in irregular borders and fragmentation (**A**), which is highlighted by CD10 staining (**B**). **C** BCL2 staining may be difficult to interpret, because of a mix of strongly positive mantle zone cells and generally less strongly positive lymphoma cells.

mesenteric and retroperitoneal presentation, may show widespread sclerosis in interfollicular regions. Some foci of sclerosis or hyalinosis may also be present within neoplastic follicles resembling the hyaline-vascular follicles of Castleman disease {3247,639}. Some cases may contain abundant intrafollicular amorphous deposits that stain strongly for CD10 and CD20, resulting from the shedding of cell membrane materials {1500}. Massive necrosis can be found in rare cases but does not necessarily indicate transformation.

In the bone marrow, paratrabecular infiltration is typical for FL, although interstitial areas may be also involved. Neoplastic follicles containing FDC are rarely encountered in the bone marrow. Lymphoma cells are usually smaller than regular centrocytes, resembling the FL cells found in the interfollicular regions of lymph nodes.

Immunophenotype

FL cells express B-cell antigens (CD19, CD20, CD22, CD79a, PAX5), in addition to surface immunoglobulin, mostly of the IgM isotype, with or without IgD; expression of IgG is less frequent, and IgA is rare. They also express the GC-associated markers CD10, BCL6, GCET1, HGAL (GCET2), LMO2, AID, MEF2B, and stathmin, with variable sensitivity and specificity of each of the markers {4513,2527,2651,2764}. Expression of CD10 and BCL6 may vary between neoplastic follicles and is usually stronger in the neoplastic follicles than in interfollicular FL cells. It may be

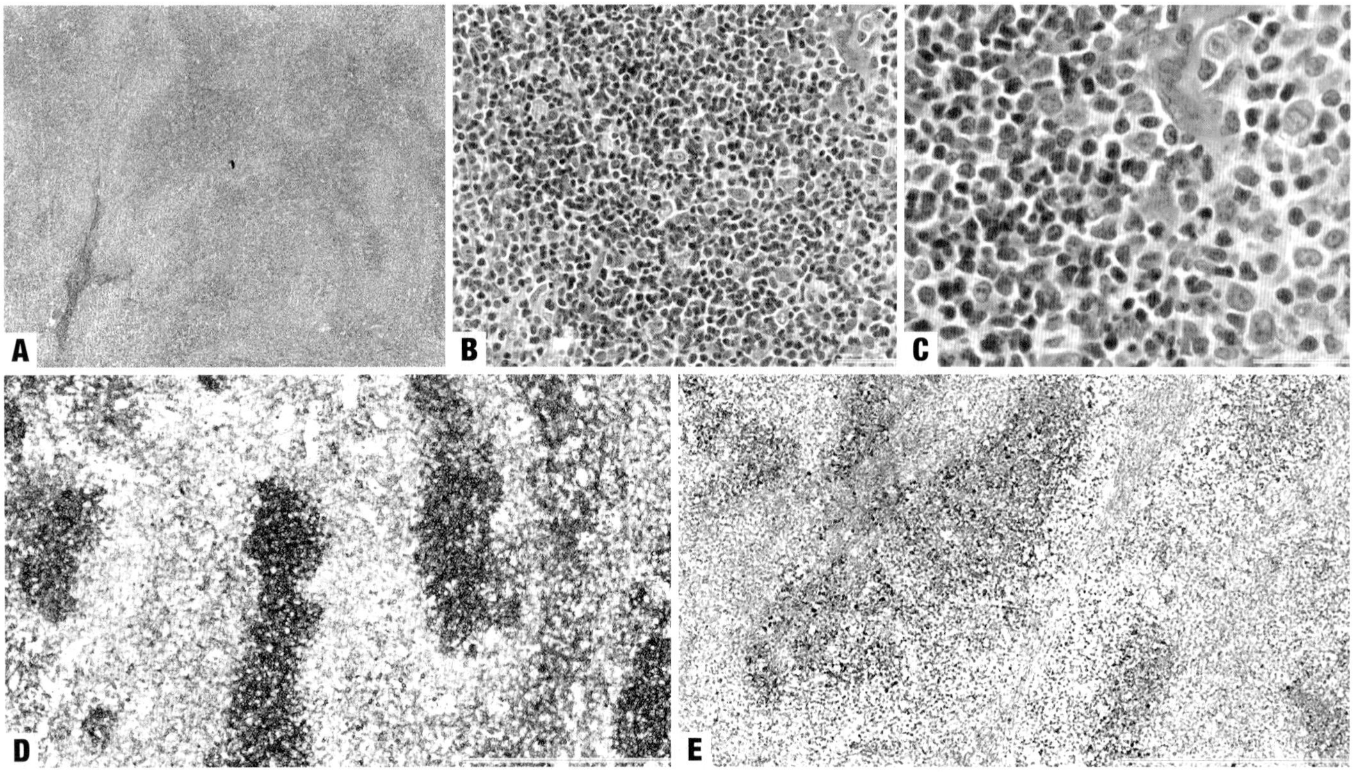

Fig. 4.112 Follicular lymphoma with marginal zone differentiation. **A** Marginal zone differentiation is characterized by neoplastic follicles surrounded by clear areas mimicking the marginal zone at low magnification. **B** High-power view shows that the clear areas contain neoplastic cells of slightly larger size and relatively abundant cytoplasm resembling monocytoid B cells, whereas centrocytes are present in the central part of the follicle (**C**). The neoplastic nature of clear cells is supported by positive CD20 (**D**) and BCL6 (**E**) immunohistochemistry, which appears weaker than in the central part of the follicles, however.

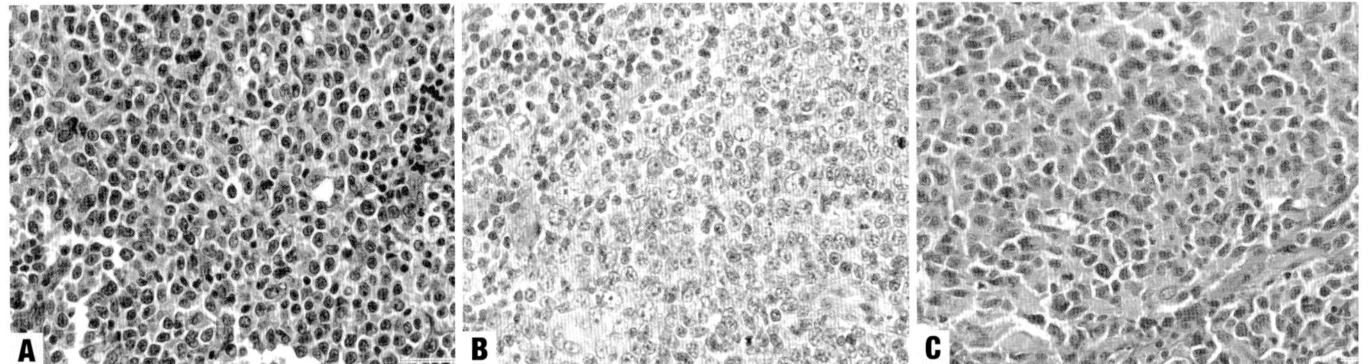

Fig. 4.113 Follicular lymphoma with unusual cytological features. **A,B** Follicular lymphoma with unusual cytological features is diagnosed in cases with a nodular pattern in which the nodules are composed of medium-sized cells with blastoid chromatin and occasional nucleoli. Scattered large centroblasts may be present (**B**). **C** The cell population may also contain cleaved cells that are larger than classic follicular lymphoma centrocytes (also known as large centrocytes).

absent in FL cells located in areas of marginal zone differentiation, peripheral blood, or bone marrow {4514}. In the rare CD10/BCL6-negative cases, the diagnosis of FL should be supported by the use of other GC-associated markers, which are commonly negative in other small B-cell lymphomas.

In most cases, the neoplastic follicles express BCL2, thus allowing their delineation from reactive follicles. The frequency of BCL2-negative cases is low in cFL (~15%). The lack of BCL2 expression may be due to mutations in *BCL2* that affect the BCL2 epitope recognized by the antibody used. If BCL2 is negative, it is recommended to use additional anti-BCL2 antibodies directed against different epitopes. Rare FL cases remain negative to multiple antibodies used, which usually corresponds to a lack of *BCL2* rearrangement {22}. In some cases, the abundance of intrafollicular BCL2-positive T cells may hamper the assessment of BCL2 expression in neoplastic FL cells. Comparison with corresponding CD3 immunohistochemistry may avoid misinterpretation. IRF4 (MUM1) is mostly negative in FL, except in occasional cases {4430,4432,1893}, which may be centroblast-rich and also lack CD10 and BCL2 expression {2898,1900}. The neoplastic follicles show highly variable Ki-67 proliferation indexes, but most cases have a proliferation index much lower than that of reactive follicles {2039}. The Ki-67+ cells are sometimes concentrated in the peripheral portions of the neoplastic follicles. Polarization characteristic of reactive follicles is not seen. A high proliferation index is often seen in cases with high numbers of centroblasts, although it can sometimes also be seen in centrocyte-rich cases {4302,4432}. CD30 positivity can be rarely observed in neoplastic follicles, some of which may also show HRS-like cells {4432}. Expression of CD5 or PD1 has rarely been reported {4431,3159}. EBV association can be detected exceptionally {2462}. FDCs in the neoplastic follicles usually express CD21, CD23, and/or CD35 but are often irregularly distributed. However, diminished expression of these markers may occur even in obviously follicular areas {1808}.

Grading

Traditionally, FL has been graded as FL1, FL2, FL3A, and FL3B, according to the quantification of absolute numbers of centroblasts / transformed cells in 10 consecutive high-power fields (HPFs) {2519}. However, there is accumulating evidence of the lack of reproducibility in counting centroblasts, and thus of grading itself {3413,2133}. Many studies have indicated no statistically significant difference in clinical outcomes between FL1, FL2, and FL3A, which are treated similarly in modern clinical trials {202,1578,2534,2802,3413}. Furthermore, there is compelling evidence that FL3A is biologically related to FL1/2, with similar immunohistochemical and genetic profiles {1631, 2072,2231} and frequent coexistence in the same affected lymph node.

At present, there is no definitive evidence to support the distinction between FL1, FL2, and FL3A, and hence to mandate grading. FL1/2 and FL3A together constitute the cFL subtype, which is defined by a mixture of centrocytes and centroblasts in various proportions, but in which centrocytes must be unequivocally present. The vast majority (90%) of FLs are cFLs {4268}, in which centrocytes are often the predominant cell population. If centrocytes are scarce, FLBCL must be excluded, and additional tissue may be required to clarify the subtype. Grading is nevertheless considered optional. If required by local clinical practice, it should be performed using conventional criteria, i.e. by counting or estimating the absolute number of centroblasts in neoplastic follicles per HPF of 0.159 mm in diameter and 0.458 mm^2 in area (see Table A in the foreword of this volume for HPF conversion). FL1/2 cases contain 0–15 centroblasts, and FL3A cases contain > 15 centroblasts per HPF of 0.159 mm in diameter and 0.458 mm^2 in area {2519,2915}. FL3 can be further subdivided according to the presence/absence of centrocytes, with centrocytes still present in FL3A but absent in FL3B (now termed FLBCL) {3087}. Rare cases of FL with a prominent diffuse pattern and an increased number of centroblasts (consistent with FL3A) have been reported, and such cases were designated as DLBCL in the previous (revised fourth) edition {2072}. Currently, it is uncertain whether such cases should be classified as FL or DLBCL. In such cases, individual treatment choices should be made in multidisciplinary conference settings, taking into consideration clinical, laboratory, and imaging parameters. However, the presence of diffuse areas composed entirely or predominantly of large cells warrants a diagnosis of DLBCL.

The reliability of subtyping/grading is highly dependent on adequate sampling. Accurate subtyping cannot be performed on FNAs and may be difficult or unreliable on core needle biopsies. Therefore, an excisional biopsy is strongly recommended for primary diagnosis. For small biopsies with no discernible follicular component but displaying features of cFL, a diagnosis of "FL, likely cFL" is advised.

FL with unusual cytological features

In rare cases, FL may be composed of predominantly medium-sized cells with immature or blastoid chromatin. Other infrequent morphologies include large cells with cleaved/irregular nuclei (large centrocytes) {1055,2231}. These uncommon morphologies often present with particular features that deserve optional specifications related to cytology, morphology, phenotype, proliferation, or genetics {2231}. They display higher Ki-67 proliferation and IRF4 (MUM1) expression in a higher proportion of cells. Furthermore, the frequency of *BCL2* rearrangement is lower. Their diagnosis may require negative *IRF4* FISH testing if IRF4 (MUM1) protein is strongly expressed. Although still largely unknown, the prognosis of these cases may differ from that of cFL {2231}. Because the data currently available on these uncommon morphologies are limited, the prognostic impact remains to be ascertained {2231}. The distinction of uFL will allow such data to be collected in the coming years, for the purposes of better risk stratification.

FL with a predominantly diffuse growth pattern

A diffuse FL subtype was initially described as being characterized by a predominantly diffuse growth pattern, CD23 expression, and absence of t(14;18)(q32;q21) {1922,3740,2895}. In such cases, a diffuse pattern is supported by the absence of demonstrable FDCs, although FDC remnants may be present in residual small follicles (microfollicles). The cell population should be composed of a vast majority of centrocytes, except in residual follicles. BCL2 immunohistochemistry is often weak to absent, especially in remnant follicles. Sclerosis and interstitial fibrosis may be observed. dFL mainly occurs in the inguinal region and may form large tumour masses, but infrequently it disseminates. Patients often present with limited-stage disease and have a favourable prognosis {1922,3740,2895}. Neoplastic cells are usually positive for CD10 and CD23, but CD10 expression may be absent. Although not specific, mutations in *STAT6* are more frequently observed in inguinal dFL than in cFL {3740, 2895}. Of note, a partly diffuse (sometimes extensive) growth pattern is a regularly encountered feature in FL in general {2267, 4539,4538,2895}. Therefore, a definite diagnosis of dFL should not be made on limited biopsy material, including core needle biopsy samples.

Follicular large B-cell lymphoma

FLBCL (formerly FL3B) is commonly regarded as a particular subtype of FL with a close clinical and biological relationship to DLBCL {3087,1632,2072,1631,2231,2073}. FLBCL is defined by the presence of a follicular pattern with follicles composed of sheets of centroblasts and an absence of centrocytes. *BCL2* translocation is uncommon {3546}. FLBCL rarely coexists with cFL but frequently coexists with DLBCL. Because of the extreme rarity of pure FLBCL {3087,1923,2072,3413,2231}, the possibility of concurrent DLBCL must be excluded by careful sampling. Therefore, a definitive diagnosis of this entity should not

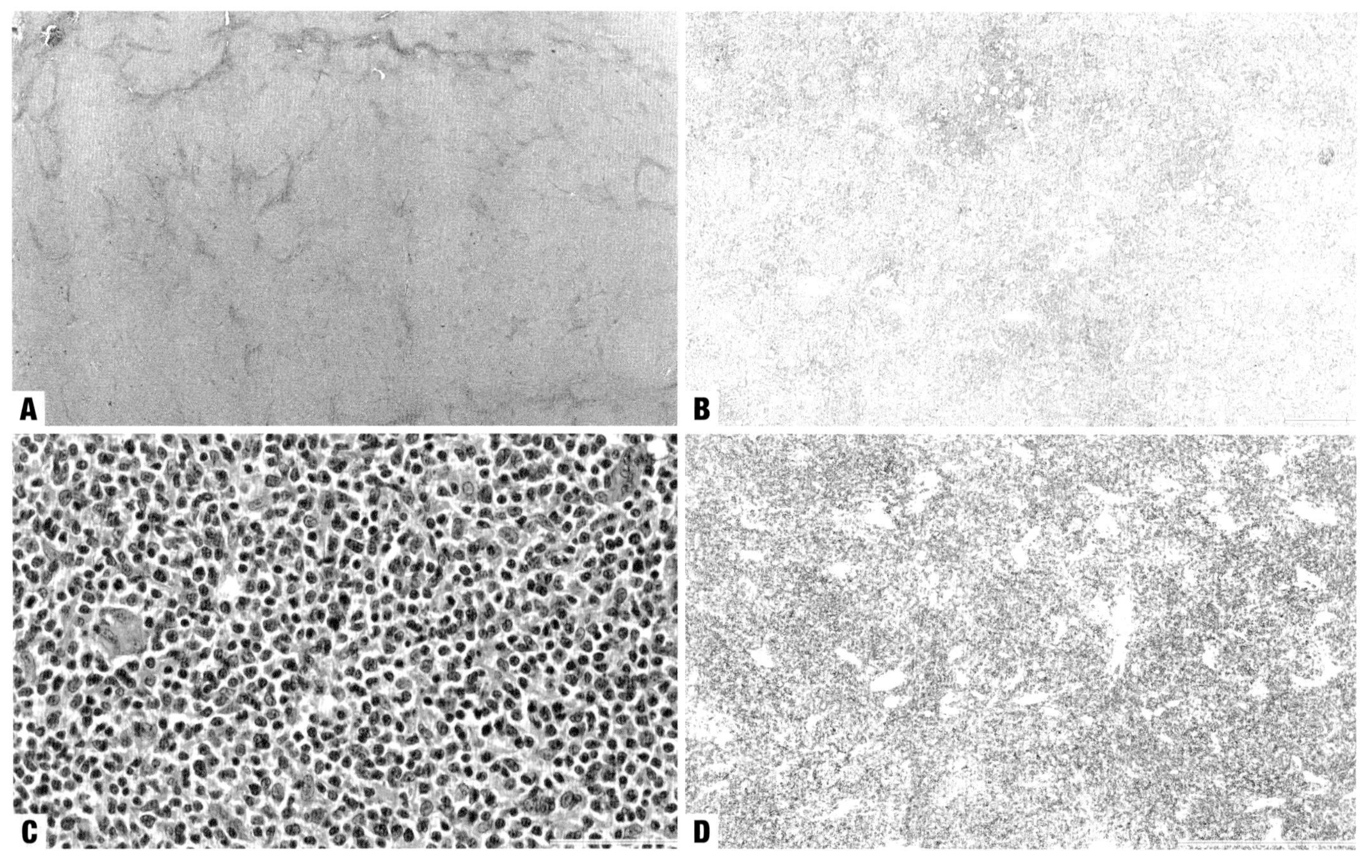

Fig. 4.114 Follicular lymphoma with a predominantly diffuse growth pattern. Follicular lymphoma with a predominantly diffuse growth pattern may show some vague nodularity (**A**), but underlying CD21+ follicular dendritic meshworks are absent or inconspicuous (**B**). **C** The cell population consists of a mixture of centrocytes and centroblasts. **D** Sheets of centroblasts are lacking. CD23 is typically expressed in most lymphoma cells.

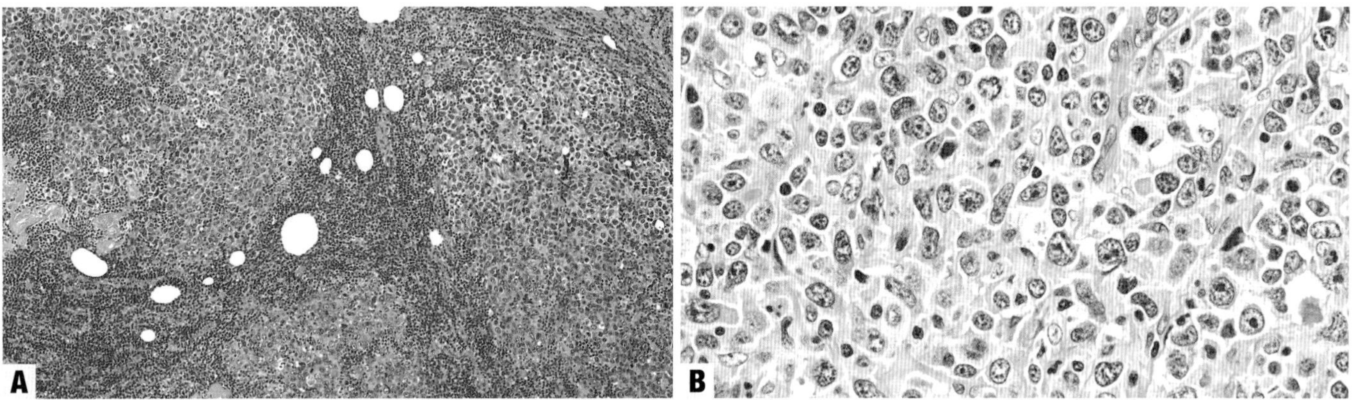

Fig. 4.115 Follicular large B-cell lymphoma. **A** Follicular large B-cell lymphoma / FL grade 3B tumours are often composed of large nodules with poorly defined borders. **B** At higher magnification, the cytological pattern is characterized by compact nests of large cells and the absence of centrocytes. Large cells may display either a typical centroblastic pattern or more variation in size, sharing a common feature of round nuclei with vesicular chromatin.

be made on a core needle biopsy. A presumptive diagnosis of FLBCL should prompt additional investigations, such as *BCL6* or *MYC* rearrangement {2072,1631,2231}. *IRF4* FISH analysis is required if IRF4 (MUM1) protein is strongly expressed, to exclude large B-cell lymphoma with *IRF4* rearrangement.

Differential diagnosis

Florid follicular hyperplasia can pose problems in the distinction from FL. Generally, follicles in florid follicular hyperplasia are widely spaced, of uneven size and shape, and contain prominent GCs with polarization and tingible-body macrophages. The GC cells are negative for BCL2 expression, and the Ki-67 proliferation index is high in florid follicular hyperplasia. It occasionally may show a clonal CD10+ population by flow cytometry, which should not be considered sufficient evidence of malignancy. Rare FL may harbour tingible-body macrophages and show BCL2 negativity that may suggest benign follicular hyperplasia. Using different BCL2 antibodies (corresponding to different clones) may be useful, because BCL2 protein may not be detectable in some FLs due to mutations in *BCL2*. The presence of B cells of GC phenotype (positive for CD10, HGAL, or MEF2B) in interfollicular areas favours a diagnosis of FL. A low Ki-67 proliferation index would favour a diagnosis of FL. Furthermore, a lack of polarization (evidenced by morphology and Ki-67) argues against a reactive lesion. In some cases, FISH (*BCL2*, *BCL6*, and IGH) and/or clonality (IGH and IGK) studies may be needed.

FL cases with marginal zone differentiation or plasmacytoid cells may mimic nodal marginal zone lymphoma (NMZL) with a predominant nodular growth pattern and/or NMZL with extensive follicular colonization. The distorted architecture of the follicles and the presence of BCL2-negative, CD10/BCL6-positive intrafollicular cells favour the diagnosis of NMZL. It should be noted that CD10 expression (in isolation) does not exclude a diagnosis of NMZL. The expression of MNDA or IRTA1 favours a diagnosis of NMZL {2668,1870}. In some cases, the histophenotypical distinction between FL and NMZL may be impossible; in such cases, the presence of *BCL2* translocation favours a diagnosis of FL, although its absence does not totally rule this out. More extensive genetic analyses may also aid in the differentiation of difficult cases {881}.

A floral pattern in FL can mimic progressive transformation of CGs. BCL2 expression may be difficult to interpret, owing to the mixing of mantle cells displaying strong BCL2 positivity with FL cells expressing BCL2 at lower levels.

FL cases harbouring CD30+ HRS-like cells may raise the suspicion of classic Hodgkin lymphoma, which can be ruled out by the atypical morphology of the surrounding lymphoid cells. However composite tumours comprising classic Hodgkin lymphoma and FL do rarely occur {4069}.

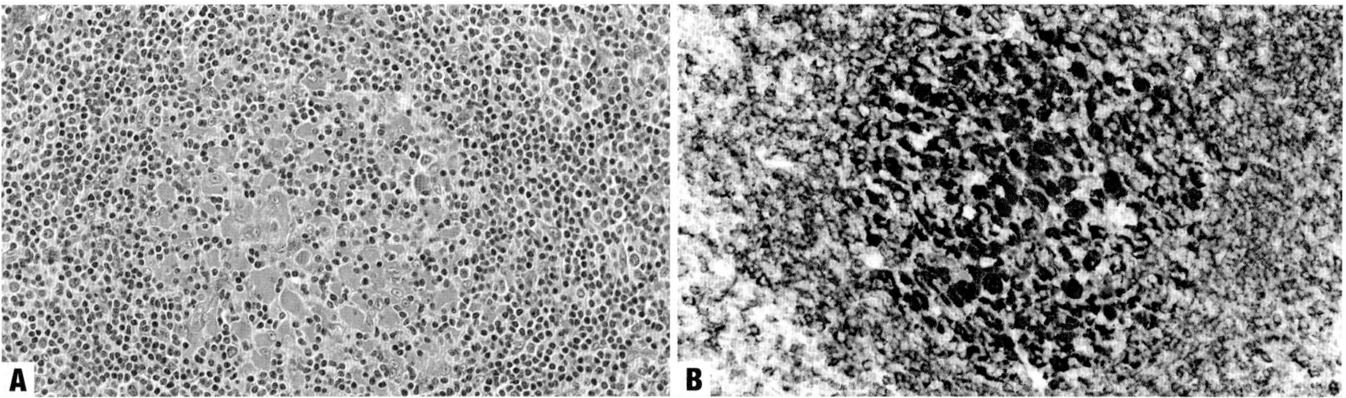

Fig. 4.116 Follicular lymphoma with follicular eosinophilic precipitates. **A** Amorphous deposits are located within the neoplastic follicles. **B** Follicular lymphoma cells are positive for CD20, and the precipitate is also positive, because it is formed of cell membrane materials.

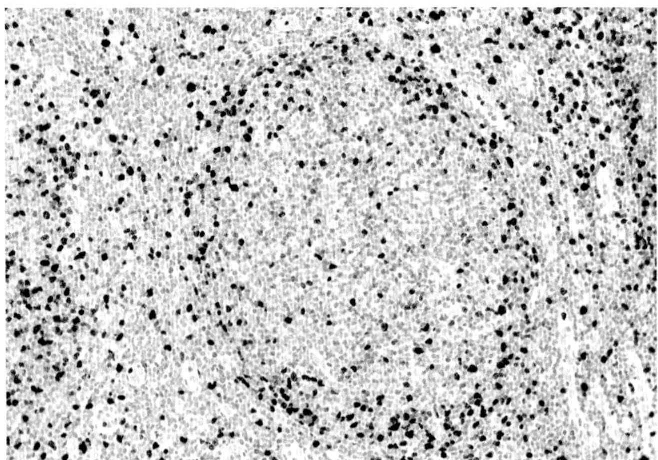

Fig. 4.117 Follicular lymphoma with a prominent interfollicular pattern. The Ki-67 index is commonly low in follicular lymphoma, and the positive cells are often concentrated in the peripheral portion of the neoplastic germinal centres.

Large B-cell lymphoma with *IRF4* rearrangement must be ruled out in cases composed of centroblasts or medium-sized blastoid cells with a partly follicular pattern {3338}, especially in children and young adults. This requires IRF4 (MUM1) testing by immunohistochemistry. If IRF4 (MUM1) is strongly and uniformly expressed, FISH studies for *IRF4* translocation should be considered.

Cytology

Cytological preparations of lymph nodes reveal typical centroblasts and centrocytes. The diagnosis of FL can be suspected if centrocytes constitute most of the cell population and macrophages are rare. However, an unequivocal diagnosis of FL should not be made on the basis of cytology alone. Cytological aspirates of lymph nodes may be used in assessing recurrence, especially when used in combination with flow cytometric analysis. It may also be a surrogate for assessing transformation in a context of strong clinical suspicion, especially in severely ill patients with poorly accessible sites.

Diagnostic molecular pathology

IG heavy chain (IGH) and light chain (IGK, IGL) genes are monoclonally rearranged in FL, which allows its distinction from reactive follicular hyperplasia. Multiplex PCR reactions using BIOMED-2 primer sets detect clonal rearrangements in > 90% of FL cases when primers targeting IGH and IGK are included. When only IGH assays are used, clonal rearrangements may be missed {326,1098,3173}.

Investigation of IGH::*BCL2* translocation may be applied in the diagnostic workup of suspected BCL2 immunohistochemistry–negative FL or dFL and to support the distinction of FL from other small B-cell lymphomas, such as NMZL. In these settings, analysis of *BCL6* translocation may have added value. FISH testing of *BCL2*, *BCL6*, and *IRF4* is recommended to distinguish unusual cases of IRF4 (MUM1)-expressing FL and FLBCL from large B-cell lymphoma with *IRF4* rearrangement {2380,3546}.

Next-generation sequencing is currently not recommended in the routine workup of FL, since the mutation profile of FL shares considerable overlap with other lymphoma entities.

Essential and desirable diagnostic criteria

Essential: B-cell lymphoma composed of varying proportions of centrocytes and/or centroblasts (large transformed cells), with a dominance of centrocytes in the overwhelming majority of cases; immunophenotype compatible with a germinal-centre B-cell origin, with positivity for markers such as CD10, BCL6, MEF2B, GCET1, HGAL (GCET2), or LMO2.

Desirable: at least partly follicular growth pattern; *BCL2* or *BCL6* rearrangements and/or a lack of *IRF4* rearrangement (in equivocal cases).

Staging

Staging is performed using the Lugano classification, a modification of the Ann Arbor staging system {687}. A complete blood count and peripheral blood smear are required. Assessment of bone marrow involvement with a bone marrow biopsy is recommended, especially when the results would alter case management. Bone marrow aspiration has a lower yield, because of the difficulty in aspirating cells from the paratrabecular locations. Conventional imaging tools such as CT are useful in assessing the degree of lymphadenopathy and the extent of disease. FDG PET has the potential to upstage 10–45% of early-stage patients to advanced-stage disease {4389,26,443}, and therefore is recommended. Functional imaging is also useful in identifying patients with suspected transformation {2988}. Biopsies are needed for confirmation and should be directed to the site of the greatest FDG avidity.

Prognosis and prediction

cFL is an indolent disease {998}, with a median survival time of > 17 years with current therapies {2818}. Progression occurs continuously over time, with no plateau in the survival curves {274}. The prognosis of FL is closely related to the disease extent at diagnosis. FLIPI, a modification of the International Prognostic Index (IPI), has a prognostic impact on outcome {3777,274}, which remains significant in the rituximab era {503, 2978}. FLIPI uses five independent adverse predictors: age > 60 years, haemoglobin < 12 g/dL, elevated serum LDH, Ann Arbor stage III/IV (disseminated disease in the Lugano system), and > 4 involved nodal areas. The presence of 0–1, 2, and 3–5 of these factors defines low-risk, intermediate-risk, and high-risk disease, respectively. In patients with progression within 24 months after diagnosis or first-line immunochemotherapy (POD24), 5-year overall survival is significantly worse {575,1838,1233}.

Other prognostic indexes, such as FLIPI-2 and PRIMA-PI, are not commonly used in daily practice, because their performance has not been sufficiently validated {201,1232}. A clinicogenetic risk model based on the mutation status of seven genes combined with FLIPI and Eastern Cooperative Oncology Group (ECOG) performance status (m7-FLIPI) for patients treated with immunochemotherapy has been established and awaits further independent validation {3154,4343, 394}.

The occurrence of *EZH2* mutations tends to have a favourable prognostic impact on patients treated with immunochemotherapy (excluding bendamustine-based treatment) {1679,3836, 3154} and may predict response to EZH2 inhibition {2803}. An association with adverse outcome has been suggested for *TP53* mutations, 2p gain, 9p21 deletion, or 17p deletion {3078,

701,2230,3154,1679,3321}. FL with double-hit *BCL2* and *MYC* rearrangements behaves more aggressively {2702,650,504, 2231}.

Gene expression and immunohistochemistry studies have examined the prognostic relevance of tumour microenvironment immune components, with no clear consensus as yet {4433,395,4028}. A gene expression signature related to dark-zone centroblasts was shown to be associated with poor outcomes under some, but not all, explored treatments {1678,1680,4433,394,4099}. The prognostic value of high Ki-67 expression has not been clarified to date, although a trend towards unfavourable evolution was observed, even in centrocyte-rich FL {4430,4432}. Overall, the prognostic value of genomic alterations, gene expression, and immunohistochemical markers currently remains controversial because of the lack of comprehensive validation, and their impact on treatment decisions in individual patients and outside clinical trials remains unanswered.

Histological transformation of FL to DLBCL occurs at a risk of 1–3% per year {2758,92,2365,1150}. The median time to transformation is 2.5–4.1 years {92,2365}. Various clinical parameters, including a high FLIPI score and resistance to first-line therapy, have been reported as risk factors for transformation {83,2819}, but reliable immunological or genetic predictive biomarkers have not been identified thus far. Transformation is often associated with a rapid increase in serum LDH, discordant progression of localized lymphadenopathy, new development of unusual extranodal disease (e.g. liver, bone, muscle, brain), new development of B symptoms, hypercalcaemia, and high uptake values on FDG PET imaging {1888,92,2988,2365}.

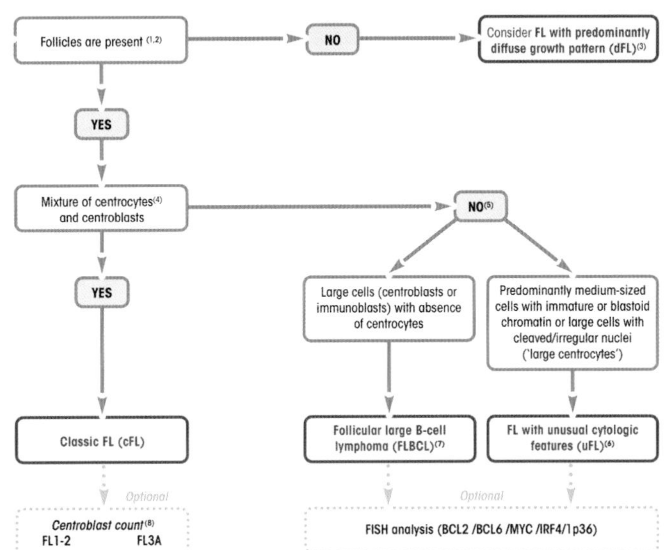

Fig. 4.118 Algorithm for follicular lymphoma (FL) subtyping and optional grading. Footnotes: (1) Subtyping/grading applies only to lymphomas already identified as FL. It should be performed on surgical biopsies for optimal accuracy. (2) To apply the algorithm, at least one evaluable neoplastic follicle that is identified either morphologically or using CD21/CD23 is required. (3) See text for the diagnostic criteria for follicular lymphoma with a predominantly diffuse growth pattern. (4) See text for centrocyte definition. "Mixture" implies a significant number of unequivocal centrocytes. (5) The lack of centrocytes renders IRF4 (MUM1) testing (at least by immunohistochemistry) mandatory. In positive cases, subsequent FISH is required to exclude large B-cell lymphoma with *IRF4* rearrangement. (6) See text for details. Optional descriptive features of follicular lymphoma with unusual cytological features include morphology (e.g. "with large centrocytes" or "with blastoid cells") and genetics (e.g. "with/without *BCL2* [or *BCL6* or *MYC*] rearrangement"). (7) See text for details about immunohistochemistry and FISH testing required for the diagnosis of follicular large B-cell lymphoma. (8) See text for details of the counting method.

Paediatric-type follicular lymphoma

Louissaint A Jr
Attarbaschi A
Burkhardt B
Klapper W
Marafioti T
Oschlies I
Siebert R
Woessmann W

Definition

Paediatric-type follicular lymphoma (PTFL) is a localized, nodal mature B-cell lymphoma occurring predominantly in the paediatric, adolescent, and young adult age group. It is characterized by a clonal proliferation of germinal-centre B cells with a pure follicular growth pattern, altered lymph nodal architecture, a high proliferation index, and an absence of *BCL2*, *BCL6*, and *IRF4* rearrangements.

ICD-O coding

9690/3 Paediatric-type follicular lymphoma

ICD-11 coding

2A80.4 Paediatric-type follicular lymphoma

Related terminology

Acceptable: paediatric follicular lymphoma.

Subtype(s)

None

Localization

Virtually all cases of PTFL manifest as limited-stage peripheral lymphadenopathy. Most patients present with a single enlarged lymph node in the head and neck region or, less commonly, an enlarged inguinal, femoral, or axillary lymph node {3077,2430}. Para-aortic and mesenteric lymph node involvement has not been reported. Extranodal presentation is excluded by definition, although rare clonal follicular proliferation with features of PTFL has been described in the conjunctiva {3047}.

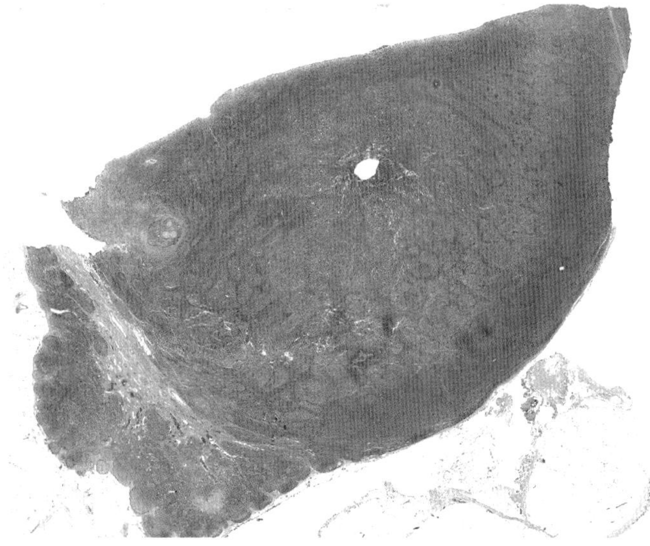

Fig. 4.119 Paediatric-type follicular lymphoma. Lymph node with partial infiltration by a proliferation of atypical follicles with a rim of reactive tissue and node-in-node phenomenon.

Clinical features

Most patients present with localized painless lymph node enlargement without B symptoms. There is no elevation of serum LDH levels {3906,169,170}. Imaging may confirm the localized nature of the disease.

Epidemiology

Most patients are children, adolescents, or young adults. In one of the earlier series, the patient age ranged from 8 to 36 years (median: 18 years) but patients aged up to 60 years have been reported {2430,2432}. There is a marked male predominance (M:F ratio: > 10:1). PTFL accounts for 1–2% of childhood non-Hodgkin lymphomas {115,44,3077,2430,2380,3906}.

Etiology

Unknown

Pathogenesis

PTFL shows low genomic complexity and lacks the translocations found in other germinal centre–derived lymphomas (e.g. *BCL2*, *BCL6*, *MYC*) {3077,2430,2558,3619,42}. The mutation pattern of PTFL is different from that of classic follicular lymphoma, and non-silent mutations in epigenetic modifier genes such as *EP300*, *CREBBP*, *EZH2*, *KMT2D*, or *ARID1A* are rare {2432}. PTFL also lacks *IRF4* rearrangements that characterize large B-cell lymphoma with *IRF4* rearrangement {3544,3542}. Recurrent alterations in PTFL include deletions and copy-neutral loss of heterozygosity at 1p36 (including *TNFRSF14*; 25–40%) and mutations of *TNFRSF14* (44–54%) and *MAP2K1* (43–49%) {2558,3619,2432,3621}. A hotspot mutation affecting *IRF8* has also been reported {3093,3621}.

Macroscopic appearance

Enlarged lymph node without sclerosis or necrosis

Histopathology

The normal lymph node architecture is extensively altered by atypical, enlarged follicles that are sometimes floral, serpiginous, or confluent. Mantle zones are attenuated or absent; germinal centres are expansile and often lack zonation, but contain tingible-body macrophages. Marginal zone differentiation might be present in some cases. A rim of residual reactive lymph nodal tissue is frequent, also described as a node-in-node appearance {3338}. PTFL usually consists of medium-sized to large blastoid cells, cytologically intermediate between centrocytes and centroblasts. Any diffuse area of large cells consistent with a diffuse large B-cell lymphoma will exclude a diagnosis of PTFL.

Immunophenotype

The neoplastic cells coexpress B-cell markers (e.g. CD20, CD79a, and PAX5) and germinal-centre markers (e.g. BCL6

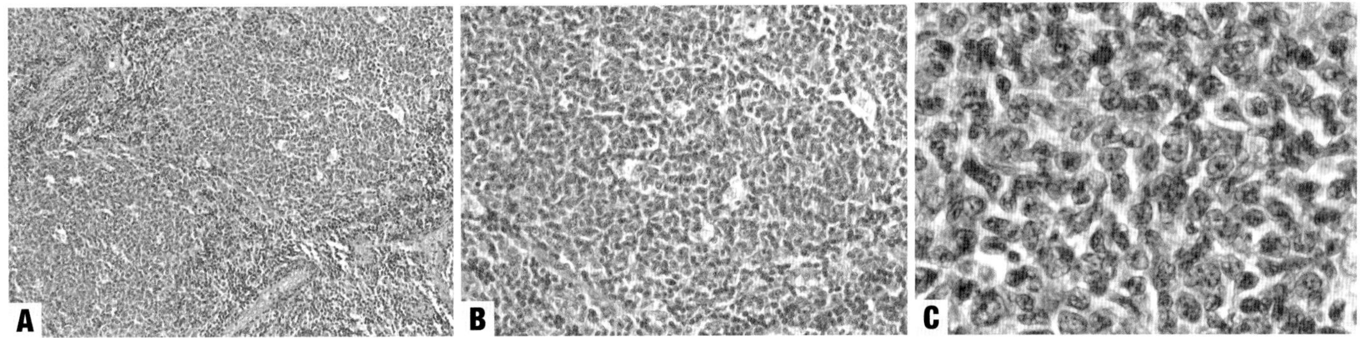

Fig. 4.120 Paediatric-type follicular lymphoma. **A** Confluent atypical follicles lacking zonation, starry-sky macrophages, and a follicle mantle. The follicles consist of intermediate-sized cells resembling larger centrocytes or small centroblasts. **B** Atypical follicles lacking zonation and mantle zones. Some starry-sky macrophages are seen. Cytology shows uniform intermediate-sized cells with features between larger centrocytes and small centroblasts. **C** Cytology, with cells intermediate between large centrocytes and smaller centroblasts.

and CD10, with CD10 expression being frequently strong). These markers, together with CD21-positive and CD23-positive follicular dendric cell meshworks, highlight the pure follicular architecture and restriction of the neoplastic cells to the follicles, and the relative absence of neoplastic cells in interfollicular areas. The neoplastic germinal centre B cells are negative for BCL2 in most cases, although weak or partial BCL2 expression might be seen. Neoplastic cells are also negative for IRF4 (MUM1). The Ki-67 proliferation index is usually > 30%, and the proliferating cells often lack polarity {2422, 3903,3077,3338,2103,42}.

Differential diagnosis

The differential diagnosis includes paediatric nodal marginal zone lymphoma, which also typically contains large germinal centres, often with changes similar to those seen in progressive transformation of germinal centres. Characteristic features supporting a diagnosis of PTFL include a lack of features of progressive transformation of germinal centres, absent interfollicular expansion of marginal zone B cells, and a diminished number of PD1+ T cells within the neoplastic germinal centres. The differential diagnosis of PTFL also includes rare cases of florid follicular hyperplasia, of which some cases may harbour

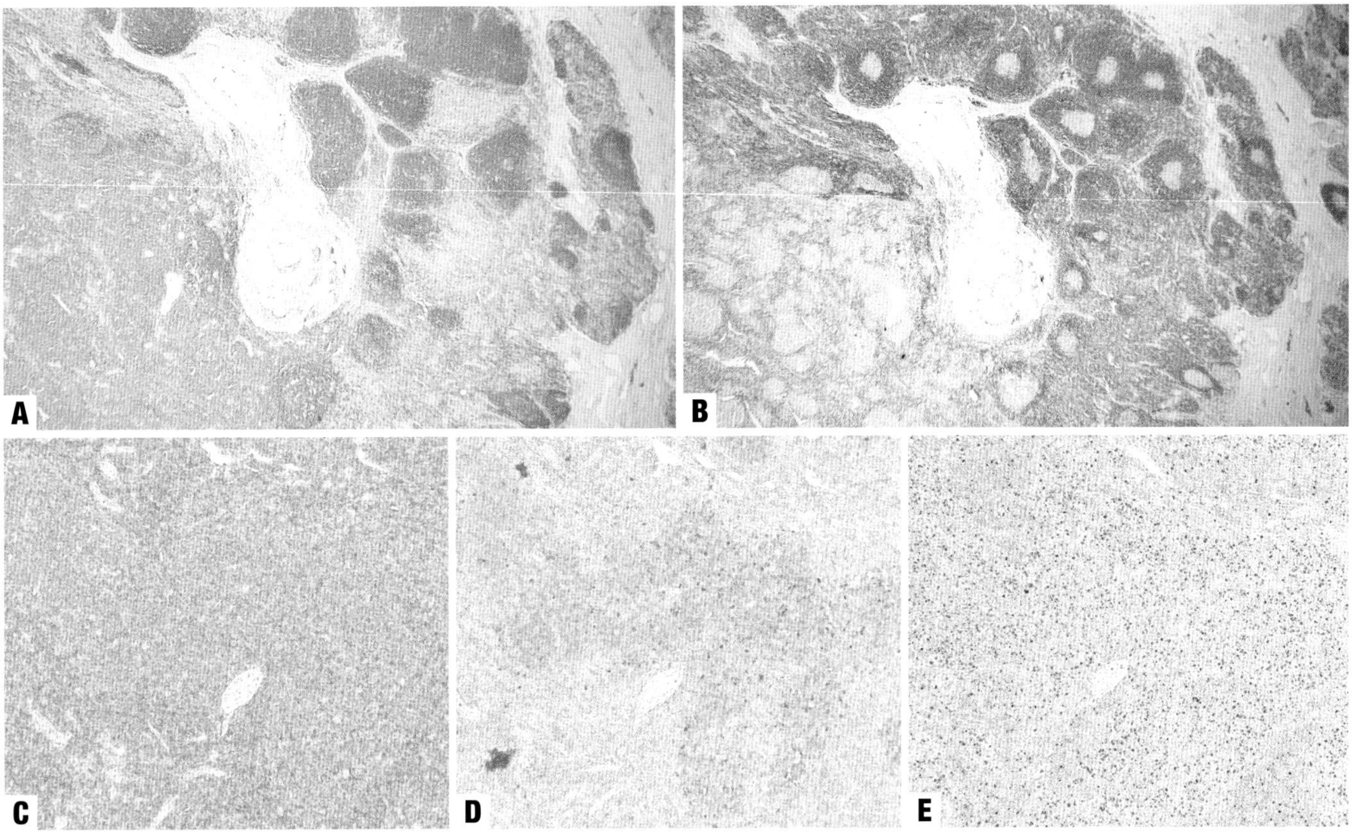

Fig. 4.121 Paediatric-type follicular lymphoma. **A** Partial infiltration of the lymph node by confluent atypical follicles expressing CD20 and a rim of preserved reactive lymph node with well-demarcated reactive follicles. **B** Very faint expression of BCL2 in the areas of atypical follicles, and sharply demarcated negativity for BCL2 in the reactive germinal centres. **C** Atypical confluent follicles with an increase in CD20-positive cells in the interfollicular areas. **D** Expression of CD10 is confined to the atypical germinal centres, and the interfollicular areas remain negative. **E** The atypical follicles lack zonation in the Ki-67 staining, and the proliferation index is slightly lower than in reactive germinal centres.

small populations of clonal B cells {2164} but do not show architectural distortion. Emerging data suggest that the expression of FOXP1 in PTFL may be helpful, as this is not seen in reactive germinal centres {42}. Finally, some cases of classic follicular lymphoma occurring in young adults lacking *BCL2* rearrangements and BCL2 expression may be challenging to distinguish from PTFL {4437,2895}. However, these cases usually fail to meet all the essential diagnostic criteria for PTFL listed below.

Cytology

The FNA cytology might resemble that of a reactive lymph node rich in large cells and is insufficient for PTFL diagnosis.

Diagnostic molecular pathology

A monoclonal IG gene rearrangement can be detected in nearly all cases and is helpful in the differential diagnosis from florid reactive follicular hyperplasia {2164,3338,3619,42}. Exclusion of *BCL2*, *BCL6*, and *MYC* translocations by FISH is required for the diagnosis of PTFL {3906}. *IRF4* FISH should additionally be performed to rule out large B-cell lymphoma with *IRF4* translocation, in cases where neoplastic cells show strong, uniform IRF4 (MUM1) protein expression.

Essential and desirable diagnostic criteria

Essential: a patient in the paediatric, adolescent, and young adult age group (usually age < 40 years, most 2–25 years); localized nodal disease; purely follicular growth with marked architectural distortion and germinal-centre marker expression; predominance of intermediate-sized to large blastoid cells and a high proliferation fraction; absence of diffuse proliferation of large cells meeting criteria for diffuse large B-cell lymphoma; evidence of B-cell monoclonality by immunophenotyping or genetics; absence of *BCL2*, *BCL6*, and *MYC* rearrangements; absence of strong, uniform IRF4 (MUM1) protein expression and/or absence of *IRF4* rearrangement.

Desirable: markedly expansile follicles; mutations in *MAP2K1* and *TNFRSF14*.

Staging

Although most patients with PTFL present with localized disease in the head and neck region, staging should be performed {3476,169}.

Prognosis and prediction

PTFL does not necessarily require chemotherapy, because it has an overall excellent outcome. Survival rates exceed 95% {167,2422,3077,3192,3254,2621,170,3796,169}. Based on the available literature, watch and wait after complete excision of localized disease (performed at diagnosis or after a diagnostic biopsy) is considered an adequate therapeutic approach, provided the resection will not cause morbidity {169}.

Duodenal-type follicular lymphoma

Karube K
Herfarth K
Lorsbach RB
Raderer M
Weigert O

Definition

Duodenal-type follicular lymphoma (DTFL) is a variant of follicular lymphoma (FL) restricted to the gastrointestinal tract, mainly to the second portion of the duodenum. It is a neoplasm of germinal-centre B cells showing a follicular architecture and is mostly limited to the mucosa. DTFLs are of low histological grade and have an indolent clinical course and excellent outcomes.

ICD-O coding

9695/3 Duodenal-type follicular lymphoma

ICD-11 coding

2A80.6 & XH9L76 Follicular lymphoma of small intestine & Follicular lymphoma, duodenal type

Related terminology

None

Subtype(s)

None

Localization

DTFL is particularly common in the second (descending) portion of the duodenum, sometimes with peripapillary clustering of lesions. In most cases, there are additional lesions throughout the small intestine and, less commonly, in the stomach, colon, and rectum {3936}.

Clinical features

In general, patients are asymptomatic, and the disease is usually incidentally discovered on endoscopy performed routinely or for other reasons. The majority have localized disease (stage IE) either within the duodenum or (less commonly) scattered along the small bowel, occasionally accompanied by regional lymphadenopathy. Endosonography is often negative or shows restriction of the process to the mucosa and submucosa {3615}.

Epidemiology

DTFL accounts for about 4% of all gastrointestinal lymphomas, and a DTFL is identified in 1 in 3000–7000 gastroduodenoscopies {3615,3936}. The median age of patients is 52–65 years in larger retrospective series. Whereas some studies show a female predominance {3936,1550}, others show no sex predilection {3615,3936,1495,2472,2250}.

Etiology

Unknown

Pathogenesis

The pathogenesis of DTFL shows many similarities with the early steps of nodal/systemic FL pathogenesis, in that t(14;18)(q32;q21) (IGH::*BCL2*) and recurrent mutations in *TNFRSF14*, *EZH2*, *KMT2D*, and/or *CREBBP* are found in almost all cases {1550}. However, DTFL displays a lower frequency of *KMT2D* mutations, especially of multiple mutations, than nodal/systemic FL, as well as a lower genetic complexity, reminiscent of in situ follicular B-cell neoplasm {2513}. Virtually all cases show decreased expression of activation-induced cytidine deaminase (AID) compared with nodal/systemic FL, indicating a premalignant character with similarities to in situ follicular B-cell neoplasm, as shown in cases with the coexistence of both lesions {3937,2894,1383}. The gene expression profile of DTFL differs from that of nodal/systemic FL, especially in the expression of chemokines. The expression of CCL20, which is involved in the recruitment of proinflammatory T helper 17 (Th17) cells, is significantly higher in DTFL than in nodal/systemic FL {3938,1550}. Together with the bias of IG gene usage towards IGHV4 (VH4) and IGHV5 (VH5), this strongly suggests a role of chronic inflammation and antigenic stimulation in the pathogenesis of DTFL {3584}.

Macroscopic appearance

Most patients present with grey to whitish granular lesions or small nodules on endoscopy. Larger polypoid lesions are rare, but lesions as large as 20 mm in diameter have been reported {2250}.

Histopathology

The lymphoid infiltrate with a follicular pattern is located mainly in the mucosa but may show minimal submucosal extension. The follicles are composed of small to medium-sized

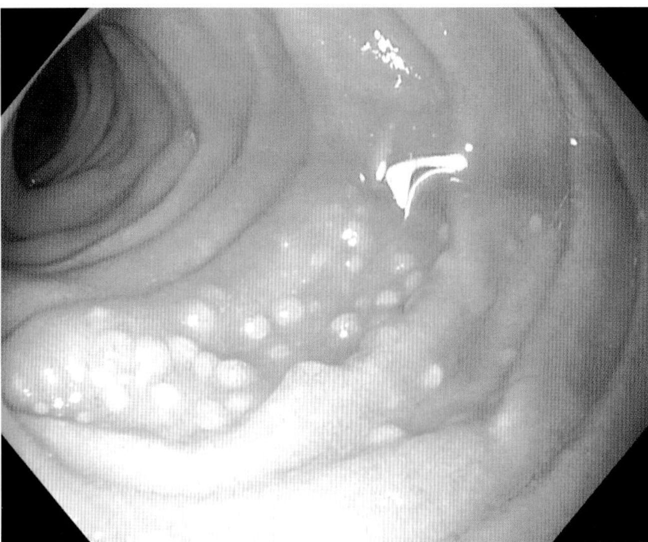

Fig. 4.122 Duodenal-type follicular lymphoma. Endoscopy shows macroscopic findings of duodenal-type follicular lymphoma with numerous whitish granules.

centrocytes, morphologically similar to those seen in classic FL. Tumour cells often invade into the villi beyond the follicles, and the enlarged villi may show a glove-balloon sign {4102}. This is a helpful diagnostic feature, especially when only a small or core needle biopsy is available in which much of the architectural information is lacking.

Immunophenotype

The tumour cells show a phenotype similar to that of nodal/systemic FL, being positive for CD10, BCL6, and BCL2, along with expression of B-cell antigens. Follicular dendritic cell meshworks (CD21/CD23/CD35+) are pushed to the periphery of the neoplastic follicles (hollow meshworks), in contrast to the preserved meshworks usually seen in nodal/systemic FL.

Differential diagnosis

Although other small B-cell lymphomas (e.g. chronic lymphocytic leukaemia / small lymphocytic lymphoma, mantle cell lymphoma, and marginal zone lymphoma) could be differential diagnoses, characteristic clinical, morphological, and immunophenotypic patterns usually distinguish DTFL from these. The glove-balloon sign (villous colonization by neoplastic lymphoid cells) is a useful histological feature for the diagnosis of DTFL.

Cytology

Not recommended

Diagnostic molecular pathology

Identification of t(14;18)(q32;q21) (IGH::*BCL2*) may aid in the diagnosis of rare equivocal cases.

Essential and desirable diagnostic criteria

Essential: germinal-centre B-cell lymphoma with tumour cells confined predominantly to the mucosa of the intestine, characterized by follicles composed predominantly of centrocytes, and with positivity for germinal-centre markers and BCL2.

Desirable: exclusion of secondary involvement from nodal/systemic FL, especially when atypical pathological features are observed.

Staging

Staging should follow the Lugano staging system for gastrointestinal lymphomas. Although the diagnosis is usually straightforward by histology, gastroduodenoscopy with multiple biopsies plus endosonography are the key components of the diagnostic workup. Clinical staging including CT and bone marrow biopsy may be useful to rule out secondary spread from nodal/systemic FL.

Prognosis and prediction

The prognosis is excellent. No disease-related death was observed in two large cohorts with a 10-year and a 77-month follow-up, respectively {3615,1550}. Retrospective data have suggested that DTFL involving the second part of the duodenum

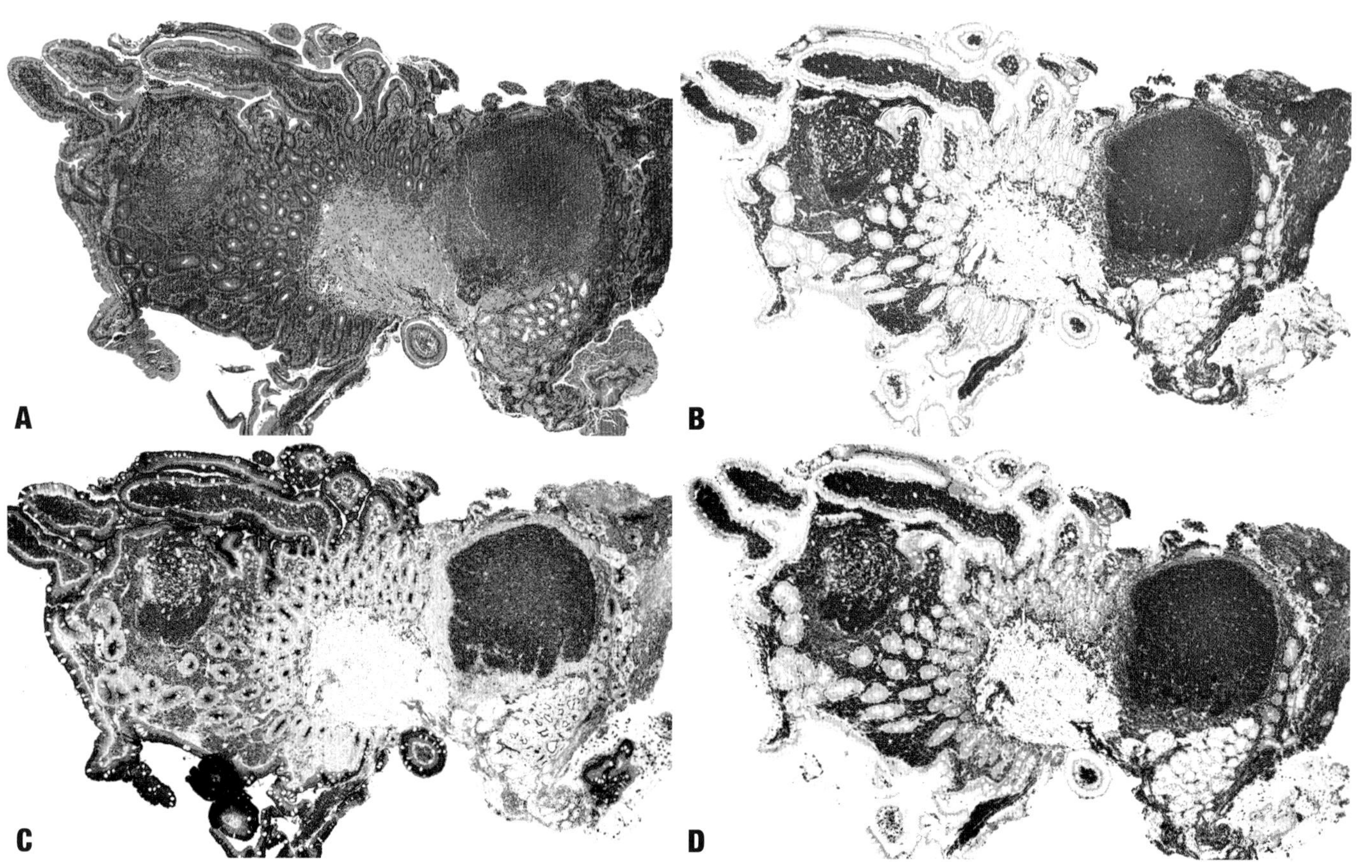

Fig. 4.123 Duodenal-type follicular lymphoma. **A** Duodenal biopsy showing abnormal lymphoid follicles as well as lamina propria infiltration by lymphoid cells. **B** Immunostaining for CD20 highlights the follicles as well as the lymphoid cells in the lamina propria. **C** A similar pattern is seen for CD10, indicating that the extrafollicular lymphoid cells show germinal centre cell differentiation. **D** The follicles show strong immunostaining for BCL2, and the extrafollicular lymphoid cells are also strongly positive.

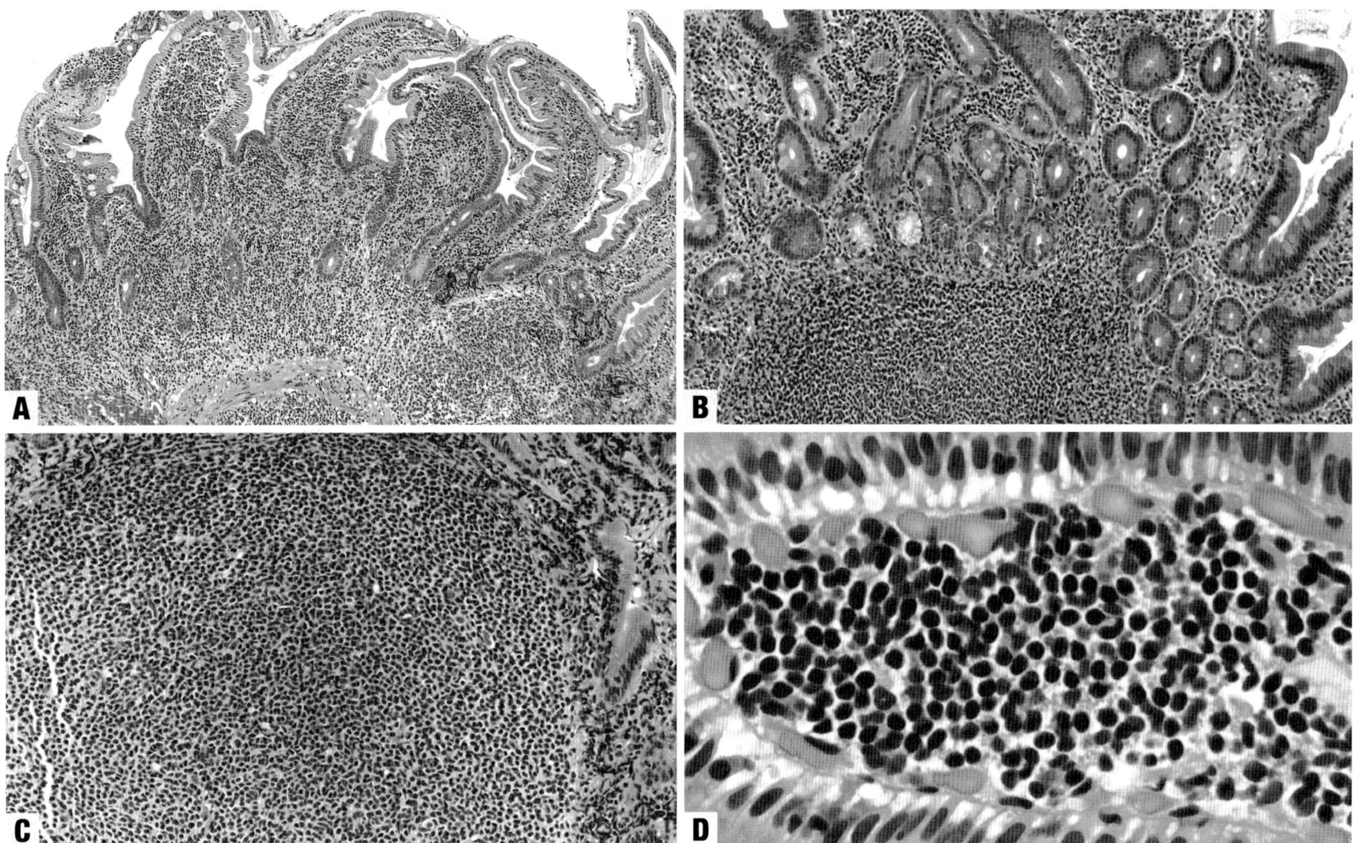

Fig. 4.124 Duodenal-type follicular lymphoma. **A** Duodenal biopsy at low magnification showing enlarged villi infiltrated by lymphoma forming a glove-balloon sign. **B** The infiltrate is composed of abnormal lymphoid follicles. **C** The follicles comprise mostly small lymphoid cells (centrocytes), with no admixed tingible-body macrophages. **D** The lamina propria also shows infiltration by a monotonous population of small lymphoid cells.

is prognostically better than cases involving other parts of the small intestine {3936}. Additional risk factors might involve age > 65 years, advanced stage, male sex, and abdominal symptoms. The preferred approach is watch and wait. Radiotherapy, rituximab monotherapy, chemotherapy (+/– rituximab), and clarithromycin have been reported as effective treatments in mostly small series or case reports, but there are no data to demonstrate a benefit from treatment in asymptomatic patients {3615,1495,3973,2250}. No benefit from surgery was found in a SEER database analysis {4578}.

Primary cutaneous follicle centre lymphoma

Louissaint A Jr
Jansen PM
Oschlies I
Pileri A
Sander CA
Santucci M
Vergier B
Vermeer MH
Willemze R

Definition

Primary cutaneous follicle centre lymphoma (PCFCL) is a tumour of follicle centre cells, including centrocytes and variable numbers of centroblasts, with a follicular, follicular and diffuse, or diffuse growth pattern, that generally occurs in the skin of the head or trunk.

ICD-O coding

9597/3 Primary cutaneous follicle centre lymphoma

ICD-11 coding

2A80.3 Primary cutaneous follicle centre lymphoma

Related terminology

None

Subtype(s)

None

Localization

PCFCL characteristically manifests with solitary or localized skin lesions on the head/neck or the trunk. Approximately 5% of patients present with skin lesions on the legs, and 15% with multifocal skin lesions {2074,4589,3679}.

Clinical features

Patients present with firm, erythematous to violaceous non-ulcerating plaques, nodules, or tumours of variable size. Particularly on the trunk, tumours may be surrounded by erythematous papules and slightly infiltrated, sometimes figurate plaques, which may precede the development of tumorous lesions by months or years {4381,3574,332}. Rare cases featuring miliary and clustered papules or macules on the head have been reported {2578,2577}. Cutaneous relapses are observed in about 30% of patients, but dissemination to extracutaneous sites including lymph nodes is uncommon (~10% of patients) {4589,3679}.

Epidemiology

PCFCL makes up approximately 50% of primary cutaneous B-cell lymphomas and 10% of all primary cutaneous lymphomas. It mainly affects middle-aged adults, with an M:F ratio of approximately 1.5:1 {4589,3679,1479}.

Etiology

Unknown

Pathogenesis

PCFCL is a monoclonal proliferation of germinal centre–derived B cells, which harbour clonally rearranged IG genes, with somatic hypermutation {2,1314,2776,1259}. In most studies, cases of PCFCL with disease limited to the skin on staging rarely show *BCL2* rearrangements {4217,1450,11,3219}. The presence of *BCL2* rearrangements at diagnosis is associated with a higher risk of later systemic spread {3219,4583}. Deletion of chromosome 14q32.33, containing the oncogene *AKT1* and the IGH locus, has been reported {959}. PCFCL harbours mutations in *CREBBP* (25%), *KMT2D* (21%), and *BCL2* (0%) much less frequently than classic follicular lymphoma, in which these genes are frequently mutated {234}. PCFCL shows the gene expression profile of germinal centre–like large B-cell lymphomas and often features amplification of *REL* {2,1606,959}. B-cell receptor genes appear to acquire N-linked glycosylation motifs similar to classic follicular lymphoma and in contrast to primary cutaneous diffuse large B-cell lymphoma (PCLBCL) {2100}. Mutations in *MYD88* and inactivation of *CDKN2A* and *CDKN2B* by deletion (9p21.3) or their promoter hypermethylation are not or only rarely found in PCFCL {959,2644}, in contrast to leg-type PCLBCL.

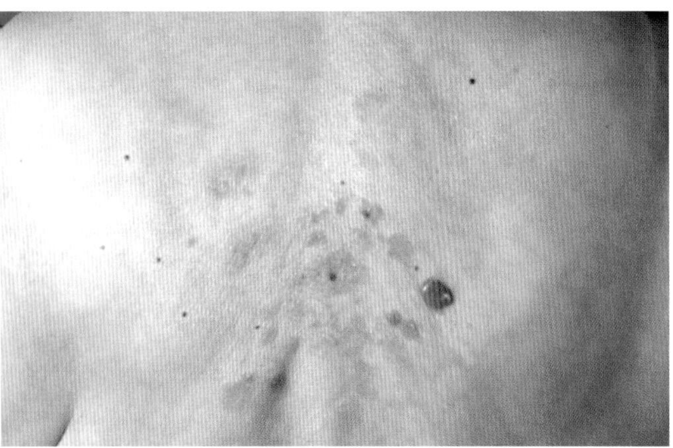

Fig. 4.125 Primary cutaneous follicle centre lymphoma. Clinical presentation with plaques and tumours on the back.

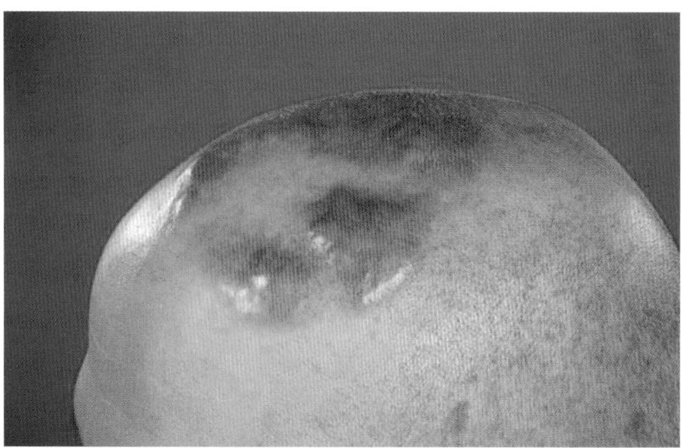

Fig. 4.126 Primary cutaneous follicle centre lymphoma. Clinical presentation with confluent tumours on the scalp.

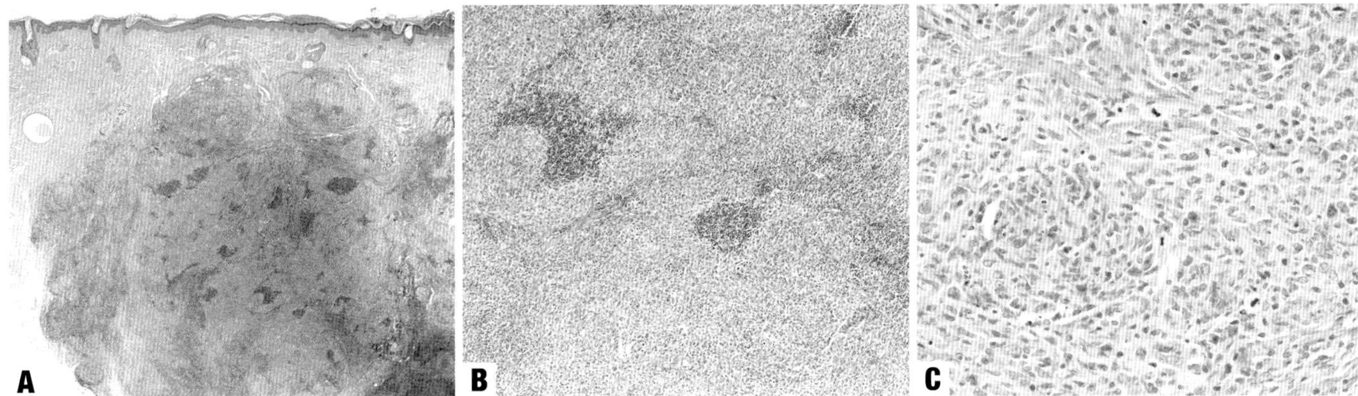

Fig. 4.127 Primary cutaneous follicle centre lymphoma. **A** The large cell / spindle cell pattern, showing cutaneous involvement by a nodular, and in part diffuse, lymphoid infiltrate extending into the subcutis. **B,C** The growth pattern shows a confluent nodular and vaguely follicular architecture (**B**), with sheets of large, and in part spindle, cells with intermingled centrocytoid cells and some polylobulated cells (**C**).

Chapter 4

Macroscopic appearance

PCFCL appears as firm, erythematous to violaceous non-ulcerating plaques, nodules, or tumours of variable size.

Histopathology

PCFCL shows perivascular and periadnexal or diffuse infiltrates with sparing of the epidermis. The infiltrates may show a follicular, follicular and diffuse, or diffuse growth pattern {3574, 4381,489}. Histological grading is not applicable in PCFCL. Cases with a follicular growth pattern show nodular infiltrates throughout the entire dermis, often extending into the subcutis. Unlike in cutaneous follicular hyperplasia, the follicles in PCFCL are often poorly defined, show a monotonous proliferation of BCL6+ follicle centre cells, lack tingible-body macrophages, generally have an attenuated or absent mantle zone, and show a variably high proliferation rate and a lack of polarization {590, 1375}. Reactive T cells may be numerous, and a prominent stromal fibroblastic/fibrohistiocytic component is usually present. Cases with a diffuse growth pattern usually show a monotonous population of large centrocytes, some of which may have a multilobated appearance, and variable numbers of admixed centroblasts {4381,3574,332,1392}. In rare cases, the large centrocytes may be spindle-shaped {591,1372,3075}. The Ki-67 proliferative fraction in diffuse PCFCLs is generally high.

Immunophenotype

The neoplastic cells express CD20 and CD79a but are usually negative for immunoglobulins. PCFCL consistently expresses BCL6. CD10 may be positive in cases with a follicular growth pattern but is generally negative in cases with a diffuse growth pattern {897, 2696,2074,3679}. A disrupted meshwork of CD21+/CD35+ follicular dendritic cells is frequently seen in the atypical follicles but might be absent in cases with a diffuse growth pattern {1450}. Most cases do not express BCL2 or show faint BCL2 staining (weaker than admixed T cells) {590,711,2074,3679}, although several studies have shown BCL2 expression in 8.5–61% of PCFCLs {47,2696, 1374,3219}. Staining for IRF4 (MUM1) and FOXP1 is negative in most cases; CD5 and CD43 are always negative {2074,3679}.

Differential diagnosis

Strong expression of both BCL2 and CD10 by the neoplastic B cells should always raise suspicion of a classic (nodal) follicular lymphoma involving the skin secondarily {1607}. PCFCL with a follicular growth pattern may be distinguished from cutaneous marginal zone B-cell lymphoma primarily on the basis of the expression of germinal-centre markers (CD10 and BCL6, and if necessary other markers such as MEF2B, LMO2, or HGAL [GCET2]), a lack of expression of MNDA, and a lack of plasmacytic differentiation in PCFCL. The main differential diagnosis in cases with a diffuse

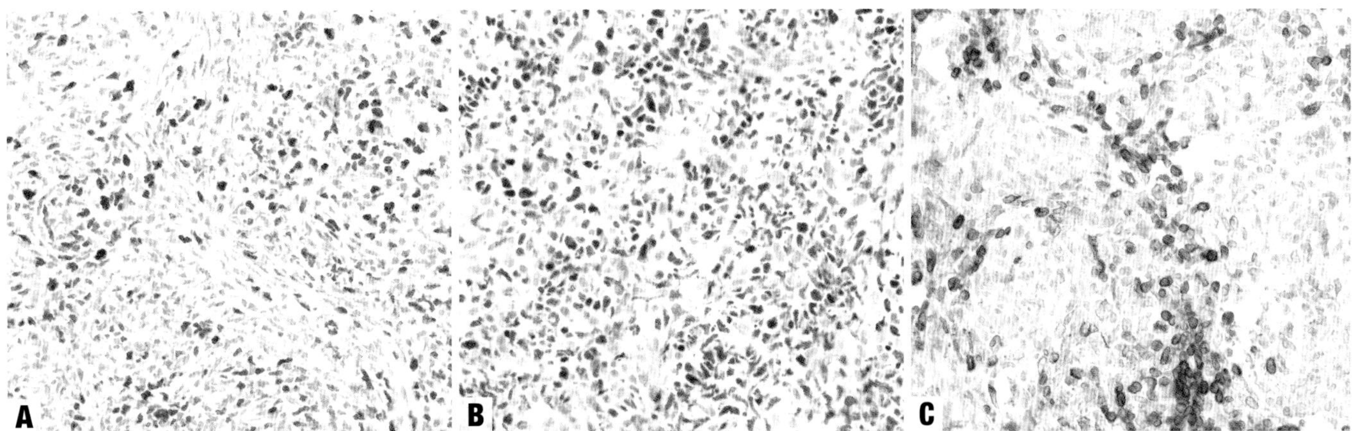

Fig. 4.128 Primary cutaneous follicle centre lymphoma. The large/spindle cell neoplastic B-cell infiltrate shows a relatively high Ki-67 proliferation index (**A**), strong staining for BCL6 (**B**), and faint staining for BCL2 (**C**).

growth pattern is PCLBCL, leg type. Unlike PCLBCL, PCFCL does not express IgM and does not show strong expression of IRF4 (MUM1), in addition to having a germinal-centre phenotype.

Cytology

Not relevant

Diagnostic molecular pathology

Clonality assays, *BCL2* analysis, and targeted sequencing may be informative for challenging cases (see *Pathogenesis*).

Essential and desirable diagnostic criteria

Essential: follicular and/or diffuse proliferation of centrocytes and admixed centroblasts (diffuse lymphomas comprising exclusively centroblasts/immunoblasts are excluded); B cells with coexpression of germinal-centre markers (BCL6 and/or CD10 or other germinal-centre markers); no extracutaneous involvement by lymphoma.

Desirable: localization to head or trunk; evidence of B-cell monoclonality; absent or weak BCL2 expression (usually); lack of IRF4 (MUM1) expression; lack of *BCL2* rearrangement (usually).

Staging

Because cases with a secondary cutaneous follicular lymphoma may have a very similar clinical presentation, staging is important to rule out systemic disease. PCFCL workup includes blood tests (including LDH) {2015} and CT/PET of the chest, abdomen, and pelvis {3680}. Bone marrow biopsy is not routinely performed.

Prognosis and prediction

Irrespective of the clinical, histological, and immunohistochemical features and the genetic aberrations, PCFCL has an excellent prognosis, with a 5-year survival rate of > 95% {3574,1392,4589,3679}. PCFCL presenting on the leg is reported to have a less favourable prognosis {2074,3679}. In patients with localized or few scattered lesions, local radiotherapy is the preferred treatment modality {3679,1479}. Cutaneous relapses, observed in about 30% of patients, do not indicate progressive disease. Systemic therapy is only required in patients with very extensive cutaneous disease or extremely thick skin tumours, or in patients who develop extracutaneous disease.

Mantle cell lymphoma: Introduction

Coupland SE

The category of mantle cell neoplasms is allocated to three individual sections: in situ mantle cell neoplasm, mantle cell lymphoma (MCL), and non-nodal MCL.

In situ mantle cell neoplasm is rare and represents a colonization of mantle zones of lymphoid follicles by B cells carrying the IGH::*CCND1* rearrangement leading to cyclin D1 overexpression. In situ mantle cell neoplasm is typically an incidental finding in lymph nodes and rarely (in < 10% of cases) progresses to MCL {3028}.

The t(11;14)(q13;q32) translocation, leading to IGH::*CCND1* fusion, is the genetic hallmark of MCL, present in ≥ 95% of cases {2302,4178}. Occasional MCLs express strong and diffuse cyclin D1 protein but lack the *CCND1* rearrangement. In these cases, cryptic rearrangements of IGK or IGL enhancers with *CCND1* result in cyclin D1 overexpression {3207,1264, 3273}. Rare cases of MCL negative for both cyclin D1 protein expression and *CCND1* rearrangements show alternative cyclin activation, mostly by IG::*CCND2* fusion {3545}. In recent years, the median overall survival of patients with MCL has substantially improved. The identification of prognostic subgroups, such as high-risk MCL, is clinically becoming more relevant. Widely available and well-established biomarkers of high-risk MCL are cytomorphology, Ki-67 proliferation index, p53 immunohistochemistry, and *TP53* mutation analysis {1642,188}.

Non-nodal MCL is characterized by the involvement of blood, bone marrow, and spleen, but little or no lymphadenopathy, and a mostly asymptomatic clinical presentation. Biologically, non-nodal MCL differs from MCL, as evidenced by (1) a lack of SOX11 expression {2924,3495}, low Ki-67 proliferation indexes {3285}, and frequently a lack of CD5 {2924}; (2) differences in the IGHV gene repertoire, with striking predominant IGHV1-8 gene usage {3285}, together with a higher somatic hypermutation load {3071,1463,2924}; (3) fewer genetic alterations and infrequent genomic complexity, despite an overall similar incidence of *TP53* aberrations {3495,2864}.

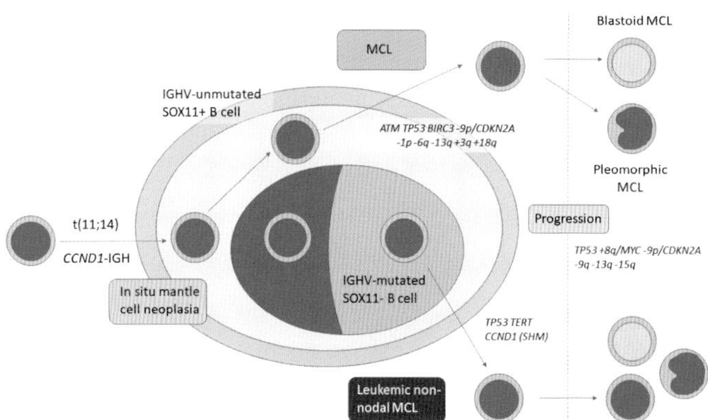

Fig. 4.129 Schematic representation of the three defined mantle cell neoplasms. In situ mantle cell neoplasm is confined to the mantle zone of the lymph node; the neoplastic cells carry the characteristic t(11;14)(q13;q32) translocation and overexpress both cyclin D1 and SOX11. The variable regions of their IG genes (IGHV) are not mutated. Mantle cell lymphoma (MCL) is characterized by lymph node effacement and the same t(11;14)(q13;q32) translocation as in situ mantle cell neoplasm in most cases, but also complex mutations and copy number variations as indicated. MCL can progress to one of its variants: blastoid or pleomorphic MCL. Leukaemic non-nodal MCL is thought to arise from an IGHV-mutated SOX11-negative cell with characteristic alterations in *TP53* and *TERT*.

In situ mantle cell neoplasm

Lazzi S
Klapper W
Naresh KN
Rosenquist R
Rule S
Wang M

Definition

In situ mantle cell neoplasm (ISMCN) is defined by the presence of cyclin D1–positive B cells, usually with *CCND1* rearrangement, restricted to usually non-expanded mantle zones of lymphoid follicles.

ICD-O coding

9673/1 In situ mantle cell neoplasm

ICD-11 coding

2A85.5 & XH8EM2 Mantle cell lymphoma & In situ mantle cell neoplasia

Related terminology

Acceptable: in situ mantle cell neoplasia.

Not recommended: in situ mantle cell lymphoma; mantle cell lymphoma–like B cells of uncertain/undetermined significance.

Subtype(s)

None

Localization

ISMCN is most often found in lymph nodes but may be seen in extranodal lymphoid tissues {564,2093,1159}. Involvement of more than one site does not exclude the diagnosis {564,101, 1831}.

Clinical features

ISMCN is typically an incidental finding in lymph nodes examined for other reasons and is characterized by indolent behaviour {3402,133,549,564}. Occasionally, ISMCN may be identified retrospectively after the diagnosis and/or treatment of overt mantle cell lymphoma (MCL) {564,1788} in previous specimens from the patients, or in association with another lymphoma, including chronic lymphocytic leukaemia / small lymphocytic lymphoma {564}, nodal or extranodal marginal zone lymphoma {564,3763}, follicular lymphoma, and/or in situ follicular B-cell neoplasm {133,3489,564,3980,4243}. ISMCN occasionally progresses to overt MCL, with an overall frequency of < 10% {3028}.

Epidemiology

ISMCN is very rare, with a prevalence of 0.35% in unselected reactive lymph nodes {3028}. It affects older adults (median age: 66 years), without a sex predilection {564,1651}.

Etiology

Unknown

Pathogenesis

ISMCN represents a colonization of the mantle zones of lymphoid follicles by B cells carrying the IGH::*CCND1* fusion, which causes the juxtaposition of *CCND1* to an IG locus, leading to cyclin D1 overexpression. In some cases, an ISMCN pattern is seen in the setting of leukaemic non-nodal MCL {2588}.

Macroscopic appearance

Not relevant

Histopathology

ISMCN generally involves multiple follicles in the same lymph node {329}. Although other pathological processes may be present, involved lymph nodes or extranodal lymphoid tissues usually show preserved histological architecture and reactive hyperplasia. The involved follicles show normal-appearing or minimally expanded mantle zone without atypical cells. Cyclin D1–positive B cells are typically restricted to the inner mantle zone, with few cells in the outer mantle zone and occasional cells in the interfollicular areas {564,1159}. Rare cases show intrafollicular spread {1044}.

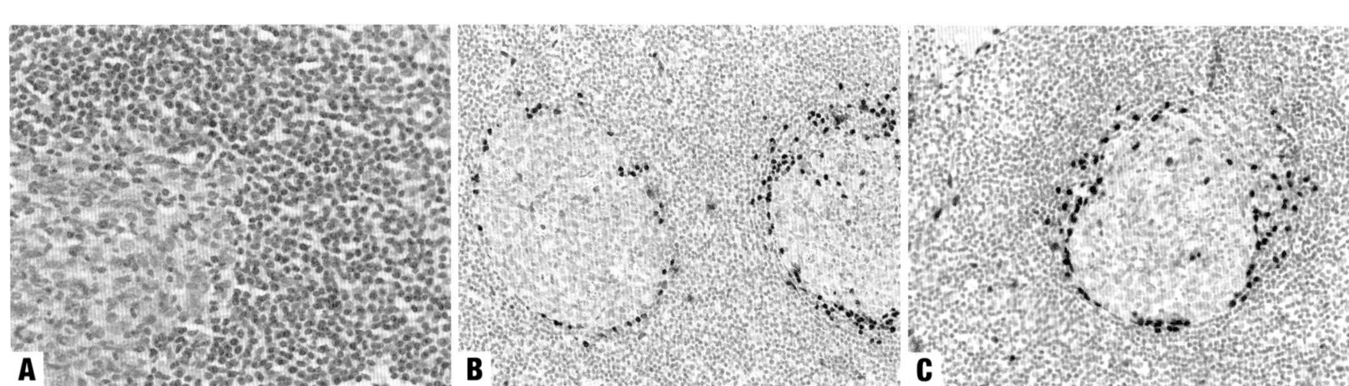

Fig. 4.130 In situ mantle cell neoplasm. **A** Lymphoid mantle cells without atypia in a mesenteric lymph node cannot be recognized without using immunohistochemistry. **B** Cyclin D1–positive cells are restricted to the inner layer of the mantle zone, with scattered cells in the reactive germinal centre. **C** The cyclin D1–positive cells coexpress SOX11.

Immunohistochemistry

Phenotypically, in addition to cyclin D1, ISMCN shows expression of pan–B-cell markers (CD19, CD20, CD79a, or PAX5), along with positivity of IgD and BCL2. It is more often negative for CD5 and CD43 than overt MCL is {3028}. SOX11 expression is variable; its prevalence and significance require further studies {564, 1159,25}.

Differential diagnosis

ISMCN must be distinguished from MCL with mantle zone growth pattern {564,4528}. This distinction may be difficult, because in some cases of MCL with mantle zone growth pattern there may be ISMCN-like foci {1159,1651,4528}. The histopathological differences are summarized in Table 4.27.

Cytology

ISMCN is usually not discernible on fine CNB.

Diagnostic molecular pathology

Detection of a *CCND1* rearrangement by FISH can confirm the immunophenotypic findings {3028,3562}.

Essential and desirable diagnostic criteria

Essential: preservation of the lymphoid architecture without expansion of the mantle zone; cyclin D1–positive B cells predominantly restricted to the inner layers of the mantle zones of lymphoid follicles; staging negative for overt MCL.

Desirable: detection of a *CCND1* rearrangement in the mantle cells.

Staging

A diagnosis of ISMCN warrants rigorous clinical staging and careful follow-up to exclude overt MCL.

Prognosis and prediction

Based on the limited number of cases observed, ISMCN is typically a stable disease with an indolent course and favourable clinical outcomes. Only rarely is there a need for therapy {1897}.

Table 4.27 Distinguishing mantle cell lymphoma (MCL) with a mantle zone pattern from in situ MCL neoplasm

Feature	Mantle zone growth of MCL	In situ MCL neoplasm
Lymph node architecture	Altered by expanded follicle mantle zones	Morphologically inconspicuous
Follicle mantle zone	Most mantle zones involved Expanded mantle zones Mantle zones mostly completely replaced by neoplastic cells	Few/focal involved mantle zones Mantle zones not expanded Partial replacement of mantle zones by neoplastic cells (mostly inner part of mantle, rarely in the germinal centre)
Accompanying growth pattern	Frequent additional nodular or diffuse growth of MCL	No other growth pattern detectable
Cyclin D1	Positive in whole follicle mantle; mostly complete replacement of mantle cells; occasionally intrafollicular and perifollicular	Restricted to the inner layer of mantle zone; not all mantle cells are positive; rare, scattered intrafollicular (germinal centre) and perifollicular
CD5	Usually positive	Variable; very difficult to evaluate
Clinical presentation	Relatively frequent presentation of MCL Mostly multifocal lymphadenopathy with or without leukaemic spread and/or bone marrow involvement	Rare Incidental finding in lymph nodes analysed because of an unrelated disease or benign hyperplasia Most cases without involvement of blood and bone marrow

Mantle cell lymphoma

Klapper W
Ferry JA
Hermine O
Li S
Lossos IS
Medeiros LJ
Naresh KN
Rosenquist R
Rule S
Stilgenbauer S

Definition

Mantle cell lymphoma (MCL) is a mature B-cell neoplasm derived from the mantle zone of lymphoid follicles and typically composed of small to medium-sized monomorphic cells expressing CD5, SOX11, and cyclin D1. It is associated with CCND-family rearrangements, most commonly *CCND1*.

ICD-O coding

9673/3 Mantle cell lymphoma
9673/3 Cyclin D1–positive mantle cell lymphoma
9673/3 Cyclin D1–negative mantle cell lymphoma

ICD-11 coding

2A85.5 Mantle cell lymphoma

Related terminology

Not recommended: centrocytic lymphoma; malignant lymphoma, lymphocytic intermediate differentiation, diffuse.

Subtype(s)

Molecular subtypes: cyclin D1–positive MCL; cyclin D1–negative MCL.
Morphological subtypes: see Table 4.28.

Localization

MCL usually involves lymph nodes, but extranodal involvement is also common, particularly of the Waldeyer ring, gastrointestinal tract, spleen, and bone marrow. Gastrointestinal tract involvement can manifest with numerous polypoid lesions. Other organs that may be involved include the skin, endocrine glands, lungs, and CNS, most often occurring as relapsing disease.

Clinical features

Most patients present with peripheral lymphadenopathy. Splenomegaly and bone marrow involvement are common. Gastrointestinal tract involvement may be associated with diarrhoea, weight loss, or bleeding. Rarely, patients with an aggressive histological variant of MCL present with a clinical picture resembling acute lymphoblastic leukaemia or an aggressive lymphoma with profound cytopenias, and/or with organ compression. MCL may rarely present as localized (stage I/II) disease

Table 4.28 Morphological subtypes of mantle cell lymphoma

Subtype	Morphology
Blastoid	Cells resemble lymphoblasts (precursor cells) with round nuclei, fine chromatin, inconspicuous nucleoli, and a narrow rim of cytoplasm
Pleomorphic	Cells are variable in size but mostly large, with irregular nuclear contours and prominent nucleoli, and with prominent, often pale cytoplasm
Small cell	Small cells with dense chromatin, round nuclei, and a narrow rim of cytoplasm resembling chronic lymphocytic leukaemia; no paraimmunoblasts
Marginal zone–like	Medium-sized cells with abundant pale cytoplasm resembling marginal zone cells and monocytoid B cells

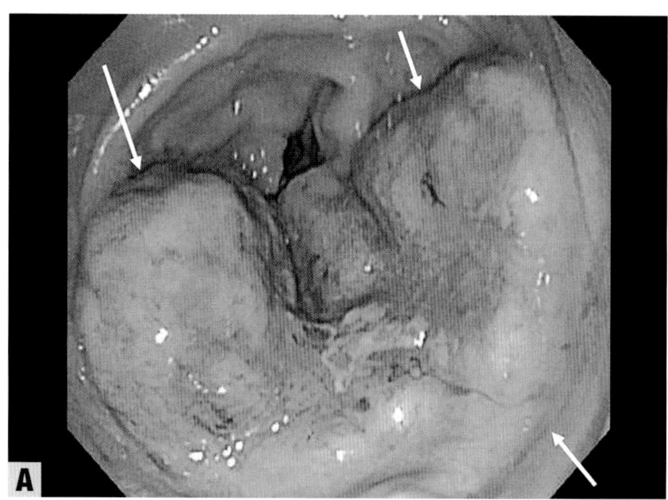

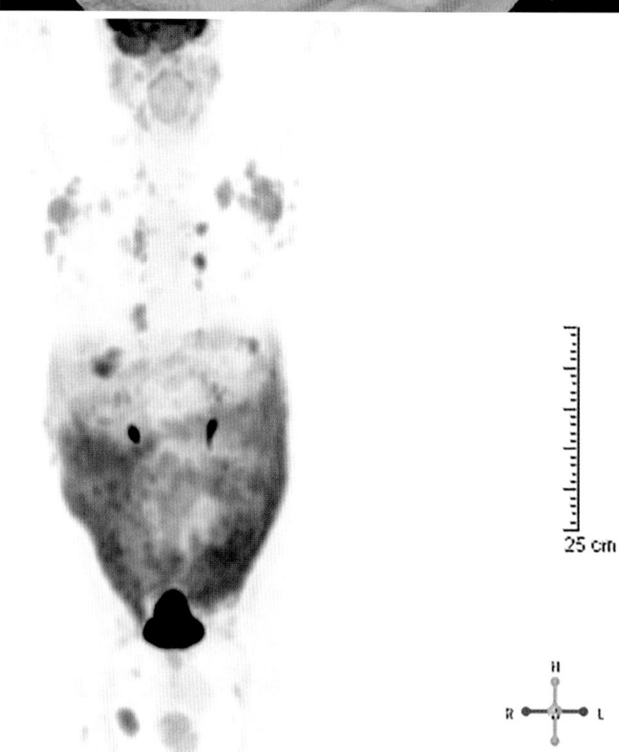

Fig. 4.131 Mantle cell lymphoma. **A** A large colonic tumour consistent with mantle cell lymphoma encompassing 50% of the circumference of the lumen, characterized by surface erythema and raised edges (arrows). **B** Advanced-stage mantle cell lymphoma with disseminated involvement of the gastrointestinal tract and omentum (PET-CT).

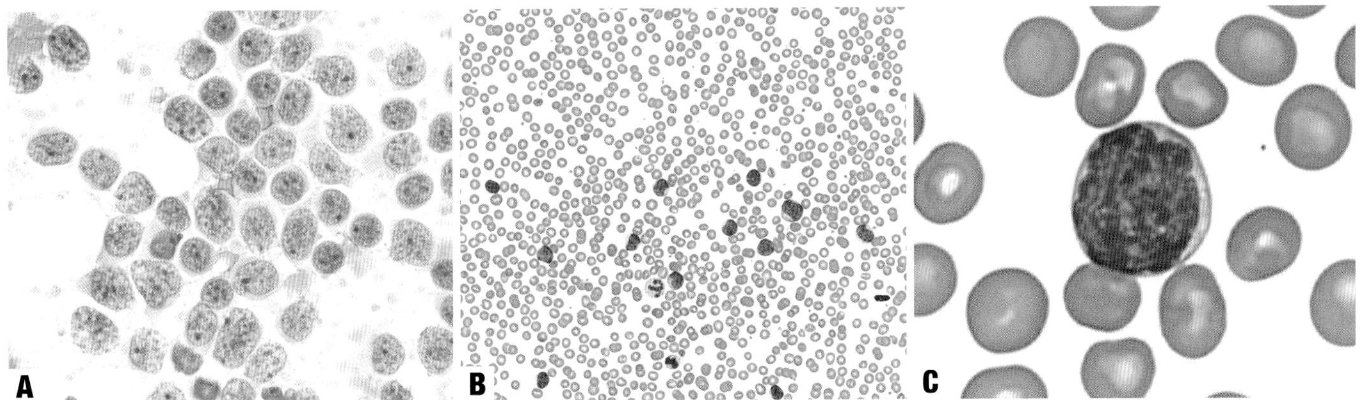

Fig. 4.132 Mantle cell lymphoma. **A** FNA of a lymph node with mantle cell lymphoma shows small to medium-sized cells with oval to irregular nuclei, fine stippled chromatin, small or absent nucleoli, and very scant cytoplasm on Pap. **B** A peripheral blood smear from a different patient with mantle cell lymphoma, blastoid variant (cyclin D1+, SOX11+), shows lymphocytosis at scanning magnification. **C** High magnification (oil immersion) shows an enlarged lymphoid cell with an irregular nucleus, stippled chromatin, and scant cytoplasm (Wright–Giemsa stain).

involving extranodal sites, mimicking extranodal marginal zone lymphoma {2781}.

Patients may present with splenic enlargement and peripheral lymphocytosis without nodal disease or cytopenias, designated leukaemic non-nodal MCL (nnMCL). These cases often follow a more indolent clinical course.

MCL that is detected incidentally during surgery for an unrelated disease, particularly involving the urogenital and digestive tract, often corresponds to in situ mantle cell neoplasm.

Epidemiology

MCL accounts for 3–10% of B-cell lymphomas worldwide. The median age of occurrence is 68–69 years {1246}. The M:F ratio is about 3–4:1 {2452}.

Etiology

The etiology is unknown. Rare familial clustering has been reported {4052}.

Pathogenesis

Most MCL cases carry unmutated or minimally/borderline-mutated IGHV genes, whereas a minority have a higher rate of somatic hypermutation, which is typically more often observed in leukaemic nnMCL {1983,1463,2924,3285}. MCL displays a distinctive IG gene repertoire, with preferential usage of distinct IGHV genes (IGHV3-21, IGHV4-34, and IGHV1-8). In 10% of MCL cases, stereotyped variable heavy chain CDR3 sequences are expressed, implying an antigen-driven selection for a proportion of MCLs {1463,35,4449,3285}.

The t(11;14)(q13;q32) translocation is the genetic hallmark and primary event in the pathogenesis of MCL, present in ≥ 95% of cases {2302,4178}. This translocation juxtaposes *CCND1* to IGH on chromosome 14q32. Occasionally, IGK or IGL serve as the *CCND1* translocation partner {3496}. In most MCLs, the translocation is acquired at the precursor B-cell stage, mediated by recombination-activating enzymes, but t(11;14) occurs in mature B cells via activation-induced cytidine deaminase in a small subset of cases {2864}. *CCND1* rearrangement results in overexpression of the cell-cycle regulatory protein cyclin D1 {886,887}. More rarely, aberrant expression of truncated transcripts with a prolonged cyclin D1 half-life occur {3474}. These transcripts, caused by genomic rearrangements at the *CCND1* 3′ untranslated region or by 3′ untranslated region mutations, are associated with higher proliferation indexes and an inferior prognosis {4372}. Constitutive overexpression of cyclin D1 activates the cyclin D1–dependent kinase pathway, which overcomes the cell-cycle suppressive effect of RB1 and p27, promotes cell growth and malignant transformation, and ultimately leads to the development of MCL {1787,3330}. In the occasional cases of MCL that strongly express cyclin D1 but do not show *CCND1* rearrangement by FISH, genomic studies have revealed cryptic rearrangements of IGK or IGL enhancers with *CCND1* {3207,1264,3273}. In a small subset of MCL negative for cyclin D1 expression and *CCND1* rearrangements (cyclin D1–negative MCL), *CCND2* and *CCND3* rearrangements have been identified as alternative mechanisms of cell-cycle dysregulation {3545}.

Clonal B cells with *CCND1* rearrangement have been detected in the blood of healthy individuals {2247}, which, together with results from mouse models, suggest that *CCND1* rearrangement alone is insufficient to cause MCL {2435,1352}. Secondary genomic alterations are present in > 90% of cases and play important roles in pathogenesis {2315}. These secondary copy-number changes include gains or amplifications of 3q, 7p, 8q (*MYC*), 15q, and 18q (*BCL2*), and losses of 1p, 2q, 6q, 8p, 9p (*CDKN2A* or *CDKN2B*, in 10–36% of cases), 9q, 10p, 11q (*ATM*, in 11–57%), 13q (*RB1*, 25–55%), 17p (*TP53*,

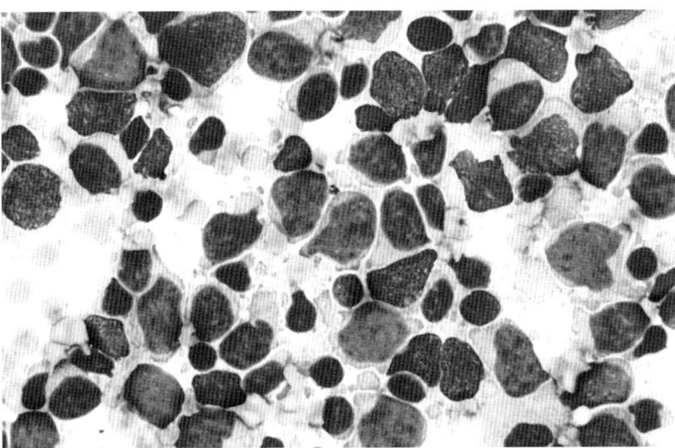

Fig. 4.133 Mantle cell lymphoma, pleomorphic variant. Cytology preparation (Giemsa).

in 21–45%), and 19p {3496,281,3468}. SNP array studies have detected copy-number neutral loss of heterozygosity in as many as 60% of cases including the 17p region (*TP53*) {282,1470, 3496}. Tetraploid chromosome clones have been detected especially in the pleomorphic variant of MCL {3086}.

Next-generation sequencing studies have shown that MCL displays a complex mutation landscape {1584}. *ATM* is most frequently mutated (41–61% of cases), followed by *TP53* (14–31%), *CCND1* (14–34%), *KMT2D* (12–23%), *NSD2* (10–13%), *SMARCA4* (8%), *UBR5* (7–18%), *BIRC3* (6–10%), *NOTCH1* (5–14%), *S1PR1* (3–15%), and *CARD11* (3–15%) {3470,3468}. These alterations involve genes encoding components of key signalling pathways in MCL pathogenesis, including (but not limited to) cell-cycle regulation (*CCND1*, *RB1*), DNA damage response (*ATM*, *TP53*), cell proliferation and apoptosis (*BCL2*, *MYC*), B-cell receptor / NF-κB signalling (*CARD11*/*BIRC3*/*MAP3K14*), and epigenetic modifiers (*KMT2D*, *NSD2*, *SMARCA4*). *MYC* translocations and *TP53* mutations are often associated with disease progression {1566,4299}.

Interestingly, the neural transcription factor SOX11 also plays an important oncogenic role in MCL. *SOX11* belongs to the SOX gene family, whose members encode transcriptional factors characterized by containing a high mobility group DNA-binding domain {281}. *SOX11* belongs to subgroup C, with high homology to *SOX4* and *SOX12*, which are essential in organogenesis and have overlapping roles in neural development and neurite growth. Contrary to SOX4, which is crucial for T- and B-lymphopoiesis, SOX11 is not known to have lymphopoietic functions and is not expressed in normal lymphoid tissues, progenitors, or normal B cells. Nonetheless, SOX11 is overexpressed in in situ mantle cell neoplasm – suggesting it plays a role in the early stage of MCL pathogenesis {564,25}. Although the causes and consequences of SOX11 expression in MCL require further investigation, it has been postulated to play an important role in multiple signalling pathways, including B-cell differentiation, and in modulating the lymphoma microenvironment, cell-cycle progression, mobility/migration, and apoptosis {4199,3114,281, 287}.

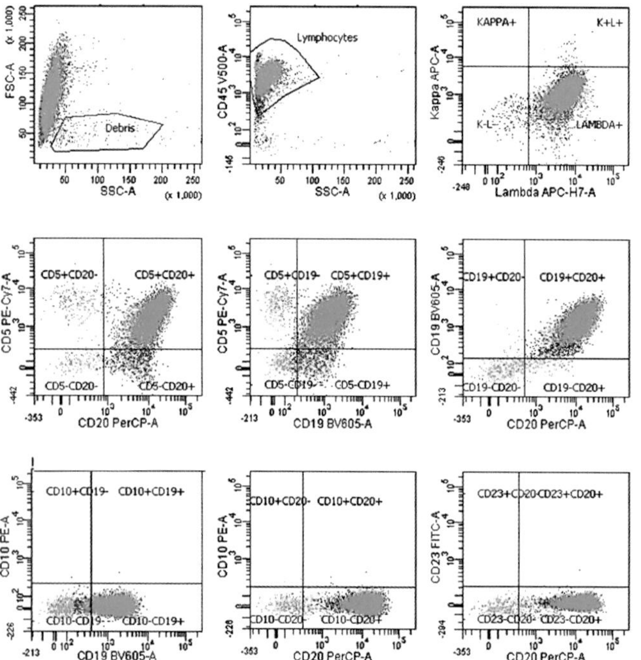

Fig. 4.134 Mantle cell lymphoma. Flow cytometric analysis of an FNAB of lymph node shows a population of neoplastic B cells expressing CD19, CD20, CD5, and monotypic lambda light chain, but not CD10 or CD23.

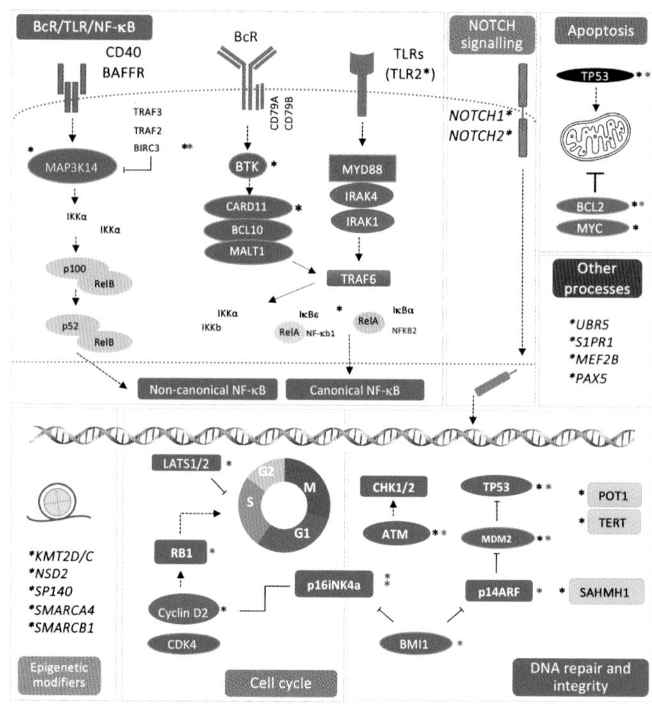

Fig. 4.135 Mantle cell lymphoma. Pathways and cellular processes involved in mantle cell lymphoma. A black asterisk denotes recurrent single nucleotide variants (SNVs) and indels; a red asterisk, deletions; and a blue asterisk, gene amplifications. BcR, B-cell receptor; NICD, NOTCH intracellular domain; TLR, toll-like receptor.

Macroscopic appearance

This is dependent on the site of involvement. Multiple polypoid lesions have been described in cases with extensive involvement of the gastrointestinal tract (previously designated multiple lymphomatous polyposis).

Histopathology

MCL shows diffuse, nodular, and (rarely) mantle zone growth patterns, and it has various cytological variants, including blastoid, pleomorphic, small cell, and marginal zone–like, which may also co-occur {2275,231,2223,4020}. MCL with a mantle zone growth pattern needs to be distinguished from in situ mantle cell neoplasm (see Table 4.27, p. 445, in *In situ mantle cell neoplasm*).

Mainstream MCL cytology is characterized by small to medium-sized cells with slightly irregular nuclear contours and scant cytoplasm {2275,3908}. Nuclear chromatin is irregularly dispersed, and nucleoli are inconspicuous. The mitotic rate and proliferation index can vary greatly among cases. Plasmacytic differentiation with mature light chain–restricted plasma cells can rarely occur {4515,4239,4464}. Pleomorphic and blastoid variants (see Table 4.28, p. 446) are usually associated with increased mitotic and proliferation indexes.

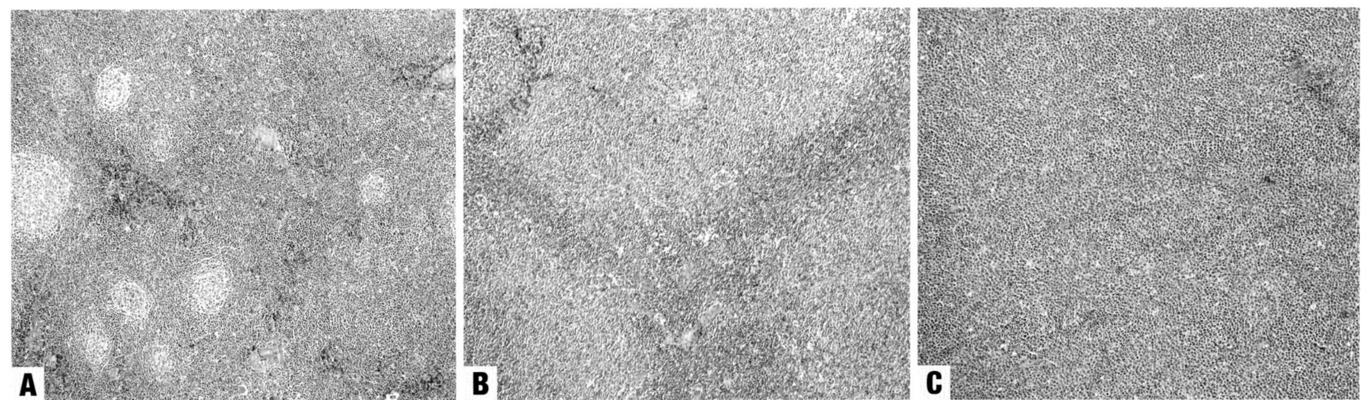

Fig. 4.136 Mantle cell lymphoma, growth patterns. **A** Mantle zone pattern. **B** Nodular pattern. **C** Diffuse pattern.

The cytology and growth pattern may vary between primary diagnosis and relapse, with a trend towards more highly proliferative variants at relapse {2979,4248}. Occasionally, cases with blastoid or pleomorphic cytology at diagnosis relapse with the more regular MCL morphology {4248}.

The microenvironment of MCL is composed of a low to moderate number of admixed T cells, hyalinized small blood vessels, and singly scattered epithelioid histiocytes. A variable number of follicular dendritic cells is present, usually associated with a mantle zone or nodular pattern {3642}. Highly proliferative MCL may show a starry-sky pattern due to the presence of tingible-body macrophages. Infiltration of glands, mimicking lymphoepithelial lesions, is rarely seen {2075}.

In the bone marrow, the pattern is variable depending on the extent of infiltration, ranging from scattered cells to dense nodular aggregates. Paratrabecular and diffuse patterns can also be seen {4324}. In the spleen, MCL infiltrates the white pulp, with variable involvement of the red pulp.

Immunophenotype

MCLs express pan–B-cell markers (CD19, CD20, CD22, CD79a). The intensity of immunoglobulin expression (most commonly IgM/IgD, and lambda light chain expression more frequent than kappa) is moderate to strong as detected by flow cytometry {4154}. CD5, FMC7, and CD43 are usually positive {609,1285}, whereas expression of CD10 or BCL6 is rare but is more commonly seen in aggressive variants {1285,527}.

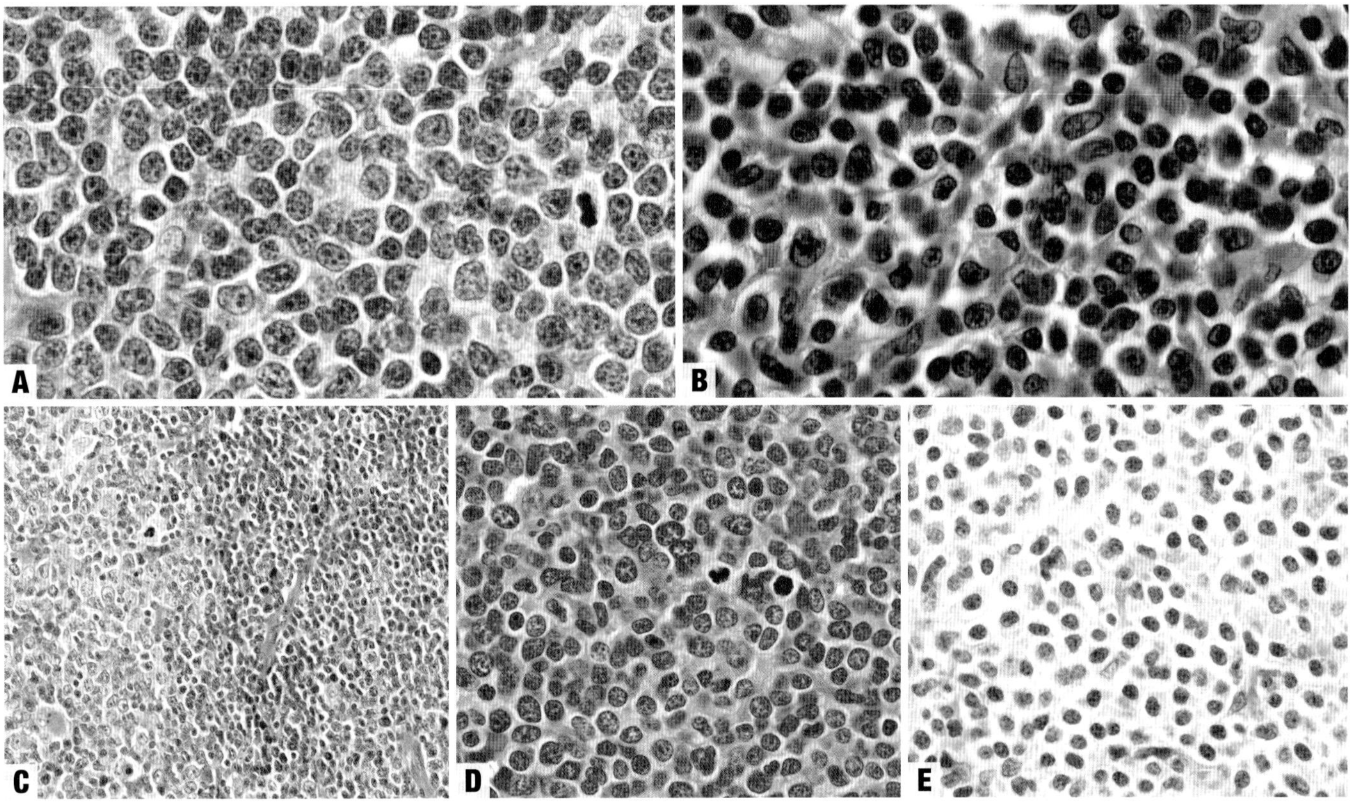

Fig. 4.137 Mantle cell lymphoma, cytological variants. **A** Classic. **B** Small cell. **C** Pleomorphic (combined with classic morphology). **D** Blastoid. **E** Marginal zone–like.

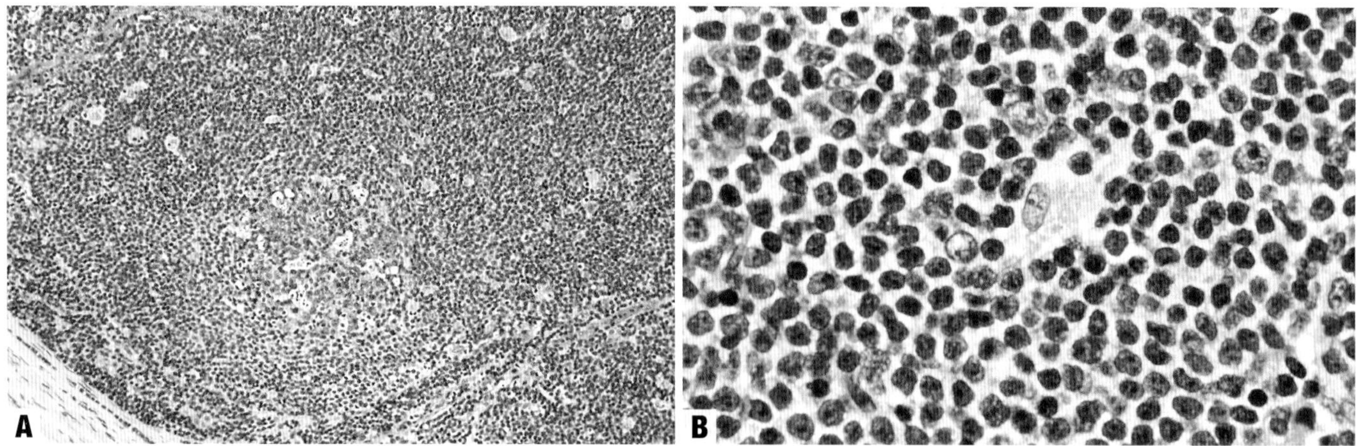

Fig. 4.138 Mantle cell lymphoma. **A** A naked germinal centre is surrounded by mantle cell lymphoma with classic cytological features. **B** The infiltrate is composed of a monotonous population of tumour cells with irregular nuclear contours. Large cells are rare. Epithelioid histiocytes are also present.

CD23 is weakly positive by flow cytometry in about 10% of cases; CD23 also labels a variable number of follicular dendritic cells within the lymphoma microenvironment {3642,1285}. An absence of CD200 expression by flow cytometry is helpful in distinguishing MCL from chronic lymphocytic leukaemia {2075, 609}. Expression of cyclin D1 is detected in > 95% of MCLs, due to *CCND1* rearrangements {697,4047}. SOX11 is detectable in > 90% of MCLs and helps in identifying CD5-negative or cyclin D1–negative MCL {4309,1053,2820,949,187}. However, SOX11 is not specific for MCL and may be expressed in other lymphoid neoplasms, such as B-lymphoblastic leukaemia/lymphoma, Burkitt lymphoma, and hairy cell leukaemia {949,674, 2264}. Of note, SOX11 is often negative in leukaemic nnMCL. Expression of the markers usually found in chronic lymphocytic leukaemia is rare, with LEF1 more likely to be seen in blastoid or pleomorphic MCL, and CD200 in leukaemic nnMCL {609,1128, 2649,3562,2654}.

Cyclin D1–negative MCL lack expression of cyclin D1 and *CCND1* rearrangements {1245,1326}. Approximately half of the cases harbour rearrangements of *CCND2*, and the remaining

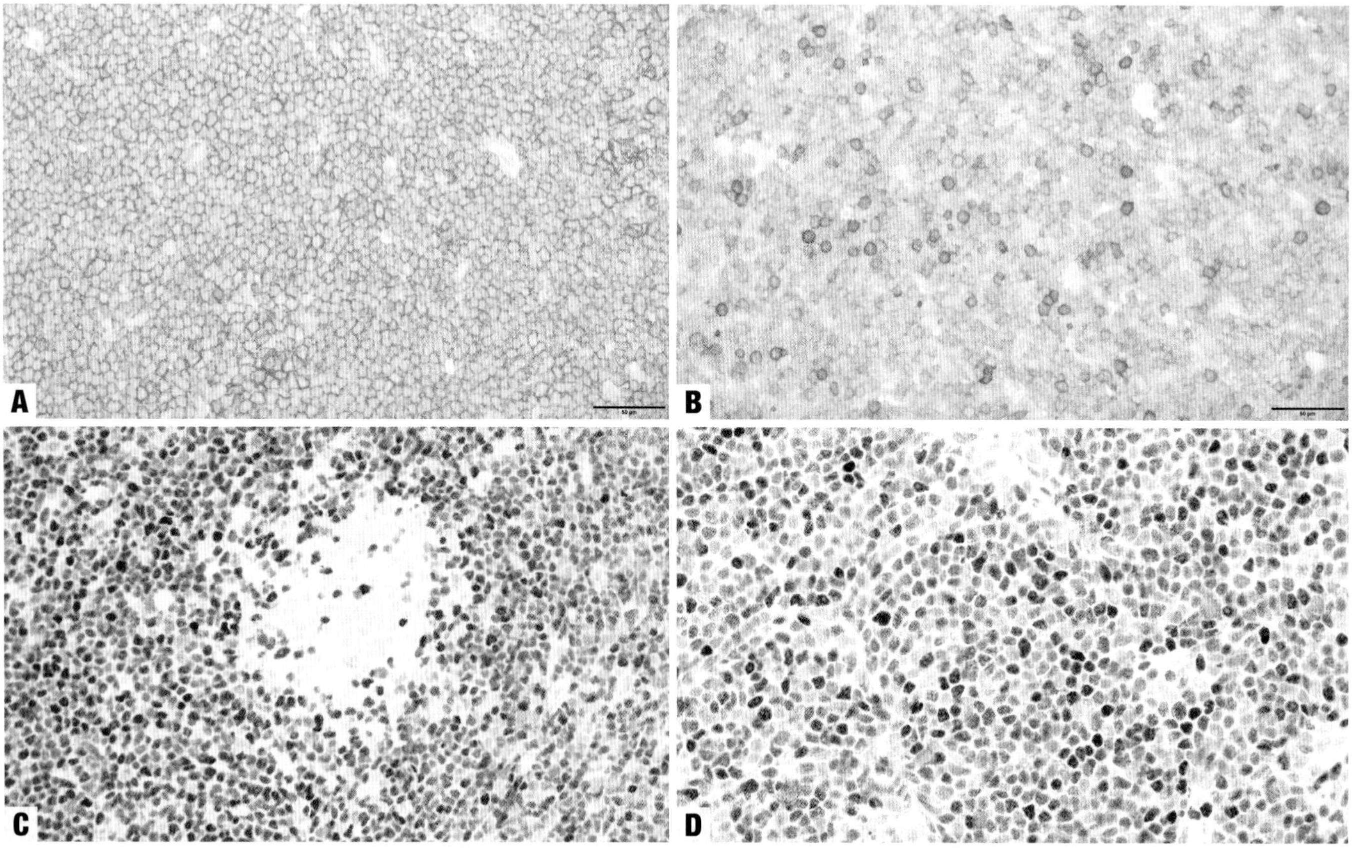

Fig. 4.139 Mantle cell lymphoma, immunophenotype. The immunophenotype is characterized by immunohistochemistry, with expression of CD20 (**A**) and CD5, which may be weaker than in the admixed T cells (**B**). Cyclin D1 (**C**) and SOX11 (**D**) expression is found in the majority of cells, with characteristic variable staining intensity.

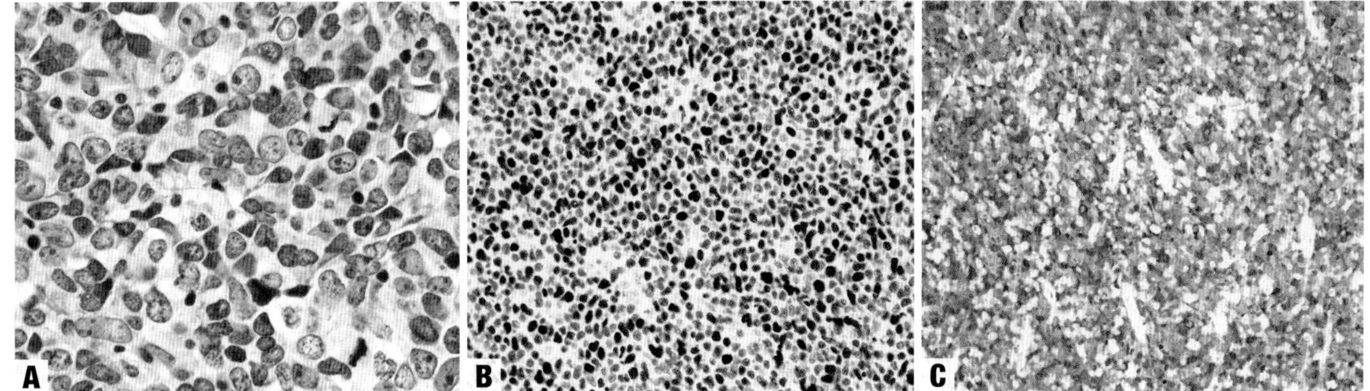

Fig. 4.140 Mantle cell lymphoma. **A** Blastoid mantle cell lymphoma cells show immature chromatin, and mitotic figures are frequent. **B** *TP53* mutation is frequently present and is reflected by strong expression of p53 by immunohistochemistry. **C** Virtually all neoplastic cells are positive for cyclin D1.

cases have other genetic alterations leading to the expression of cyclin D2 or cyclin D3 {1264,3545,2557}. In contrast to cyclin D1, cyclin D2 and cyclin D3 are expressed in normal lymphocytes and, therefore, are also observed in other small B-cell lymphomas originating from lymphocytes of corresponding developmental stages {2669}. CD5, SOX11, and p27 expression is useful for identifying cyclin D1–negative MCL {3330,3562}. Rare cases of MCL lack cyclin D1 immunoreactivity despite the presence of *CCND1* rearrangements. In such cases, lack of immunoreactivity is due to mutations in *CCND1* or truncated cyclin D1 mRNA {1699,2471}.

Differential diagnosis

This includes other small to medium-sized B-cell lymphomas that can express cyclin D1, such as plasma cell myeloma, which also can have *CCND1* rearrangements, as well as neoplasms that do not carry *CCND1* rearrangements, such as chronic lymphocytic leukaemia (weakly in proliferation centres), diffuse large B-cell lymphoma, and hairy cell leukaemia. Pleomorphic and blastoid variants of MCL must be differentiated from diffuse large B-cell lymphoma, B-lymphoblastic leukaemia/lymphoma, and Burkitt lymphoma, among others.

Cytology

Distinguishing MCL from other types of small cell lymphoma on the basis of cytomorphology alone, without ancillary investigations, is very difficult {2851}. Cytological specimens typically show a monomorphic proliferation of lymphoid cells that are slightly larger and have more open chromatin than normal small lymphocytes. Neoplastic cells often have slightly to prominently irregular nuclei, although occasional cases of MCL have tumour cells with round nuclei. Nucleoli are usually (but not always) inconspicuous {2851}. The blastoid variant of MCL is characterized by larger nuclei with fine chromatin, whereas the pleomorphic variant shows large cells with irregular nuclei, and sometimes bizarre cells {1221}.

FNAB may be a useful technique to establish a diagnosis of MCL, with high sensitivity and specificity, when combined with flow cytometric immunophenotypic analysis, particularly when a cell block is available for immunohistochemistry {1221,248}. Evaluation using FISH to detect *CCND1* rearrangement can also be helpful for diagnosis {248}. FNAB is particularly useful in the setting of relapsed MCL {1221,248}.

Diagnostic molecular pathology

In the context of routine diagnostics, in a neoplasm with appropriate morphology and immunophenotype, demonstration of uniform nuclear overexpression of cyclin D1 is sufficient to confirm the diagnosis {697,4047,3305}. If the morphology or the immunophenotype deviates from the expected features of MCL, demonstration of *CCND1* rearrangement or IGH::*CCND1* fusion and an extended immunohistochemistry panel is recommended, to exclude lymphomas that can express cyclin D1 (see *Differential diagnosis*). In the absence of cyclin D1 expression and *CCND1* rearrangements, cyclin D1–negative MCL may be confirmed by testing for *CCND2* translocations.

TP53 mutation analysis may help to define a high-risk MCL cohort {1642,188}.

Essential and desirable diagnostic criteria

Cyclin D1–positive MCL

Essential: lymphoma cells of B lineage (positive for CD20 and usually CD5); morphology of classic variant (monomorphic and centrocyte-like) or, less often, variant morphology; cyclin D1 positivity and/or detection of *CCND1* rearrangement.

Desirable: SOX11 expression positivity.

Cyclin D1–negative MCL

Essential: lymphoma cells of B lineage (positive for CD20 and usually CD5); morphology of classic variant (monomorphic and centrocyte-like) or, less often, variant morphology; immunophenotype consistent with MCL, including SOX11 expression; absence of cyclin D1 expression and *CCND1* rearrangement.

Desirable: *CCND2* rearrangement.

Staging

Staging is performed according to the Lugano criteria {688} and includes clinical examination, routine laboratory tests (including white blood cell count and LDH levels), bone marrow aspiration / blood smear and biopsy, and immunophenotyping. It includes CT of the head and neck, cervical, thoracic, abdominal, and pelvic regions.

FDG PET might be used at diagnosis for prognosis and staging, although it may be insensitive to gastrointestinal tract involvement. Patients with gastrointestinal symptoms may require endoscopy (upper and lower). CNS investigation is

Box 4.01 Prognostic markers in mantle cell lymphoma (MCL) (modified according to Dreyling and Silkenstedt {3746})

Current clinical use

- Age
- Performance status
- CNS involvement at diagnosis
- Stage of disease (I and II vs III and IV)
- Serum level of B2M
- Serum level of LDH
- Morphology (classic vs blastoid)
- MCL International Prognostic Index (MIPI)
- Ki-67 (< 30% vs ≥ 30%) and inclusion into combined-MIPI
- p53 expression by immunohistochemistry
- *TP53* mutations/deletions by sequencing analysis

Potential future use

- MCL35 RNA expression analysis
- Measurable residual disease testing
- Somatic mutations (e.g. in *NOTCH1* and others)
- FDG PET

indicated in patients with neurological symptoms and could be considered in patients with aggressive variants.

Prognosis and prediction

Prognosis

MCL used to be considered an incurable disease. However, with current therapeutic approaches, the median overall survival time has increased dramatically, from 3 years to more than 5–10 years, and some patients may eventually be cured. A variety of prognostic markers have been evaluated, some of which are well established and may be applied in daily practice (see Box 4.01). Of note, these prognostic biomarkers are established for conventional MCL, but not for in situ mantle cell neoplasm or leukaemic nnMCL. Because of the rarity of cyclin D1–negative MCL, it is uncertain whether prognostic markers may also apply to this subtype. MCLs presenting with isolated or predominant extranodal manifestations are reported to have a more favourable outcome than nodal MCL {2781}.

The MCL International Prognostic Index (MIPI) {1640,1641} defines risk groups but so far does not govern treatment approaches for individual patients. Clinical trials using biomarkers to identify and stratify high-risk MCL are currently in progress to establish a future default set of markers for clinical application. Widely available and established biomarkers from retrospective studies are cytomorphology, Ki-67, and p53 staining (see Box 4.01). *TP53* mutation analysis may help to define a high-risk MCL cohort {1642,188}. Detailed guidelines for Ki-67 and p53 assessment in MCL have been established {2038,188,791,840}. The currently accepted Ki-67 cut-off point for prognostic stratification is 30%, with Ki-67 expression > 30% being associated with worse outcome and is included in the MIPI in a combined index (MIPI-c) {791, 3611}. High p53 expression has been defined as at least 50% positive lymphoma cells (uniformly strong nuclear staining) and is associated with a poor overall survival (median: 2 years) {188}.

Prediction

At first diagnosis, MCL is positive for surface B-cell markers (CD20, CD19) that might serve as therapeutic targets. Retesting for these therapeutic targets at relapse is recommended in order to identify mutations associated with drug resistance, for example against BTK inhibitors {715,1776} and other drugs {4577}. However, there is a lack of formal predictive marker analyses guiding treatment.

Leukaemic non-nodal mantle cell lymphoma

Calaminici M
Klapper W
Rosenquist R
Schuh A
Stamatopoulos KE
Stilgenbauer S

Definition
Leukaemic non-nodal mantle cell lymphoma (nnMCL) is characterized by the involvement of blood, bone marrow, and spleen by neoplastic cells with morphological and immunophenotypic similarities to nodal mantle cell lymphoma (MCL), with absent or minimal evidence of lymphadenopathy, and usually with an asymptomatic presentation.

ICD-O coding
9673/3 Leukaemic non-nodal mantle cell lymphoma

ICD-11 coding
2A85.5 Mantle cell lymphoma

Related terminology
None

Subtype(s)
None

Localization
The most commonly involved sites are the peripheral blood, bone marrow, and spleen, typically with absent or minimal lymphadenopathy {3071,1168,3067}. Gastrointestinal involvement at presentation has also been reported {124,3071,1168}.

Clinical features
Most patients present with incidental, stable, or slowly increasing lymphocytosis and are otherwise asymptomatic. Nodal involvement is minimal or absent {1092}.

Epidemiology
The age at presentation (typically in the sixth decade of life) and male predominance are similar to MCL {1168,3067}.

Etiology
Unknown

Pathogenesis
Like MCL, nnMCL is characterized by cyclin D1 overexpression, mostly as a result of a t(11;14)(q13;q32) translocation, which juxtaposes *CCND1* with the IGH locus {4244,4178,2864}. Moreover, nnMCL and MCL share similar global gene expression profiles {1168}. However, nnMCL displays significant biological differences from MCL, as evidenced by: (1) distinct immunophenotypic characteristics, such as a lack of SOX11 expression {3495,2924}, low Ki-67 index {3285}, and frequent expression of DBA44 {3285}; (2) distinct immunogenetic features, exemplified by differences in the IGHV gene repertoire, with striking predominant usage of IGHV1-8 {3285}, together with a significantly higher load of somatic hypermutations {3071,1463, 2924}; and (3) fewer genetic alterations and infrequent genomic complexity, despite an overall similar incidence of *TP53* aberrations {3495,3536,2864}. Taken together, these findings suggest that the microenvironment impacts the pathogenesis of nnMCL, shaping clonal evolution and, hence, clinical presentation and outcome.

Macroscopic appearance
Not relevant

Histopathology
Peripheral blood smears show slightly atypical small to medium-sized lymphoid cells with hyperchromatic nuclei and nuclear clefts. Some cases demonstrate chronic lymphocytic leukaemia–type small cell morphology. Flow cytometry reveals the presence of neoplastic cells in percentages ranging from 11% to 76%, with lower expression of CD38 than in MCL, and expression of CD200 and CD23 in a subset of cells, which are features in common with chronic lymphocytic leukaemia {3067, 1092}.

The bone marrow is always involved. In most cases, the marrow is normocellular with trilineage haematopoiesis and minimal or no lymphomatous involvement evident on routine stains. Immunohistochemistry highlights a population of small lymphoid cells with interstitial and/or sinusoidal growth patterns. Neoplastic cells may form small aggregates or infiltrate as single cells in low percentages varying between 1% and 10–20%.

Immunophenotype
The neoplastic cells express CD20 and cyclin D1. CD5 positivity is seen in most cases, with variable intensity; however, negative cases have been described. SOX11 expression tends to be low or negative, an important feature to differentiate nnMCL from MCL and to confirm the diagnosis of nnMCL in combination with the clinical presentation {1168}. In cases with splenic or extranodal involvement, CD20+/cyclin D1+ neoplastic cells are observed in small lymphoid aggregates or confined to mantle zones of secondary follicles in a pattern overlapping with that of in situ mantle cell neoplasm {3067,1092}.

Differential diagnosis
It is essential to exclude other small cell lymphomas, including chronic lymphocytic leukaemia and splenic marginal zone lymphoma.

Cytology
See *Histopathology*, above.

Diagnostic molecular pathology
Detection of *CCND1* rearrangements may be helpful in differentiating nnMCL from other types of leukaemic small B-cell lymphomas, particularly if the cyclin D1 immunohistochemistry is equivocal.

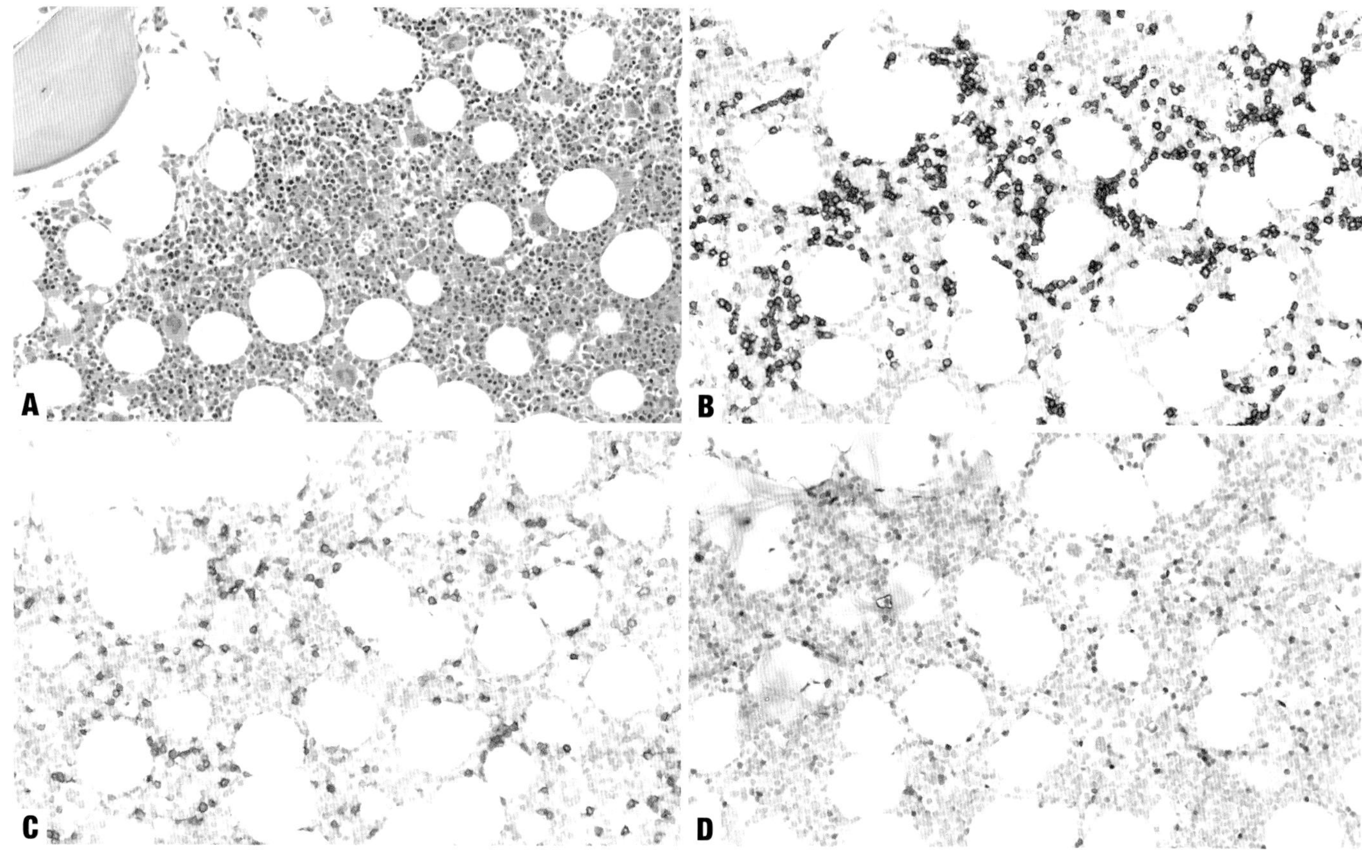

Fig. 4.141 Leukaemic non-nodal mantle cell lymphoma. **A** Subtle interstitial bone marrow infiltration by small neoplastic lymphoid cells. **B** CD20 immunohistochemistry highlights neoplastic cells in an interstitial pattern. **C** The majority of CD20-positive small lymphoid cells also express CD5. **D** Cyclin D1 is expressed by > 30% of CD20+/CD5+ small lymphoid cells. The t(11;14) translocation was demonstrated by FISH. SOX11 was negative (not shown).

Essential and desirable diagnostic criteria

Essential: typical asymptomatic clinical presentation with lymphocytosis and absence of (or insignificant) nodal involvement; monomorphic small to medium-sized cells of B lineage; cyclin D1 positivity and/or detection of *CCND1* rearrangement.

Desirable: absent or very weak expression of SOX11.

Staging

Staging is recommended according to the guidelines for MCL.

Prognosis and prediction

The clinical course is more favourable than that of MCL, so nnMCL is sometimes managed with a watch-and-wait approach or with treatment approaches that are much less intensive {2545,1769}. Studies show that the median survival is significantly longer for patients with nnMCL than for those with MCL (e.g. 79 months [range: 22–136 months] in nnMCL vs 30 months [range: 10–50 months] in MCL, $P = 0.005$ {3071}). Even in the presence of splenomegaly and gastrointestinal involvement, patients remain asymptomatic and do not require treatment for long periods of time {3071,1168}.

In some cases, however, aggressive disease may develop, with a rapidly enlarging spleen, lymphadenopathy, and morphological progression to an aggressive variant (i.e. blastoid or pleomorphic variants). The acquisition of genetic lesions, such as *TP53* aberrations, may be related to such an aggressive clinical course {3495,535,766}. Aggressive nnMCLs respond poorly to standard chemotherapy; immunotherapy and targeted agents may have a role in improving outcome.

Transformations of indolent B-cell lymphomas: Introduction

de Jong D

High-grade transformation of an indolent B-cell lymphoma into an aggressive lymphoma represents one of the hitherto unmet challenges in the clinical care of patients. It is part of the natural clinical course of various indolent B-cell lymphomas, albeit occurring with varying frequency. Ultimately, the diagnosis and clinical consequences are a frequent subject of discussion during multidisciplinary tumour board meetings in daily practice. However, the diagnostic criteria and the spectrum of manifestations of transformation have so far not been addressed as a separate subject in previous editions of the WHO classification of lymphomas.

Clinically, transformation in the setting of a known B-cell lymphoma is associated with symptoms and signs of rapid disease progression and poor prognosis. The actual frequency of transformation in the different types of indolent B-cell lymphomas is difficult to assess, because the diagnosis is not always proved by biopsy or at autopsy. Furthermore, the clinical signs indicating transformation may also be noted in cases in which the biopsy only reveals morphological features of disease progression rather than transformation {2427,401}.

Histological transformation may be defined as the emergence of a morphologically aggressive lymphoma type in a patient with a previously or synchronously diagnosed indolent non-Hodgkin lymphoma {2832}. In exceptional cases, the aggressive lymphoma is the first diagnosis, the small B-cell lymphoma being diagnosed subsequently. The morphology is most often that of diffuse large B-cell lymphoma, more rarely of intermediate/blastoid type, and infrequently of other tumour types (e.g. classic Hodgkin lymphoma {1772} or plasmablastic lymphoma {2549}), and it is indistinguishable from the corresponding de novo lymphoma type. The transformed lymphoma has the same cell lineage and is clonally related to the indolent B-cell lymphoma. In the setting of transformed follicular lymphoma, a high proportion of the cases are predicted, on the basis of mutation patterns, to branch from a common (mutated) ancestor cell, rather than to derive from linear progression from a manifest follicular lymphoma {3040,3152,432}. The current definition of transformed lymphoma may be too simple, as various more complex situations will require more analysis and deliberation. First, not all changes in morphology reflect true transformation. Cases that largely maintain features of the pre-existing lesion, such as a change in growth pattern (e.g. follicular to diffuse), an increase in the number of large lymphoid cells, an increase in size/number of proliferation centres, increased nuclear polymorphism or acquisition of more blastoid features, or a higher proliferation rate, are commonly encountered and are related to disease progression rather than to transformation {2832}. Clinical decisions in such cases should be supported by multidisciplinary discussions, especially to avoid overinterpretation. Second, in 10–20% of cases, an aggressive lymphoma, such as diffuse large B-cell lymphoma, arises in the setting of an indolent lymphoma without a clonal relationship. This situation is well known in the setting of a diffuse large B-cell lymphoma arising in chronic lymphocytic leukaemia {4022,2526}. Conceptually, a de novo secondary malignancy, therapy-unrelated or therapy-related (due to direct cytotoxic damage or multichemotherapy-related relative immunodeficiency), should be considered. The distinction is important, because clonally related transformed lymphomas have an inferior prognosis to those that are clonally unrelated and arise de novo {1840,1839}. Cases of transdifferentiation, in which the subsequent neoplasm is of a different cell lineage than the presenting indolent B-cell lymphoma, have been excluded; this subject is covered in the chapter on histiocytic and dendritic cell neoplasms.

Transformations of indolent B-cell lymphomas

Ott G
Coupland SE
Delabie J
Geddie WR
Naresh KN
Schuh A
Siebert R

Definition

Transformation is defined as the emergence of an aggressive lymphoma type in a patient with a previously or synchronously diagnosed clonally related indolent B-cell lymphoma. Transformed lymphomas should be reported according to their aggressive lymphoma entity, followed by adding the term "transformed from" and the denominator of the indolent lymphoma from which they have evolved.

ICD-O coding

See indolent lymphoma type

ICD-11 coding

See indolent lymphoma type

Related terminology

None

Subtype(s)

None

Localization

Transformed lymphomas may manifest at nodal or extranodal sites.

Clinical features

High-grade transformation (HGT) from a low-grade lymphoma should be suspected from rapidly enlarging lymph nodes and the development or worsening of B symptoms. Disease progression to extranodal sites, including the CNS, contributes to the wide range of clinical manifestations observed. Typical laboratory features heralding HGT include a rise in LDH to greater than twice the upper limit of normal as a reflection of total tumour burden, the emergence of hypercalcaemia due to increased bone turnover, and the rapid development or worsening of cytopenias indicating bone marrow infiltration by high-grade disease. The diagnosis of HGT must be confirmed by tissue biopsy, ideally from a site with high PET-CT uptake, defined as a maximum standardized uptake value (SUV) of > 5 {480,2983}.

Epidemiology

The incidence of HGT varies widely among the different indolent entities (see Table 4.29).

Etiology

Currently, it is thought that the process of transformation is mediated – and ultimately caused – by the progressive or parallel acquisition of genetic alterations that confer increased

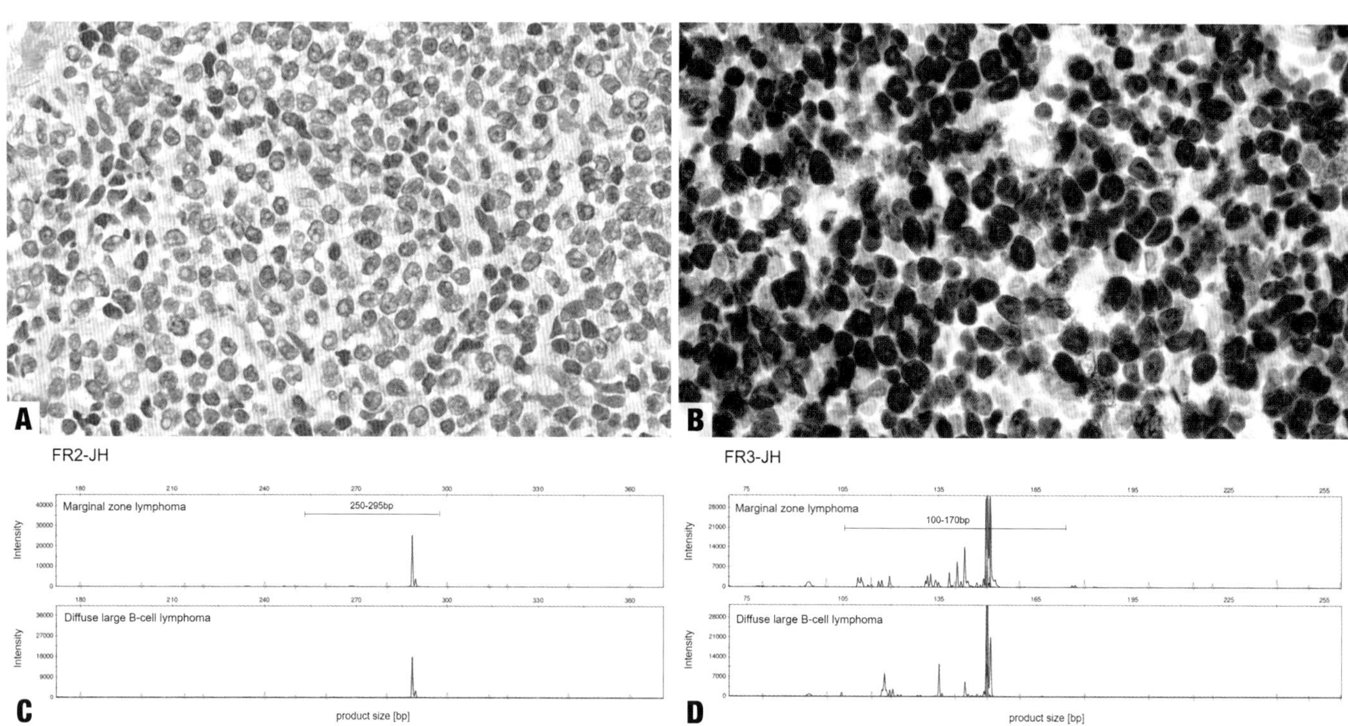

Fig. 4.142 Transformations of indolent B-cell lymphomas: diffuse large B-cell lymphoma NOS transformed from nodal marginal zone lymphoma. **A** The transformed component shows a centroblastic morphology. **B** The Ki-67 proliferation index is high. **C,D** PCR amplification of the JH segments in the FR2A (**C**) and FR3A (**D**) regions shows identical amplification in both the indolent marginal zone and the transformed aggressive lymphoma. Sequencing of the PCR products further proved the clonal identity suggested by the PCR results for FR3-JH and FR2-JH.

Table 4.29 Rates of transformation, genetic predictors, and genetic events at transformation of indolent B-cell lymphomas

Indolent B-cell lymphoma	Rate of transformation			Clinical predictive scores	Genetic predictors of transformation	Genetics present at transformation	References
	DLBCL	Hodgkin lymphoma	B-ALL/LBL				
CLL	2–8% 2.8% cumulative incidence at 5 years	< 1%	Not described	None	CD38 genotype, absence of del(13q14), IGHV4-39 usage, stereotyped B-cell receptor	*TP53* mutation and/or del(17p) (60–70% of cases), *NOTCH1* mutations (30% of cases), activation of *MYC* by translocation, amplification or mutation (30% of cases), and 9p21 deletion affecting *CDKN2A* (20% of cases); genomic complexity and dysregulation in DNA damage response pathway BTK and PLCG2 (patients on covalent-binding BTK inhibitors)	{3481,1102, 1103,706, 3480,2052, 3478,1847, 2469,1861, 1563,116}
MZL	7.5–8% 2.4% cumulative incidence at 1 year	Not described	Not described	Failure to achieve CR after initial treatment, elevated LDH, and more than four nodal sites at the time of MZL diagnosis are the main predictors of increased risk of HGT	Not known	Not known	{1614,64, 2473,2671}
LPL	5–13% 1% cumulative incidence at 5 years	Not described	Not described	Not known	Not known	Complex karyotype (90% of cases) Deletion of chromosome 17p (30%) *MYC* rearrangement (38%)	{1031,2358, 2186}
FL	14.3% 8% cumulative incidence at 5 years	< 1%	1%	High FLIPI score	*TP53, BTG1, MKI67, XBP1*	Co-occurrence of *MYC, BCL2,* and *BCL6* translocations Mutation/loss of *CDKN2A/B* and *TP53* Deletions and gains: del(1q), del(6q), +2, +3q, +5 Loss of B2M; *TP53, PIM1, B2M* mutations Mutations in *EBF1* and regulators of NF-κB signalling (*MYD88* and *TNFAIP3*) Mutations in *TP53, B2M, CCND3, GNA13, S1PR2,* and *P2RY8*	{4267,3152, 274,3041, 3040,2127}

B-ALL/LBL, B-lymphoblastic leukaemia/lymphoma; CLL, chronic lymphocytic leukaemia; CR, complete remission; DLBCL, diffuse large B-cell lymphoma; FL, follicular lymphoma; HGT, high-grade transformation; LPL, lymphoplasmacytic lymphoma; MZL, marginal zone lymphoma.

proliferation and an aggressive phenotype to the neoplastic cells when compared with the indolent counterpart.

Pathogenesis

The pathogenesis of HGT is poorly understood. Clonally related HGT leading to a disease that histopathologically resembles diffuse large B-cell lymphoma is driven by genomic instability causing rapid acquisition of additional genetic aberrations. In addition to identical IG gene rearrangements, transformed cells also carry some or all the driver mutations identified in the low-grade lymphoma or its ancestor neoplastic cell population. In the setting of transformed follicular lymphoma, the mutation landscape suggests that a high proportion of cases derive from a common (mutated) ancestor cell by early or late branching rather than linear progression {3040,3152,432}. This means that the genetic features of transformed lymphoma are diverse and certainly very different from those of de novo diffuse large B-cell lymphoma (see Table 4.29). In instances in which the diagnosis of the aggressive lymphoma precedes the diagnosis of the clonally related indolent counterpart, HGT can only be recognized in retrospect.

Clonally unrelated disease is excluded from the "high-grade transformation of indolent B-cell lymphoma" class. It is often associated with EBV infection and occurs more frequently in the context of immune deficiency/dysregulation, which can either be from an existing underlying condition (e.g. an autoimmune disease) or more generally be caused by the chemotherapy for the previous low-grade lymphoma. Immunomodulatory agents, such as fludarabine, and intensified schemes that involve high-dose chemotherapy and bone marrow rescue are most often implicated.

Macroscopic appearance

Enlarged lymph nodes or extranodal masses

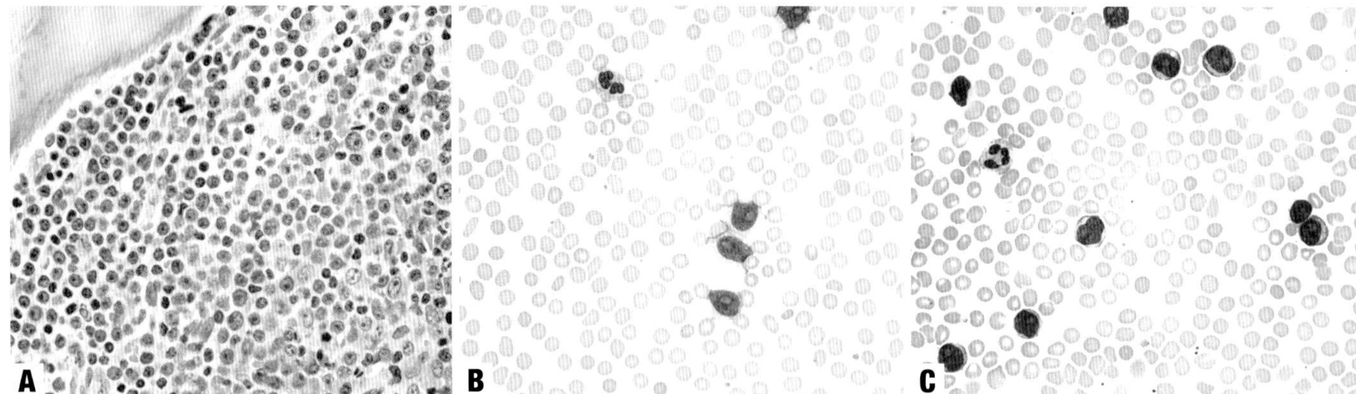

Fig. 4.143 Transformations of indolent B-cell lymphomas: diffuse large B-cell lymphoma NOS transformed from lymphoplasmacytic lymphoma. **A** Bone marrow trephine shows infiltration with medium-sized transformed cells. Peripheral blood (**B**) and bone marrow (**C**) smears show a similar cell type with prominent nucleoli.

Histopathology

Large B-cell lymphomas transformed from indolent B-cell lymphomas are virtually indistinguishable from their de novo counterparts. They usually form sheets of blasts with centroblastic, immunoblastic, or anaplastic morphology. In the setting of chronic lymphocytic leukaemia, Richter transformation (RT) characterizes transformation to either diffuse large B-cell lymphoma or classic Hodgkin lymphoma (CHL) and must be differentiated from histologically aggressive chronic lymphocytic leukaemia with larger proliferation centres and higher mitotic count or Ki-67 index {3775}. Clinical decision-making may also regard transition from classic follicular lymphoma (FL grades 1, 2, or 3A) to follicular large B-cell lymphoma (FL grade 3B) as transformation. The cytomorphological appearance of transformed lymphomas usually does not inform about the underlying disease. In the setting of follicular lymphoma (but not only limited to this entity), the acquisition of an additional *MYC* rearrangement may lead to the emergence of an aggressive lymphoma. In this type of transformation, the morphology varies. There may be a diffuse proliferation of either large and pleomorphic cells or intermediate cells with scant basophilic cytoplasm and slightly irregular nuclei, or, alternatively, by a monotonously appearing blastoid proliferation with finely dispersed chromatin and inconspicuous nucleoli mimicking lymphoblasts {3906}. These should be classified as diffuse large B-cell lymphoma or, alternatively, as high-grade B-cell lymphoma with *MYC* and *BCL2* rearrangements transformed from follicular lymphoma.

Immunophenotype

Often, the transformed blasts retain immunophenotypic features of their low-grade counterparts, such as CD10 and BCL6 expression in cases transformed from follicular lymphoma, or CD5 or CD23 expression in RT; however, diverging immunophenotypes with variable antigen loss may be seen. Transformed lymphoma cells of RT more often express PD1 than do chronic lymphocytic leukaemia cells {1542,288}. In rare cases of transformation from small B-cell lymphoma, the tumour cells may express TdT at varying levels and frequencies (ranging from 2% to 100%) and show additional features of immature cells, such as loss of CD45, CD20, and/or BCL6 {345}. Since the underlying biology and the overall immunophenotype are essentially different from those of de novo lymphoblastic B-cell leukaemia/lymphoma, these proliferations should not be classified as such. CHL arising in the setting of transformation is indistinguishable from de novo disease, although increased numbers of mixed-cellularity CHL cases may be observed in this setting. However, many CHL cases (mostly EBV-associated) are clonally unrelated to the preceding lymphoma and hence may arise in the background of immunodeficiency.

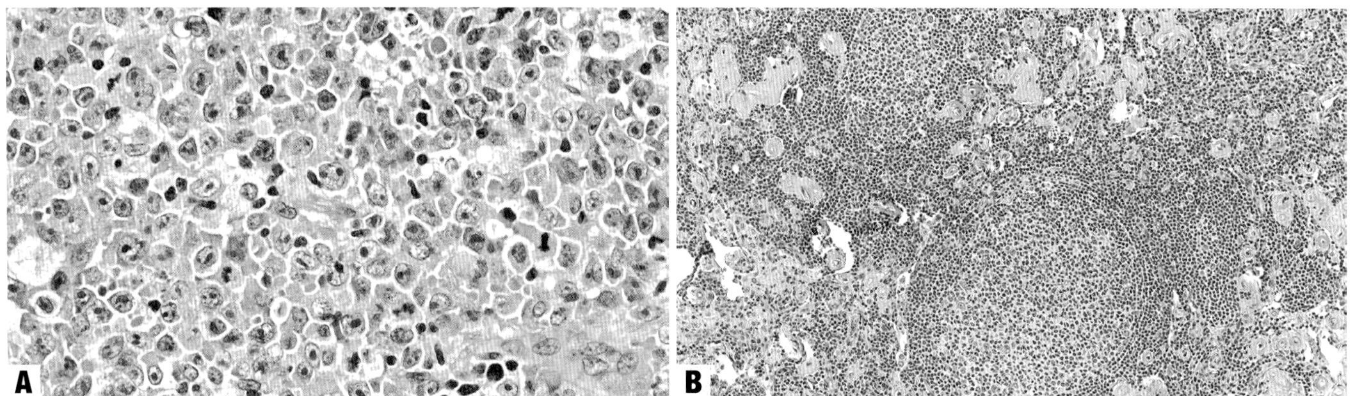

Fig. 4.144 Transformations of indolent B-cell lymphomas: diffuse large B-cell lymphoma with *MYC* and *BCL2* rearrangements transformed from follicular lymphoma. **A** A lymph node showing a large B-cell infiltrate with a large component of immunoblasts. **B** Adjacent to the diffuse large B-cell lymphoma, the indolent component of classic follicular lymphoma is present.

Because these lymphomas are clonally unrelated, they are not included in the present definition of HGT of indolent B-cell lymphomas.

Differential diagnosis

Large B-cell lymphoma transformation from marginal zone lymphoma (MZL) may occasionally be more difficult to diagnose. MZL usually shows the presence of scattered large cells among small B cells. An increased number of scattered large cells or small clusters may raise the question of transformation to large B-cell lymphoma. There is no agreement regarding the clinical relevance associated with increased numbers of large cells {2291,4065} or with the cell proliferation rate {528}. Although no quantitative criteria have been established and few studies have addressed the issue, the presence of large, confluent sheets of large cells are usually accepted as evidence of HGT {981}. The presence of clusters (> 20 cells) of large cells has also been used as a criterion for transformation {981}; however, such clusters should be differentiated from clusters of large cells colonizing residual germinal centres that are often observed in MZL without clinical evidence of transformation {4065}. Monocytoid differentiation in nodal MZL with often medium-sized cells and irregular nuclei should also not be overinterpreted as transformation. Demonstration of a nodular pattern and an absence of sheets of large cells precludes a diagnosis of large cell lymphoma in this setting {4065}.

Cytology

In general, FNAB alone is not adequate for the diagnosis and characterization of lymphomas including transformation, because the tissue architecture is essential for establishing a definite diagnosis. However, in patients with indolent lymphoma and suspected transformation, FNAB of enlarging nodes or an extranodal mass is of value for establishing a preliminary diagnosis, excluding other pathologies, gathering material for ancillary testing, and guiding site selection for subsequent core or excisional biopsy. The predictive value of FNAB in the setting of suspected transformation is dependent on adequacy of sampling, availability of ancillary techniques, and the experience of the laboratory. In those instances where other means of obtaining tissue for histological examination have failed or are not possible, a diagnosis of transformation on FNAB is acceptable if supported by immunophenotyping on a cell block preparation by flow cytometry.

Diagnostic molecular pathology

Specifically for RT, it is important to demonstrate the clonal relationship between the aggressive lymphoma and its low-grade counterpart, because prognosis and management differ between clonally related and unrelated RT {790A,1102,2052}.

Essential and desirable diagnostic criteria

Essential: emergence of an aggressive lymphoma in a patient in the setting of a previously known or synchronously diagnosed

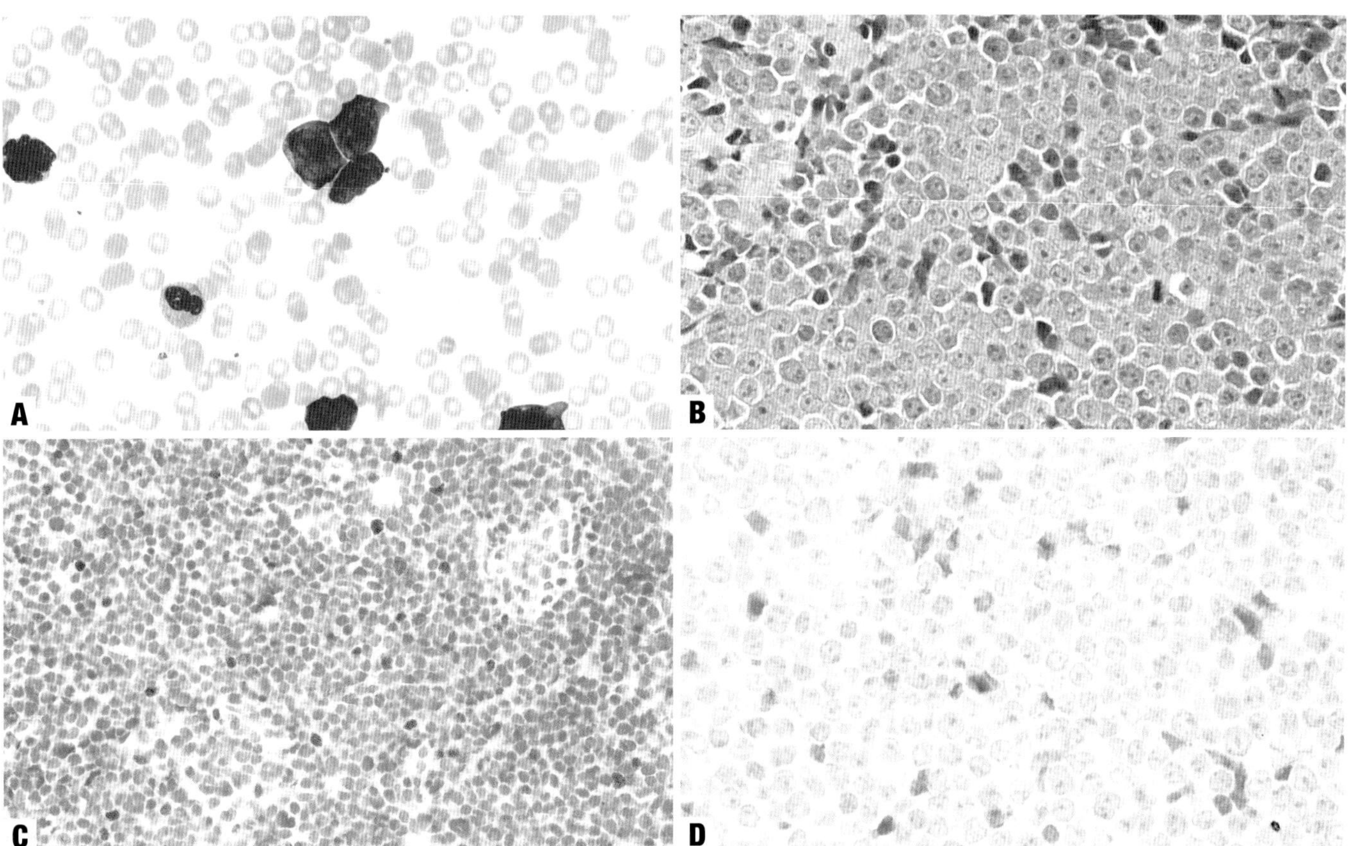

Fig. 4.145 Transformations of indolent B-cell lymphomas: high-grade B-cell lymphoma NOS transformed from follicular lymphoma. **A** Bone marrow aspirate shows a transformed B-cell population with medium-sized blastoid morphology (Giemsa). **B** The tumour cells of the transformed component have the morphology of medium-sized blastoid cells. **C** The tumour cells are partly TdT-positive. **D** CD20 is not expressed.

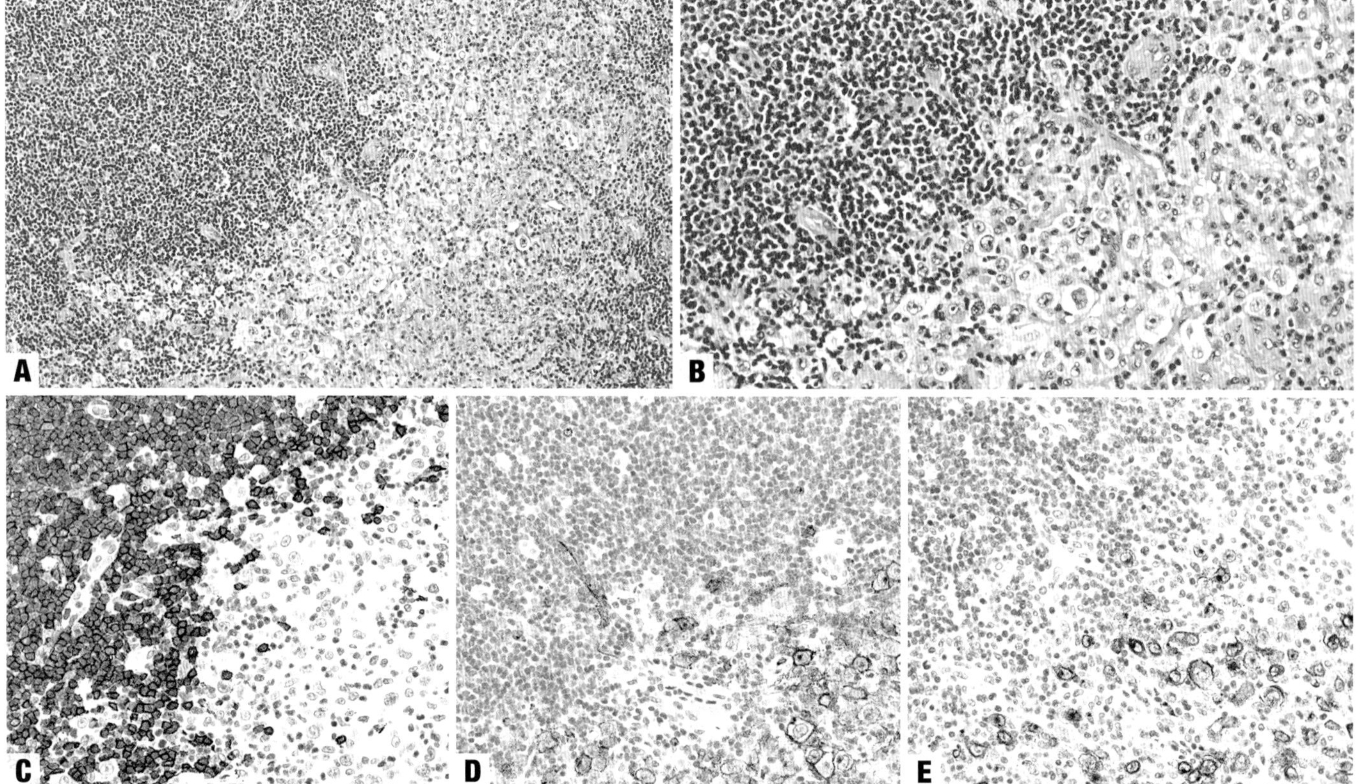

Fig. 4.146 Transformations of indolent B-cell lymphomas: classic Hodgkin lymphoma transformed from chronic lymphocytic leukaemia. **A** The chronic lymphocytic leukaemia component is seen on the left side, and the transformed component is seen to the right side as a more polymorphous infiltrate. **B** HRS cells are seen in the polymorphous infiltrate. **C** The chronic lymphocytic leukaemia cells are strongly positive for CD20, whereas the transformed component is negative. **D** The HRS cells in the polymorphous infiltrate to the right are strongly positive for CD30. **E** They also express LMP1, as is often the case in Hodgkin-type Richter transformation. Depending on the clinical context, association with immunodeficiency/dysregulation should be considered.

indolent lymphoma; proof of clonal identity of the indolent and aggressive tumours in RT.

Desirable: clinicopathological correlation.

Staging

Not relevant

Prognosis and prediction

Irrespective of the underlying histopathology, HGT always carries an inferior prognosis as compared with its de novo counterpart. The incidence of transformation and genetic predictors of transformation vary depending on the underlying pathology (see Table 4.29, p. 457).

Large B-cell lymphomas: Introduction

Ott G
Alaggio R
Dave SS
de Jong D
Naresh KN
Siebert R

The family/class of large B-cell lymphomas comprises a spectrum of tumours with varying morphologies, genetic features, and clinical behaviours. Diffuse large B-cell lymphoma (DLBCL) NOS represents the largest entity and is defined by morphology and a mature B-cell phenotype. This edition retains continuity with the revised fourth edition in that only large B-cell lymphomas that do not meet criteria for a more specific entity are classified as DLBCL-NOS. DLBCL-NOS is very heterogeneous, from a morphological, phenotypical, genotypic, and – maybe most importantly – clinical point of view. Therefore, distinction of subtypes that address any of these aspects in a meaningful way is justified.

Most cases of DLBCL-NOS broadly recapitulate the differentiation and maturation mechanisms active in normal B-cell development, so two main subtypes previously defined in the revised fourth edition continue to be recognized: the germinal-centre B-cell subtype and the activated B-cell subtype. More recent data from next-generation sequencing studies have illustrated that – despite the use of different sequencing approaches and various clustering algorithms – the genetic landscape of DLBCL-NOS can be used for subclassification with broad concordance, suggesting that the underlying disease biology may indeed be captured by comprehensive genetic landscapes.

This new edition recognizes 17 specific entities as large B-cell lymphomas outside DLBCL-NOS, grouped according to their genetic characteristics, specific clinical context, or particular site of (extranodal) origin. In most of these categories, biological concepts and diagnostic strategies have remained largely unchanged; however, some of the names have been changed from the revised fourth edition, such as "diffuse large B-cell lymphoma" to "large B-cell lymphoma", acknowledging the fact that a diffuse growth pattern does not necessarily make part of the definition of the disease, or that a growth pattern cannot be assessed in some entities (e.g. in fibrin-associated large B-cell lymphoma and in fluid overload–associated large B-cell lymphoma). High-grade B-cell lymphoma (HGBCL) with dual rearrangements of *MYC* and *BCL2* and/or *BCL6* has been conceptionally reframed and reassigned. HGBCL with *MYC* and *BCL2* and/or *BCL6* rearrangement, from the revised fourth edition, has been restricted in this new edition to only those cases with *MYC* and *BCL2* rearrangements. According to the most recent literature, cases with *MYC* and *BCL2* rearrangements form a homogeneous class with a distinct morphological spectrum and exclusive, uniform dark zone genetic and gene expression characteristics, whereas cases with *MYC* and *BCL6* rearrangements represent a more diverse spectrum with varying gene expression profiles and mutation spectra. These latter are now included within DLBCL-NOS or, in rare cases, within HGBCL-NOS. Cases with *MYC* and *BCL2* rearrangements may be composed of large or intermediate/blastoid cells; hence, the primary morphological (root) categorization of the neoplasm may be maintained and the tumours designated either as diffuse large B-cell lymphoma with *MYC* and *BCL2* rearrangements or as HGBCL with *MYC* and *BCL2* rearrangements. The preferred abbreviation of high-grade B-cell lymphoma has been changed to "HGBCL" for consistency throughout all volumes of the fifth-edition WHO Classification of Tumours series.

More recent studies have shown that the mutation spectrum of Burkitt-like lymphoma with 11q aberration (as this entity was called in the revised fourth edition), despite similarities to Burkitt lymphoma in morphology, immunophenotype, and gene expression profile, is clearly different from that of Burkitt lymphoma, justifying its name change in this new edition to HGBCL with 11q aberration. Various alterations in 11q have also been described in DLBCL; however, these differ at the molecular level from the characteristic aberrations that define HGBCL with 11q aberration, precluding the integration of aggressive lymphomas with large B-cell lymphoma morphology and alterations in the long arm of chromosome 11 at this stage.

Studies from the past few years have revealed the common biological ground of aggressive B-cell lymphomas that arise as primary tumours in the CNS, vitreoretina, and testes of immunocompetent patients. All of these arise in immune sanctuaries created by their anatomical and functional immune regulatory barriers (e.g. the blood–brain, blood–retinal, and blood–testicular barriers) and share immunophenotypic, molecular, and clinical features. This now justifies grouping these tumours under the umbrella term "primary large B-cell lymphoma of immune-privileged sites". In the future, as further data accumulate, various other site-specific large B-cell lymphomas (e.g. breast, ovary, adrenal, skin) may be added to this umbrella category.

Mediastinal grey zone lymphoma is now restricted to B-cell lymphomas with overlapping features between primary mediastinal B-cell lymphoma and classic Hodgkin lymphoma, especially nodular sclerosis classic Hodgkin lymphoma. This category replaces the term "B-cell lymphoma, unclassifiable, with features intermediate between DLBCL and classic Hodgkin lymphoma" of the last edition, taking into account that lymphomas with these features are specific to the mediastinum. Current evidence supports the notion that cases with morphological and immunophenotypic features similar to mediastinal grey zone lymphoma but occurring outside and without involvement of the mediastinum are characterized by different genetic and molecular features. The preferred abbreviation for primary mediastinal B-cell lymphoma has been changed to "PMBCL" for consistency with other large B-cell lymphoma entities throughout all volumes of the fifth-edition WHO Classification of Tumours series.

Lymphoma types/entities are defined by morphological, immunophenotypic, and clinical criteria, but none of these are absolutely specific and defining. Therefore, a hierarchical line of decision-making is inevitable. For example, it should be noted that concurrent *MYC* and *BCL2* rearrangements may be encountered in the context of other lymphoma entities/types, such as follicular lymphoma, fluid overload–associated large B-cell lymphoma, or large B-cell lymphoma of immune-privileged sites, although such events are rare. The morphological and/or clinical settings defining the different entities/types overrule the genetic characteristics in such cases. Similarly, a setting of immune deficiency/dysregulation overrules other defining parameters (e.g. the IDD setting overrules a primary CNS localization as entity/type-defining parameter in cases of diffuse large B-cell lymphoma in a patient with AIDS).

Together, the choices that have been made to update the classification of large B-cell lymphomas are based on studies by many groups around the world and published in peer-reviewed journals. Classification should be regarded as a snapshot in time. In a few years, the next update (the sixth edition) will implement and formalize the available and probably essentially changed and increased state of knowledge. It may be foreseen that by that time, the gap between biological disease classification and treatment consequences will be further closed.

Diffuse large B-cell lymphoma NOS

Rosenwald A
Barrans SL
Calaminici M
Corboy GP
Davies AJ
Delabie J
Dunleavy K
Farinha P
Gopal AK
Gujral S
Klapper W
Lenz G
Medeiros LJ
Nair R
Naresh KN
Sabattini E
Slack GW
Wang Z

Definition

Diffuse large B-cell lymphoma (DLBCL) NOS is a lymphoma consisting of medium-sized to large B cells with a diffuse growth pattern. This is a morphologically and molecularly heterogeneous entity that does not meet the diagnostic criteria for specific large B-cell lymphoma neoplasms.

ICD-O coding

9680/3 Diffuse large B-cell lymphoma, NOS
9680/3 Diffuse large B-cell lymphoma, centroblastic subtype
9684/3 Diffuse large B-cell lymphoma, immunoblastic subtype
9680/3 Diffuse large B-cell lymphoma, anaplastic subtype
9680/3 Diffuse large B-cell lymphoma, germinal-centre B-cell subtype
9680/3 Diffuse large B-cell lymphoma, activated B-cell subtype
9680/3 Diffuse large B-cell lymphoma with MYC and BCL6 rearrangements

ICD-11 coding

2A81.Z Diffuse large B-cell lymphoma, NOS

Box 4.02 Types and subtypes of diffuse large B-cell lymphoma

Diffuse large B-cell lymphoma NOS
- Morphological subtypes
  - Centroblastic subtype
  - Immunoblastic subtype
  - Anaplastic subtype
  - Other rare variants
- Molecular subtypes
  - Germinal-centre B-cell–like subtype
  - Activated B-cell–like subtype
- Genetic subtype
  - Diffuse large B-cell lymphoma with *MYC* and *BCL6* rearrangements

Other lymphomas of large B cells (see the relevant sections within this volume)
- T-cell/histiocyte–rich large B-cell lymphoma
- Diffuse large B-cell lymphoma / high-grade B-cell lymphoma with *MYC* and *BCL2* rearrangements
- ALK-positive large B-cell lymphoma
- Large B-cell lymphoma with *IRF4* rearrangement
- High-grade B-cell lymphoma with 11q aberration
- Lymphomatoid granulomatosis
- EBV-positive diffuse large B-cell lymphoma NOS
- Diffuse large B-cell lymphoma associated with chronic inflammation
- Fibrin-associated large B-cell lymphoma
- Fluid overload–associated large B-cell lymphoma
- Plasmablastic lymphoma
- Primary large B-cell lymphoma of immune-privileged sites
- Primary cutaneous diffuse large B-cell lymphoma, leg type
- Intravascular large B-cell lymphoma
- Primary mediastinal large B-cell lymphoma
- Mediastinal grey zone lymphoma
- High-grade B-cell lymphoma NOS

Related terminology

None

Subtype(s)

See Box 4.02.

Localization

The majority of patients with DLBCL-NOS present with nodal disease. About 30–40% of patients present with disease confined to extranodal sites at diagnosis {2976,115}. Virtually any site can be involved, but common extranodal sites include the gastrointestinal tract (stomach and ileocaecal region), head and neck (salivary glands, thyroid gland, ocular adnexa), bone, liver, kidney, and the adrenal gland. Kidney or adrenal gland involvement is associated with an increased risk of spread to the CNS. Involvement of the CNS by DLBCL-NOS is uncommon at diagnosis but may occur, particularly in some high-risk clinical settings. Bone marrow involvement is seen in 15–20% of patients at diagnosis, which may represent either DLBCL-NOS (concordant involvement) or indolent lymphoma (discordant involvement) {115,531,3140,3667}.

Clinical features

Patients usually present with rapidly enlarging lymph nodes or mass(es) at a single site or multiple sites. They may be otherwise asymptomatic, exhibit symptoms and signs specific to the site(s) of involvement, and/or exhibit constitutional B symptoms

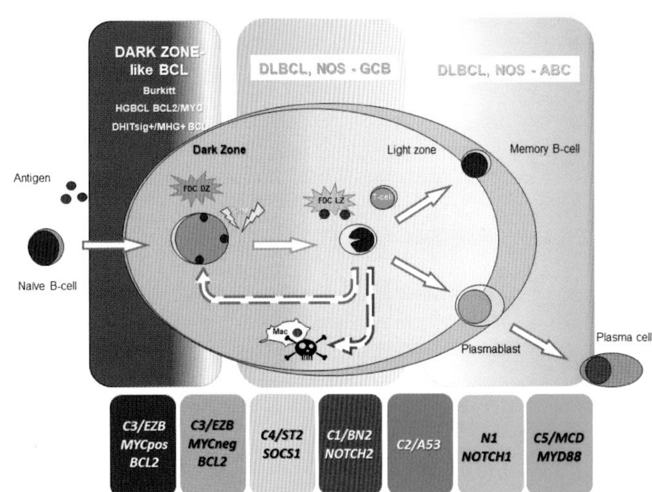

Fig. 4.147 Diffuse large B-cell lymphoma (DLBCL) NOS and related aggressive B-cell lymphoma entities. Major gene expression signatures and LymphGen and Harvard molecular subtypes of DLBCL-NOS and related aggressive B-cell lymphoma entities in relation to the normal germinal-centre reaction. ABC, activated B cell; DZ, dark zone; FDC, follicular dendritic cell; GCB, germinal-centre B cell; LZ, light zone; Mac, macrophage; SHM, somatic hypermutation.

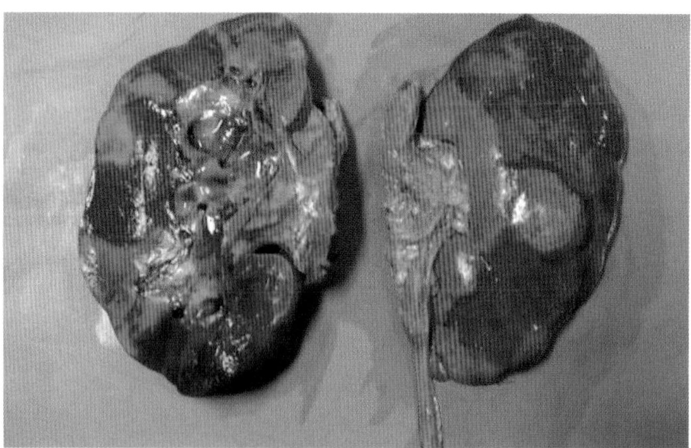

Fig. 4.148 Diffuse large B-cell lymphoma NOS, macroscopic presentation. Diffuse large B-cell lymphoma NOS presenting as a tumour mass and a component of diffuse parenchymal infiltration in the kidney.

(fever, weight loss, night sweats). Approximately half of patients present with early-stage (I/II) disease; however, the use of FDG PET imaging in staging, which is the current standard in many countries, may upstage cases or result in stage migration due to its increased sensitivity compared with CT.

Epidemiology

DLBCL-NOS represents 30% of adult lymphoma cases. There are an estimated 150 000 new cases globally each year, with low-/middle-income countries reporting higher incidence rates {3666,4505}. In the USA, the incidence varies among ethnic groups, with White populations demonstrating higher rates than Black, Asian, and Native American populations {3227}. DLBCL-NOS can be diagnosed at any age but develops more commonly with increasing age, peaking in the elderly population. It occurs in men slightly more frequently than in women {2976,3453}.

Etiology

The etiology is unknown in the majority of cases. Risk factors may include genetic features or immune dysregulation, as well as viral, environmental, or occupational exposures {588}. Genome-wide association studies have identified multiple susceptibility loci for DLBCL involving genes in immune function pathways {586}. Although DLBCL-NOS typically arises de novo, it may also present as transformation from an underlying known or occult indolent B-cell lymphoma, such as chronic lymphocytic leukaemia / small lymphocytic lymphoma, follicular lymphoma, marginal zone lymphoma, or nodular lymphocyte-predominant Hodgkin lymphoma. DLBCL arising in the setting of immune deficiency/dysregulation (e.g. related to HIV infection or immunosuppressive treatment for inflammatory/autoimmune disorders, or after solid-organ or bone marrow transplantation) is classified separately.

Pathogenesis

DLBCL-NOS is highly heterogeneous. It can either arise de novo or transform from an indolent B-cell lymphoma. In both circumstances, evolution from a clonally related (common) B-cell

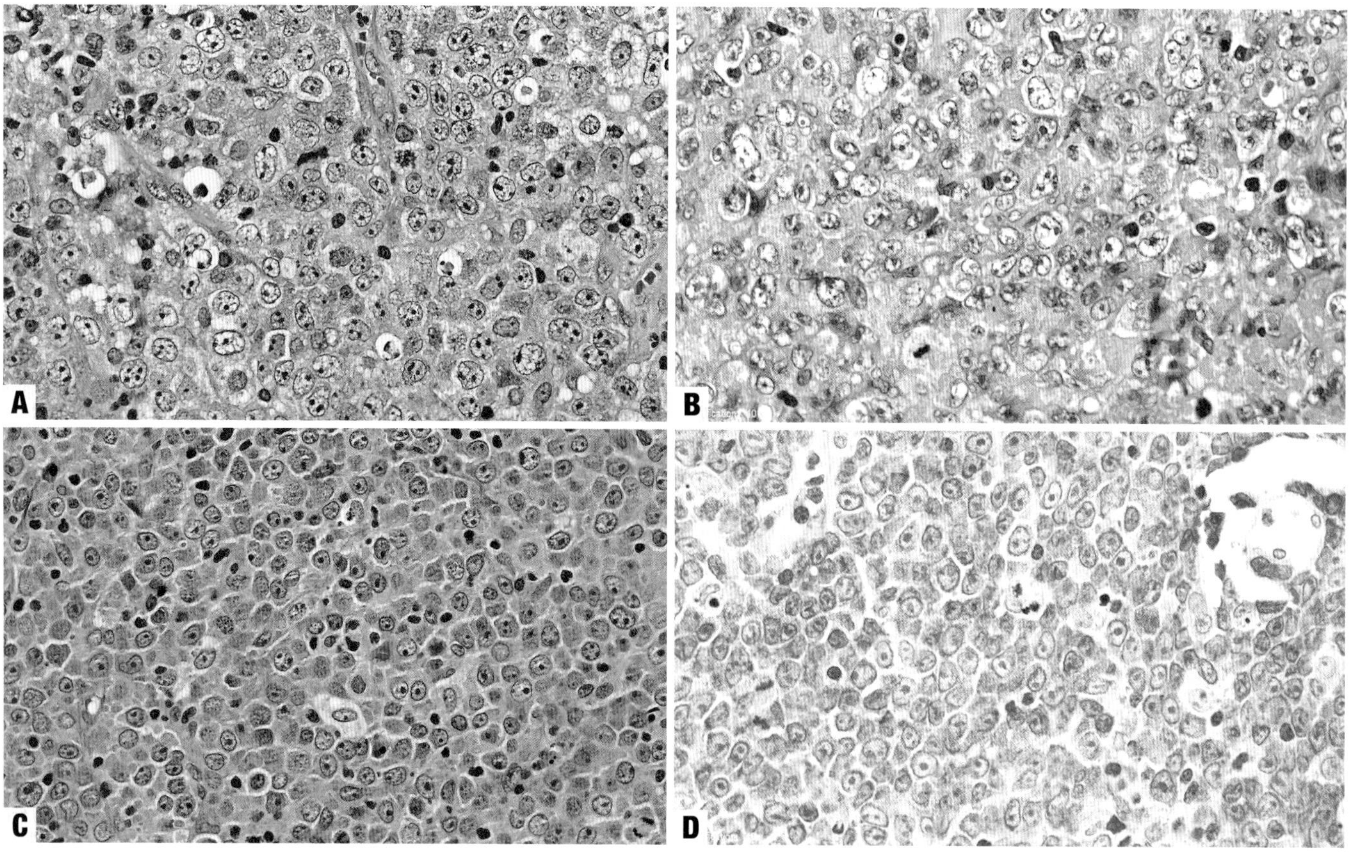

Fig. 4.149 Diffuse large B-cell lymphoma NOS, common morphological subtypes. The centroblastic subtype (**A,B**) and the immunoblastic subtype, shown here with H&E staining (**C**) and Giemsa staining (**D**), are characterized by sheets of tumour cells.

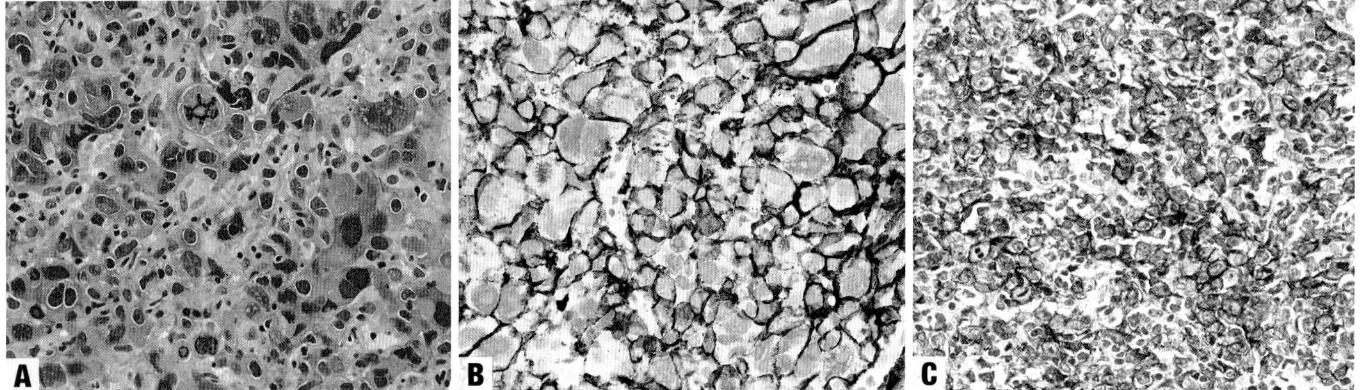

Fig. 4.150 Diffuse large B-cell lymphoma NOS, morphological subtypes. Anaplastic subtype. **A** This is characterized by nuclear pleomorphism and often shows abnormal mitotic figures. Tumour cells are uniformly positive for CD20 (**B**) and often positive for CD30 (**C**).

ancestor, such as those harbouring a *BCL2* translocation, is possible {3152}. DLBCL-NOS derives from mature B cells that have undergone IG V(D)J gene rearrangement with subsequent surface immunoglobulin expression in the bone marrow, as well as proliferation and blastic transformation after exposure to antigen in the peripheral lymphoid tissues. Like in normal B-cell differentiation, most maturation events take place in the germinal centres (GCs) of lymphatic tissues where somatic hypermutation, heavy chain class-switch recombination, and increased p53 DNA damage tolerance co-occur to produce long-lived T-cell–dependent plasma or memory B cells {936}. The proliferative larger centroblasts form the dark zone (DZ) of the GC. After several rounds of proliferation, somatic hypermutation – through the action of activation-induced cytidine deaminase (AID) – leads to clonal diversity, with ongoing IG (and other) gene mutations generating different, potentially higher, B-cell receptor (BCR) affinity for antigen {936}. From the DZ, centroblasts move to the light-zone (LZ) area as smaller centrocytes expressing surface BCR and in a BCL2-negative proapoptotic state. These cells capture antigen presented by follicular dendritic cells and crosstalk with T follicular helper (TFH) cells that provide cell fate signals. Depending on the affinity of the BCR, B cells are either eliminated or rescued and re-enter the DZ for additional rounds of mutations. The transient activation of the MYC pathway proportional to the amount of antigen and TFH help is a key element regulating the number of B-cell divisions {1192}. Finally, after several DZ–LZ selection cycles, B cells that express a high-affinity BCR exit the GC as plasma cells or as memory B cells {3786}. Specialized stromal reticular cells, notably follicular dendritic cells, provide the architectural framework that facilitates the special organization needed for GC responses. Functionally distinct follicular dendritic cell subsets populate the DZ and LZ {1961}.

Transcription factors are vital to GC initiation and maintenance, most notably BCL6 and its regulators, i.e. IRF4, MEF2B, Blimp1, BACH2, and p53. GC development in the proliferative DZ requires multiple transcription factors, such as PAX5, E2A, IRF8, FOXO1, YY1, and cyclin D3. The maturing/differentiating LZ shows increasing NF-κB–driven activation of *IRF4* and *PRDM1* (encoding Blimp1) in plasma cells or *SPI1* (encoding PU.1), *IRF8*, *PAX5*, and *BACH2* in memory B cells, along with suppression of BCL6 or MYC re-expression and return to the DZ {3786,519,988,1549}.

Epigenetic mechanisms (e.g. involving EZH2) are significant to GC responses as well. Upon activation by antigens, GC B cells highly express EZH2, in both the LZ and DZ, which plays a pivotal role in GC formation, B-cell differentiation, and inhibition of terminal B-cell differentiation {4156}. In the GC, both proliferative centroblasts and centrocytes strongly express

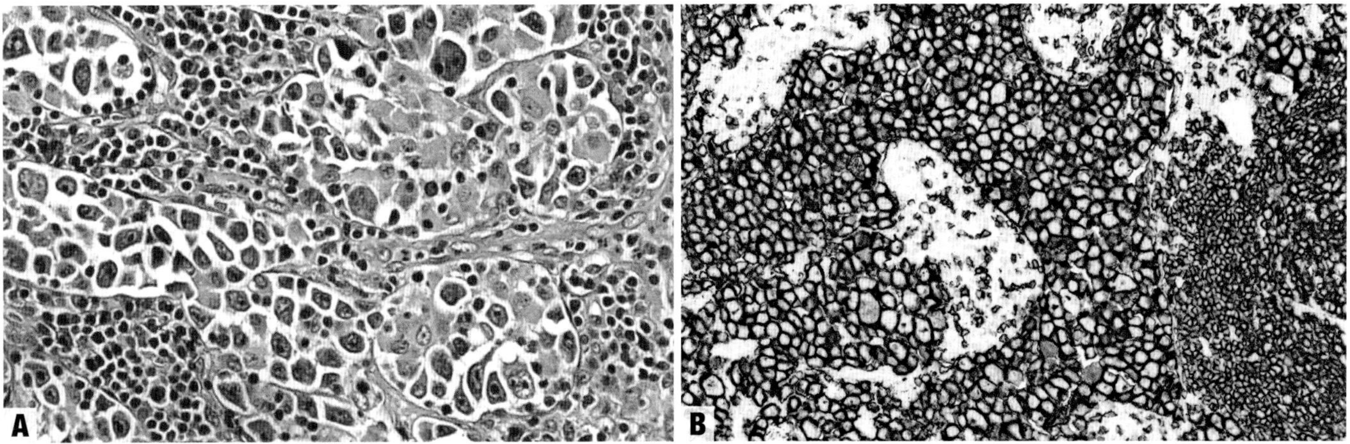

Fig. 4.151 Diffuse large B-cell lymphoma NOS, morphological subtypes. Predominantly intravascular pattern. **A** Some cases of diffuse large B-cell lymphoma NOS exhibit an intravascular component in combination with more common infiltration of large tumour cells forming sheets. **B** The intravascular component is highlighted by CD20. Cases in which tumour cells are exclusively restricted to the lumina of blood vessels should be classified as intravascular large B-cell lymphoma.

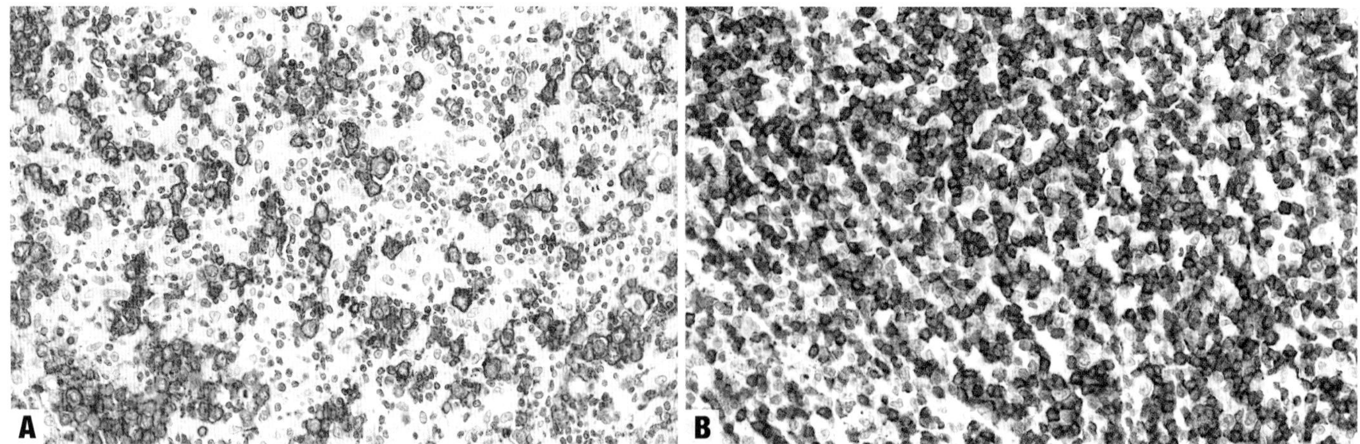

Fig. 4.152 Diffuse large B-cell lymphoma NOS, morphological subtypes. Prominent T-cell infiltrate. In some cases of diffuse large B-cell lymphoma NOS, the malignant B-cell population is largely obliterated by a dense T-cell infiltrate. **A** CD20 is very helpful for recognizing the large B cells. **B** CD5 highlights the T-cell infiltrate. By definition, cases in which the malignant B-cell component is < 10% and that lack areas with common diffuse large B-cell lymphoma NOS morphology are classified as T-cell/histiocyte–rich B-cell lymphoma.

the GC markers CD10, BCL6, and LMO2; limited IRF4 (MUM1) (encoded by *IRF4*) and MYC; and no BCL2. As plasmablastic B cells leave the GC, they express BCL2 and IRF4 (MUM1), and they downregulate GC markers.

Most DLBCL-NOS cases broadly recapitulate the GC differentiation/maturation mechanisms. They are composed of large cells, often resembling centroblasts, derived from the GC and showing mutation signatures of the somatic hypermutation machinery. Gene expression and genomic studies have delineated different molecular subtypes that broadly correlate with the different stages of B-cell differentiation (cell of origin [COO]) {3472}. One subset has a gene expression profile related to an active GC COO (germinal-centre B cell [GCB]), with common expression of GC markers (CD10, BCL6, and LMO2) {1490}. These tumours are enriched for mutations of driver genes responsible for GC development, DZ and LZ transitions, and microenvironment interactions (e.g. *EZH2*, *GNA13*, *MEF2B*, *KMT2D*, *TNFRSF14*, *B2M*, and *CREBBP*) {3151}. Within the GCB molecular subtype, a distinct subset characterized by a dual rearrangement of *MYC* and *BCL2* shows distinct molecular and clinical features {1080,3686}. Therefore, despite often showing similar morphology to DLBCL-NOS, these cases are separately classified {3657,1080,3686}.

Another DLBCL-NOS subset relates to activated B cell (ABCs), the majority with a post-GC origin, with either GC-exit or early plasmablastic phenotypes, and is characterized by constitutive activation of the BCR signalling and NF-κB pathways. These lymphomas can show variable numbers of immunoblasts and/or plasmacytoid cells and are negative for most GC markers and often positive for IRF4 (MUM1; encoded by *IRF4*) {1490}. They are enriched for BCR pathway mutations, such as in *MYD88*, *CD79B*, *PIM1*, and *PRDM1* (encoding Blimp1) {3151}. Extranodal DLBCL-NOS is more frequently associated with the ABC-DLBCL subtype.

In addition, recurrent gene rearrangements add to the molecular heterogeneity in DLBCL. The t(14;18)(q32;q21) translocation involving *BCL2*, the formation of which precedes GC exposure, is present in a quarter of cases and enriched in GCB-DLBCL (approximately 40%, compared with 5% in ABC-DLBCL {1081, 780}). In contrast, *BCL6* rearrangement is associated with AID activity and is more predominant in ABC-DLBCL (30%, compared with 10% in GCB-DLBCL {1732}).

Rearrangements of the *MYC* gene, the majority of which occur in the GC, are present in both GCB- and ABC-DLBCL {3471} and usually deregulate *MYC* via enhancer hijacking. The *MYC* translocation partner is commonly an IG gene, but DLBCLs with *MYC* rearrangements involving non-IG genes represent approximately 45% of cases {3471}. Non-IG partner genes include *BCL6*, *BCL11A*, *IKZF1*, *PAX5* (including its enhancer in *ZCCHC7*), *TFN1*, *CD96*, *SOCS1*, and *ZBTB5* {337,732}. The breakpoint, when translocated to IGH, occurs upstream (5′) of *MYC* or within exon or intron 1 but is mostly downstream (3′) of *MYC* in non-IGH translocations {732}. In contrast to DLBCL with *MYC* and *BCL2* rearrangements, cases with dual rearrangements of *MYC* and *BCL6* are molecularly heterogeneous {848}. A subset of cases with *BCL6*::*MYC* translocations as a result of t(3;8)(q27;q24) {1815} occur predominantly in GC-type DLBCL and may represent a genetic subset of DLBCL that is biologically and clinically heterogeneous. It remains to be clarified how such genomic fusion between the *BCL6* and *MYC* loci affects their protein expression {4555}.

Recent (targeted) next-generation sequencing of large numbers of DLBCL-NOS cases has revealed a highly heterogeneous molecular landscape, with about 150 protein-coding targets that are recurrently mutated or are functional targets of copy-number change, with a mean of approximately 8% of genes mutated per patient {3386}. Several groups have proposed different molecularly defined DLBCL subtypes that further subdivide the COO classification or are COO-independent {3629,644,2191,4417, 1673}. Despite using different platforms for sequencing and different cluster algorithms, these studies independently resulted in classification schemes that were broadly overlapping, suggesting that the underlying disease biology can be captured by mutation analysis, with similar mutation patterns to other lymphoma entities {4417,2793}. However, despite the overall similar clustering of cases, no unified concept for proposed clusters and their significant genetic drivers has been established so far, precluding the definition of a unified genetic framework of DLBCL-NOS at the present time. In addition, further complexity derives from a high number of non-coding mutations and focal aberrations more recently obtained from whole-genome sequencing {153,1673}.

Macroscopic appearance

Involved lymph nodes are enlarged, and the cut surface reveals a homogeneous, whitish, fleshy appearance with hilum obliteration. Grey areas that indicate necrosis and areas with adherence of a tumour mass to the surrounding soft tissue that indicate extracapsular spread are often seen. When present at extranodal sites, DLBCL-NOS tends to form large, confluent tumour masses or multiple nodules with discrete contours. In the gastrointestinal tract, gross examination shows submucosal masses presenting as exophytic growth, or ulcerated solid transmural growth with areas of haemorrhage and necrosis.

Histopathology

The tissue architecture of lymph nodes or extranodal sites is partially or totally effaced by medium-sized to large lymphoid cells (with large cells defined as having a nucleus the same size or larger than a macrophage nucleus, or more than twice the size of a small lymphocyte nucleus) that are arranged in a diffuse or vaguely nodular pattern. Interfollicular or rarely intrasinusoidal infiltration can also be observed {4452}, as well as perinodal tissue involvement. The cytological features are diverse: three common and several rare variants are described (see below). Cases with poorly classifiable cytology are sometimes observed, often due to technical issues and/or suboptimal tissue preservation. The mitotic rate is usually high, and single-cell apoptosis can be prominent. Tingible-body macrophages are present in some cases, imparting a starry-sky appearance at low power. Thick or fine fibrosis with possible compartmentalization of small groups of lymphoma cells can also be seen, and areas of geographical necrosis may be present. Variable numbers of reactive small T cells and histiocytes compose the tumour microenvironment. Cases with abundant T cells and histiocytes should not be classified as T-cell/histiocyte–rich large B-cell lymphoma unless the strict criteria for this entity are met {4442}. Diagnosis of DLBCL-NOS by morphology alone is not possible; the use of ancillary studies is required, to exclude other diseases with shared morphological features (see Table 4.30, p. 469).

Common morphological subtypes

See Box 4.02 (p. 463).

Centroblastic

The centroblastic subtype is the most common, accounting for approximately 80% of cases. Centroblasts are large lymphocytes with variable amounts of cytoplasm, round to oval nuclei, fine to vesicular chromatin, and several small to medium nucleoli often adjacent to the nuclear membrane. Monomorphic cases are composed predominantly (> 90%) of centroblasts, whereas polymorphic tumours consist of a mixture of centroblasts (< 90%), large centrocytes, and immunoblasts {1076,950,2316}. Cases with many large lymphocytes with multilobated nuclei and clear cytoplasm can be observed, particularly at extranodal sites {3005,950}. Features of plasmacytic differentiation can be rarely seen.

Immunoblastic

This subtype is less common, representing 8–10% of all cases, and is traditionally defined by ≥ 90% immunoblasts in the cell composition of the lymphoma. Immunoblasts are large lymphocytes with moderate to abundant basophilic cytoplasm and a single prominent, centrally located nucleolus. Cytological variability occurs, which may account for the variable intraobserver and interobserver reproducibility in the diagnosis of this variant {3088,4442}. In some cases, the immunoblasts show plasmacytic differentiation. Tumours where immunoblasts and plasmacytoid cells represent > 90% of all cells (but with classic immunoblasts failing to reach the 90% threshold) can be included in this subtype, provided that typical centroblasts account for < 10% {3088}. This variant has been associated

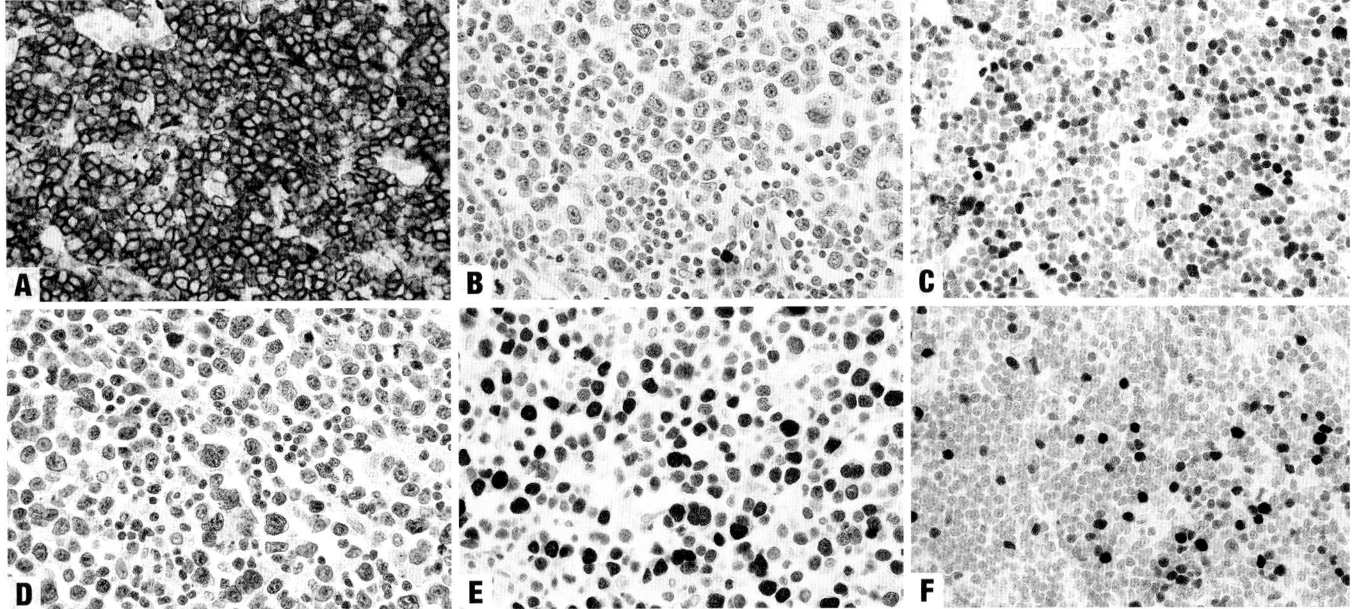

Fig. 4.153 Diffuse large B-cell lymphoma NOS, germinal-centre B-cell and non–germinal-centre B-cell subtypes. The germinal-centre B-cell–like and activated B-cell–like subtypes of diffuse large B-cell lymphoma NOS can be determined using immunohistochemistry, for example according to the Hans algorithm, based on CD10-positive (**A**) or CD10-negative (**B**) status, BCL6-positive (**C**) or BCL6-negative (**D**) status, and IRF4 (MUM1)-positive (**E**) or IRF4 (MUM1)-negative (**F**) status using an arbitrary cut-off point of 30% positive cells for BCL6 and IRF4 (MUM1) expression.

with an inferior prognosis compared with other DLBCL variants and is characterized by frequent IGH::*MYC* translocations {331, 3088,189,1633}.

Anaplastic

This subtype is rare and accounts for about 3% of all DLBCL cases. It is characterized by large to very large lymphoma cells, with pleomorphic or bizarre nuclei, usually abundant cytoplasm, and frequent cohesive sheet-like growth, and partial or extensive sinusoidal involvement. This variant often expresses CD30 and has frequent *TP53* mutations {2196,1496,2305, 2628}. These pathological features may mimic those of classic Hodgkin lymphoma with syncytial growth, anaplastic large cell lymphoma, ALK-positive large B-cell lymphoma, or undifferentiated carcinoma.

Rare morphological subtypes form < 1% of cases of DLBCL-NOS and have cells with a signet ring (mimicking gastric carcinoma) or spindle cell (mimicking sarcoma) appearance {4442}. Pseudorosetting or pseudoacinar arrangement is exceptionally observed. Other cases may show cytoplasmic granules, microvillous projections (sea anemone tumour), cytoplasmic vacuoles, or intercellular junctions as observed by electron microscopy {4442}.

Immunohistochemistry

Lymphoma cells express CD45 and pan–B-cell markers (CD19, CD20, CD22, CD79a, and PAX5) but may lack one or more of the B-cell markers, and the use of more than one B-cell marker may be necessary to confirm B-cell lineage and support the diagnosis (see Table 4.30). Rare cases may show aberrant CD3 expression, confounding lineage assignment {4419}. Light chain expression/restriction can be documented in a subset of cases; similarly, expression of IgM or IgG can be identified in a proportion of cases.

Subtyping of DLBCL-NOS according to COO using gene expression profiling is recognized as the gold standard. However, this is mostly unavailable in standard clinical practice and immunohistochemistry surrogates have been developed, the precise use of which has been challenging. Numerous subtyping systems using different markers have been explored but show limited concordance compared with gene expression. The markers used include CD10, BCL6, IRF4 (MUM1), FOXP1, GCET1, LMO2, BCL2, and cyclin D2 {1490,247,105,2917}. The Hans algorithm, which uses three markers to distinguish the GCB subtype from the non-GCB subtype is the most popular algorithm, but concordance with gene expression is only 72–86% {3224,10,841,724}. Using the Hans algorithm, CD10, BCL6, and IRF4 (MUM1) are each considered positive if ≥ 30% of the tumour cells stain positive {1490}. Overall, CD10 is positive in 30–50% of cases, BCL6 in 60–90%, and IRF4 (MUM1) in 35–65% {783,327,2850}. GCET1, a GC marker, is expressed in 40–50% of cases and correlates highly with the GCB type {2756}.

The majority of DLBCL-NOS cases express BCL2, and the intensity of expression is variable. Similarly, expression of MYC protein is highly variable. In most studies, BCL2 is considered positive if ≥ 50% of the tumour cells are positive, and MYC is considered positive if ≥ 40% of the tumour cell nuclei are positive {2059,1813, 1406,1634,4139,2483,754,2653,3657,102}. The reproducibility of MYC scoring is higher with a cut-off point of 70% {102}.

DLBCL-NOS may express CD5 in 5–10% of cases {4471, 4456}. CD5+ DLBCL-NOS can be distinguished from the pleomorphic variant of mantle cell lymphoma by the absence of cyclin D1 and SOX11 expression {4471}. A small subset of DLBCL-NOS cases express cyclin D1 in the absence of *CCND1* translocation, and most of these are negative for SOX11 expression. Cyclin D1 expression is weaker and heterogeneous in DLBCL compared with mantle cell lymphoma {3440,4201,

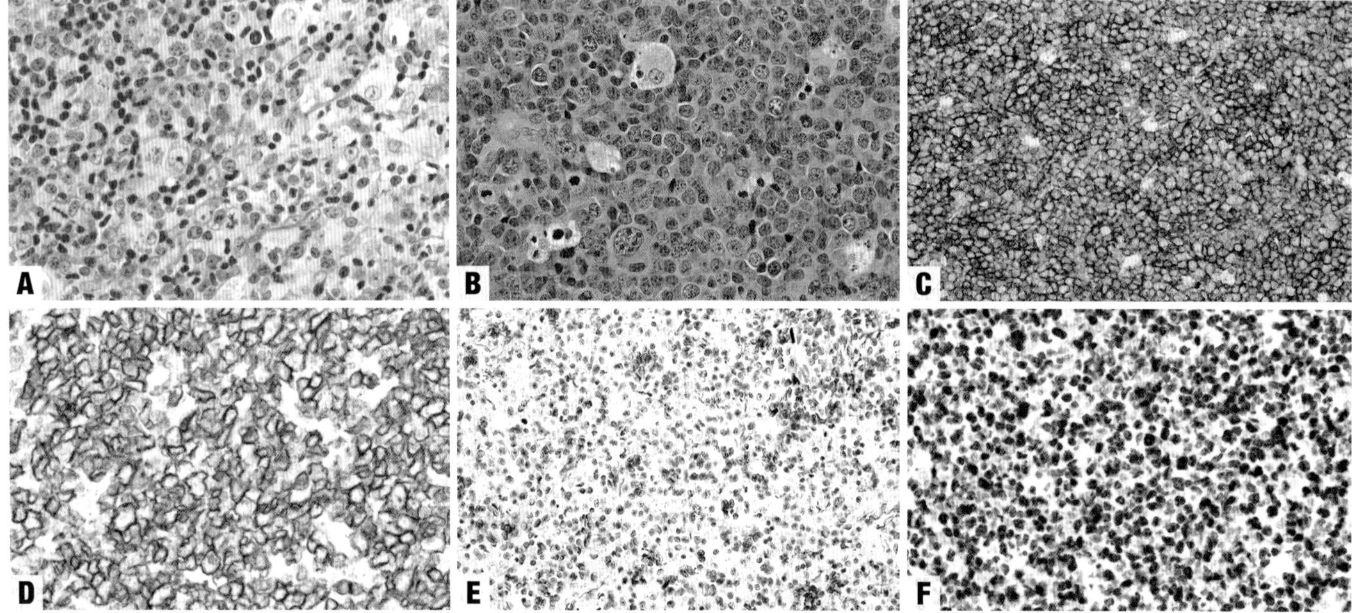

Fig. 4.154 Diffuse large B-cell lymphoma NOS, immunophenotypic variants. CD5-positive. Diffuse large B-cell lymphoma NOS expresses CD5 in tumour cells in 5–10% of cases. Such cases should be distinguished from pleomorphic and blastoid types of mantle cell lymphoma. The morphology is heterogeneous, varying from centroblastic (**A**) to remarkably pleomorphic (**B**). CD5 expression is strong and uniform (**C**) in CD20-positive tumour cells (**D**). Cyclin D1 (**E**) and SOX11 are negative. The Ki-67 index is often high (**F**).

Table 4.30 Differential diagnosis of diffuse large B-cell lymphoma (DLBCL)

Entities in differential diagnosis of DLBCL	Anatomical/morphological features	Helpful immunophenotypic markers	Molecular markers
Follicular large B-cell lymphoma	Follicular growth pattern (at least partial)	CD21, CD23, or CD35 highlights follicular dendritic cell networks	*BCL2* (~10%) or *BCL6* (10–15%) rearrangement
Mantle cell lymphoma	Pleomorphic or blastoid morphology	CD5+, cyclin D1+, SOX11+	*CCND1* (~95%) or rare *CCND2* rearrangements
DLBCL arising in CLL (Richter syndrome)	CLL component may be present	Often CD5+, CD23+, LEF1+, PD1+ in large-cell component	Alterations in *TP53* and *CDKN2A/B* are common
B-lymphoblastic leukaemia/ lymphoma	Small to medium-sized cells with lymphoblastic morphological features	CD10+, CD79a+, CD34–/+, CD20–/+, mostly TdT+	Various
T-cell/histiocyte–rich large B-cell lymphoma	Scattered tumour cells (< 10%) in a dense background of reactive T cells and histiocytes	PD1+ T cells and PDL1+ macrophages surround neoplastic B cells	*CD274* (*PDL1*) / *PDCD1LG2* (*PDL2*) copy number gains or amplification in ~65%
Primary cutaneous DLBCL, leg type	Skin; uniform large cells with prominent nucleoli	BCL2+, IRF4 (MUM1)+, MYC+, BCL6–, cytoplasmic IgM+	*MYC* rearrangements (40–50%) Amplifications of *BCL2* and *MALT1* (30–50%)
EBV-positive DLBCL-NOS	Polymorphous or monomorphic; rich in plasma cells and/or small B cells	EBER+; mostly CD20+; CD30+/–, CD79a+	*MYC* rearrangements are rare
Pyothorax-associated DLBCL	Chest wall; medical history	EBER+	Not applicable
Lymphomatoid granulomatosis, grade 3	Lungs; angiocentric and angiodestructive with geographical necrosis	EBER+, CD30–/+	Not applicable
Large B-cell lymphoma with *IRF4* rearrangement	May have a partially follicular pattern	Strong IRF4 (MUM1)+, BCL6+, CD10+/–, BCL2+/–	*IRF4* rearrangements
Primary mediastinal large B-cell lymphoma	Younger patient age; mediastinum and/or thymus location	CD23 (75%), CD30+ (75%), MAL+, PDL1/PDL2+/–	*CD274* (*PDL1*) / *PDCD1LG2* (*PDL2*) gains *CIITA* rearrangements JAK/STAT aberrations
ALK-positive large B-cell lymphoma	Immunoblastic or plasmablastic features	ALK+; plasmablastic immunophenotype (CD138+, IRF4 [MUM1]+, CD20–)	*ALK* rearrangements
Plasmablastic lymphoma	Plasmablastic features	CD138+, IRF4 (MUM1)+, CD20–, EBER+/–	*MYC* rearrangements (~50%)
KSHV/HHV8-positive large B-cell lymphoma	Immunoblastic or plasmablastic features	KSHV/HHV8+, CD138+, IRF4 (MUM1)+, CD20–, EBER+/–	Not applicable
Primary effusion lymphoma	Immunoblastic or plasmablastic features	KSHV/HHV8+, CD138+, IRF4 (MUM1)+, CD20–, EBER+/–	Not applicable
High-grade B-cell lymphoma with *MYC* and *BCL2* rearrangements	Can have DLBCL-like, Burkitt-like, or small blastoid features	BCL2+, MYC+, TdT+/–	*MYC* and *BCL2* rearrangements required for diagnosis
High-grade B-cell lymphoma NOS	Burkitt-like or small blastoid features	MYC–/+, Ki-67 high, TdT–, cyclin D1–	*MYC* rearrangements (20–35%)
Mediastinal grey zone lymphoma	Tumour cell–rich with PMBCL-like or CHL-like morphology or transitional features; cellular pleomorphism	Variable expression of B-cell markers; CD15+ (50%), CD30+, EBER–	Partial overlap with PMBCL and CHL
Burkitt lymphoma	Starry-sky pattern, intermediate-sized cells, basophilic cytoplasm, multiple small nucleoli	CD10+, BCL6+, Ki-67 high, BCL2–, MYC+	*MYC* rearrangements in > 95%; partnered with IGH or light chain loci in 100%
High-grade B-cell lymphoma with 11q aberration	Burkitt-like morphology but more polymorphic, nodular pattern can be present	CD10+, BCL2–/+, Ki-67 high	Proximal gains and telomeric losses of 11q required Complex karyotype No *MYC* rearrangements
DLBCL in association with nTFHL-AI or other T-cell lymphomas	Background T cells are atypical; increased vascularity and particularly high endothelial vessels; increased eosinophils	TFH marker expression in T-cell lymphomas with TFH phenotype; EBER+/– in B cells	Clonal TR gene rearrangements Mutations of *TET2*, *DNMT3A*, *RHOA*, *IDH2*

CHL, classic Hodgkin lymphoma; CLL, chronic lymphocytic leukaemia; EBER, EBV-encoded small RNA; nTFHL-AI, nodal T follicular helper cell lymphoma, angioimmunoblastic type; PMBCL, primary mediastinal large B-cell lymphoma; TFH, T follicular helper.

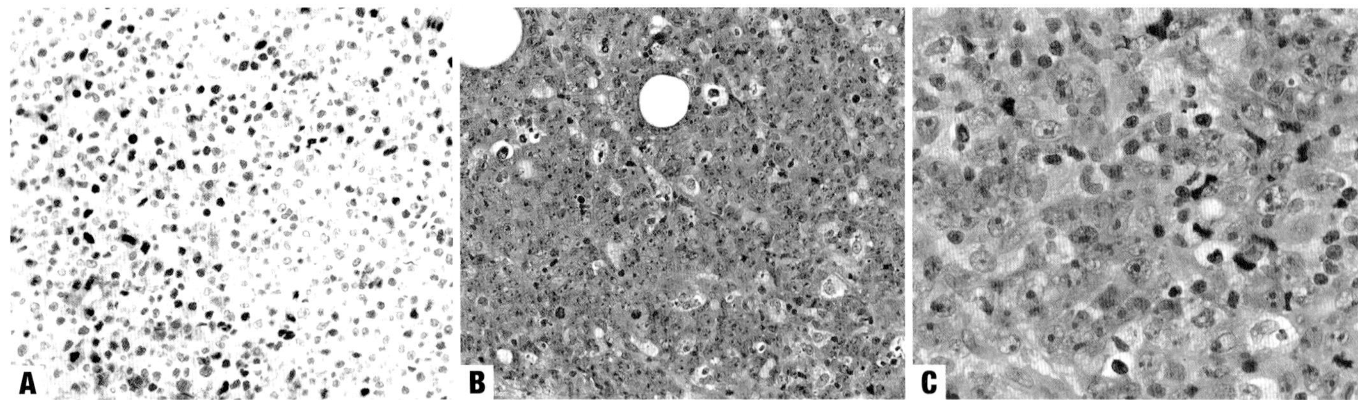

Fig. 4.155 Diffuse large B-cell lymphoma NOS, immunophenotypic variants. Cyclin D1–positive. Rare cases of diffuse large B-cell lymphoma NOS express cyclin D1 (**A**). The morphology is generally centroblastic (**B,C**). Negative SOX11 expression helps to distinguish it from mantle cell lymphoma.

1650}. Most DLBCL-NOS cases are negative for CD138. CD30 expression in a significant proportion of cells is seen in 10–20% of cases, especially in the anaplastic variant {1656,3759}. In one study, 19% of cases expressed CD30 in > 20% cells and an additional 31% of cases showed CD30 expression in a smaller proportion of cells {3540}. The presence of EBV (as identified by EBV-encoded small RNA [EBER] in situ hybridization and/or LMP1 expression) in the majority of the cells excludes DLBCL-NOS and should lead to a diagnosis of EBV-positive DLBCL; high levels of CD30 expression may point to the diagnosis of EBV-positive DLBCL, but they are not specific {428}.

Almost all cases of DLBCL lack expression of TdT. Expression of TdT in an otherwise typical DLBCL-NOS should warrant evaluation for rearrangements in *MYC* and *BCL2*. If both rearrangements are present, these cases are classified as diffuse large B-cell lymphoma with *MYC* and *BCL2* rearrangements rather than DLBCL-NOS {345,3033}. Of note, TdT expression alone does not justify classification as B-lymphoblastic leukaemia/lymphoma.

The Ki-67 proliferation index is high (≥ 80%) in most DLBCLs, although rare cases may show a lower proliferation index (closer to 40%) {1533,2083,4506}. Expression of p53 is seen in 20–60% of cases, and the proportion of positive cells and the intensity of expression are variable. However, p53 expression is not a good surrogate marker for *TP53* mutations, because p53 expression is seen in cases without *TP53* mutations {4516,700,4457,2324}.

Differential diagnosis

The differential diagnosis includes malignancies with a diffuse growth pattern and a medium to large cell type, including a wide variety of B- and T-cell lymphomas, as well as haematological malignancies such as histiocytic sarcoma and myeloid sarcoma, and non-haematological malignancies such as metastatic poorly differentiated carcinoma, metastatic melanoma, and seminoma (see Table 4.30, p. 469) {830}.

Cytology

The cytological diagnosis of DLBCL-NOS through FNA of superficial and deep-sited lymph nodes and extranodal tumour masses is a well-established, safe, efficient methodology and may represent a valid additional (although not alternative) tool to core needle and excisional biopsies in an integrated multidisciplinary diagnostic approach {192,1921,1353,2343,569}.

Smear preparations and cell blocks are highly cellular and contain numerous medium-sized to large atypical lymphoid cells in a monotonous pattern. Occasionally, cohesive clusters of atypical lymphoid cells are identified, mimicking carcinomas. Lymphoglandular bodies are numerous in the background. Cell cytology recapitulates the features described in *Histopathology*.

Diagnostic molecular pathology

Interphase cytogenetic testing is strongly recommended in order to exclude the diagnosis of diffuse large B-cell lymphoma with *MYC* and *BCL2* rearrangements. Most often, but not exclusively, FISH techniques are applied to screen for rearrangements of the *MYC* locus and, if positive, subsequently for the *BCL2* (and potentially for the *BCL6*) locus. It is important to be aware of the coverage of the different *MYC* break-apart probes used for analysis of *MYC* rearrangement, because not all probes cover the whole spectrum of potential breakpoints at the *MYC* locus {2841,732}. Cryptic *MYC* rearrangements such as small insertions into *MYC* and of *MYC* into other loci or uncommon breakpoints might escape break-apart probe design and require fusion probe assays. Likewise, rare *MYC*, as well as *BCL2*, rearrangements may be cytogenetically cryptic and thus fail to be detected by conventional FISH {2030,1587}.

Cases displaying an isolated *MYC* rearrangement or dual rearrangements of *MYC* and *BCL6* do fall within the spectrum of DLBCL-NOS; if a *MYC* rearrangement or simultaneous *MYC* and *BCL6* rearrangements are detected, the case should be reported as DLBCL-NOS with *MYC* rearrangement or with *MYC* and *BCL6* rearrangements. DLBCL-NOS in younger patients that is localized to the head and neck region and shows strong and uniform IRF4 (MUM1) expression suggests large B-cell lymphoma with *IRF4* rearrangement; *IRF4* rearrangement should be evaluated in such cases and, if present, excludes DLBCL-NOS. In occasional cases, clonality analysis and/or genetic profiling may be helpful if clinically relevant. In particular, the presence of individual mutations, such as *MYD88*, might aid in reaching a diagnosis, especially in small biopsies from extranodal sites.

Gene expression profiling is the gold standard for COO determination for DLBCL-NOS.

Because detailed mutation spectra as obtained by targeted panel and/or whole-exome/genome sequencing currently have very limited consequences for treatment decisions outside clinical trials, such analyses have little role at present in routine practice. However, this situation may be subject to change in the coming few years as more knowledge and diagnostic assays become available.

Essential and desirable diagnostic criteria

Essential: a large B-cell lymphoma with a diffuse or vaguely nodular growth pattern; mature B-cell phenotype; exclusion of other specific entities of large B-cell lymphoma.

Desirable: COO subtyping; reporting of isolated *MYC* or dual *MYC* and *BCL6* rearrangements; genetic testing, if relevant for clinical decision-making.

Staging

Approximately 50% of patients have stage I or II disease. PET-CT imaging is commonly performed at diagnosis and has resulted in stage migration, owing to its improved sensitivity compared with CT alone. In cases where PET-CT imaging can be performed, bone marrow aspiration and biopsy may not be routinely needed. However, although PET imaging is effective for detecting concordant bone marrow involvement, it is unreliable for picking up discordant disease and this may be missed where PET interpretation replaces bone marrow biopsy {688, 472}. Evaluation of the CNS should be considered where clinical characteristics predict a higher risk of involvement.

Prognosis and prediction

Clinical features

After R-CHOP therapy, the 5-year progression-free and overall survival rates are about 70% {2277,3658,4512,256,879, 2985}. The International Prognostic Index (IPI), which incorporates five clinical variables, continues to be a very valuable prognostic tool. Newer and revised versions of the IPI may improve identification of high-risk subsets of patients {3666}. Other clinical prognostic factors associated with an inferior outcome include tumour bulk (masses ≥ 100 mm), male sex, and concordant bone marrow biopsy involvement. Concordant bone marrow involvement and involvement of a high number of extranodal sites and various specific extranodal localizations have been associated with an increased risk of CNS dissemination and dictate the need for CNS prophylaxis in some centres.

Morphology

The prognostic impact of morphological subtypes of DLBCL-NOS remains uncertain. Some studies found the immunoblastic and/or anaplastic variants to be associated with inferior survival {331,3088,2305}, whereas many other studies did not. In the subgroup of immunoblastic variants with expression of CD10, *MYC* rearrangements are frequently detectable {1633}.

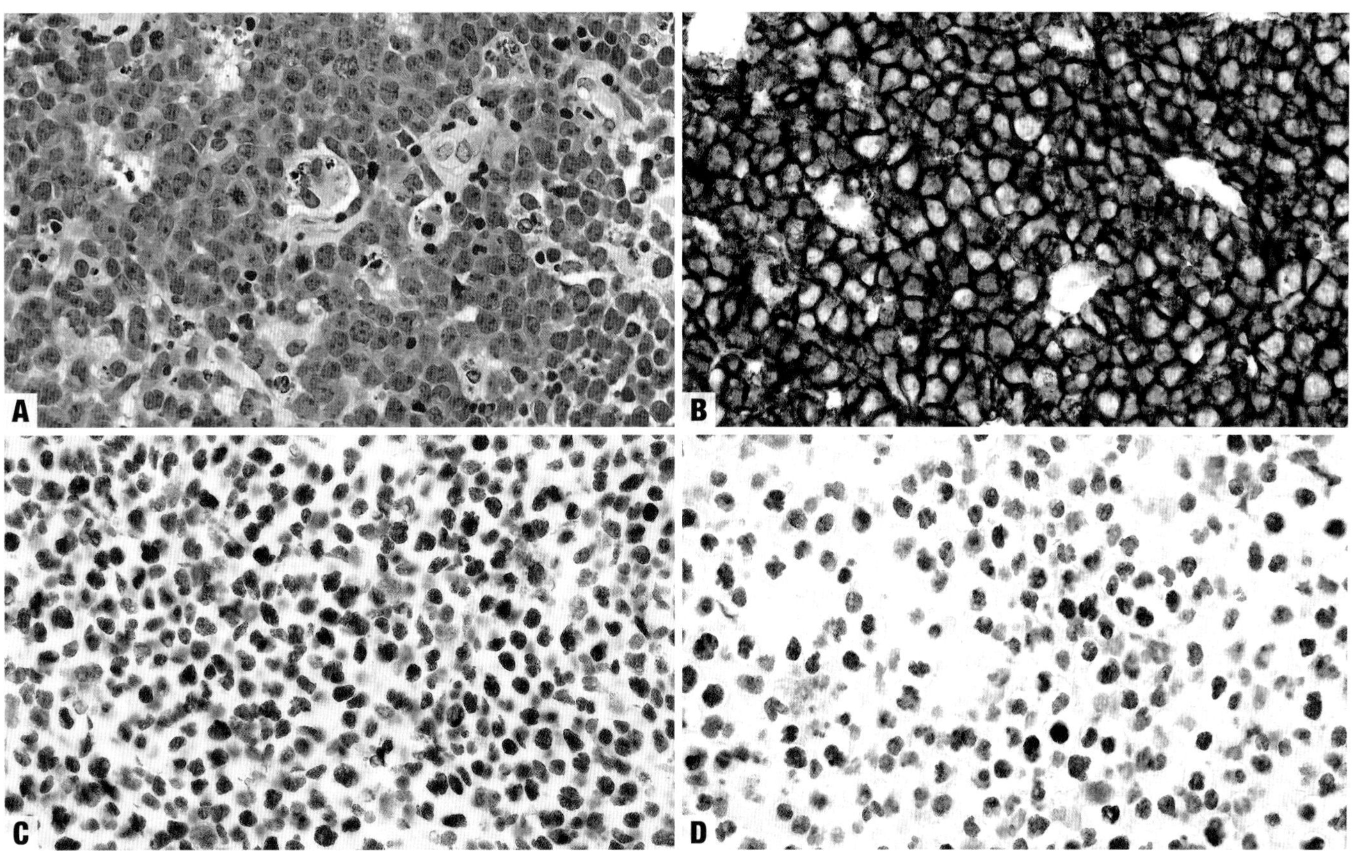

Fig. 4.156 Diffuse large B-cell lymphoma NOS, immunophenotypic variants. TdT-positive. Expression of TdT in an otherwise typical diffuse large B-cell lymphoma NOS is rare and does not justify a diagnosis of B-lymphoblastic leukaemia/lymphoma. **A** A TdT-positive case of diffuse large B-cell lymphoma NOS shows a diffuse proliferation of large atypical lymphoid cells with vesicular nuclei containing prominent nucleoli. Many mitotic figures and single cell necrosis are noted. **B** The tumour cells are strongly positive for CD20. The neoplastic cells were also positive for BCL6, IRF4 (MUM1), BCL2, and MYC (40%), and negative for CD10 (non–germinal-centre B-cell phenotype). **C** Uniform strong nuclear positivity for TdT is seen. **D** TdT expression can be more variable in other cases, however.

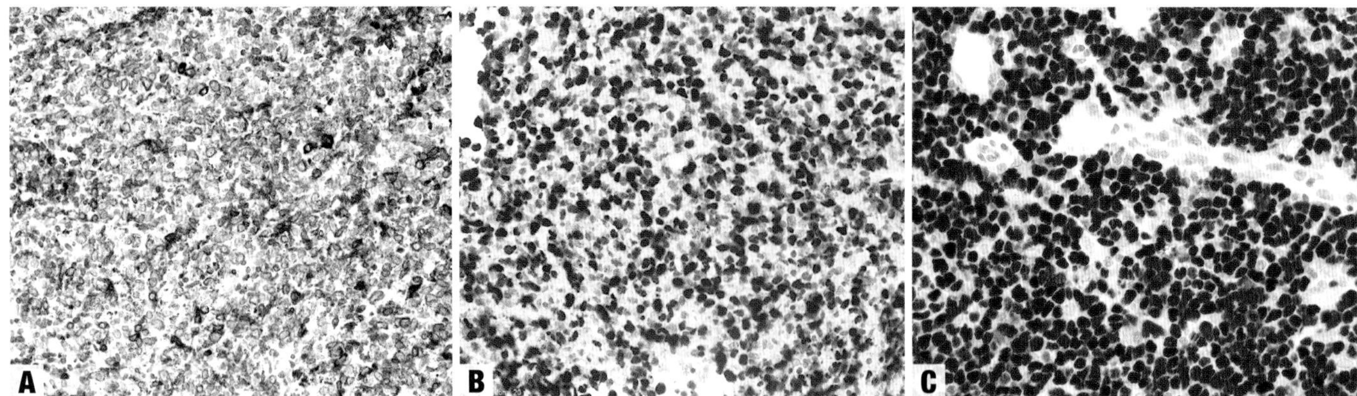

Fig. 4.157 Diffuse large B-cell lymphoma NOS, immunophenotypic characteristics associated with prognosis. Concurrent high protein expression of BCL2 (**A**) and MYC (**B**) by immunohistochemistry in diffuse large B-cell lymphomas NOS (dual-expressers) and strong expression of p53 (**C**) are associated with an adverse outcome.

Cell of origin

ABC-DLBCL-NOS has an inferior outcome in response to standard therapies when compared with the GCB group in most but not all clinical cohorts. Studies comparing COO classification by gene expression with the Hans criteria have shown that gene expression profiling has superior performance in the prediction of overall survival {3552,3815,3224,10,724,841}, and cases with the most confident COO calls by gene expression profiling are associated with the strongest survival differences {246}. However, COO classification has shown a disappointing lack of impact as a predictive marker in targeted approaches in clinical trials, specifically those directed to ABC-DLBCL.

Double-hit signature–positive / molecular high grade

Cases with a positive double-hit signature (DHITsig) / molecular high-grade (MHG) signature, both reflecting DZ biology, are a poor-prognostic molecular subgroup within DLBCL-NOS, and particularly of GCB-DLBCL, with an inferior response to standard treatment {1080,3686,65}, and they may be a target for alternative therapies.

Gene rearrangements

The overall deleterious effect of *MYC* rearrangements on DLBCL-NOS survival is pronounced when *MYC* is rearranged to an IG gene partner {3471}. Similarly, *TP53* mutation in combination with *MYC* can result in a poor outcome {764}. DLBCL with *MYC* rearrangements involving non-IG genes may result in variable MYC expression {337,4555}. The prognostic impact of a given non-IG partner of *MYC* deserves further investigation {3471,4555}. *BCL2* rearrangements in DLBCL may indicate transformation of follicular lymphoma, which may be subclinical.

Copy-number abnormalities

An increased *MYC* copy number occurs in as many as 20% of patients with DLBCL-NOS {1081,780}, but in most studies it has no impact on outcome {4139,1537}; this may be explained by the lack of correlation with MYC expression {1081,780}. Amplification of a non-rearranged *MYC* locus has been variably defined and needs further standardization; however, the prognostic impact of copy-number gain in published studies has been controversial {4139,716,2215,1081,3326,2085,3281}.

Molecular subtypes of DLBCL

The proposed molecular subtypes in DLBCL-NOS have different impacts on the prognosis {3629,644,2191,4417,1673}; however, there is currently no consensus as to how this additional information might aid in treatment decision-making. Before meaningful introduction in practice, harmonization is needed between the different proposed molecular classifications, including technical and bioinformatic aspects, as well as availability of assays under good laboratory practice standards. Thereafter, clinical trials are required before the clinical utility of the subgroups can be fully elucidated. The prognostic impact of non-coding mutations is as yet unexplored.

Protein expression and prognosis

Expression of CD5 has been linked to an adverse prognosis, especially in Asian patients, and is more often seen in ABC-DLBCL-NOS {4471,1082,2962}. Concurrent high protein expression of BCL2 and MYC in diffuse large B-cell lymphoma NOS (dual expressers) carries an adverse prognosis {1406,1813,1634,3815}. However, this may not be independent of the prognostic impact of mutation subgroups {2659}. Increased CD30 expression and strong p53 expression may also have an impact on outcome.

Therapy

The standard immunochemotherapy approach for the treatment of DLBCL-NOS is R-CHOP. Recent randomized studies have investigated whether there is a benefit to more dose-intensive regimens than R-CHOP, and the results have not demonstrated a survival advantage. Strategies targeting the COO have added agents with differential activity in the ABC-DLBCL subtype, but recently reported randomized results have not shown a clear advantage over R-CHOP in these trials {2280,4512,879,2985}.

T-cell/histiocyte–rich large B-cell lymphoma

Hartmann S
Fromm JR
Medeiros LJ
Natkunam Y
Nicolae A

Definition

T-cell/histiocyte–rich large B-cell lymphoma (THRLBCL) is an aggressive B-cell lymphoma with < 10% large neoplastic B cells, scattered in a diffuse background rich in T cells and histiocytes, and with a virtual absence of small B cells. A subset of cases show marked clinical, immunophenotypic, and molecular overlap with nodular lymphocyte-predominant Hodgkin lymphoma (NLPHL).

ICD-O coding

9688/3 T-cell/histiocyte–rich large B-cell lymphoma

ICD-11 coding

2A81.4 T-cell/histiocyte–rich large B-cell lymphoma

Related terminology

None

Subtype(s)

T-cell/histiocyte–rich large B-cell lymphoma, de novo; T-cell/histiocyte–rich large B-cell lymphoma progressed from nodular lymphocyte-predominant Hodgkin lymphoma

Localization

THRLBCL usually affects lymph nodes, often below the diaphragm. There is frequent involvement of spleen, liver, and bone marrow at diagnosis {20}.

Clinical features

THRLBCL commonly manifests as stage III–IV systemic disease. Patients typically present with B symptoms, splenomegaly, and/or hepatomegaly, often with elevated serum LDH. Imaging studies by FDG PET show a maximum standardized uptake value similar to that in diffuse large B-cell lymphoma (DLBCL) NOS, but a total metabolic tumour volume 10 times as high as that of DLBCL has been reported {3625,239}. The disease follows a heterogeneous clinical course {20}.

Epidemiology

THRLBCL accounts for < 10% of large B-cell lymphomas. It preferentially affects middle-aged or older adults (age range: 18–90 years), with rare cases affecting children {2404,4019}. There is a slight male predominance (M:F ratio: 1.7–2.6:1) {3053, 20,19,2345,1226,1157}. The sociodemographic characteristics

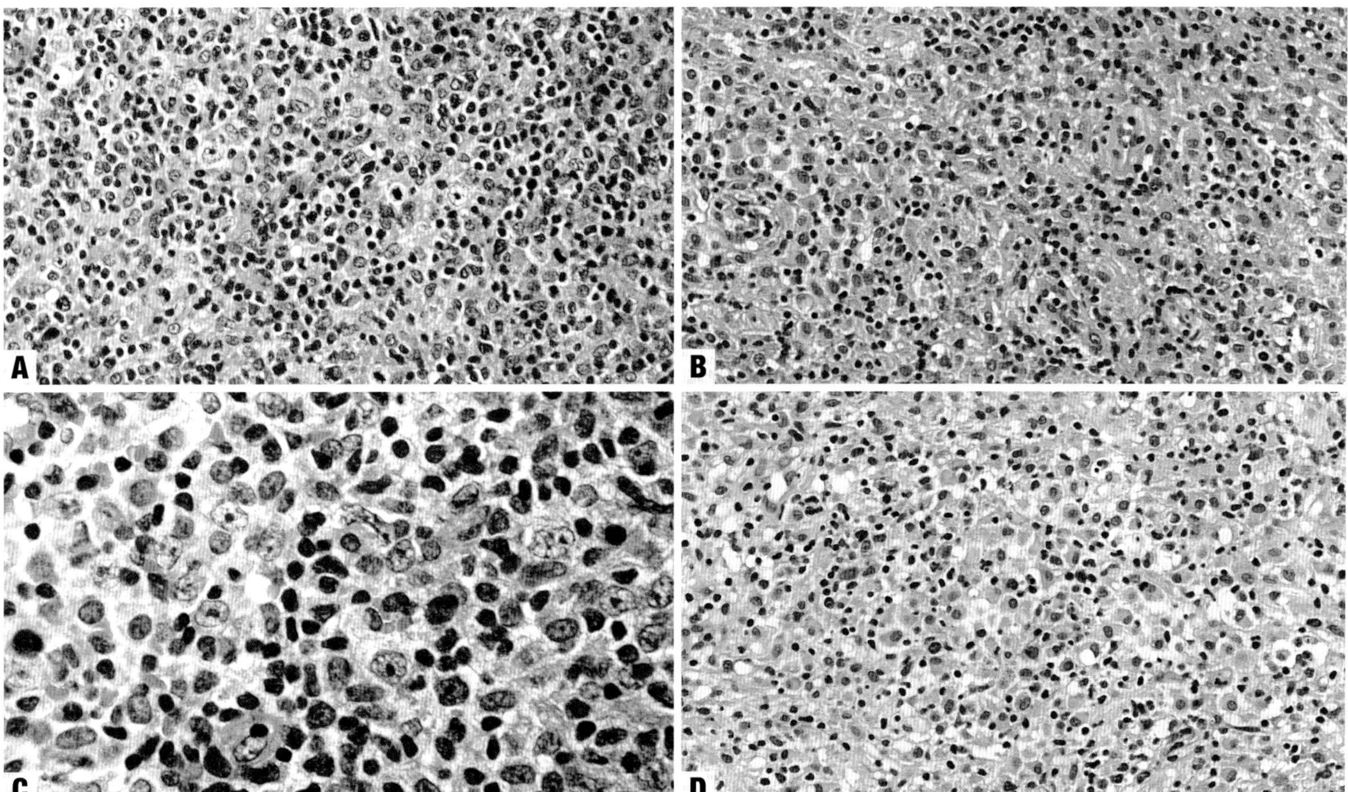

Fig. 4.158 T-cell/histiocyte–rich large B-cell lymphoma. **A** Single scattered large neoplastic cells with prominent nucleoli and partly with multilobated nuclear morphology are seen in a dense, non-neoplastic, lymphohistiocytic background. **B** Pink-appearing histiocytes mask the few pleomorphic tumour cells present. **C** Higher magnification shows pleomorphic tumour cells with atypical, partly multilobated nuclei. **D** There are abundant histiocytes, in this case with few T lymphocytes and neoplastic cells.

resemble NLPHL more than DLBCL-NOS {3053}. SEER data from the USA show a higher incidence among African Americans than among White and Asian Americans {3053}.

Etiology

Unknown

Pathogenesis

THRLBCL is derived from germinal-centre B cells with ongoing somatic hypermutation of IG genes and intraclonal diversity {449}. NLPHL and THRLBCL have been reported to occur synchronously and metachronously in occasional patients. Familial clustering of these lymphoma entities has also been reported {3500}. Microdissected tumour cells of both entities demonstrate a comparable gene expression profile {1514,477}. Recurrent genomic imbalances, such as gains of 2p16.1 (*REL* locus), are observed in both. Similarly to NLPHL variants, THRLBCL presents an overall higher number of genomic imbalances than conventional NLPHL by array comparative genomic hybridization {1515}. Both NLPHL and THRLBCL harbour mutations recurrently affecting *JUNB*, *DUSP2*, *SGK1*, *SOCS1*, and *CREBBP*, in the majority as a result of aberrant somatic hypermutation {3647, 1524}. Taken together, these data support a close pathogenetic relationship between NLPHL and THRLBCL.

The high content of macrophages/histiocytes and dendritic cells in the THRLBCL background is attributable to a tolerogenic host immune response with a prominent proinflammatory, interferon-dependent signature (IDO1, CCL8, VSIG4, STAT1, CD54 [ICAM1], CD64, and CXCL10), high IL-4 levels, and expression of metal-binding proteins (e.g. MT2A) {2466,690,4161,1525}. Although the reactive T-cell infiltrate was previously described as being composed predominantly of non-activated cytotoxic T cells {1157,424}, more recent studies using flow cytometry demonstrate a predominance of CD4+ T cells in most THRLBCLs, with a T follicular helper (TFH)-like signature observed in a subset {2155,4422}. By immunohistochemistry, the CD4:CD8 ratio of de novo THRLBCL is variable, ranging from 0.06:1 to 14.4:1 {1417,1514}, with frequent cell–cell contacts of CD8+ T cells and tumour cells {3516}. In a recent study, 64% of cases showed *CD274* (*PDL1*) / *PDCD1LG2* (*PDL2*) copy-number gains or amplifications and increased PDL1 expression {1417}.

Macroscopic appearance

The lymph node is enlarged, with a homogeneous greyish appearance and without an evident nodular pattern.

Histopathology

There is diffuse or vaguely nodular effacement of the lymph node architecture {19}. At low magnification, the involved tissue has a characteristic pale eosinophilic appearance attributable to the background histiocytic population that is also mixed with small T cells. In contrast, eosinophils and plasma cells are rarely encountered. The neoplastic large B cells are randomly scattered, without formation of aggregates or sheets. They range in

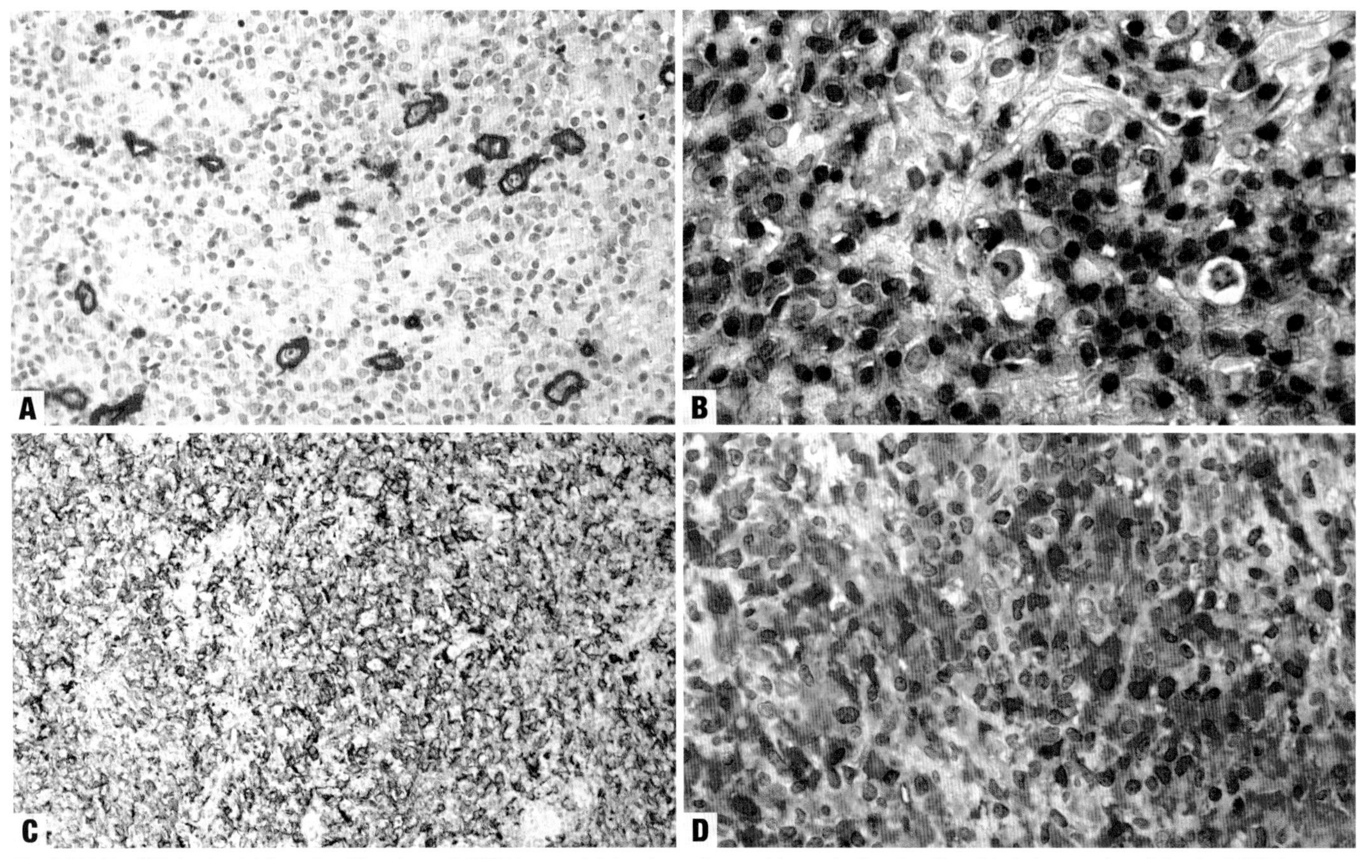

Fig. 4.159 T-cell/histiocyte–rich large B-cell lymphoma. **A** CD20 immunostaining shows pleomorphic neoplastic cells with a virtual absence of small B cells. **B** CD3 immunostaining highlights abundant small reactive T cells in the microenvironment. **C** Abundant CD163-positive macrophages. **D** Histiocytes express nuclear and cytoplasmic MT2A, indicating the metal-binding properties of these particular histiocytes.

appearance from lymphocyte-predominant cells, centroblasts, and immunoblasts to HRS-like cells {20,2345,4053}. Foci of necrosis with large cells persisting in perivascular locations and marked fibrosis may be seen. Bone marrow involvement by THRLBCL can be diffuse or show a nodular, intertrabecular or paratrabecular pattern. In the spleen, a micronodular pattern of white pulp involvement, sometimes with coalescent nodules in a fibrotic stroma, has been described {979}. In the liver, portal tracts are infiltrated and irregularly expanded.

Immunophenotype

The neoplastic cells express pan–B-cell markers (CD20, CD79a, PAX5, OCT2), CD45, MEF2B, and BCL6, and variably express IRF4 (MUM1) and EMA {2765,2345,19}. CD30, CD10, CD15, PU.1, and IgD are rarely positive {3292,2528}, and EBV is absent. Cases formerly labelled as EBV-positive THRLBCL should be diagnosed as EBV-positive diffuse large B-cell lymphoma {2954}.

The microenvironment contains high numbers of CD68+ and CD163+ histiocytes {1525}, as well as CD3+ T cells. Characteristically, there is a virtual absence of small B cells (typically < 5%, although no validated cut-off point has been established). Follicular dendritic cell (FDC) meshworks (CD21+ or CD23+) are absent.

Differential diagnosis

The main differential diagnoses of THRLBCL includes NLPHL, EBV+ DLBCL, peripheral T-cell lymphoma, and classic Hodgkin lymphoma (CHL). Distinction of THRLBCL from NLPHL can be impossible in core needle biopsy specimens. There is no immunophenotypic or molecular marker that specifically distinguishes between these entities, and their separation largely relies on the clinical presentation and the presence of at least one unequivocal nodule in NLPHL. The presence of residual IgD+ mantle cells, an abundant population of T cells expressing TFH markers (PD1, CD57) with rosettes around neoplastic B lymphocytes, and partially preserved CD21/CD23+ FDC meshworks favour NLPHL over THRLBCL. Composite cases that contain unequivocal areas of NLPHL should be classified as NLPHL variant. Cases that do not have evidence of NLPHL may still have an unsampled NLPHL component.

EBV+ DLBCL can be morphologically indistinguishable from THRLBCL. It may show scattered or small clusters of EBV+ cells resembling immunoblasts, lymphocyte-predominant cells, or HRS-like cells in a background rich in histiocytes and T cells {2755,3034,2954,3092,1612}. Thus, EBV-encoded small RNA (EBER) in situ hybridization or at least LMP1 immunohistochemical staining is mandatory in the workup of patients with suspected THRLBCL.

In the distinction of THRLBCL from nodal peripheral T-cell lymphoma with TFH phenotype, special attention should be given to the morphological atypia of T cells, the presence of numerous CD30+ T cells in the microenvironment {1520}, the expression of CD10 {2795} and other TFH markers by T cells, a hyperplastic FDC meshwork, and demonstration of a monoclonal TR gene rearrangement to substantiate the diagnosis of a nodal TFH cell lymphoma.

THRLBCL may also mimic CHL, mainly lymphocyte-depleted or mixed-cellularity subtypes, which often contain abundant histiocytes. Staining for CD20 and CD15 is helpful, because HRS cells of CHL are CD20− or variably weakly CD20+ and variably CD15+, as opposed to the neoplastic cells in THRLBCL, which are homogeneously CD20+/CD15− and additionally express other B-cell antigens. Furthermore, MEF2B, BCL6, and weak/variable IRF4 (MUM1) positivity, as well as an absence of GATA3, are helpful in the diagnosis of THRLBCL. In addition, THRLBCL lacks eosinophils and remnants of B-cell nodules often present in CHL.

Cytology

The diagnosis of THRLBCL cannot be reliably made on cytological specimens.

Diagnostic molecular pathology

The neoplastic B cells show monoclonally rearranged IG genes, although these may not be demonstrable in cases with low numbers of neoplastic B cells. TR genes are in the germline configuration.

Essential and desirable diagnostic criteria

Essential: diffuse effacement of lymph node architecture; singly scattered large B cells, without formation of aggregates or sheets; reactive background rich in histiocytes and small T cells, with no (or few) scattered small B cells; absence of FDC meshworks by CD21 or CD23 stain; absence of NLPHL.

Desirable: lymph node excision is preferred; exclude EBV association.

Staging

Staging is performed using the Lugano classification.

Prognosis and prediction

THRLBCL is an aggressive lymphoma, often refractory to chemotherapy, with a 5-year overall survival of 66% {1960,1517,1129}. The International Prognostic Index (IPI) score is highly correlated with the prognosis. Heterogeneous clinical behaviour has been described in the literature, probably due to heterogeneous diagnostic criteria.

Diffuse large B-cell lymphoma / high-grade B-cell lymphoma with *MYC* and *BCL2* rearrangements

Tooze RM
Barrans SL
Davies AJ
Dunleavy K
Gopal AK
Lenz G
Leoncini L
Li S
Macon WR
Momose S
Rosenwald A
Tamaru J

Definition

Diffuse large B-cell lymphoma / high-grade B-cell lymphoma with *MYC* and *BCL2* rearrangements (DLBCL/HGBCL-*MYC/BCL2*) is an aggressive mature B-cell lymphoma with structural chromosomal aberrations with breakpoints at both *MYC* and *BCL2* loci.

ICD-O coding

9680/3 Diffuse large B-cell lymphoma / high grade B-cell lymphoma with *MYC* and *BCL2* rearrangements

ICD-11 coding

2A81.Y & XH23Z3 Other specified diffuse large B-cell lymphomas & High-grade B-cell lymphoma with *MYC* and *BCL2* and/or *BCL6* rearrangements

Related terminology

Acceptable: high-grade B-cell lymphoma with *MYC* and *BCL2* rearrangements; high-grade B-cell lymphoma with *MYC*, *BCL2*, and *BCL6* rearrangements.

Subtype(s)

DLBCL/HGBCL-*MYC/BCL2* without *BCL6* rearrangement; DLBCL/HGBCL-*MYC/BCL2* with *BCL6* rearrangement; DLBCL/HGBCL-*MYC/BCL2* (with or without *BCL6* rearrangement) with TdT expression

Localization

Advanced-stage disease at diagnosis occurs in the majority of patients {189,3471}. Although the lymph nodes are most commonly involved, a high proportion (30–88%) of cases show in addition involvement of more than one extranodal site. Bone marrow and CNS dissemination is not infrequent.

Clinical features

A high proportion of patients present with a high International Prognostic Index (IPI) score due to advanced-stage disease (stage III–IV according to the Lugano system) {688}, a high LDH level, and extranodal involvement {2310,2228}. Clinical features may reflect extranodal site involvement (e.g. bone marrow and CNS). Adoption of routine FISH testing for DLBCL/HGBCL at many institutes has identified increased numbers of patients with DLBCL/HGBCL-*MYC/BCL2*, including some with earlier stage and lower-risk disease who probably have a less adverse outcome {245,3177,3326,4046}.

Epidemiology

In European and North American cohorts, *MYC*-rearranged diffuse large B-cell lymphoma (DLBCL) represented 11–12% of DLBCL cases, of which 39% were DLBCL/HGBCL-*MYC/BCL2* and 12–14% DLBCL/HGBCL-*MYC/BCL2* with an additional *BCL6* rearrangement {3657,3471}. DLBCL/HGBCL-*MYC/BCL2* represents 3.5–9.9% of DLBCL cases {3657,189,2135,3471}. The relative frequency may differ in other populations, but evidence is limited {4560,4083}. Most patients with DLBCL/

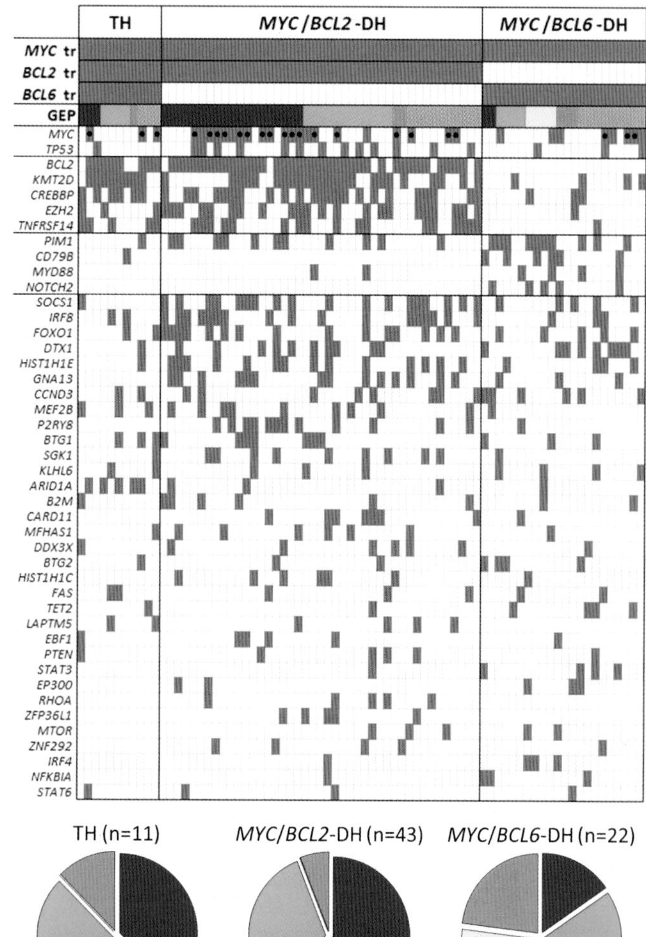

Fig. 4.160 Diffuse large B-cell lymphoma / high-grade B-cell lymphoma with *MYC* and *BCL2* rearrangements. The mutation and gene expression features are displayed, based on modified cell-of-origin classification of a representative cohort of diffuse large B-cell lymphomas with double-hit (DH) or triple-hit (TH) status. The upper panel displays the division of cases by translocation status into triple-hit, double-hit *MYC/BCL2*, and double-hit *MYC/BCL6*, as indicated. Beneath this is the gene expression–based classification per case into cell-of-origin classes, including molecular high-grade classification, followed by the mutation pattern for a lymphoma target gene panel as indicated on the left (red squares identify the presence of mutation, and black dots identify hotspot mutations in *MYC*). The pie charts beneath illustrate the relative proportions of cell-of-origin and molecular high-grade (MHG) classifications as identified in the colour code beneath {848}. ABC, activated B-cell–like gene expression signature; GCB, germinal centre B-cell–like gene expression signature; GEP, gene expression profiling; Mut/tr, mutation/translocation; N/A, not available; UNC, unclassified gene expression signature.

HGBCL-*MYC/BCL2* are in their seventh decade of life and beyond, and younger adults are affected less frequently. There is a male preponderance. The incidence is approximately 0.3–0.8 cases per 100 000 person-years {2310,189,3471}.

Etiology

Unknown

Pathogenesis

DLBCL/HGBCL-*MYC/BCL2*, by definition, harbours two oncogenic rearrangements: one targeting *MYC* and one targeting *BCL2*. Their often aggressive behaviour is postulated to be the result of aberrant expression of BCL2, leading to increased apoptotic resistance, and MYC activation, driving proliferation. The normal counterpart of DLBCL/HGBCL-*MYC/BCL2* is postulated to be a mature germinal centre–experienced B cell, with a high IGHV mutation load {189}. *BCL2* (18q21) is primarily translocated to IGH (14q32) {189,644,732}. *MYC* (8q24) translocation is more diverse and is to IG loci in 55–58% of cases – predominantly IGH, alternatively IGL via t(8;22)(q24;q11), or, more rarely, IGK via t(2;8)(p11;q24) {644,1815,732,3471}. *MYC* non-IG partners include *BCL6*, the *PAX5* enhancer region of *ZCCHC7*, and *RFTN1* {337,1815,732}. *BCL6*::*MYC* reciprocal translocations are of note, because these represent a proportion of the cases previously designated as having triple-hit status (now considered pseudo–triple-hit) as well as some cases of DLBCL/HGBCL with *MYC* and *BCL6* rearrangements (pseudo–*MYC/BCL6* double-hit) {1815}. However, the relative frequency of reciprocal *BCL6*::*MYC* translocations and the impact on *MYC* and *BCL6* locus regulation remain undetermined {4555}. *MYC* translocation to IG or non-IG loci is secondary to *BCL2* translocation and is most likely acquired in the germinal-centre reaction, but evidence of established follicular lymphoma is reported in only 20–35% {2310,189,3176,848,4245}.

Complex karyotypes are common {2241,388,3769,189,2135}. By sequencing, DLBCL/HGBCL-*MYC/BCL2* shows frequent mutations of genes typically altered in follicular lymphoma, such as *BCL2*, *KMT2D*, *CREBBP*, *EZH2*, and *TNFRSF14*, as well as *MYC* {848}. Consequently, DLBCL/HGBCL-*MYC/BCL2* is mostly concordant with the DLBCL molecular subgroups referred to as EZB cluster, C3 cluster, or BCL2 cluster in the respective molecular classification systems {3629,644,2191,4417}. DLBCL/HGBCL-*MYC/BCL2* mutation features are shared with follicular lymphoma and transformed follicular lymphoma {3040,848}.

Related gene expression signatures such as the double-hit signature (DHITsig) and molecular high-grade (MHG) signature have been shown to identify DLBCL/HGBCL-*MYC/BCL2* {1683,3686,1080}. They are also expressed in Burkitt lymphoma, pointing to the fact that they capture particular biological features related to the dark zone of the germinal centre, recently also corroborated by single-cell transcriptomic analyses {1618,4077}. Therefore, it was proposed that the DHIT signature be renamed the "dark-zone signature" {65}. Of interest, only 50% of dark-zone and MHG signature–positive cases harbour the *MYC/BCL2* double hit. In some of these cases, tumours with cryptic translocations have been identified, but in the majority a *MYC/BCL2* dual translocation or an evident surrogate thereof is absent {1587,848}.

Diffuse large B-cell lymphoma / high-grade B-cell lymphoma NOS with MYC and BCL6 rearrangements

DLBCL/HGBCL-*MYC/BCL2* represents a homogeneous pathological entity whose pathogenesis has a close relationship to that of follicular lymphoma and related molecular DLBCL subtypes {3657,1080,848,4417}. In contrast, DLBCL/HGBCL with *MYC* and *BCL6* translocations, but lacking *BCL2* translocation, diverges from DLBCL/HGBCL-*MYC/BCL2* in patterns of presentation {3241,3640,2643,2443}, frequent non–germinal-centre B-cell immunohistochemistry phenotypes, and activated

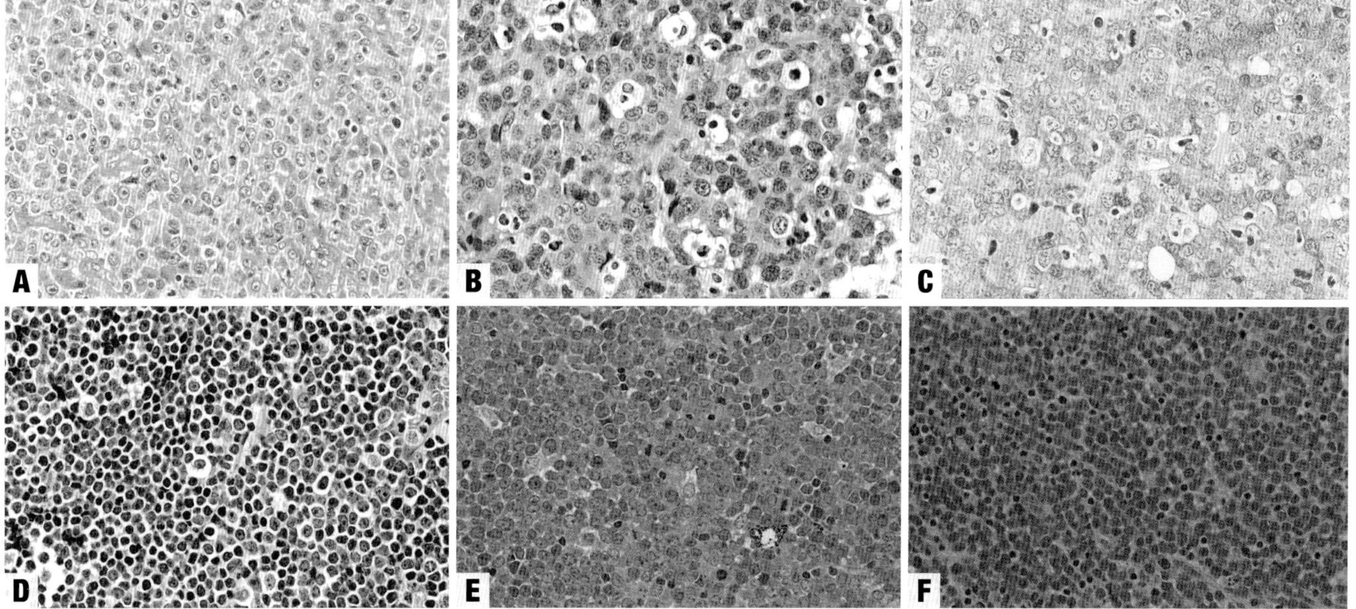

Fig. 4.161 Diffuse large B-cell lymphoma / high-grade B-cell lymphoma with *MYC* and *BCL2* rearrangements. Diffuse large B-cell lymphoma / large cell morphology seen with H&E at lower (**A**) and higher (**B**) magnification, and with Giemsa (**C**). High-grade B-cell lymphoma morphology with a monotonous appearance and tumour cells of intermediate size seen at lower (**D**) and higher (**E**) magnification. A monotonous blastoid morphology with an intermediate tumour cell size is observed (**F**).

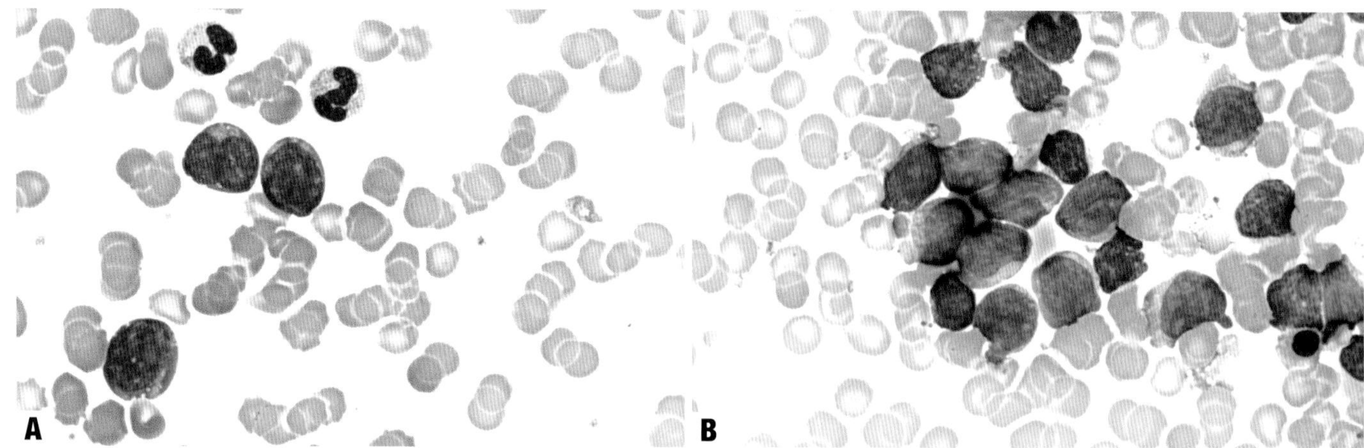

Fig. 4.162 Diffuse large B-cell lymphoma / high-grade B-cell lymphoma with *MYC* and *BCL2* rearrangements. Cytological smears show large blastoid cells in the peripheral blood (**A**) and a dense infiltrate in the bone marrow (**B**).

B-cell–like gene expression profiles {189,2216,3657,848}. In addition, it shows infrequent mutations of epigenetic regulators linking DLBCL/HGBCL-*MYC/BCL2*, follicular lymphoma, and the EZB DLBCL cluster, but instead shows a more varied pattern, including mutations in genes such as *PIM1* and *CD79B* that have been linked to the ABC-DLBCL subtype {644,848}. Because the current evidence points to a heterogeneous biology with variable gene expression profiles and mutation spectra, these cases are excluded from the DLBCL/HGBCL-*MYC/BCL2* entity and are included in DLBCL-NOS or HGBCL-NOS. Their presence, however, should be reported to allow for their inclusion into ongoing clinical trials. In addition, such cases have shown variable risk association in different series {797, 2307,2216,4494,764,2624,3471}.

Other double hits and copy-number aberrations without rearrangements

MYC translocations in the absence of a *MYC/BCL2* double-hit context occur in various lymphoma entities in isolation or with other events, such as *CCND1* translocations in mantle cell lymphoma or gain of non-rearranged *BCL2* or mutation/deletion of *TP53* {764,3657,3471} in DLBCL-NOS. Multiple characteristics linked to *MYC* translocation, such as *MYC* hotspot mutations that enhance MYC protein stability, identify high-risk disease {3471,764,3657,1080,3686,848}. Similarly, amplification of *BCL2* in the context of *MYC* translocation and low- or high-level amplifications of the *MYC* locus in cases with *BCL2* translocations enrich for high-risk DLBCL {2314,3326,2135}. Nevertheless, neither single-nucleotide nor copy-number variants constitute oncogenic hits defining this entity in the absence of a bona fide chromosomal breakpoint, because, for example, *MYC* amplifications are not associated with equivalent mRNA or protein expression to that of *MYC*-translocated cases and therefore do not justify classification as DLBCL/HGBCL-*MYC/BCL2* {780}.

Macroscopic appearance

Not applicable

Histopathology

The growth pattern is diffuse and the underlying tissue architecture is effaced. A DLBCL morphology is most frequent, and a starry-sky pattern is present in some cases. Mitotic figures and apoptosis are variable. Some cases show a morphology intermediate between that of DLBCL and Burkitt lymphoma, characterized by medium-sized to large cells showing prominent mitotic and apoptotic figures, often accompanied by starry-sky macrophages. Other cases represent the blastoid variant, which resemble lymphoblasts with medium-sized cells, scant cytoplasm, round nuclei with finely distributed chromatin, and occasional small nucleoli {1972}. Relative to DLBCL morphology, a higher frequency of dual *MYC* and *BCL2* translocations has been reported in intermediate or blastoid morphologies (reported ranges: 23–50% and 64–75% of cases, respectively) {189,2724, 1862,2763}. However, because the distinction between the intermediate and blastoid morphologies is not highly reproducible, these alternative morphologies can be grouped under the single term "intermediate/blastoid". Reporting should be performed according to a layering strategy, with morphological classification as the root and genetic information added when this becomes available in the diagnostic process: diffuse large B-cell lymphoma with *MYC* and *BCL2* rearrangements or high-grade B-cell lymphoma with *MYC* and *BCL2* rearrangements.

Immunohistochemistry

DLBCL/HGBCL-*MYC/BCL2* expresses the pan–B-cell antigens CD19, CD20, CD79a, and PAX5. CD10 is positive in 88–98%, BCL6 in 75–89%, and IRF4 (MUM1) in 17–42% {190}. Consequently, 91–99% of these tumours have a germinal-centre B-cell (GCB)-like phenotype, according to the Hans cell-of-origin classifier {1490,190,1666,2624}. Most express MYC (78–86%) and BCL2 (90–95%) proteins, with 71–81% expressing both (dual-expressers), based on thresholds of ≥ 40% and ≥ 50%, respectively, to define positivity {190,4311,1666,2624}. The Ki-67 (MIB1) proliferation index is high (range: 50–100%, median: 90%) {190}, but a low proliferation index does not exclude DLBCL/HGBCL-*MYC/BCL2* {2763}. EBV infection and varying amounts of EBER-positive tumour cells do not exclude the diagnosis, but they are rare {2377}. Approximately 2% of DLBCL/HGBCL-*MYC/BCL2* cases have been reported to contain TdT-positive tumour B cells ranging from rare positive cells to near-uniform expression. Such cases may be CD20-weak/negative and lack expression of BCL6 and/or light chains, indicating a more immature phenotype {2381,4265,345}.

Differential diagnosis

Cases of DLBCL/HGBCL-*MYC/BCL2* may morphologically resemble Burkitt lymphoma, which is excluded by identification of a *MYC* and *BCL2* dual translocation.

There are no reliable criteria for predicting DLBCL/HGBCL-*MYC/BCL2* by DLBCL morphology. Therefore, evaluation of *MYC* and *BCL2* (and *BCL6*) translocation status is advocated in all aggressive B-cell lymphomas.

Follicular lymphomas with coincident *MYC* and *BCL2* translocations are by definition excluded from this category, as are rare cases of other defined large B-cell lymphoma entities with incidental *MYC* and *BCL2* translocations {2677,2702,650}. Cases of DLBCL/HGBCL-*MYC/BCL2* with antecedent or concurrent follicular lymphoma should be reported as "DLBCL/HGBCL with *MYC* and *BCL2* rearrangements, transformed from follicular lymphoma" {345}.

Very rare B-lymphoblastic leukaemias/lymphomas (B-ALL/LBLs) have *MYC* and *BCL2* dual translocations and are seen particularly in the paediatric / young adult setting {2381,4265}. Young age is more suggestive of B-ALL/LBL, but the differentiation from DLBCL/HGBCL-*MYC/BCL2* remains challenging. Distinction on immunohistochemistry phenotype alone is not advised, but flow cytometric phenotyping to distinguish between the precursor and mature B-cell states (e.g. CD34) may be helpful {4265}. Molecular analysis may support the distinction, because *MYC*-rearranged B-ALL/LBL shows IG::*MYC* translocations, implicating V(D)J recombination at the IGH locus, and carries unmutated IGHV rearrangements and *NRAS* or *KRAS* mutations while lacking mutations observed in Burkitt lymphoma and DLBCL/HGBCL-*MYC/BCL2* {4265}. The blastoid variant may raise the differential diagnosis of mantle cell lymphoma, and immunostaining for CD5 and cyclin D1/SOX11 should be performed to exclude it.

The occurrence of a dual *MYC* and *BCL2* translocation in primary CNS large B-cell lymphomas is extremely uncommon {2981}. Therefore, exclusion of secondary involvement of the CNS from systemic disease is essential.

MYC translocations and MYC/BCL2 dual expression are reported in some cases of primary cutaneous DLBCL, leg type. However, those cases predominantly show dual *MYC* and *BCL6* translocations and therefore do not form part of the DLBCL/HGBCL-*MYC/BCL2* {2643,3640,2443}.

Chapter 4

Cytology

There are no specific cytological features of DLBCL/HGBCL-*MYC/BCL2* relative to DLBCL or HGBCL lacking translocations. Aspiration cytology, therefore, is not advised for diagnosis.

Diagnostic molecular pathology

Because DLBCL/HGBCL-*MYC/BCL2* is a genetically defined tumour, all B-cell lymphomas that could potentially fall within this category should be evaluated for gene rearrangement status. A sequential strategy starting with evaluation of *MYC* translocation is advised. If FISH is applied, a low (< 5%) false negative rate has to be acknowledged {3657} (e.g. attributable to incomplete probe coverage of *MYC* breakpoints or cryptic rearrangements with variant molecular configurations) {2841, 732}. The finding of a *MYC* rearrangement should then trigger

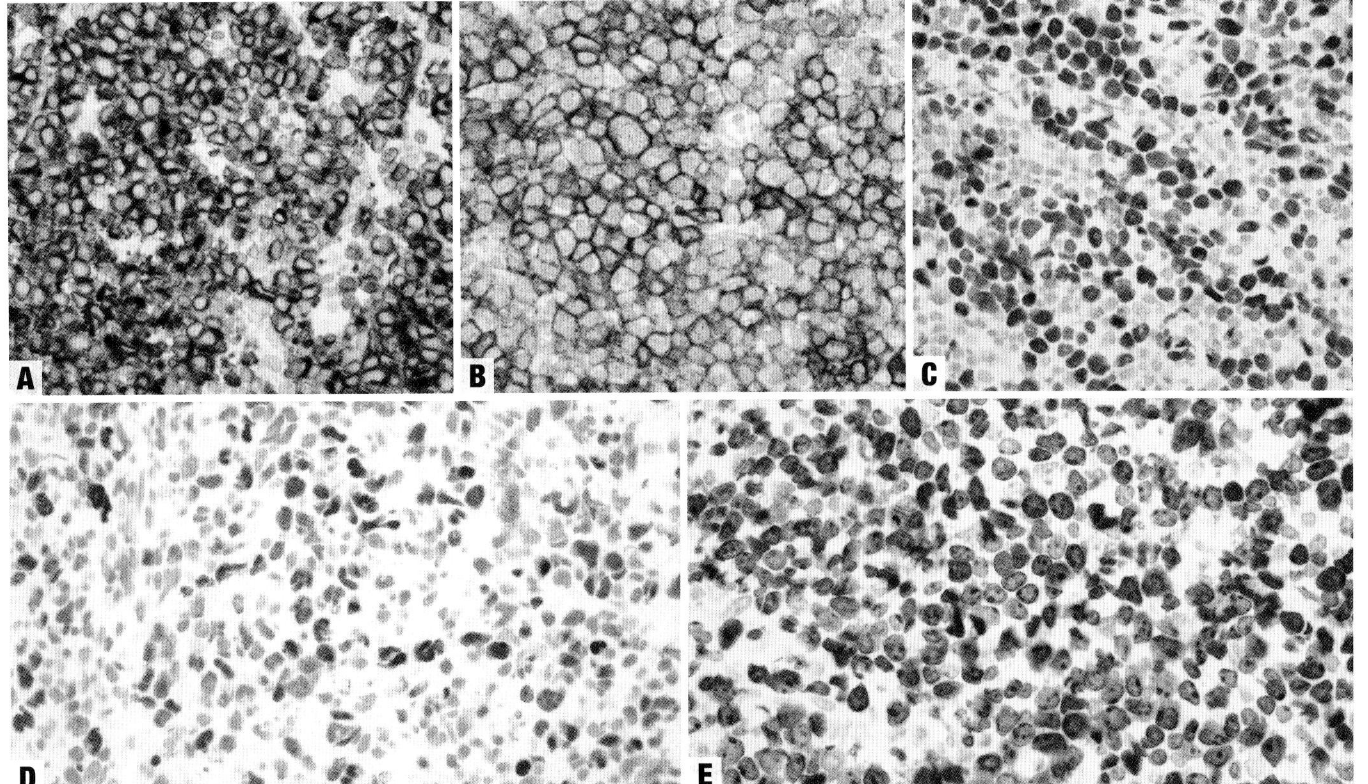

Fig. 4.163 Diffuse large B-cell lymphoma / high-grade B-cell lymphoma with *MYC*, *BCL2*, and *BCL6* rearrangement and *MYC* translocated to non-IG partner. Immunohistochemistry showing diffuse BCL2 expression (**A**), CD10 expression (**B**), BCL6 expression (**C**), and MYC expression in part of the tumour cells with varying intensity (**D**). **E** A high Ki-67 proliferation index is seen.

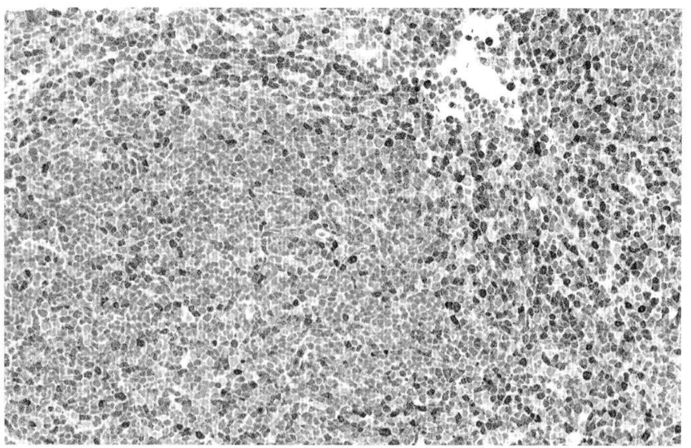

Fig. 4.164 Diffuse large B-cell lymphoma / high-grade B-cell lymphoma with *MYC* and *BCL2* rearrangements. TdT expression can be observed in tumour cells in some cases.

the evaluation of: (1) *BCL2* (and *BCL6*) rearrangement status, (2) *MYC* translocation partner {3471}.

Immunohistochemical pre-screening strategies

There is no current universally accepted and highly predictive immunohistochemical screening tool for determining which DLBCL/HGBCL cases should undergo *MYC* translocation analysis. Using GCB cell-of-origin immunohistochemistry testing would reduce *MYC* testing to about 52% of all DLBCLs while potentially detecting ≥ 99% of DLBCL-*MYC/BCL2* cases {3657}. Using GCB cell-of-origin immunohistochemistry testing together with MYC and BCL2 dual expression as a selection criterion for *MYC* FISH testing would reduce testing to 13% of DLBCL cases and achieve a 35% positive predictive value {3657}. Moderate to strong MYC protein expression in > 70% of neoplastic cells has been reported to be highly predictive of presence of *MYC* translocation {102,3176,4587}. However, false negative immunohistochemistry can occur, due to weak MYC mRNA expression despite translocation or due to genetic polymorphisms {780}.

Adverse risk in DLBCL/HGBCL-*MYC/BCL2* has been linked to IG::*MYC* translocations {3471}. Depending on the clinical consequences, testing for fusion of *MYC* to IGH, if negative, can be followed by testing of fusions to IGK or IGL loci. *MYC* translocation to a non-IG partner can be reported where all three IG loci have been excluded as fusion partners of *MYC*, with an optional statement that this may indicate a less adverse outcome.

Essential and desirable diagnostic criteria

Essential: morphology and phenotype consistent with an aggressive B-cell lymphoma; evidence of concurrent *MYC* and *BCL2* rearrangements (with or without *BCL6* rearrangement).

Desirable: GCB phenotype; TdT protein expression status; determination of *MYC* fusion partner.

Staging

The Lugano system is used to stage these lymphomas {688}.

Prognosis and prediction

DLBCL/HGBCL-*MYC/BCL2* is characterized by an aggressive clinical course. Immunochemotherapy with R-CHOP is associated with poor outcomes, with 4/5-year overall survival rates of about 40–50% {2191,2228}. As a result, there are advocates for dose-intensified regimens, but there is a paucity of prospective and randomized studies to inform optimal approaches {3213, 2313,2214,1020,4046,610,2228}. The *MYC* translocation partner (IG::*MYC*), TdT expression, and *MYC* hotspot mutation may select further for higher risk within DLBCL/HGBCL-*MYC/BCL2* {1080,3686,3471,848}, but their impact on treatment choice is unclear.

ALK-positive large B-cell lymphoma

Medeiros LJ
Delabie J
Farinha P
Molina TJ
Sengar M
Takeuchi K
Wang HY

Definition

Anaplastic lymphoma kinase–positive large B-cell lymphoma (ALK+ LBCL) is a diffuse, monomorphic neoplasm of large B cells with a plasmablastic immunophenotype and ALK expression due to *ALK* rearrangement.

ICD-O coding

9737/3 ALK-positive large B-cell lymphoma

ICD-11 coding

2A81.8 ALK-positive large B-cell lymphoma

Related terminology

Not recommended: ALK-positive plasmablastic B-cell lymphoma; ALK-positive diffuse large B-cell lymphoma (obsolete).

Subtype(s)

None

Localization

ALK+ LBCL arises in lymph nodes in roughly 75% of cases, with frequent involvement of cervical lymph nodes. A variety of extranodal sites have been reported, among them the upper aerodigestive tract, brain, gastrointestinal tract, liver, and spleen {1804,571}.

Clinical features

Patients may present with asymptomatic lymphadenopathy or may have symptoms attributable to a tumour mass {2234, 3121,3876,571}. Approximately half to two thirds of patients have B symptoms. Serum LDH and B2M levels are commonly elevated. Patients may have localized or widely disseminated disease. Staging bone marrow evaluation is positive in 25–35% of patients, and two thirds of patients have a high International Prognostic Index (IPI) score {2234,571}.

Epidemiology

ALK+ LBCL is uncommon and represents < 1% of large B-cell lymphomas. Since its original description in 1997 {926}, a total of 184 cases have been reported, as summarized in a recent review {571}. There is a wide age range (9–85 years), with a median of 35–38 years {3121,571}. The M:F ratio is 3–4:1 {3876, 571}. There is no known association with immunodeficiency.

Etiology

Unknown

Pathogenesis

Translocations, inversions, and insertions involving *ALK* at chromosome 2p23 play an essential role in pathogenesis. A total of 10 molecular alterations have been described, and seven partners of *ALK* translocation are known {3064,3485,3945,2261, 3533,1739} (see Table 4.31, p. 431). By far the most common is t(2;17)(p23;q23), involving clathrin (*CLTC*). ALK is a tyrosine kinase that is constitutively activated by these molecular alterations. Activated ALK triggers many cellular signalling pathways involved in transformation, growth, and inhibition of apoptosis, including the JAK/STAT, PI3K/AKT, MAPK/ERK, and PLCG2 pathways {4138,571}. Gains or amplifications of *MYC* occur in about 50% of cases {4138}.

Macroscopic appearance

ALK+ LBCL appears as a tumour mass that has a fish-flesh appearance. Haemorrhage and/or necrosis can be present.

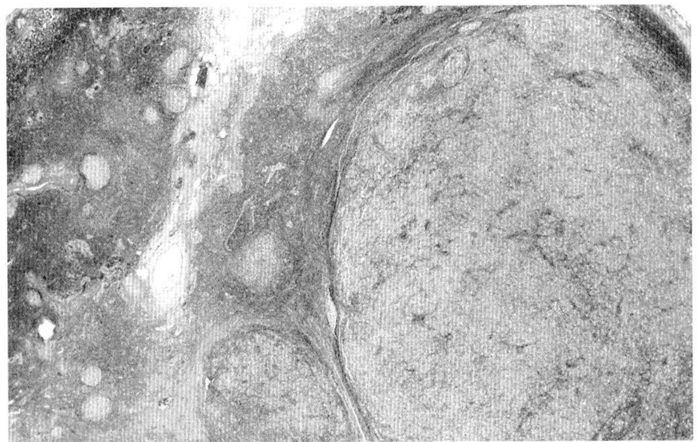

Fig. 4.165 ALK-positive large B-cell lymphoma. The neoplastic infiltrate partially replaces the lymph node parenchyma (right side).

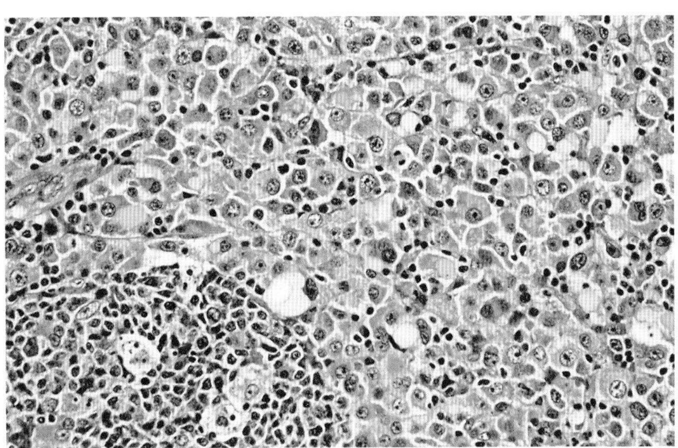

Fig. 4.166 ALK-positive large B-cell lymphoma. The neoplastic cells extensively replace lymph node structures (reactive germinal centre at lower left). They show plasmablastic features with abundant eosinophilic cytoplasm and eccentrically located nuclei.

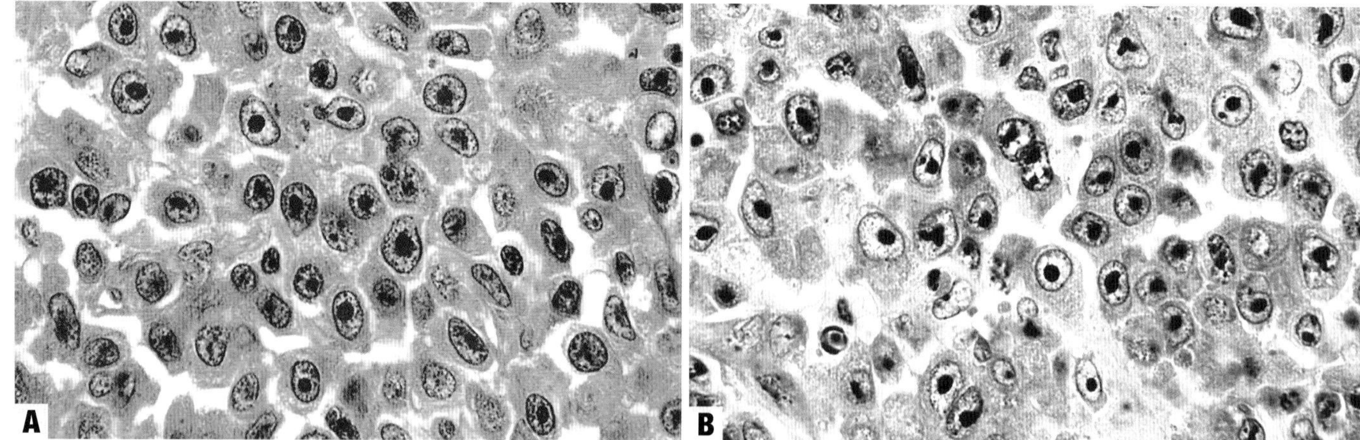

Fig. 4.167 ALK-positive large B-cell lymphoma. High magnification shows neoplastic cells with large central nuclei, prominent nucleoli, and abundant cytoplasm. **A** H&E. **B** Giemsa.

Histopathology

ALK+ LBCL usually replaces the normal architecture diffusely, but in lymph nodes one third of cases show a sinusoidal pattern of involvement {3121,3876}. The neoplastic cells are monomorphic and large, with abundant amphophilic or eosinophilic cytoplasm. These cells can have central nuclei and prominent nucleoli resembling immunoblasts, or they can have abundant cytoplasm with eccentrically located nuclei more in keeping with plasmablasts. Infrequently, the lymphoma cells show anaplastic features, and giant HRS-like cells can be present {3121}. Apoptosis is often brisk and mitotic figures numerous. Necrosis is present in about 20% of cases.

Immunohistochemistry

The neoplastic cells are positive for ALK and the pattern of staining correlates with the type of *ALK* rearrangement (see Table 4.31), with cytoplasmic granular staining being most common.

The neoplastic cells have a plasmablastic immunophenotype: positive for plasma cell markers such as CD138, IRF4 (MUM1), VS38c, Blimp1, and XBP1 and most often negative for CD20. CD20 can be variable, however, and is weakly positive in 10–15% of cases. The lymphoma cells also express EMA, BOB1, OCT2, CD45RB (can be weak), cytoplasmic immunoglobulin (IgA > IgG; lambda > kappa), MYC, and activated STAT3 (nuclear and/or phosphorylated) {2234,4138,3533,571}. CD4, CD10, CD38, CD43, and/or CD57 have been reported in 40–50% of cases, but often variably and/or weakly. Infrequently, cases can be positive for PAX5 (~20%), CD79a (~20%), BCL6 (~20%), CD15 (~20%), CD30 (~15%), and keratins (~15%). Perforin has been positive in a few cases assessed {3814,4325}. The lymphoma cells are negative for CD19, CD22, cyclin D1, and BCL2. There is no evidence of infection by EBV or KSHV/HHV8 {3533,571}.

Table 4.31 *ALK* abnormalities and immunohistochemical staining pattern in ALK+ large B-cell lymphoma

Known or theoretical cytogenetic abnormality	*ALK* partner	ALK immunostaining pattern
t(2;17)(p23;q23)	*CLTC*	Cytoplasmic; granular
t(2;5)(p23;q35.3)	*SQSTM1*	Cytoplasmic; diffuse
t(2;5)(p23;q35)	*NPM1*	Nuclear and cytoplasmic
inv(2)(p23q13) or t(2;2)(p23;q13)	*RANBP2*	Nuclear membrane and perinuclear punctate
inv(2)(p21p23)	*EML4*	Cytoplasmic; diffuse
inv(2)(p21q31.1) or t(2;2)(p23;q31.1)	*GORASP2*	Cytoplasmic; diffuse
Cryptic	*SEC31A*	Cytoplasmic; granular
t(X;2)(q21;q23)	Unknown	Cytoplasmic; granular
t(2;12)(p23;q24.1)	Unknown	Cytoplasmic; granular
Insertion of 3′ *ALK* into 4q22-24	Unknown	Cytoplasmic; granular

Differential diagnosis

The differential diagnosis includes other lymphomas with plasmablastic features, such as plasmablastic lymphoma, KSHV/HHV8-positive diffuse large B-cell lymphoma, and primary effusion lymphoma.

Cytology

In FNA smears the neoplastic cells are large and have abundant cytoplasm, large nuclei, and macronucleoli {3537}. Mitotic

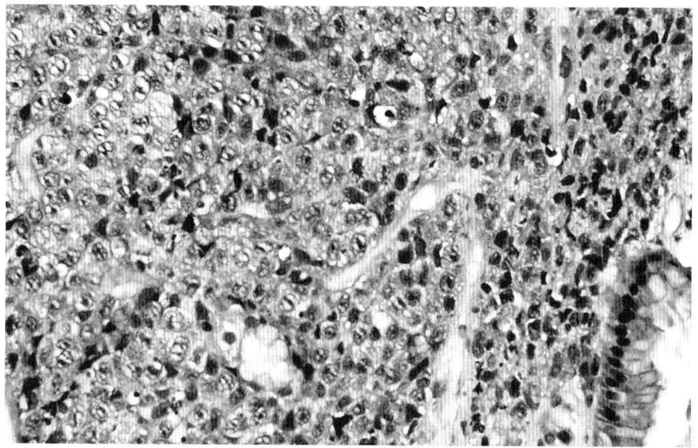

Fig. 4.168 ALK-positive large B-cell lymphoma. A case presenting in the gastrointestinal tract (benign epithelium at lower right of field) shows a large component of tumour cells with immunoblast-like features.

figures are usually present, and the lymphoma cells often appear cohesive.

Diagnostic molecular pathology

The IG genes are monoclonally rearranged in most cases, and the TR genes are germline. *ALK* is rearranged.

Essential and desirable diagnostic criteria

Essential: large cell morphology; plasmablastic immunophenotype; ALK expression.

Desirable: *ALK* genetic alterations (usually translocations); no EBV association.

Staging

The Lugano system is used to stage lymphomas and has been adopted by the Union for International Cancer Control (UICC) TNM classification {688}. About 40% of patients have localized disease (stage I or II) and 60% have advanced disease (stage III or IV).

Prognosis and prediction

Patients are treated with systemic chemotherapy, usually the CHOP (cyclophosphamide, doxorubicin, vincristine, and prednisone) regimen {2234,571}. As these neoplasms are usually CD20-negative, rituximab is not indicated. There is likely to be a role for ALK inhibitors in future therapeutic regimens, but at present, experience using ALK inhibitors is mostly anecdotal {4325,4562}.

The median overall survival time of patients with ALK+ LBCL is < 2 years, and the 5-year overall survival rate is 28% {571}. Children and patients with localized disease have a better survival. Older patients, those with advanced-stage disease, and those with combined nodal and extranodal disease have a poorer prognosis {2234,571}.

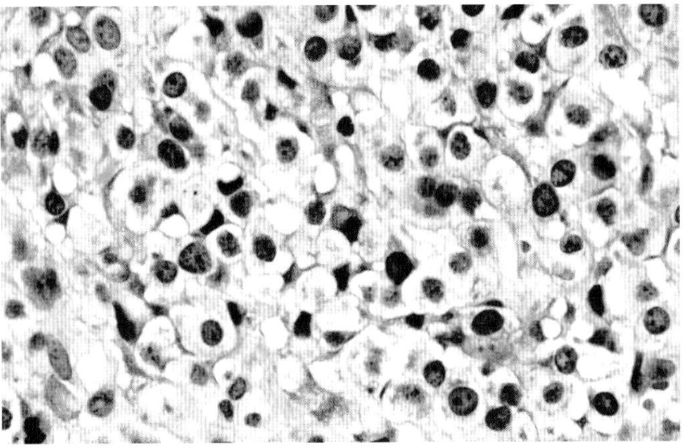

Fig. 4.169 ALK-positive large B-cell lymphoma. A case presenting in the oral cavity shows neoplastic cells with abundant pale cytoplasm.

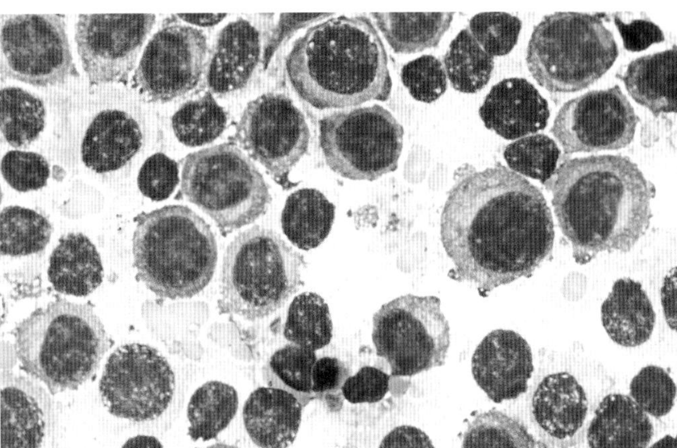

Fig. 4.170 ALK-positive large B-cell lymphoma. FNA smear: the neoplastic cells are large, with round nuclei and abundant cytoplasm.

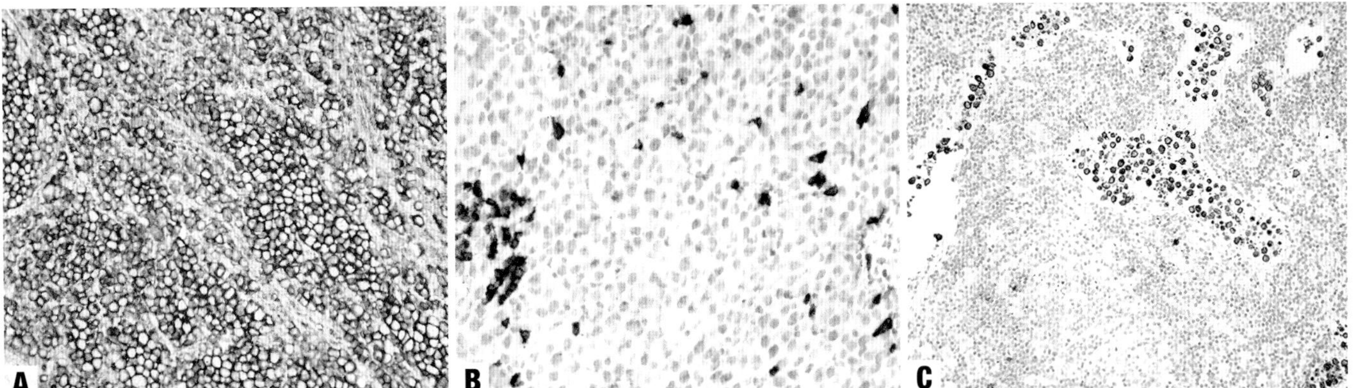

Fig. 4.171 ALK-positive large B-cell lymphoma. **A** Neoplastic cells show a plasmablastic immunophenotype, positive for CD138 and other plasma cell markers. **B** Immunohistochemistry for CD20 is negative. **C** Immunohistochemistry for ALK highlights neoplastic cells in a sinusoidal pattern.

Large B-cell lymphoma with *IRF4* rearrangement

Oschlies I
Burkhardt B
Schafernak KT
Siebert R
Woessmann W

Definition

Large B-cell lymphoma (LBCL) with *IRF4* rearrangement (LBCL-*IRF4*-R) is a de novo mature B-cell lymphoma with a follicular and/or diffuse growth pattern, defined by strong expression of IRF4 (MUM1), usually due to an IG::*IRF4* translocation.

ICD-O coding

9698/3 Large B-cell lymphoma with *IRF4* rearrangement

ICD-11 coding

2A81.Y & XH6SU8 Other specified diffuse large B-cell lymphomas & Large B-cell lymphoma with *IRF4* rearrangement

Related terminology

None

Subtype(s)

None

Localization

LBCL-*IRF4*-R typically involves the Waldeyer ring or cervical lymph nodes, less commonly Peyer patches or intestinal lymph nodes, and exceptionally other sites {3544,895,717,3361,2753, 193}. The majority of patients have localized disease.

Clinical features

Most patients present with asymmetrical tonsillar enlargement or isolated cervical lymphadenopathy without B symptoms {4396,193}.

Epidemiology

Overall, LBCL-*IRF4*-R is rare, representing < 0.1% of LBCLs. The relative incidence of LBCL-*IRF4*-R among LBCLs strongly decreases with age, and most reported patients are children and young adults. There is a slight male predominance {3544, 2040,3361}. Whereas 6–20% of paediatric mature B-cell lymphomas with diffuse large B-cell lymphoma and/or follicular large cell lymphoma morphology represent LBCL-*IRF4*-R {717, 193}, the prevalence is very low in adult patients with lymphomas with comparable morphology {3544,1632}.

Etiology

Unknown

Pathogenesis

A structural variant juxtaposes *IRF4* next to an IG locus, leading to pathognomonic overexpression of IRF4 (MUM1) {3544, 193}. Additional structural and nucleotide variants in *BCL6* (most within the *IRF4*-binding site) and mutations in *IRF4* result in disruption of the physiological BCL6–IRF4 interaction {3544,3361}. Losses of 17p/*TP53* (25–39%) and gains of chromosomes 7 (26–45%) and 11q (35–40%) are recurrent, as are mutations of genes related to the NF-κB pathway (*CARD11*, *CD79B*, *MYD88*), which are observed in about 35% of cases. Ongoing somatic hypermutation and gene expression profiling of LBCL-*IRF4*-R suggest a germinal-centre B-cell origin with features distinct from diffuse large B-cell lymphoma NOS {3542,3544,3361}. LBCL-*IRF4*-R seems to harbour low genomic complexity overall, especially in cases arising at a young age {1231}.

Macroscopic appearance

Not relevant

Histopathology

LBCL-*IRF4*-R has a purely follicular, purely diffuse, or combined follicular and diffuse architecture, resembling follicular large cell lymphoma (mostly follicular lymphoma grade 3B) and/or diffuse large B-cell lymphoma. The follicular component consists of enlarged, round, and in part confluent follicles without zonation. Follicular and diffuse areas consist of sheets of typical centroblasts and (less frequently) medium-sized blastic cells with smaller nucleoli. A starry-sky pattern is usually absent. Intermingled small T cells are scarce {3544,169}.

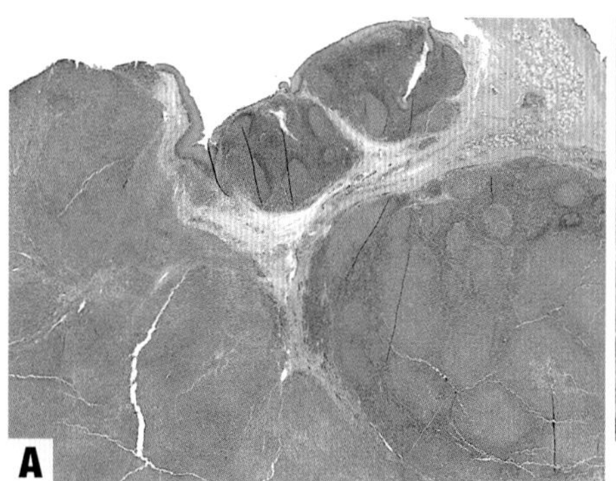
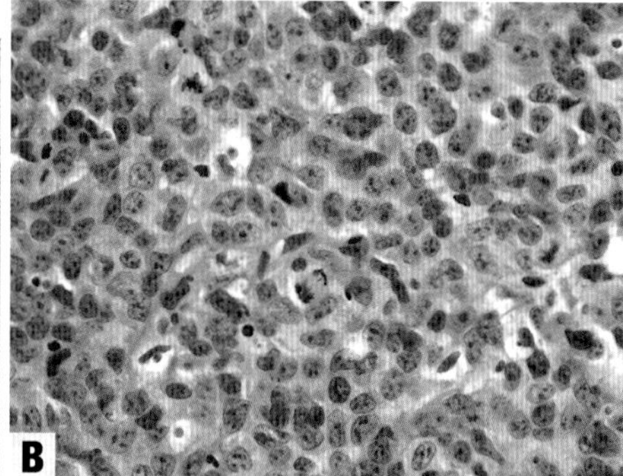
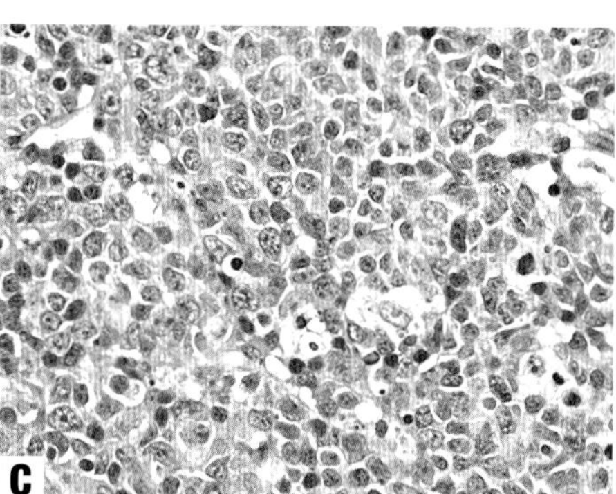

Fig. 4.172 Large B-cell lymphoma with *IRF4* rearrangement. **A** Partial infiltration of the tonsil by a lymphoma with a diffuse and follicular growth pattern. High magnification shows sheets of tumour with centroblastic large cell morphology (**B**) and blastoid large cell morphology with smaller nucleoli (**C**).

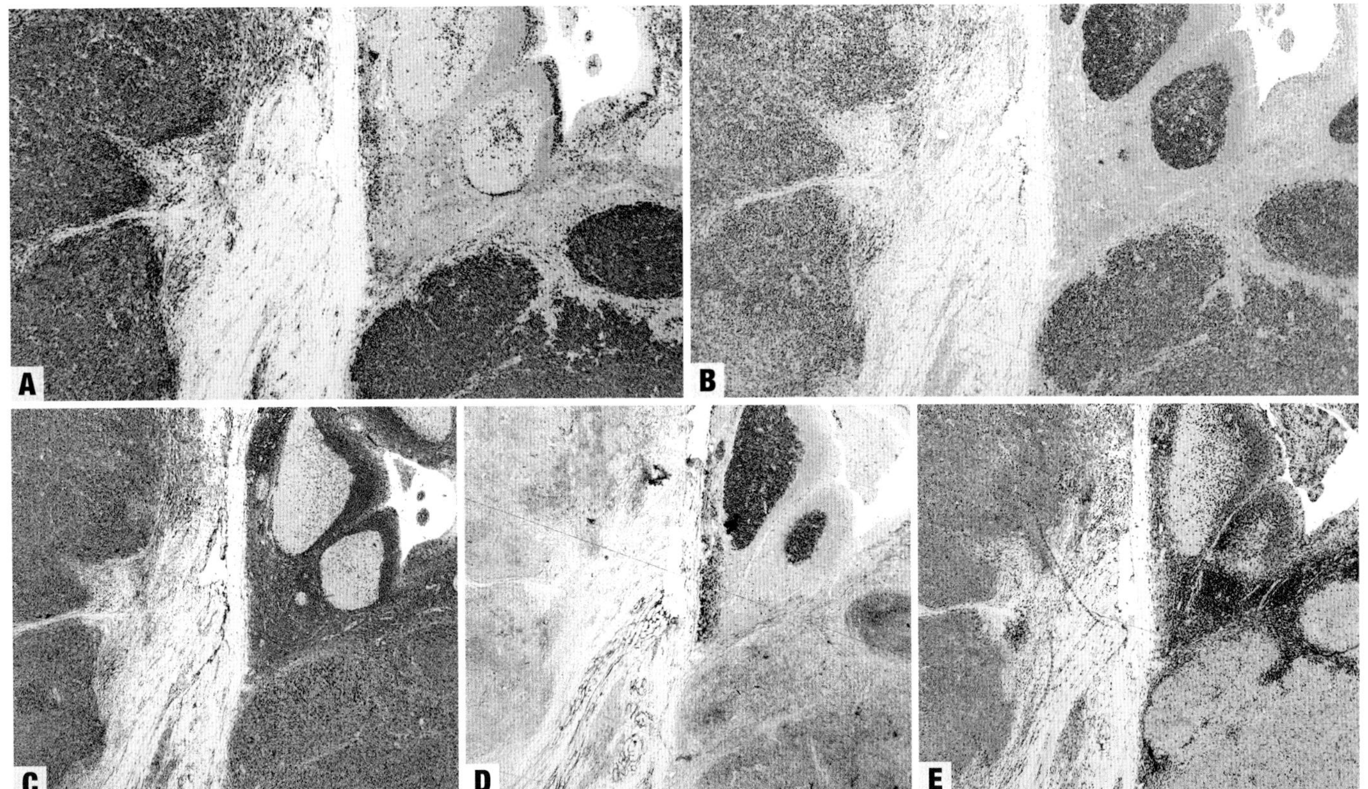

Fig. 4.173 Large B-cell lymphoma with *IRF4* rearrangement. **A** Strong IRF4 (MUM1) expression in the follicular and diffuse growth tumour components. **B** BCL6 is positive in reactive and neoplastic follicles and within the diffuse component. **C** The neoplastic follicles and the diffuse component express BCL2, while reactive germinal centres remain negative. **D** CD10 is strongly expressed in reactive germinal centres and shows weak expression within the lymphoma. **E** The lymphoma cells show coexpression of CD5.

Immunophenotype

A mature B-cell phenotype with strong expression of both IRF4 (MUM1) and BCL6 is characteristic. CD10 and BCL2 are expressed in 50–60% of cases, and CD5 is observed in about 30%. Therefore, screening for *IRF4* translocations is especially indicated in LBCLs with simultaneous expression of BCL6 (and CD10) and IRF4 (MUM1) {1231}. Blimp1 is negative, and the Ki-67 proliferation index is high {3544,668,3361}.

Differential diagnosis

Paediatric-type follicular lymphoma by definition lacks *IRF4* translocation and involvement of extranodal tissue; furthermore, follicular large B-cell lymphoma morphology and strong expression of IRF4 (MUM1) are rare {3338}. Follicular large cell lymphoma in adults aged > 40 years might express IRF4 (MUM1) but usually lacks the *IRF4* translocation {1632}. Other neoplasms with *IRF4* translocation, such as plasma cell myeloma, chronic lymphocytic leukaemia, and several T-cell neoplasms, display a different histopathology {686,4260,3780,816}.

Cytology

Not relevant

Diagnostic molecular pathology

The main feature of LBCL-*IRF4*-R is a chromosomal translocation of *IRF4* (6p25.3), most frequently with the IGH locus, or rarely with IGK or IGL {3544,3361}. A lack of this alteration should lead to the consideration of various differential diagnoses, although in rare cases *IRF4* rearrangement might be cryptic to molecular cytogenetic methods. *BCL2* and *MYC* are virtually never rearranged, whereas chromosomal breaks affecting the *BCL6* locus have been reported {3544,3361,670,4580}.

Essential and desirable diagnostic criteria

Essential: intermediate or large cell morphology and a follicular and/or diffuse growth pattern; mature B-cell phenotype with coexpression of BCL6 and IRF4 (MUM1); *IRF4* translocation; if *IRF4* rearrangement analysis cannot be performed, the proper clinical setting in combination with a typical immunophenotype allows the diagnosis, but as "not molecularly confirmed".

Desirable: evidence of the IG::*IRF4* translocation; absence of *BCL2* and *MYC* gene rearrangement.

Staging

Staging is performed according to the revised International Pediatric Non-Hodgkin Lymphoma Staging System (IPNHLSS) {3476} or the Lugano staging system {688}.

Prognosis and prediction

The overall outcome seems favourable, with rare relapses after risk-adapted chemotherapy in paediatric/young patients {3544, 3361,193}. Limited data are available to consider treatment de-escalation; nevertheless, several paediatric cases of localized, entirely follicular, disease have been described as apparently cured by resection only {2380,3338,4527,193,1389}.

High-grade B-cell lymphoma with 11q aberration

Klapper W
Burkhardt B
d'Amore ESG
Leoncini L
Rymkiewicz G
Siebert R
Woessmann W

Definition

High-grade B-cell lymphoma with 11q aberration (HGBCL-11q) is an aggressive mature B-cell lymphoma with a morphology similar to that of Burkitt lymphoma or showing an intermediate to blastoid appearance in most cases and a characteristic chromosome 11q-gain/loss pattern. Cases with concomitant *MYC* rearrangements are excluded.

ICD-O coding

9687/3 High-grade B-cell lymphoma with 11q aberration

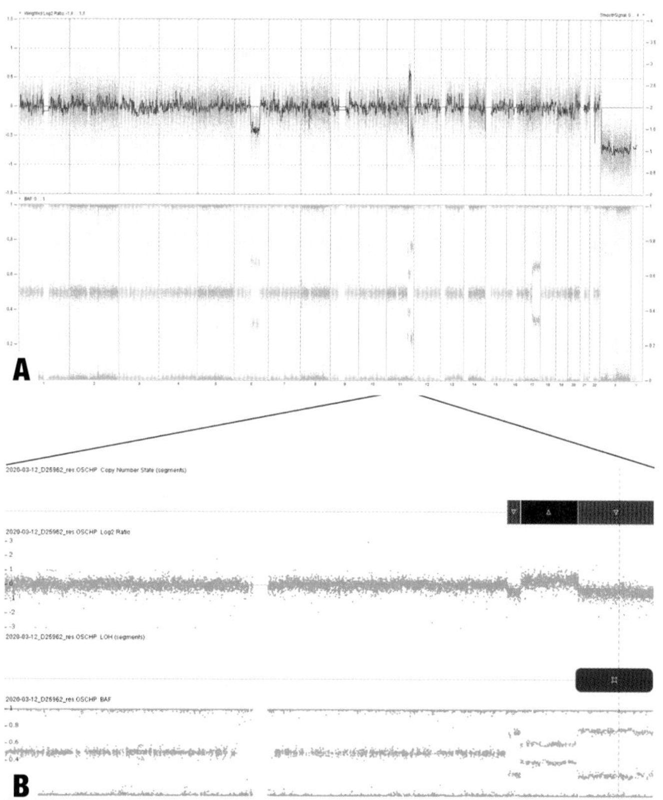

Fig. 4.174 High-grade B-cell lymphoma with 11q aberration: OncoScan analysis showing the typical 11q aberration pattern. **A** Genome-wide view of the imbalances (upper) and B-allele frequencies (lower) along all chromosomes ordered along the *x* axis from 1p (left) to Yq (right). Chromosomes are separated by different colours. The zero line indicates a balanced copy number status (i.e. two copies). Gains are indicated by positive values on the *y* axis, and losses by negative values. Besides the typical 11q gain/loss pattern a deletion in 6q can be seen in the copy-number plot resulting in an altered B-allele frequency in the lower plot. Here, 1 and 0 indicate homozygosity for the (germline) B and A alleles, respectively, whereas 0.5 indicates heterozygosity AB. Deviation from that due to imbalances (chromosomes 6q and 11q) or copy-neutral loss of heterozygosity (chromosome 17q) result in aberrant B-allele frequencies. **B** High-resolution view of chromosome 11 in the same case. On top of the copy-number track, losses (red) and gains (blue) are indicated, pointing to the typical 11q aberration pattern, with gain in 11q23 and loss in 11q23.3-qter. The latter is detected as loss of heterozygosity (LOH) because one allele is lost.

ICD-11 coding

2A85.6 & XH8NN2 Burkitt lymphoma including Burkitt leukaemia & Burkitt-like lymphoma with 11q aberration

Related terminology

Acceptable: large B-cell lymphoma with 11q aberration.

Not recommended: Burkitt-like lymphoma with 11q aberration; *MYC*-negative Burkitt lymphoma (obsolete).

Subtype(s)

None

Localization

About 75–80% of lymphomas manifest as localized nodal or extranodal disease in the head and neck area (60%) or gastrointestinal tract (30–40%) {1429,1371}.

Clinical features

Presenting signs and symptoms are related to the localization of tumour masses. Patients usually do not present with B symptoms {1429,1371,193}. Rare cases have been described in immunocompromised patients {1174}.

Epidemiology

HGBCL-11q is rare. Most cases reported so far have been diagnosed in Europe and the USA and in children/adolescents and patients aged < 60 years {3543,1429,1371,193}.

Etiology

Unknown

Pathogenesis

The defining genetic event is a complex aberration involving the long arm of chromosome 11 (11q) with a minimal region of gain in 11q23.3 and a minimal region of loss at 11q24.1-qter in the absence of a *MYC* translocation {3543}. A subset of cases show no 11q23.3 gain but only telomeric loss and/or solely telomeric loss of heterozygosity (LOH) {3543}. The presence of the 11q gain is less specific for HGBCL-11q than the telomeric loss / LOH and may also occur in other mature aggressive B-cell lymphomas {1535,1429,193,1630}. The minimal regions of gains and losses contain, among others, the genes *KMT2A* and *ETS1*. Their impact as driver alterations, however, is yet unclear. Mutations in *ID3*, *TCF3*, *SMARCA4*, and *CCND3*, as usually encountered in Burkitt lymphoma, are rare. *GNA13* mutations have been observed in about 50% of cases {4266,1371}. This mutation spectrum is more similar to that encountered in diffuse large B-cell lymphoma of germinal-centre type. Unlike in Burkitt lymphoma, the ID3/TCF3 pathway (one of the biological hallmarks of Burkitt lymphoma) is not affected in HGBCL-11q to a similar extent. These data, along with the absence of the IG::*MYC* rearrangement, suggest that HGBCL-11q, despite its similar gene expression profile with

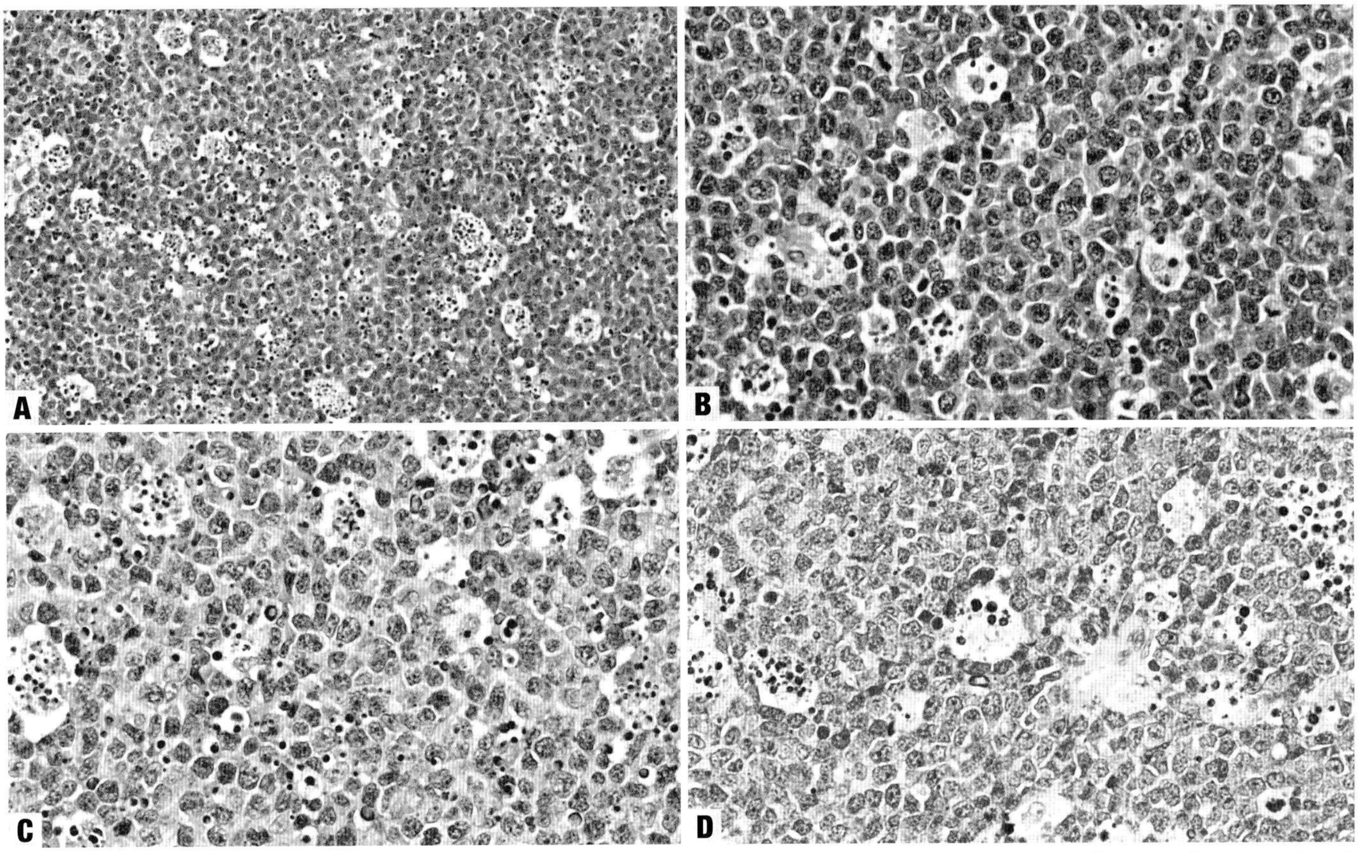

Fig. 4.175 High-grade B-cell lymphoma with 11q aberration. **A** Diffuse effacement of the lymph node parenchyma and a starry-sky pattern. **B** Higher magnification reveals medium-sized blastic cells and starry-sky macrophages. **C** A cohesive growth pattern is appreciated. **D** Giemsa highlights the cellular detail of medium-sized tumour cells with a small rim of moderately basophilic cytoplasm and round to oval nuclei with finely dispersed chromatin.

Burkitt lymphoma {3543}, represents a mature aggressive B-cell lymphoma distinct from Burkitt lymphoma.

Macroscopic appearance

HGBCL-11q may present with large tumours, depending on the site of origin. A fish-flesh cut surface is characteristic.

Histopathology

HGBCL-11q usually shows a diffuse, cohesive lymphomatous infiltrate, comprising medium-sized lymphoid cells with dense nuclear chromatin and multiple nucleoli reminiscent of Burkitt lymphoma or an intermediate or blastoid appearance. Compared with Burkitt lymphoma, HGBCL-11q often shows more cellular pleomorphism, some variation in nuclear size and shape, and larger nucleoli {3543}. A starry-sky pattern is commonly present, with the macrophages displaying coarse apoptotic debris {3543,1630}.

Immunophenotype

HGBCL-11q is characterized by the expression of B-lineage markers, CD10, and BCL6; a high proliferation index (Ki-67

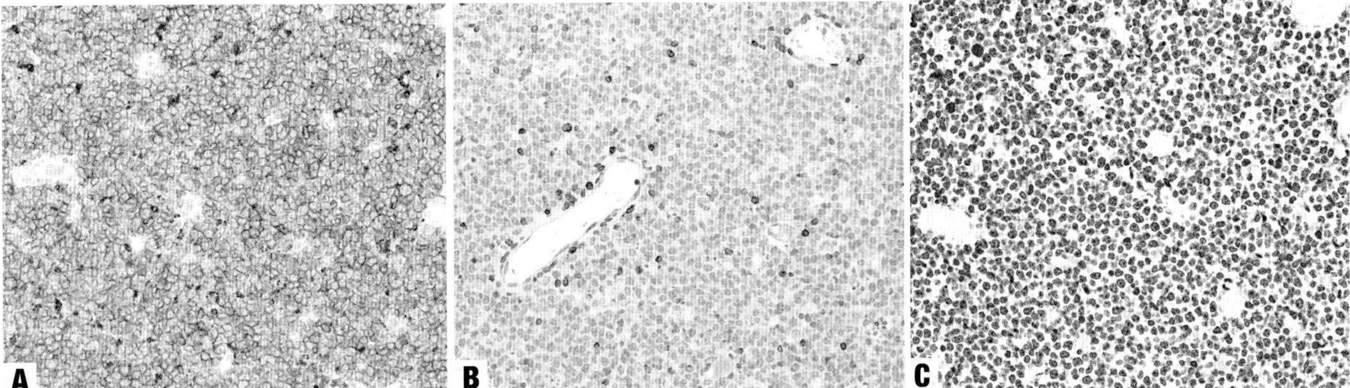

Fig. 4.176 High-grade B-cell lymphoma with 11q aberration. The tumour cells are strongly positive for CD10 (**A**) and negative for BCL2 (**B**). **C** There is a high Ki-67 proliferation index.

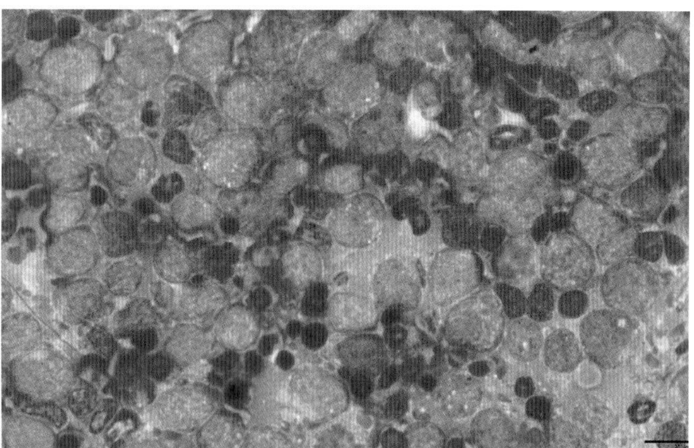

Fig. 4.177 High-grade B-cell lymphoma with 11q aberration. Cytology specimen shows medium-sized blastoid cells without cytoplasmic vacuoles (Giemsa).

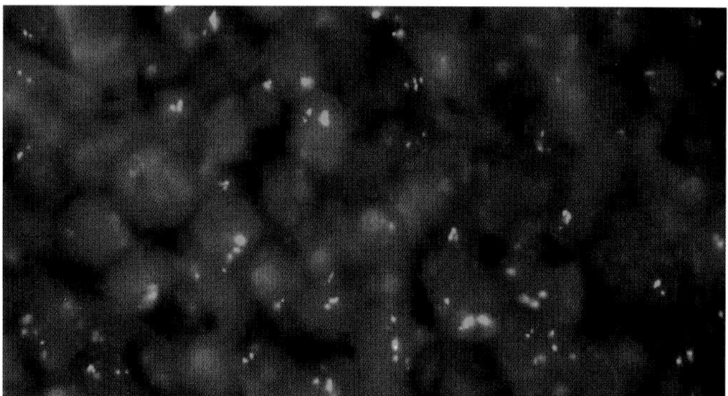

Fig. 4.178 High-grade B-cell lymphoma with 11q aberration. FISH indicating the typical centromeric gain (green) and telomeric loss (red) pattern.

≥ 90%); and negativity for BCL2 (with few exceptions) {3543}. There may be variable, sometimes high, expression of MYC protein despite an absence of *MYC* rearrangement {3510}. The lymphoma cells show LMO2 and sometimes CD56 expression. Flow cytometric detection of CD16 and CD56 or expression of CD8 is highly characteristic of HGBCL-11q, as is absence of strong CD38 expression in this context {3510}.

Differential diagnosis

The main differential diagnoses are Burkitt lymphoma, aggressive B-cell lymphomas with intermediate or blastoid cytology (e.g. HGBCL with *MYC* and *BCL2* rearrangements), or HGBCL-NOS, especially when a germinal centre phenotype is demonstrated {3543}. It is currently unclear whether tumours with diffuse large B-cell lymphoma morphology and an 11q-gain/loss pattern belong to this entity. No EBV-encoded small RNA (EBER)-positive HGBCL-11q cases have been reported thus far.

Cytology

Cytology shows medium-sized to large lymphoid cells with scant basophilic cytoplasm and usually no cytoplasmic vacuoles.

Diagnostic molecular pathology

The diagnosis relies on the detection of the typical molecular aberration in concert with matching cytomorphology and an absence of a *MYC* translocation. Next-generation sequencing techniques and high-resolution array-based comparative genomic hybridization are considered the most reliable techniques to identify the detailed genomic alterations, including variant patterns of telomeric loss and/or solely telomeric LOH in the absence of gains {3543}. Interphase FISH is commonly used as a diagnostic test, but it cannot detect LOH {1429,3510}. Generally, testing for 11q loss/gain to confirm a diagnosis of HGBCL-11q is useful only in lymphomas with the morphology, immunophenotype, or gene expression profile described above {1630}.

Essential and desirable diagnostic criteria

Essential: lymphoma with an intermediate/blastoid or Burkitt-like morphology; typical immunophenotype (B-cell markers+, CD10+, BCL6+, BCL2–); chromosome 11q gain/loss, telomeric loss, or telomeric LOH pattern; exclusion of a *MYC* translocation.

Desirable: expression of CD56 in the absence of CD38-high by flow cytometry.

Staging

Staging is performed according to the revised International Pediatric Non-Hodgkin Lymphoma Staging System (IPNHLSS) {3476} in children and adolescents and the Lugano criteria in adults {688}.

Prognosis and prediction

Almost no recurrence has been reported so far in young patients treated according to protocols designed for Burkitt lymphoma {1371,193}. Limited experience with adult patients undergoing therapy designed for diffuse large B-cell lymphoma suggests a favourable outcome {1429,3510,1371}.

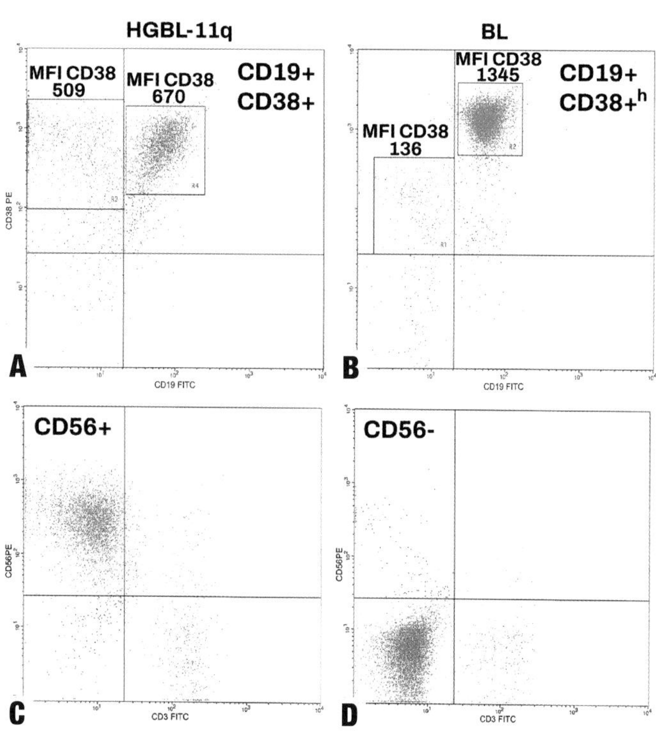

Fig. 4.179 High-grade B-cell lymphoma with 11q aberration (HGBCL-11q). Flow cytometry–based analysis of median fluorescence intensity (MFI) of CD38 expression (**A,B**) and CD56 (**C,D**) in HGBCL-11q and Burkitt lymphoma (BL). MFI of CD38 expression in HGBCL-11q is similar to normal T lymphocyte expression (CD38+, **A**), and in BL it is higher (CD38+^{h}, **B**). The absence of CD38+^{h} (**A**) and CD56+ (**C**) characterize HGBCL-11q. CD38+^{h} (**B**) and the lack of CD56 (**D**) characterize BL.

Lymphomatoid granulomatosis

Anagnostopoulos I
Deckert M
Nicholson AG
Siebert R

Definition

Lymphomatoid granulomatosis (LYG) is an EBV-associated angiocentric and angiodestructive B-cell lymphoproliferative disorder involving extranodal sites, composed of EBV-positive atypical large B cells usually admixed with a large number of reactive T cells. It occurs in patients lacking evidence of inborn or acquired immune deficiency/dysregulation other than immunosenescence.

ICD-O coding

9766/1 Lymphomatoid granulomatosis, NOS
9766/1 Lymphomatoid granulomatosis, grade 1
9766/1 Lymphomatoid granulomatosis, grade 2
9766/3 Lymphomatoid granulomatosis, grade 3

ICD-11 coding

2A81.3 Lymphomatoid granulomatosis

Related terminology

Acceptable: EBV-positive diffuse large B-cell lymphoma (for grade 3 LYG only).
Not recommended: angiocentric lymphoproliferative lesion.

Subtype(s)

Lymphomatoid granulomatosis, grade 1; lymphomatoid granulomatosis, grade 2; lymphomatoid granulomatosis, grade 3

Localization

LYG always involves the lung, and frequently involves the CNS (40%), skin (34%), kidneys (19%), and liver (17%), but it can occur in essentially any organ {1925,3783,652}. Lymph node and/or bone marrow involvement is rare and, therefore, if encountered, should raise suspicion for an alternative diagnosis {2110}.

Clinical features

Despite universal lung involvement, only 30–60% of patients present with overt respiratory symptoms, and the remaining

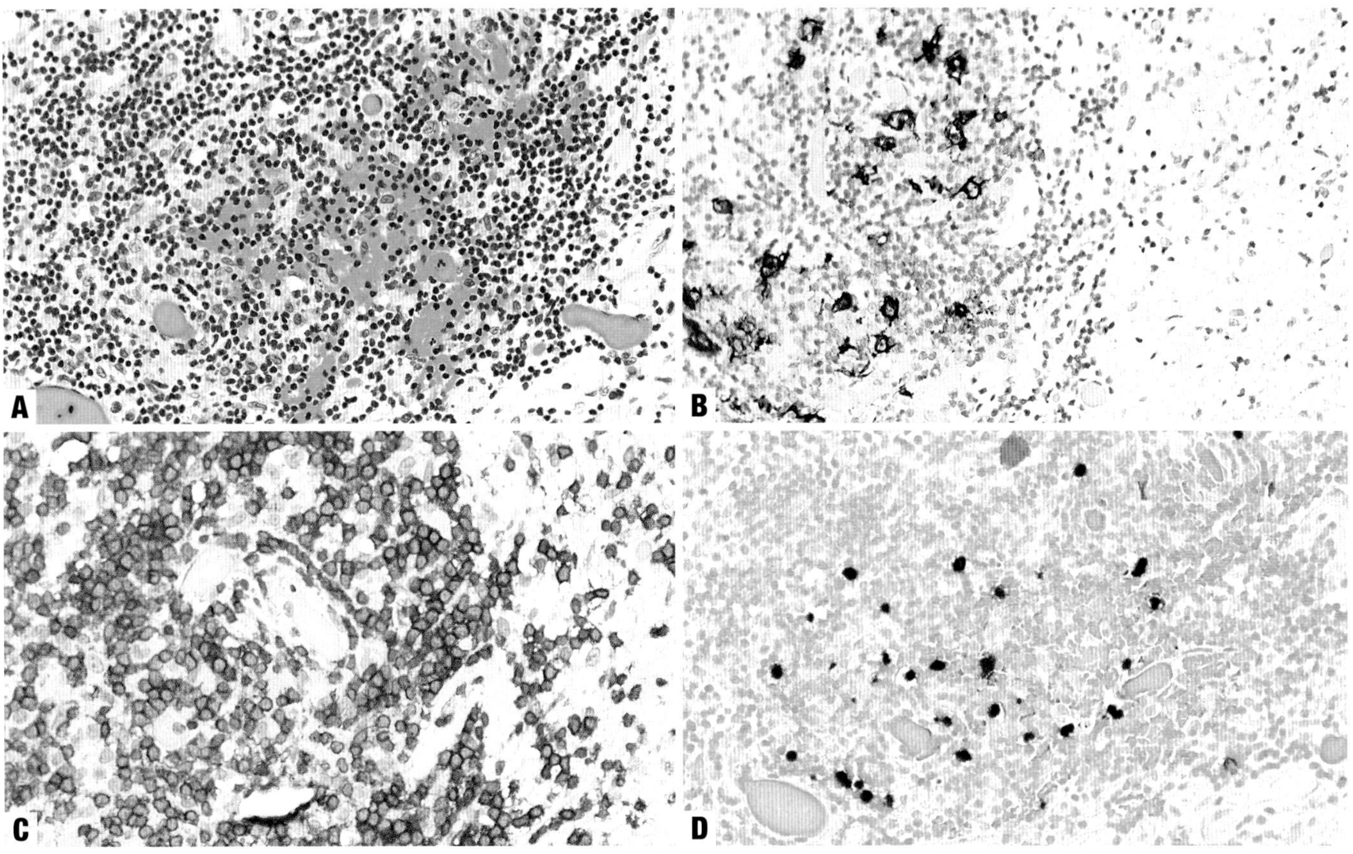

Fig. 4.180 Lymphomatoid granulomatosis, grade 2. **A** The infiltrate in brain is composed of numerous small lymphoid cells and only a few large transformed cells. **B** There are a few large transformed CD20-positive B cells. **C** The majority of the lymphoid cells correspond to CD3-positive T cells. **D** A small number of latently EBV-infected lymphoid cells as shown by in situ hybridization for EBV-encoded small RNA (EBER).

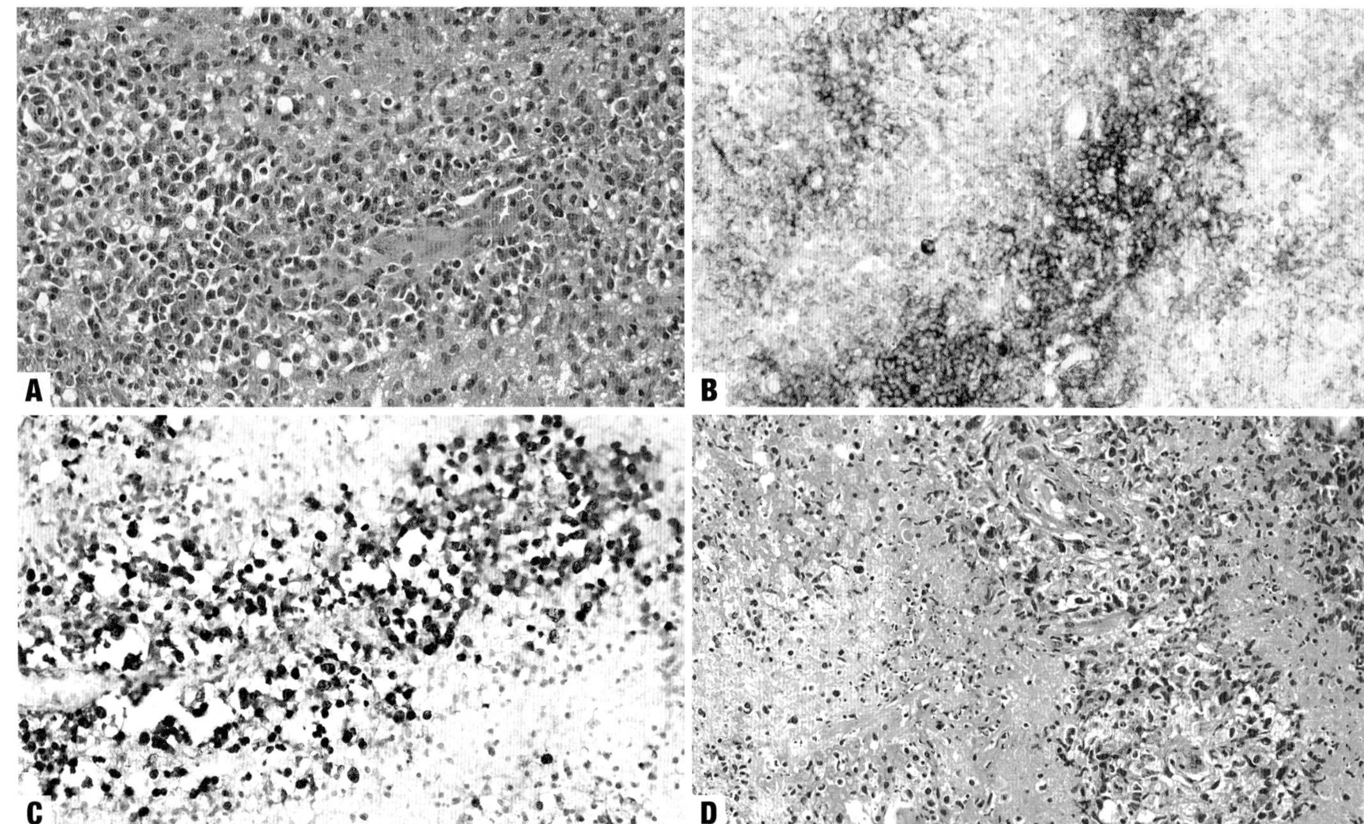

Fig. 4.181 Lymphomatoid granulomatosis. **A** Lymphomatoid granulomatosis, grade 3, in the brain exhibits polymorphic angiocentric infiltrates. **B** CD20 shows clusters of viable CD20+ B cells at the edge of a necrotizing lesion. Cellular debris and lymphoid cells within the necrosis exhibit weak immunoreactivity. **C** In situ hybridization for EBV-encoded small RNA (EBER) highlights the fact that the majority of the large transformed cells are EBV-positive. **D** In a case in the skin, the angiocentric infiltrate contains numerous large transformed lymphoid cells and is accompanied by fibrinoid necrosis of the affected blood vessels. There are also large necrotic areas.

cases are identified on imaging {652}. Presenting symptoms include cough, dyspnoea, and chest pain, and these may be accompanied by constitutional symptoms (i.e. fever, weight loss, malaise, and fatigue) {3463,652}. Cutaneous lesions can occur at any stage of the disease process, with approximately one third of patients having lesions at initial presentation, but rarely precede pulmonary manifestations {1924,283,1925,3783}. Neurological symptoms depend on the involved CNS site and are therefore highly variable. They may include hemiparesis, ataxia, disorientation, and cranial nerve palsies, as well as hearing loss, diplopia, dysarthria, and atonic bladder {3164,1925,3783}.

Epidemiology

The disease is rare and exact data on its prevalence do not exist. LYG is more common in North American populations and rare in Asian populations {1925,2632}. The median age is between the fourth and sixth decades of life. The M:F ratio is 2:1.

Etiology

The etiology is unknown.

Pathogenesis

Current hypotheses include defective immunosurveillance of EBV-infected B cells and an abnormal immune response to EBV, because previously healthy individuals with LYG have shown various defects in cell-mediated and/or humoral immunity {3795,4386, 3994} but no overt immunodeficiency state. Functional impairment of CD8+ cytotoxic T cells accounts for the diminished immune control of EBV-infected B cells and is thought to be an important factor in the development of this disease {3795,4386}.

Macroscopic appearance

The lung shows multiple nodules of variable sizes, with and without central necrosis. The lesions are most often bilateral, predominantly arising in the middle to lower lung fields. Occasionally there is only a solitary lung nodule. Nodular lesions are also found in the involved kidneys and brain, usually associated with central necrosis. Skin lesions are in the form of multiple erythematous dermal papules and/or subcutaneous nodules with or without ulceration, or (less commonly) multiple indurated, erythematous to whitish plaque-like lesions. They are frequently disseminated and are less commonly confined to the extremities, trunk, or head and neck {1783,283}.

Histopathology

LYG is characterized by an angiocentric and angiodestructive, polymorphous lymphoid infiltrate with involvement of small- to large-calibre vessels. Small lymphocytes predominate and are admixed with variable numbers of histiocytes, plasma cells, and large atypical cells. The background small lymphocytes (predominantly T cells) may show some atypia or nuclear irregularities but do not appear overtly neoplastic. The large atypical cells may resemble immunoblasts or have a more pleomorphic appearance, resembling Hodgkin cells. Multinucleated forms may be seen, but classic Reed–Sternberg cells are generally not present. Neutrophils and eosinophils are usually inconspicuous. Central necrosis is often, although variably, present. Despite the name of the lesion ("granulomatosis"), well-formed granulomas are typically absent. In the skin, lymphohistiocytic infiltration can be seen in the subcutaneous fatty tissue, with secondary granulomatous reaction around fat necrosis. Dermal involvement is variable.

Grading

LYG is graded by comparing the proportion of EBV-positive B cells and their degree of cytological atypia to the background population of reactive T cells. Three grades are recognized, notwithstanding issues with reproducibility and the possibility of underestimating the number of EBV+ cells in the presence of extensive necrosis.

Grade 1 lesions are composed of a polymorphous lymphoid infiltrate without significant atypia; necrosis is absent or focal. Large EBV-positive lymphoid cells are rare and can be better identified by CD20 and in situ hybridization for EBV-encoded small RNA (EBER).

In grade 2 lesions, large EBV-positive B cells are typically present (usually in the range of ~40–400/mm^2, equating to 5–50/HPF of 0.12 mm^2 in area); necrosis is more commonly seen.

Grade 3 lesions are characterized by a larger number of EBV-positive B cells (generally > 400/mm^2, equating to > 50/HPF of 0.12 mm^2 in area) {3783}. Necrosis is common and often extensive {3783}. The large atypical cells may occur in clusters. However, if there is a uniform population of large atypical cells, a diagnosis of EBV-positive diffuse large B-cell lymphoma is warranted.

Immunohistochemistry

The atypical large B cells express pan–B-cell markers, are variably positive for CD30, and are negative for CD15. A subset of these cells may express EBV LMP1. EBNA2 is also frequently positive, consistent with type III EBV latency. Staining for kappa and lambda light chains is of limited value, although rare cases may show light chain restriction in plasma cells. The majority of lymphoid cells in the background are CD3-positive T cells, with CD4-positive cells out numbering CD8-positive cells {3783}.

Differential diagnosis

The differential diagnosis includes other forms of EBV-positive B-cell lymphoproliferative disorders and can be challenging, particularly when extranodal sites are involved (see Table 4.32, modified according to {2632}).

Whereas previously the incidence of LYG was reported to be higher in patients with immunodeficiencies (i.e. Wiskott–Aldrich syndrome, HIV infection, high-dose chemotherapy) {1494,3661, 960}, according to the current definition, a history of inborn or acquired immune deficiency/dysregulation other than immunosenescence excludes the diagnosis of LYG. In such cases, the diagnosis should follow the guidelines outlined in the sections on lymphoid proliferations and lymphomas associated with immune deficiency and dysregulation (p. 549) and can be designated as "polymorphic lymphoproliferative disorder, LYG type, EBV+", followed by the specified immune deficiency/dysregulation setting (e.g. HIV, iatrogenic/methotrexate) and in the case of grade 3–type lesions as "diffuse large B-cell lymphoma, LYG type, EBV+", followed by the specified immune deficiency/dysregulation setting.

Cytology

The use of FNAB alone is not recommended in this condition.

Diagnostic molecular pathology

The large atypical cells are positive for EBV by in situ hybridization using EBER probes. EBER-positive cells usually show

Table 4.32 Comparison of clinicopathological features of lymphomatoid granulomatosis, immune deficiency/dysregulation–associated polymorphic B-cell lymphoproliferative disorder, and EBV-positive diffuse large B-cell lymphoma

Features	Lymphomatoid granulomatosis	Polymorphic lymphoproliferative disorder	EBV+ diffuse large B-cell lymphoma NOS
Clinical features			
	By definition immunocompetent, but immunosenescence may play a role	Immunodeficient state known	Often immunocompetent, but immunosenescence may play a role
	Extranodal involvement frequent, most commonly lung, CNS, and skin	Extranodal involvement frequent, most commonly gastrointestinal, lung, CNS, kidney, heart, and liver, including the allograft in posttransplant cases	Extranodal involvement less common and involves different sites
	Lymph node and/or bone marrow involvement extremely rare	Lymph node involvement very common, and bone marrow may be extensively involved in posttransplant cases	Lymph node involvement common, bone marrow involvement uncommon
Histological features			
	EBV+ large B cells do not predominate in lesions of grade 1 and grade 2 but can predominate in grade 3	EBV+ large and small B-cell population is variable	EBV+ large B-cell population is variable (minority or predominant)
	Background rich in small lymphocytes (predominantly T cells) including some plasma cells and histiocytes	Polymorphic infiltrate with variable proportion of cells exhibiting full spectrum of B-cell differentiation, including T cells and histiocytes	Polymorphic background infiltrate can be prominent (in polymorphic variant) including small lymphocytes, plasma cells, and histiocytes
	Angiocentric and angioinvasive infiltrate typically present at least in some areas	Infiltrate typically not angiocentric or angioinvasive	Angiocentric and angioinvasive infiltrate can be present
	Various degrees of coagulative necrosis	Coagulative necrosis may be present	Various degrees of coagulative necrosis
EBV viral load	Often low to negative	Often significantly elevated	Often significantly elevated

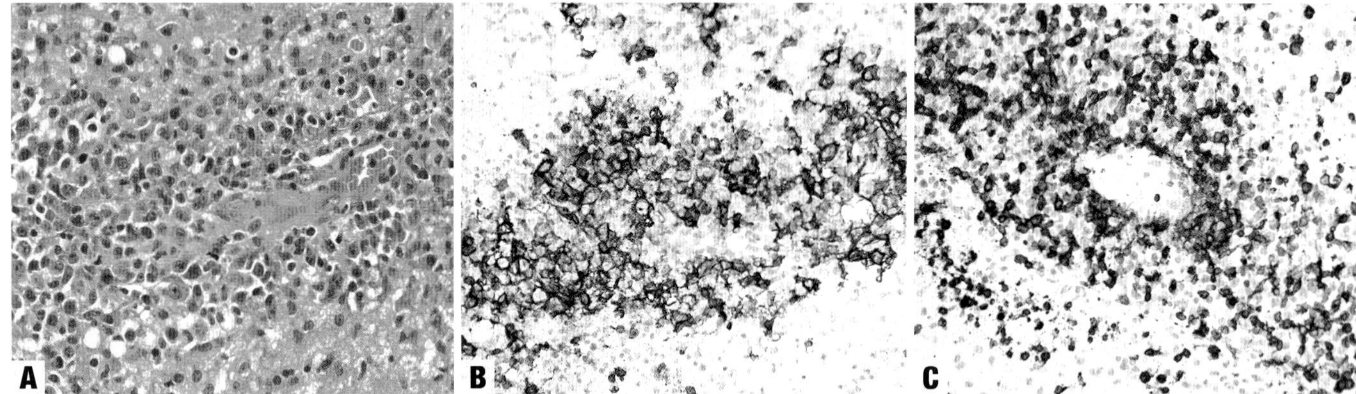

Fig. 4.182 Lymphomatoid granulomatosis, grade 3. **A** A case localized to the brain. Higher magnification shows that the infiltrate is composed of numerous large transformed lymphoid cells admixed with small lymphoid cells and plasma cells. **B** CD20 immunostaining highlights the large number of B cells. **C** CD3 highlights the angiocentric and angioinvasive distribution of T cells.

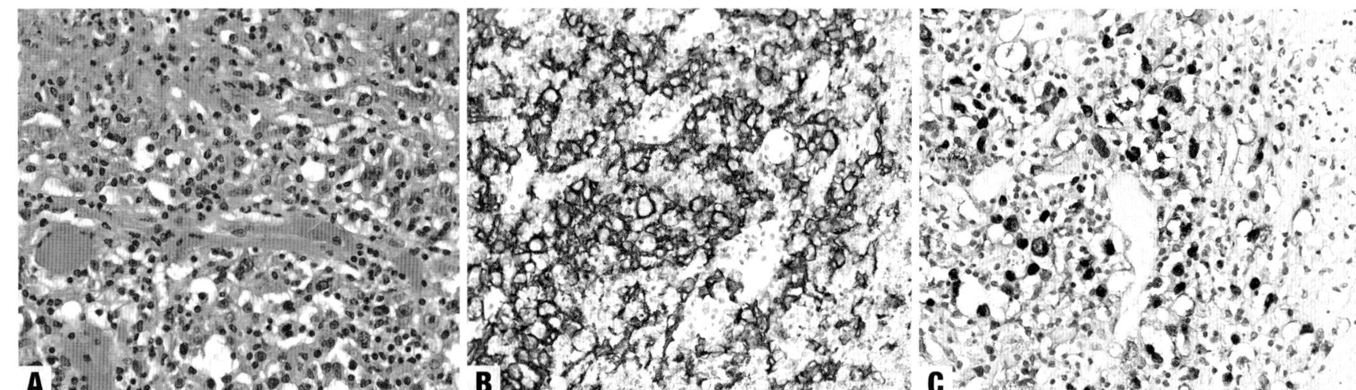

Fig. 4.183 Lymphomatoid granulomatosis, grade 3. **A** At higher magnification, the infiltrate in this case localized to the lung is composed of numerous large transformed lymphoid cells admixed with small lymphoid cells and plasma cells. **B** CD20 is positive in large transformed B cells. **C** The spectrum of larger and smaller EBV-encoded small RNA (EBER)-positive cells is seen.

a spectrum in cell size, with numerous small B cells being positive as well. Monoclonal IG gene rearrangements may be identified in most grade 2 and grade 3 lesions, and different clonal rearrangements may be present in different lesions or from different sites of involvement. B-cell clonality may not be detected in grade 1 lesions, most likely because of the paucity of EBV-infected cells. Clonal TR gene rearrangements are usually not present, although restricted patterns may be observed {3783}.

Essential and desirable diagnostic criteria

Essential: extranodal disease; polymorphous lymphoid infiltrate with striking angiocentricity; transmural involvement of small to medium-sized vessels by variable numbers of EBV+ large B cells admixed, with abundant small T lymphocytes; exclusion of immunodeficiency other than immunosenescence.

Staging

The disease is usually extranodal, therefore conventional staging (i.e. Lugano classification, a modification of the Ann Arbor staging system {688}) is not informative.

Prognosis and prediction

The clinical behaviour of LYG varies widely; the disease ranges from an indolent process to an aggressive B-cell lymphoma. Accurate histological grading is essential in predicting disease course and guiding therapy. Accordingly, grade 1 and 2 lesions are commonly treated by immune modulation (e.g. interferon), and grade 3 lesions are treated as aggressive lymphoma with chemotherapy.

In the largest retrospective series, 63% of the patients died, most of them within the first year of diagnosis, with a median overall survival of 14 months. However, 30% of patients experience spontaneous remission without treatment. The cause of death is related to extensive lung involvement or the destruction of other involved organs {2632}.

EBV-positive diffuse large B-cell lymphoma

Anagnostopoulos I
Asano N
Chapman JR
de Jong D
Klapper W
Lenz G
Medeiros LJ
Miles RR
Steidl C

Definition

Epstein Barr virus (EBV)-positive diffuse large B-cell lymphoma (DLBCL) is a large B-cell lymphoma in which the majority of the neoplastic cells harbour EBV. Affected patients do not have a history of lymphoma or underlying immune deficiency/dysregulation (other than immunosenescence). The neoplasm should not fulfil criteria for other EBV+ lymphoproliferative disorders or lymphomas.

ICD-O coding

9680/3 EBV-positive diffuse large B-cell lymphoma

ICD-11 coding

2A81.Y & XH1QK0 Other specified diffuse large B-cell lymphomas & EBV-positive diffuse large B-cell lymphoma

Related terminology

Acceptable: EBV-positive diffuse large B-cell lymphoma NOS.

Not recommended: EBV-positive diffuse large B-cell lymphoma of the elderly; senile EBV-associated B-cell lymphoproliferative disorder; age-related EBV-positive lymphoproliferative disorder.

Subtype(s)

None

Localization

Nodal and extranodal sites can be involved. Cases in younger patients (aged < 45 years) often show predominantly nodal involvement, which can be localized or generalized; about 10% of patients present with extranodal disease {4112,2954}. Extranodal manifestations are more frequent (40%) in elderly patients, usually involving the lungs, gastrointestinal tract, skin, and bone marrow {3091,3142,984,3034,4055,428}. Approximately 5–10% of patients present with both nodal and extranodal involvement.

Clinical features

The clinical presentation is variable {3091,3092,984,1612,2954, 428}. B symptoms are common. More than 50% of patients have a high or high-intermediate age-adjusted International Prognostic Index (aaIPI) score and an Eastern Cooperative Oncology Group (ECOG) performance status score of > 2 {428}. In most patients, EBV DNA is detectable in serum or blood, although

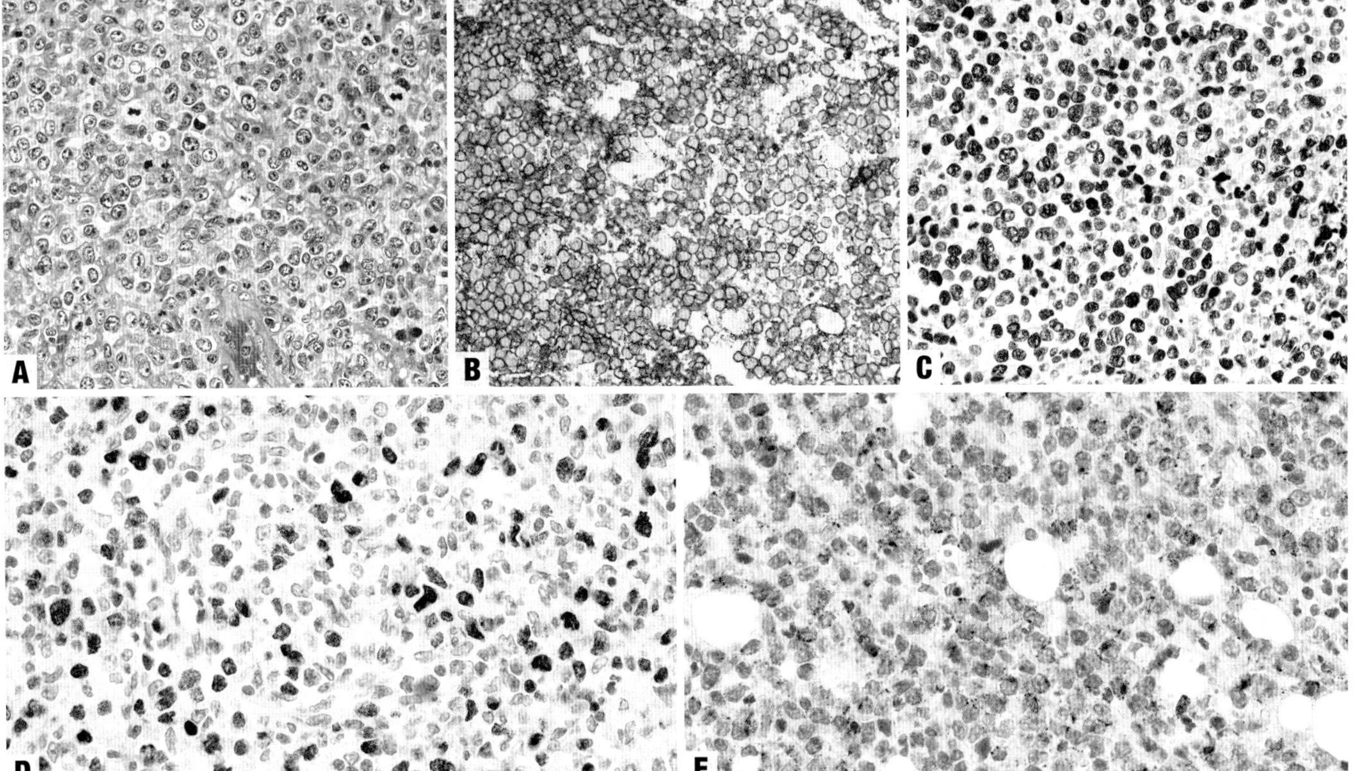

Fig. 4.184 EBV-positive diffuse large B-cell lymphoma. **A** A monomorphic lesion is composed of a monotonous proliferation of centroblast-like cells. **B** The lymphoma cells are strongly and uniformly positive for CD20. **C** In situ hybridization for EBV-encoded small RNA (EBER) highlights the fact that almost all tumour cells are latently infected. **D** The tumour cells express EBNA2. **E** The majority of the tumour cells express EBV-encoded LMP1.

this finding is not specific for the disease {2334,3037}. According to one European study, haemophagocytic lymphohistiocytosis can occur at a high rate {428}.

Epidemiology

EBV+ DLBCL is infrequent in high-income countries, accounting for < 6% of all DLBCLs {4055,3031,2868,1609}, but is more prevalent in Africa, Asia, and Latin America (4.7–28%) {3142, 1612,3037,2438,3006,1695,568,2893}. Most cases occur in patients aged ≥ 50 years, with a peak in the seventh or eighth decade of life, and a smaller incidence peak in the third decade of life {2954}. The M:F ratio is 1.2–3.6:1.

Etiology

The etiology is unknown. By definition, lymphoproliferative disorders and lymphomas arising in the setting of inborn or acquired immune deficiency/dysregulation are specifically excluded.

Pathogenesis

Immunosenescence has been suggested to play a role in the development of EBV+ DLBCL in older patients. EBV+ DLBCL shows a lower mutation burden than EBV– DLBCL, compatible with the hypothesis that EBV-driven pathogenesis requires fewer driver mutations or oncogenic events {1308}. The presence of EBV has been reported to be mutually exclusive with either *MYD88* and/or *CD79A* mutations {4223}. The mutation landscape is dominated by recurrent alterations in the NF-κB, WNT, and IL-6/JAK/STAT pathways {4584,1308} and differs from that of EBV– DLBCL-NOS. A set of mutated genes possibly specific for this disease, including *CCR6*, *CCR7*, *DAPK1*, *TNFRSF21*, *CSNK2B*, and *YY1*, has been reported {1308}. 6q deletions are recurrent and lead to loss of *PRDM1* and *TNFAIP3* {1308}.

PDL1 overexpression is mediated by LMP1, which activates the transcription factor AP-1 and the JAK/STAT and NF-κB pathways {3034,2755,1405,1134,353}, or through structural variations in genes including *CD274* (*PDL1*) / *PDCD1LG2* (*PDL2*) {1909}. PDL1 expression has been reported in 95% of cases {428}. However, the frequency in elderly patients seems to be low (11%), in contrast to the higher occurrence {3925} in younger patients {2954}, suggesting that immune escape may be more important in younger patients than in older patients.

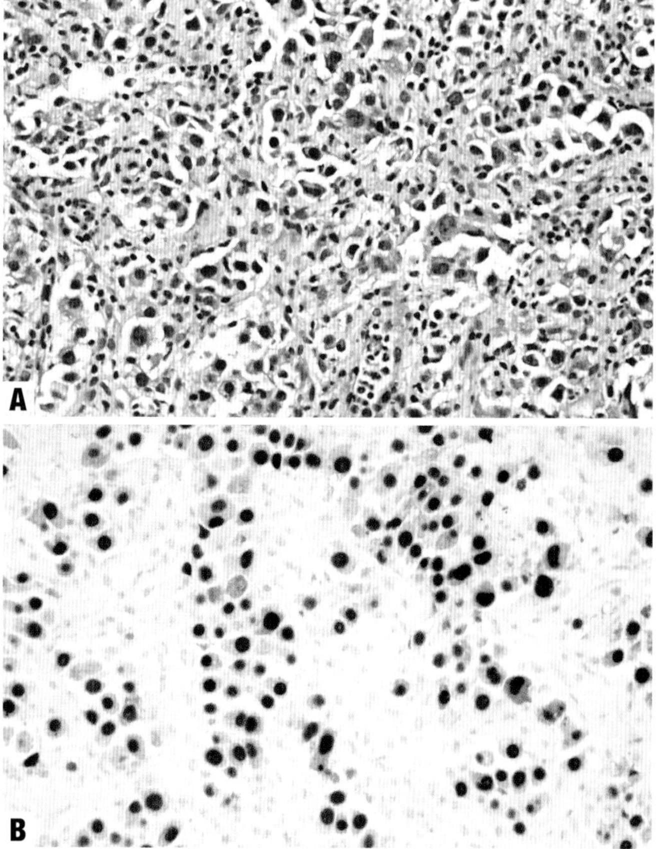

Fig. 4.185 EBV-positive diffuse large B-cell lymphoma. **A** Large neoplastic cells are located within sinusoids. **B** They are strongly positive for IRF4 (MUM1).

Macroscopic appearance

Lymphadenopathy or tumours/masses

Histopathology

Histological features encompass a broad spectrum, based on the density of tumour cells and the quality of the immune microenvironment, that has been subdivided into polymorphic versus monomorphic types {3092,161,984,2755}. In polymorphic cases, large transformed cells/immunoblasts, HRS-like and lymphocyte-predominant–like cells are scattered in a reactive background including small lymphocytes, plasma cells, and histiocytes (including epithelioid histiocytes) and can resemble T-cell/histiocyte–rich large B-cell lymphoma. Monomorphic cases, which are less common, comprise sheets of atypical large lymphoid cells and are indistinguishable from EBV– DLBCL without ancillary studies to demonstrate EBV. Some cases show a mixture of polymorphic and DLBCL-like areas. Angiocentric/angiodestructive lesions and extensive coagulative geographical necrosis are other characteristic findings, although these are not invariably found.

Immunophenotype

The neoplastic cells are positive for the pan–B-cell antigens CD19, CD20, CD22, CD79a, and PAX5 and usually show an activated B-cell–like immunophenotype, with positivity for IRF4 (MUM1) and a lack of CD10; BCL6 is variably positive. Most cases are CD30-positive, with staining ranging from partial and weak to diffuse and strong. The neoplastic cells express CD15 in a few cases, but other immunophenotypic features of classic Hodgkin lymphoma are usually absent {984,2954}.

LMP1 is expressed in most cases (> 90%) and EBNA2 in only a subset (7–36%); thus type II EBV latency is more frequent than type III. The tumour cells often express PDL1 and PDL2, especially in younger patients {2954,655}.

Differential diagnosis

The differential diagnosis can be challenging, particularly regarding the overlap with EBV+ mucocutaneous ulcer and lymphomatoid granulomatosis. There is morphological and immunophenotypic overlap between EBV+ DLBCL and the spectrum of B-cell lymphoproliferations in patients with immune deficiency/dysregulation, including polymorphic B-cell lymphoproliferative disorders, and the distinction should be made on the basis of the clinical context (see Table 4.33).

Cytology

FNAB can be of value in this condition by establishing the diagnosis and allowing for flow cytometry, but it should be followed up by tissue excision.

Diagnostic molecular pathology

In situ hybridization for EBV-encoded small RNA (EBER) is mandatory for the diagnosis, and the majority of the large atypical cells should be positive, although this is arbitrary. Of note, low numbers (< 10% of all B cells) of EBER-positive bystander small lymphocytes can occur in conventional DLBCL and should not lead to a diagnosis of EBV+ DLBCL {1612,3857,3006}. In selected circumstances, identification of monoclonal rearrangements of the IG genes is helpful for distinguishing EBV+ DLBCL from EBV+ reactive hyperplasias and infectious mononucleosis, although clonality may not be detectable in all cases {984, 2954}.

Essential and desirable diagnostic criteria

Essential: partial or total architectural effacement of affected tissue; atypical lymphoid infiltrate composed of either sheets of large malignant cells or many scattered large transformed cells of variable morphology, including HRS-like cells, in a richly cellular reactive background, often accompanied by necrosis; large cells confirmed to be of B-cell lineage (e.g. CD20, PAX5, CD79a); EBV present in the majority of large B cells; absence of inborn or acquired immunodeficiency or a history of lymphoma; exclusion of

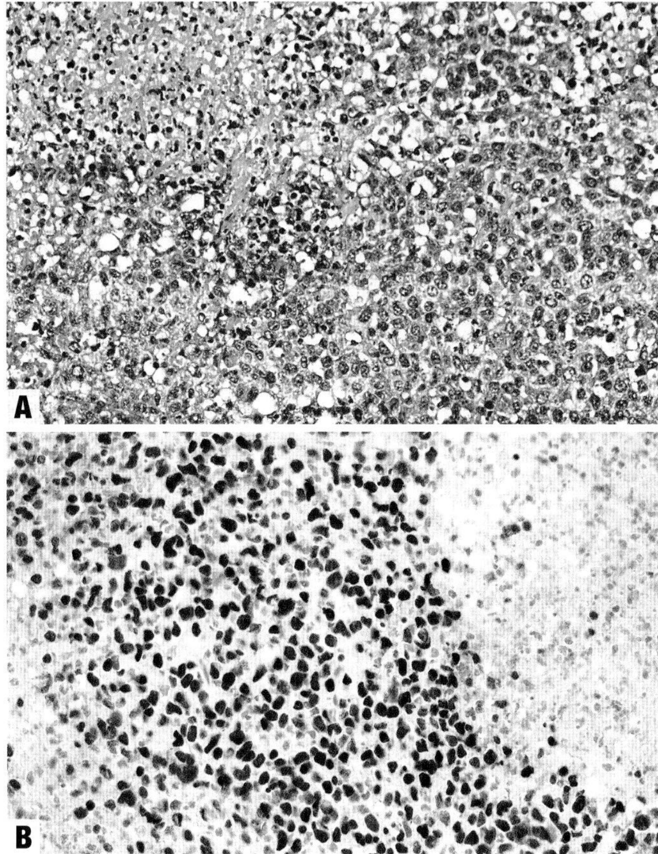

Fig. 4.186 EBV-positive diffuse large B-cell lymphoma. **A** This monomorphic lesion shows geographical necrosis. **B** The majority of the tumour cells express EBV-encoded EBNA2.

Table 4.33 Comparison of clinicopathological features of EBV-positive diffuse large B-cell lymphoma, EBV-positive mucocutaneous ulcer, and lymphomatoid granulomatosis

Features	EBV+ diffuse large B-cell lymphoma	EBV+ mucocutaneous ulcer	Lymphomatoid granulomatosis
Clinical features			
	By definition immunocompetent, but immunosenescence may play a role	Immunodeficient state known, immunosenescence may play a role	By definition immunocompetent, but immunosenescence may play a role
	Extranodal involvement less common and involves different sites	Restricted to extranodal sites, usually unifocal, superficial, and circumscribed, most commonly in the oral mucosa, tonsils, palate, and gastrointestinal tract	Extranodal involvement frequent, most commonly lung, CNS, and skin
	Lymph node involvement common and bone marrow involvement uncommon	Lymphadenopathy due to other lymphoid proliferations caused by the underlying immune deficiency/dysregulation may be present	Lymph node and/or bone marrow involvement extremely rare
Histological features			
	EBV+ large B-cell population is variable (minority or predominant)	EBV+ large B-cell population is variable (minority or predominant)	EBV+ large B cells do not predominate in lesions of grade 1 and grade 2, and predominate in grade 3
	Polymorphic background infiltrate can be prominent (in polymorphic variant) including small lymphocytes, plasma cells, and histiocytes	Polymorphic background infiltrate prominent, including small lymphocytes, plasma cells, eosinophils, and histiocytes Deepest margin of lesion contains a band-like infiltrate of small lymphocytes	Background rich in small lymphocytes (predominantly T cells) including some plasma cells and histiocytes
	Angiocentric and angioinvasive infiltrate can be present	Angiocentric or angioinvasive infiltrate can be present	Angiocentric and angioinvasive infiltrate typically present at least in some areas
	Various degrees of coagulative necrosis	Various degrees of coagulative necrosis	Various degrees of coagulative necrosis
EBV viral load	Often significantly elevated	Typically negative	Often low to negative

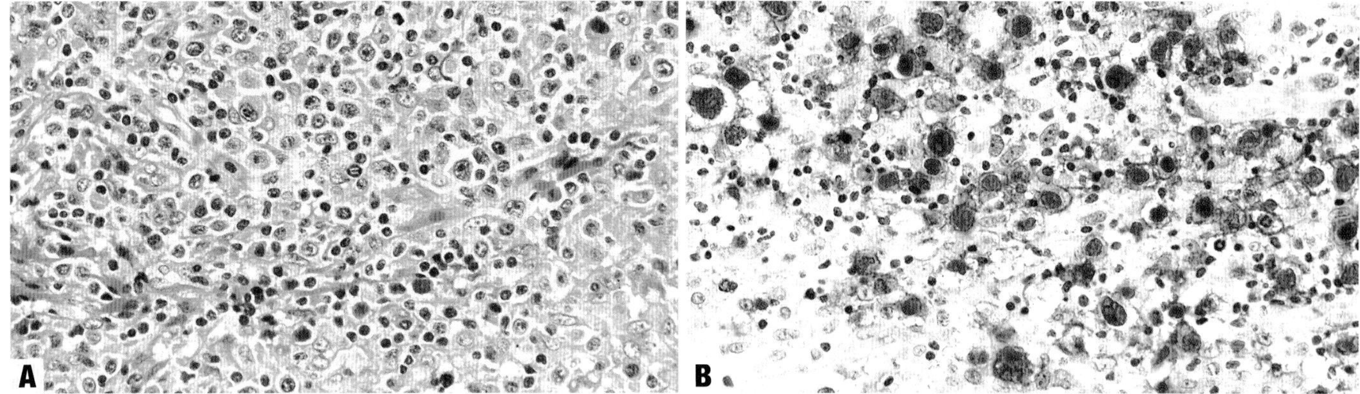

Fig. 4.187 EBV-positive diffuse large B-cell lymphoma. **A** A polymorphic lesion is composed of a mixed proliferation of large transformed cells, numerous reactive small lymphocytes, occasional plasma cells, and some histiocytes. **B** Double labelling employing in situ hybridization for EBV-encoded small RNA (EBER, brown nuclear stain) and for CD20 (red membranous stain) highlights the fact that the scattered large neoplastic B cells are EBV-positive.

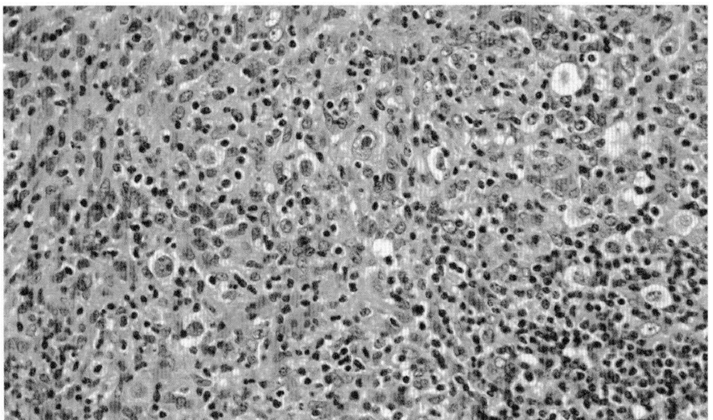

Fig. 4.188 EBV-positive diffuse large B-cell lymphoma. In polymorphic cases, HRS-like cells are scattered in a background of reactive cells.

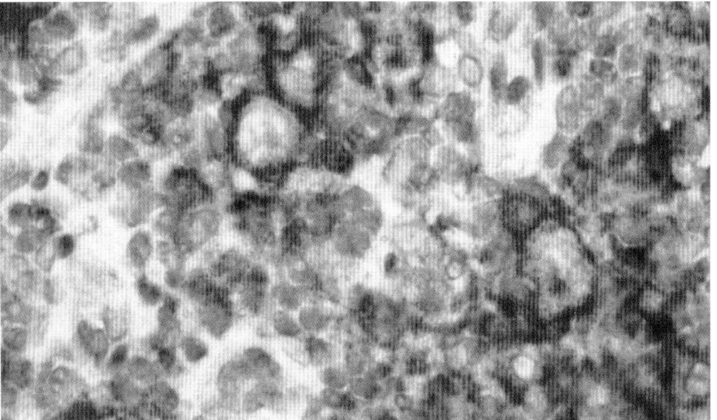

Fig. 4.189 EBV-positive diffuse large B-cell lymphoma. PDL1 in EBV diffuse large B-cell lymphoma NOS in a young patient, with a polymorphic / T-cell/histiocyte–rich background and with a positive B-cell clone by PCR.

other EBV-related lymphomas and lymphoproliferative disorders.

Desirable: EBV DNA detectable in serum or whole blood (in selected cases).

Staging

The stage of the disease is determined using the Lugano classification, a modification of the Ann Arbor staging system {688}.

Prognosis and prediction

The prognostic impact of EBV infection in DLBCL is variable according to Asian, European, and US studies. Although most studies in Asian populations have demonstrated inferior outcomes after treatment including R-CHOP {51,3583,2438,2893}, several studies in European and US populations did not find any correlation between EBV positivity and prognosis {3031,4055, 4390}, particularly in younger patients {2954}; however, some studies in European and US patients showed that EBV had a negative impact in elderly patients {428}. An adverse impact of CD30 expression on both overall survival and progression-free survival has been observed {3031,4390,303}. Some reported poor prognostic factors include type III EBV latency (EBNA2 expression) {3856}, and the presence of secondary haemophagocytic lymphohistiocytosis at diagnosis or during treatment {428}.

Diffuse large B-cell lymphoma associated with chronic inflammation

Xerri L
Aozasa K
Chan JKC
Gopal AK

Definition

Diffuse large B-cell lymphoma (DLBCL) associated with chronic inflammation (CI-DLBCL) is an EBV-associated neoplasm occurring in the setting of longstanding chronic inflammation involving confined natural body spaces or acquired tissue spaces. Pyothorax-associated lymphoma (PAL) is the prototypical form, developing in the pleural cavity of patients with longstanding pyothorax.

ICD-O coding

9680/3 Diffuse large B-cell lymphoma associated with chronic inflammation

ICD-11 coding

2A81.7 Diffuse large B-cell lymphoma associated with chronic inflammation

Related terminology

Acceptable: pyothorax-associated lymphoma.

Subtype(s)

None

Localization

The most frequently reported sites are the pleural cavity, bone (especially the femur), joints, and periarticular soft tissue {692}.

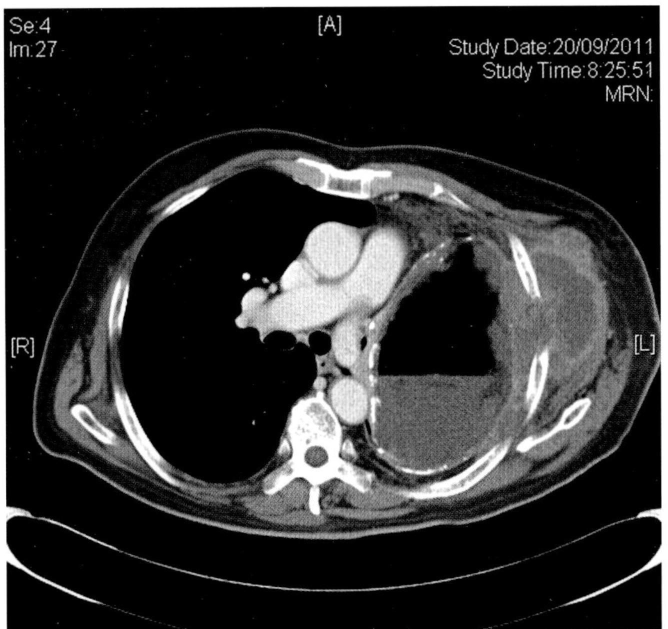

Fig. 4.190 Diffuse large B-cell lymphoma associated with chronic inflammation. Pyothorax-associated lymphoma. CT shows a tumour mass involving the pleura on the left side, accompanied by an effusion. The tumour invades through the chest wall into the soft tissues.

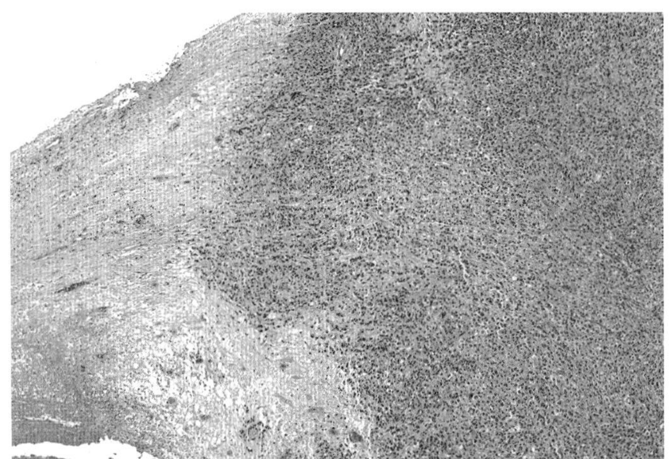

Fig. 4.191 Diffuse large B-cell lymphoma associated with chronic inflammation. Pyothorax-associated lymphoma. The tumour comprises sheets of lymphoma cells, with large areas of coagulative necrosis.

Clinical features

Symptoms of PAL include chest and back pain; fever; and respiratory symptoms, such as cough, haemoptysis, and dyspnoea. Radiological examination reveals a tumour mass in the pleura (in 80% of cases), pleura and lung, or lung near the pleura. Serum LDH is commonly elevated {3210,2889}. CI-DLBCL lesions in the bone, joint, periarticular soft tissue, or skin usually present with pain and/or a mass lesion. The involved bone shows lytic lesions.

Epidemiology

PAL develops after a long history (median: 37 years) of pyothorax, often resulting from artificial pneumothorax for the treatment of tuberculosis {3210,2889,130,2905}. As this procedure is no longer practised, the incidence of PAL has drastically decreased. Cases have been reported mostly in Japan, and rarely elsewhere. Patient age at diagnosis ranges from the fifth to eighth decade of life {2889,2905}. The M:F ratio is 12:1 {2544, 3210}.

For CI-DLBCL arising in other settings, such as chronic osteomyelitis, metallic implant insertion, surgical mesh implantation, and chronic skin venous ulcer, the interval following the predisposing event is usually > 10 years (range: 1.2–57 years) {800,692,1253}.

Etiology

CI-DLBCL develops in patients without recognized immunodeficiency, with the possible exception of immunosenescence {1875,663}.

Pathogenesis

CI-DLBCL is strongly associated with EBV infection {3582,3210, 3930,3929}. Chronic inflammation in a confined space probably induces local immunodeficiency by the production of IL-10, favouring escape from immunosurveillance of EBV-transformed B cells, which are also stimulated via autocrine or paracrine IL-6R engagement {1880,1877,800,692}.

Immunoglobulin genes are clonally rearranged and hypermutated but lack ongoing mutations {2700,3932}. Cytogenetics show complex karyotypes with numerous abnormalities {3930}. *TP53* mutations are found in about 70% of cases {1625}. *TNFAIP3* (*A20*) is often deleted {119}.

The gene expression profile of PAL is distinct from that of nodal DLBCL, at least partly due to EBV infection {2969}. Downregulation of HLA class I expression and mutations of cytotoxic T-lymphocyte epitopes in EBNA3B might contribute to the immune escape of lymphoma cells {1879,1878}. The latter process also involves regulatory T cells, which are abundantly present in PAL {1582}.

Macroscopic appearance

PAL lesions are usually large (often > 100 mm). Few data, however, exist for CI-DLBCL at other sites {130}.

Histopathology

Most cases show a centroblastic or immunoblastic morphology, with round nuclei and large nucleoli {3876,2027}. Massive necrosis and angiocentric growth may be present.

Immunophenotype

Most cases express B-lineage markers, such as CD20 and CD79a. Some cases may show plasmablastic differentiation, manifesting as variable loss of CD20 and/or CD79a, and variable expression of IRF4 (MUM1) and CD138. Lymphoma cells exhibit an activated B-cell–like phenotype. CD30 may be expressed. Occasional cases aberrantly express one or more T-cell antigens (CD2, CD3, CD4, CD7), causing problems in lineage assignment {3210,2889}. Type III EBV latency (i.e. positivity for LMP1 and EBNA2) is characteristic {3210,1253}.

Differential diagnosis

Cases showing plasmablastic differentiation must be distinguished from plasmablastic lymphoma on the basis of clinical context. CI-DLBCL and fibrin-associated large B-cell lymphoma (FA-LBCL) have overlapping cytological and phenotypic features. Their distinction, however, is important because of the aggressive nature of CI-DLBCL compared with the rather indolent nature of FA-LBCL. At least focal infiltration in pre-existing structures or the formation of a mass lesion distinguishes CI-DLBCL from FA-LBCL. Fibrin deposits are common in FA-LBCL but rare in CI-DLBCL. The distinction between the two is especially difficult, if possible at all, on small specimens such as core needle biopsies. Clinicopathological correlations and imaging studies are highly contributory to making the distinction.

PAL differs from primary effusion lymphoma, which is KSHV/HHV8-positive and in most cases presents with effusions in the absence of a tumour mass.

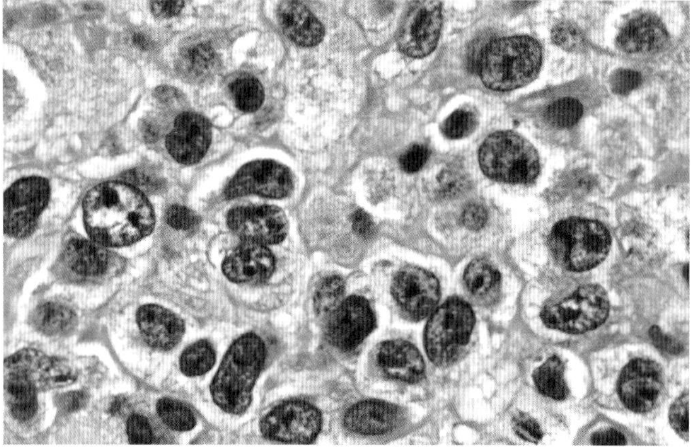

Fig. 4.192 Diffuse large B-cell lymphoma associated with chronic inflammation. Pyothorax-associated lymphoma. The large lymphoma cells have round or irregularly folded nuclei and distinct nucleoli.

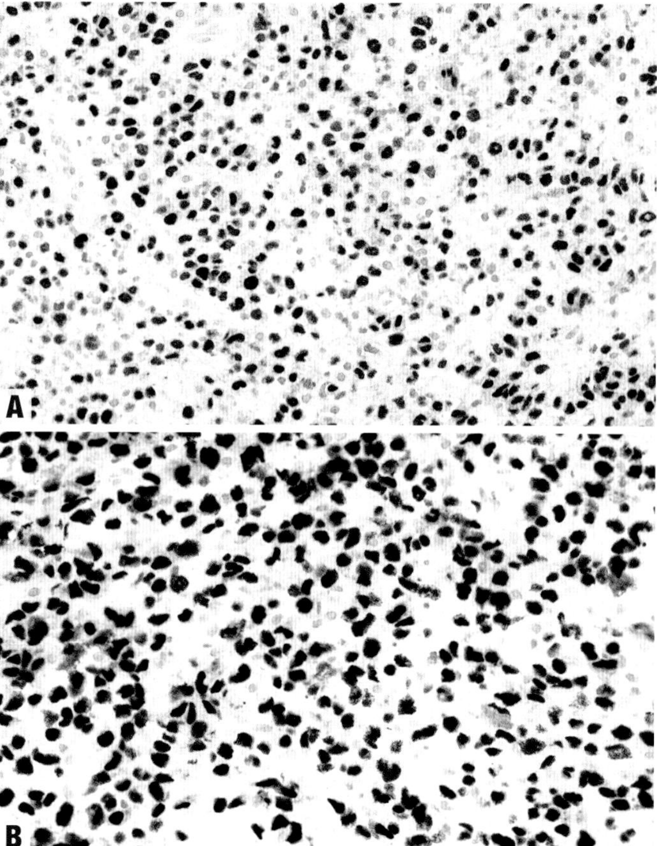

Fig. 4.193 Diffuse large B-cell lymphoma associated with chronic inflammation. **A** Pyothorax-associated lymphoma with positive immunohistochemistry for PAX5, supporting a B-cell lineage. **B** Positive nuclear staining for EBNA2 indicates type III EBV latency.

Cytology

The diagnosis is very difficult to make on FNAB and requires ancillary methods.

Diagnostic molecular pathology

In situ hybridization for EBV-encoded small RNA (EBER) is positive in tumour cells.

Essential and desirable diagnostic criteria

Essential: large B-cell lymphoma; setting of local chronic inflammation; EBV association; exclusion of other EBV-associated neoplasms.

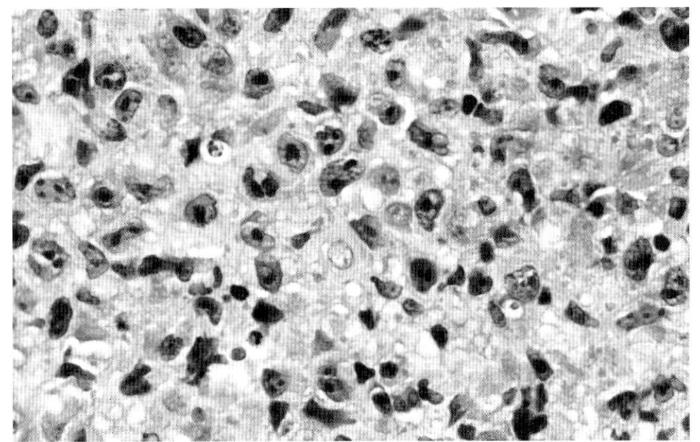

Fig. 4.194 Diffuse large B-cell lymphoma associated with chronic inflammation. In this case, arising in a longstanding anal fissure, the large lymphoma cells have irregularly folded nuclei and large nucleoli.

Desirable: occurrence in a natural or acquired confined body or tissue space.

Staging

CI-DLBCL is staged according to the Lugano classification {688}. PAL tumours are often confined to the thoracic cavity at diagnosis {2889}.

Prognosis and prediction

CI-DLBCL is an aggressive lymphoma. The 5-year overall survival rate of PAL is 20–35% {2889,2905}. Poor performance status, high LDH levels, and high clinical stage are unfavourable factors {2905}. Outcome data are limited for CI-DLBCL other than PAL.

Fibrin-associated large B-cell lymphoma

Boyer DF
Cheuk W
Coupland SE
Ferry JA
Maleszewski JJ
Shimada K

Definition

Fibrin-associated large B-cell lymphoma (FA-LBCL) is a neoplasm of large B cells found incidentally at sites of chronic fibrin deposition in confined natural or acquired anatomical spaces and sites.

ICD-O coding

9678/3 Fibrin-associated large B-cell lymphoma

ICD-11 coding

2A81.Y & XH0RM6 Other specified diffuse large B-cell lymphomas & Fibrin-associated EBV-positive diffuse large B-cell lymphoma

Related terminology

Acceptable: fibrin-associated diffuse large B-cell lymphoma.

Not recommended: microscopic/incidental diffuse large B-cell lymphoma associated with chronic inflammation; EBV-positive large B-cell lymphoma arising in atrial myxoma; microscopic diffuse large B-cell lymphoma occurring in pseudocyst.

Subtype(s)

None

Localization

FA-LBCL arises in sites of chronic fibrin deposition including cyst and pseudocyst cavities {416}, in the peri-implant space of breast implants {3443}, and in chronic haematomas {4544}, as well as in intravascular or intracardiac locations, such as the surface of cardiac myxomas {440}, endovascular grafts, and prosthetic cardiac valves {2685} (see Table 4.34). Embolization of fibrinous material from intravascular or cardiac sites involved by FA-LBCL may carry the lymphoma cells along with the embolus {440}.

Clinical features

The clinical presentation depends on the underlying anatomical lesion involved by FA-LBCL and can be asymptomatic. Some patients with FA-LBCL in atrial myxoma or endovascular grafts present with thromboembolic events; however, it is unknown whether the risk of thromboembolism differs from similar vascular grafts or myxomas without FA-LBCL.

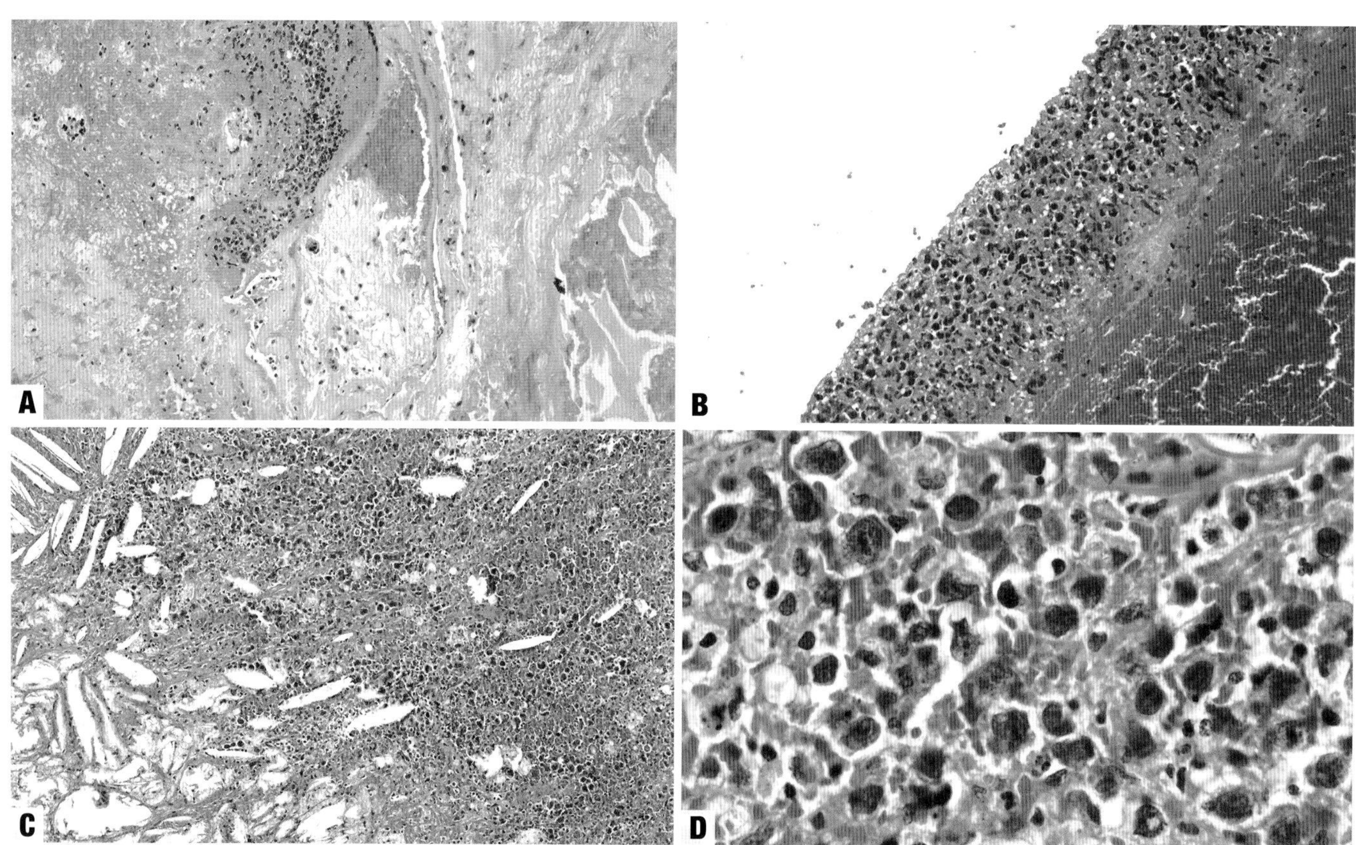

Fig. 4.195 Fibrin-associated large B-cell lymphoma. **A** An aggregate of large lymphocytes within fibrin in a cardiac myxoma. **B** Large lymphocytes on the surface of a femoral artery embolus. **C** Large lymphocytes associated with chronic haemorrhage and cholesterol clefts in a hydrocoele. **D** High magnification of the hydrocoele specimen shows atypical immunoblasts with frequent mitotic figures and apoptotic bodies.

Epidemiology

The overall incidence is unknown. FA-LBCL is diagnosed in adults, with a wide age range (25–91 years; median: 59.5 years). Some anatomical localizations of the disease (breast-implant associated, testicular haematoma-associated) have an obvious sex bias (see Table 4.34).

Etiology

The etiology is unknown. Patients rarely have evidence of recognized immunosuppression, with the possible exception of immunosenescence.

Pathogenesis

FA-LBCL is associated with EBV infection, but rare EBV-negative cases have also been described {2027,279}. The local microenvironment is hypothesized to create a form of local immune escape excluding EBV+ B cells from immunosurveillance {2408}. Dense fibrin around the tumour cells, upregulation of PDL1 {440}, and production of IL-6 by cardiac myxomas have been implicated in creating a permissive environment {45}. FA-LBCL is usually negative for rearrangements of *BCL2*, *BCL6*, and *MYC*, but rare cases with *BCL6* or *MYC* rearrangement have been reported {4480,2666}.

Macroscopic appearance

Not applicable

Histopathology

Aggregates of large lymphoid cells, often of atypical immunoblastic type, are surrounded by fibrin and cellular debris. There may be focal infiltration of myxomatous stroma (e.g. in cardiac myxoma) or fibrous capsular tissue (e.g. in breast implant–associated cases) but infiltration into pre-existing normal parenchymal tissue or mass formation is absent. Mitotic figures and apoptotic changes are frequent. Associated inflammation is usually sparse, although a prominent lymphoplasmacytic infiltrate may be found in some cases {440}. Rare EBV-negative cases have a presentation and histology identical to those of the EBV-positive cases {2027,279}.

Immunohistochemistry

The immunophenotype usually resembles activated B cells: the tumour cells are positive for pan–B-cell markers (CD20, CD79a, and PAX5). CD10 is negative. IRF4 (MUM1) is positive. BCL2, BCL6, and CD30 are variable. A minority have plasmablastic features, including intracytoplasmic positivity for monotypic light chain, positive CD138, and decreased expression of CD20 and PAX5. Aberrant expression of T-cell markers, typically CD3, CD4, or CD43, is occasionally present. Ki-67/MIB1 staining shows a high proliferation index, usually > 90%. Most cases have type III EBV latency, signified by positivity for LMP1 and EBNA2 and negativity for BZLF1 {440}. KSHV/HHV8 (by latency-associated nuclear antigen [LANA] immunohistochemistry) is negative.

Differential diagnosis

The lack of mass formation and infiltrative growth distinguishes this entity from EBV-positive diffuse large B-cell lymphoma (DLBCL) and DLBCL associated with chronic inflammation.

Cytology

Lymphoma cells are large with narrow to broad basophilic cytoplasm and round or irregular nuclei with coarse chromatin.

Table 4.34 Localization and clinical characteristics of reported cases of fibrin-associated large B-cell lymphoma

Site	Number of cases	Median age (range), years	M:F ratio	Foreign body	Persistent or recurrent disease / reported cases with follow-up
Cardiac					
Atrial myxoma	17	54 (46–70)	6:11	0/17	1/16
Atrial thrombus	2	42.5 (29–56)	2:0	0/2	0/2
Cardiac valve	5	66 (50–80)	3:2	4/5	0/5
Cyst/pseudocyst					
Adrenal	5	70 (48–71)	3:2	0/5	0/5
Kidney	2	53.5 (46–61)	2:0	0/2	0/1
Spleen	2	33 (29–37)	1:1	0/2	0/2
Retroperitoneum	2	58.5 (44–73)	2:0	0/2	0/2
Ovary	2	56.5 (56–57)	0:2	0/2	0/2
Testis	2	57.5 (27–88)	2:0	0/2	0/1
Breast implant					
Periprosthetic space	10	65 (46–83)	0:10	10/10	0/9
Haematoma/thrombus					
Endovascular graft	6	62 (48–79)	5:1	6/6	3/5
Intracranial	4	70.5 (25–81)	3:1	1/4	0/3
Large-artery aneurysm	2	82.5 (74–91)	5:1	1/2	0/2
Testicular haematoma	1	79	1:0	0/1	0/1

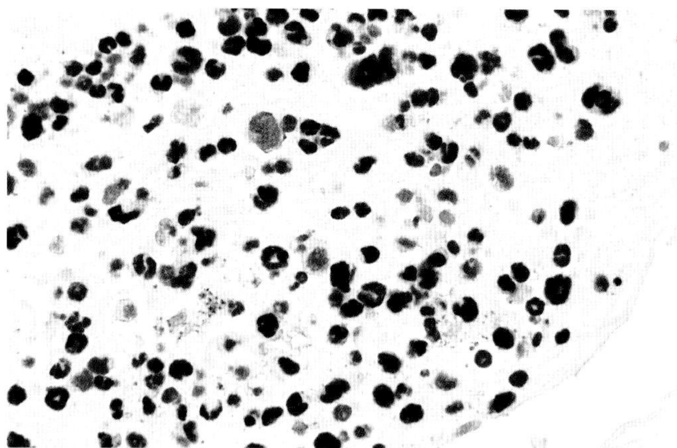

Fig. 4.196 Fibrin-associated large B-cell lymphoma. EBV-encoded small RNA (EBER) in situ hybridization in a cardiac myxoma reveals EBV infection of the tumour cells.

Diagnosis of FA-LBCL is not possible from cytological material alone.

Diagnostic molecular pathology

In situ hybridization for EBV-encoded small RNA (EBER) is nearly always positive.

Essential and desirable diagnostic criteria

Essential: microscopic aggregates of atypical large B lymphocytes in a background of fibrinous debris; presentation at sites of chronic fibrin deposition in confined natural or acquired anatomical spaces and sites; no mass-forming lymphoma lesion; no infiltration into pre-existing normal parenchymal tissue.

Desirable: non–germinal-centre B-cell immunophenotype; EBV positivity.

Staging

All reported cases have been localized to a single extranodal site, consistent with stage IE of the Lugano classification {688}.

Prognosis and prediction

No cases of biopsy-proven FA-LBCL with subsequent development of infiltrative or disseminated lymphoma have been identified so far. Retrospective reports show no difference in outcomes between patients treated with chemotherapy, chemoimmunotherapy, or surgical excision {440}. No deaths directly attributable to FA-LBCL have been reported {440,4480,4544}. When the underlying lesion cannot be completed excised, persistence or local regrowth of FA-LBCL has been reported {403,440}.

Fluid overload–associated large B-cell lymphoma

de Jong D
Chapuy B
Said JW
Truemper LH

Definition
Fluid overload–associated large B-cell lymphoma (FO-LBCL) is a B-cell neoplasm presenting as serous effusions without detectable tumour masses, often in patients with fluid overload states. It is not associated with KSHV/HHV8.

ICD-O coding
9678/3 Fluid overload–associated large B-cell lymphoma

ICD-11 coding
2A81.Y Other specified diffuse large B-cell lymphomas

Related terminology
Acceptable: fluid-overload effusion lymphoma; KSHV/HHV8-negative effusion-based lymphoma.
Not recommended: PEL-like effusion lymphoma; HHV8-negative PEL; HHV8-unrelated PEL-like lymphoma.

Subtype(s)
None

Localization
The majority of the reported cases have occurred in the pleural cavity (70%), followed by the pericardial and abdominal cavities. Pleural effusions often accompany effusions in other sites (~40%) {1850}. A single case of scrotal involvement has been described {4426}. No manifestations outside body cavities or mass formation are detected at presentation, but they can occur at relapse. Extranodal sites such as the pleura, CNS, and abdominal organs may then become involved {68}.

Clinical features
Patients with FO-LBCL typically present with unilateral or bilateral pleural, pericardial, or abdominal effusions, without detectable tumour masses. More than 50% of patients have an identified underlying condition causing fluid overload, such as chronic heart failure, renal insufficiency, protein-losing enteropathy, or liver failure / cirrhosis. Symptoms are commonly related to the effusions and to the underlying disorder.

Epidemiology
FO-LBCL is very rare, with < 100 cases reported in the literature {2071,68,4426,2641,1850}. Patients are usually elderly (median age: 70–77 years) and predominantly male (M:F ratio: 2:1). The disease seems to be more prevalent in Asia, especially in Japan, where 46–60% of the cases were reported and where this disease forms the large majority of effusion-related lymphomas {2071,1850}.

Etiology
Unknown

Pathogenesis
In 50% of patients, FO-LBCL is associated with an underlying medical condition leading to fluid overload. Although KSHV/HHV8 infection does not play a role, a significant proportion of cases are associated with other viruses, such as HCV (most prevalent in ascites-based cases; 20–40%) and HBV (10%) {68, 4426,2137}. EBV association is reported in 13–30% of cases {68,2137}. FO-LBCL is not associated with overt immunodeficiency and is rarely (~5%) associated with HIV. Predominance in elderly patients suggests that immunosenescence may play a role in pathogenesis.

Limited information is available on the genomic landscape and molecular oncogenesis. Genetic studies have shown an overall complex copy-number landscape. Frequent recurrent focal deletions are reported in 3p14.2 and 6q21 {2641,3019}. Structural alterations at the *MYC* locus, including translocations

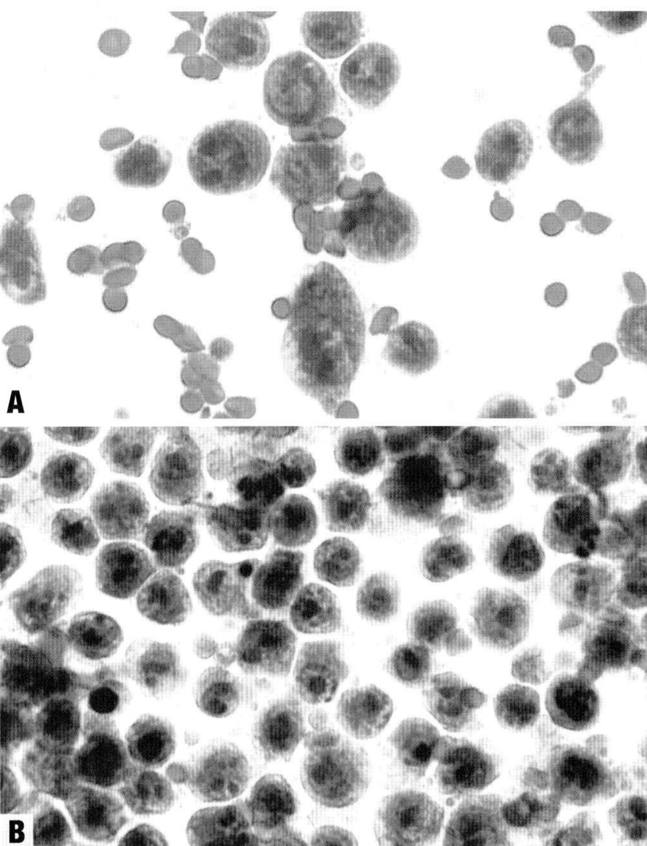

Fig. 4.197 Fluid overload–associated large B-cell lymphoma. Ascitic fluid from an HIV-negative 30-year-old man with congenital heart disease, congestive cardiac failure, ascites, and lower-extremity oedema. Cytology revealed large malignant lymphoid cells with prominent nucleoli, highlighted in Pap (**A**) and Giemsa (**B**) stains. The tumour cells were positive for CD79a and negative for CD20, KSHV/HHV8, and EBV-encoded small RNA (EBER). There was a clonal IG gene rearrangement.

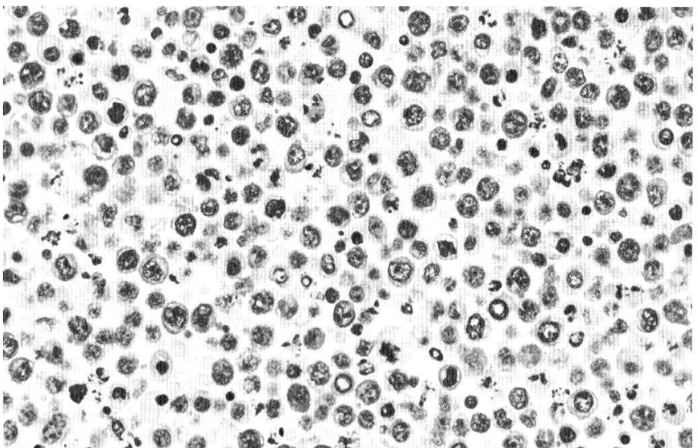

Fig. 4.198 Fluid overload–associated large B-cell lymphoma. A cytoblock from pleural fluid shows medium-sized to large lymphoid cells with basophilic cytoplasm (Giemsa).

and amplifications, are reported in as many as 50% of cases {2641,4426}. *MYC* translocations may have IG or non-IG gene partners, and cases with concurrent *MYC* and *BCL2* translocations have been reported. The mutation spectrum is marked by features of activation-induced cytidine deaminase (AID)-mediated non-IG somatic hypermutation. Mutations have been reported to recurrently affect *MYD88*, *H1-4* (*HIST1H1E*), *BTG1*, *BTG2*, *IRF4*, and chromatin modifying genes (e.g. *CREBBP*, *KMT2D*, and *MEF2B*) {2641}.

Macroscopic appearance

Not relevant

Histopathology

See *Cytology* for morphological appearances.

Immunophenotype

The tumour cells usually express a complete B-cell phenotype (CD20, CD79a, and CD19). Pan–B-cell markers may not be expressed in a small percentage of cases; in particular, CD20 can be negative in approximately 20% of FO-LBCL. A non–germinal-centre cell phenotype is most common. CD138 is infrequently expressed (10%) and CD30 is variably expressed (20–30%). Rare cases are positive for CD10 (~10%) {1850} but lack expression of other germinal-centre markers (GCET1, LMO2) {68,4426,656,2641}.

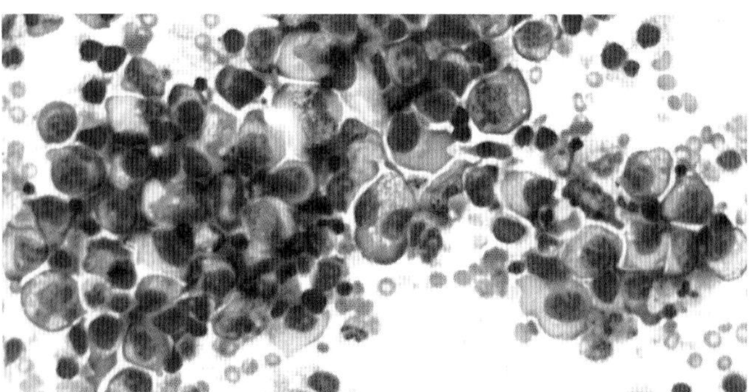

Fig. 4.199 Fluid overload–associated large B-cell lymphoma. A 51-year-old man with alcoholic cirrhosis presented with lower-extremity oedema and dyspnoea, bilateral pleural effusions, and ascites. Pleural fluid revealed large malignant lymphoid cells with prominent nucleoli and basophilic cytoplasm (Giemsa).

Differential diagnosis

FO-LBCL must be differentiated from primary effusion lymphoma, which as a rule is diagnosed in patients with immune deficiency/dysregulation (mostly frequently in those positive for HIV) and generally at a younger age. Primary effusion lymphoma is a proliferation of mature B cells that lack pan–B-cell markers and is KSHV/HHV8-positive by definition. Pyothorax-associated lymphomas arise in the pleural cavity after long-standing inflammation, usually due to tuberculosis or chronic pneumothorax, and are mass-forming. These B-cell lymphomas are usually associated with dense inflammatory infiltrates and are associated with EBV. Secondary effusion-based localizations from primary diffuse large B-cell lymphoma should be excluded primarily on clinical grounds by complete staging procedures.

Rare cases of large B-cell lymphoma arising in pleural effusions in patients treated with dasatinib have been described {740,1193}. All cases had expression of mature B-cell markers (CD20, PAX5, CD79a) and were KSHV/HHV8-negative, whereas EBV was positive in some of the reported cases. In line with the nomenclature of immune deficiency/dysregulation (IDD)-associated B-cell lymphoproliferative disorders, such cases may be reported as IDD-associated FO-LBCL, EBV-positive or -negative, iatrogenic setting (post-dasatinib). EBV-positive cases of FO-LBCL seem to be preferentially observed in IDD settings, including in post–liver transplant, HIV, common variable immunodeficiency, and autoimmune disease settings {68,2137}. Also in such cases, the nomenclature for IDD-associated lymphoproliferative disorders should be applied and may also be considered in elderly patients (presumed immunosenescence). Especially in EBV-positive cases, more aggressive manifestations of IDD-associated B-cell lymphoproliferative disorder (EBV-positive diffuse large B-cell lymphoma) should be excluded {2372}.

Cytology

The diagnosis is commonly made on cytological material (smears, cytocentrifuge preparations, cytoblock sections). The atypical cells show a wide morphological spectrum, ranging from centroblastic or immunoblastic to anaplastic with prominent nucleoli. Less commonly, a small to medium-sized or plasmacytoid morphology is reported. The cytoplasm is commonly abundant. Admixture of histiocytes is common, but significant inflammatory infiltrates are lacking {2071,68}.

Diagnostic molecular pathology

Monoclonal heavy or light chain IG gene rearrangement can be demonstrated in the majority of cases. *MYC* translocations are reported at high frequency. Concurrent *MYC* and *BCL2* translocation does not exclude the diagnosis. According to the current published literature, EBV-encoded small RNA (EBER) may be positive in FO-LBCL {68,2137}.

Essential and desirable diagnostic criteria

Essential: a large cell lymphoma restricted to body cavity effusions; exclusion of secondary involvement by systemic lymphoma; B-cell phenotype; KSHV/HHV8-negative.
Desirable: clonal IG gene rearrangement.

Staging

Staging should be performed to exclude secondary malignant body cavity effusion by primary systemic indolent and aggressive B-cell lymphomas.

Prognosis and prediction

The prognosis of FO-LBCL is favourable in most cases and is largely determined by comorbidity. Most patients are treated with CHOP(-like) therapy with or without rituximab and show a favourable outcome. Several cases with spontaneous regression without any systemic treatment, or with lasting remission after pleurodesis only, have been described {68}. Two-year overall survival and progression-free survival rates are > 85% and 70%, respectively {2137,1850}. Information on prognostic factors is limited and may include age < 70 years, poor performance status, presence of ascites, and lack of CD20 expression as unfavourable factors {2137}.

Plasmablastic lymphoma

Montes-Moreno S
Leoncini L
Louissaint A Jr
Miranda RN
Montes-Moreno S
Sengar M

Definition

Plasmablastic lymphoma (PBL) is an aggressive lymphoid neoplasm composed of large atypical B cells with plasmablastic or immunoblastic morphology and a terminal B-cell differentiation phenotype, predominantly arising at extranodal sites.

ICD-O coding

9735/3 Plasmablastic lymphoma

ICD-11 coding

2A81.2 Plasmablastic lymphoma

Related terminology

None

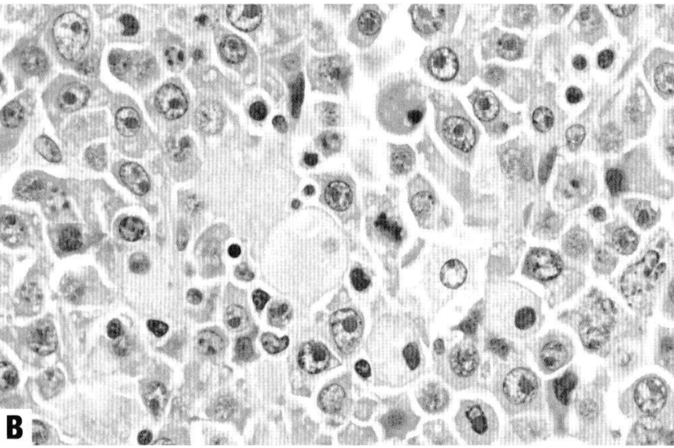

Fig. 4.200 Plasmablastic lymphoma. **A** A case showing a diffuse large cell neoplasm with a prominent starry-sky pattern. **B** The cells are large and non-cohesive, with abundant basophilic cytoplasm, a central or eccentric large vesicular nucleus, and a distinct single nucleolus. Note the presence of histiocytes.

Subtype(s)

None

Localization

PBL usually involves extranodal sites, such as the nasal/oral cavity (~50%), digestive system (~20%), bone and soft tissues (~15%), and skin (~5%). Nodal involvement can also occur without apparent extranodal disease.

Clinical features

Clinical features of PBL depend on the site involved and the extent of involvement. In the oral cavity, the gingiva and palate are the most commonly affected sites. The tumour induces painful swelling, and features rapid growth with frequent ulceration and necrosis and common bone destruction {438,1207}. PBL usually arises de novo in patients with immune deficiency/dysregulation {923} (see Table 4.42, p. 550, in *Lymphoid proliferations and lymphomas associated with immune deficiency and dysregulation: Introduction*). PBL can also arise secondarily as a transformation of follicular lymphoma or chronic lymphocytic leukaemia / small lymphocytic lymphoma (CLL/SLL) {2549,3122,1096}.

Epidemiology

PBL is rare, accounting for 1% of large B-cell lymphomas {3339} and 2% of HIV-related lymphomas {572}. There is a male predominance (M:F radio: 3:1) {572}. The disease occurs more often in adults than in children {2374,572}.

Etiology

The etiology is unknown. PBL occurring in the setting of immune deficiency/dysregulation are generally, but not invariably, associated with EBV. PBL has been reported to occur in the context of newly emerging iatrogenic immune deficiency/dysregulation settings, such as anti-CD19 chimeric antigen receptor (CAR) T-cell therapy {1096}.

Pathogenesis

Most PBLs occur in the context of immune deficiency/dysregulation (e.g. HIV infection; 31–62%) or immunosuppressive therapy for bone marrow transplant, solid-organ transplantation, or autoimmune diseases (3–7%). PBL may also occur in elderly adults without overt immunodeficiency; in these cases, immunosenescence may contribute to the pathogenesis {2806,572, 2397,2236,2754}. EBV reactivation, with type I and occasionally type II latency, is observed {572}. The presence of an EBV abortive lytic cycle profile has been described as a feature {100, 2390}.

Complex karyotypes are common. MYC overexpression is found in as many as 80% of the cases. *MYC* rearrangements, usually with IG genes, are reported in about 60% of cases {1243}. Lymphomas with plasmablastic features carrying dual

MYC and *BCL2* translocations have been exclusively seen in cases transformed from follicular lymphoma {3919,391,3089}. Chromosomal translocations commonly encountered in plasma cell myeloma other than *MYC* rearrangements have not been described in de novo PBL. EBV-negative PBL cases show a higher mutation load and more frequent *TP53*, *CARD11*, and *MYC* mutations, whereas EBV-positive PBLs tend to have more mutations affecting the JAK/STAT pathway {3362}. Somatic mutations involving JAK/STAT, MAPK/ERK, and NOTCH pathways are frequently detected {3362,2390,1297,1243} together with *TP53* mutations (see Table 4.35). The microRNA expression profile of PBL reveals a number of EBV-encoded microRNAs, suggesting a pathogenetic role of EBV-encoded microRNAs in the lymphomagenesis of EBV-positive cases {103}. Gene expression profiling has demonstrated downregulation of B-cell receptor signalling and upregulation of plasma cell differentiation–associated genes and *MYC* {638}.

Macroscopic appearance

Not relevant

Histopathology

PBL demonstrates a destructive infiltrate composed of large immunoblastic and plasmablastic cells. A starry-sky pattern and brisk mitotic activity may be identified. Intermediate-sized lymphoplasmacytoid cells and plasma cells constitute a minor component of the infiltrate in rare cases.

Immunohistochemistry

Immunohistochemistry demonstrates absent CD20 expression and reduced/absent expression of PAX5 and CD45 (LCA). CD79a is positive in 40% of cases. Expression of markers associated with plasma cell differentiation, such as CD138, CD38, VS38c, Blimp1, and XBP1, are found in most cases. IRF4 (MUM1) is always positive {923,2752,2754,2236}. Immunoglobulin light chain restriction is usually demonstrable by immunohistochemistry or by flow cytometry. MYC protein is often expressed. Significantly higher levels of MYC protein expression are found in cases with MYC translocation or amplification {1297}. Ki-67 is usually positive in > 90% of cells {2397, 2754}. PDL1 overexpression {2236,1297} and loss or aberrant expression of MHC class II have been demonstrated {3616}. CD10, CD56, and CD30 are positive in 20–30% of cases, whereas BCL6 is rarely positive. EBV association is demonstrable in 60% of cases {1243} and is more frequent in patients with HIV (82%). ALK and KSHV/HHV8 latency-associated nuclear antigen (LANA) are negative. Rare cases with aberrant weak to moderate cytoplasmic expression of CD3 have been reported {3120}. Rarely (< 10%), aberrant cytokeratin expression warrants a differential diagnosis with (undifferentiated) carcinoma {1681}.

Differential diagnosis

PBL shows morphological and phenotypical overlap with diffuse large B-cell lymphoma (DLBCL) NOS with immunoblastic morphology {3088,1681}, DLBCL with partial plasmablastic phenotype {2752}, EBV-positive DLBCL {2384}, and *MYC*-and *BCL2*-rearranged large B-cell lymphomas with plasmablastic features transformed from follicular lymphoma. ALK-positive large B-cell lymphoma and extracavitary/solid primary effusion lymphoma should be excluded. Expression of CD20 and/or PAX5 favours DLBCL over PBL, whereas expression of XBP1, Blimp1, and CD138 supports a diagnosis of PBL. Plasmablastic transformation of plasma cell myeloma (PCM) is usually heralded by a previous diagnosis of PCM, the presence of CRAB clinical features (hypercalcaemia, renal insufficiency, anaemia, and bone lesions) {4194,100, 2384}, and bone marrow infiltration by mature clonal plasma cells. Genetic features of PCM (e.g. typical translocations or mutation spectrum) favour plasmablastic transformation of PCM over de novo PBL. Rare cases of PBL in HIV-positive individuals may show overlapping clinical features with PCM {3919}. However, the distinction may not be made unequivocally in all cases.

Table 4.35 Frequency of genetic alterations in plasmablastic lymphoma at diagnosis

Gene / chromosomal region	Frequency of genetic lesion	Type of genetic lesion
	70%	Translocation
MYC	10%	Gain/amplification
	10%	Mutation
JAK/STAT pathway		
STAT3	16–42%	Mutation
JAK1	5–14%	Mutation
SOCS1	10–12%	Mutation
MAPK/ERK pathway		
***RAS* (*NRAS, KRAS, HRAS*)**	12–33%	Mutation
MAP2K1	7%	Mutation
BRAF	5–7%	Mutation
NOTCH pathway		
NOTCH1	7%	Mutation
SPEN	8%	Mutation
NOTCH4	6%	Mutation
NCOR2	12%	Mutation
TP53	6–30%	Mutation
17p	10%	Deletion
***IRF4* (6p25.3)**	29%	Gain
***MCL1* (1q21.3)**	32–43%	Gain
***CD44* (11p13)**	37%	Gain

STAT3 mutations are found in as many as 42% of cases, particularly in patients with HIV and EBV, involving the SH2 domain and associated with increased phosphorylated STAT3 expression {1297} and JAK/STAT pathway signature overexpression {3362, 2390}. Other JAK/STAT pathway components such as *JAK1* and *SOCS1* are also recurrently mutated in 5–15% of the cases {3362,2390,1243}. MAPK/ERK pathway mutations include *NRAS* (30%), *KRAS* (12%), *HRAS* (2%), *BRAF* (7%), and *MAP2K1* (7%) mutations. Other genetic events include *TP53* mutation, 17p deletion / loss of heterozygosity, *IRF4* (6p25.3) amplification (29%) {1243}, 11p13 gain (including *CD44*) (37%) {2390}, and 1q21.3 gain (including *MCL1*, *IL6R*) (43%) {2390,1243}.

Cytology

Cells are large and non-cohesive, with abundant basophilic cytoplasm and central to eccentric large vesicular nuclei with distinct single nucleoli.

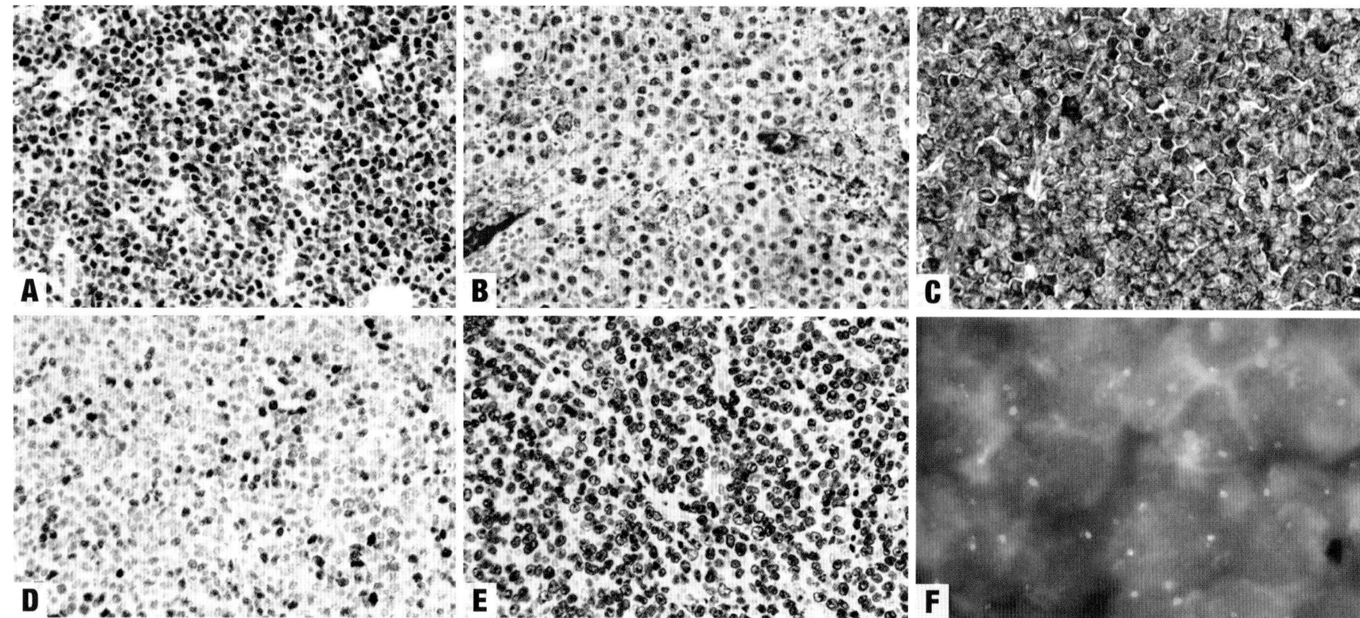

Fig. 4.201 Plasmablastic lymphoma. **A** The tumour cells are strongly positive for IRF4 (MUM1). **B** Most tumour cell nuclei express Blimp1. **C** CD138 is expressed in all tumour cells. **D** MYC is variably expressed in the tumour cell nuclei. **E** The Ki-67 proliferation index is very high in this case. **F** FISH for *MYC* translocation shows split signals using break-apart probes.

Diagnostic molecular pathology

Monoclonal IG rearrangements can be demonstrated in PBL.

Essential and desirable diagnostic criteria

Essential: lymphoma with plasmablastic/immunoblastic morphology; expression of plasma cell–associated antigens (e.g. IRF4 [MUM1], CD138, Blimp1); negativity for CD20, PAX5, ALK, and KSHV/HHV8.

Desirable: EBV positivity (EBV-encoded small RNA [EBER]) in about 60% of cases; detection of *MYC* rearrangements; detection of monoclonal IG rearrangements.

Staging

The Lugano system is used to stage lymphomas and has been adopted by the Union for International Cancer Control (UICC) TNM classification {688}.

Prognosis and prediction

The prognosis of PBL is poor, with a median overall survival time of 6–32 months with conventional chemotherapy. Patients diagnosed with low clinical stage have shown more favourable outcomes {2397,3253}. A high International Prognostic Index (IPI) score and the presence of *MYC* translocations or gain have a negative impact on outcome {2806}.

Primary large B-cell lymphoma of immune-privileged sites

Coupland SE
Batchelor T
Calaminici M
Chapuy B
Deckert M
Dunleavy K
Elenitoba-Johnson KSJ
Ferry JA
Hoang-Xuan K
Jeon YK
Kuzu I
Lenz G
Nagane M
Soffietti R

Definition

Primary large B-cell lymphomas (LBCLs) of immune-privileged sites (IP-LBCLs) comprise LBCLs that arise as primary tumours in the CNS, vitreoretina, and testis of immunocompetent patients. Excluded from this category are the lymphomas that arise in the dura and the choroid, lymphomas secondarily involving these sites, and lymphomas occurring in immune deficiency/dysregulation–related settings.

ICD-O coding

9680/3 Primary large B-cell lymphoma of immune-privileged sites
9680/3 Primary large B-cell lymphoma of the CNS
9680/3 Primary large B-cell lymphoma of vitreoretina
9680/3 Primary large B-cell lymphoma of the testis

ICD-11 coding

2A81.Y Other specified diffuse large B-cell lymphomas
2481.5 Primary diffuse large B-cell lymphoma of the central nervous system

Related terminology

Acceptable: primary diffuse large B-cell lymphoma of the CNS; primary diffuse large B-cell lymphoma of the vitreoretina; primary diffuse large B-cell lymphoma of the testis.
Not recommended: primary CNS lymphoma; primary intraocular lymphoma; primary testicular lymphoma.

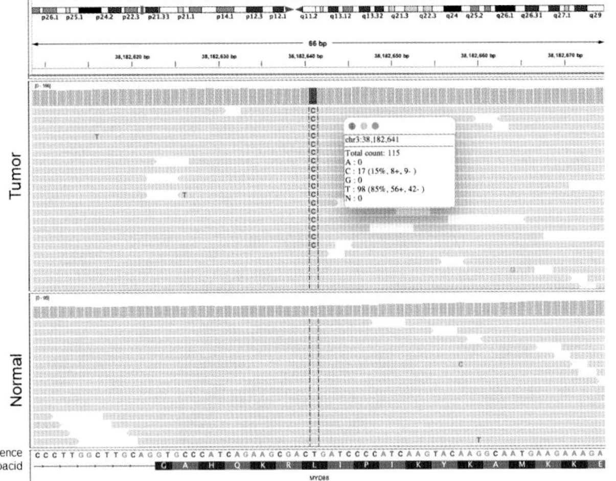

Fig. 4.202 *MYD88* mutation in a case of diffuse large B-cell lymphoma arising in an immune-privileged site. Depicted is an Integrative Genomics Viewer (IGV) screenshot of a somatic mutation in *MYD88*. Reads in the tumour and patient-matched normal sample are depicted at the top and bottom, respectively. Nucleotides matching the reference sequence are in grey, nucleotides different from the reference are colour-coded. Reference DNA and the corresponding amino acid sequence are at the bottom. Specifically, this tumour sample has a somatic mutation on chromosome 3 at positions 38, 182, and 641 in *MYD88* from a T to a C that gives rise to a change in the amino acid sequence from a lysine to a proline (*MYD88* p.L265P).

Subtype(s)

Primary large B-cell lymphoma of the CNS (PCNS-LBCL); primary large B-cell lymphoma of the vitreoretina (PVR-LBCL); primary large B-cell lymphoma of the testis (PT-LBCL)

Localization

PCNS-LBCL is solitary (65% of cases) or multifocal. Tumours are mainly located in the cerebral hemispheres (38%), thalamus / basal ganglia (16%), corpus callosum (14%), periventricular region (12%), or cerebellum (9%) {2144}. The leptomeninges may be involved, but exclusive meningeal involvement is unusual. PVR-LBCL is typically located in the subretinal space (between the photoreceptors and the retinal pigment epithelium overlying the Bruch membrane). Tumour cells are also found around vessels in the retina and scattered in the vitreous. With advanced disease, the tumour infiltrates the aqueous, forming deposits on the posterior surface of the cornea (keratic precipitates). Very rarely, PVR-LBCL involves the vitreous only, without retinal invasion. Optic nerve involvement is infrequent {819}. PT-LBCL involves the testicular parenchyma and adjacent structures, such as the epididymis.

Clinical features

PCNS-LBCL and PVR-LBCL develop insidiously, typically mimicking other conditions and thus causing delays in diagnosis. Patients with PCNS-LBCL have focal neurological deficits (50–80%), as well as headache, nausea, and cranial neuropathies; neuropsychiatric symptoms are common {3614,3080}. In rare instances, PCNS-LBCL can relapse outside the CNS {1186,410,3158}.

PVR-LBCL may occur independently of, concurrently with, or after PCNS-LBCL, with patients presenting with blurred vision, posterior uveitis (masquerade syndrome), floaters, and retinal haemorrhage and/or detachment. It is bilateral in 60% of cases {819,3313}.

PT-LBCL manifests with a painless unilateral testicular mass; occasionally (6–10%), bilateral disease is present at diagnosis. PT-LBCL often relapses in the CNS or in the contralateral testis.

Epidemiology

PCNS-LBCL represents 2–3% of all brain malignancies, with an incidence of 0.47 cases per 100 000 person-years {4233}. The incidence rate has inexplicably increased over the past two decades in patients aged > 60 years. PVR-LBCL represents 1% of all ocular malignancies and has a similar incidence to PCNS-LBCL, also with an increased occurrence over the past two decades {819,3313}. Both occur in the fifth to seventh decade of life (median ages: 66 and 68 years, respectively). There is a slight male predominance in both disorders (M:F ratio: 3:2). PT-LBCL represents 5% of all testicular malignancies and arises in men aged > 60 years, with an incidence of 0.09–0.26 cases per 100 000 person-years {1186}.

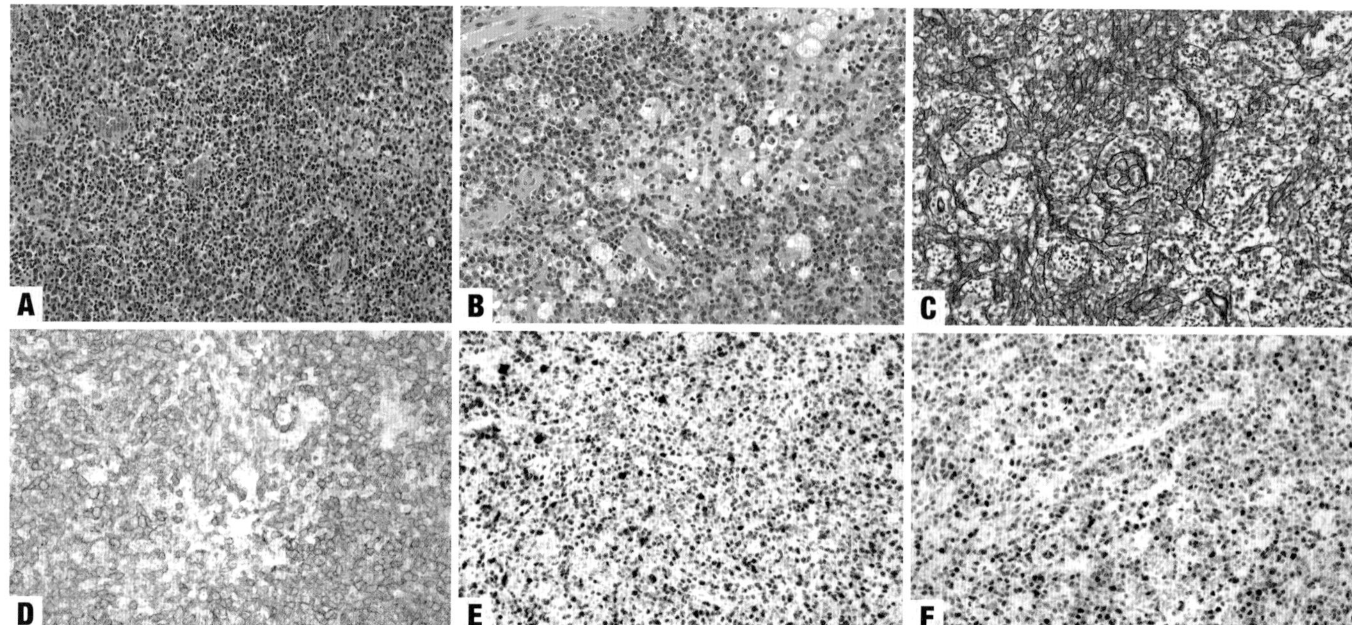

Fig. 4.203 Primary large B-cell lymphoma of immune-privileged sites. **A** A highly cellular primary large B-cell lymphoma of the CNS (PCNS-LBCL) shows large cells admixed with reactive lymphocytes and histiocytes. In addition to a patternless growth, a blood vessel wall is infiltrated by tumour cells. **B** A PCNS-LBCL showing large tumour cells admixed with reactive lymphocytes and histiocytes. **C** Tumour cells infiltrate blood vessel walls, distending the network of reticulin fibres. **D** The tumour cells strongly express CD20. **E,F** The majority of the tumour cells express BCL6 (**E**) and IRF4 (MUM1) (**F**).

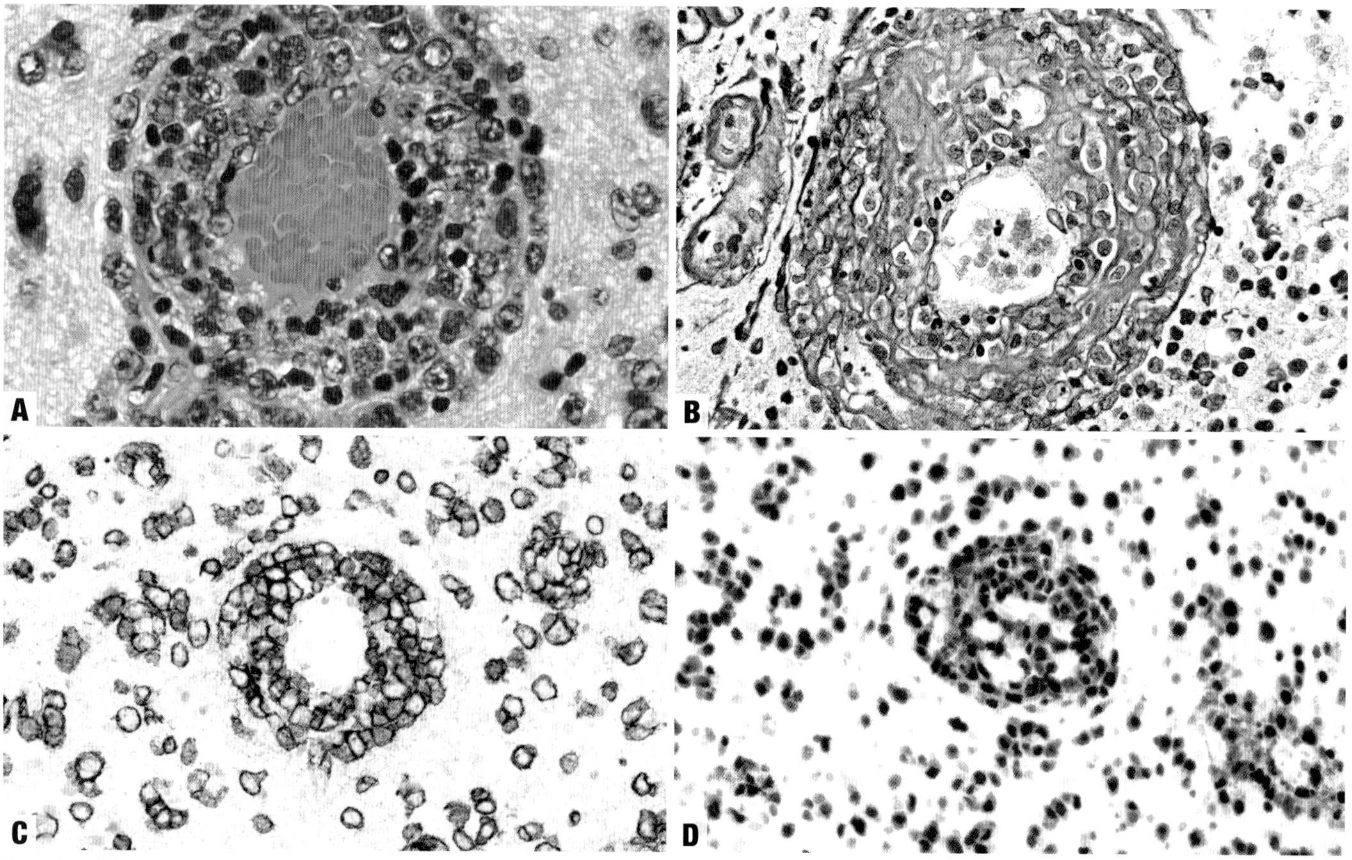

Fig. 4.204 Primary large B-cell lymphoma of immune-privileged sites. The large lymphoma cells of primary large B-cell lymphoma of the CNS show a predilection for infiltrating the walls of blood vessels. They often have vesicular chromatin, distinct nucleoli, and amphophilic cytoplasm (**A**). Infiltration of lymphoma cells into the blood vessel wall is accompanied by reduplication of the reticulin fibres of the vessel (reticulin stain) (**B**). Immunostaining for CD20 (**C**) and IRF4 (MUM1) (**D**) highlights the large lymphoma cells, including those accentuated in the blood vessel walls.

Etiology

Unknown

Pathogenesis

PCNS-LBCL, PVR-LBCL, and PT-LBCL share morphological, immunophenotypic, and molecular features. They are grouped as one category because they arise in immune sanctuaries created by their respective anatomical structures (e.g. the blood–brain, blood–retinal, and blood–testicular barriers), and target organ immune regulation, which in turn determines their molecular biology and clinical behaviour. It remains unclear at present where the originating precursor neoplastic B cells arise before proliferating in these organs, as all three sites normally lack regular lymphoid tissue within them. Whether lymphoma arises in situ or outside these organs, subsequently homing to them, is an area of debate and continuing research {2737,4012,2745}. However, PCNS-LBCL, PVR-LBCL, and PT-LBCL cells all demonstrate features corresponding to mature germinal centre (GC)-exit B cells {4004,2740,296}, which have undergone a prolonged GC reaction with evidence of ongoing somatic hypermutation in their rearranged IG genes {4004,2740,296} (see Table 4.36).

Our understanding of immune privilege is a rapidly evolving field in current research {3407,2027,60}, adding to what already is known from anatomical structures and target organ immune regulation, and hence this "immune-privileged lymphoma" grouping is likely to evolve with time. Indeed, supported by shared molecular features, discussions are underway as to whether primary LBCL of the ovary, breast, and even skin should be included in this group.

PCNS-LBCL and PVR-LBCL preferentially rearrange the IGHV4-34 gene, which is implicated in autoimmune diseases, in 36–80% and 55% of cases, respectively {2740,820,2742,296}. This preferential usage of the IGHV4-34 gene in PCNS-LBCL {4004,2740,2742} together with IGH somatic hypermutation results in auto-immunity, whereby the tumour B-cell receptor is directed to multiple autoantigens on resident CNS cell populations {1768,478,2743,2741,2745,4012}. This mechanism supports that immunological drive plays a role in at least a phase of the oncogenesis of these lymphomas.

PCNS-LBCL, PVR-LBCL, and PT-LBCL also possess common genetic alterations that enable immune escape and downregulation of specific immune reactions {3407,1830,1829,409, 2424}. This includes, for example, genetic inactivation of MHC class I and II and of *B2M*, with subsequent loss of protein

Table 4.36 Molecular alterations of primary large B-cell lymphoma of immune-privileged sites: primary CNS large B-cell lymphoma (PCNS-LBCL), primary vitreoretinal large B-cell lymphoma (PVR-LBCL), and primary testicular large B-cell lymphoma (PT-LBCL)

Characteristic	PCNS-LBCL	PVR-LBCL	PT-LBCL
Developmental stage of tumour cell	Late GC-exit B cell	Late GC-exit B cell	Late GC-exit B cell
Phenotype	PAX5+, CD19+, CD20+, CD22+, CD79a+, IgM+, IgD+, BCL2+, MYC+, BCL6+ IRF4 (MUM1)+, CD38−, CD138−, Ki-67 high	PAX5+, CD19+, CD20+, CD79a+, IgM+, Ki-67 high	PAX5+, CD19+, CD20+, CD79a+, IgM+, Ki-67 high
Cell of origin	Self-reactive/polyreactive B cell	Unknown	Unknown
Antigen recognized by the tumour cell	GRINL1A, ADAP2, BAIAP2, neurabin-1/SAMD14, MPZL1, S100, MOBP, MBP, galectin-3, endoglin	Unknown	Unknown
IGHV rearrangement	IGHV4-34	IGHV4-34	IGHV4-34
SHM	+, ongoing	+	+, ongoing
SHM targets	IG	IG	IG
Aberrant SHM	*BCL6, PIM1, PAX5, RHOH, KLHL14, SUSD2, IGLL5, MYC, BCL2, IRF4, SOCS1*	*BCL6, PIM1, IGLL5, IRF4*	*BCL6, IGLL5, PIM1, BTG2, BTG1, IRF4, SBPL10*
Translocations	IG, *BCL6, CD274, PDCD1LG2*	IG	*BCL6, FOXP1, CD274, PDCD1LG2*
Mutations (non-SHM)	*MYD88* p.L265P, *CD79B* p.Y196, *INPP5D* (*SHIP*), *CBL, BLNK, TBL1XR1, PRDM1, OSBPL10, B2M, BTG1, FAS* (*CD95*), *ETV6*	*MYD88* p.L265P, *CD79B, TBL1XR1, BTG2, BTG1, ETV6*	*MYD88* p.L265P, *CD79B* p.Y196, *TBL1XR1, ETV6*
Chromosomal gains	18q21.22-q23 (*BCL2, MALT1*), chromosome 12, 9p13 (*PAX5*), 9p24.3 (*CD274* [*PDL1*]), 19q13.43	2q35, 12q12, 18q	18q21.22-q23 (*BCL2, MALT1*), 3q12.3 (*NFKBIZ*), 9p24.3 (*CD274*), 19q13
Chromosomal losses	6q21 (*PRDM1*), 6p21 (*MHC* locus), 8q12.1-q12.2 (*TOX*), 9p21 (*CDKN2A*), 10q23.21 (*PTEN*), 15q21 (*B2M*)	9p21 (85%, *CDKN2A*)	6p21 (MHC locus), 9p21 (*CDKN2A*), 15q21 (*B2M*)
Epigenetic silencing	*RFC, DAPK1* (*DAPK*), *CDKN2A, MGMT*	Unknown	Unknown
Signalling pathways activated/dysregulated	TLR, BCR, NF-κB, PI3K, JAK/STAT	TLR, BCR	TLR, BCR, NF-κB, PI3K, JAK/STAT
Protein expression	BCL2^{high}, BCL6^{high}, MYC^{high}, FOXP1^{high}, loss of HLA class I and II, loss of B2M	BCL2^{high}, BCL6^{high}, MYC^{high}	pSTAT3^{high}, FOXP1^{high}, PDL2 (PDCD1LG2)^{high}, loss of HLA class I and II, loss of B2M
Diffuse large B-cell lymphoma molecular subtypes	MCD, C5 (i.e. gains in *BCL2* and/or mutations in *MYD88* [p.L265P], *CD79B, ETV6, PIM1, GRHPR, TBL1XR1*, and *BTG1*)	MCD, C5	MCD, C5

BCR, B-cell receptor; GC, germinal centre; MBP, myelin basic protein; p, phosphorylated; SHM, somatic hypermutation; TLR, toll-like receptor; +, present.

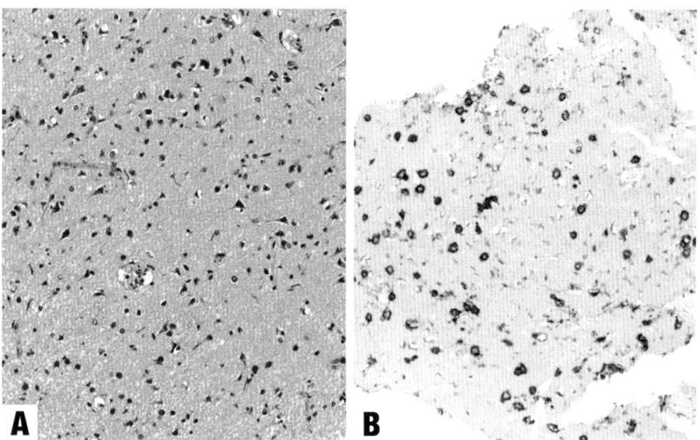

Fig. 4.205 Primary large B-cell lymphoma of immune-privileged sites. **A** The neoplastic lymphocytes in primary large B-cell lymphoma of the CNS can be difficult to recognize on H&E-stained sections, especially when limited tissue is present in stereotactic biopsies. **B** CD20 staining is helpful for recognizing scattered neoplastic B cells among the glial cells.

expression {411,3653}, leading to escape recognition by cytotoxic T cells {3278,2424}.

The overall genomic signature of PCNS-LBCL, PVR-LBCL, and PT-LBCL resembles the C5/MCD/MYD88 signature found in diffuse large B-cell lymphoma NOS {405,641,3629,644,2191, 4417,1673}. This signature emphasizes the common genomic heritage of these lymphomas and further underscores why they have been grouped here.

The most frequent common genetic hallmarks of PCNS-LBCL, PVR-LBCL, and PT-LBCL, which are also the hallmarks of the C5/MCD/MYD88 signature mentioned above, are the concordant *MYD88* (p.L265P) and *CD79B* mutations {2739, 2744,653,4190,641,1213,385}, which are probably acquired early in lymphomagenesis {644,2424}.

Additionally, PCNS-LBCL, PVR-LBCL, and PT-LBCL foster B-cell receptor and toll-like receptor signalling leading to constitutional NF-κB activation, thus facilitating escape from apoptosis and supporting survival. The footprints of aberrant somatic hypermutation, targeting genes implicated in lymphomagenesis, including *BCL2*, *MYC*, *PIM1*, *PAX5*, *RHOH*, *KLHL14*, *IRF4*, *BTG1*, *BTG2*, *IGLL5*, and *SUSD2*, are consistently present {2746,4190,2424}.

PRDM1 and *TBL1XR1* mutations {823,1367,641} also contribute to the GC-exit phenotype by blocking terminal B-cell differentiation and by inducing pre-memory transcriptional reprogramming {4212,4213}. Persistent BCL6 activity together with MYC expression fosters cyclic re-entry into the GC, thus supporting a prolonged GC reaction. The oncogenesis most probably follows a stepwise course in which the various alterations leading to constitutional NF-κB activation and GC trapping predominate in the early phases, only subsequently followed by alterations leading to immune escape {2424}.

Translocations target the IG genes and *BCL6* in PCNS-LBCL, PVR-LBCL, and PT-LBCL {2747,2736,3652,513,2650}. Genetic imbalances are frequent, particularly gains of 18q21 (*BCL2*, *MALT1*) and 9p24.3 (*CD274* [*PDL1*]) and losses of 6q21 (*PRDM1*) and 6p21 (HLA locus). In addition, losses of 15q21 (*B2M*), 10q23.21 (*PTEN*), and 9p21 (*CDKN2A*) are recurrent {767,3653,641,408,3407,1830,1828,411}.

In PCNS-LBCL, DNA methylation has been more extensively studied than PVR-LBCL and PT-LBCL. The DNA methylome does not unequivocally distinguish PCNS-LBCL from non-CNS LBCL {4247}.

Macroscopic appearance

In PCNS-LBCL, single or multiple grey to yellow masses are seen within the parenchyma, with varying degrees of demarcation. The lesions are of variable consistency, often with haemorrhage and necrosis. In PVR-LBCL, enucleation samples are rarely received; these are only seen in advanced cases where no definitive diagnosis could be reached via vitrectomy or aqueous tap, with complete painful vision loss. Such specimens demonstrate a detached, necrotic, and possibly haemorrhagic retina with dense vitreous strands. In PT-LBCL, well demarcated, tan, grey, or white tumour masses of variable consistency and dimensions are easily identified.

Histopathology

The histopathology of PCNS-LBCL, PVR-LBCL, and PT-LBCL is similar, comprising neoplastic medium-sized to large cells with pleomorphic nuclei, vesicular chromatin, and prominent nucleoli surrounded by a narrow rim of eosinophilic to basophilic cytoplasm. Mitotic figures are often brisk, with scattered apoptotic bodies.

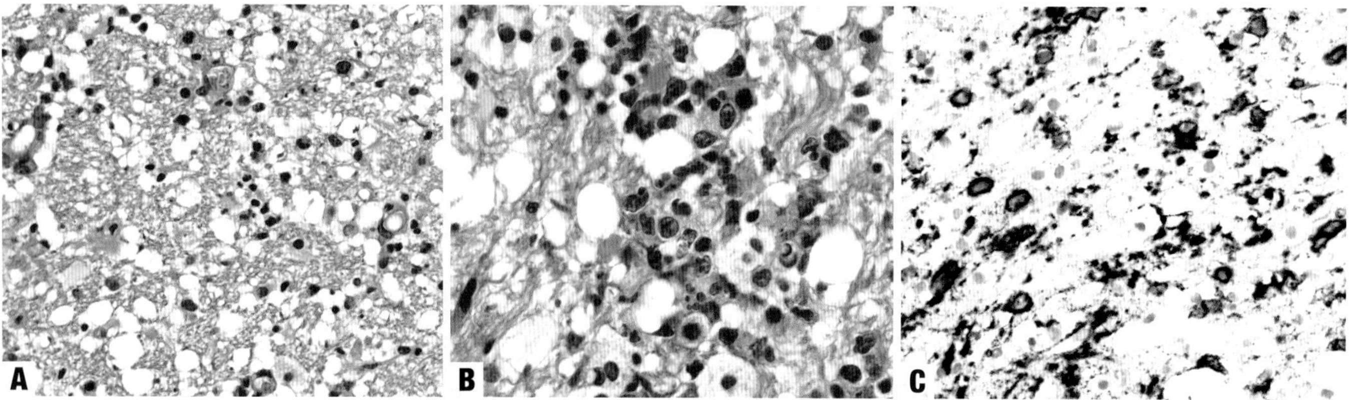

Fig. 4.206 Primary large B-cell lymphoma of immune-privileged sites. **A** High-dose steroid treatment prior to biopsy in primary large B-cell lymphoma of the CNS can result in tumour cell apoptosis, making a definitive diagnosis of lymphoma challenging; the apoptotic lymphoma cells appear as nuclear debris scattered in the brain parenchyma. **B** Although most areas of the brain biopsy are not diagnostic, there can be foci where some viable large lymphoma cells can be identified. **C** Tumour cells can be highlighted by immunostaining for CD20.

In PCNS-LBCL, the infiltration type is typically diffuse, patternless, and perivascular, with areas of necrosis. Reactive gliosis and reactive T cells, small B cells, macrophages, and activated microglia are present {912,1337}. Splitting of the vessel walls due to tumour cell infiltration is highly characteristic of PCNS-LBCL.

In PVR-LBCL, the neoplastic cells are typically located in the subretinal space or show a perivascular infiltration of the retina, with spillover into the vitreous. The B cells are often observed on a lytic (necrotic) cellular background with macrophages.

PT-LBCL cells also show a diffuse infiltrate, leading to obliteration of the seminiferous tubules with associated intertubular spread. Epididymal involvement is usually seen {1186}.

Tissue limitations

Steroid treatment before biopsy of PCNS-LBCL and PVR-LBCL often causes various morphological changes, including significant apoptosis, lysis of neoplastic cells, and increased numbers of macrophages, leading to false negative samples. Therefore, to allow diagnosis, steroids should be withheld whenever possible. Preoperative and intraoperative consultation is key in yielding successful biopsies that enable morphological, immunohistochemical, and molecular analyses {1337,1160}.

In some cases, a histological biopsy may not be possible for various reasons (e.g. poor condition of the patient; deeply seated CNS tumour; or a lymphoma located near fragile anatomical structures, e.g. blood vessels or detached retina), and hence alternative diagnostic methods must be considered. These include cytological examination of the vitreous or cerebrospinal fluid (CSF), or even detailed radiographic imaging only, although these procedures as such preclude definitive lymphoma classification.

Immunophenotype

The immunoprofile of the cells in these tumours is similar. They express mature B-cell markers (CD20, CD22, CD79a, CD19, and PAX5), IRF4 (MUM1), BCL2, BCL6, and IgM, and they show a high Ki-67 proliferation index (> 80–90%) {2747,58, 3653,2296,479,1343,408}. CD10 can be expressed in < 10% of cases {912}; however, it should raise the suspicion of disseminated systemic diffuse LBCL and prompt appropriate investigations. Immunophenotyping may be undertaken by flow cytometry in vitreous and CSF samples {882,3644,148}. Positivity for EBV is not typical and should prompt consideration of an immune deficiency/dysregulation–associated lymphoma.

Differential diagnosis

In immunocompetent patients, the relevant differential diagnosis of lymphomas presenting with CNS localization is broad (see Table 4.37).

When reviewing biopsies from the eye, the possibility of other primary tumours (e.g. primary choroidal lymphoma and non-pigmented choroidal melanoma with retinal infiltration) should be considered {819}. Similarly, metastatic carcinomas and skin melanomas should also be excluded.

Table 4.37 Differential diagnosis of primary large B-cell lymphoma of the CNS with the other primary CNS lymphomas[a]

Entity	Clinical presentation and imaging	Morphology	Phenotype	Molecular features	Clinical behaviour	References
Primary CNS parenchymal EMZL and LPL	> 92% supratentorial > 65% single lesion MRI hyperintense Isolated to CNS	Small mature lymphoid and/or lymphoplasmacytic cells Perivascular or diffuse infiltration pattern	MZL/LPL: CD20, CD79a, PAX5, CD38, CD138, IRF4 (MUM1), lambda or kappa light chain restriction Ki-67 index very low	*MYD88* mutation (LPL)	Indolent	{2349, 3132,2974}
Primary dura EMZL	Solitary localized nodular mass with intradural involvement	Small mature monocytoid lymphocytes, with or without plasmacytic differentiation Some cases accompanied by amyloid deposition	CD20, CD79a, PAX5, CD38, CD138, IRF4 (MUM1), light chain restriction frequent IgG4+ plasma cells present in some patients Ki-67 index very low	IGH clonal *TNFAIP3* *NOTCH2* *TBL1XR1* Trisomy 3	Indolent	{1281, 4103,4210, 2974}
Primary CNS parenchymal Burkitt lymphoma	Isolated mass	Typical small to medium-sized lymphoid cells with high apoptosis and mitosis	CD20, PAX5, CD10, BCL6, MYC; Ki-67 index very high (> 90%)	*MYC* translocation	Very aggressive	{3206,435, 2349}
Primary CNS PTCL and ALK-negative ALCL	Solitary or multiple lesions	PTCL-NOS: small to medium-sized cells ALK-negative ALCL: large atypical cells	PTCL: CD3, CD4 or CD8, CD5, CD7; Ki-67 index moderate ALCL: CD30, CD4, TIA1, perforin, granzyme; Ki-67 index high	Clonal TRB (TCRB), TRG (TCRG)	Very aggressive	{2349, 2648,2349, 3710}
IV-LBCL[b]	Perivascular leukoencephalopathy–like features No mass	Intravascular large pleomorphic lymphoid cells without parenchymal invasion	CD45, CD20, CD79a, PAX5, IRF4 (MUM1); Ki-67 index very high (> 80%)	*MYD88*, *CD79B* mutations	Very aggressive	{3724, 2586}

ALCL, anaplastic large cell lymphoma; DLBCL, diffuse large B-cell lymphoma; EMZL, extranodal marginal zone lymphoma; IV-LBCL, intravascular large B-cell lymphoma; LPL, lymphoplasmacytic lymphoma; MZL, marginal zone lymphoma; PTCL, peripheral T-cell lymphoma.

[a]The main differential diagnostic issue for any putative primary CNS lymphoma type remains exclusion of secondary CNS involvement of a primary systemic lymphoma (DLBCL, LPL, EMZL, PTCL-NOS, ALK-negative ALCL, and others). [b]IV-LBCL is not really a primary CNS lymphoma, but it is mentioned in this table because of its frequent CNS involvement, often as a presenting symptom.

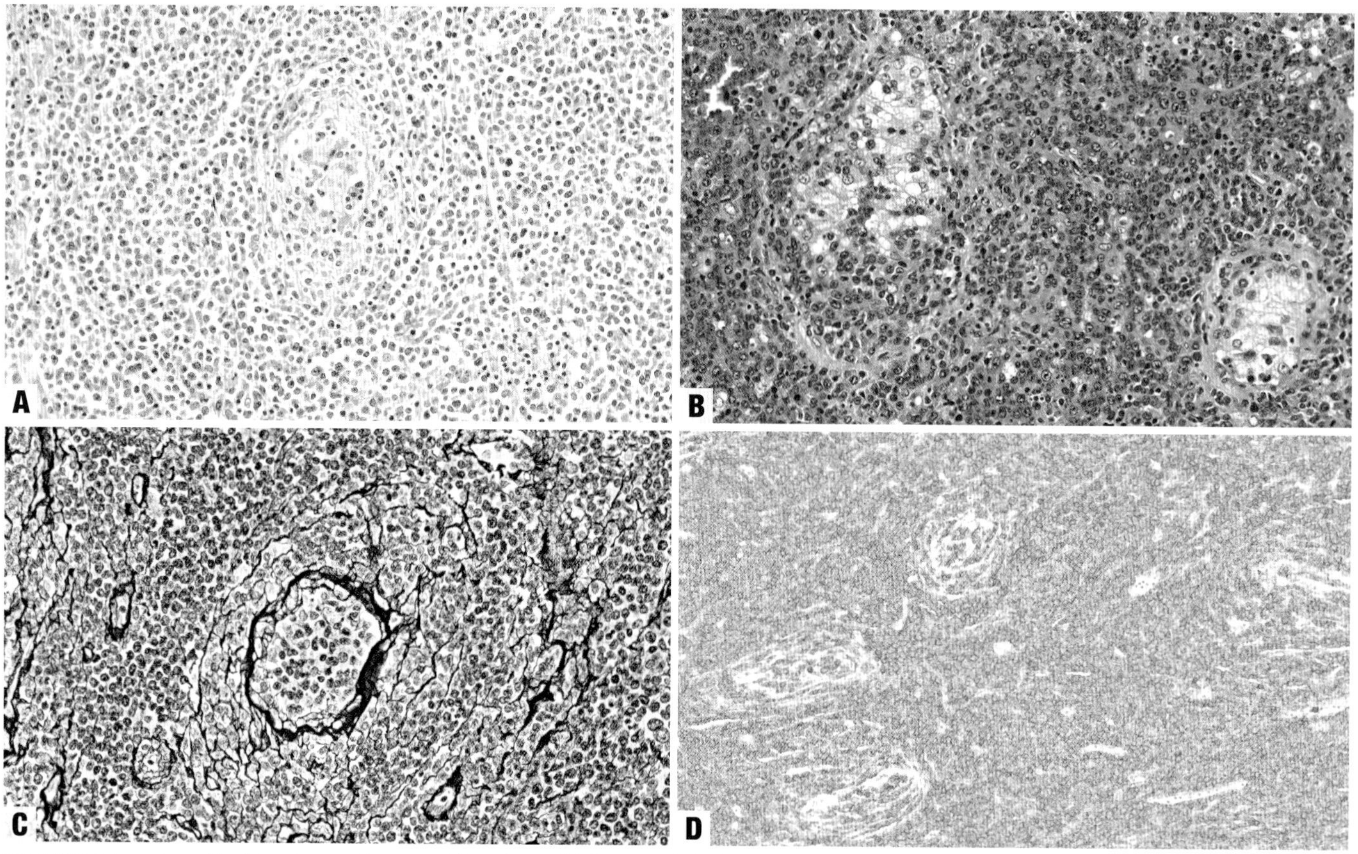

Fig. 4.207 Primary large B-cell lymphoma of immune-privileged sites. **A** Primary testicular large B-cell lymphoma showing neoplastic cells infiltrating seminiferous tubules. **B** At high power, neoplastic cells infiltrating seminiferous tubules can be appreciated. **C** Infiltration results in reduplication of their basal laminae (reticulin stain). **D** CD20-positive neoplastic cells surround and infiltrate seminiferous tubules.

In PCNS-LBCL, autoimmune CNS inflammation (including multiple sclerosis and acute demyelinating encephalomyelitis) is an important differential diagnosis; furthermore, sentinel lesions and brain abscess need to be considered. Finally, especially in the context of any potential immunosuppression, infectious conditions due to viruses (e.g. EBV) and microorganisms (e.g. *Toxoplasma gondii*, *Mycobacterium tuberculosis*, *Cryptococcus*, *Aspergillus*, and *Nocardia*) must be excluded.

In testicular samples, B-lymphoblastic leukaemia/lymphoma, Burkitt lymphoma, and diffuse large B-cell lymphoma / high-grade B-cell lymphoma with *MYC* and *BCL2* rearrangements need to be excluded.

Cytology

Leptomeningeal dissemination of PCNS-LBCL results in the presence of lymphomatous cells in CSF samples. Morphological examination can be challenging, because their recognition

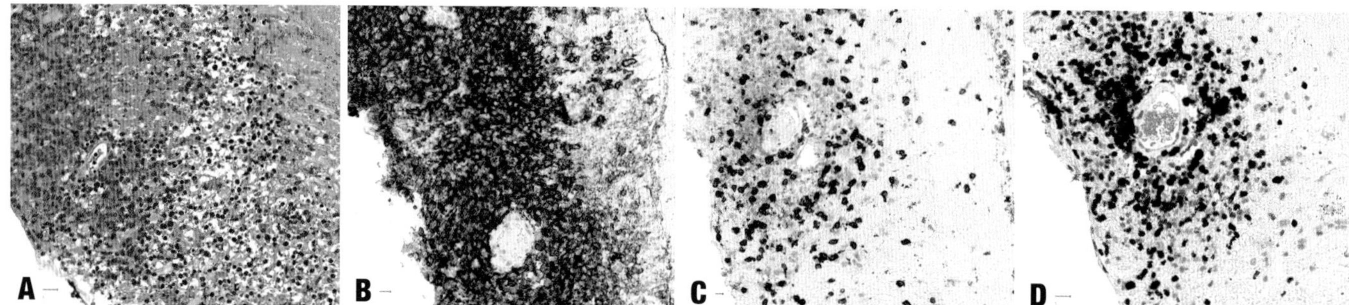

Fig. 4.208 Primary large B-cell lymphoma of immune-privileged sites. **A** A chorioretinal biopsy demonstrating a dense infiltration by atypical lymphocytes on a background of cellular debris and apoptotic cells, with associated haemorrhage and necrosis of the retina. The scattered pigmented epithelial cells represent the retinal pigment epithelial layer that has been completely disrupted by the tumour cells. The photoreceptors are no longer discernible. **B** CD20 immunostain (DAB) highlighting the neoplastic B cells within the retina, with the intraretinal blood vessels almost being consumed by the tumour cells. The fine linear stippling (upper right) is background, highlighting the inner surface of the Bruch membrane where the retinal pigment epithelial layer should be attached. **C** Contrasting CD3 immunostain (DAB) showing only scattered reactive T lymphocytes within the primary large B-cell lymphoma of the vitreoretina. **D** Ki-67 (MIB1, DAB) highlighting the viable and strongly proliferating neoplastic B cells within the chorioretinal biopsy.

is highly dependent on the number of neoplastic cells present and the degree of preservation. Similarly, vitrectomy samples in PVR-DBLCL vary in the degree of their cellularity but are composed of scattered medium-sized B cells with large polymorphic nuclei and small basophilic cytoplasmic rims. Typically, there is a dirty background composed of lytic cells, macrophages, and scattered small T cells.

Diagnostic molecular pathology

Clonality analysis of IG genes enables the differentiation of LBCL from reactive inflammatory lesions. In rare cases where infiltrates are dominated by atypical T cells, clonality analysis of TR genes is also of value.

Mutation analysis

MYD88 and *CD79B* hotspot mutations are highly recurrent in PCNS-LBCL, PVR-LBCL, and PT-LBCL. Detection of these can aid in the diagnosis, if the number of tumour cells is too low for clonality analysis {2746,2739,405,4032,136,3313,1579,2738,3959,408}, and potentially in future studies or clinical trials, using cell-free DNA {408,3057}.

Detection of pathognomonic oncogene rearrangements associated with systemic aggressive lymphomas, such as *ALK*, *CCND1*, *BCL2*, *MYC*, and 11q rearrangements, renders a diagnosis of IP-LBCL improbable.

Essential and desirable diagnostic criteria

Essential: large B-cell lymphoma primarily confined to the CNS, vitreoretina, or testis at presentation; exclusion of secondary involvement by other entities of large B-cell lymphoma; exclusion of immune deficiency/dysregulation–related settings.

Desirable: post–germinal-centre B-cell phenotype (IRF4 [MUM1]+, BCL6+, CD10−); absence of EBV (in > 97% of cases); demonstration of a clonal B-cell population or *MYD88* and/or *CD79B* hotspot mutations in cases in which histology is not definitive (e.g. corticosteroid-mitigated PCNS-LBCL or PVR-LBCL).

Staging

This varies according to the primary site of involvement but essentially follows the Lugano lymphoma staging system {688}.

Baseline staging for PCNS-LBCL should include contrast-enhanced MRI of the brain, contrast-enhanced MRI of the spine (if spinal symptoms are present), and ophthalmological and CSF evaluations. To detect systemic dissemination, FDG body PET-CT (versus CT alone) is the preferred imaging modality; bone marrow biopsy is rarely indicated if PET-CT is performed.

For PVR-LBCL, examination of the contralateral eye and brain imaging should be undertaken {1160}.

For PT-LBCL, ultrasonography and MRI of the testes may be helpful for evaluation of primary disease. The recommended staging is the same as for other aggressive non-Hodgkin lymphomas, with FDG PET-CT or CT imaging and bone marrow evaluation as indicated. Additionally, MRI of the brain and CSF evaluation by cytology and flow cytometry are recommended. Analysis of the CSF for the presence of circulating tumour DNA is currently being explored as an ultrasensitive technology to detect CNS involvement {3057}.

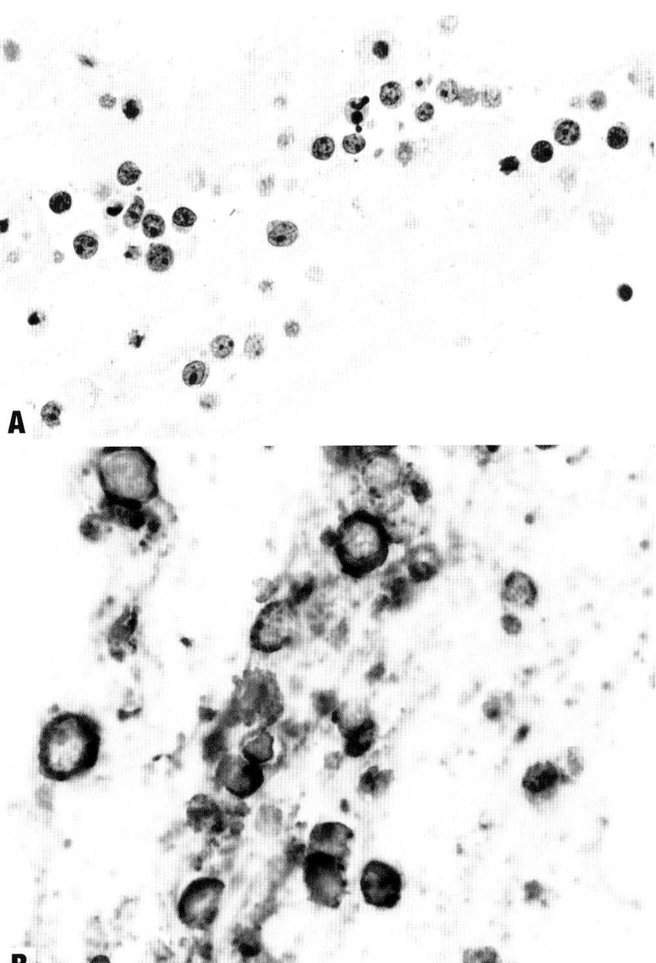

Fig. 4.209 Primary vitreoretinal large B-cell lymphoma. **A** Cell block produced from an aspirate of the vitreous shows loose clusters of atypical large lymphoid cells consistent with lymphoma. **B** The atypical large lymphoid cells are immunoreactive for CD20.

Prognosis and prediction

PCNS-LBCL

In population-based series, immunocompetent adults with PCNS-LBCL have 5-year overall survival rates of 30–40% {3719,1643}, whereas long-term survival for younger patients with PCNS-LBCL treated with modern immunochemotherapy and consolidated with autologous transplants is achievable in 15–20% of patients {1714,1325,1904,2798,1177}.

In addition to high International Prognostic Index (IPI) scores, a high CSF protein concentration and involvement of deep brain structures are independent unfavourable predictors of survival {1175}. Increased age is particularly associated with shorter survival and an increased risk of neurotoxicity {16,2105}. The missense variant Tc2c.C776G of *TCN2* (transcobalamin C) has been shown to be associated with neurotoxicity and reduced survival {2367}. The presence of reactive perivascular CD3 T-cell infiltrates in PCNS-LBCL biopsies is associated with improved survival {3278}. BCL6 expression as a prognostic parameter is controversial {3368,2725,3294,3785}. Del(6q22) is associated with inferior overall survival {513}.

PCNS-LBCL only rarely spreads outside the CNS. Two prognostic scoring systems are widely applied to better predict clinical outcome and for patient stratification in clinical trials: (1) the International Extranodal Lymphoma Study Group (IELSG) score {1175} and (2) the Memorial Sloan Kettering Cancer Center (MSKCC) score {15}.

PVR-LBCL

The treatment and prognosis are very much dependent on the disease extent, meaning unilateral or bilateral ocular involvement, with or without CNS involvement. Generally, patient survival is very poor {1160}. Treatment protocols vary and usually include intravitreal injections of methotrexate and rituximab, rituximab-based systemic chemotherapy, radiotherapy, and haematopoietic stem cell transplantation {1160,1350}.

PT-LBCL

The prognosis of PT-LBCL with rituximab-based chemotherapies is comparable to that of systemic nodal diffuse large B-cell lymphoma {1709,2455}. The 5-year progression-free survival and overall survival rates have been reported to be about 75% and 85%, respectively {4242}. Prognostic factors have been derived from retrospective series rather than clinical trials. Like for other aggressive B-cell lymphomas, IPI characteristics are prognostic. A unique prognostic characteristic of PT-LBCL is the propensity for late relapses involving sanctuary sites, and this should be considered in primary therapy decisions and surveillance strategies {653}. CNS relapse is a specific challenge that limits the overall outcome.

Primary cutaneous diffuse large B-cell lymphoma, leg type

Oschlies I
Battistella M
Chapuy B
Jansen PM
Kempf W
Parrens M
Vergier B
Vermeer MH
Willemze R

Definition
Primary cutaneous diffuse large B-cell lymphoma, leg type (PCLBCL-LT), is a lymphoma composed exclusively of centroblasts and immunoblasts, most commonly arising in the leg.

ICD-O coding
9680/3 Primary cutaneous diffuse large B-cell lymphoma, leg type

ICD-11 coding
2A81.A Primary cutaneous diffuse large B-cell lymphoma, leg type

Related terminology
Acceptable: primary cutaneous diffuse large B-cell lymphoma.

Subtype(s)
None

Localization
PCLBCL-LT preferentially affects the lower legs, but 10–25% of cases arise at other sites such as the trunk or arms; presentation in the head is exceptional {2074,4589,3679,2536}.

Clinical features
Patients with PCLBCL-LT present with red or bluish-red, often rapidly growing and ulcerating, localized or multiple skin tumours most frequently affecting one or both (lower) legs {1392,2074,4589,3679}. These lymphomas frequently disseminate to extracutaneous sites, such as lymph nodes, CNS, lung, and other visceral organs.

Epidemiology
PCLBCL-LT accounts for 3–4% of all primary cutaneous lymphomas and 10–20% of primary cutaneous B-cell lymphomas {4379,4377,973}. It typically occurs in elderly patients (median age: ~75 years), and it is more common in women, with an M:F ratio of 1:2–4 {4224,973}.

Etiology
Unknown

Pathogenesis
PCLBCL-LT is thought to arise from a germinal centre–experienced B-cell with high level of IGHV somatic hypermutation. Molecular features of the IGH switch μ region indicate a class-switch recombination defect {3221}. Chromosomal translocations involving IGH, *MYC*, and *BCL6* occur in 50%, 5–43%, and 23–50%, respectively; and concomitant *MYC* and *BCL6* translocations are observed in 4–19%. Translocations of *BCL2* are exceptional {1473,3220,2536,3640,2645,2443}. The characteristic strong BCL2 expression of PCLBCL-LT despite the lack of *BCL2* translocations may be related to high-level amplifications in 18q21.3 (in 67% of cases), which encompass the *BCL2* and

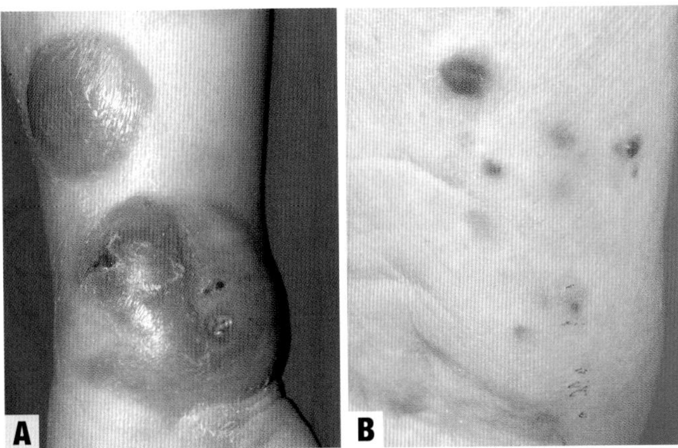

Fig. 4.210 Primary cutaneous diffuse large B-cell lymphoma, leg type. Typical clinical presentations with large and confluent tumours of the leg (**A**) and with multiple red to bluish nodules and indurated round patches (**B**).

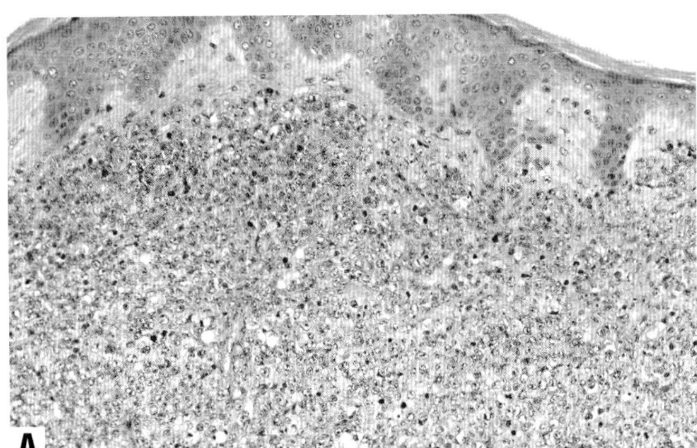

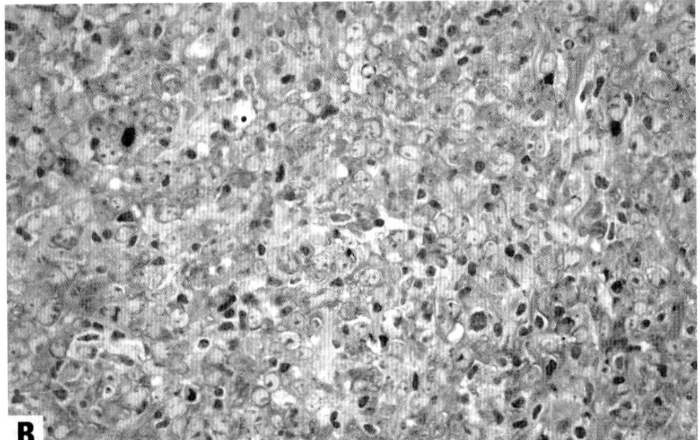

Fig. 4.211 Primary cutaneous diffuse large B-cell lymphoma, leg type. **A** Pandermal dense diffuse infiltration by large cells, sparing the epidermis. **B** At high magnification, sheets of centroblasts and immunoblasts are seen (Giemsa stain).

MALT1 loci {959,2536}. Recurrent genetic losses include *PRDM1* (described in 15% of cases), *TNFAIP3* (in 25%), and *CDKN2A* and *CDKN2B* on chromosome 9p21 (in 67–75%), this last genetic loss correlating with adverse prognosis {959,3681,2536}.

Highly recurrent hotspot mutations in the adaptor molecule of the toll-like receptor MYD88 are found in approximately 70–75% of cases. PCLBCL-LT also exhibits mutations recurrently affecting *CD79B*, *TNFAIP3*, and *CARD11*, deregulating the NF-κB and B-cell receptor signalling pathways, as well as frequent mutations in *PIM1* (reported in 70%) {3218,2078, 3220,3217,2536,4582,1014}. Genetic alterations in immune evasion pathways, such as deletions of the HLA class I and II loci and the gene encoding MHC regulator CIITA (C2TA) and rearrangements of the *CD274* (*PDL1*) and *PDCD1LG2* (*PDL2*) loci, have been described {2536,4582}. The gene expression profile of PCLBCL-LT resembles activated B-cell–like diffuse large B-cell lymphoma (ABC-DLBCL) {1606}. The molecular features of PCLBCL-LT share similarities with the genetic profile proposed to define the molecular C5/MCD DLBCL-NOS clusters {3629,642,4417} and resemble those of primary large B-cell lymphoma of immune-privileged sites {3220,2536,4582}. Of note, the gene expression profiles and genetic landscape of PCLBCL-LT are completely different from those of primary cutaneous follicle centre lymphomas (PCFCLs), a cutaneous B-cell lymphoma that may also be rich in large cells {1606,2644,3075, 3639}.

Macroscopic appearance

See *Clinical features*.

Histopathology

PCLBCL-LT shows diffuse monotonous, non-epidermotropic infiltrates in the dermis and subcutis, with confluent sheets of centroblasts and immunoblasts {4224,1392}. Mitotic figures are frequent.

Immunophenotype

The neoplastic B cells are positive for pan–B-cell markers, including CD20 and CD79a. PCLBCL-LTs strongly express BCL2, IRF4 (MUM1), FOXP1, MYC, and cytoplasmic IgM with monotypic light chains. BCL6 is variably expressed, whereas CD10 is negative in most cases {1374,1607,1395,2074,2077, 928}. The proliferation index is high (Ki-67 > 40%).

Approximately 10% of cases show deviations from this typical immunophenotype (e.g. BCL2–, IRF4 [MUM1]–, or weak CD10+), but they can still be diagnosed as PCLBCL-LT if other characteristic features of the entity are present {2074,3679, 2642}. Small B cells and CD21+/CD35+ follicular dendritic cell meshworks are absent. Reactive T cells are relatively sparse and are often confined to perivascular areas.

Differential diagnosis

The main differential diagnoses, especially with lymphomas at non-leg sites, are variants of PCFCL with diffuse growth rich in large or spindled cells {4377}. Table 4.38 summarizes the main distinguishing features. Very rare cases that do not meet the diagnostic criteria for either PCLBCL-LT or PCFCL might be diagnosed as PCLBCL-NOS.

Secondary cutaneous infiltration by systemic large B-cell lymphomas and transformed indolent lymphomas must be excluded

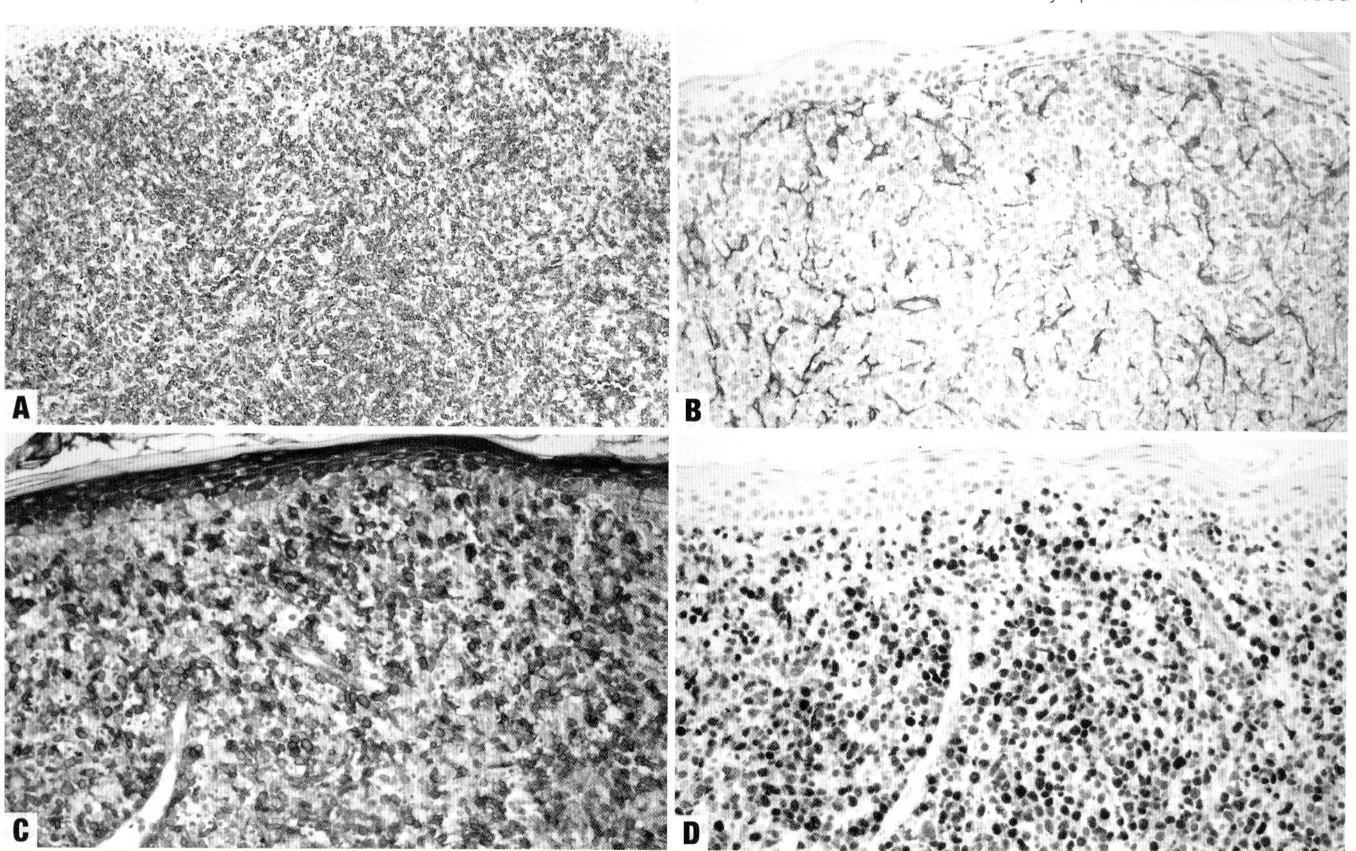

Fig. 4.212 Primary cutaneous diffuse large B-cell lymphoma, leg type. **A** Strong cytoplasmic staining for BCL2. **B** CD10 is typically negative. Note that intermingled stromal fibres may be mistaken for CD10 expression in lymphoma cells. **C** Strong cytoplasmic staining for IgM. **D** Strong nuclear staining for IRF4 (MUM1).

Table 4.38 Differential diagnosis of diffuse variants of primary cutaneous follicle centre lymphomas (PCFCLs) rich in large/spindled cells versus primary cutaneous diffuse large B-cell lymphoma, leg type (PCLBCL-LT)

Feature	PCFCL diffuse large cell / spindle cell variants	PCLBCL-LT
Histopathology		
Morphology of tumour cells	++ Predominance of large centrocytes including multilobated and spindle cells; centroblasts may be present, but not in confluent sheets	++ Predominance or confluent sheets of round centroblasts and/or immunoblasts, rare blastoid cells
High proliferative rate	+, in diffuse PCFCL ++	++
Diffuse growth	–/+	++
Follicular growth	+/–	– (nodules possible)
Reactive T cells	++	+
Immunophenotype		
IRF4 (MUM1)	–/+	++[a]
BCL2	–/+	++[a]
IgM	–	++[a]
CD10	–/+	–[a]
BCL6	+	+/–
Cell-of-origin algorithm	GCB	Non-GCB[a]
CD21 FDC networks	+/–	–
Molecular alterations (in diagnostic setting)	*MYD88* mutation is absent *BCL2* breaks ~10% No *MYC* breaks	*MYD88* and/or *CD79B* mutation ~70% *MYC* breaks ~30% No *BCL2* breaks
Clinical presentation	Scalp, upper body Exceptional at leg Rare systemic progression	Leg, lower body, (arms) Exceptional at head/neck Most cases with systemic progression
Treatment and outcome	Local treatment, 95% DSS	Systemic treatment, ~50% DSS

DSS, disease-specific survival; FDC, follicular dendritic cell; GCB, germinal-centre B cell.
[a]Rare deviation from the typical immunophenotype (e.g. weak CD10 expression, absence of BCL2 or IgM / IRF4 [MUM1]) is acceptable, if the other criteria are consistent with PCLBCL-LT).

by staging in all cases. Rarely, the skin might be the first presentation of blastic variants of mantle cell lymphoma mimicking PCLBCL-LT and should be excluded by cyclin D1 staining {4337,1997}.

In situ hybridization for EBV-encoded small RNA (EBER) is recommended in order to exclude EBV-associated lymphoproliferations and lymphomas, including EBV-positive mucocutaneous ulcers and plasmablastic lymphomas, especially in patients with immune deficiency/dysregulation {2952,782,3663,2076}.

Cytology

Not relevant

Diagnostic molecular pathology

Most cases can be diagnosed without additional molecular tests. In cases in which the differential diagnosis with PCFCL is difficult, the presence of *MYD88* and/or *CD79B* mutations favours PCLBCL-LT.

Essential and desirable diagnostic criteria

Essential: dermal and/or subcutaneous infiltration by sheets of large cells (centroblasts, immunoblasts, blastoid cells); mature B-cell phenotype; diffuse growth with absence of follicular dendritic cell meshworks; skin-confined disease at presentation.

Desirable: strong BCL2 expression; expression of IgM and IRF4 (MUM1), non–germinal-centre B-cell phenotype.

Staging

Staging should be performed according to the International Society for Cutaneous Lymphomas (ISCL) / European Organisation for Research and Treatment of Cancer (EORTC) guidelines for primary cutaneous lymphomas other than mycosis fungoides {2015}.

Prognosis and prediction

Some studies have shown a 5-year overall survival rate of approximately 50% {4224,1392,1393}; however, more recent studies show a significantly better clinical outcome for patients when rituximab is added to multiagent (CHOP or CHOP-like) chemotherapy regimens {1479,1394}. Involved field radiation might be added for localized initial disease or relapses {4373}. Multiple skin lesions at diagnosis, inactivation of *CDKN2A* (either by deletion or by promoter hypermethylation), and the presence of *MYC* rearrangements have been reported to be associated with an inferior prognosis {1392,959,3679,1393,3681,3640}.

Intravascular large B-cell lymphoma

de Jong D
Batchelor T
Deckert M
Ferry JA
Hoang-Xuan K
Nagane M
Shimada K
Soffietti R
Takeuchi K

Definition

Intravascular large B-cell lymphoma (IVLBCL) is an aggressive extranodal B-cell lymphoma characterized by the proliferation of large neoplastic B cells virtually exclusively within the lumina of blood vessels.

ICD-O coding

9712/3 Intravascular large B-cell lymphoma

ICD-11 coding

2A81.1 Intravascular large B-cell lymphoma

Related terminology

Not recommended: angiotropic lymphoma; intravascular lymphomatosis.

Subtype(s)

Classic IVLBCL; cutaneous IVLBCL; haemophagocytic IVLBCL

Localization

IVLBCL may involve virtually any organ. Lymph nodes are usually spared.

Clinical features

Classic subtype

Most patients present with fever of unknown origin (50–70%), pain, local organ-specific symptoms, or multiorgan failure. CNS symptoms (30–40% of patients) mimic those of cerebral infarction and other neurological disorders {1309}. The skin is the most common site of presentation (30–40%), but is by definition associated with the involvement of other organs. Other manifestations include renal and adrenal insufficiency, pulmonary hypertension, hypoxaemia, and pulmonary embolism.

A random skin biopsy (even in the absence of clinically overt cutaneous lesions), bone marrow evaluation, and transbronchial lung biopsy are helpful in establishing the diagnosis of suspected IVLBCL {1087,2585}. Despite the intraluminal location of the neoplastic cells, they are uncommonly (5–10% of cases) identified in peripheral blood smears.

Cutaneous subtype

The cutaneous subtype is by definition restricted to the skin at presentation. A wide range of appearances, including peau d'orange–like lesions, marked blue-red discolouration, solitary or clustered plaques, and ulcerating nodules and tumours, is described. In the cutaneous subtype, patients present with more favourable clinical features, including an Eastern Cooperative Oncology Group (ECOG) performance status score of ≤ 1 and normal blood counts, although systemic symptoms may be present in as many as 30% of patients. The clinical course is less aggressive than for the classic subtype.

Haemophagocytic subtype

The presenting symptoms are dominated by those related to haemophagocytic syndrome, hepatosplenomegaly, and thrombocytopenia (> 75%). Bone marrow and peripheral blood evaluation may show tumour cells. The onset and clinical course are very rapid.

Epidemiology

The classic subtype of IVLBCL occurs in adults, with a median age of 70 years and with no sex predilection. The cutaneous subtype occurs in patients with a median age of 59 years, is virtually restricted to women, and is more frequent in North America and western Europe. The haemophagocytic subtype is predominantly reported in Asia and arises at a similar mean age and with a similar sex distribution to the classic subtype {1179,

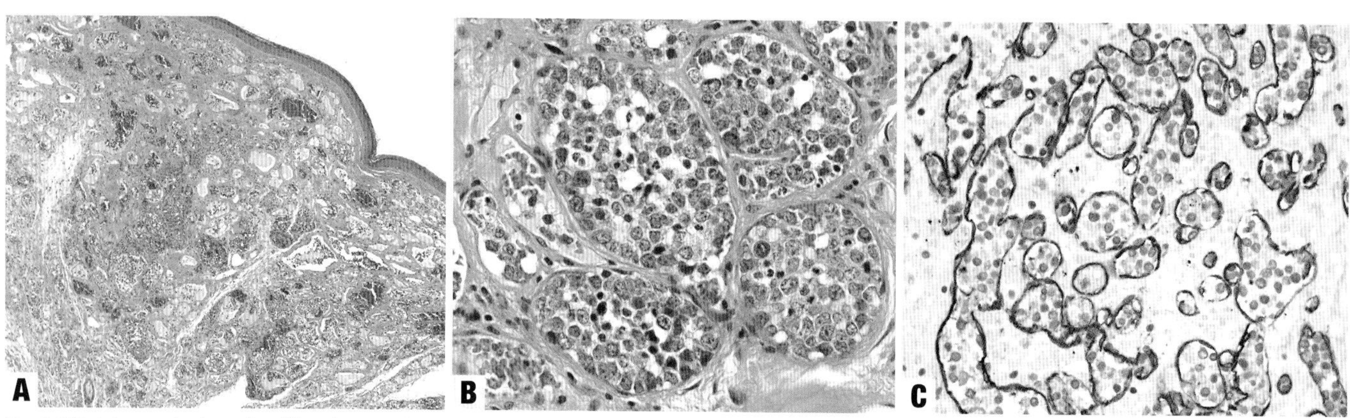

Fig. 4.213 Intravascular large B-cell lymphoma. **A** Intravascular large B-cell lymphoma involving a cutaneous haemangioma, showing capillaries distended by tumour cells. **B** Higher-magnification view shows large tumour cells with vesicular chromatin and several small nucleoli filling vascular spaces. Apoptotic tumour cells are present. **C** CD34 immunohistochemistry highlighting large tumour B cells restricted to intravascular spaces.

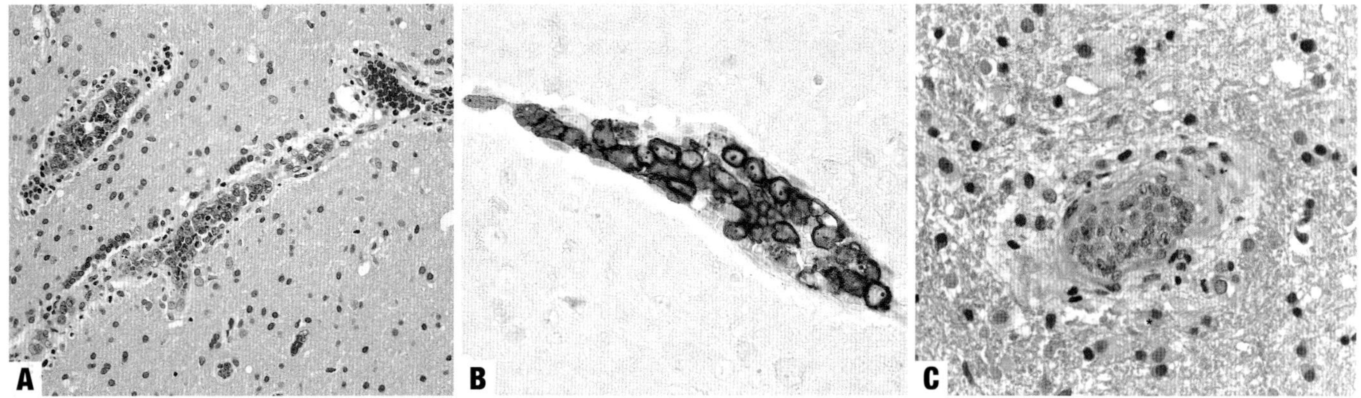
Fig. 4.214 Intravascular large B-cell lymphoma. **A** Intravascular large B-cell lymphoma in the cerebral white matter. **B** Tumour cells are highlighted by CD20 immunohistochemistry. **C** Perivascular microglia and astrocytes are activated.

3279,2391}. Overall, the incidence of the disease is 0.095 per million {710,3354} without overall essential geographical differences, but rather with different clinical patterns of presentation {1179}.

Etiology

The etiology is unknown. Viral associations are not described.

Pathogenesis

The mechanisms by which tumour cell proliferations are confined to the intravascular space are numerous and involve regulation of lymphocyte trafficking, vascular adhesion, and transvascular migration. The neoplastic cells lack adhesion molecules, including CD29 (integrin beta-1) and CD54 (ICAM1) {3277}. Various chemokine receptors (CXCR5, CCR6, CCR7) and matrix metalloproteinases involved in transvascular migration are absent or expressed at low levels {2032,82,1906,3725}. Thus, the tumour cells are capable of adhering to endothelial cells but unable to migrate across the blood vessel wall. *MYD88* and *CD79B* hotspot mutations are reported in about half of cases and one third to two thirds of cases, respectively. *SETD1B* (57%) and *HLA-B* (57%) mutations are also common {3641,3869,3727,1370}. Structural variants affecting *CD274* (*PDL1*) and *PDCD1LG2* (*PDL2*) are reported to be recurrent {3727}. Overall, the genetic landscape suggests that constitutive NF-κB activation and immune evasion are dominant pathogenetic mechanisms in IVLBCL; thus, there are biological similarities to primary large B-cell lymphoma of immune-privileged sites (IP-LBCL). This entity thus far accommodates cases presenting in the CNS, testis, and vitreoretinal space. As further evidence becomes available, IP-LBCL may absorb other biologically similar site-specific large B-cell lymphomas, including IVLBCL.

Macroscopic appearance

Cutaneous involvement may present with peau d'orange–like lesions, discolouration, plaques, and ulcerating nodules and tumours. In the brain, macroscopy may demonstrate acute and/or old infarction, haemorrhage, and necrosis; however, CNS lesions are usually inconspicuous.

Histopathology

Large lymphoid cells with vesicular nuclei and single or multiple prominent nucleoli, often showing mitotic figures, are observed within the lumina of small vessels, especially capillaries. A free-floating (discohesive), cohesive, or marginating/adherent growth pattern may be observed. Rarely, the lymphoid cells can be anaplastic. In certain organs, such as the brain, there can be features related to the occlusion of vascular lumina, such as haemorrhage and infarction. In the haemophagocytic subtype, a varying infiltrate of non-neoplastic histiocytes with signs of haemophagocytosis is present. The liver, spleen, and bone marrow are most frequently involved. In the bone marrow, the intravascular infiltrate may be sparse {2847}.

Immunophenotype

Pan–B-cell markers (CD20, CD79a) are expressed, often with coexpression of CD5 and PDL1 (CD274) (20–40%) {3531,1454}. Most cases express IRF4 (MUM1) (75–80%) and have a non–germinal-centre B-cell immunophenotype; however, approximately 13% are CD10-positive {2848}.

Differential diagnosis

Various B- and T-cell lymphomas, including peripheral T-cell lymphomas, NK/T-cell lymphomas, and KSHV/HHV8-positive diffuse large B-cell lymphoma, may occur with a dominant intravascular presentation. These, however, should be classified according to their primary entity {1187}.

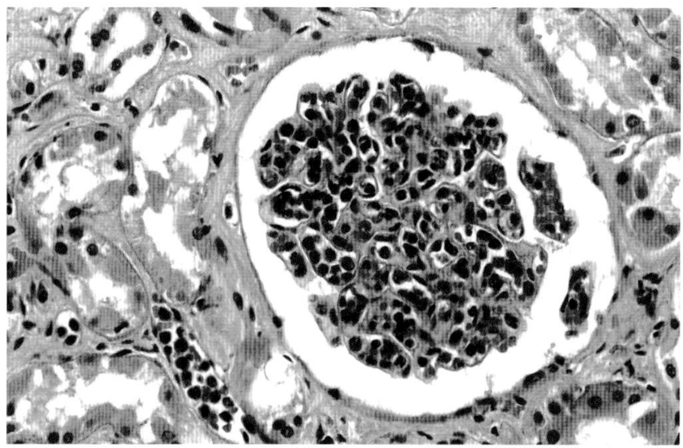
Fig. 4.215 Intravascular large B-cell lymphoma involving the kidney shows large, dark-staining lymphoid cells in glomerular capillaries and in a peritubular capillary.

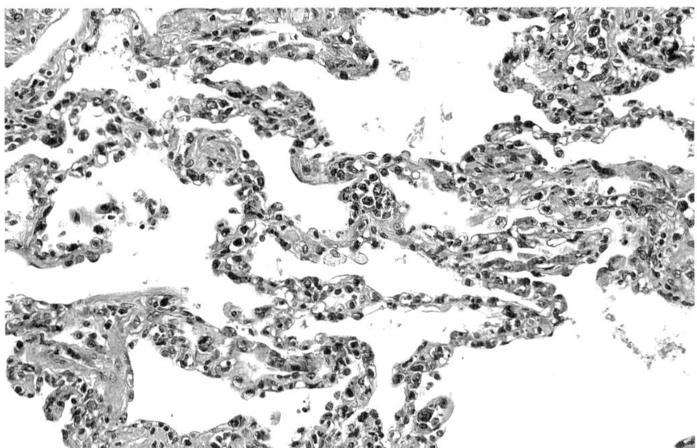

Fig. 4.216 Intravascular large B-cell lymphoma involving the lung, showing alveolar capillaries distended by tumour cells.

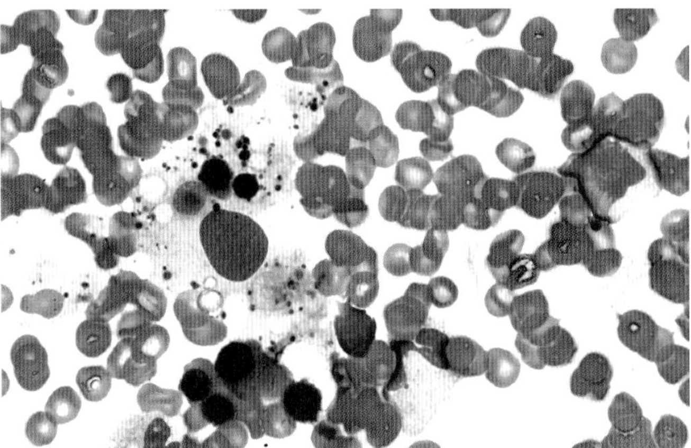

Fig. 4.217 Intravascular large B-cell lymphoma. Remarkable haemophagocytosis by a macrophage is shown in the bone marrow in a patient with haemophagocytic subtype (May–Grünwald–Giemsa).

Cytology

Neoplastic cells are only rarely detected in the cerebrospinal fluid.

Diagnostic molecular pathology

Diagnostic molecular pathology is not needed in the majority of cases. In equivocal cases, cell-free DNA can be interrogated by liquid biopsy for genes recurrently mutated or for clonality {3869,3727}.

Essential and desirable diagnostic criteria

Essential: large lymphoid cells with centroblastic, immunoblastic, or (rarely) anaplastic morphology; restricted to intravascular spaces, especially capillaries (a minimal extravascular component is acceptable); pan–B-cell markers positive.

Desirable: KSHV/HHV8-negative by latency-associated nuclear antigen (LANA) immunohistochemistry; EBV-negative by EBV-encoded small RNA (EBER) in situ hybridization.

Staging

Staging is performed according to the Lugano modification of the Ann Arbor staging system (although it is not optimally suited to or correlated with outcome for IVLBCL).

Prognosis and prediction

IVLBCL is an aggressive lymphoma. Increasingly, the diagnosis is now made during life. The poor prognosis is still often caused by delayed diagnosis, however. The cutaneous subtype has a better outcome, possibly related to earlier detection, whereas the haemophagocytic subtype follows a very aggressive course (median survival time: 2–8 months) {1176,3721}. Chemotherapy with rituximab has improved outcome, with a 3-year overall survival rate of 60–81% {3723,1178,1180,3721,3726,3897,402}. In cases with CNS involvement, methotrexate-based chemotherapy may improve outcome {1940,3722}.

Primary mediastinal large B-cell lymphoma

Traverse-Glehen A
Fromm JR
Klapper W
Lacasce AS
Nicolae A
Rosenwald A
Sarkozy C
Siebert R
Steidl C

Definition

Primary mediastinal large B-cell lymphoma (PMBCL) is a mature aggressive B-cell lymphoma of putative thymic B-cell origin, arising in the anterior mediastinum with distinctive clinical, immunophenotypic, and molecular features.

ICD-O coding

9679/3 Mediastinal large B-cell lymphoma

ICD-11 coding

2A81.0 Primary mediastinal large B-cell lymphoma

Related terminology

Not recommended: primary mediastinal clear cell lymphoma of B-cell type; mediastinal diffuse large cell lymphoma with sclerosis.

Subtype(s)

None

Localization

PMBCL typically arises in the anterior-superior mediastinum (thymic niche) with variable extension to the lung, pleura, or pericardium. Regional lymph nodes are frequently involved, most commonly the supraclavicular lymph nodes. Bone marrow involvement is uncommon at presentation. Extranodal localization is rare at diagnosis but can been seen at relapse, at which time CNS, adrenal, liver, and/or kidney localization may occur {3592}.

Clinical features

Patients commonly present with cough and/or dyspnoea and superior vena cava syndrome, particularly when the disease is bulky. Most patients have stage I or II disease. The mediastinal tumour commonly invades the lung and cardiac structures, which may be accompanied by pleural and/or pericardial effusions in approximately 30%. Serum LDH is elevated in the majority (80%) of patients {128}.

Epidemiology

PMBCL accounts for 2–4% of all non-Hodgkin lymphomas and 6–12% of large B-cell lymphomas. It occurs predominantly in young adults (third decade of life), with a female predominance (M:F ratio: 1:2). It can occur in children. PMBCL may occur before, simultaneously with, or at relapse of nodular sclerosing classic Hodgkin lymphoma {3239,4066}. It is uniformly distributed around the world. Familial clustering has been described, based on shared gene mutations identified in affected families {3512}.

Etiology

Unknown

Pathogenesis

Gene expression profiling has established PMBCL as a distinct B-cell lymphoma entity characterized by a signature that significantly overlaps with nodular sclerosis classic Hodgkin lymphoma (CHL) and that is markedly distinct from other aggressive B-cell lymphomas, in particular activated B-cell–like and germinal-centre B-cell–like diffuse large B-cell lymphoma (DLBCL) {3473,3594,2814}. Molecular hallmarks of PMBCL include deregulation of NF-κB {1189}, JAK/STAT signalling pathways {1448}, and various mechanisms of immune escape {3429,1404,2813}. These hallmarks are underpinned by numerous gene mutations, leading to constitutive pathway activation and somatically acquired immune privilege {1013,2811,846}. The most frequent gene alterations include point mutations of *SOCS1*, *GNA13*, *STAT6*, *CD58*, *B2M*, *ITPKB*, *TNFAIP3*, and *IL4R*; copy-number gains of 2p16 (harbouring *REL*) {4355} and 9p24 (harbouring *CD274* [*PDL1*] and *PDCD1LG2* [*PDL2*]) {1404}; deletions of 6q23 (harbouring *TNFAIP3*), 9p21 (harbouring *CDKN2A*), and 17p13 (harbouring *TP53*) {2535}; and

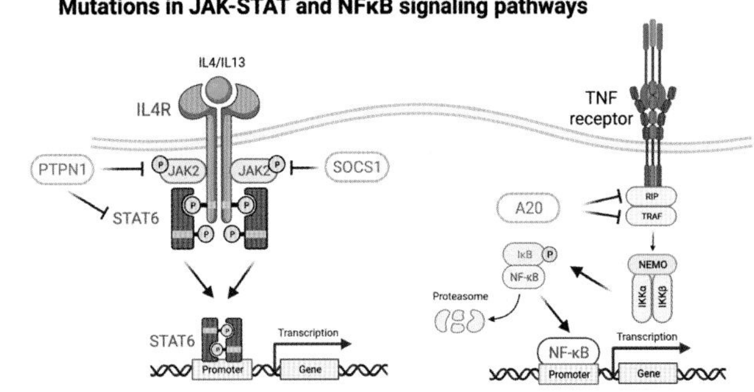

Gain of function: IL4R, JAK2, STAT6, REL (part of NF-κB complex)

A **Loss of function:** PTPN1, SOCS1, A20, NFKBIA/E (part of IκB)

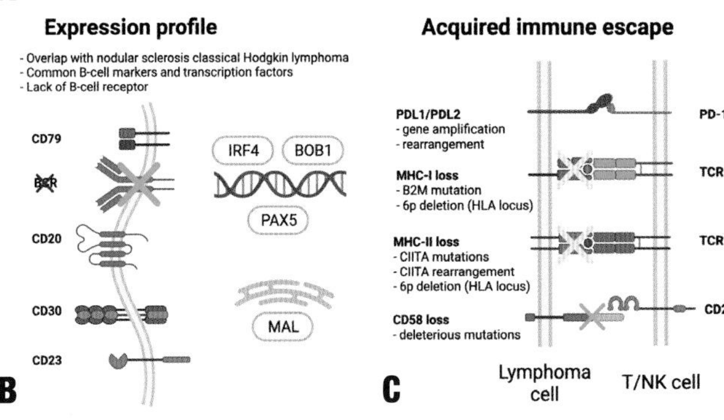

Fig. 4.218 Molecular pathogenesis of primary mediastinal large B-cell lymphoma. Three molecular hallmarks are depicted. **A** Frequent mutations in the JAK/STAT and NF-κB signalling pathways. Gain-of-function mutations are highlighted in green, loss-of-function mutations are highlighted in red. **B** The distinctive expression profile. **C** Mechanisms of somatically acquired immune escape. Figure created with BioRender.com.

chromosomal rearrangements targeting the MHC class II master regulator gene *CIITA* (*C2TA*) and the programmed death ligand genes *CD274* (*PDL1*) and *PDCD1LG2* (*PDL2*) {3824, 4110}. In a subset of PMBCL these mutations arise in a setting of aberrant somatic hypermutation, likely mediated by activation-induced cytidine deaminase (AID) {3282,643}. Rearrangements of *BCL2*, *BCL6*, and *MYC* are rare to absent. The mature B-cell phenotype can often be incomplete (e.g. immunoglobulin expression is frequently absent) {2269}. The variable and sometimes prominent T-cell microenvironment in PMBCL, a feature that is shared with mediastinal grey zone lymphoma and CHL, underscores the pathogenetic importance of a permissive

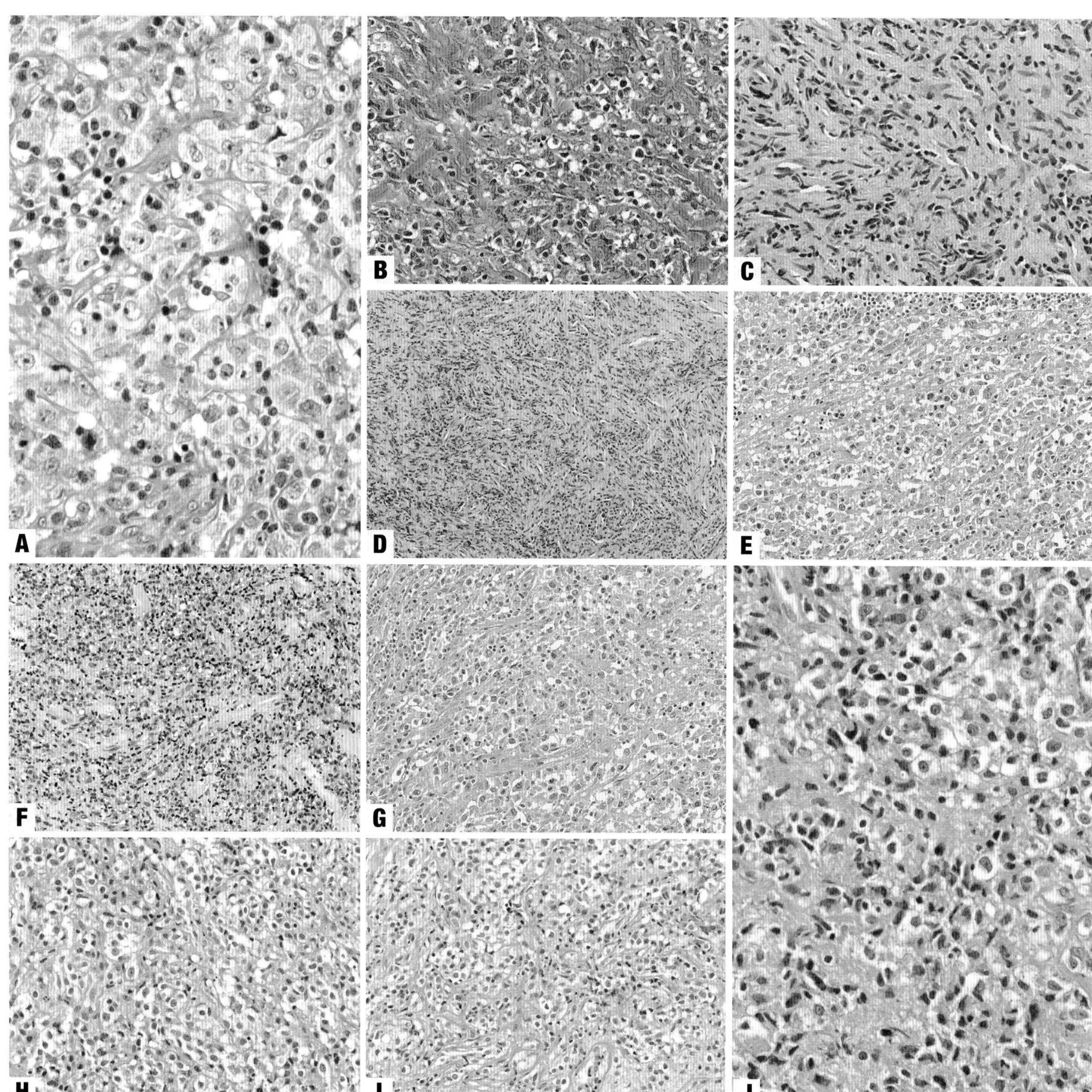

Fig. 4.219 Primary mediastinal large B-cell lymphoma. There is wide morphological and cytological variation from case to case. **A** Diffuse infiltration of large clear cells with abundant cytoplasm and alveolar compartmentalizing by fine fibrosis. **B** Diffuse infiltration of large clear cells with coarse collagenous fibrosis. **C** Neoplastic cells with spindle cell morphology in a dense sclerotic background. Higher magnification highlights polymorphic nuclear features. **D** Neoplastic cells with spindle cell morphology in a dense sclerotic background. **E** A cohesive proliferation of large neoplastic cells. **F** A cohesive sheet of small to medium-sized neoplastic cells in a collagenous background. **G** Large polymorphic neoplastic cells, including multinucleated tumour cells, resembling HRS cells. **H** Sheets of medium to large atypical lymphoid cells with round nuclei, small nucleoli, and abundant pale cytoplasm. **I** Delicate reticular fibrosis with compartmentalization of groups of neoplastic tumour cells. **J** Numerous neoplastic cells show crush artefacts, which hamper the morphological evaluation of the specimen.

niche for oncogenesis {2813}. Loss of MHC molecules, in part explained by underlying genetic events, is a common feature of PMBCL {3409,3429}.

Macroscopic appearance

PMBCL presents as a solid mass, tan to light brown, sometimes with foci of necrosis.

Histopathology

PMBCL presents as a diffuse infiltration of neoplastic lymphoid cells distributed in clusters or sheets, often in a fibrotic background. The amount of fibrosis ranges from fine reticular, with alveolar compartmentalization of neoplastic cells, to coarse collagenous. The neoplastic cells exhibit broad cytological diversity but are usually medium-sized to large, with abundant pale cytoplasm and round or ovoid nuclei with small nucleoli {4518, 2720,3169}. There may be a cohesive proliferation of immunoblasts, pleomorphic cells ranging in size with vesicular nuclei, scattered cells resembling HRS cells, or a paucicellular infiltrate in a dense sclerotic stroma {3169,4066}. A variable number of admixed reactive lymphocytes, histiocytes, and (more rarely) granulocytes may be seen. Remnants of thymic epithelium and foci of necrosis may be present. PMBCL usually involves the lymph node in a carcinoma-like pattern, with initial colonization of marginal sinuses, subsequent perifollicular involvement, and eventual total effacement of nodal structures, without a stromal component {3169}.

Immunophenotype

The lymphoma cells express CD45 and B-cell lineage antigens, such as CD19, CD22, CD20, and CD79a. They typically lack surface and cytoplasmic immunoglobulin expression, despite the presence of functional rearrangements of IG genes and expression of B-lineage transcription regulators such as BOB1, PU.1, OCT2, and PAX5 {1865,3236,2396}. Most PMBCLs (> 80%) are positive for CD30, but, unlike in CHL, the staining intensity is often heterogeneous and weak {1580,3236}. The neoplastic cells frequently (75–95%) express IRF4 (MUM1) and have variable expression of BCL6 and BCL2; CD10 expression is uncommon (< 30% of cases) {896,3236,520,374}. Biomarkers with high specificity and sensitivity > 70% for PMBCL include CD23, MAL, CD200, PDL1, and PDL2 {799,3236,520,995,3716, 1316}. Of note, CD23 and MAL are expressed by a subset of normal thymic medullary B-cell lymphocytes {799,520}. As a result of NF-κB, TNF, and JAK/STAT signalling pathway activation, expression of c-REL (65–77%), TRAF1 (62–86%), TNFAIP2 (87%), and phosphorylated STAT6 (73%) is frequently observed {1448,3435,2097,995}. PMBCL often lacks expression of HLA class I and/or class II molecules {2721,2720}. Rare cases are CD15-positive, often with a small dot-like paranuclear pattern {374}. EBV is encountered only in exceptional cases {582} but does not absolutely exclude the diagnosis.

Differential diagnosis

DLBCL-NOS involving the mediastinum is particularly challenging to distinguish from PMBCL on the basis of histological and routine immunophenotypic criteria. Knowledge of the clinical findings is essential, given that DLBCL-NOS may show involvement of mediastinal lymph nodes, often with widespread extrathoracic disease (rather than the thymic area). Remnants of thymic epithelium in the biopsy provide support for PMBCL. For small needle biopsies, expression of CD30, CD23, MAL, CD200, or PDL1/PDL2 can be helpful to exclude DLBCL-NOS. In difficult cases, ancillary gene expression testing, detection of *CIITA* (*C2TA*) rearrangements/mutations, copy-number gains of *CD274* (*PDL1*) and *PDCD1LG2* (*PDL2*), or gene mutations (i.e. *SOCS1*, *STAT6*) can be useful in the differential diagnosis {1404, 4110,2813,643,2814}.

According to current evidence, cases with features reminiscent of PMBCL {2814,4314} presenting outside the mediastinum should be classified as DLBCL-NOS (with distinct phenotypic and genetic features) {1022}. Whether very rare cases of true "extramediastinal PMBCL" exist awaits further studies.

The distinction of mediastinal grey zone lymphoma from PMBCL is problematic on core biopsies and a larger (incisional) biopsy is usually required. As opposed to PMBCL, mediastinal grey zone lymphoma with PMBCL-like morphology is defined as being strongly and uniformly positive for CD30 with partial or complete loss of the B-cell programme and/or strong CD15 expression {3578,3239} (see *Mediastinal grey zone lymphoma*, p. 527).

CHL can be considered in the differential diagnosis of PMBCL when abundant fibrosis and scattered pleomorphic/multilobated nuclei resembling HRS cells are encountered. Absence of CD45 and B-cell antigens like CD79a, CD19, and transcription factors, and strong expression of CD30 in all tumour cells, favour CHL over PMBCL {4066,3074}. EBV positivity favours the diagnosis of CHL but it can be observed in very rare cases of PMBCL. Although CHL and PMBCL share many similarities in their gene expression profiles, MAL expression is very rare in CHL. Composite or synchronous cases of CHL and PMBCL have been described.

Cytology

FNA has a place as the first screening procedure to distinguish lymphoma from other malignant tumours. However, a diagnosis of PMBCL is not advised on FNA alone, and a tissue biopsy is recommended. In cases where clinical circumstances preclude a tissue biopsy (e.g. severe superior vena cava syndrome), FNA can support the diagnosis of PMBCL, provided that the specimen is adequate and the immunophenotype and clinical presentation are consistent with a diagnosis of PMBCL.

Diagnostic molecular pathology

The diagnosis of PMBCL usually does not require ancillary molecular studies. In difficult cases, knowledge of the mutation profile may help in the distinction between PMBCL and DLBCL-NOS. In addition, gene expression profiling can identify PMBCL with high accuracy (85%) {2814}.

Studies to detect rearrangements of *CIITA* (*C2TA*) and abnormalities of the *JAK2*/*PDCD1LG2*/*CD274* locus at 9p24.1 that are recurrently found in PMBCL can also be useful.

Rearrangements of *BCL2*, *BCL6*, and *MYC* are rare to absent, and their assessment has no added value in the context of PMBCL.

Essential and desirable diagnostic criteria

Essential: large B-cell lymphoma in the anterior mediastinum; mature B-cell phenotype; at least partial expression of CD23 and/or CD30.

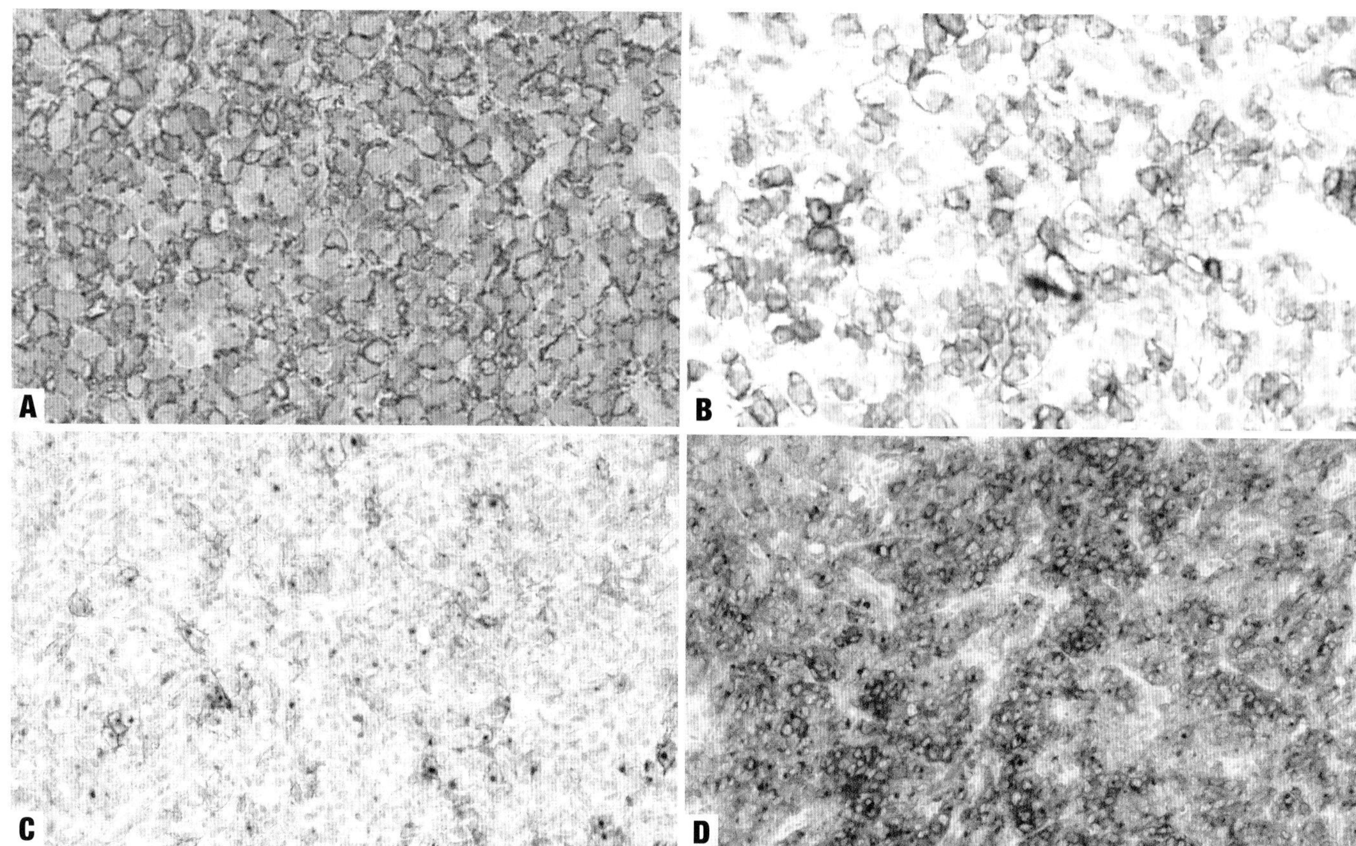

Fig. 4.220 Primary mediastinal large B-cell lymphoma. The tumour cells are positive for CD20 (**A**), show heterogeneous CD30 expression (**B**), and are varyingly positive for CD23, sometimes with only focal expression (**C**). MAL shows cytoplasmic and Golgi accentuation (**D**).

Desirable: distinctive stromal sclerosis; expression of at least one of the following markers: MAL, CD200, PDL1, and PDL2; copy gain or rearrangement of the *CD274/PDCD1LG2* locus and/or rearrangement involving *CIITA* (*C2TA*).

Staging

Staging is performed according to the Lugano classification, adapted from the Ann Arbor staging system with Cotswold modifications {688}.

Prognosis and prediction

The prognosis of PMBCL is favourable, with 85–90% of patients achieving durable remission with anthracycline-based chemo-immunotherapy. Intensified chemotherapy regimens, such as dose-adjusted EPOCH-R, are associated with higher complete remission rates and reduced need for consolidative radiotherapy than R-CHOP at the expense of increased toxicity without overall survival benefit {1021,565,3592,537}. No biological features are clearly associated with outcomes. A high International Prognostic Index (IPI) score and metabolic heterogeneity on baseline PET are associated with an inferior prognosis {577,589}. The positive predictive value of end-of-treatment PET-CT is low, and a biopsy is strongly recommended to confirm persistent disease if suspected on radiographic grounds. As many as 10% of patients may have primary refractory PMBCL, but a few will be chemo-sensitive to second-line therapy, and hence may benefit from autologous haematopoietic stem cell transplant. Chimeric antigen receptor (CAR) T-cell therapy and the use of PD1 inhibitors with or without brentuximab vedotin are therapeutic options for relapsed/refractory patients {2927,2395,4590}.

Mediastinal grey zone lymphoma

Sarkozy C
Hansmann ML
Klapper W
Lacasce AS
Marx A
Nicolae A
Rosenwald A
Traverse-Glehen A

Definition

Mediastinal grey zone lymphoma (MGZL) is a B-cell lymphoma with overlapping clinical, morphological, immunophenotypic, and molecular features between primary mediastinal B-cell lymphoma (PMBCL) and classic Hodgkin lymphoma (CHL), particularly nodular sclerosis CHL (NSCHL).

ICD-O coding

9596/3 Mediastinal grey zone lymphoma

ICD-11 coding

2A86.Y Other specified B-cell lymphoma, mixed features

Related terminology

Not recommended: B-cell lymphoma, unclassifiable, with features intermediate between diffuse large B-cell lymphoma and classic Hodgkin lymphoma; Hodgkin-like anaplastic large cell lymphoma.

Subtype(s)

None

Localization

MGZL typically presents as a localized anterior mediastinal mass, with frequent involvement of the supraclavicular lymph nodes and invasion of the lung or pleura. Dissemination below the diaphragm and to other extranodal sites is uncommon {1292,4066,3239,3577}. Rare cases without anterior mediastinal involvement are referred to as grey zone lymphoma with primary extramediastinal presentation (PEMGZL). Such cases present generally as disseminated disease with lymph node, spleen, liver, and/or bone marrow involvement. There is no consensus on the precise definition of PEMGZL, however.

Clinical features

A localized, bulky, anterior mediastinal mass is the most common clinical presentation, and patients often present with a cough and dyspnoea {1292,4066,3239,3577}. Extension to the pleura/lung and superior vena cava syndrome are observed in a substantial number of patients, who also often present with B symptoms and elevated serum LDH.

Epidemiology

MGZL presents in young patients (as NSCHL and PMBCL), preferentially male (as opposed to PMBCL, which is more frequent in young female patients), with a median age of 30 years {4066,1038,4387,3579}. Rare cases have been reported in children {3074}. Most published series of MGZL are from Europe and North America, and insufficient epidemiological data are available from other parts of the world.

Presumed PEMGZL cases are rare {1292,4066,3239,3577}; it is reported to occur in older patients (median age: 65 years), with no sex predilection.

Etiology

Unknown

Pathogenesis

MGZL shares genetic, epigenetic, and phenotypic features with its related entities NSCHL and PMBCL, suggesting derivation from thymic B cells and/or (post–)germinal-centre B cells {1037, 3259,3579}. Structural chromosomal aberrations involving 9p24.1 (*JAK2/CD274/PDCD1LG2*) and 16p13.13 (*CIITA* [*C2TA*]), as well as frequent deleterious *B2M* mutations and loss of MHC class I and MHC class II expression indicate that somatically acquired immune escape plays an important role in pathogenesis {1038,3579}. MGZL shares genomic aberrations with classic Hodgkin lymphoma and PMBCL, including alterations in the JAK/STAT, NF-κB (including 2p16.1 and *REL* copy-number variations), and nuclear transport pathways. The most frequently mutated genes include *SOCS1*, *TNFAIP3*, *NFKBIE*, *GNA13*, and *XPO1* {3579}. Mutation features exclusively occurring in MGZL have not been described; *BCL2* and *BCL6* rearrangements are absent {1038,3579,3578}.

The pathobiology of PEMGZL differs essentially from that of MGZL. Gene expression studies support the concept of MGZL being closely related to PMBCL, whereas PEMGZL shows features that are more related to DLBCL-NOS {3577}. Like DLBCL-NOS, PEMGZL has frequent alterations of *TP53*, *BCL2*, *BIRC6*, and *CREBBP* {3579}, with *BCL2* and *BCL6* rearrangements (41% and 18%, respectively). *JAK2/CD274/PDCD1LG2* gain/amplification have also been reported in PEMGZL {1038,3579, 3578}. Therefore, a diagnosis of PEMGZL should be applied very restrictively. Cases that share morphological and/or immunophenotypic features with MGZL outside the mediastinum are generally better classified as DLBCL-NOS.

Macroscopic appearance

The tumour has a tan, fish-flesh aspect. Necrosis and fibrosis leading to nodularity may be seen.

Histopathology

MGZL is a challenging diagnosis that should be considered after exclusion of CHL and PMBCL. The defining feature of MGZL is a mismatch between morphological and immunophenotypic findings, whose integration is critical to the diagnosis (see Table 4.39, p. 528). Needle biopsy specimens may be inadequate, and obtaining large pieces of tissue (preferably by incisional biopsy), together with an appropriate panel of stains, is typically required {4066,3239}. Furthermore, given the treatment implications and lack of precise diagnostic criteria, an expert pathological review to confirm the diagnosis and multidisciplinary integration of findings is recommended.

The morphological spectrum of MGZL is broad, and divergent or transitional morphological areas may be seen within the same tumour specimen. The majority (70%) of MGZLs closely

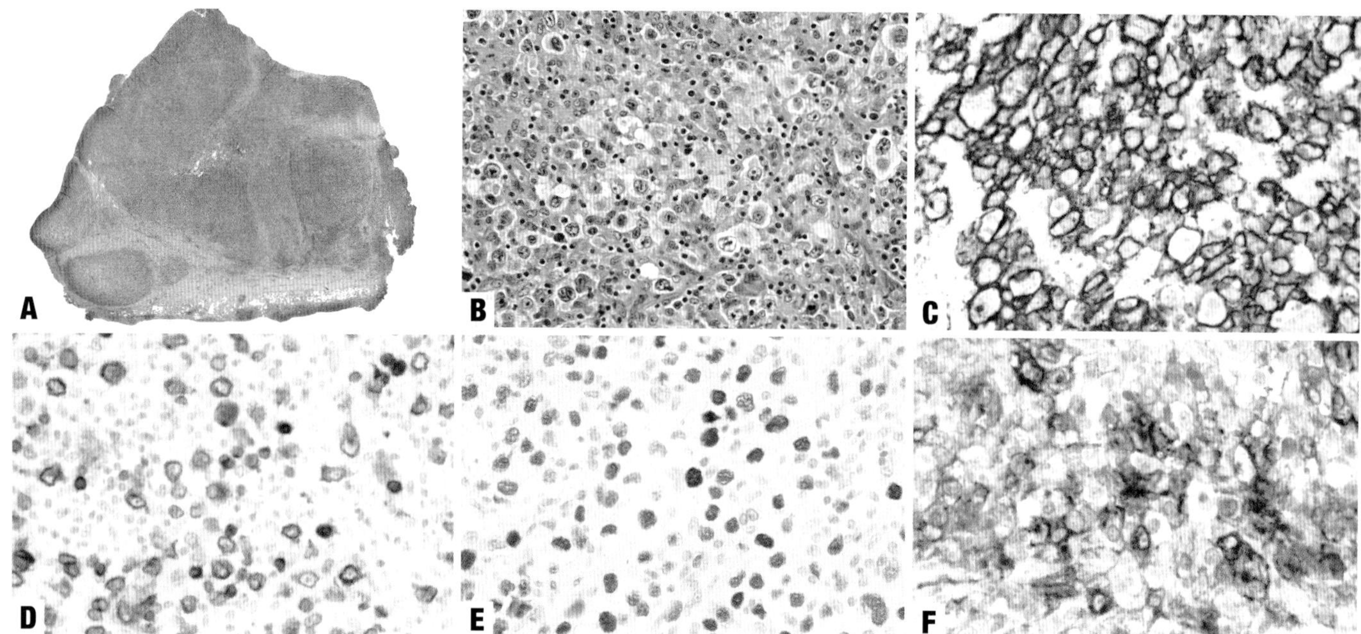

Fig. 4.221 Mediastinal grey zone lymphoma with classic Hodgkin-like morphology. **A** The excisional biopsy was taken from a 22-year-old with a mediastinal mass showing a nodular proliferation with fibrous septa. **B** Higher magnification shows sheet-like growth of pleomorphic cells often resembling lacunar cells, with an inflammatory background. The tumour cells are strongly positive for CD20 (**C**), and positive for CD79a (**D**) and OCT2 (**E**). **F** There is a heterogeneous positivity for CD30. CD15 is negative (not shown).

resemble NSCHL and are called CHL-like, whereas the remainder mimic PMBCL and are called PMBCL-like.

MGZL CHL-like cases often show confluent growth of pleomorphic neoplastic cells within a variably abundant microenvironment and dense fibrotic stroma. Cases with only scattered HRS-like cells and an absence of confluent neoplastic cells are less common. The neoplastic cells show a broad spectrum of cytological features, resembling typical HRS cells, lacunar cells, centroblasts, or immunoblasts. The background inflammatory infiltrate may include eosinophils, lymphocytes, plasma cells, and histiocytes, like in NSCHL. Some fibrous bands with nodular demarcation and scarce areas of necrosis, which lack neutrophilic infiltrate, may be seen {4066,3239,3578}.

MGZL PMBCL-like cases show a rather monomorphic appearance, with sheets of medium-sized to large neoplastic cells within a variably dense fibrotic stroma, usually containing a paucicellular inflammatory infiltrate. Marked pleomorphism and some HRS-like cells may be encountered.

Immunophenotype

CHL-like MGZL cases show a well-preserved B-cell programme, unlike CHL. The exact number of B-cell markers required to be expressed for a diagnosis of MGZL remains controversial. In this context, the uniform and strong expression of B-cell markers (CD20, CD19, and CD79a) is considered a more robust indicator of a conserved B-cell programme than the expression of nuclear transcription factors (PAX5, OCT2, and BOB1). In practice, besides the strong and uniform expression of PAX5 and CD20, at least one additional B-cell marker should be strongly positive in the majority of neoplastic cells to support the diagnosis. If additional B-cell markers are negative (solely CD20 and PAX5 positive on the majority of neoplastic cells), a diagnosis of CHL is favoured. CD30 is typically positive, whereas CD15 is present in a minority of cases. In addition, IRF4 (MUM1), BCL6, and fascin are commonly expressed; CD10 and ALK are negative; and CD45 is variably expressed. EBV assessed by EBV-encoded small RNA (EBER) in situ hybridization is negative in the vast majority of cases.

PMBCL-like MGZL demonstrates variable loss of the B-cell programme, with frequent strong and uniform positivity for CD30

Table 4.39 Differential diagnosis between mediastinal grey zone lymphoma (MGZL), classic Hodgkin lymphoma (CHL) expressing CD20 and/or strong PAX5 in HRS cells, and primary mediastinal large B-cell lymphoma (PMBCL)

Criterion	Consider CHL	Consider MGZL	Consider PMBCL
CD30	Uniform in HRS cells	Mostly heterogeneous in HRS-like cells	Can be positive
CD15	Positive in at least some HRS cells	Usually negative	Usually negative
B-cell programme	Defective B-cell programme with lack of expression of other B-cell markers	Retained B-cell programme with uniform and strong expression of CD20 and PAX5 in combination with at least one additional B-cell marker (CD19 and CD79a or OCT2 and BOB1)	Retained B-cell programme with uniform and strong expression of CD20 and PAX5, and additional B-cell marker
EBV (LMP or EBER)	Supports the diagnosis	Exceedingly rare in a mediastinal presentation Precludes the diagnosis in non-mediastinal sites	Exceedingly rare

EBER, EBV-encoded small RNA.

and/or CD15 {4066,3239,3578}. Therefore, when dealing with a case of PMBCL-like morphology and uniform CD30 expression, a diagnosis of MGZL should be considered, supported by partial or complete loss of B-cell markers or strong CD15 expression. Conversely, a typical PMBCL morphology with preservation of B-cell markers but with an intense and diffuse expression of CD30, without CD15 expression, is not consistent with MGZL, and a diagnosis of PMBCL is preferred. Finally, when assessed using EBER in situ hybridization, EBV is negative in the vast majority of cases.

Differential diagnosis

The diagnosis of MGZL should only be considered after careful exclusion of other entities, in particular CHL, PMBCL, EBV+ DLBCL, and B-cell lymphoproliferative disorders in immunodeficiency settings {3239}, as well as T-cell lymphomas with HRS-like cells / transformed cells. EBV+ MGZL is extremely rare, and alternative differential diagnoses should be seriously considered in these cases {3579}.

In view of the different genetic features at both the gene expression and DNA levels, the vast majority of cases of PEMGZL are likely better classified as DLBCL-NOS {3579}, and it is recommended that the diagnosis be made sparingly outside of (clinical) research studies in routine practice.

Composite cases with areas consistent with PMBCL and NSCHL in a single tumour can be observed. Moreover, some patients present with an unambiguous diagnosis of CHL and PMBCL sequentially during the course of the disease (e.g. at primary diagnosis and at relapse, termed sequential/metachronous) in the same or different anatomical sites. The phenomenon of composite and sequential/metachronous PMBCL and CHL suggests plasticity across these entities, and a clonal relation between the PMBCL and NSCHL presentations has been demonstrated in selected cases. However, these cases should not be classified as MGZL – both components should be named separately {4066,3331,1038,191}.

Composite lymphomas (diagnosed at any site) composed of DLBCL and CHL should also not be classified as MGZL and should be reported with the components named separately. It should be noted that these are in general not biologically or clonally related.

Cytology

The cytological features observed in FNAB are not reliable for distinguishing this tumour from other mediastinal lymphomas.

Diagnostic molecular pathology

Clonal IG gene rearrangement is usually present.

The genomic alterations described in *Pathogenesis* are not specific; many are also detected in entities representing differential diagnoses, particularly PMBCL and CHL. Therefore, detection of genomic features is currently not required for the diagnosis of MGZL.

Essential and desirable diagnostic criteria

Essential for CHL-like MGZL: confluent growth of pleomorphic cells within a variably abundant microenvironment and dense fibrotic stroma; uniform strong expression of CD20, PAX5, and at least one additional B-cell marker (CD19, CD79a, BOB1, OCT2); positive expression of CD30, with varying intensity.

Essential for PMBCL-like MGZL: monomorphic sheets of medium-sized to large neoplastic cells within a variably dense fibrotic stroma; strong and uniform positive expression of CD30 and partial or complete loss of B-cell markers, or strong CD15 expression.

Desirable for both: because the complex histological features are often not reliably identifiable in core needle biopsies, a larger biopsy is strongly preferred for the diagnosis; absence of EBV.

Staging

The Lugano classification, adapted from the Ann Arbor staging system with Cotswold modifications, is used for staging {688}.

Prognosis and prediction

Retrospective series report about 35% of primary refractory cases and a lower response rate to regimens effective in CHL, such as ABVD {1292,1434,3580,709,3239}. Detection of strong and diffuse expression of CD20 provides a rationale to add rituximab to CHL-type polychemotherapy or to treat with a PMBCL-like regimen. In the only prospective trial to date, the outcome of MGZL was inferior to that of PMBCL {4387}. Predictive factors, such as lymphocyte count, Eastern Cooperative Oncology Group (ECOG) performance status, anaemia, B symptoms, albumin level, CD15 expression, DC-SIGN–positive cells, and mutation burden, have mainly been reported in univariate analyses and/or in retrospective series {4387,3580,3239,3579} and are not currently included in clinical decision-making.

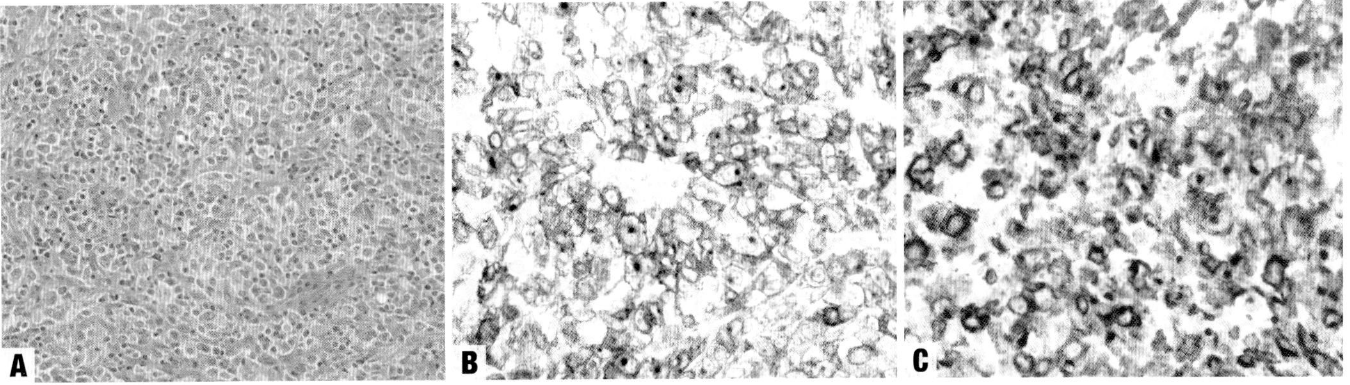

Fig. 4.222 Mediastinal grey zone lymphoma with primary mediastinal large B-cell lymphoma–like morphology. **A** Primary mediastinal large B-cell lymphoma–like mediastinal grey zone lymphoma showing sheets and nests of large tumour cells with clear cytoplasm. Fine fibrous bands are appreciated. **B** The tumour cells are positive for CD30. **C** The tumour cells show CD15 expression.

High-grade B-cell lymphoma NOS

Leoncini L
Dave SS
Delabie J
Dunleavy K
Ennishi D
Li S
Naresh KN
Rosenwald A
Siebert R

Definition
High-grade B-cell lymphoma (HGBCL) NOS represents a heterogeneous type of aggressive mature B-cell lymphoma composed of medium-sized or blastoid cells that does not fulfil the diagnostic criteria for other defined lymphoma entities.

ICD-O coding
9680/3 High-grade B-cell lymphoma, NOS
9680/3 High-grade B-cell lymphoma, NOS, with *MYC* and *BCL6* rearrangements

ICD-11 coding
2A81.Z & XH2WM7 Diffuse large B-cell lymphoma, NOS & High-grade B-cell lymphoma, NOS

Related terminology
None

Subtype(s)
High-grade B-cell lymphoma NOS with *MYC* and *BCL6* rearrangements

Localization
Most patients present with widespread disease involving lymph nodes and extranodal sites {3411,3059}.

Clinical features
Generalized lymphadenopathy is common. Bone marrow infiltration with various degrees of cytopenia is often present. Serum LDH levels are usually high. Patients usually have a high-intermediate or high International Prognostic Index (IPI) score {3411,3059}.

Epidemiology
Limited data are available for HGBCL-NOS specifically, in part because the nomenclature and definition of these lymphomas have been subject to change in successive editions of the WHO classification. The incidence generally increases with age and, consequently, elderly patients are affected most often. No sex predilection has been reported {3411,3059}.

Etiology
Unknown

Pathogenesis
Limited data are available for HGBCL-NOS, and those that are in the literature indicate that this is a heterogeneous tumour category. Isolated *MYC* rearrangements are reported in 8–58% of cases {1694,2763,780,1366,2312}, and *MYC* amplifications in 32% {2763}. *MYC* amplification concurrent with IGH::*BCL2* translocations or amplification of both oncogenes has been described {2314}. Translocations of *BCL2* and *BCL6* are each reported in 10–18% of HGBCL-NOS cases {1366,780,2312}. Recent sequencing data suggest (although based on a small number of cases) that the most commonly mutated genes are *TP53* (30–36%), *KMT2D* (33–42%), and *MYC* and *TNFSF14* (both 33%) {2312}. Other EZB/C3-cluster mutations are also described {780, 2312}. The mutation spectrum and gene expression signatures suggest that HGBCL-NOS contains more than one biological subgroup. By the LymphGen algorithm, most cases of HGBCL-NOS are grouped into the unclassified category, and the remainder as EZB (13%), MCD (9%), ST2 (7%), and BN2 (4%) {780}. Gene expression profiling shows that 54% of cases of HGBCL-NOS harbour the double-hit/dark-zone signature (DZsig) that was initially developed to identify diffuse large B-cell lymphoma / HGBCL with *MYC* and *BCL2* rearrangements {780,2312}.

Macroscopic appearance
Not relevant

Histopathology
HGBCL-NOS generally shows a diffuse proliferation of intermediate or blastoid cells with sparsely admixed small lymphocytes. A starry-sky pattern caused by macrophages with apoptotic bodies may be present. Cohesive growth is usually not prominent. There

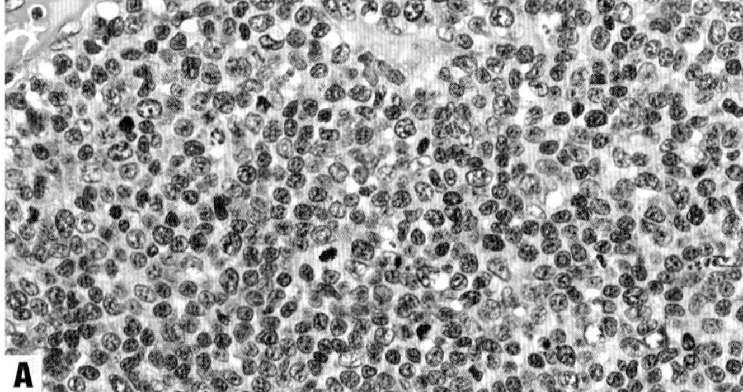

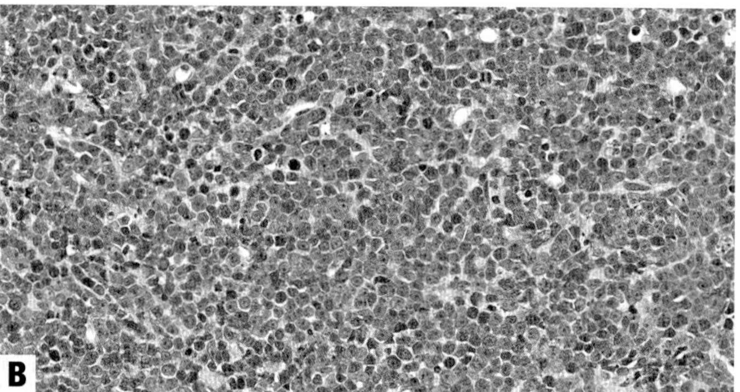

Fig. 4.223 High-grade B-cell lymphoma NOS. **A** The morphology varies, with some cases showing a heterogeneous infiltrate of small to medium-sized blastoid tumour cells. **B** Other cases show uniform tumour cells with blastoid features.

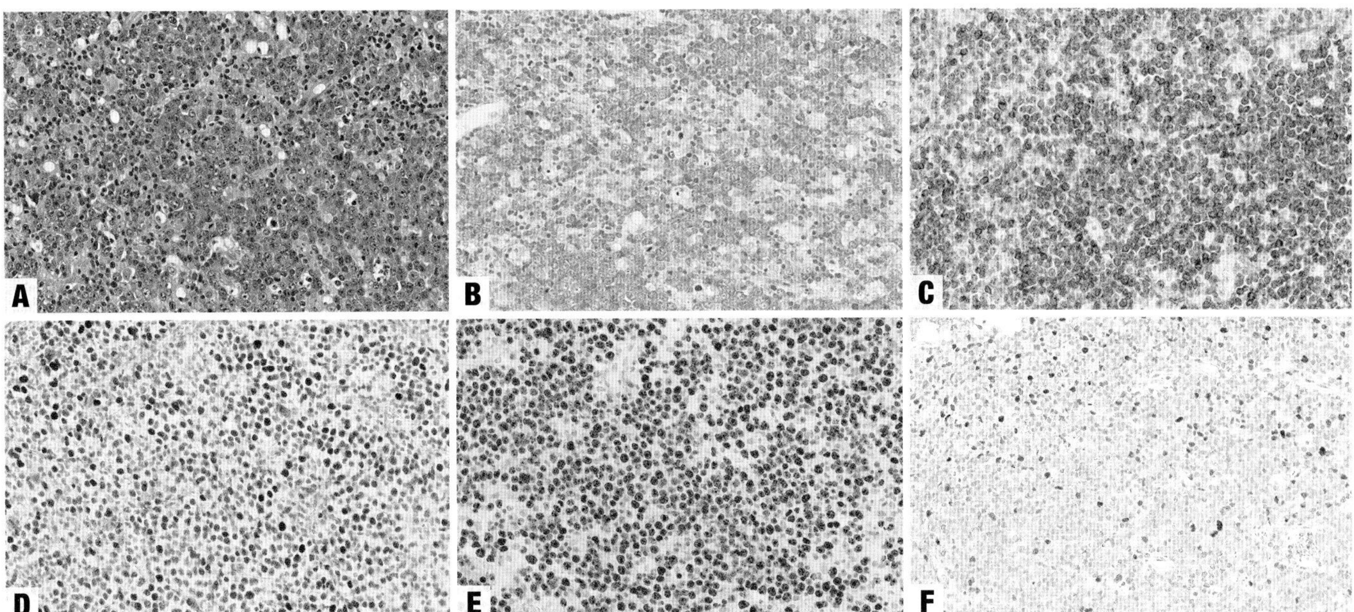

Fig. 4.224 High-grade B-cell lymphoma NOS. **A** Morphology intermediate between diffuse large B-cell lymphoma and Burkitt lymphoma, characterized by a diffuse proliferation of medium-sized to large cells with a few admixed small lymphocytes. The cellular morphology is variable, exhibiting more variation in nuclear size and nucleolar content than generally acceptable for Burkitt lymphoma (H&E stain). **B** The cytomorphological detail is better appreciated in a Giemsa stain. **C** The neoplastic cells strongly express BCL2. **D** MYC is variably expressed by the neoplastic cells. **E** The proliferative rate is generally (but not always) high, here showing a Ki-67 proliferation index of > 90%. **F** MYC may be expressed at low levels, here in < 10% of the neoplastic cells.

is variable cellular and nuclear pleomorphism, usually more than is generally acceptable for Burkitt lymphoma. The cytoplasm is usually less basophilic than in Burkitt lymphoma {3411,2299}. The rare blastoid variant has small to intermediate-sized cells with a small rim of cytoplasm, round nuclear contours, inconspicuous nucleoli, and finely dispersed chromatin {1862,2763}.

Immunophenotype

HGBCL-NOS expresses the pan–B-cell markers CD20, CD19, and CD22 and lacks expression of CD34 and TdT. Many cases show expression of CD10, BCL6, and BCL2. IRF4 (MUM1) expression is variable. According to the Hans classifier, HGBCL-NOS often shows a germinal-centre B-cell–like phenotype, but some are non–germinal-centre B-cell–like. The Ki-67 proliferation index is variable (40–90%) {3085}. MYC expression is variable, partially depending on the presence of a *MYC* translocation, and roughly half of the cases are dual-expressers of MYC and BCL2 {1694,3032}. High p53 expression in most cells correlates with *TP53* mutations {2311,2299}.

Differential diagnosis

Burkitt lymphoma is distinguished by its pathognomonic cytomorphology and immunophenotype. FISH analysis or another technique is required to exclude HGBCL with *MYC* and *BCL2* rearrangements and HGBCL with 11q aberration. B-lymphoblastic leukaemias/lymphomas express TdT and other markers related to immature phenotypes. The blastoid variant of mantle cell lymphoma expresses cyclin D1, SOX11, and often CD5.

Cytology

The diagnosis of HGBCL-NOS cannot be made on the basis of cytological (fine core needle specimens) alone. Cytoplasmic vacuoles are few or absent in cytological imprints.

Diagnostic molecular pathology

The diagnosis of HGBCL-NOS requires the exclusion of dual rearrangements of *MYC* and *BCL2*, and of the characteristic 11q aberration pattern typical of HGBCL with 11q aberration. In HGBCL-NOS with a *MYC* single hit, differentiation from Burkitt lymphoma may be supported by mutation analyses; genes such as *ID3*, *TCF3*, *SMARCA4*, and *CCND3* are typically mutated in Burkitt lymphoma but not in HGBCL-NOS.

Essential and desirable diagnostic criteria

Essential: intermediate or blastoid cytomorphology not consistent with either diffuse large B-cell lymphoma or Burkitt lymphoma; lack of TdT and CD34 expression (to exclude lymphoblastic lymphoma); lack of cyclin D1 expression (to exclude mantle cell lymphoma); absence of a dual translocation involving *MYC* and *BCL2*; absence of the 11q23.2-q23.3 gain and 11q24.1-qter deletion pattern of HGBCL with 11q aberration.

Desirable: double-hit/dark-zone B-cell lymphoma gene expression signature; *KMT2D* and *TP53* mutations.

Staging

Staging is done according to the Lugano criteria.

Prognosis and prediction

Because of the rarity of HGBCL-NOS, no reliable data on prognostic or predictive features are available. Treatment is generally undertaken according to established guidelines for aggressive lymphomas. Intermediate-intensity or dose-intensive treatment approaches are currently favoured {3059}.

Burkitt lymphoma

Sayed S
Cheuk W
d'Amore ESG
Dave SS
Ferry JA
Gopal S
Klapper W
Leoncini L
Mbulaiteye SM
Medeiros LJ
Naresh KN
Rochford R
Siebert R

Definition

Burkitt lymphoma (BL) is a mature aggressive B-cell neoplasm composed of monomorphic, medium-sized cells with basophilic cytoplasm, multiple small nucleoli, a germinal-centre B-cell phenotype, a high proliferation index, and an IG::*MYC* rearrangement.

ICD-O coding

9687/3 Burkitt lymphoma

Traditional subtypes
9687/3 Endemic Burkitt lymphoma
9687/3 Sporadic Burkitt lymphoma
9687/3 Immunodeficiency-associated Burkitt lymphoma

Recommended subtypes
9687/3 EBV-associated Burkitt lymphoma
9687/3 EBV-negative Burkitt lymphoma

ICD-11 coding

2A85.6 Burkitt lymphoma including Burkitt leukaemia

Related terminology

Not recommended: Burkitt cell leukaemia; atypical Burkitt lymphoma; Burkitt-like lymphoma.

Subtype(s)

Traditional subtypes
Endemic BL; sporadic BL; immunodeficiency-associated BL.

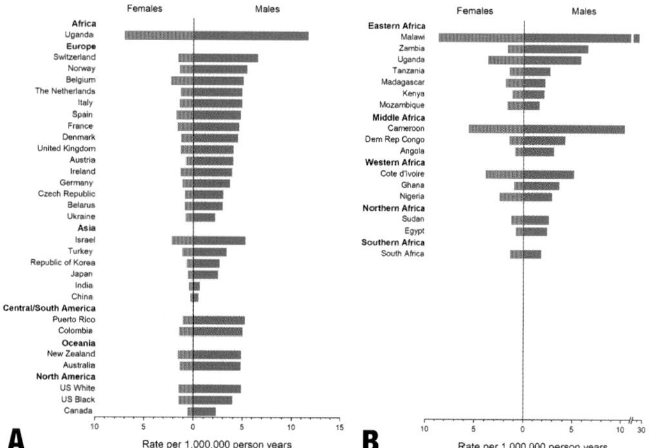

Fig. 4.225 Burkitt lymphoma. Age-standardized Burkitt lymphoma incidence rates per 1 million person-years (World Standard Population) for males and females for countries with ≥ 60 cases total. **A** Rates for the 28 countries included in *Cancer Incidence in Five Continents*, Volume XI (CI5-XI). **B** Rates for 16 countries included in the African Cancer Registry Network (AFRCN) data. The *x*-axis scale for Malawi is broken to accommodate the higher male Burkitt lymphoma rate in that country.

Recommended subtypes
EBV-associated BL; EBV-negative BL.

Localization

Extranodal sites are most commonly involved. However, there is geographical variation in the sites of involvement. In endemic BL, the mandible and maxilla, as well as other facial bones, were traditionally reported as most frequently involved {111,1852}. More recent literature typically describes frequent abdominal presentations {1377}. Sporadic BL commonly involves the abdomen, soft tissues of the orbit, Waldeyer ring, gingiva, thyroid gland, ovary, testis, and breast {233,3324}. BLs arising in immune deficiency/dysregulation settings more commonly have nodal involvement, although extranodal involvement is also frequent {166}. Patients with any BL subtype are at high risk of CNS disease {3555,1377}. Although population-based studies show a low incidence of CNS involvement {2615}, clinical studies from Malawi {3817} and the USA {3462} suggest its frequency ranges from 10% to 30% of cases.

Clinical features

Patients with BL commonly present with a high tumour burden, widely disseminated disease, and rapidly growing tumours due to the short doubling time of BL cells. Site-specific symptoms include altered vision, nasal obstruction, enlarged tonsil(s), dental/jaw pain (often with loss of teeth), abdominal masses (ileocaecal lesions, retroperitoneal nodes), renal lesions, and testicular masses. Breast involvement is uncommon except in pregnant and lactating women, in whom the disease is usually bilateral. Lymphadenopathy mainly occurs in BL arising in immune deficiency/dysregulation settings. Systemic symptoms occur in a subset of patients. Leukaemic presentation / bone marrow infiltration occurs in as many as 20% of cases, especially in BL arising in immune deficiency/dysregulation settings {3070}; however, it is rare in patients with endemic BL, although its occurrence may be underestimated in limited-resource settings.

Epidemiology

Three subtypes of BL, historically recognized as endemic, non-endemic (sporadic), and immunodeficiency-associated, have traditionally been used to describe the epidemiology of BL {1503}. BL is the most common childhood cancer in many countries in equatorial Africa and in Papua New Guinea, where it is considered endemic and is associated with EBV in > 90% of the cases {3839}. Elsewhere, BL is less common in children, where it is considered sporadic and is associated with EBV in about 20% of the cases {2290}. Immunodeficiency-associated BL is more common in the setting of HIV infection than in other forms of immunosuppression {2290}.

However, the designation of endemic or sporadic BL subtypes is problematic, because it is primarily based on variations

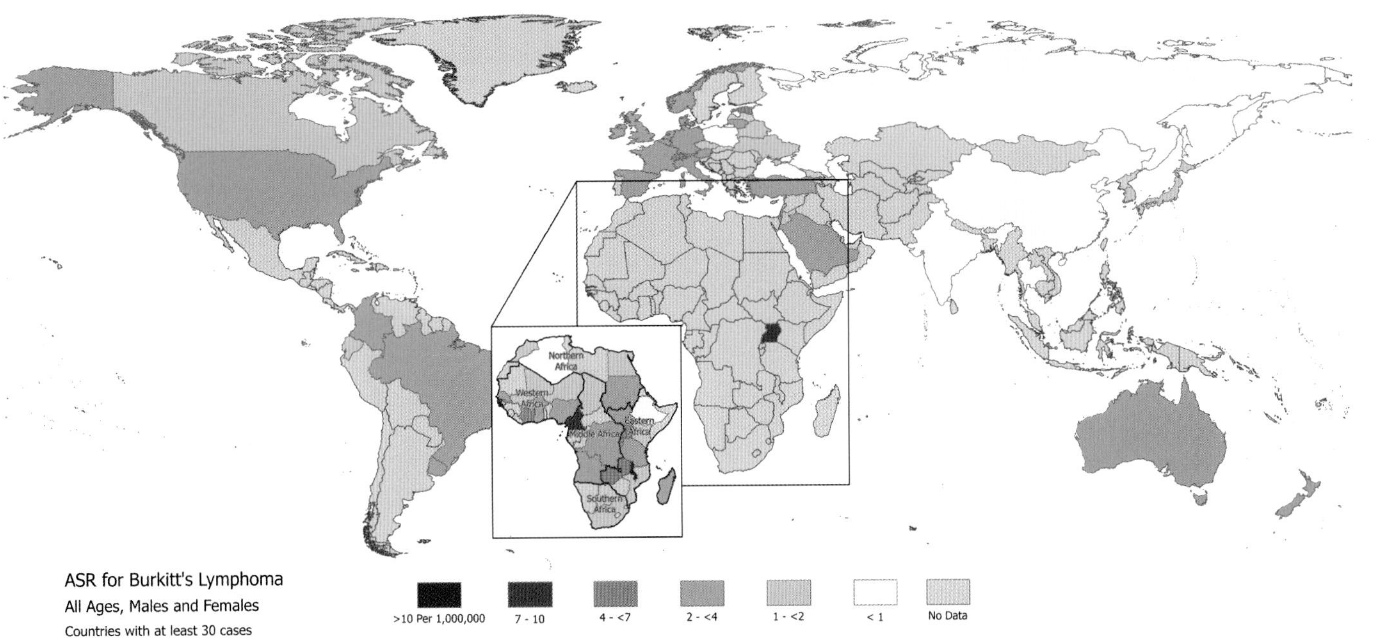

Fig. 4.226 Burkitt lymphoma. Age-standardized Burkitt lymphoma incidence rates per 1 million person-years (World Standard Population) for males and females combined in 38 countries with ≥ 30 cases during 2008–2012, using data from *Cancer Incidence in Five Continents*, Volume XI (CI5-XI). **Inset:** Data for 27 African countries with ≥ 30 cases during 2018 from the African Cancer Registry Network (AFRCN).

in geographical incidence and epidemiology, and there is no molecular pathological definition of each traditional subtype {4416}. It is probable that sporadic BL also occurs in Africa and may account for the rare EBV-negative cases of BL reported from that continent {4416}. Indeed, recent research data suggest that EBV-positive BL and EBV-negative BL form discrete groups with similar molecular features, regardless of epidemiological context and geographical region {299,3,1938,1391, 3405,2281}. Thus, EBV may be the defining etiological feature of the subtypes of BL {3434}, and EBV-positive and EBV-negative BL have been shown to differ in their underlying cell biology and pathogenetic mechanisms, justifying a new approach to their designation {552,1766,4416,2281,3434}.

BL rates vary widely (2- to 50-fold) in different populations worldwide {1482,1816}. The highest age-standardized rates (ASRs) of BL are observed in sub-Saharan Africa, Malawi, Uganda, and Cameroon, consistent with the high malaria prevalence there, but rates are lower in subtropical regions of Africa or in countries at high altitude. BL rates are much lower in Central and South America, Europe, North America, and Asia, but variability is observed within regions. BL incidence rates appear lowest in Asia, being 20 times lower in China than in Uganda {1816}.

In general, the M:F ratio of BL is 2–4:1 {3002,2613,2614, 1816}. The M:F ratio is highest before puberty and decreases with age {2613}. The ratio appears to be higher (as high as 10:1) for tumours involving the face or head structures {2615}. In the USA, 50% of all BL cases occur in adults aged 20–59 years, 28% occur in adults aged ≥ 60 years, and 22% occur in the paediatric age group (0–19 years). Adult BLs represent 1–2% of non-Hodgkin lymphomas in adults or elderly patients {2722}. The age-specific incidence of BL shows a bimodal pattern, with distinct peaks at about 10 years and about 60 years {3002, 2613,2614}, suggesting that there might be biological differences in BL diagnosed at different ages {3405}.

Etiology

Risk factors for endemic BL are *Plasmodium falciparum* (malaria) and EBV infections (for details, see *Pathogenesis*). Factors causing BL in low-incidence areas, such as Europe, Asia, and South America, are not well understood. EBV is reported in at most 20% of sporadic BL cases {2290}, although the incidence of EBV-positive BL increases with age in central Europe {3405}. Genetic factors appear to be important. This is supported by a consistent finding of a high M:F ratio in children, particularly prepubescent children {2688}. Other clues about genetic contribution come from reports of familial BL clusters, including two recent cases in whom germline variants in *TCF4* and *CHD8* were reported {1381}. Reports of a high BL risk in rare inherited disorders, including inborn errors of immunity (e.g. X-linked lymphoproliferative syndrome 1 [XLP1], MIM number: 308240; X-linked immunodeficiency with magnesium

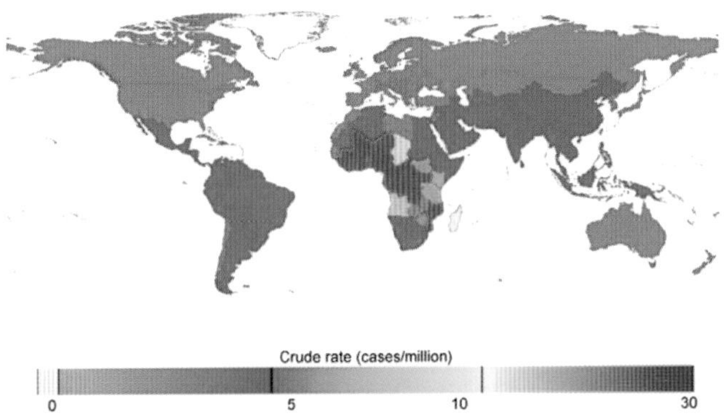

Fig. 4.227 Burkitt lymphoma. Estimated Burkitt lymphoma incidence in children aged < 15 years in 2015, as reported in the Baseline Model, which is based on data from the SEER Program, GLOBOCAN 2018, and International Incidence of Childhood Cancer (IICC-3), as well as estimates from the Global Childhood Cancer (GCC) model {1816}.

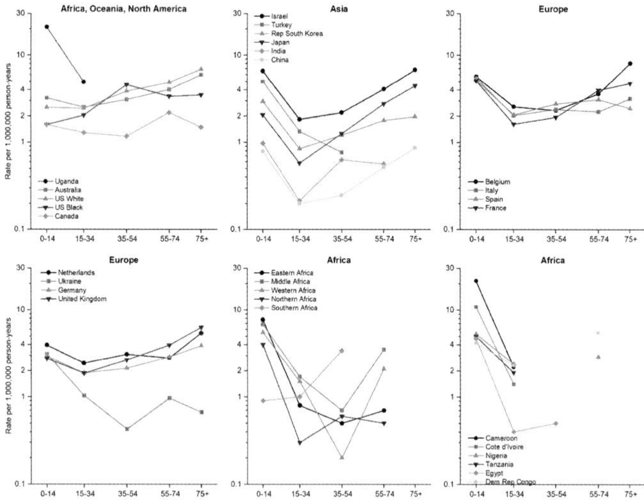

Fig. 4.228 Burkitt lymphoma. Incidence rates for 5 age groups for countries with ≥ 100 total cases. Rates for 18 countries in 5 continents are based on *Cancer Incidence in Five Continents*, Volume XI (CI5-XI) data for 2008–2012, and rates for Africa are supplemented with data reported to the African Cancer Registry Network (AFRCN) for 2018 by region and separately for 6 countries with cases in both the 0–14 years and the 15–34 years age groups. Rates based on < 10 cases are not shown. Horizontal lines for Burkitt lymphoma rates = 2 and 4 cases per million divide the graph space into three areas corresponding to low, intermediate, and high Burkitt lymphoma rates.

defect, EBV infection, and neoplasia [XMEN], MIM number: 300853) and DNA repair disorders (e.g. ataxia–telangiectasia, MIM number: 208900) also support a genetic predisposition to (EBV-positive) BL.

Pathogenesis

Malaria

Several studies have shown an association between the complexity of infection and BL risk {1074,1817,147}. According to these recent data, children who are exposed to mixed *P. falciparum* infection have a higher risk for BL than those exposed to infection of a single *P. falciparum* variant, which could explain why *P. falciparum* may be associated with BL in some but not all areas. Children can be repeatedly infected with *P. falciparum*–associated malaria, resulting in chronic stimulation of B cells, suppression of T-cell immunity, and induction of activation-induced cytidine deaminase (AID), an enzyme associated with the formation of the *MYC* translocation typical of BL {3424}. Consistent with this, EBV-positive BL shows AID-mediated somatic hypermutation with features of antigen selection in their rearranged IG genes {98,1391}, as well as loss of T-cell responses to the EBV EBNA1 protein in patients with BL {2771}.

Immunodeficiency

BL occurring in HIV-positive individuals tends to present in patients with relatively high CD4 counts and is frequently the first manifestation of HIV infection. As a consequence, the widespread introduction of combination antiretroviral therapy (cART) has had less effect on the incidence of BL than on the incidence of other types of lymphoma {3357}. The association with EBV in this special setting is variable. Similarly, BL also occurs later in posttransplant cases when the immunosuppressive medication has been reduced and chronic immune stimulation is prolonged.

EBV

A challenge in understanding the role of EBV in the etiology of BL is the ubiquity of the virus in the human population. Primary infection can occur at < 1 year of age in sub-Saharan Africa, resulting in a loss of viral control and a high burden of infected cells {363,937,3257}, thus potentially increasing the risk of malignant transformation. EBV encodes several transforming proteins, but only EBNA1 is consistently detected in EBV-positive BL {3492}. Abrogation of apoptotic pathways is required in B cells to tolerate constitutive *MYC* activation, suggesting that such pathogenetic events must occur before *MYC* translocation. EBV, therefore, may be essential early in pathogenesis by allowing B cells to evade apoptosis {76,1200} and impact host cell homeostasis in various ways, by epigenetic modification of host genes and by interfering with cellular microRNA expression {2278,3229,2923}. EBV variants in BL that have deletions of *EBNA2* are also linked to the suppression of apoptosis {1943}. A hit-and-run mechanism in EBV infection has been proposed {2839} and is supported by recent evidence suggesting that EBV plays an initiating role in oncogenesis, but the viral genome is subsequently lost with the acquisition of stable (epi)genetic changes by the neoplastic cells {2838}.

Molecular pathogenesis

The primary genetic event in BL is the IG::*MYC* translocation juxtaposing *MYC* either to the IGH locus by the t(8;14)(q24;q32) translocation (in 80% of cases) or, less commonly, to the IGL or IGK locus by the t(8;22)(q24;q11) and t(2;8)(p12;q24) translocations, resulting in constitutive MYC expression. Breakpoints of *MYC* in the IGH::*MYC* are nearby upstream (5′) or within the first exon or intron of *MYC* in most sporadic and immune deficiency/dysregulation–related BLs, but in endemic BL they can map over hundreds of kilobases upstream from the *MYC* basal promoter {3181,2118}. In IGK::*MYC* and IGL::*MYC*, the breakpoints in 8q24 are usually downstream (3′) of *MYC*, even up to 2 Mb. Other *MYC* translocations with non-IG genes have not been definitively demonstrated in BL but may be associated with other high-grade B-cell lymphomas (HGBCLs) and diffuse large B-cell lymphomas {1683}. Conventional cytogenetic or molecular methods may miss some IG::*MYC* translocations {3634}. Cryptic insertions of *MYC* into IGH have been described {4264}. Alternative mechanisms that dysregulate

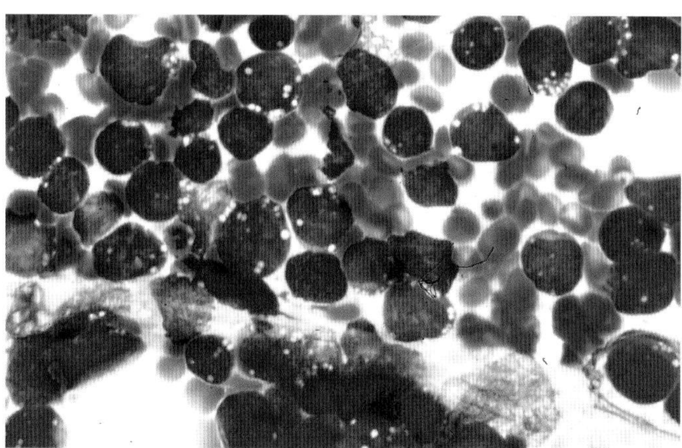

Fig. 4.229 Burkitt lymphoma. In cytological preparations, the lymphoma cells have deeply basophilic cytoplasm with many large, characteristic lipid vacuoles.

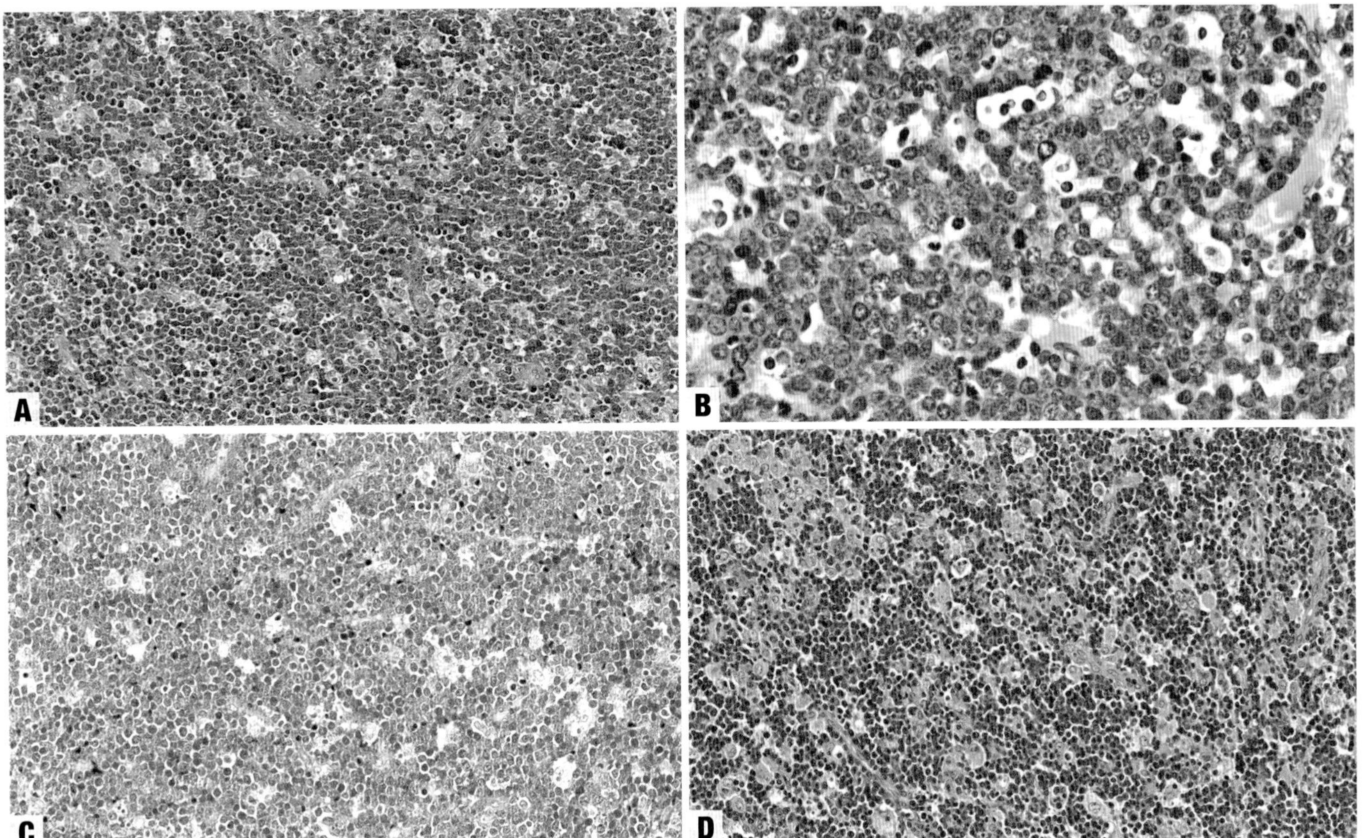

Fig. 4.230 Burkitt lymphoma. **A** Diffuse growth pattern composed of monomorphic medium-sized lymphoid cells with basophilic cytoplasm, squared-off cytoplasmic borders, round nuclei with finely clumped and dispersed chromatin, and multiple basophilic and paracentrally located nucleoli. The cells display some degree of cohesion, with abundant mitoses and apoptosis. There is a starry-sky pattern due to the presence of many macrophages with phagocytic activity containing apoptotic debris. **B** Higher magnification shows medium-sized tumour cells with a coarse chromatin pattern. **C** The cytonuclear detail is better appreciated in Giemsa-stained preparations. **D** Some Burkitt lymphoma cases may have a florid granulomatous reaction, sometimes even causing problems in the recognition of the tumour.

MYC have been described in a small subset of cases but should foster consideration of the differential diagnosis {2283, 1391,4264,2837}. A complex karyotype or multiple imbalances are uncommon at initial diagnosis in BL and should challenge the diagnosis and may require additional testing. The IG::*MYC* translocation is thought to be mediated by aberrant activation of AID {3424}. Mutations in genes controlling cell proliferation, growth, and survival have been identified in BL, but there is no consistent oncogene besides *MYC* that characterizes all BLs. A characteristic molecular BL (mBL) signature is identified by gene expression profiling studies {1683,877}. Slightly different signatures occur in endemic BL and sporadic BL {3229}, and in adult sporadic BL {431,2041}.

Next-generation sequencing has documented a high frequency of mutations in *TCF3* (which encodes a transcription factor) and its negative regulator *ID3*, which activates both the PI3K pathway (promoting cell survival) and cell cycle–related genes such as *CCND3* (activating cell proliferation) {3406, 3630,2434,3}. Mutations in *TCF3* or its repressor *ID3* that result in tonic activation of B-cell receptor signalling are among the predominant coding mutations found in EBV-negative BL, although they are also frequently seen in EBV-positive cases {1391}. Other common pathways affected by mutations include B-cell receptor and PI3K signalling, apoptosis, SWI/SNF signalling, and G protein–coupled receptor signalling {1408,1391, 3125}. Of note, *TP53* mutations/deletions occur in 25–50% of cases and are also enriched in EBV-negative BL {1391,2411, 3125,2939}.

In comparison with EBV-negative BL, EBV-positive cases show significantly higher levels of AID (*AICDA*) mRNA expression and somatic hypermutation activities, particularly in non-coding sequences close to the transcription start site {1391}. Despite this, EBV-positive BL harbours fewer driver mutations, particularly in the apoptosis pathway, than EBV-negative BL {1391}, further corroborating the pathogenetic role of EBV in lymphomagenesis. Thus, the emerging evidence from in-depth genetic analysis suggests a dual mechanism of BL pathogenesis: mutational versus virally driven {3}.

Macroscopic appearance

There is often a bulky mass comprising contiguous lymph nodes and surrounding tissue. The cut surface has a fish-flesh appearance with focal necrosis and haemorrhage. In some cases, jaw excisions are undertaken, revealing a maxilla or mandible with a large necrotic and destructive mass.

Histopathology

BL shows a diffuse growth pattern and is composed of monomorphic medium-sized lymphoid cells with basophilic cytoplasm, squared-off cytoplasmic borders, round nuclei with finely clumped and dispersed chromatin, and multiple basophilic and paracentrally located nucleoli. The cells display some degree of cohesion, with abundant mitoses and apoptosis. Many macrophages with phagocytic activity containing apoptotic debris are seen in the background. A sprinkling of tingible-body macrophages in a background of cohesive blue cells results in the classic – albeit not specific – starry-sky pattern. Coagulative necrosis is common. Reactive small lymphocytes are rare.

Some EBV-positive cases may have a florid granulomatous reaction obscuring the tumour. These cases are characterized by a proinflammatory microenvironment, typically present with limited-stage disease, and have an especially good prognosis, sometimes even with spontaneous remission {1615,1497,1390}. Some cases of BL show greater nuclear pleomorphism despite clinical, immunophenotypic, and molecular features characteristic of typical BL. In these cases, the nucleoli may be more prominent and fewer in number. In other cases, particularly in adults with immune deficiency/dysregulation, the tumour cells may exhibit plasmacytoid differentiation with eccentric basophilic cytoplasm and often a single central nucleolus {3449}. These morphological features are in line with gene expression profiling studies suggesting that the morphological spectrum of BL is broader than generally thought {1683}.

Immunohistochemistry

BL expresses pan–B-cell antigens (CD19, CD20, CD79a, CD22, and PAX5) and germinal centre–associated antigens (CD10 [particularly strong], BCL6, CD38, HGAL, and MEF2B). The cells are variably positive for the germinal-centre marker GCET1 and consistently negative for LMO2, and they frequently show strong expression of IgM. Aberrant expression of CD43, LEF1, and TCL1A is seen {2197,297,254,3436,2901,2651}. Intense nuclear MYC expression in > 80% cells is noted in almost all cases; very rare cases lack MYC positivity despite the presence of *MYC* rearrangement due to mutations of the gene or other mechanisms {3972,102}. Ki-67 expression is typically > 95%. Cytoplasmic lipid vacuoles can be demonstrated by staining with adipophilin antibody {104}. Neoplastic cells are usually negative for CD5, CD23, and CD138, and are characteristically negative for BCL2, CD44, and TdT. However, weak BCL2 expression can be seen in about 20% of cases and does not exclude the diagnosis. Strong expression of BCL2 and expression of cyclin D1 or TdT is not compatible with a diagnosis of BL; a lack of MYC expression would make the diagnosis of BL not very likely.

Flow cytometry

Characteristically, BL tumour cells are CD45-low. They express CD19, CD20, CD10, CD38, CD43, CD81, FMC7, and monotypic surface kappa or lambda light chain; expression of CD38 and CD81 is particularly bright. They lack expression of BCL2, CD44, and TdT {2516,556,4080}.

Differential diagnosis

Cases whose morphology and immunophenotype diverges from what is expected for BL (more frequently seen in the context of immune deficiency/dysregulation settings, particularly HIV) warrant investigations for an alternative diagnosis (see Table 4.40). On the other hand, cases with some variation in the size and shape of the nuclei can still be diagnosed as BL if they show a combination of an isolated IG::*MYC* translocation with

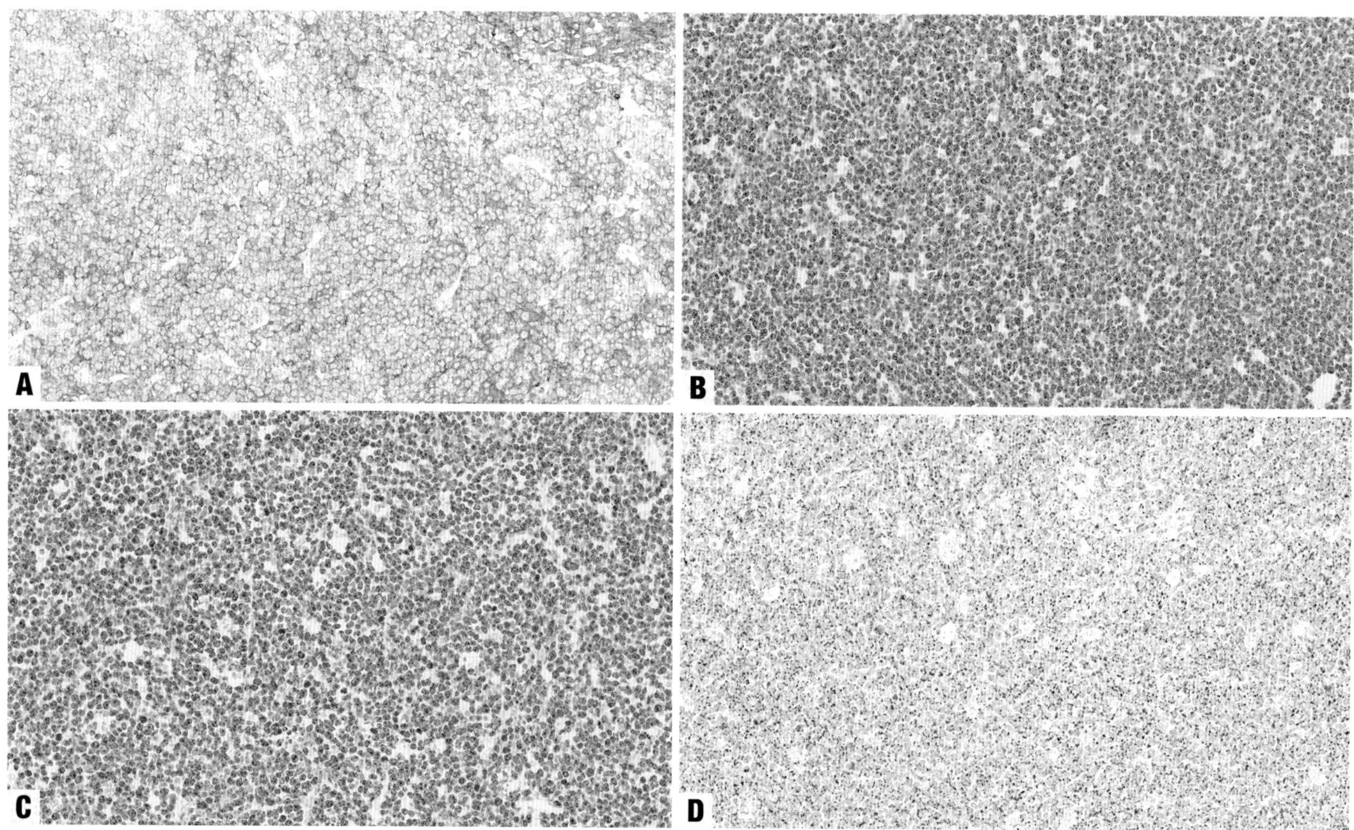

Fig. 4.231 Burkitt lymphoma. **A** The neoplastic cells are CD10-positive. **B** Immunohistochemistry shows intense MYC expression in > 80% of the cells. **C** Ki-67 expression is typically > 95%. **D** Cytoplasmic lipid vacuoles can be demonstrated by staining with adipophilin antibody.

a typical immunophenotype (CD10+, BCL6+, BCL2–, Ki-67 > 95%) {1694}.

The differential diagnosis includes B-lymphoblastic leukaemia/lymphoma; HGBCL with *MYC* and *BCL2* rearrangements (predominantly in adults); HGBCL-NOS; HGBCL with 11q aberration, and – on small biopsies – paediatric-type follicular lymphoma (predominantly in paediatric patients).

Lymphoblastic lymphoma is excluded by its morphology (fine chromatin, scant cytoplasm), strong expression of TdT, and presence of additional markers of immaturity (e.g. CD34).

Some cases of HGBCL-NOS have histological features similar to those of BL, and some have *MYC* rearrangement, heightening the similarity to BL. However, cases of HGBCL-NOS usually lack expression of CD10 and show strong expression of BCL2. Dual rearrangements of *MYC* and *BCL2* with or without *BCL6* rearrangement exclude a diagnosis of BL; such cases are diagnosed as HGBCL with *MYC* and *BCL2* rearrangements, and cases with concurrent *MYC* and *BCL6* rearrangements are classified as a genetic subtype of HGBCL-NOS with *MYC* and *BCL6* rearrangements. Evaluation of these translocations, therefore, is recommended in adult patients. Cases that lack rearrangements of *MYC* should be evaluated for the 11q gain/loss pattern associated with HGBCL with 11q aberration {1630}.

Embryonal rhabdomyosarcoma can occur in the head and neck and, on cytology preparations, can show vacuolization of cytoplasm; it should be ruled out by the polygonal or spindle shape of some cells, the prominent nucleoli, the lack of deeply basophilic cytoplasm, and the characteristic immunophenotype with expression of desmin and myogenin.

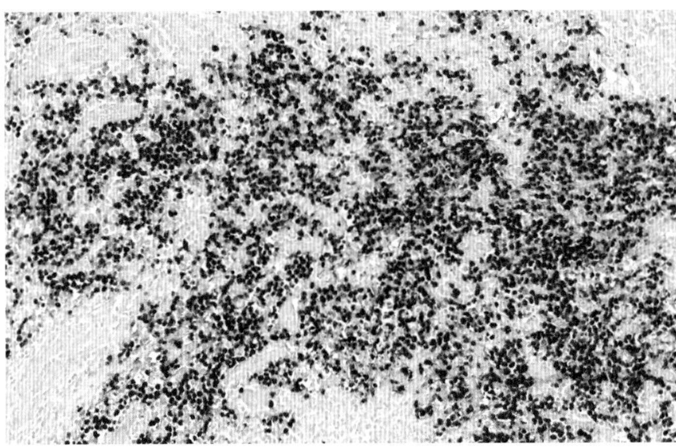

Fig. 4.232 Burkitt lymphoma. EBV-positive Burkitt lymphoma is strongly and uniformly positive for EBV-encoded small RNA (EBER).

Performing genetic studies requires good infrastructure along with good technical and analytical expertise, which is currently not available in many parts of the world with a high incidence of BL. To address this, a refined algorithm for the diagnosis of BL has been proposed, to be used in resource-challenged settings. The diagnosis of BL requires the typical morphological features, characteristic phenotype (expression of CD20, CD10, and CD38; negative or very weak BCL2 expression; lack of CD44), intense MYC expression in > 80% cells, and a Ki-67 index of ≥ 95%. In a resource-limited setting, such a constellation of morphology and immunophenotype in

Table 4.40 Differential diagnosis of Burkitt lymphoma (BL)

Diagnosis	Morphology	Immunophenotype/immunohistochemistry	Genetics
Burkitt lymphoma	Cohesive monomorphic, medium-sized cells with multiple small nucleoli and basophilic cytoplasm	B cells positive for CD10, BCL6, CD38, and MYC; Ki-67 index > 95%; negative for BCL2, TdT, CD44, and cyclin D1	IG::*MYC* translocations Absence of *BCL2* or *BCL6* translocation(s)
B-lymphoblastic leukaemia/ lymphoma	Finer nuclear chromatin; nucleoli often less conspicuous	Uniform expression of TdT in most cases; CD34 expression in a subset of cases	Lack of *MYC* translocation; presence of other key defining rearrangements/translocations
High-grade B-cell lymphoma with *MYC* and *BCL2* rearrangements	Variable: intermediate between BL and DLBCL, DLBCL, or blastoid	Most express BCL2; some cases show variable expression of TdT	*BCL2* translocation in addition to *MYC* translocation
High-grade B-cell lymphoma NOS	Medium to large cells; variation in nuclear size and nucleolar content; cohesive growth is usually absent	Most express BCL2; variable MYC expression dependent on *MYC* abnormalities	Can show isolated *MYC*, isolated *BCL2*, or *BCL2* and *BCL6* translocation(s) Does not show dual *BCL2* and *MYC* translocations or 11q aberration Can show *MYC*/*BCL6* translocations
Large B-cell lymphoma with 11q aberration	Some resemblance to BL, but often shows more pleomorphism with some variation in nuclear shape/size and presence of larger nucleoli	Variable MYC expression	Gain in 11q23.3 and the minimal region of loss at 11q24.1-qter; lack of *MYC* translocation
Diffuse large B-cell lymphoma NOS	Larger cells; nucleoli more prominent; peripherally located nucleoli; pleomorphism	Majority express BCL2; can lack CD10, BCL6, CD38, or MYC expression; can show expression of CD44	Majority lack *MYC* translocation Variable presence of *BCL2* or *BCL6* translocation(s)
Paediatric-type follicular lymphoma (particularly in a core needle biopsy)	Intermediate to large blastoid cells, cytologically between centrocytes and centroblasts Follicular pattern may not be apparent in a core needle biopsy	B cells positive for CD10 and BCL6; Ki-67 index > 30%; BCL2 negative/weak; negative for MYC and cyclin D1 CD21/CD23-positive follicular dendritic cell meshworks	Absence of *MYC*, *BCL2*, *BCL6*, and *IRF4* translocations

BL, Burkitt lymphoma; DLBCL, diffuse large B-cell lymphoma.

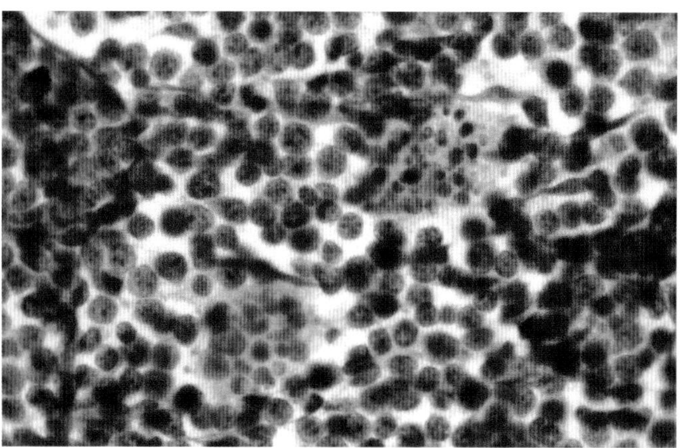

Fig. 4.233 Burkitt lymphoma. A smear of an FNA from a Burkitt lymphoma. The lymphoid population is monotonous and consists of intermediate-sized lymphocytes with regular nuclei and characteristically coarse chromatin with multiple basophilic nucleoli. The cytoplasm is basophilic, and small lipid vacuoles are identified in Giemsa-stained specimens. Apoptotic debris is often seen scattered or in the form of macrophages with tingible bodies, seen in the centre of this image.

concert with a typical clinical context would suffice for a diagnosis of BL {2901,2903}.

Cytology

In cytological preparations of FNAs, medium-sized lymphoid cells have deeply basophilic cytoplasm that often contains some fine lipid vacuoles. Nuclei are round, and multiple basophilic nucleoli are noted {2478,2479,3802}.

Diagnostic molecular pathology

Demonstration of *MYC* breakage or IG::*MYC* translocation, preferably with absence of *BCL2* and *BCL6* translocation, may support the diagnosis of BL in the appropriate morphological and immunophenotypic context. Documented absence of an IG::*MYC* fusion argues against the diagnosis of typical BL.

Essential and desirable diagnostic criteria

Essential: medium-sized, monomorphic lymphoma cells with basophilic cytoplasm and multiple small nucleoli; CD20 and CD10 positivity, absence or (rarely) weak expression of BCL2, Ki-67 index > 95%; usually strong expression of MYC (in > 80% of cells) and/or demonstration of *MYC* breakage or IG::*MYC* translocation.

Desirable: starry-sky pattern, cohesive growth pattern; BCL6 positivity, TdT negativity, CD38 positivity; exclusion of *BCL2* and *BCL6* rearrangements (mainly required in adult BL).

Staging

The predominantly extranodal distribution of BL makes Ann Arbor staging suboptimal. The system proposed by Murphy and revised in 2015 is used routinely for children {3476}.

Prognosis and prediction

The prognosis for all patients with BL treated with contemporary immunochemotherapy regimens including rituximab in high-resource settings is excellent. The overall survival rate exceeds 90% in children and 80% in adults {88,3547,3058} in contemporary multicentre clinical trials. The recently proposed BL-IPI subdivides patients into low-, intermediate-, and high-risk groups, with overall survival rates of 96%, 76%, and 59%, respectively {3058}. Also, patients with HIV-associated BL are currently successfully treated with similar immunochemotherapy regimens.

In low/middle-resource settings, outcomes for patients with BL have been less good, in part because of inadequate resources for diagnosis and treatment {1377,3096} and a lack of awareness in the population and among health care workers, leading to delays in presentation and diagnosis. Results have improved since the introduction of more intensive regimens in sub-Saharan Africa {805} and improvements in the comprehensive cancer care delivery infrastructure, but BL still poses a huge burden on cancer care.

KSHV/HHV8-associated B-cell lymphoid proliferations and lymphomas: Introduction

Naresh KN

Kaposi sarcoma–associated herpesvirus / human herpesvirus 8 (KSHV/HHV8) is transmitted by saliva and is acquired primarily in childhood in highly endemic areas or through sex (predominately in men who have sex with men). KSHV/HHV8 is etiologically related to a spectrum of unique clinicopathological entities. Most of these KSHV/HHV8-associated lymphoid proliferations, which include multicentric Castleman disease, KSHV/HHV8-positive germinotropic lymphoproliferative disorder (KSHV/HHV8-positive GLPD), primary effusion lymphoma (PEL) / extracavitary PEL (EC-PEL), and KSHV/HHV8-positive diffuse large B-cell lymphoma (KSHV/HHV8-positive DLBCL), occur in patients with an immunodeficiency. PEL/EC-PEL and KSHV/HHV8-positive DLBCL are characteristically seen in the setting of severe immunodeficiency, such as HIV infection or posttransplant. KSHV/HHV8-positive GLPD, in contrast, is reportedly more prevalent in immunocompetent patients. However, KSHV/HHV8-positive GLPD occurs more frequently in older individuals, which may suggest that relative immunodeficiency caused by immunosenescence may play a role in some. It is remarkable that in contrast to EBV, KSHV/HHV8 is not involved as a driver of lymphoid proliferations among patients with inborn errors of immunity.

Major progress has been made in understanding the biology of KSHV/HHV8 and recognizing the morphological and clinical spectrum of lymphoid proliferations caused by this virus. In this fifth edition of the WHO classification of haematolymphoid tumours, such novel information is included, and definitions have been refined on the basis of the current state of knowledge. Clinical, morphological, and immunophenotypic criteria defining the various entities are listed in Table 4.41. In keeping

Table 4.41 Clinicopathological features of KSHV/HHV8-positive germinotropic lymphoproliferative disorder (GLPD), KSHV/HHV8-positive diffuse large B-cell lymphoma (DLBCL), and KSHV/HHV8-associated multicentric Castleman disease (MCD)

Feature	KSHV/HHV8-associated MCD	PEL/EC-PEL	KSHV/HHV8-positive DLBCL	KSHV/HHV8-positive GLPD
Clinical	M:F ratio: ~2.2:1 Age: 40–45 years ~80% are HIV+; HIV– patients older (in their sixties) Frequently associated with Kaposi sarcoma in HIV+ patients	Male predominance Age: 20–50 years Immunosuppressed (HIV, posttransplant) Frequently associated with Kaposi sarcoma or KSHV/HHV8-associated MCD	Male predominance Age: 30–40 years Often HIV+ patients with KSHV/HHV8-associated MCD	M:F ratio: 1.5:1 Age: 30–90 years (median: 60 years) Most are HIV–
Site	Lymph nodes, spleen	PEL involves serous cavities, including pleural, pericardial, and abdominal EC-PEL in lymph nodes or extranodal sites (gastrointestinal tract, skin, etc.)	Lymph nodes, spleen, peripheral blood, extranodal sites	Lymph nodes, usually localized; sometimes multifocal (more common in HIV+ patients)
Cytomorphology	Medium to large cells with plasmablastic or immunoblastic appearance	Large pleomorphic cells with plasmablastic, immunoblastic, or anaplastic morphology	Large cells with plasmablastic or immunoblastic appearance	Large cells with plasmablastic, immunoblastic, or anaplastic morphology
Histology	Involuted to hyperplastic follicles; interfollicular vascular proliferation and plasmacytosis	Sheets of large cells effacing architecture; may be focal in lymph nodes (EC-PEL)	Sheets of large cells effacing architecture	Variable replacement of germinal centres without significant nodal architectural effacement; may have scattered cells in interfollicular areas or sinuses
Phenotype	CD20–/+ IRF4 (MUM1)+ IgM lambda+ CD138– vIL-6+ in a large proportion of cells	Few or no B-cell antigens expressed; rare aberrant T-cell antigen expression CD30+, IRF4 (MUM1)+, CD138+/– Most negative for immunoglobulin vIL-6 variably positive	CD20+/–, IRF4 (MUM1)+, IgM lambda+ CD138–; vIL-6+ in a large proportion of tumour cells	Usually B-cell antigen–negative Most CD138–, CD30–; IRF4 (MUM1)+; immunoglobulin can be positive or negative vIL-6 variably positive
KSHV/HHV8 LANA	Positive	Positive	Positive	Positive
EBV (EBER)	Usually negative	Positive > 80%	Usually negative	Positive > 90%
IG gene rearrangement and hypermutation	Polyclonal; lacks somatic hypermutations	Monoclonal; usually with somatic hypermutations	Monoclonal; lacks somatic hypermutations	Most polyclonal or oligoclonal, with few monoclonal; with somatic hypermutations

EBER, EBV-encoded small RNA; EC-PEL, extracavitary primary effusion lymphoma; LANA, latency-associated nuclear antigen; PEL, primary effusion lymphoma.

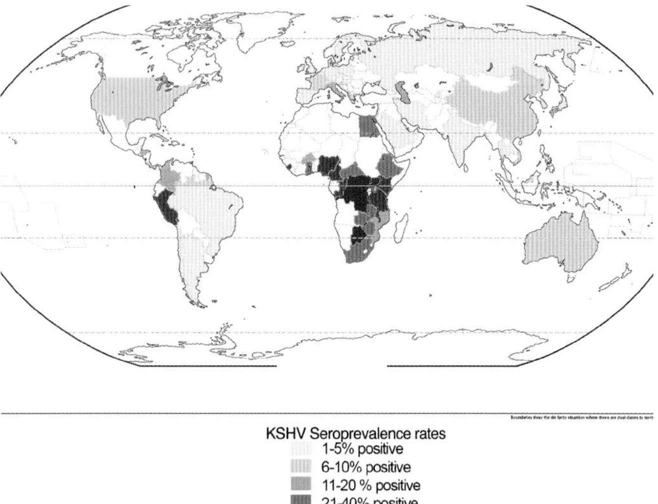

Fig. 4.234 Geographical seroprevalence of KSHV/HHV8. The KSHV/HHV8 seroprevalence in sub-Saharan Africa (> 40%) is significantly higher than in northern Europe, Asia, and the USA (< 10%). However, distributions vary regionally both in Africa and in Europe: in southern Italy, including Sicily and Sardinia, the seroprevalence is significantly higher (intermediate levels of 10–30%) (figure modified from {596}).

with the terminology for other herpesviruses, the name "KSHV/HHV8" is now preferred, to accommodate the common practices of both haematopathologists and virus researchers. It should be noted that KSHV/HHV8-associated lymphoid proliferations are discussed in a dedicated section rather than included in the sections on immune deficiency/dysregulation (IDD)-associated proliferations. KSHV/HHV8 biology is recognized as the unique common driver, whereas an association with IDD is variable between the KSHV/HHV8-associated entities, justifying this choice. In overt IDD settings, however, the formal three-part nomenclature for IDD-associated proliferations is preferred (e.g. "primary effusion lymphoma, KSHV/HHV8+, EBV+, HIV setting").

The insight that the various KSHV/HHV8-associated entities may not be as distinct as previously assumed impacts the current WHO classification. The morphological spectrum of some entities has been recognized to be broader than previously appreciated. Examples are intravascular localization and classic Hodgkin lymphoma–like morphology in KSHV/HHV8-DLBCL and EC-PEL. Furthermore, clinical, phenotypic, viral status (KSHV/HHV8 with or without EBV), and morphological overlap between entities is increasingly appreciated. It is not always possible to differentiate between KSHV/HHV8-positive DLBCL and EC-PEL, although the expression of IgM/lambda may favour the former. Moreover, EC-PEL and KSHV/HHV8-positive GLPD with plasmablastic aggregates may overlap morphologically, precluding their distinction, particularly as both entities are usually positive for both KSHV/HHV8 and EBV.

It is likely that KSHV/HHV8 biology underlies the overlapping features described above but that this biology may not be adequately captured by our current disease-defining criteria. This notion of a likely common underlying pathogenesis is underpinned by the observation that both PEL and KSHV/HHV8-positive DLBCL may occur together with or be preceded by KSHV/HHV8-associated multicentric Castleman disease, and cases of KSHV/HHV8-positive DLBCL may be preceded by KSHV/HHV8-positive GLPD. Currently, the rarity of such reported cases precludes the ability to determine biologically defined boundaries between the entities, if indeed such boundaries exist. While more knowledge may accumulate over the coming years to resolve such issues, discussion in a multidisciplinary setting is essential in difficult cases to decide on the best classification and treatment for individual patients. Ultimately, from better knowledge about the underlying biology, improved and targeted therapeutic interventions may result for KSHV/HHV8-associated lymphoid proliferations.

Primary effusion lymphoma

Said JW
Bacon CM
Bower M
Cesarman E
Chadburn A
Du MQ
Medeiros LJ
Michelow P

Definition

Primary effusion lymphoma (PEL) is a large B-cell lymphoma presenting as a pleural, pericardial, and/or peritoneal serous effusion in the absence of lymph node involvement or an extranodal mass lesion, except for the rare presence of a body cavity–related tumour mass. It is consistently associated with Kaposi sarcoma–associated herpesvirus / human herpesvirus 8 (KSHV/HHV8) and usually coinfected with EBV. Extracavitary PEL (EC-PEL) is a related entity presenting with a tumour mass, often at extranodal sites.

ICD-O coding

9678/3 Primary effusion lymphoma
9678/3 Extracavitary primary effusion lymphoma

ICD-11 coding

2A81.9 Primary effusion lymphoma

Related terminology

Not recommended: body cavity–based lymphoma.

Subtype(s)

Primary effusion lymphoma; extracavitary primary effusion lymphoma

Localization

Pleural, pericardial, and abdominal body cavities are typically involved in PEL. EC-PEL involves lymph nodes and extranodal sites.

Clinical features

Most patients with PEL present with lymphomatous effusions involving serous cavities including the peritoneum, pericardium, or pleura, rarely accompanied by a tumour mass directly related to the body cavity {595}. Most patients with PEL are HIV-positive with a low CD4 cell count (≤ 200 × 10^6/L) {1439}. Other manifestations of KSHV/HHV8 infection, including Kaposi sarcoma and multicentric Castleman disease, are present in approximately 50% of patients at presentation. EC-PEL manifests as solid tumours without an effusion, involving lymph nodes or extranodal sites including the gastrointestinal tract, lung, and skin, and rarely the CNS or bone marrow, or it exhibits intravascular localization {2129,471,1431}.

Epidemiology

PEL presents most commonly in patients with HIV/AIDS, and less commonly in other immunosuppressed individuals, including transplant recipients {4542}. PEL represents approximately 4% of HIV-related lymphomas and < 1% of non–HIV-associated lymphomas {3483}. The proportion of PEL among AIDS-related lymphomas has increased in the era of antiretroviral therapy (ART) {3357}. PEL also occurs rarely in elderly patients with no evidence of immunosuppression other than immunosenescence {3483}. Patients from KSHV/HHV8-endemic areas (sub-Saharan Africa and Mediterranean countries) are typically older than HIV-positive patients.

Etiology

The main etiological agent is KSHV/HHV8 infection, with coinfection by EBV in approximately 80% of cases, in association with immunosuppression (usually HIV, or rarely posttransplant).

Pathogenesis

PEL appears to be largely driven by KSHV/HHV8, where all tumour cells contain naked viral episomes {1220,594}. Although the KSHV/HHV8 viral genome encodes for more

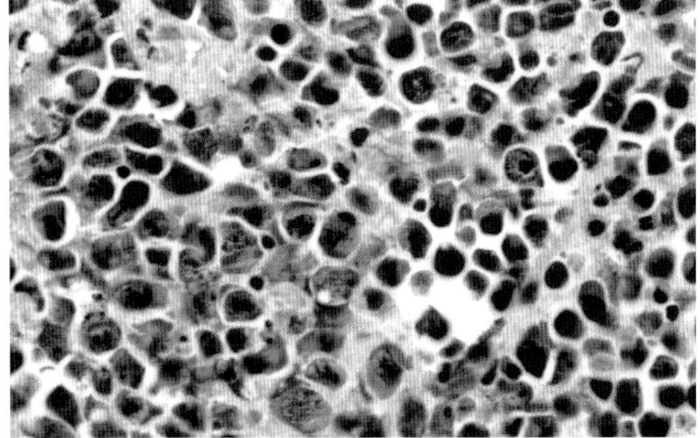

Fig. 4.235 Primary effusion lymphoma. Cell block from a patient with HIV and a malignant pleural effusion. The cells have a plasmablastic/immunoblastic appearance with abundant amphophilic cytoplasm.

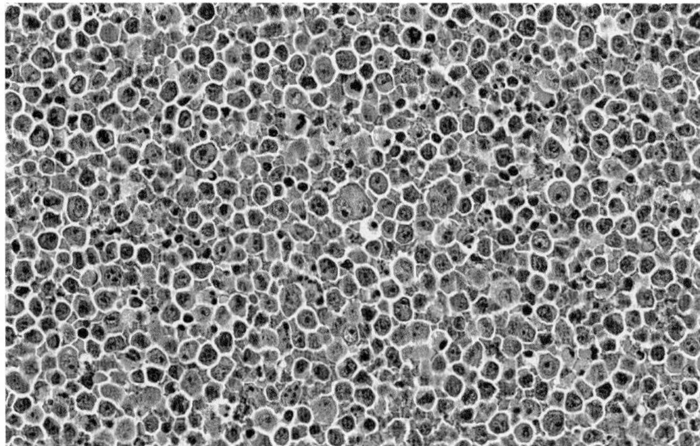

Fig. 4.236 Primary effusion lymphoma. Cell block from the pleural fluid of an 86-year-old patient with primary effusion lymphoma. The infiltrate includes Reed–Sternberg–like cells with prominent nucleoli.

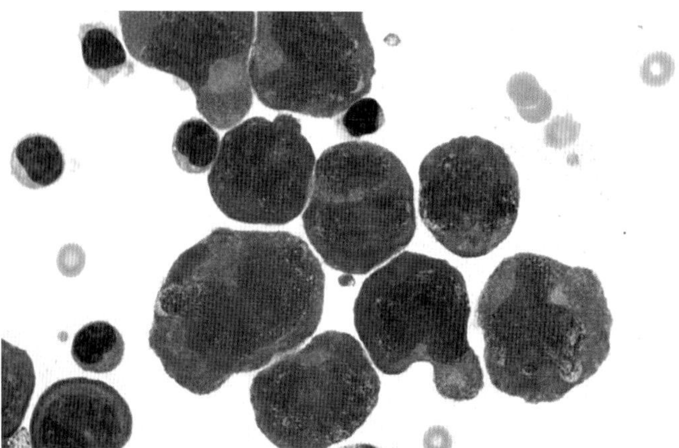

Fig. 4.237 Primary effusion lymphoma. Pleural fluid cytology from a patient with primary effusion lymphoma. There is marked pleomorphism with prominent nucleoli and abundant cytoplasm (Giemsa).

than 80 proteins, only a small number are expressed in PEL, where a latent pattern of gene expression is seen. The virus can undergo lytic viral replication in a small proportion of the PEL cells, where most viral genes are expressed, leading to infectious virus production. The viral proteins expressed in PEL are latency-associated nuclear antigen (LANA), vCyclin, vFLIP, vIRF3, and kaposin B {594}. LANA is diagnostically important as a target for immunohistochemistry but may have important pathogenetic roles by binding a number of tumour suppressor proteins (p53, RB1, and GSK3B). vCyclin is a homologue of human cyclin D with effects on the cell cycle. vFLIP activates the transcription factor NF-κB, which controls the expression of a number of cytokines and growth factors, as well as antiapoptotic proteins. vFLIP protein is essential for PEL cell survival. vIRF3 is homologous to cellular IRFs (including IRF4, important in B-cell differentiation and germinal-centre formation) and is a negative regulator of interferon responses. Kaposin B can bind and activate MK2, and through that mechanism it can stabilize the mRNA of a number of cytokines, growth factors, and oncogenes. In addition, KSHV/HHV8 encodes a number of microRNAs; one of these in particular, KSHV/HHV8 miR-K11, may have a potential lymphogenic effect. Despite the number of potential viral oncogenic products, KSHV/HHV8 does not transform B cells in culture, in contrast with EBV. EBV may contribute to transformation in the cases with both viruses, but in these, EBV has a restricted (type I latency) expression pattern.

Limited genomic studies exist, but it appears that there are no recurrent alterations of oncogenes and tumour suppressor genes that are common in other lymphomas. However, PEL depends on the expression of a number of cellular proteins, including cyclin D2 (encoded by *CCND2*), cFLIP, and MCL1 {2524}. Recurrent cytogenetic alterations include trisomy 7, trisomy 12, and aberrations in the proximal long arm of chromosome 1 (1q) {4385}.

Macroscopic appearance

Not relevant

Histopathology

PEL tumour cells are large with immunoblastic, plasmablastic, or anaplastic features. Malignant cells usually lie singly in a background of apoptotic debris. Nuclei have irregular outlines with coarse chromatin. They have prominent nucleoli, and abundant basophilic or amphophilic cytoplasm with or without vacuoles. The cells may be multinucleated resembling Hodgkin or Reed–Sternberg cells {874,459}.

EC-PEL consists of sheets of large pleomorphic, immunoblastic, plasmablastic, or anaplastic cells with cytological features similar to those of PEL cells (see below). In lymph nodes there are sheets of large pleomorphic cells, which may completely efface the architecture, show partial involvement, or be sinusoidal.

Immunophenotype

PEL and EC-PEL lymphoma cells are derived from B cells, but they may lack CD45 and therefore can be misdiagnosed as other tumours {603}. They lack the common B-cell markers CD19, CD20, CD22, PAX5, OCT2, BOB1, and CD79a {2062, 2866}. Surface and cytoplasmic immunoglobulin is usually absent. The malignant cells lack germinal-centre markers (CD10 and BCL6) but often express markers of terminal B-cell differentiation (HLA-DR, CD30, EMA, CD38, VS38c, CD138,

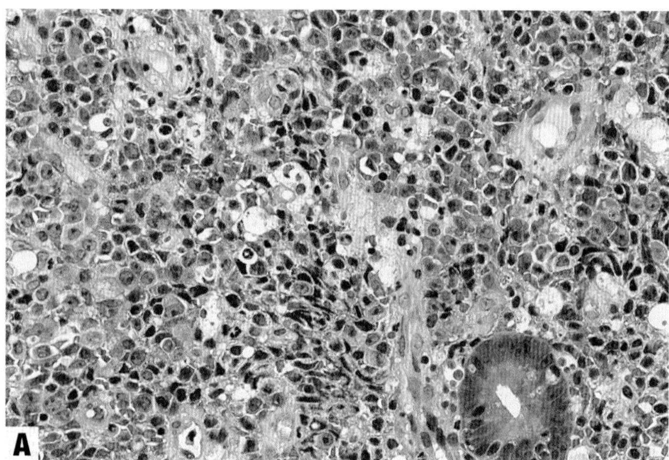

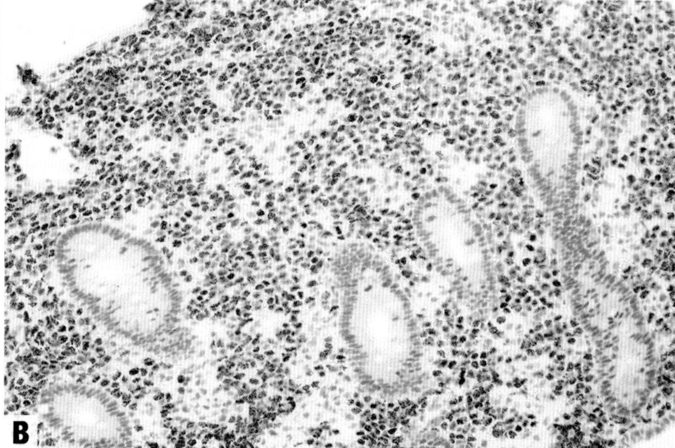

Fig. 4.238 Primary effusion lymphoma, extracavitary. **A** Biopsy of a jejunal mass from a 38-year-old man with HIV, Kaposi sarcoma, and a circumferential mass in the small bowel. **B** Cells are positive for EBV-encoded small RNA (EBER) by in situ hybridization (not shown) and for KSHV/HHV8 latency-associated nuclear antigen (LANA).

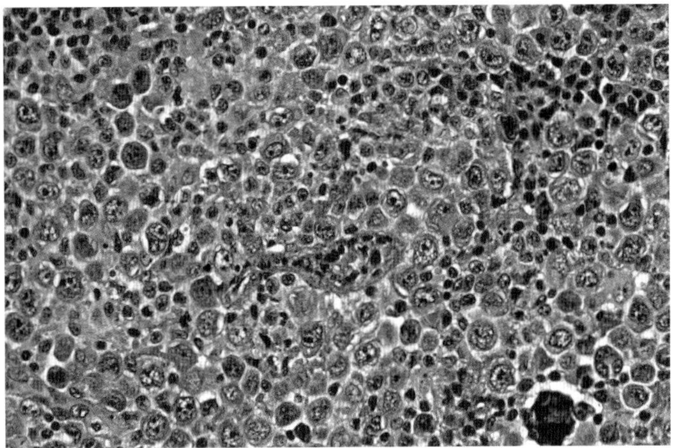

Fig. 4.239 Primary effusion lymphoma, extracavitary. Extracavitary primary effusion lymphoma at higher magnification showing sheets of large pleomorphic malignant cells.

IRF4 [MUM1], and Blimp1). The cells usually lack T- or NK-cell antigens, but aberrant expression of T-cell markers occurs in as many as 30% of cases {3527,426,1439}. Demonstration of KSHV/HHV8 (usually performed by immunohistochemistry using an antibody to KSHV/HHV8 LANA [ORF73]) is essential for the diagnosis. Most, if not all, PEL cases in the HIV-positive population are positive for EBV-encoded small RNA (EBER) but lack LMP1. vIL-6 as demonstrated by immunohistochemistry is variably positive. EC-PELs more often express B-cell–associated antigens and/or immunoglobulin {603}.

Differential diagnosis

The differential diagnosis includes fluid overload–associated large B-cell lymphoma, which may share cytological features and (rarely) association with EBV but is negative for KSHV/HHV8. EC-PEL may have overlapping features with germinotropic lymphoproliferative disorder and KSHV/HHV8-positive diffuse large B-cell lymphoma (see Table 4.41, p. 539, in *KSHV/HHV8-associated B-cell lymphoid proliferations and lymphomas: Introduction*).

Cytology

The cytological features of PEL cells are described in *Histopathology*. Flow cytometry is helpful in the diagnosis, and characteristic features include large cell size; high cellular complexity; dim expression of CD45; and expression of CD38, CD138, VS38c, and HLA-DR. Cells are negative for B-cell–associated markers including CD19, CD20, and surface and cytoplasmic light chains {1273}.

Diagnostic molecular pathology

The monoclonal B-cell nature can be demonstrated by IG rearrangement analysis in most cases {603,1483}. PCR for the presence of KSHV/HHV8 and EBV would also support the diagnosis of PEL.

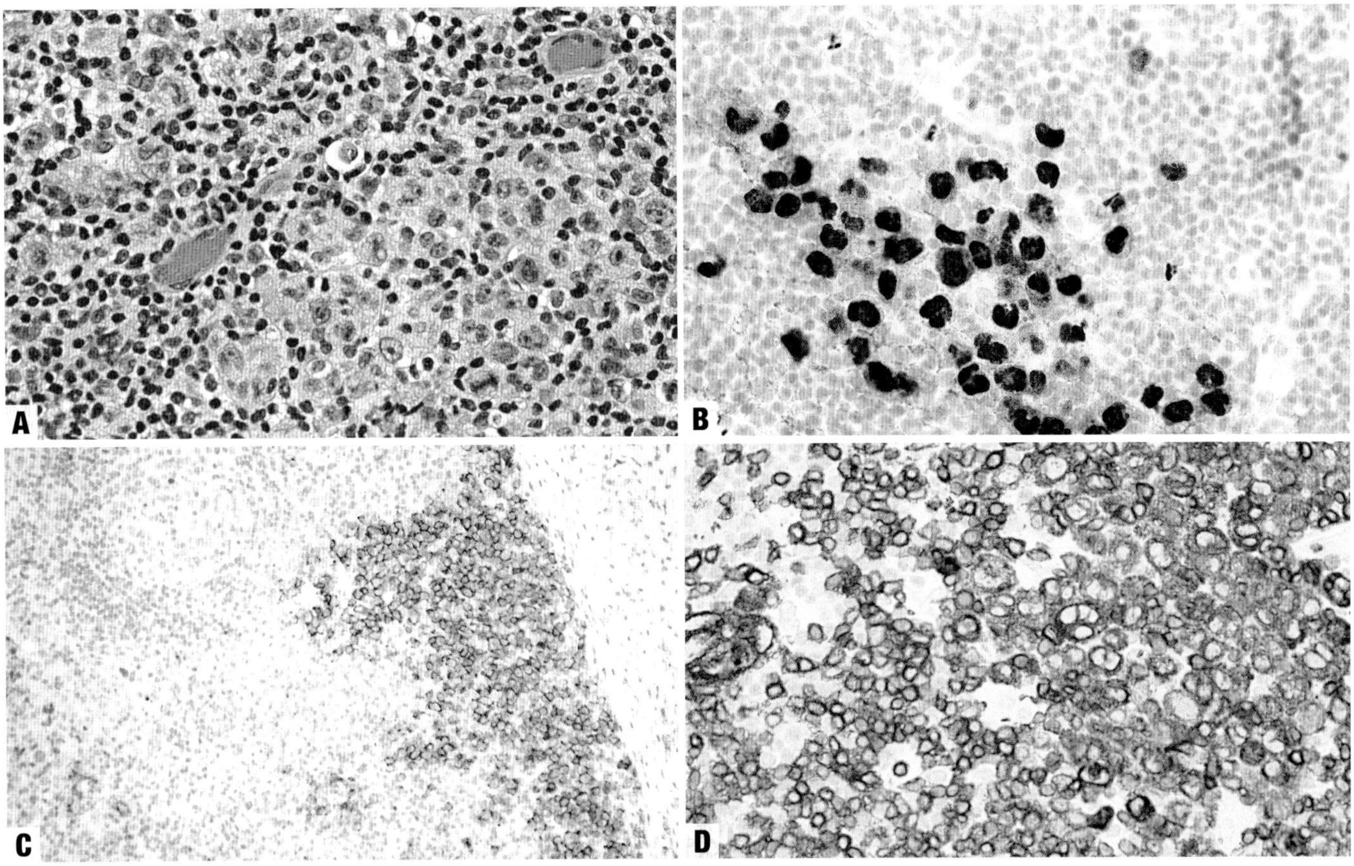

Fig. 4.240 Primary effusion lymphoma, extracavitary. **A** Lymph node with partial involvement by extracavitary primary effusion lymphoma. **B** Malignant cells show strong nuclear staining for KSHV/HHV8 latency-associated nuclear antigen (LANA). **C** The cells are positive for CD138, highlighting preferential localization in the lymph node sinus. **D** Aberrant expression of the T-cell marker CD3 can be seen.

Essential and desirable diagnostic criteria

Essential for PEL: large B-cell lymphoma presenting as a serous effusion in the pleural, pericardial, or abdominal cavity; a tumour mass directly associated with the effusion is accepted; absence of lymph node or other extranodal involvement; large pleomorphic malignant cells with the immunophenotype of terminally differentiated B cells; KSHV/HHV8 positivity (usually by LANA immunohistochemistry).

Essential for EC-PEL: large B-cell lymphoma presenting with nodal or extranodal involvement without an associated effusion; large pleomorphic malignant cells with the immunophenotype of terminally differentiated B cells; KSHV/HHV8 positivity (usually by LANA immunohistochemistry).

Desirable for both: the presence of EBV, although neither necessary nor sufficient, is supportive of the diagnosis.

Staging

EC-PEL is usually stage I or II at presentation.

Prognosis and prediction

PEL is an aggressive lymphoma with a relatively poor prognosis despite the overall improvement in outcome of HIV-related lymphomas {1439,1557,1658,46}. Remissions and prolonged survival have been reported with chemotherapy and (in the HIV-related cases) ART {3415,963}. More favourable outcomes have been reported in patients with EBV-positive PEL {2450}. The prognosis of extracavitary or solid PEL is somewhat more favourable than that of PEL, with fewer relapses in patients who achieve complete remission {603,1439}.

KSHV/HHV8-positive diffuse large B-cell lymphoma

Vega F
Bower M
Cesarman E
Chadburn A
Du MQ
Said JW

Definition

Kaposi sarcoma–associated herpesvirus / human herpesvirus 8 (KSHV/HHV8)-positive diffuse large B-cell lymphoma (DLBCL) is a large B-cell lymphoma consistently associated with KSHV/HHV8, in general arising in patients with profound immunodeficiency, but it may occur in non-immunocompromised patients. The tumour cells morphologically resemble plasmablasts or immunoblasts and have abundant cytoplasmic IgM.

ICD-O coding

9738/3 KSHV/HHV8-positive diffuse large B-cell lymphoma

ICD-11 coding

2A81.Y & XH5HJ5 Other specified diffuse large B-cell lymphomas & Large B-cell lymphoma arising in HHV8-associated multicentric Castleman disease

Related terminology

Acceptable: HHV8-positive diffuse large B-cell lymphoma NOS.
Not recommended: large B-cell lymphoma arising in HHV8-associated multicentric Castleman disease (obsolete).

Subtype(s)

None

Localization

KSHV/HHV8-positive DLBCL characteristically involves the lymph nodes and/or spleen, but it can disseminate to extranodal sites and can also manifest with peripheral blood involvement {3042,1024}. Rarely, the lymphoma is limited to the spleen {4307}.

Clinical features

Patients with KSHV/HHV8-positive DLBCL usually present with profound immunodeficiency, and they are most often HIV-seropositive and have KSHV/HHV8-positive multicentric Castleman disease (MCD). However, similar lymphomas have been reported in the absence of MCD, in patients with KSHV/HHV8-positive germinotropic lymphoproliferative disorder or in apparently non-immunocompromised patients, including HIV-negative patients {1078,824,1369}. Patients present with generalized lymphadenopathies and splenomegaly.

Epidemiology

KSHV/HHV8-positive DLBCL is very rare. The majority of patients are HIV-positive men aged between 30 and 40 years. Because of its rarity, however, formal and reliable data on geographical distribution are lacking. The geographical distribution is assumed to mirror the geographical prevalence of KSHV/HHV8, specifically that of KSHV/HHV8-MCD {4104, 606}.

Etiology

KSHV/HHV8 is transmitted by saliva and is acquired primarily in childhood in highly endemic areas, or through sex, predominately in men who have sex with men {594}. KSHV/HHV8-positive DLBCL is associated with KSHV/HHV8 infection. Co-infection with EBV is rare and occurs in association with profound immunosuppression that is most generally mediated by HIV. The risk of developing KSHV/HHV8-positive DLBCL in people living with HIV is 15 times as high in those also diagnosed with MCD than in those without MCD {3042}. It has been suggested that the treatment of MCD with rituximab reduces this risk of lymphoma {1322}.

Pathogenesis

The pathogenesis of KSHV/HHV8-positive DLBCL is related to the expression of a few transforming viral genes that affect cellular proliferation and survival, including vIL-6, latency-associated nuclear antigen (LANA; ORF73), and viral cyclin, among others. Thereby, LANA contributes by dysregulating cell growth and survival and plays a role in viral persistence, as it tethers the KSHV/HHV8 episomes to the chromosomes during cell division {594} (see *Primary effusion lymphoma*, p. 541, for more detail).

The cells infected by KSHV/HHV8 correspond to naïve, IgM-producing B cells without IG somatic hypermutations, unlike extracavitary primary effusion lymphoma, in which IG genes are hypermutated {1011}. No specific information on molecular pathogenesis is available.

Macroscopic appearance

Involved lymph nodes are enlarged, and the cut surface reveals a homogeneous whitish and fleshy appearance with hilum obliteration. Necrosis may be observed. At extranodal sites, including the spleen, the lymphoma presents as large confluent tumour masses or multiple nodules with discrete contours.

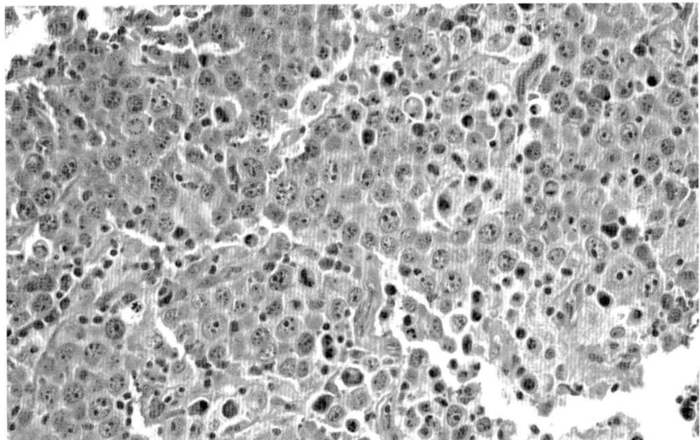

Fig. 4.241 KSHV/HHV8-positive diffuse large B-cell lymphoma. KSHV/HHV8-positive diffuse large B-cell lymphoma involving lymph node. There are sheets of large neoplastic cells, some of which resemble plasmablasts.

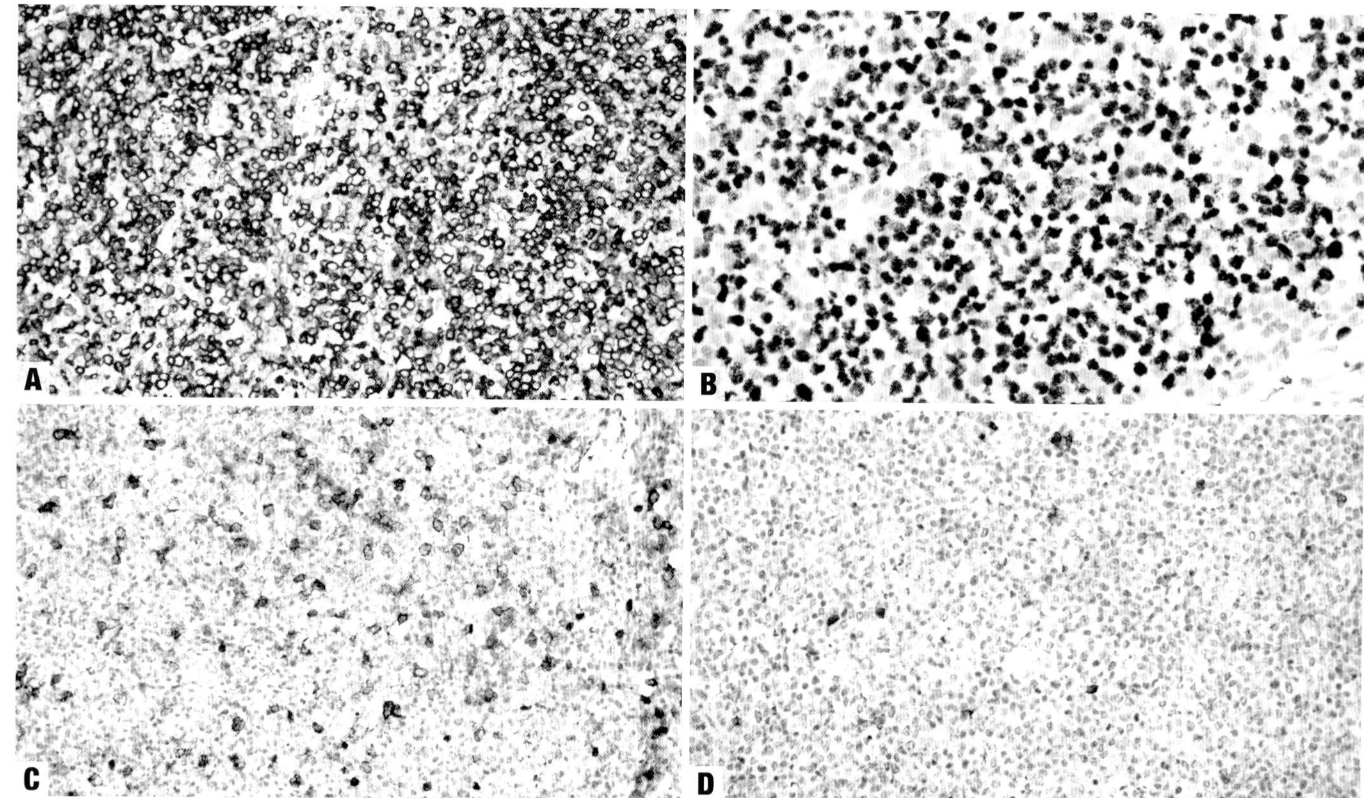

Fig. 4.242 KSHV/HHV8-positive diffuse large B-cell lymphoma. Lymph node involvement. The tumour cells are strongly positive for IgM (**A**) and latency-associated nuclear antigen (LANA) (**B**). **C** A small subset are weakly positive for CD20. **D** The tumour cells are negative for CD138.

Histopathology

KSHV/HHV8-positive DLBCL is characterized by coalescent sheets of intermediate to large lymphoid cells that efface the nodal or splenic architecture. The tumour cells have vesicular, often eccentrically placed nuclei containing one or two prominent nucleoli and amphophilic cytoplasm, often resembling plasmablasts or immunoblasts. Rare cases morphologically resemble intravascular large B-cell lymphoma {1187,824} or Hodgkin lymphoma {1187,3559}.

Immunophenotype

The lymphoma is characterized by a monoclonal proliferation of KSHV/HHV8-infected B cells expressing cytoplasmic IgM and usually lambda light chain. The tumour cells are positive for LANA (KSHV/HHV8), vIL-6, and IRF4 (MUM1), and are often negative for CD79a, CD38, CD27, and CD138 {3042}. The lymphoma cells are usually variably positive for CD45 and CD20. EBV-encoded small RNA (EBER) is usually negative, but some cases are double-positive for KSHV/HHV8 and EBV {1369,4307}.

Differential diagnosis

KSHV/HHV8 positive lymphoid cells can be seen in reactive lymph nodes without features of MCD from asymptomatic HIV-positive or negative individuals {1369}. Expression of IgM and positivity for LANA (KSHV/HHV8) help to distinguish KSHV/HHV8-positive DLBCL from solid primary effusion lymphoma and DLBCL-NOS, respectively.

Cytology

Although a diagnosis of KSHV/HHV8-positive DLBCL can be suggested from cytological specimens, a biopsy is recommended for a definite diagnosis, including evaluation for changes of KSHV/HHV8-positive MCD and KSHV/HHV8-positive germinotropic lymphoproliferative disorder.

Diagnostic molecular pathology

Demonstration of KSHV/HHV8 infection (by immunohistochemistry or other appropriate molecular methods)

Essential and desirable diagnostic criteria

Essential: presentation with primary nodal and/or splenic involvement; effacement of architecture by large blasts / transformed B cells with generally plasmablastic, immunoblastic, or anaplastic morphology; positive immunostaining for LANA (KSHV/HHV8) and IgM.

Desirable: absence of immunoglobulin somatic hypermutations; EBER in situ hybridization (usually negative but can be positive in some cases).

Staging

The Lugano classification is used as adapted from the Ann Arbor staging system with Cotswold modifications {688}.

Prognosis and prediction

KSHV/HHV8-positive DLBCL is an extremely aggressive lymphoma. In cases arising on a background of KSHV/HHV8-positive MCD in HIV-positive people, the prognosis is poor, with a median survival of a few months {3296,3358}.

KSHV/HHV8-positive germinotropic lymphoproliferative disorder

Chadburn A
Du MQ
Said JW
Vega F

Definition

Kaposi sarcoma–associated herpesvirus / human herpesvirus 8 (KSHV/HHV8)-positive germinotropic lymphoproliferative disorder (KSHV/HHV8-positive GLPD) is characterized by KSHV/HHV8-positive and usually EBV-positive large atypical lymphoid cells that predominantly colonize germinal centres. These lesions are usually polyclonal and classically arise in elderly, immunocompetent patients.

ICD-O coding

None

ICD-11 coding

2A81.Y Other specified diffuse large B-cell lymphoma

Related terminology

Acceptable: HHV8-positive germinotropic lymphoproliferative disorder.

Subtype(s)

None

Localization

KSHV/HHV8-positive GLPD occurs in lymph nodes, most frequently in the neck. The disease may be localized or involve multiple sites based on clinical or radiographic examination. The bone marrow is not involved {4543,1333}.

Clinical features

Most patients present with lymphadenopathy, sometimes longstanding, without B symptoms. Only rarely are significant laboratory abnormalities present {4543,1333}.

Epidemiology

KSHV/HHV8-positive GLPD is very rare. The majority of patients are elderly (median age: 60 years, range: 20–86 years), immunocompetent individuals, and there is a slight male predominance {606,4543,1333}. Cases have occurred in HIV-positive individuals, who are generally younger male patients with B symptoms {1369,346}.

Etiology

The etiology is related to KSHV/HHV8 infection.

Pathogenesis

The presence KSHV/HHV8 indicates a pathogenetic role. The proliferating cells are positive for KSHV/HHV8-associated vIL-6, which is a driver of cell growth. The exact role of EBV in the development of the proliferation is unclear {1010,649,660, 3454,3003,4543}. Approximately 85% of cases are polyclonal B-cell proliferations, according to IG gene rearrangement studies, with rare monoclonal cases in HIV-positive patients {1010, 1369,4543}. The abnormal B cells have somatic hypermutations consistent with a germinal-centre origin {1010}. The single case

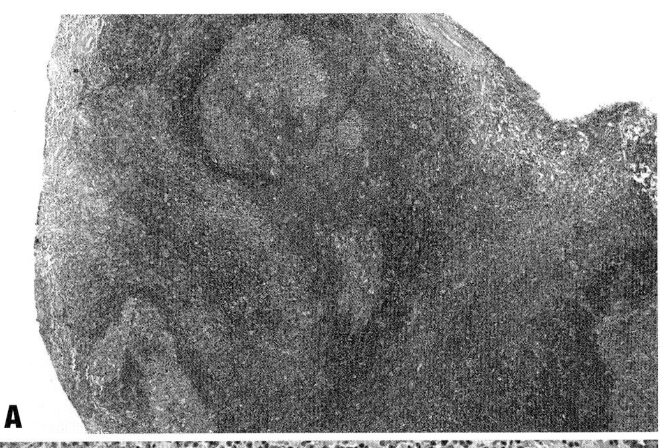

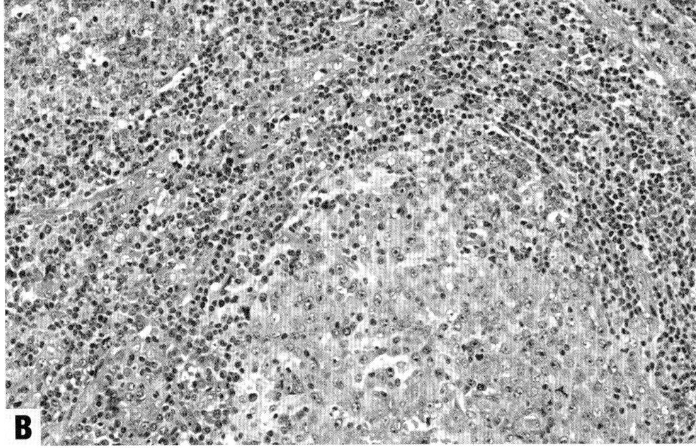

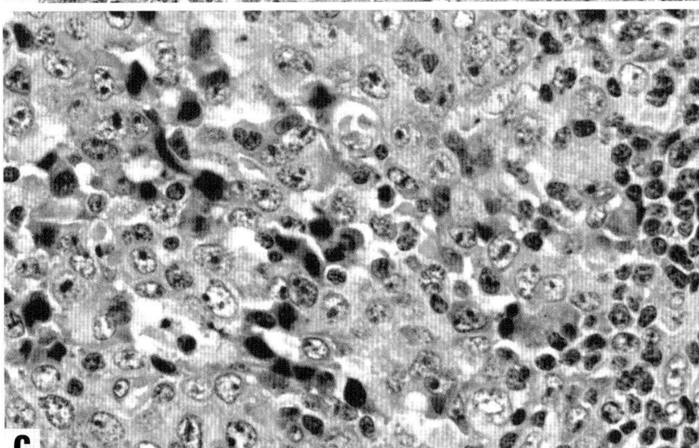

Fig. 4.243 KSHV/HHV8-positive germinotropic lymphoproliferative disorder. **A** There is overall retention of the lymph node architecture; focal involvement of the follicles can be seen. **B** The abnormal cell population variably involves the germinal centres. **C** The germinotropic lymphoproliferative disorder cells are immunoblastic, plasmablastic, and/or anaplastic in appearance. Multinucleated cells may be present. Often mitotic figures and apoptotic debris can be seen.

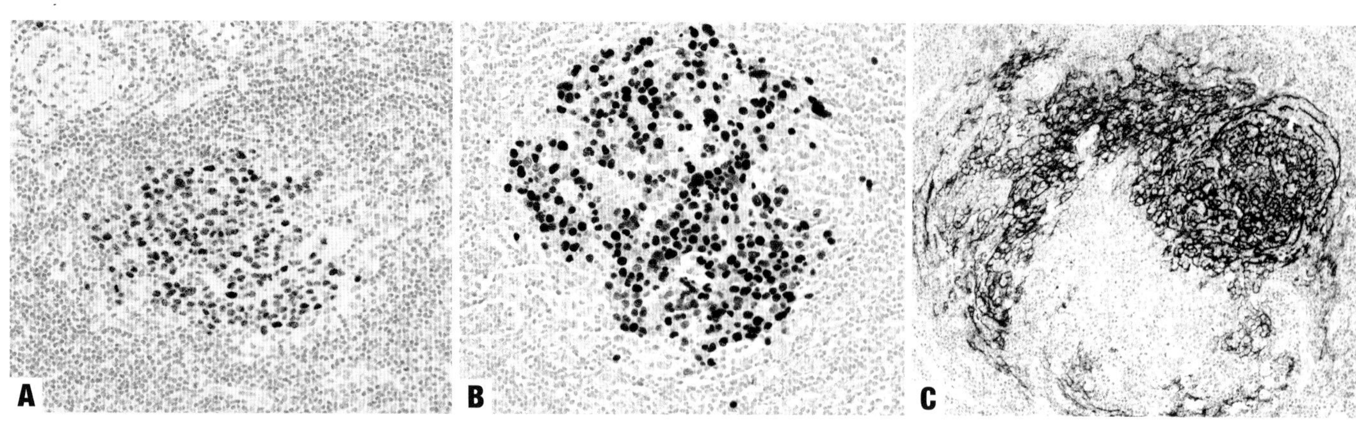

Fig. 4.244 KSHV/HHV8-positive germinotropic lymphoproliferative disorder. **A** The germinotropic lymphoproliferative disorder cells are positive for KSHV/HHV8 by immunostaining for latency-associated nuclear antigen (LANA). **B** They are usually positive for EBV-encoded small RNA (EBER) by in situ hybridization. **C** Immunostaining for CD21 confirms the presence of germinotropic lymphoproliferative disorder cells in the germinal centres.

evaluated by targeted next-generation sequencing did not contain pathogenic mutations {3454}.

Macroscopic appearance

The lymph nodes range from 20 to 75 mm, with matted node groups as large as 260 mm reported {4543}.

Histopathology

Lymph nodes show retention of architecture. A variable number of germinal centres exhibit partial or complete replacement by clusters or sheets of plasmablastic, immunoblastic, and/or anaplastic-appearing cells. These cells have large nuclei with round, oval, or irregular nuclear borders, vesicular chromatin, and one to two prominent nucleoli. Multinucleated cells may be seen. The cells have relatively abundant, usually amphophilic, cytoplasm. The abnormal cells may also be seen in the mantle zones, interfollicular areas, or sinuses. The uninvolved follicles are often atrophic or, less often, hyperplastic. There is usually polytypic plasmacytosis in the interfollicular areas {1010,346, 4543,1333}.

KSHV/HHV8-positive GLPD is positive for KSHV/HHV8 by immunostaining for latency-associated nuclear antigen (LANA) and vIL-6. Most cases are positive for EBV-encoded small RNA (EBER) but lack LMP1 {1010,1369,346,3454,200}. GLPD typically lacks expression of pan–B-cell antigens and is negative for germinal-centre markers. KSHV/HHV8-positive GLPD is positive for IRF4 (MUM1), variably positive for CD38 and EMA, and occasionally positive for CD138, with rare expression of CD3 and CD30 reported. Monotypic immunoglobulin expression is seen in approximately two thirds of cases {1010,1369, 346,606,4543,1333}. The KSHV/HHV8-positive GLPD cells are usually enmeshed in CD21+ follicular dendritic cell meshworks {1010,867,1333,824,200,3454}. GLPD is negative for ACVRL1 (ALK1), CD15, CD56, cyclin D1, and BCL2. Expression of CD45 is rare. The Ki-67 proliferation index is high {1010,3454,4543, 1333}.

The differential diagnosis of KSHV/HHV8-positive GLPD includes the other KSHV/HHV8-positive lesions (see Table 4.41, p. 539, in *KSHV/HHV8-associated B-cell lymphoid proliferations and lymphomas: Introduction*). GLPDs can be separated from EBV+ B-cell lymphomas that may show areas of colonization of germinal centres by immunostaining for LANA (KSHV/ HHV8) {2420}.

Cytology

The diagnosis of KSHV/HHV8-positive GLPD cannot be made on cytology alone. An adequate excisional or incisional tissue biopsy is required for a definite diagnosis, including differentiation from other KSHV/HHV8-positive lymphoid proliferations.

Diagnostic molecular pathology

Molecular studies are not essential for the diagnosis, but the polyclonal nature of KSHV/HHV8-positive GLPD can be helpful in separating this disease from extracavitary primary effusion lymphoma.

Essential and desirable diagnostic criteria

Essential: retained lymph node architecture, with some germinal centres partially or completely replaced by clusters or sheets of plasmablastic, immunoblastic, and/or anaplastic cells; positive immunostaining for LANA (KSHV/HHV8).

Desirable: positive in situ hybridization for EBV (EBER) and polyclonal B-cell gene rearrangement.

Staging

Formal staging as for malignant lymphoma is not routinely required.

Prognosis and prediction

Most patients have no evidence of disease or have stable disease with either no treatment or radiation therapy or chemotherapy with or without rituximab, with survival times as long as 15 years reported {4543,1333}. Rare patients may develop aggressive KSHV/HHV8-positive or EBV-positive diffuse large B-cell lymphoma {824,346}.

Lymphoid proliferations and lymphomas associated with immune deficiency and dysregulation: Introduction

de Jong D
Chan JKC
Coupland SE
Naresh KN
Siebert R

Chapter 4

Immune deficiency and dysregulation–associated lymphoproliferative disorders (IDD-LPDs) form a heterogeneous group, both clinicopathologically and etiologically. IDD-LPDs have traditionally been classified according to the immunodeficiency background in which they arise, with separate sections in previous editions of the WHO classification of haematolymphoid tumours covering four major backgrounds: primary immunodeficiencies, HIV infection, posttransplantation status, and other iatrogenic immunodeficiencies. Although this approach has served its purpose well for many years, the inconsistent terminology and diagnostic criteria for similar lesions in different immunodeficiency settings, and the imprecise definitions within some of these, as well as the inability to absorb new knowledge outside the preset immunodeficiency settings, indicate that the limits of this approach have been reached.

Initiated at the 2015 workshop of the Society for Hematopathology / European Association for Haematopathology and since explored by various researchers in the haematopathology and haematology community, evidence has accrued to justify a novel approach to the classification of immunodeficiency-associated lymphoproliferative disorders {2919}. This new overarching framework accommodates both commonalities in histology and variations in frequency, distinct causal associations of specific lesions, involvement of various oncogenic viruses, and specific clinical and/or therapeutic consequences. To that end, a unifying, standardized nomenclature has been designed, based on a three-part approach to accommodate (1) the name of the histological lesion, (2) the presence or absence of one or more oncogenic viruses, and (3) the clinical setting / immunodeficiency background. This integrated nomenclature will allow the comparison of clinicopathological studies across different types of IDD-LPDs, to better define the underlying shared and/or unique pathogenetic mechanisms. Because the mechanism of lymphoproliferation includes not just immune deficiency but also immune dysregulation and even inappropriate hyperactivation, the term "immune deficiency and dysregulation–associated lymphoproliferative disorders" was introduced. And because primary immunodeficiencies have been renamed "inborn errors of immunity" by the International Union of Immunological Societies (IUIS), this nomenclature has been adopted to replace the term "primary immunodeficiency".

The observation of a higher frequency of EBV-positive diffuse large B-cell lymphoma in elderly patients without any known cause of immunodeficiency led to the concept of immunosenescence as a source of immune deficiency/dysregulation (IDD), which predisposes to the development of IDD-LPDs; it is now considered a valid IDD context, albeit the immunodeficiency as such cannot be substantiated in an objective manner. As a consequence, EBV-positive diffuse large B-cell lymphoma is also discussed as a separate entity in this edition, although similar proliferations in the present chapter share essential pathological criteria and the distinction is not absolute. Another acquired IDD setting that has recently gained attention occurs in patients treated with multichemotherapy regimens for previous solid cancers or haematological malignancies, who experience significant immune dysregulation leading to IDD-LPDs. The spectrum of iatrogenic causes that result in IDD-LPDs is still expanding. Atypical lymphoproliferative disorders following treatment with newly developed compounds for various indications are increasingly described: in the context of novel immunotherapy (e.g. anti-CD20, anti-CD38, chimeric antigen receptor [CAR] T-cell therapy, BTK inhibitors), after immunomodulatory treatments (e.g. as induction strategies for immune tolerance in solid-organ transplantation), after next-generation immunosuppression in autoimmune and inflammatory diseases (e.g. asthma), and in the context of more effective antiretroviral treatment strategies in patients with HIV. The recognition that acquired somatic mutations and anti-cytokine antibodies may lead to phenotypes identical to those seen in specific inborn errors of immunity is emerging and requires further study. For further details, see Table 4.42 (p. 550), Table 4.43 (p. 552), and Table 4.44 (p. 554).

The unifying framework and nomenclature in this edition will allow the integration of emerging knowledge and enable standardized and meaningful comparisons for clinical diagnosis and studies worldwide. Improved definitions of IDD-LPDs bring increasing awareness. In suspected cases, a multidisciplinary approach, including a careful assessment of the patient's clinical history and immune status, is considered mandatory for optimal patient care.

Table 4.42 Lymphoproliferative disorders and lymphomas arising in immune deficiency/dysregulation (IDD) settings, and their relative frequency[a] (continued on next page)

Type of lesion	Subtype	Type of immunodeficiency setting					Viral status[c]	Main section(s) within this volume
		Acquired errors of immunity				Inborn errors of immunity		
		Posttransplant	HIV infection	Autoimmune/ therapy-related[b]	Immunosenescence			
Hyperplasias								
	Follicular hyperplasia	+++	+	+++	+	+	EBV+/−	*Hyperplasias arising in immune deficiency/dysregulation* (p. 555)
	Infectious mononucleosis–like hyperplasia	++	+	+	−	+	EBV+/−	*Hyperplasias arising in immune deficiency/dysregulation* (p. 555)
	Plasmacytic hyperplasia	+	+	+	+	+	EBV+/−	*Hyperplasias arising in immune deficiency/dysregulation* (p. 555)
	KSHV/HHV8-positive multicentric Castleman disease	−	+++	−	−	−	KSHV/HHV8+	*KSHV/HHV8-associated multicentric Castleman disease* (p. 325)
	Other types of hyperplasias and involutions[d]	+	+	+	+	++	EBV−/+	*Hyperplasias arising in immune deficiency/dysregulation* (p. 555)
Lymphoproliferative disorders of varied malignant potential[e]								
	Polymorphic lymphoproliferative disorder	+++	+	+++	++	+	EBV+	*Polymorphic lymphoproliferative disorders arising in immune deficiency/dysregulation* (p. 561)
	EBV+ mucocutaneous ulcer	++	+	+++	+++	+	EBV+	*EBV-positive mucocutaneous ulcer* (p. 565)
	KSHV/HHV8-positive germinotropic lymphoproliferative disorder	−	−	−	+	−	KSHV/HHV8+ EBV+	*KSHV/HHV8-positive germinotropic lymphoproliferative disorder* (p. 547)
Lymphomas								
	Small (low-grade) B-cell lymphomas	+	+	+	+	+	EBV+/−	*Extranodal marginal zone lymphoma of mucosa-associated lymphoid tissue* (p. 401)
	Diffuse large B-cell lymphoma	+++	+++	+	+	+++	EBV−/+	*Diffuse large B-cell lymphoma NOS* (p. 463) *Diffuse large B-cell lymphoma / high-grade B-cell lymphoma with MYC and BCL2 rearrangements* (p. 476) *EBV-positive diffuse large B-cell lymphoma* (p. 493)
	Burkitt lymphoma	+	++	−	+	+	EBV−/+	*Burkitt lymphoma* (p. 532)
	Classic Hodgkin lymphoma	+	++	+	+	++	EBV+/−	*Classic Hodgkin lymphoma* (p. 580)
	KSHV/HHV8-positive diffuse large B-cell lymphoma NOS	+	+	−	+	−	KSHV/HHV8+	*KSHV/HHV8-positive diffuse large B-cell lymphoma* (p. 545)

[a]Relative frequencies are estimated and cannot be directly compared across all IDD settings. With evolution of more effective treatments, frequencies of specific lesions have changed over time. With standardized nomenclature and diagnostic criteria, it is anticipated that more homogeneous comparisons will be made in the future. [b]"Therapy-related" refers to the prior use of immunosuppressive or immunomodulatory medications and includes multiagent chemotherapy used in the treatment of solid and haematopoietic malignancies. [c]Viral status: EBV-negative hyperplasias and lymphoproliferative disorders occur in various IDD settings; however, a relationship with IDD cannot be substantiated in some settings because no marker other than EBV currently exists to confirm a relationship to IDD. Clinical correlation is essential to exclude other etiologies of lymphoid hyperplasias and to provide pathogen- or cause-specific treatment. [d]Includes several categories of EBV-negative and EBV-positive lesions in patients with IDD, such as EBV-negative follicular involutions and immune reconstitution inflammatory syndrome (IRIS) in HIV infection, EBV-negative T-cell and NK-cell proliferations and histiocytic proliferations that may be triggered by other infectious or inflammatory etiologies, and EBV reactivation in posttransplant and other settings. [e]T-cell and NK-cell proliferations of varied malignant potential include chronic active EBV infection (see *Systemic chronic active EBV disease*, p. 777).

Table 4.42 Lymphoproliferative disorders and lymphomas arising in immune deficiency/dysregulation (IDD) settings, and their relative frequency[a] (continued)

Type of lesion	Subtype	Type of immunodeficiency setting					Viral status[c]	Main section(s) within this volume
		Acquired errors of immunity				Inborn errors of immunity		
		Posttransplant	HIV infection	Autoimmune/ therapy-related[b]	Immunose-nescence			
	Primary effusion lymphoma	+	++	–	+	–	KSHV/HHV8+ EBV+	*Primary effusion lymphoma* (p. 541)
	Plasmablastic lymphoma	+	+	+	+	+	EBV+/–	*Plasmablastic lymphoma* (p. 506)
	Plasma cell neoplasms	+	+	+	+	–	EBV–/+	*Plasma cell neoplasms: Introduction* (p. 621) *Plasmacytoma* (p. 622) *Plasma cell myeloma / multiple myeloma* (p. 625) *Plasma cell neoplasms with associated paraneoplastic syndrome* (p. 631)
	T-cell and NK-cell lymphomas	+	+	+	+	+	EBV–/+	*NK-large granular lymphocytic leukaemia* (p. 665) *Aggressive NK-cell leukaemia* (p. 677) *Intestinal T-cell and NK-cell lymphoid proliferations and lymphomas: Introduction* (p. 710) *Indolent T-cell lymphoma of the gastrointestinal tract* (p. 712) *Indolent NK-cell lymphoproliferative disorder of the gastrointestinal tract* (p. 715) *Enteropathy-associated T-cell lymphoma* (p. 717) *Monomorphic epitheliotropic intestinal T-cell lymphoma* (p. 722) *Intestinal T-cell lymphoma NOS* (p. 725) *Extranodal NK/T-cell lymphoma* (p. 765)

[a]Relative frequencies are estimated and cannot be directly compared across all IDD settings. With evolution of more effective treatments, frequencies of specific lesions have changed over time. With standardized nomenclature and diagnostic criteria, it is anticipated that more homogeneous comparisons will be made in the future. [b]"Therapy-related" refers to the prior use of immunosuppressive or immunomodulatory medications and includes multiagent chemotherapy used in the treatment of solid and haematopoietic malignancies. [c]Viral status: EBV-negative hyperplasias and lymphoproliferative disorders occur in various IDD settings; however, a relationship with IDD cannot be substantiated in some settings because no marker other than EBV currently exists to confirm a relationship to IDD. Clinical correlation is essential to exclude other etiologies of lymphoid hyperplasias and to provide pathogen- or cause-specific treatment. [d]Includes several categories of EBV-negative and EBV-positive lesions in patients with IDD, such as EBV-negative follicular involutions and immune reconstitution inflammatory syndrome (IRIS) in HIV infection, EBV-negative T-cell and NK-cell proliferations and histiocytic proliferations that may be triggered by other infectious or inflammatory etiologies, and EBV reactivation in posttransplant and other settings. [e]T-cell and NK-cell proliferations of varied malignant potential include chronic active EBV infection (see *Systemic chronic active EBV disease*, p. 777).

Table 4.43 Epidemiological and clinical manifestations of lymphoproliferative disorders (LPDs) and lymphomas arising in immune deficiency and immune dysregulation settings (continued on next page)

Feature	Posttransplant-related LPD		HIV-related LPD	Autoimmune/therapy-related LPD			Immunosenescence-related LPD	IEI-related LPD
	After allogeneic HSCT	After SOT		Systemic disorder (autoimmune)-related LPD	Immunosuppression/ immunomodulator-related LPD	Polychemotherapy-related LPD		
Epidemiology	Incidence ranges from 0.5% to 17% depending on type of donor and conditioning	SIR: 3.5 (CHL) to 10 (NHL) Incidence ranges from 1.5% to 20% depending on transplanted organ	Before cART era: • SIR: 60–200 (DLBCL and BL) • After cART era: • > 50% decrease DLBCL • Smaller effect on BL • No effect on CHL (relative increase in incidence)	Association between some autoimmune/ systemic disorders and lymphoma, although prevalence of different disorders in the total lymphoma population remains low (0.3–5%) Some are phenocopies of IEIs due to acquired somatic mutations (e.g. ALPS-sFAS)	No specific data available	No specific data available	Median age for most B-cell lymphomas is > 70 years	Overall incidence unknown; lifetime incidence ranges from 4% to 70% depending on underlying immunodeficiency
Most important risk factors	Donor type (HLA mismatch) Higher recipient age Conditioning regimen (T-cell depletion)	Transplant type (highest in multiorgan, lowest in kidney transplantation) EBV mismatch (R–/D+) at time of transplantation Induction regimen (early cases) / maintenance therapy (late cases)	HIV is associated with a high risk of BL, CHL, and KSHV/HHV8+ MCD; these frequently occur in patients with relatively high CD4 T-cell counts who may be on cART Large B-cell lymphomas including those associated with KSHV/HHV8 and PEL are associated with more severe immunosuppression, low CD4 T-cell counts, high HIV viral load and among those not on cART	Underlying disease (highest risk in RA, Sjögren syndrome, SLE, coeliac disease, dermatitis herpetiformis, Hashimoto thyroiditis, AIHA) Severity / inflammatory activity of the disease	Duration of therapy (most evidence with methotrexate)	T-cell–depleting agents Profound immunosuppressive chemotherapy (including autologous HSCT)	Ageing Several hypotheses: • Age-related clonal haematopoiesis • Age-related epigenetic changes • Increased sensitivity to infections, including EBV	IEI with associated chromosomal instability IEI with associated susceptibility to EBV infection and B-LPD
Timing	> 95% early (6–12 months posttransplant)	30–40% early (< 1 year posttransplant) 60–70% late (> 1 year posttransplant)	High-grade B-cell lymphomas are AIDS-defining illnesses The incidence of CHL rises after initiation of cART, in particular if ongoing moderate immunosuppression	Lifelong additional risk if treated with immunosuppressive and/ or immunomodulation treatment	Shorter mean duration between start and LPD for immunosuppressive agents (71–92 months) Longer mean duration between start and LPD for immunomodulation agents (28 months)	Can be both early and late after initiation of therapy	Typically > 45–50 years of age (median: 70–75 years), but data are scarce given the lack of immunosenescence markers	Most occur in early childhood, but among patients with CVID these can occur in adulthood

AIHA, autoimmune haemolytic anaemia; ALPS-sFAS, autoimmune lymphoproliferative syndrome with somatic *FAS* mutation; BL, Burkitt lymphoma; cART, combination antiretroviral therapy; CHL, classic Hodgkin lymphoma; CVID, common variable immunodeficiency; DLBCL, diffuse large B-cell lymphoma; GLPD, germinotropic lymphoproliferative disorder; HLH, haemophagocytic lymphohistiocytosis; HSCT, haematopoietic stem cell transplantation; IEI, inborn error of immunity; MCD, multicentric Castleman disease; NHL, non-Hodgkin lymphoma; PEL, primary effusion lymphoma; PCNS-LBCL, primary large B-cell lymphoma of the CNS; RA, rheumatoid arthritis; SIR, standardized incidence ratio; SLE, systemic lupus erythematosus; SOT, solid-organ transplant.

Table 4.43 Epidemiological and clinical manifestations of lymphoproliferative disorders (LPDs) and lymphomas arising in immune deficiency and immune dysregulation settings (continued)

Feature	Posttransplant-related LPD		HIV-related LPD	Autoimmune/therapy-related LPD			Immunosenescence-related LPD	IEI-related LPD
	After allogeneic HSCT	After SOT		Systemic disorder (autoimmune)-related LPD	Immunosuppression/ immunomodulator-related LPD	Polychemotherapy-related LPD		
EBV association	> 95% EBV-associated	60% EBV-associated	60–100% EBV-associated KSHV/HHV8-associated LPDs include PEL, GLPD, MCD, and some DLBCLs Dual infection with EBV and KSHV/HHV8 associated with PEL and GLPD	Not known (EBV association higher if immunosuppressive medication)	As many as 30% EBV-associated	As many as 80–90% EBV-associated	Varies depending on geographical location (e.g. 3–14% EBV+ DLBCL)	Varies depending on underlying IEI; B-cell lymphomas often EBV+, T-cell lymphomas and LPDs usually EBV−
Clinical features	Two types of presentation: • Nodal, with lymphadenopathies, hepatomegaly, and/or splenomegaly; often also lung and gastrointestinal involvement • Fulminant course with bone marrow involvement, multiorgan failure, and HLH	60–90% extranodal involvement (gastrointestinal tract, lung, bone marrow, allograft, CNS)	50–60% NHL > 1 extranodal site 30–40% CHL > 1 extranodal site 1–2% NHL are PCNS-LBCL, usually associated with profound immunosuppression and untreated advanced HIV infection	Probably not different from lymphomas in immunocompetent patients	Extranodal presentation more frequent than lymphoma in immunocompetent patients, but dependent on LPD subtype	60% extranodal involvement	As many as 80% may show extranodal involvement	Nodal and extranodal presentations; in immune dysregulation subset, EBV may be associated with fulminant course including HLH
First-line treatment	Rituximab	Reduction of immunosuppression (may be sufficient for hyperplasias) Rituximab (PTLD-1 trial) Lymphoma-specific therapy for rare subtypes	Start cART for all Lymphoma-specific therapy Opportunistic infection prophylaxis and careful attention to pharmacokinetic interactions are necessary	Lymphoma-specific therapy Rituximab (treatment lymphoma + underlying disorder)	Withdrawal of immunosuppression Rituximab Lymphoma-specific therapy for rare subtypes	Lymphoma-specific therapy	Treatment options often limited because of comorbidities and poor performance state Lymphoma-specific therapy if indicated and possible	Lymphoma-specific chemotherapy Radiotherapy should be avoided in IEI with DNA repair errors Rituximab (if EBV-associated) Allogeneic HSCT may be curative for both lymphoma and underlying IEI (in particular if also HLH)
References	{3858,2211,71,3370, 662,661,1084}	{916,954,2029,4058, 369,517}	{2986,569,2631,1380,253, 63,551}	{206,1941,1973,3398, 3720,2417,3753}	{2532,2723,2658, 2160,4033,1347, 3590,4034}	{3248,2056,2804, 1294}	{3517,3733,4525, 1778,3417}	{3969,1464,4465, 1558,3400}

AIHA, autoimmune haemolytic anaemia; ALPS-sFAS, autoimmune lymphoproliferative syndrome with somatic *FAS* mutation; BL, Burkitt lymphoma; cART, combination antiretroviral therapy; CHL, classic Hodgkin lymphoma; CVID, common variable immunodeficiency; DLBCL, diffuse large B-cell lymphoma; GLPD, germinotropic lymphoproliferative disorder; HLH, haemophagocytic lymphohistiocytosis; HSCT, haematopoietic stem cell transplantation; IEI, inborn error of immunity; MCD, multicentric Castleman disease; NHL, non-Hodgkin lymphoma; PEL, primary effusion lymphoma; PCNS-LBCL, primary large B-cell lymphoma of the CNS; RA, rheumatoid arthritis; SIR, standardized incidence ratio; SLE, systemic lupus erythematosus; SOT, solid-organ transplant.

Table 4.44 Comparison of prior and current nomenclature of lymphoproliferative disorders and lymphomas arising in immune deficiency and dysregulation settings

Type of lesion	Immunodeficiency setting	Nomenclature in previous editions of the WHO classification	Three-part nomenclature (name of lesion, virus status, type of immunodeficiency)[a]
Hyperplasias	Posttransplantation	Non-destructive posttransplant lymphoproliferative disorder, name of hyperplasia[b]	Name of hyperplasia, EBV+/–, type of immunodeficiency
	Settings other than posttransplantation	No specific name	
Lymphoproliferative disorders of varied malignant potential	Posttransplantation	Polymorphic posttransplant lymphoproliferative disorder[b]	Polymorphic lymphoproliferative disorder, EBV+, type of immunodeficiency
	Settings other than posttransplantation	Polymorphic/lymphoplasmacytic infiltrate resembling polymorphic posttransplant lymphoproliferative disorder	
	All settings	EBV+ mucocutaneous ulcer	EBV+ mucocutaneous ulcer, type of immunodeficiency
Lymphomas	Posttransplantation	Monomorphic posttransplant lymphoproliferative disorder, name of lymphoma according to immunocompetent patient[b]	Name of lymphoma according to immunocompetent patient, EBV+/– and/or KSHV/HHV8+/–, type of immunodeficiency
	Settings other than posttransplantation	Name of lymphoma according to immunocompetent patient	
	Posttransplantation	Classic Hodgkin lymphoma posttransplant lymphoproliferative disorder[b]	
	Settings other than posttransplantation	Classic Hodgkin lymphoma	

[a]If immunodeficiency or immune dysregulation is suspected but not specifically diagnosed, the term "suspected" can be used (e.g. suspected immunosenescence setting). [b]Nomenclature specific to the posttransplant setting is not recommended. The three-part nomenclature common to all settings of immunodeficiency and dysregulation is recommended for diagnosis.
References: {2919,2920,606,1396,1397,2918,891}.

Hyperplasias arising in immune deficiency/dysregulation

Natkunam Y
Bhagat G
Bower M
Chadburn A
Chan JKC
Dierickx D
Gratzinger D
Michelow P
Naresh KN
Sato Y
Satou A

Definition

Hyperplasias arising in settings of immune deficiency/dysregulation (IDD) are heterogeneous, non-clonal lymphoid and/or plasmacytic proliferations with preservation of the underlying tissue architecture. They are usually, but not exclusively, driven by EBV or KSHV/HHV8.

ICD-O coding

None

ICD-11 coding

2B32.3 & XH2R75 Polymorphic posttransplant lymphoproliferative disorder & Posttransplant lymphoproliferative disorder, NOS

Related terminology

Not recommended: non-destructive posttransplant lymphoproliferative disorder.

Note: in the posttransplant setting only, it is acceptable to include "posttransplant lymphoproliferative disorder (PTLD)" as an addendum.

Subtype(s)

Follicular hyperplasia (FH); infectious mononucleosis–like hyperplasia (IMH); plasmacytic hyperplasia (PCH); KSHV/HHV8-positive multicentric Castleman disease (see *KSHV/HHV8-associated multicentric Castleman disease*, p. 325).

For a complete list of IDD-associated hyperplasias, involutions, and related lesions, see Table 4.45 (p. 556).

Localization

The localization of hyperplasias varies with the underlying IDD. Hyperplasia in the posttransplant setting usually involve the tonsils and adenoids, and less commonly involve lymph nodes and mucosal sites {2061,4136}. Most patients with HIV infection {600} and autoimmune diseases {2089,2090} present with generalized lymphadenopathy. Autoimmune/therapy-related hyperplasias may manifest as localized or multisite lymphadenopathy {3490,3094,2160}. Inborn error of immunity (IEI)-related hyperplasias involve nodal, splenic, and extranodal sites.

Clinical features

Adenoid-tonsillar hypertrophy manifests with breathing and/or feeding difficulties, rhinorrhoea, sinusitis, otalgia, and recurrent middle ear infections. Lymphadenopathy and splenomegaly are often accompanied by pain, tenderness, and constitutional symptoms, although symptoms can be variable or nonspecific. Hyperplasias may occur early or late after organ transplantation (median: 17–50 months) {602,2929}, and usually 8–10 years after HIV infection {2089,2090}. Autoimmune/therapy-related hyperplasias develop approximately 2.5 years after commencing therapy {3490,2160}. Lymphadenopathy and splenomegaly are presenting features of some IEIs.

Epidemiology

The incidence of hyperplasias in IDD settings is unknown. Adenoid-tonsillar hypertrophy, primarily due to follicular hyperplasia (FH), is most common in children and young adults after solid-organ transplantation, with young age and EBV seronegativity conferring an increased risk {3699}. Infectious mononucleosis–like hyperplasia (IMH) and plasmacytic hyperplasia (PCH) account for 10–20% of lesions in the posttransplant setting {2734,2494}. The age range of patients with HIV and autoimmune/therapy-related hyperplasias is broad {600,3490,2160}. The incidence of hyperplasias in the context of autoimmune diseases ranges from 26% to 82%, and they are more common in rheumatoid arthritis and childhood-onset systemic lupus erythematosus, and in patients with higher disease activity {3698,521,

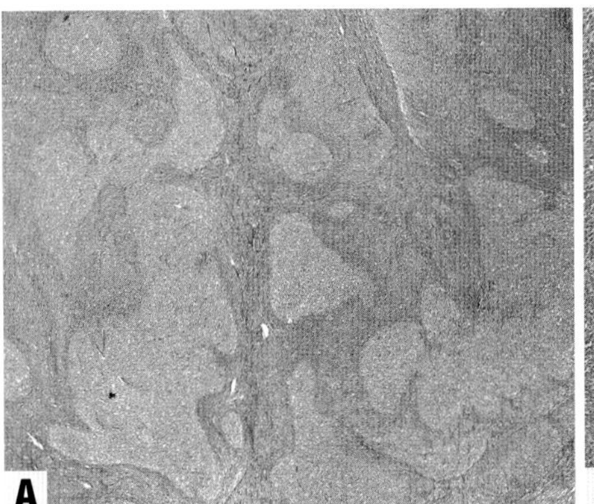
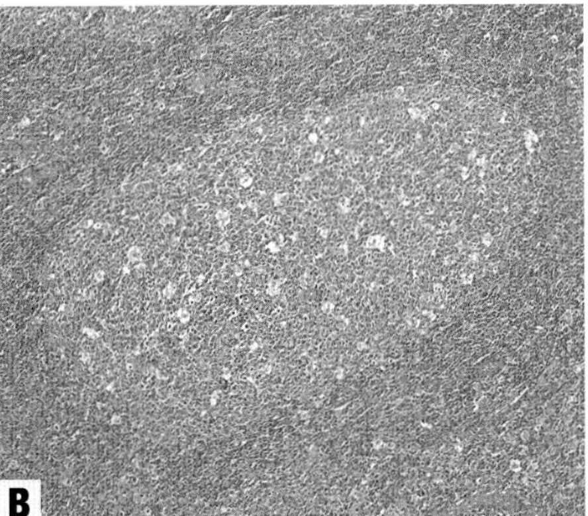
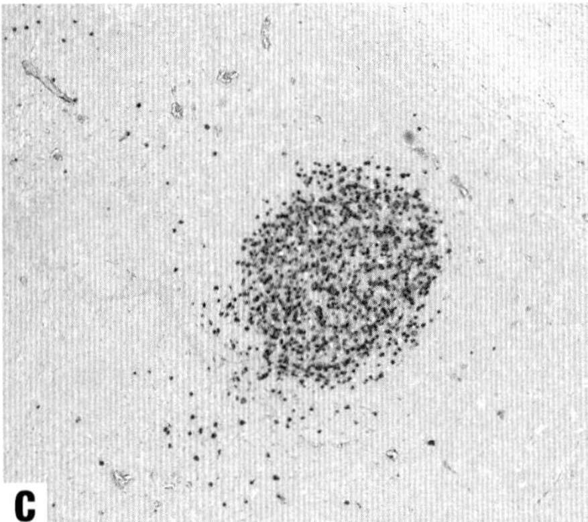

Fig. 4.245 Hyperplasias arising in immune deficiency/dysregulation. **A** Florid follicular hyperplasia in a patient after haematopoietic stem cell transplant. **B** A single follicle in florid follicular hyperplasia shows reactive changes with numerous tingible-body macrophages. **C** Focal follicles show positivity for EBV by in situ hybridization for EBV-encoded small RNA (EBER).

2392}. Hyperplasias account for 14% of methotrexate-related lymphoproliferative disorders {2160}. Autoimmune-related hyperplasias more commonly occur in young adults (median age: 35–38 years) {2089,2090}. Immunosenescence-related hyperplasia occurs in older patients (median age: 67 years) {984}; however, there are no objective criteria defining this presumed category.

Table 4.45 Hyperplasias and involutions arising in immune deficiency/dysregulation (IDD) settings (continued on next page)

Diagnosis	Characteristic features
Follicular proliferations	
Follicular hyperplasia	Follicular hyperplasia is commonly seen in lymph nodes and tonsils Outside the HIV setting, EBV+ cells are typically scattered or in large numbers in the interfollicular areas and occasional GCs EBV− cases occur, which, outside the IEI or HIV settings, are impossible to separate from sporadic follicular hyperplasias {2918} Follicular hyperplasia in the HIV setting occurs primarily in lymph nodes and glandular tissue (benign lymphoepithelial lesion) Early in HIV infection, there is prominent follicular hyperplasia characterized by follicles of variable shapes, some showing progressive transformation of GCs, with numerous mitotic figures and tingible-body macrophages, attenuated mantle zones, and monocytoid B-cell hyperplasia {600}
Follicle lysis/involution	Lymph nodes in untreated patients living with HIV can show follicle lysis in the background of follicular hyperplasia; these follicles may show haemorrhage and attenuated mantle zones The follicular dendritic cell meshworks crumble (highlighted by CD21), resulting in fragmentation of the follicles The GCs typically have serrated borders The follicles often show a paucity of GC cells, with FDCs having more abundant cytoplasm; follicles show encroachment by T cells and other B cells {600} In later stages, there can be complete collapse of the follicular structures (follicular involution) with replacement by PAS-positive amorphous material, hypervascularity, or lymphocyte depletion Follicular involution is characterized by small, involuted, hypocellular GCs and relatively expanded interfollicular areas with increased plasma cells and decreased lymphocytes In the cART era, follicular involution has become less frequent and is typically not biopsied
Lymphoid / lymph node depletion	Lymph nodes in untreated patients living with HIV can eventually lead to lymphoid depletion The lymph nodes show relative or pseudoparacortical expansion (in comparison with follicles or cortical areas) and increased vascularity, with appearances similar to vascular transformation of sinuses The paracortical areas show prominent histiocytes Most of the lymphoid cells present in the paracortical areas are CD8+ small lymphoid cells
Progressive transformation of germinal centres	This is characterized by expanded follicles whose GCs are infiltrated by mantle zone B cells (see *Reactive B-cell–rich lymphoid proliferations that can mimic lymphoma*, p. 309)
Castleman disease–like changes	Lymphoid follicles may show an increased density of follicular dendritic cells, mantle zone onion-skinning, decreased density of GC B cells, twinning of follicles, and penetrating vessels (see *Unicentric Castleman disease*, p. 319)
Interfollicular and paracortical proliferations	
Infectious mononucleosis–like hyperplasia	This commonly involves lymph nodes and tonsils in adolescents and young adults, characterized by paracortical expansion by immunoblasts, some with HRS-like morphology, in a mixed inflammatory background, and typically a lack of architectural destruction The differential diagnoses include polymorphic LPD, EBV+ DLBCL, EBV+ CHL, and EBV+ mucocutaneous ulcer
Plasmacytic hyperplasia	Plasmacytic hyperplasia is characterized by an interfollicular infiltrate of polytypic plasma cells Differential diagnoses include EBV+ marginal zone lymphoma, plasma cell neoplasm, and plasmablastic lymphoma A lack of kappa/lambda light chain restriction aids in distinguishing plasmacytic hyperplasia from these entities {2918}
Other paracortical hyperplasias	Paracortical hyperplasias, including T-zone hyperplasias, may be seen with or without accompanying follicular hyperplasia and typically consist of T cells admixed with antigen-presenting cells, variably prominent vasculature, and variably increased immunoblasts and/or plasma cells {2090,2087} These hyperplasias may mimic T-cell lymphomas; however, the T cells in the hyperplasia do not show cytological atypia or aberrant expression of T-cell antigens, except for ALPS (see *Autoimmune lymphoproliferative syndrome*, p. 646)
EBV reactivation	IDD facilitates virus reactivation, leading to unchecked proliferation of EBV-infected B lymphocytes and eventual development of EBV+ LPDs Histologically, EBV reactivation can resemble follicular hyperplasia, paracortical hyperplasia, infectious mononucleosis–like hyperplasia, or plasmacytic hyperplasia

ALPS, autoimmune lymphoproliferative syndrome; cART, combined antiretroviral therapy; CHL, classic Hodgkin lymphoma; DLBCL, diffuse large B-cell lymphoma; DNT cells, CD4/CD8 double-negative T cells; FDC, follicular dendritic cell; GC, germinal centre; IEI, inborn error of immunity; LGL, T-large granular lymphocytic leukaemia; LPD, lymphoproliferative disorder.

Table 4.45 Hyperplasias and involutions arising in immune deficiency/dysregulation (IDD) settings (continued)

Diagnosis	Characteristic features
Immune reconstitution inflammatory syndrome (IRIS)	IRIS is an inflammatory condition arising in HIV-infected patients where there is a paradoxical worsening of pre-existing opportunistic infections after initiation of cART, usually in patients with low pretreatment CD4 counts Regained capacity to mount an inflammatory response after cART results in inflammatory response Morphological features in the lymph node depend on the associated infective etiology, including viral, bacterial, fungal, or parasitic Although the morphological features of these infectious pathologies are like those without IRIS, the level of host response may far exceed what is expected for the histological changes or the number of organisms There may be prominent necrotizing inflammation (often granulomatous) with few or no organisms {2928}
T-cell and histiocytic proliferations	
Haemophagocytic lymphohistiocytosis	Bone marrow and spleen may be involved in haemophagocytic lymphohistiocytosis with many phagocytic histiocytes in patients living with HIV and in posttransplant settings; these are often driven by accompanying EBV or KSHV/HHV8 infections and can occur in the background of an accompanying lymphoproliferative disorder or lymphoma {3820,4204,3660}
Extranodal T-cell proliferation/ expansions (e.g. CD8, LGL, DNT cells)	See *Autoimmune lymphoproliferative syndrome* (p. 646) and *Inborn error of immunity-associated lymphoid proliferations and lymphomas* (p. 573)
Chronic active EBV disease	See *Systemic chronic active EBV disease* (p. 777)

ALPS, autoimmune lymphoproliferative syndrome; cART, combined antiretroviral therapy; CHL, classic Hodgkin lymphoma; DLBCL, diffuse large B-cell lymphoma; DNT cells, CD4/CD8 double-negative T cells; FDC, follicular dendritic cell; GC, germinal centre; IEI, inborn error of immunity; LGL, T-large granular lymphocytic leukaemia; LPD, lymphoproliferative disorder.

Etiology

EBV is almost always positive in hyperplasias in the posttransplant setting. In autoimmune/therapy-related or HIV-related hyperplasias, scattered EBV-positive cells may be seen and may indicate the underlying IDD, although their contribution to the development of hyperplasias is unknown. Roles for other viruses have been suggested in EBV-negative hyperplasias, but not proved. Without EBV, the relationship between the hyperplasia and IDD is difficult to confirm and other causes of hyperplasias must be excluded.

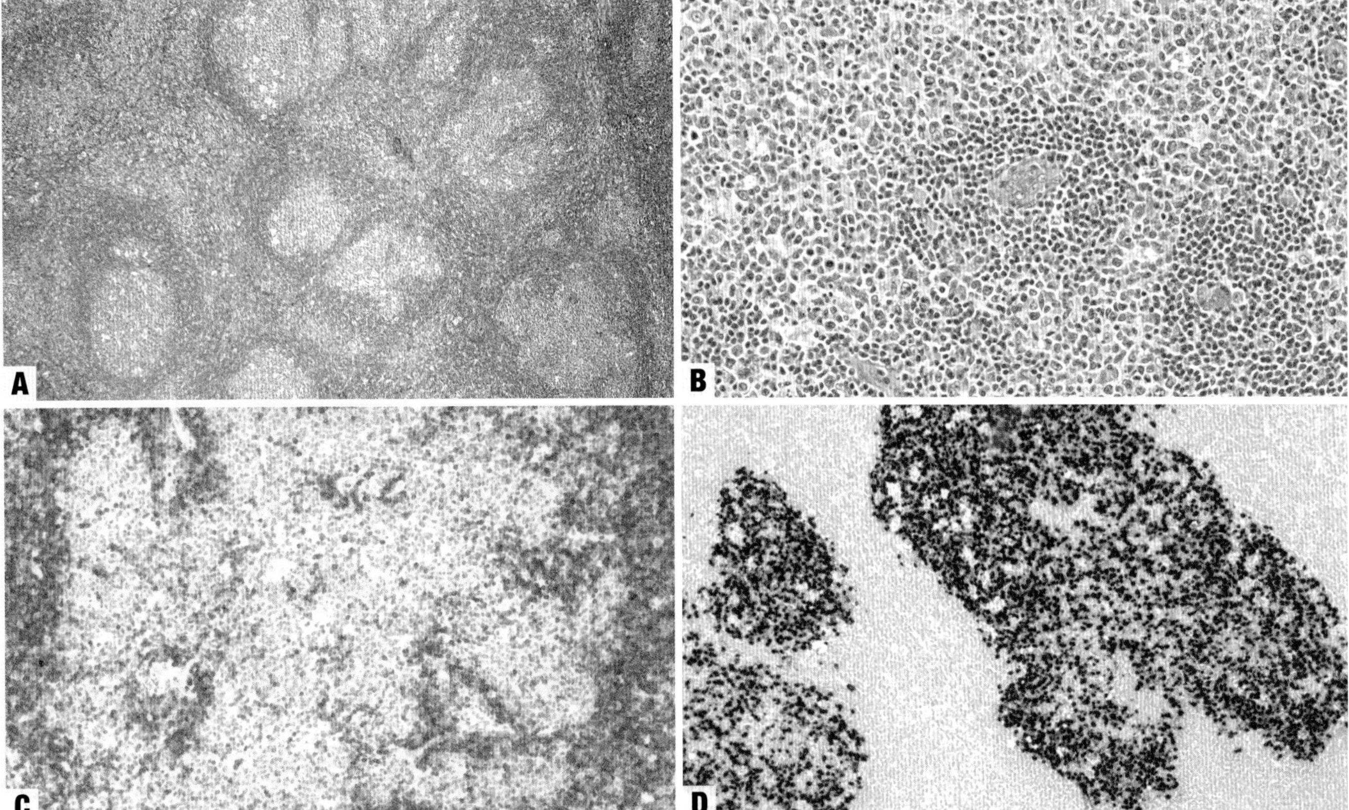

Fig. 4.246 Hyperplasias arising in immune deficiency/dysregulation. **A** Dasatinib-related hyperplasia in a patient with *BCR::ABL1*-positive chronic myeloid leukaemia treated with the tyrosine kinase inhibitor dasatinib. There is preserved lymph node architecture with enlarged secondary follicles with infiltration of mantle zone B cells into germinal centres and prominent penetrating vessels. **B** Involved follicles showing mantle zone B cells disrupting germinal centres. **C** Immunohistochemistry for BCL2 highlights cuffs of mantle zone B cells around the vessels that penetrate the germinal centre. **D** EBV-encoded small RNA (EBER) in situ hybridization detects EBV within occasional follicles.

Pathogenesis

T-cell immunosurveillance

IDD-associated hyperplasias arise due to disruption of T-cell immunosurveillance / immune function, resulting in uncontrolled expansion of EBV and/or other viruses, chronic immune stimulation, and ineffective clearance by apoptosis of autoreactive B cells in germinal-centre reactions. T follicular helper (TFH) cell hyperactivation due to cytokine stimulation is thought to contribute to the aberrant germinal-centre responses and lymphoid hyperplasia in autoimmune diseases {2087,3901,4115}. Additional pathogenetic mechanisms may underlie hyperplasias in other IDD settings.

Clonality and genetic alterations

B-cell hyperplasias typically lack monoclonal IG rearrangements, but both minor (oligo)clonal IG rearrangements and a few karyotypic abnormalities can be detected in some cases {4136,3684}. TR rearrangement studies may show clonal peaks, usually within a polyclonal background, which have been attributed to restricted reactive T-cell repertoires {2918}.

Macroscopic appearance

Hypertrophic adenoids and/or tonsils and enlarged lymph nodes have a tan, fish-flesh appearance.

Histopathology

All types of hyperplasias may be seen in various IDD settings, although their relative frequencies and characteristic associations may vary (see Table 4.45, p. 556). Typically, the architecture of the affected lymphoid organ is preserved, although tissue distortion may occur. The lymphocytic and/or plasma cell infiltrates display a spectrum of cytomorphological changes. Some examples are discussed below.

FH can be florid and is characterized by enlarged lymphoid follicles that have expanded dark zones, attenuated or absent mantle zones, and reduced interfollicular areas {4136}. In autoimmune/therapy-related, IEI, and immunosenescence settings, FH may be accompanied by paracortical hyperplasia with increased plasma cells and/or immunoblasts and increased vascularity and necrosis is occasionally present. Castleman disease–like changes may also be seen in this setting {2089, 2090,2160,984}. For HIV-related hyperplasias, see Table 4.45 (p. 556) {600}.

In IMH, there is marked paracortical expansion with increased immunoblasts on a background of small lymphoid cells, plasma cells, and histiocytes. In some cases, increased large or HRS-like cells can mimic diffuse large B-cell or classic Hodgkin lymphoma, respectively. PCH shows permeation of interfollicular areas by plasma cells or plasmacytoid cells. Hyperplastic follicles are usually retained in all types of B-cell hyperplasias.

In autoimmune disease–related hyperplasias of mucosa-associated lymphoid tissues, there can be lymphoid infiltration of the proliferated epithelial component, forming lymphoepithelial lesions (epimyoepithelial islands), such as in Sjögren syndrome–related lymphoepithelial sialadenitis

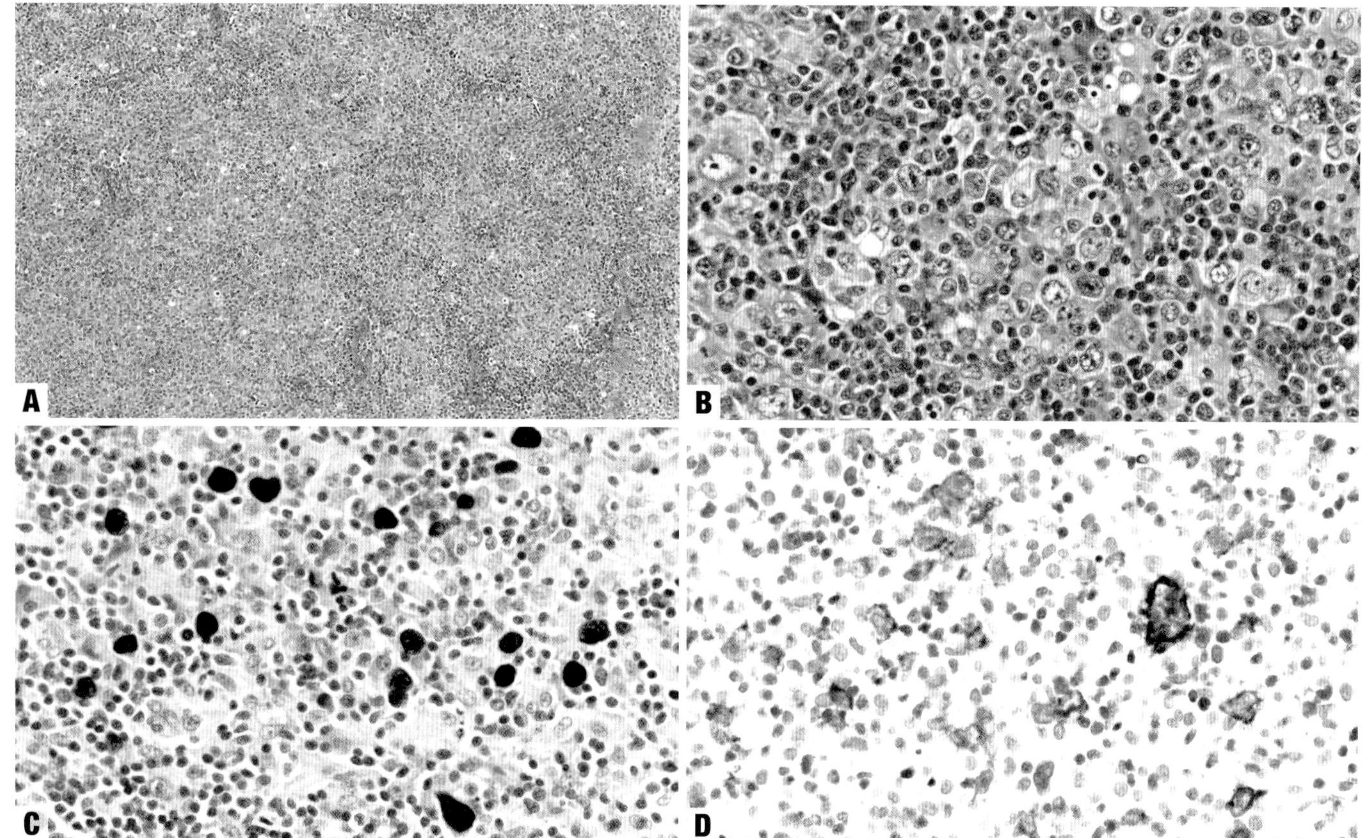

Fig. 4.247 Hyperplasias arising in immune deficiency/dysregulation. Infectious mononucleosis–like hyperplasia. **A** Low magnification shows preservation of tissue architecture with paracortical expansion. **B** At high magnification there is a mixed infiltrate rich in immunoblasts within the expanded paracortex. **C** In situ hybridization for EBV-encoded small RNA (EBER) highlights variably sized cells, including large immunoblasts. **D** Immunohistochemistry for CD20 highlights variably sized B cells, including large immunoblasts.

{1502}. Some autoimmune hyperplasias are characterized by abundant small T cells without cytological atypia, intermingled with plasma cells and immunoblasts, accompanied by an increased vascularity of interfollicular areas {2090}. The histology of autoimmune lymphoproliferative syndrome (ALPS) and IEI-associated lymphoproliferative disorders is described in the respective sections.

Immunophenotype

B-cell hyperplasias in patients with IDD are recognized by their association with EBV. FH shows a normal immunoarchitecture with reactive germinal centres (CD10+, BCL6+, BCL2−). Scattered EBV+ lymphocytes are seen in the interfollicular areas and occasionally within reactive follicles. In HIV-related FH, CD8+ T cells are increased within the lymphoid follicles. In IMH, the B cells show variable expression of CD20 and other B-cell markers and transcription factors, admixed with T cells showing CD8+ cells predominating over CD4+ cells. EBV is present in B cells of variable sizes. The immunoblasts and HRS-like cells express CD30, CD45, and IRF4 (MUM1), but typically lack CD15. Immunoblasts in IMH may be of both B-cell and T-cell lineages. Immunoglobulin light chain protein expression is polytypic in the small and large B cells and plasma cells. Most of the plasma cells express CD19 in PCH, and they display a polytypic profile. In T-cell hyperplasias, aberrant loss of T-cell antigens or CD4/CD8 double-negative T (DNT) cell populations may be present (see *Reactive B-cell–rich lymphoid proliferations that can mimic lymphoma*, p. 309, and *Autoimmune lymphoproliferative syndrome*, p. 646).

Differential diagnosis

The differential diagnosis of hyperplasias includes a variety of entities that range from nonspecific hyperplasias, infectious mononucleosis, IgG4-related disease, and polymorphic lymphoproliferative disorders, to large B-cell lymphomas and classic Hodgkin lymphoma. Progressive transformation of germinal centres and Castleman-like change can be seen in the background of ALPS.

Cytology

FNAC shows heterogeneous lymphocytes, plasma cells, histiocytes, and tingible-body macrophages without atypia. IMH in addition contains variable proportions of large immunoblasts and HRS-like cells. A predominance of plasma cells may be seen in PCH. Flow cytometry typically shows a heterogeneous lymphoid population and polyclonal B cells; T cells may exhibit the phenotype of T-large granular lymphocytic leukaemia or show aberrant immunophenotypes such as DNT cells in ALPS with somatic *FAS* mutation (ALPS-sFAS). Given the broad spectrum of presentations, cytology is usually not sufficient, and a histological biopsy is preferred for definitive diagnosis.

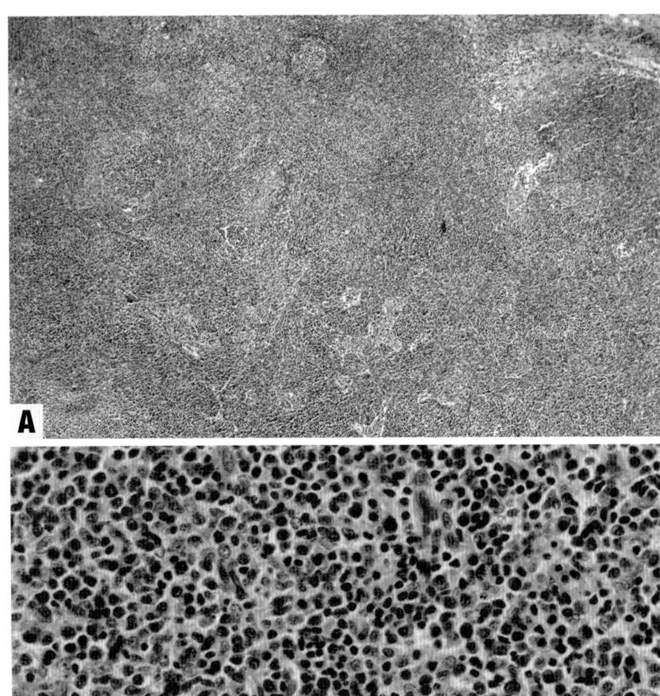

Fig. 4.248 Hyperplasias arising in immune deficiency/dysregulation. **A** Plasmacytic hyperplasia involving multiple lymph node sites in the posttransplant setting shows marked paracortical expansion. **B** There is a predominance of plasma cells within medullary cords that expand the interfollicular/paracortical regions of an involved lymph node.

Diagnostic molecular pathology

Molecular assays are in general not required. A lack of monoclonal IG or TR gene rearrangements may be helpful to rule

Table 4.46 Examples of prior and current nomenclature of hyperplasias arising in immune deficiency/dysregulation (IDD) settings

Immunodeficiency setting	Nomenclature in previous editions of the WHO classification	Three-part nomenclature (name of lesion, virus status, type of immunodeficiency)
Posttransplantation	Infectious mononucleosis–like hyperplasia posttransplant lymphoproliferative disorder	Infectious mononucleosis–like hyperplasia, EBV+, posttransplant setting
HIV infection	KSHV/HHV8+ multicentric Castleman disease	KSHV/HHV8+ multicentric Castleman disease, HIV setting
Autoimmune/therapy-related	Follicular hyperplasia	Follicular hyperplasia, EBV+, autoimmune setting
Immunosenescence (not recognized in prior editions)	Plasmacytic hyperplasia	Plasmacytic hyperplasia, EBV+, presumed immunosenescence
Inborn error of immunity	Granulomatous/CD8+ T-cell–rich lesions	Granulomatous/CD8+ T-cell–rich lesions, EBV−, common variable immunodeficiency

out lymphomas in challenging cases. Expansion of restricted subsets of T and B cells could potentially produce misleading results {3475,4191}.

EBV association should preferably be demonstrated by EBV-encoded small RNA (EBER) in situ hybridization.

Essential and desirable diagnostic criteria

Essential: setting confirmed or highly suspicious for IDD; lack of architectural effacement; heterogeneous lymphoid and/or plasmacytic proliferations without atypia; one of the following three features: (1) detection of EBV/EBER in tissue in the majority of hyperplasias, (2) detection of KSHV/HHV8 in multicentric Castleman disease, (3) other specific features related to IDD (e.g. DNT cell proliferations in ALPS).

Staging

Not applicable

Prognosis and prediction

The clinical management of hyperplasias and involutions (see Table 4.46, p. 559, for previous nomenclature) may vary according to the specific type of lesion and the immunodeficiency setting. Typically, hyperplastic lesions are self-limiting and resolve spontaneously, or in some cases may require immune reconstitution and/or discontinuing therapy, usually with complete resolution.

Polymorphic lymphoproliferative disorders arising in immune deficiency/dysregulation

Natkunam Y
Bhagat G
Bower M
Chadburn A
Chan JKC
Dierickx D
Gratzinger D
Michelow P
Naresh KN
Sato Y
Satou A

Definition

Polymorphic lymphoproliferative disorders (LPDs) arise in patients with immune deficiency or dysregulation and are composed of a heterogeneous lymphoid cell infiltrate with variable numbers of B cells exhibiting a full spectrum of B-cell differentiation that efface the architecture of involved tissues. Large B cells, including HRS-like cells, may be present. Polymorphic LPDs are monoclonal or oligoclonal, usually EBV-driven B-cell proliferations that have no or only a few genetic alterations.

ICD-O coding

9971/1 Polymorphic lymphoproliferative disorders arising in immune deficiency/dysregulation

ICD-11 coding

2B32.3 Polymorphic posttransplant lymphoproliferative disorder

Related terminology

Not recommended: polymorphic lymphoma; polymorphic posttransplant lymphoproliferative disorder (P-PTLD); P-PTLD–like lymphoproliferative disorder.

Note: in the posttransplant setting only, it is acceptable to include "posttransplant lymphoproliferative disorder (PTLD)" as an addendum.

Subtype(s)

None

Localization

Polymorphic LPDs mainly involve lymph nodes, although other lymphoid organs (e.g. tonsils) and a variety of extranodal sites (e.g. lung, gastrointestinal tract, liver, and CNS) can be involved {602,984,3248,2160}. The bone marrow may be involved {2733}.

Clinical features

Polymorphic LPDs are associated with a broad range of clinical features. Haemophagocytic lymphohistiocytosis may be present {2918} (see Table 4.43, p. 552, in *Lymphoid proliferations and lymphomas associated with immune deficiency and dysregulation: Introduction*).

Epidemiology

Polymorphic LPDs can arise in any immunodeficiency setting {602,4400,984,3248,2918} (see Table 4.47, p. 562) but have been best described following transplantation. Polymorphic LPDs account for 20–80% of posttransplant LPDs in haematopoietic stem cell and solid-organ transplant recipients {2061,545,516,4135} and are the most common posttransplant LPDs in children {4331}. The frequency of polymorphic LPDs in autoimmune/therapy-related immunodeficiency related to methotrexate is 15–30% {4400,4401}, and in the HIV setting is < 5% {2867,509}. Because of the general lack of recognition of polymorphic LPDs outside the transplant setting, the true incidence in other immunodeficiency settings may be higher than stated above.

Etiology

EBV is etiologically associated with the majority of polymorphic LPDs. In the absence of EBV, the relationship with immune deficiency/dysregulation may be difficult to recognize. Polymorphic LPDs associated with other viruses have not been defined {606}.

Pathogenesis

T-cell immunosurveillance

Polymorphic LPDs arise when the immunodeficient status of the patient causes a disruption in T-cell immunosurveillance. The lesions have no or only a few genetic alterations and therefore

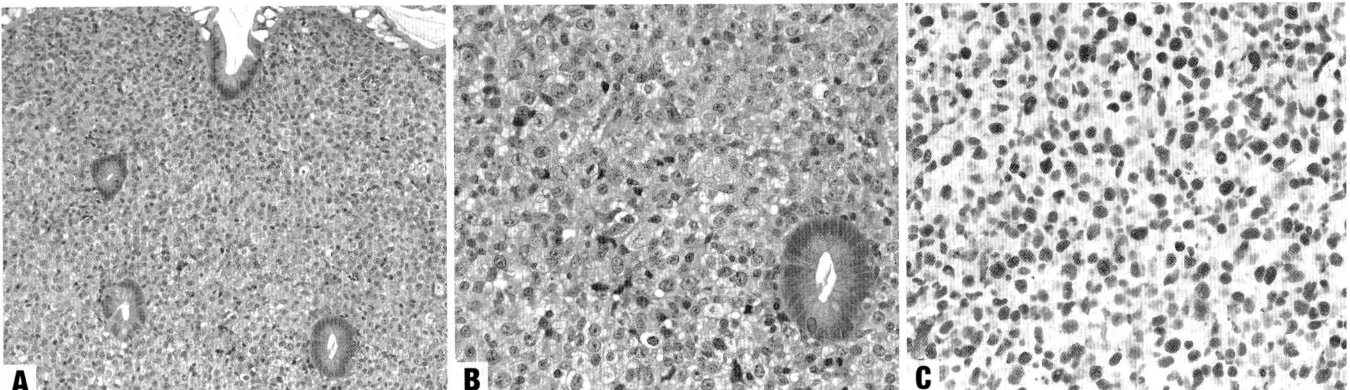

Fig. 4.249 Polymorphic lymphoproliferative disorder arising in immune deficiency/dysregulation. **A** Stomach biopsy in a haematopoietic stem cell transplant recipient shows a polymorphic lymphoproliferative disorder with diffuse effacement of the architecture (EBV+, posttransplant setting). **B** The polymorphic infiltrate is characterized by a range of B-cell differentiation stages admixed with plasma cells and histiocytes. **C** In situ hybridization for EBV-encoded small RNA (EBER) shows EBV positivity in the majority of the cells, which range in size from small to large.

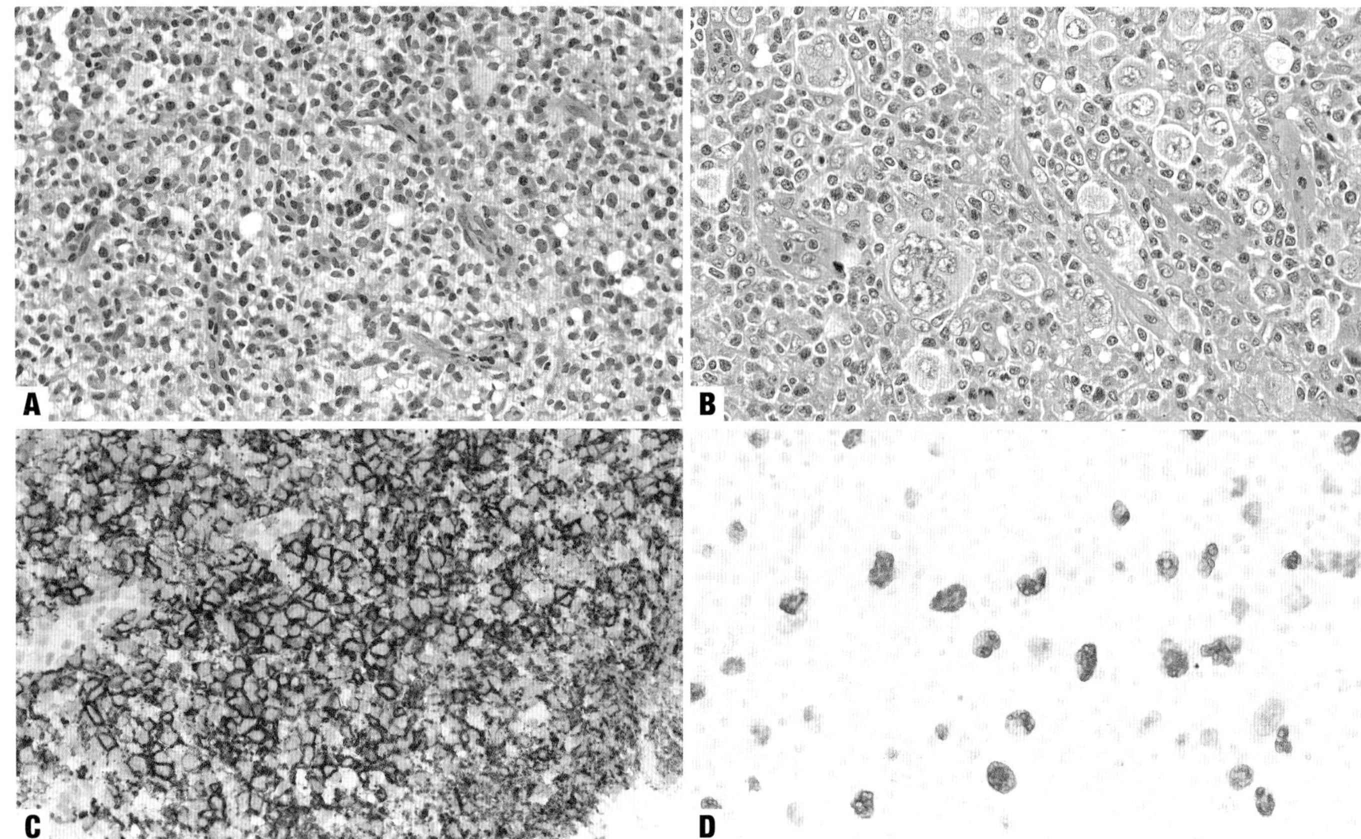

Fig. 4.250 Polymorphic lymphoproliferative disorder arising in immune deficiency/dysregulation. **A** Polymorphic lymphoproliferative disorder in a patient with rheumatoid arthritis treated with methotrexate. This lesion resolved upon withdrawal of methotrexate. There is a heterogeneous infiltrate of small and large lymphoid cells and immunoblasts admixed with plasma cells, histiocytes, and eosinophils. **B** There are atypical large cells including those resembling HRS cells in a mixed inflammatory background. **C** The atypical cells show a range of sizes and strong expression of B-cell markers (CD20 shown here). **D** In situ hybridization for EBV-encoded small RNA (EBER) at high magnification highlights EBER-positive HRS-like cells, together with numerous EBV-positive cells ranging in size from small to large.

may regress upon restoration of the immune response {2340, 4007,3399,2845}. Additional pathogenetic mechanisms may vary according to immunodeficiency settings (e.g. the severity and duration of autoimmune disease predispose to polymorphic LPDs, in addition to the immunosuppressive medication) {4400} (see Table 4.47).

EBV latency

EBV plays a multifactorial role in immune deficiency/dysregulation (IDD)-associated LPDs. In infected B cells, the EBV latent membrane proteins LMP2A and LMP1 provide survival signals mimicking, respectively, B-cell receptor and CD40 signalling and activation of NF-κB, which induces cell proliferation. The EBV nuclear antigen EBNA1 regulates viral DNA replication, transcription, and immune evasion from cytotoxic T cells, whereas EBNA2 regulates several viral and cellular genes {2340,4007,3399,2845}. EBV exhibits a range of transcriptional programmes, with latency patterns II (LMP1+/EBNA2−) and III (LMP1+/EBNA2+), being the most common in IDD-associated LPDs. Polymorphic LPDs in the posttransplant setting typically show type III EBV latency or an admixture of type II and type III latency, whereas the majority of methotrexate-associated polymorphic LPDs show type II EBV latency {2160} (Table 4.48). Occasionally, expression of lytic proteins is also seen.

Clonality and genetic alterations

Polymorphic LPDs show monoclonal or oligoclonal IG rearrangements {2061,545,4135}. In some cases, multiple synchronous

Table 4.47 Comparison of polymorphic lymphoproliferative disorders arising in various immunodeficiency settings

Feature	Posttransplant (PTLD)	HIV	Autoimmune/iatrogenic	Immunosenescence
Prevalence	20–80%	< 5%	15–30%	Unknown
Timing	Early after transplantation (~1 year)	Late associated with more severe immunosuppression	A few months to > 10 years	Advanced age
Risk factors	EBV seronegativity at the time of transplantation	Absence of cART; low CD4 counts	Severity and duration of autoimmune disease; cessation of immunosuppressive medication	Risk increases with advancing age

cART, combination antiretroviral therapy; PTLD, posttransplant lymphoproliferative disorder.

Table 4.48 EBV latency types and associated lymphoproliferative disorders (LPDs)

Latency	EBER	LMP1	EBNA2	Typical examples of LPDs
Latency I	+	–	–	Burkitt lymphoma Primary effusion lymphoma Plasmablastic lymphoma
Latency II	+	+	–	Polymorphic LPD, iatrogenic setting (methotrexate) Immunodeficiency-associated large B-cell lymphoma Classic Hodgkin lymphoma Extranodal NK/T-cell lymphoma Nodal T follicular helper cell lymphoma, angioimmunoblastic type
Latency III	+	+	+	Polymorphic LPD, posttransplant setting Immunodeficiency-associated large B-cell lymphoma

EBER, EBV-encoded small RNA

lesions are seen and each disease site may contain a different clone {601}. Posttransplant polymorphic LPDs show monoclonal IG rearrangements in all cases {2061}. Among methotrexate-associated polymorphic LPDs, 50–70% show monoclonal IG gene rearrangements {1708,4474}. Small monoclonal T-cell populations, as reflected by TR gene rearrangements, may be detected and are attributed to reactive T-cell populations {2918}. Various cytogenetic abnormalities are found in 15–30% of cases {3269,971,4136} and do not preclude a diagnosis of polymorphic LPD.

Macroscopic appearance

Mass-forming lesions with or without ulceration and necrosis

Histopathology

The morphological spectrum of polymorphic LPDs is broad. Typically, there is architectural destruction by a heterogeneous infiltrate of cells. There are variable proportions of B cells, which can exhibit a full spectrum of B-cell differentiation, including small lymphoid cells, plasmacytoid cells, plasma cells, plasmablasts, and immunoblasts, as well as T cells and histiocytes. The number and cytomorphology of the immunoblasts are also variable and may include pleomorphic and/or HRS-like cells. Diffuse sheets of large B cells are absent. Morphological features may vary within an involved site and between sites within the same patient. The bone marrow may show mild to extensive involvement by polymorphic infiltrates and/or haemophagocytic lymphohistiocytosis {2733,2918,891}.

Immunophenotype

The small B-cell component may show a range of expression of CD20, CD19, CD22, and CD79a, as well as B-cell transcription factors such as PAX5, OCT2, and BOB1, according to the proportion of cells with plasmacytoid differentiation. The large B cells and HRS-like cells variably express CD45, CD30, and B-lineage markers; IRF4 (MUM1) is frequently expressed, and rare cases may be CD15-positive. A subset of polymorphic LPDs may lack surface immunoglobulin expression. EBV is seen in variable proportions of both small and large cells. Immunoglobulin light chain restriction may be dissimilar within and among sampled sites and may not correlate with clonality studies. In some cases, T cells and histiocytes may predominate, imparting a T-cell/histiocyte–rich or Hodgkin lymphoma–like background {2918}.

Differential diagnosis

The differential diagnosis of polymorphic LPDs covers a broad range of entities (see Table 4.49, p. 564). The presence and variable number of EBV-positive cells overlaps with features of infectious mononucleosis–like hyperplasia, EBV-positive mucocutaneous ulcer, classic Hodgkin lymphoma, and EBV-positive diffuse large B-cell lymphoma. Currently, there are no objective data to support a specific cut-off point for the number of large transformed cells in any of these entities and therefore the boundaries remain indistinct.

According to the current definition, a history of IDD other than immunosenescence excludes the diagnosis of lymphomatoid granulomatosis. Cases with angiotropism and angiodestruction with necrosis suggestive of lymphomatoid granulomatosis, grades 1 and 2, in IDD settings should be classified as polymorphic LPD, lymphomatoid granulomatosis type, and further reported according to the guidelines for IDD-associated LPDs.

EBV-positive mucocutaneous ulcer is localized to specific extranodal cutaneous and mucosal sites.

Small B-cell lymphomas (especially those with prominent plasmacytoid differentiation, such as marginal zone lymphoma) and plasmacytomas may be difficult to separate from polymorphic LPDs when EBV-positive {1339,891,1362,3589}. The distinction of such B-cell lymphomas from polymorphic LPDs may be arbitrary, and the appropriate nomenclature may be challenging or may vary according to the clinical context.

A polymorphous lymphoproliferation with a range of morphological features should prompt workup for an underlying immunodeficiency, if the immune status of the patient is unknown.

Cytology

Cytological smears show all lymphoid populations as described in *Histopathology*. Flow cytometry may detect either polytypic or monotypic B and/or plasma cells and is of little added value. Given the overlap of polymorphic LPD with both hyperplastic and neoplastic lymphoid lesions, an incisional or excisional biopsy is required for a definitive diagnosis. Core needle biopsies may be acceptable when an optimal incision/excision biopsy is precluded for medical reasons. In such cases, interventional radiology-guided methods are preferred.

Diagnostic molecular pathology

Clonality analysis of IG gene rearrangement contributes to the diagnosis of polymorphic LPD and some of the differential

Table 4.49 Differential diagnosis of polymorphic lymphoproliferative disorders (LPDs)

Diagnosis	Distinctive features and criteria for separation
Infectious mononucleosis–like hyperplasia	Infectious mononucleosis–like hyperplasia commonly involves lymph nodes and tonsils in adolescents and young adults, with paracortical expansion by immunoblasts, some with HRS-like morphology in a mixed inflammatory background; they do not show a spectrum of B-cell differentiation stages and they lack architectural destruction, which allows their separation from polymorphic LPDs
EBVMCU	EBVMCU is a polymorphic lesion confined to the oral mucosa, skin, or gastrointestinal tract and is a sharply circumscribed ulcerative lesion Separation from polymorphic LPDs may require clinical staging and demonstration of clonal IG gene rearrangements in polymorphic LPDs
Small (low grade) B-cell lymphomas	Small B-cell lymphomas, particularly NMZL and EMZL, show strong overlap with polymorphic LPDs in morphology and sites of involvement (skin, gastrointestinal tract, lung, lymph nodes) The presence of lymphoepithelial lesions in EMZL is helpful to separate them from polymorphic LPDs Mutations in *MYD88* and *CXCR4* in lymphoplasmacytic lymphomas allow their separation from polymorphic LPDs EBV– small B-cell lymphomas should be classified as in immunocompetent patients
EBV-positive DLBCL	EBV-positive DLBCL may overlap with polymorphic LPDs, especially those with a T-cell/histiocyte–rich morphology and polymorphous background Unlike polymorphic LPD, EBV-positive DLBCL lacks the spectrum of B-cell differentiation stages, although plasmacytoid differentiation or admixed immunoblasts or HRS-like cells may be present In polymorphic LPD, EBV is typically positive in a range of cell sizes; polymorphic LPD lacks sheets of large atypical B cells
Classic Hodgkin lymphoma (CHL)	Diagnostic criteria for CHL must be strictly applied, although atypical phenotypes (i.e. CD20, CD79a, and T-cell marker expression) are more often seen in CHL occurring in immunodeficiency settings In EBV+ CHL, most EBV+ cells should be HRS-like; scattered small EBV+ lymphocytes may be seen in the background The typical nodular sclerosis architecture or mixed cellularity background favours CHL CHL usually involves lymph nodes, whereas many polymorphic LPDs involve extranodal sites
Plasmablastic lymphoma	Plasmablastic lymphoma demonstrates a diffuse proliferation of large immunoblastic or plasmablastic cells with a plasmacytic phenotype (e.g. CD20–, PAX5–, CD138+, IRF4 [MUM1]+), often with *MYC* rearrangement, which is lacking in polymorphic LPDs
Nodal T follicular helper (TFH) cell lymphoma, angioimmunoblastic type (nTFHL-AI)	nTFHL-AI is typified by a proliferation of variably sized lymphoid cells with clear cytoplasm, a prominent proliferation of high endothelial venules, and follicular dendritic cell meshworks A TFH phenotype, TR rearrangements, *RHOA* and other somatic mutations, and other epigenetic alterations are typically found in nTFHL-AI but are lacking in polymorphic LPDs Secondary EBV+ B-cell proliferations in nTFHL-AI may mimic polymorphic LPD, and recognition of the underlying T-cell lymphoma serves to separate them from polymorphic LPDs

DLBCL, diffuse large B-cell lymphoma; EBVMCU, EBV-positive mucocutaneous ulcer; EMZL, extranodal marginal zone lymphoma; NMZL, nodal marginal zone lymphoma.

diagnostic alternatives, including hyperplasias and lymphomas. Results should always be interpreted in the context of all morphological and immunophenotypic information. EBV-encoded small RNA (EBER) in situ hybridization is preferred for demonstrating an EBV association.

Essential and desirable diagnostic criteria

Essential: setting confirmed or highly suspicious for IDD; architectural effacement; polymorphous infiltrate with a spectrum of B-cell differentiation stages; atypical large cells positive for CD20 (variable), CD30 (variable), and PAX5; EBV positivity demonstrated in tissue (EBV viral load measurements in the blood are not sufficient for diagnosis).

Desirable: IG gene rearrangement studies to support exclusion of hyperplasias.

Staging

Staging with PET-CT is necessary for polymorphic LPDs and follows the Lugano (modified Ann Arbor) staging system {688}. Although metabolic quantification shows differences between polymorphic LPDs and more aggressive subtypes, standardized uptake value–based parameters cannot be used as a diagnostic tool or replace histological classification given the significant overlap between the different subtypes of immunodeficiency-associated LPDs {2735}.

Prognosis and prediction

Polymorphic LPDs follow a highly variable clinical course. There are no well-defined histopathological, immunophenotypic, or molecular prognostic/predictive factors within the polymorphic LPD group. Clinical management varies according to the specific immunodeficiency setting. Treatment options range from immune reconstitution by reducing immunosuppression or antiviral therapy and immunotherapy, to reduction of the EBV-infected B-cell reservoir with immunotherapy, to cytoreduction with immunochemotherapy. An incremental approach to management is most effective, with aggressive treatments reserved for patients with refractory disease. Response may be seen in solid-organ transplant recipients and therapy-related immunodeficiency upon reduction or withdrawal of immunosuppression {3418,3586, 2160}. HIV-positive patients may respond to the initiation of antiretroviral therapy (ART), with complete resolution in some patients {2867,509}. Patients may develop recurrent disease, which may span the entire spectrum of immunodeficiency-associated LPDs.

EBV-positive mucocutaneous ulcer

Natkunam Y
Bhagat G
Bower M
Chadburn A
Chan JKC
Dierickx D
Gratzinger D
Michelow P
Naresh KN
Sato Y
Satou A

Definition

EBV-positive mucocutaneous ulcer (EBVMCU) is a lymphoproliferative disorder (LPD) with a polymorphous lymphoid infiltrate including EBV-positive atypical large B cells and/or HRS-like cells, which typically involves mucosal and cutaneous sites in patients with immune deficiency/dysregulation (IDD).

ICD-O coding

9680/1 EBV-positive mucocutaneous ulcer

ICD-11 coding

2A85.Y & XH3SG2 Further specified mature B-cell neoplasms or lymphoma & EBV-positive mucocutaneous ulcer

Related terminology

None

Subtype(s)

None

Localization

EBVMCU involves the skin and mucosal sites, including the oral mucosa, tonsils, palate, and gastrointestinal tract {852,985,873, 3586}.

Clinical features

EBVMCU typically presents as a well-circumscribed, often painful ulcer in mucosal or cutaneous sites, without systemic symptoms, lymphadenopathy, hepatosplenomegaly, or bone marrow involvement {985,172,1511,3300,1713}. Multifocal lesions within one anatomical region may be seen {985,3300}.

Epidemiology

No reliable data are available on the incidence of EBVMCU. Presentation is generally in elderly patients (aged > 70 years). EBVMCU occurs in a variety of inborn or acquired IDD contexts, including autoimmunity, therapy-related immune suppression/dysregulation, immunosenescence, HIV infection, and post–organ transplantation settings {985,172,1511,873,1713}.

Etiology

EBV is present in all cases and is probably etiologically associated.

Pathogenesis

The pathogenesis is probably related to alterations in the cytotoxic T-cell repertoire and functionality in response to EBV in immunosuppressed patients. IG gene rearrangements are detected in 50% of cases and are probably due to clonal expansions of EBV-infected B cells; rare clonal T-cell expansions may also lead to the detection of TR gene rearrangements {985,2918}.

Macroscopic appearance

Shallow ulcer without an associated mass

Histopathology

Mucosal and cutaneous lesions show well-circumscribed ulcers with a polymorphous infiltrate of lymphoid cells ranging in size from small to large, variable numbers of immunoblasts, and HRS-like cells. There are admixed plasma cells, histiocytes, and eosinophils. Angioinvasion, thrombosis, and necrosis are often prominent; apoptotic cells may be seen. The overlying epithelium may show pseudoepitheliomatous hyperplasia. The base of the lesion is sharply demarcated by a dense rim of small lymphocytes. Small lymphocytic infiltrates predominate in some cases {1254}.

The polymorphic infiltrate consists of a mixture of CD20-positive and CD3-positive lymphoid cells. CD8-positive T cells may predominate in some cases. The atypical large B cells and HRS-like cells are EBV-positive, express B-cell markers, and are frequently CD30 positive, but they only rarely express CD15

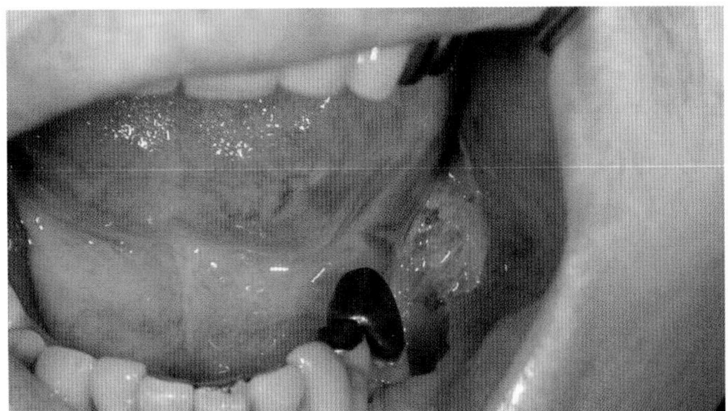

Fig. 4.251 EBV-positive mucocutaneous ulcer. A well-circumscribed ulcerated lesion involving the oral mucosa.

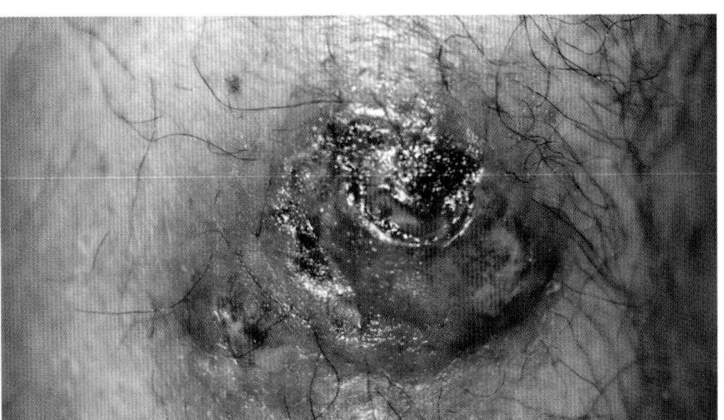

Fig. 4.252 EBV-positive mucocutaneous ulcer. Macroscopic image shows a well-circumscribed ulcerated lesion involving the skin.

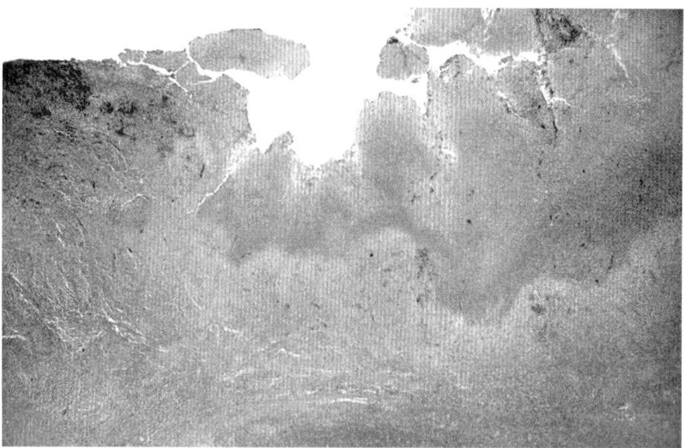

Fig. 4.253 EBV-positive mucocutaneous ulcer. Extensive surface ulceration and necrosis overlying a polymorphous infiltrate in a case of EBV-positive mucocutaneous ulcer involving the tonsil.

{985,1511,2918,3300}. Small CD3-positive T cells typically form a boundary with the uninvolved adjacent tissue and lack EBV.

The differential diagnosis of EBVMCU includes polymorphic LPDs, EBV-positive diffuse large B-cell lymphoma (DLBCL), and classic Hodgkin lymphoma (CHL), especially when there are increased large immunoblasts and HRS-like cells. EBV is typically detected in a range of cell sizes in EBVMCU and polymorphic LPDs. The circumscription and localization to cutaneous and mucosal sites of EBVMCU are unlike polymorphic LPDs, DLBCL, or CHL, and a good overview of the tissue architecture is important. The diagnosis may be challenging in superficial, small, or core needle biopsies. The presence of necrosis and angiocentric infiltrates containing EBV in nasal or oropharyngeal locations may morphologically mimic extranodal NK/T-cell lymphoma; immunohistochemistry showing an NK/T-cell phenotype excludes EBVMCU.

Cytology

Cytological features of FNA samples may show a polymorphous lymphoid infiltrate with necrosis. Given the overlap of EBVMCU with polymorphic LPDs and neoplastic lymphoid lesions, histological assessment is required for a definitive diagnosis.

Diagnostic molecular pathology

Monoclonal B-cell receptor or TR gene rearrangements are found in more than 30–35% of cases and therefore do not separate EBVMCU from polymorphic LPDs and overt lymphomas {985}.

Essential and desirable diagnostic criteria

Essential: setting confirmed or highly suspicious for IDD; well-circumscribed shallow ulcer in mucosal or cutaneous sites

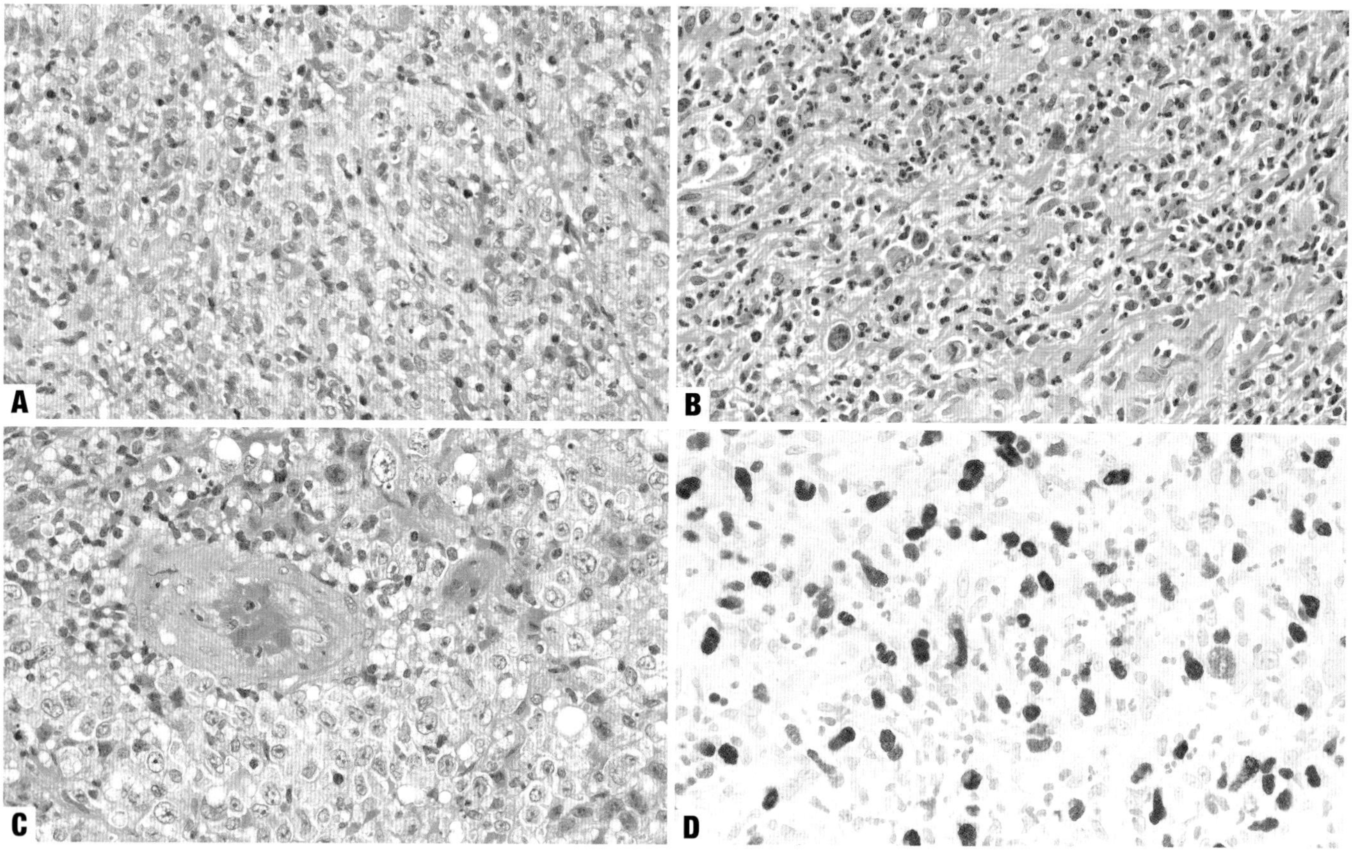

Fig. 4.254 EBV-positive mucocutaneous ulcer. **A** The polymorphic infiltrate of EBV-positive mucocutaneous ulcer exhibits a mixture of cell types including small lymphocytes, plasma cells, histiocytes, eosinophils, and large transformed cells resembling HRS cells. **B** Large immunoblasts and HRS-like cells in a mixed inflammatory background may be a prominent feature of EBV-positive mucocutaneous ulcer (cutaneous localization). **C** Angioinvasion can be present (oral cavity localization). **D** In situ hybridization for EBV-encoded small RNA (EBER) shows the presence of numerous EBV-positive cells in small and large lymphoid cells, highlighting HRS-like cells (cutaneous localization).

with a polymorphous lymphoid infiltrate; atypical large cells positive for CD20 (variable), CD30 (variable), and PAX5; EBV positivity in tissue (EBV viral load measurements in blood are not sufficient for diagnosis).

Desirable: band of CD3+ T cells at the periphery and at the base of the lesion.

Staging

Formal staging procedures for EBVMCU are not indicated; however, when there is clinical suspicion of more extensive LPDs in a patient with known or suspected IDD, including a suspected inborn error of immunity, staging workup should be performed to exclude additional and/or more aggressive LPDs at other sites. Imaging should also be undertaken to exclude mass lesions or deep-seated lesions.

Prognosis and prediction

The majority of EBVMCUs regress spontaneously or respond to withdrawal of immunosuppression where immune reconstitution is possible. Localized therapy may be needed in some cases. Occasional cases may have a relapsing and remitting course, without progression {852,985,172,3515,1511,2918}.

Lymphomas arising in immune deficiency/dysregulation

Naresh KN
Bhagat G
Bower M
Chadburn A
Chan JKC
Dierickx D
Gratzinger D
Michelow P
Natkunam Y
Sato Y
Satou A

Definition

Lymphomas arising in patients with immune deficiency or immune dysregulation cover a spectrum of lymphoma types. They are frequently, but not exclusively, associated with EBV and/or KSHV/HHV8.

ICD-O coding

Code as type of lymphoma.

ICD-11 coding

Code as type of lymphoma.

Related terminology

Not recommended: monomorphic posttransplant lymphoproliferative disorder (PTLD); monomorphic PTLD–like lymphoproliferative disorder; classic Hodgkin lymphoma, PTLD

Note: in the posttransplant setting only, it is acceptable to include "posttransplant lymphoproliferative disorder (PTLD)" as an addendum.

Subtype(s)

See Table 4.44 (p. 554) in *Lymphoid proliferations and lymphomas associated with immune deficiency and dysregulation: Introduction*, and Table 4.50.

Localization

Lymphomas arising in the immune deficiency/dysregulation (IDD) setting (IDD-lymphomas) may involve lymph nodes and extranodal sites including an allograft. Extranodal presentation is generally more frequent than for similar lymphomas in immunocompetent patients {516,956,2024,2734,369,2029}. In some IDD settings, lymphomas may characteristically arise at extranodal sites. Localization of extranodal marginal zone lymphoma is most prevalent in the skin and subcutaneous soft tissue, but bronchial, gastric, breast, and orbital presentations are also documented {272,4222,2997,1339,2911,163,891,567}. In Sjögren syndrome, a salivary gland presentation is most common {1054}. CNS localization of diffuse large B-cell lymphoma (DLBCL) is typically seen in mycophenolate mofetil–treated kidney transplant recipients {1100,832}. In HIV settings, primary CNS lymphoma more frequently manifests with multiple lesions in the cerebrum {3530}; Burkitt lymphoma (BL) often has a leukaemic presentation; and classic Hodgkin lymphoma (CHL) may have an atypical clinical presentation with advanced-stage bone marrow or liver involvement {2759,814,340,3798,2856,3070}.

Clinical features

IDD-lymphomas are associated with a large range of clinical features similar to those of corresponding lymphomas in immunocompetent patients, as well as characteristics specific for IDD, which may vary according to the specific settings, as summarized in Table 4.42 (p. 550) and Table 4.43 (p. 552) in *Lymphoid proliferations and lymphomas associated with immune deficiency and dysregulation: Introduction*).

The morphological presentation as DLBCL, CHL, or other lymphomas and the time to development of lymphoma largely depend on the severity of immunodeficiency and the particular dysregulations of specific immune cell populations. Some examples of setting-specific features are given below.

In the solid-organ transplant setting, as many as 15% of the cases show (often isolated) involvement of the allograft. In contrast to the more frequent recipient-derived solid-organ transplant–related lymphomas, these cases are mainly donor-derived and EBV-associated, and they present early (< 1 year) after transplantation. In these cases, donor lymphoid cells (in particular in organ transplants with a high lymphoid load, including lung, liver, and bowel transplants) can rapidly proliferate in a tolerant environment {3209,2245,2551}. Hepatosplenic T-cell lymphoma represents another unique presentation. Although most cases occur de novo, as many as 20–30% of cases present in patients with immune disorders, including prior transplantation. Hepatosplenic T-cell lymphoma typically occurs in young patients, with a clear male predominance. As the name implies, hepatomegaly and splenomegaly are typical. Cytopenias, which may be due to splenomegaly, bone marrow

Table 4.50 Examples of prior and current nomenclature of lymphomas arising in immune deficiency/dysregulation settings

Immunodeficiency setting	Nomenclature in previous editions of the WHO classification	Three-part nomenclature (name of lesion, virus status, type of immunodeficiency)
Posttransplantation	Monomorphic posttransplant lymphoproliferative disorder, Burkitt lymphoma	Burkitt lymphoma, EBV−, posttransplant setting
HIV infection	Classic Hodgkin lymphoma	Classic Hodgkin lymphoma, EBV+, HIV setting
Autoimmune/therapy-related	Diffuse large B-cell lymphoma	Diffuse large B-cell lymphoma, EBV+, autoimmune setting
Immunosenescence (not recognized in prior editions)	Diffuse large B-cell lymphoma	Diffuse large B-cell lymphoma, EBV+, presumed immunosenescence setting
Inborn error of immunity	Extranodal marginal zone lymphoma	Extranodal marginal zone lymphoma, EBV−, hyper-IgM syndrome

involvement, and/or haemophagocytosis, are frequent {1137, 3302,1304}.

Similarly, in the HIV setting, people living with HIV (PLWH) often present at an advanced clinical stage; bulky disease with a high tumour burden is frequent. LDH is usually markedly elevated. Primary CNS lymphoma and DLBCL more often occur in the setting of longstanding HIV infection and AIDS and are associated with higher rates of opportunistic infections and lower CD4+ T-cell counts (mean: < 100 × 10^6/L). In contrast, BL and CHL occur in less immunodeficient patients with significantly higher CD4+ T-cell counts (> 200 × 10^6/L) {547,339, 2016,1671}. KSHV/HHV8-associated lymphomas, such as primary effusion lymphomas and KSHV/HHV8-positive DLBCL, typically occur in the HIV setting.

Epidemiology

IDD-lymphomas may occur in any immune deficiency or immune dysregulation setting and cover a spectrum of morphologies, including small B-cell lymphoma, DLBCL, BL, CHL, and T- and NK-cell lymphomas, as well as various specific entities. Because the diagnostic criteria have been subject to change and are inconsistent across IDD settings in prior editions of the WHO classification, published data on epidemiological aspects of IDD-lymphomas are difficult to compare. Moreover, changes in clinical management, such as the development of more effective combination antiretroviral therapy (cART) in PLWH and newer pretransplantation conditioning and induction regimens in posttransplantation settings, have impacted epidemiological features. A broad summary is provided in Table 4.43 (p. 552) in *Lymphoid proliferations and lymphomas associated with immune deficiency and dysregulation: Introduction*, and specific examples are discussed in detail below.

In the HIV setting, the incidence of lymphoma is reportedly increased 60–200 times in PLWH. Before cART was available, the incidence rates of primary CNS lymphoma and BL were 1000 times as high as in the age- and sex-matched general population {2288,318}. Since the introduction of cART, the incidence of non-Hodgkin lymphoma has decreased by 50%, mainly due to decreases in primary CNS lymphoma and DLBCL {339,1077,362,2016}. cART has had little effect on the incidence of Burkitt lymphoma {3357}. In contrast, the risk of HIV-associated CHL has remained stable, and the incidence of CHL in PLWH has increased, with the highest risk occurring in the first few months after starting cART {2220,1380}.

In autoimmune/therapy-related settings, the risk and the specific type of lymphoma vary depending on the type of immunosuppressive or immunomodulatory agent, the degree of immune deficiency, and the nature and severity of the underlying autoimmune/rheumatological disorder being treated {2657,206, 1125,1124,1529,3753,870,1941}. Although the epidemiological aspects have been best described in patients with rheumatoid arthritis treated with methotrexate {1638,2961,1708,1499}, treatment protocols have become more diverse and have impacted the spectrum of associated lymphomas {4401,499,2418,2407, 2693,483,2532}. Moreover, with the increasing use of novel immunomodulatory drugs and other forms of immunotherapy (chimeric antigen receptor [CAR] T-cell therapy) for cancer and autoimmune/inflammatory diseases, new types of lesions are emerging and their incidence may increase in the future. In particular the increasing use of T-cell depleting agents (including the purine analogue fludarabine, which is also part of the conditioning regimen for CAR T-cell therapy), may lead to long-lasting T-cell depletion and hence loss of immunosurveillance and the development of EBV-associated lymphomas {2056,1294,2804}.

Other suggested associations include an increased risk of hepatosplenic T-cell lymphoma in patients with Crohn disease or inflammatory bowel disease treated with infliximab and/or other TNF antagonists (adalimumab and etanercept); however, the data require further validation {2112}.

Etiology

EBV and KSHV/HHV8 are associated with a significant proportion of IDD-lymphomas. The rate of EBV involvement varies across different IDD settings and depends in part on the severity and type of immunosuppression. Since the introduction of more effective treatment (cART) for HIV patients and novel pretransplantation conditioning regimens, the rate of EBV association in IDD-lymphomas has significantly declined overall and differs according to lymphoma type {595,1480,529,184,3807}.

The etiology of EBV-negative and KSHV/HHV8-negative IDD-lymphomas is unknown. In some cases, a viral-specific epigenetic signature (imprint) of prior EBV infection with only part of the viral genome being retained can be demonstrated with highly sensitive techniques (RNAscope), but it may no longer be detectable at the time of diagnosis of the lymphoma (hit-and-run theory) {3810,2964}. There is little in vivo evidence supporting this hypothesis to date. Other unknown viruses and chronic antigenic stimulation (such as the antigenicity of the transplanted graft itself) have been hypothesized as driving agents {367}.

In patients with inflammatory bowel disease, thiopurines and/or TNF antagonists may increase the risk of developing hepatosplenic T-cell lymphoma, but this association has been debated more recently {3865}.

Pathogenesis

The pathogenetic aspects of some specific lymphoma entities, including plasmablastic lymphoma, primary effusion lymphoma, KSHV/HHV8-positive DLBCL, and extranodal NK/T-cell lymphomas are discussed in the respective sections. Although IDD-associated B-cell lymphomas share some underlying pathogenesis, mechanisms specific to the immunodeficiency settings also play a role. The most detailed information available thus far is for posttransplantation, HIV infection, and immunosenescence settings.

EBV association and EBV latency

EBV serves as a major driver in the pathogenesis of IDD-lymphomas. Various EBV proteins have been reported to be essential for efficient B-cell transformation, including LMP1, LMP2A, EBNA2, EBNALP, EBNA3A, and EBNA3C. Of these, LMP1, LMP2A, and EBNA2 are the most widely acknowledged to have oncogenic potential, and they can interact with the cellular mechanisms of the host cell {811,3524,278}. LMP1 can mimic CD40-mediated B-cell activation, whereas LMP2A can simulate B-cell receptor signalling, thus enhancing the two major survival signals important for germinal-centre B cells {1995,2514}. EBNA2 acts as a master transcriptional regulator of both viral and cellular genes. Mutations in the EBV genome can further potentiate the viral lymphomagenic ability {1942,4364,2748}. EBV-encoded small RNAs (EBERs) are expressed throughout all phases of the viral cycle. Although they provide a reliable marker for EBV infection, EBERs are not transforming by themselves. Based on the pattern of expression, three different latency expression profiles are recognized, and these are differentially associated with particular IDD-lymphomas (see Table 4.48, p. 563, in *Polymorphic lymphoproliferative disorders arising in immune deficiency/dysregulation*). EBV+ DLBCLs arising in patients with IDD are mostly associated with the type II and type III latency patterns, whereas EBV+ BL generally expresses a type I latency pattern. These patterns are relatively consistent across IDD settings {2539}. In posttransplantation and HIV settings, EBV+ DLBCL and CHL are characterized by a lower somatic mutation burden than similar lymphomas without EBV association, further supporting the added oncogenic potential of the latent EBV genes/proteins in lymphomagenesis {2652,640,1173}.

Genetic alterations

Overall, EBV+ DLBCLs arising in patients with IDD are most frequently of activated B-cell–like subtype {2805,825}. Although the frequencies of gene mutations related to NF-κB signalling are lower than in DLBCLs in immunocompetent patients, the NF-κB signalling pathway is constitutively activated in EBV+ DLBCLs in patients with IDD {2652,640}. Instead of gene mutations, LMP1 and LMP2A are strongly associated with activation of the NF-κB pathway. EBV+ HIV-associated DLBCLs are characterized by frequent *STAT3* mutations {2652,640}. In EBV+ DLBCLs in the

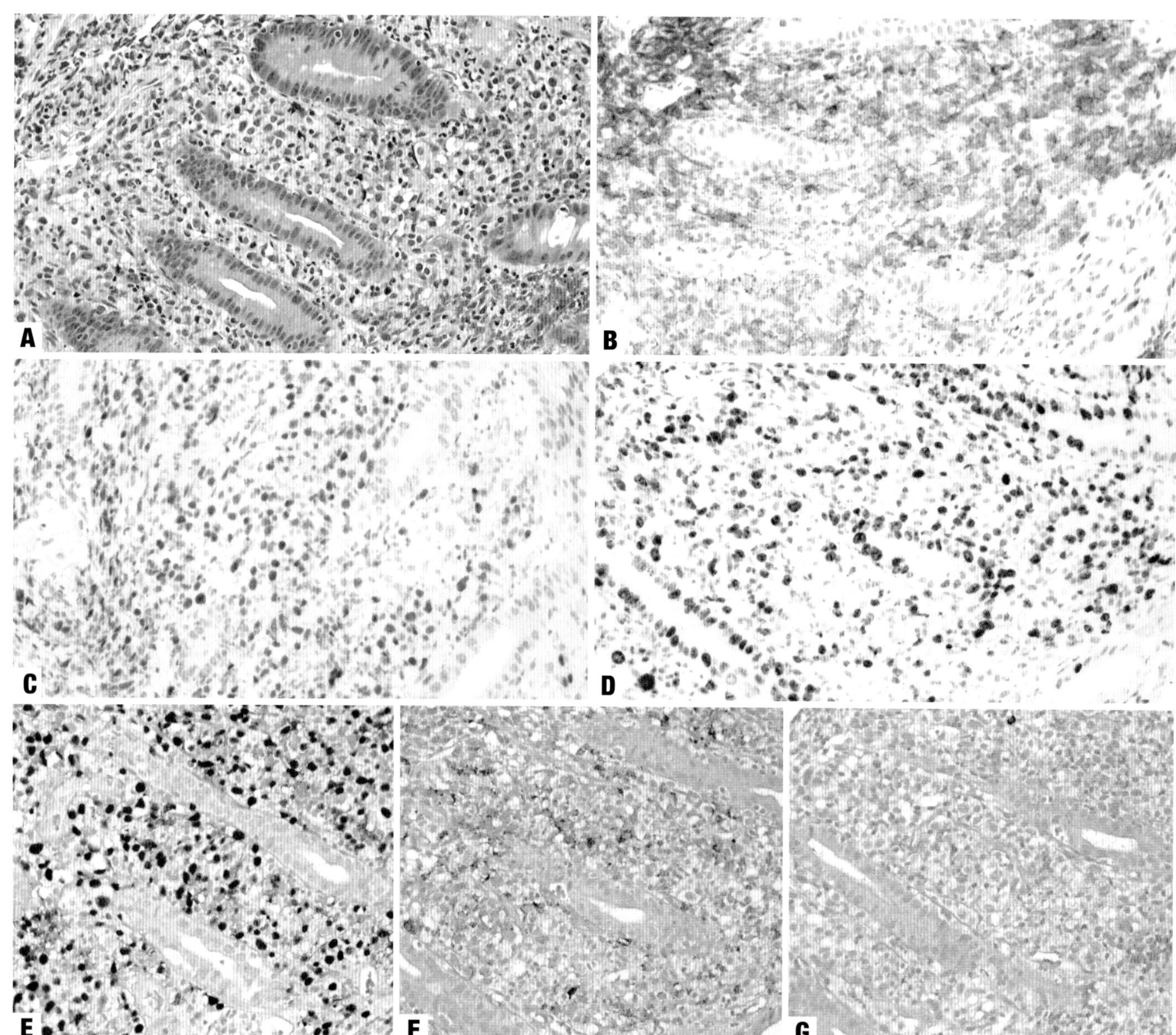

Fig. 4.255 Lymphomas arising in immune deficiency/dysregulation. EBV-positive diffuse large B-cell lymphoma in the post–chimeric antigen receptor (CAR) T-cell therapy setting. Circumferential obstructive mass lesion presenting in the colon of a patient who received CAR T-cell therapy for diffuse large B-cell lymphoma. **A** Pleomorphic large cells and admixed plasma cells fill the lamina propria of this superficial biopsy. **B,C** The infiltrate is positive for CD22 (**B**) and PAX5 (**C**). **D** The Ki-67 proliferation index is high. **E** Pleomorphic large cells and admixed plasma cells are positive for EBV-encoded small RNA (EBER). **F** Kappa light chain in situ hybridization shows weak monotypic expression. **G** Lambda light chain in situ hybridization shows an absence of immunoglobulin lambda light chain expression, mirroring kappa light chain restriction in this proliferation. The original diffuse large B-cell lymphoma showed opposite light chain restriction, lacked plasmacytic differentiation, was predominantly nodal, and was EBV-negative.

posttransplant setting, a gain/amplification in 9p24.1, containing *CD274* (*PDL1*), *PDCD1LG2* (*PDL2*), and *JAK2*, was detected in 24% of the cases {1173}. Most methotrexate-associated CHLs and some methotrexate-associated DLBCLs express PDL1 in tumour cells {2084,1346}. The alterations in 9p24.1 and PDL1 overexpression contribute to immune evasion in DLBCL and CHL. EBV-negative DLBCLs presenting in patients with IDD frequently have *TP53* mutations, but they are more often genetically similar to lymphomas in immunocompetent patients and also more often of germinal-centre B-cell–like type {2805,1173, 2652,640}.

Some recurrent copy-number variations overlap with those in immunocompetent patients, whereas others are relatively specific {1173}. Genetic abnormalities of *MYC* and *BCL6* may be observed in DLBCL arising in patients with immune deficiency/dysregulation, but *BCL2* translocations are usually not seen {1268,4134,2481,640}. Thus far, no information is available on the genomic landscape of EBV+ indolent B-cell lymphomas and plasma cell neoplasms in IDD settings and to what extent they differ from other EBV-negative lymphomas in immunocompetent patients.

Microenvironment

In HIV-associated CHL, there may be decreased numbers of nodal CD4+ T cells and a lack of CD4+ rosetting around HRS cells, and the lymph nodes may show a higher density of CD8+ T cells and FOXP3+ T cells {1521,2114}. HIV-associated DLBCLs have reduced CD4+ and FOXP3+ T cells, increased activated cytotoxic cells and tumour-associated macrophages, and a higher blood vessel density {2337,637}. EBV+ posttransplant DLBCLs show clonally expanded populations of CD8+ T cells and CD163+ M2 macrophages, and this is particularly frequent in EBV+ cases {1707,2807}. A higher density of infiltrating CD8+ T cells may be associated with reduced mortality from lymphoma in patients with HIV {637}.

Macroscopic appearance

Discussed under specific sections for each tumour type

Histopathology

Various lymphoma types that occur in IDD settings are described in separate sections. Most IDD-lymphomas also occur in immunocompetent patients, but they may differ in some morphological, immunophenotypic, and/or pathogenetic aspects that impact differential diagnostic considerations. Pathology reports for IDD-lymphomas should follow the three-part nomenclature provided {2919}.

Small B-cell lymphomas

Extranodal marginal zone lymphoma, nodal marginal zone lymphoma, lymphoplasmacytic lymphoma, and plasmacytoma are described in various IDD settings. Criteria for the specific lymphoma types as described for immunocompetent patients should be met. If EBV is positive in the lesional cells, an etiological relationship to an underlying IDD is apparent, but when EBV is negative an etiological link is unclear. Nodal marginal zone lymphoma in IDD settings exhibits prominent plasmacytic differentiation and generally contains class-switched B/plasmacytic cells. There is extensive overlap with polymorphic lymphoproliferative disorders (LPDs), and the boundary between the two may be impossible to distinguish; features such as lymphoepithelial lesions may help in diagnosing an extranodal marginal zone lymphoma {891}.

Diffuse large B-cell lymphoma

DLBCLs arising in the IDD setting are indistinguishable histologically from DLBCL-NOS or EBV+ DLBCL-NOS, and the diagnostic criteria are identical except for the critical clinical setting of underlying IDD. In addition to large transformed cells/immunoblasts and reactive components, HRS-like cells are seen in some cases. In addition to EBER, expression of LMP1 and (less often) EBNA2 is seen. Polymorphic LPD is a major differential diagnostic consideration. The presence of diffuse sheets of large B cells supports the diagnosis of DLBCL. In some patients with IDD a T-cell/histiocyte–rich microenvironment may be prominent, resembling T-cell/histiocyte–rich large B-cell lymphoma. Given the difficulty related to the somewhat indistinct boundaries, multidisciplinary discussion to reach an optimal diagnosis based on pathological features and the clinical context is advised in those patients in whom the border between polymorphic LPD, DLBCL, and CHL is unclear.

According to the current definition, a history of IDD other than immunosenescence excludes the diagnosis of lymphomatoid granulomatosis. Lymphomas with angiotropism and angiodestruction with necrosis in an IDD context may be classified as lymphomatoid granulomatosis–type DLBCL, and further reported according to the guidelines for IDD-associated LPD. Detailed descriptions and criteria for KSHV/HHV8-associated lymphoid proliferations are provided in the dedicated sections. In IDD settings, reporting guidelines for IDD-associated proliferations should be used (e.g. primary effusion lymphoma, KSHV/HHV8+, EBV+, HIV setting).

Burkitt lymphoma

BL is much more common in PLWH than in other IDD settings. The diagnostic criteria are the same as for sporadic BL occurring in immunocompetent patients, with some notable differences. BL arising in patients with IDD may show greater variation in cell size and shape. Best known in HIV infection, BL may have plasmacytoid differentiation with eccentrically placed nuclei, a single central nucleolus, and abundant cytoplasm that contains immunoglobulin {3449}. The plasmacytoid subset of BL shows a stronger association with EBV (50–70%) than does the non-plasmacytoid subset (~30%) {1353,2366}.

Classic Hodgkin lymphoma

The morphological features of CHL in IDD settings are usually of the mixed-cellularity or nodular sclerosis subtype {21}. Almost all cases are EBV-associated {1569}. In IDD settings, the immunophenotype of HRS-like cells is frequently more variable and not fully consistent with the criteria defined for CHL (see respective section). Particularly, the expression of CD20 may be stronger and more uniform, and the expression of CD79a and CD19 is more often seen {2954,891}. This reflects the presence of a continuum between DLBCL and CHL in large B-cell proliferations in IDD settings. However, contrary to similar phenotypes in immunocompetent patients, the clinicopathological context is not that of mediastinal grey zone lymphoma (see respective section). Therefore, in IDD settings, the diagnostic criteria for CHL should be applied very strictly. Classification as mediastinal grey zone lymphoma is not recommended in IDD settings, except when EBV is negative and the lesion is restricted to the mediastinum with or without intrathoracic extension. IDD-associated polymorphic LPD and EBV-positive mucocutaneous ulcer may contain varying proportion of HRS-like cells with typical or aberrant immunophenotypes. If there is involvement of sites that are unusual for CHL, such as primary nodal involvement below the diaphragm, non-contiguous nodal involvement, or extranodal sites (including the mucosa, skin, or gastrointestinal tract), a polymorphic LPD or EBV-positive mucocutaneous ulcer should be diagnosed.

T-cell lymphomas

Rare cases of T-cell and NK/T-cell lymphomas have been reported in IDD settings, including peripheral T-cell lymphoma, anaplastic large cell lymphoma, angioimmunoblastic-type nodal T follicular helper cell lymphoma, hepatosplenic T-cell lymphoma, mycosis fungoides, and extranodal NK/T-cell lymphoma {4024,1616,1262,342,495,1442,1800,538,155,1572, 1396,3588,3590}. Adult T-cell leukaemia/lymphoma is rare but is known to occur in IDD settings. Outside the context of inborn errors of immunity, T-cell lymphomas in IDD settings are extremely rare, precluding the collection of convincing epidemiological evidence of a causal relationship with IDD. Moreover, with the exception of extranodal NK/T-cell lymphoma and systemic T-cell lymphomas in which EBV positivity is part of the disease definition, the majority of described T-cell lymphomas in IDD settings are EBV-negative {1396,3590}.

Cytology

In immunodeficient patients, FNAB can be useful for the assessment of lymphadenopathy and other masses when the differential diagnosis includes infectious processes, metastatic carcinomas, and lymphomas. The precise diagnosis and subclassification of lymphoma by FNA alone is not advisable {608,2622,2134}.

Diagnostic molecular pathology

Discussed in specific sections

Essential and desirable diagnostic criteria

Essential: setting confirmed or highly suspicious for IDD; meets diagnostic criteria for corresponding lymphomas in immunocompetent patients.

Desirable: detection of EBV (EBER) and/or KSHV/HHV8 (latency-associated nuclear antigen [LANA]) in tissue (EBV viral load measurements in the blood are not sufficient for diagnosis); demonstration of clonal B- or T-cell populations by molecular techniques in challenging cases.

Staging

Discussed in specific sections

Prognosis and prediction

Treatment of lymphoma in IDD largely depends on the specific immunodeficiency setting, in particular in those instances in which the immune defect may be (in part) correctable. In patients with HIV, any lymphoma-directed treatment should be complemented by effective cART. Withdrawal or reduction of immunosuppression may be the first-line approach in immune suppression / immune modulator–related lymphomas and in patients after solid-organ transplantation, followed by rituximab monotherapy in selected cases {3553,1425,735,1073,736,1638, 1368,1708,80,1583}. This may result in lymphoma regression in a minority of the patients. In most instances, lymphoma-specific therapy is required for disease control. Although several prognostic scores have been proposed for lymphomas occurring in the solid-organ transplantation setting, the majority have not been validated. In general, poor-prognostic factors in patients with immunocompetent lymphoma also apply to patients presenting with lymphoma after solid-organ transplantation. In fact, the International Prognostic Index (IPI), which includes older age, decreased performance state, extranodal involvement, elevated LDH, and advanced stage, seems to be a very powerful prognostic score in this population, too. An inadequate response to rituximab and thoracic transplants are also important poor-prognostic factors {1727,955,4057}. For lymphomas occurring in the haematopoietic stem cell transplant setting, a new prognostic score was recently introduced, which includes three pretransplant prognostic factors: the use of ATG in the conditioning regimen, the type of donor, and aplastic anaemia as the underlying disorder {1251}. The expression of MYC in DLBCL is associated with a worse prognosis in PLWH {636, 637}. Before the ART era, the prognosis of PLWH who developed lymphoma was closely related to the severity of immunodeficiency {425}. Effective ART has reduced the impact of HIV-related prognostic factors and now allows curative therapy for most patients with aggressive lymphomas, resulting in survival comparable to that of lymphoma occurring in the general population {2348,3635,4119,253,2987,63}.

Inborn error of immunity–associated lymphoid proliferations and lymphomas

Gratzinger D
Chan JKC
Dierickx D
Natkunam Y
Pan-Hammarström Q
Satou A

Definition

Inborn error of immunity (IEI)-associated lymphoproliferative disorders (IEI-LPDs) are mass-forming or infiltrative proliferations of B or (more rarely) T cells that arise as a result of the underlying IEI.

ICD-O coding

Code as type of lymphoma.

ICD-11 coding

4A01 Primary immunodeficiencies due to disorders of adaptive immunity

Related terminology

Not recommended: primary immunodeficiency; fatal infectious mononucleosis; monomorphic lymphoproliferative disorder.

Subtype(s)

Lymphoid hyperplasias in the IEI setting; polymorphic lymphoproliferative disorders in the IEI setting; EBV-positive mucocutaneous ulcer in the IEI setting; lymphomas in the IEI setting

Localization

IEI-associated lymphoid proliferations and lymphomas arise in lymph nodes and extranodal sites, including the gastrointestinal tract, skin, lungs, and bone marrow.

Clinical features

Clinical features according to the underlying IEI are summarized in Table 4.51 (p. 574) {3968,3969}. The incidence of lymphomas in the IEI setting peaks during the first and third decades of life; 67% are stage III or IV. Patients with X-linked lymphoproliferative syndrome 1 (XLP1) and familial haemophagocytic lymphohistiocytosis syndromes are at increased risk of EBV+ lymphoproliferative disorder (LPD)-associated haemophagocytic lymphohistiocytosis. Granulomatous/CD8+ T-cell–rich lesions can result in significant respiratory, gastrointestinal, and other complications in common variable immunodeficiency (CVID) (see Table 4.52, p. 576) {3669}.

Epidemiology

The exact prevalence of IEIs is unknown. Estimates suggest the prevalence is increasing as more IEIs are molecularly

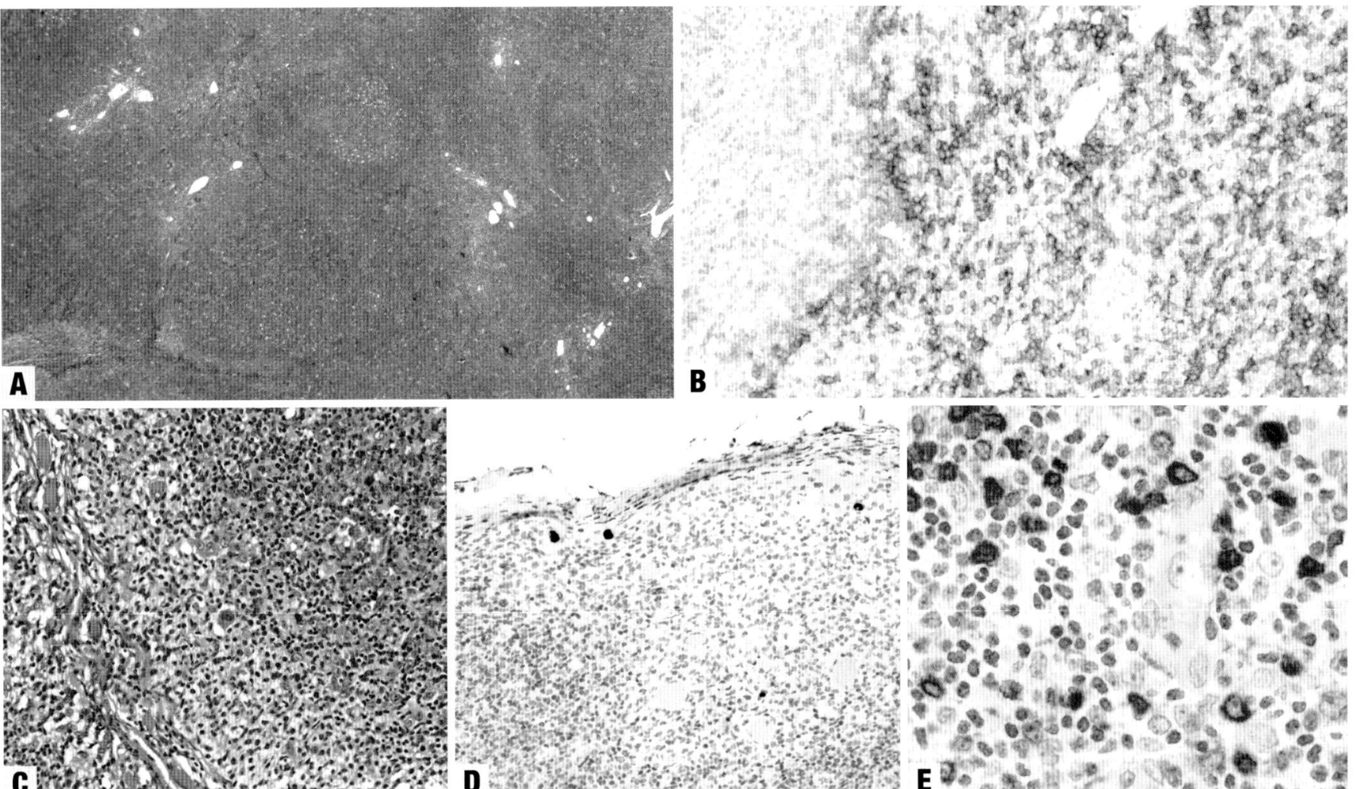

Fig. 4.256 Activated PI3Kδ syndrome (APDS)-associated lymphadenopathy. **A** APDS-associated lymphadenopathy with enlarged germinal centres lacking well-formed mantle zones. **B** Increased T follicular helper (TFH) cells within the poorly defined germinal centres as shown by PD1 immunohistochemistry. **C** At higher power, CMV inclusions are observed. Expanded monocytoid B-cell areas contain occasional large cells with prominent nucleoli. **D** Immunohistochemistry for CMV highlights scattered large infected cells. **E** Scattered variably sized EBV+ lymphoid cells (brown, EBV-encoded small RNA [EBER] in situ hybridization) are B lineage (red, CD79a immunohistochemistry).

Table 4.51 Pathogenesis, clinical features, and associated lymphoproliferative disorders across major categories of inborn errors of immunity (IEIs) of T and B cells {3967, 3969} (continued on next page)

IEI subtype	Pathogenesis	Clinical features	Lymphoproliferative disorders
Predominantly antibody deficiencies: 52% of IEIs worldwide {13}			
Common variable immunodeficiency (~35% of PIDs) {2611}	Marked decrease in at least two immunoglobulin subsets (IgG and either IgA or IgM or both) often due to defects in B-cell development and maturation; altered T-cell repertoire {3475,999,14,3597}	Infections, autoimmunity, lymphoproliferation; lymphoma and gastric cancer predisposition	EBV+/− DLBCL > EBV+ CHL > EMZL > T-LGLL {4465,3767,4338}; cutaneous and other extranodal CD8+ T-cell–rich lymphoid or lymphohistiocytic infiltrates
Activated PI3Kδ syndrome (APDS)	Abnormal T-lymphocyte signalling due to gain-of-function mutations in *PIK3CD* {2439} or loss-of-function mutations in *PIK3R1*, *PTEN* {1781}	Lymphadenopathy, hepatosplenomegaly, nodular mucosal lymphoid hyperplasia, herpesvirus infections, (EBV, CMV, HSV)	DLBCL > CHL > EMZL > others; majority of DLBCL and CHL cases are EBV+ {818, 1066,1029}
Hyper-IgM syndrome	Defective class-switch recombination, lack of germinal centres, e.g. AID deficiency {4496}	Bacterial infections, lymphadenopathy, plasmacytosis	DLBCL, CHL, EMZL {1278}
Agammaglobulinaemia	Decreased to absent B cells, e.g. mutations in *BTK* (X-linked agammaglobulinaemia) {1568}	Severe bacterial infections	Lymphoma uncommon {3376}; rare cutaneous granulomatous CD8+ T-cell lymphoproliferative disorder {1280}
Combined immunodeficiencies: 10.8% of IEIs worldwide {13}			
Syndromic combined immunodeficiencies with predisposition to malignancy (AT, NBS)	Pleiotropic DNA repair defects, e.g. *ATM* deficiency (AT) {3863,3596}	Infection, developmental abnormalities, radiation sensitivity (see *Ataxia–telangiectasia*, p. 810)	AT: DLBCL, BL, CHL, T-LBL, rarely T-PLL {3863,3400} NBS: DLBCL > T-LBL > PTCL > others {3702}
SCIDs	Defects in core T-cell development and signalling pathways or DNA recombination repair, e.g. *DCLRE1C* (*ARTEMIS*) deficiency {2808}	Severe infection susceptibility; subset radiosensitive	Lymphoma rarely reported; usually EBV+ DLBCL {3400}
Leaky SCID, Omenn syndrome	Hypomorphic versions of SCID e.g. *DCLRE1C* (*ARTEMIS*) deficiency {4250}	Infection, adenopathy, rash, eosinophilia, granulomatous lesions	EBV+ DLBCL {3400}; rare cutaneous granulomatous CD8+ T-cell lymphoproliferative disorder {195}
Combined immunodeficiencies	Defects in less critical or downstream T-cell signalling pathways or cytoskeletal proteins, e.g. *WAS* {1027,2094}; CD154 (CD40L) deficiency {77,154}	Infection, autoimmunity; subset with thrombocytopenia (Wiskott–Aldrich syndrome)	DLBCL > BL > CHL > other, often EBV+ {3400}
Thymic defects with additional congenital abnormalities	Lack of thymic development with associated developmental abnormalities, e.g. del22q11.2 {752}	Infections, developmental abnormalities (e.g. velocardiofacial/ DiGeorge syndrome)	Rare case report of EBV+ B-cell lymphoma {3400}
Immuno-osseous dysplasias	Pleiotropic cellular defects, e.g. mutations in *RMRP* (cartilage-hair hypoplasia) {4001}	Skeletal abnormalities, bone marrow failure, and immunodeficiency	B-cell lymphoma {3400}
Hyper-IgE syndromes	T-cell subset defects with dysregulated IgE production, e.g. *STAT3* (Job syndrome) {4395}	High IgE, pyogenic infections, skeletal/dental abnormalities	DLBCL > CHL > BL > T-cell lymphoma; minority EBV+ {2148}
Immune dysregulation			
Familial HLH syndromes {1265}	T-cell hyperactivation leading to histiocyte activation, e.g. mutations in *PRF1* (familial HLH type 2), *LYST* (Chédiak–Higashi syndrome) {1799}	HLH, hepatosplenomegaly; Chédiak–Higashi syndrome: hypopigmentation, platelet and neutrophil defects	Predominance of HLH; lymphoma rare
Autosomal dominant immune dysregulation syndrome	*CTLA4* dominant negative loss of function {3645}	Autoimmunity, lymphoproliferation, infections	Enriched for EBV+ CHL; CD4+ T-cell–rich extranodal infiltrates {1047}
Regulatory T-cell defects	Lack or dysfunction of CD4+ CD25+ regulatory T cells, increased autoreactive T cells, e.g. *FOXP3* deficiency (IPEX) {1279}	Autoimmunity, lymphoproliferation, infections, inflammatory bowel disease	Predominance of HLH; lymphoma rare

AID, activation-induced cytidine deaminase; ALPS, autoimmune lymphoproliferative syndrome; ALPS-FAS, ALPS with germline *FAS* variants; AT, ataxia–telangiectasia; BL, Burkitt lymphoma; CAEBV, chronic active EBV; CHL, classic Hodgkin lymphoma; DLBCL, diffuse large B-cell lymphoma; EMZL, extranodal marginal zone lymphoma; HLH, haemophagocytic lymphohistiocytosis; HSV, herpes simplex virus; IM, infectious mononucleosis; IPEX, immunodysregulation, polyendocrinopathy, and enteropathy, X-linked; LPD, lymphoproliferative disorder; NBS, Nijmegen breakage syndrome; NLPHL, nodular lymphocyte-predominant Hodgkin lymphoma; PID, primary immunodeficiency disorder; PTCL, peripheral T-cell lymphoma; SCID, severe combined immunodeficiency; SPTCL, subcutaneous panniculitis-like T-cell lymphoma; T-LBL, T-lymphoblastic lymphoma; T-LGLL, T-large granular lymphocyte leukaemia; T-PLL, T-prolymphocytic leukaemia; XLP1, X-linked lymphoproliferative syndrome 1; XMEN, X-linked immunodeficiency with magnesium defect, EBV infection, and neoplasia.

Table 4.51 Pathogenesis, clinical features, and associated lymphoproliferative disorders across major categories of inborn errors of immunity (IEIs) of T and B cells {3967, 3969} (continued)

IEI subtype	Pathogenesis	Clinical features	Lymphoproliferative disorders
ALPS (see *Autoimmune lymphoproliferative syndrome*, p. 646)	Defective T-cell apoptosis, e.g. *FAS* (*TNFRSF6*) deficiency (ALPS-FAS) {1464}; many other mutations result in ALPS-like phenotype {2417}; *KRAS* and *NRAS* somatic mutations can produce an ALPS-like phenotype {3924} as well as myeloid manifestations {525,2938} (see *RASopathies*, p. 812)	Splenomegaly, lymphadenopathy, autoimmunity, lymphoproliferation	CHL, NLPHL, DLBCL, others {3848,2937, 3298,4208}
EBV susceptibility, B lymphoproliferation	Impaired elimination of proliferating EBV+ B cells and *MYC*-rearranged B cells, e.g. *SH2D1A* (XLP1) {770}, ITK deficiency {1674}, CD70 deficiency, CD27 deficiency, MAGT1 deficiency (XMEN) {3372}, CD137 (41BB) deficiency {3779}	Severe primary EBV infection (IM) with HLH; CAEBV	XLP1: BL {2876}, ITK deficiency: EBV+ CHL {3400}, polymorphic or Hodgkin-like LPD often involving lung {361}, CD70 and CD27 deficiency, EBV+ CHL > EBV+ DLBCL {3400,1335}, XMEN: EBV+ DLBCL, CHL, BL {3400}
Other			
SPTCL with germline *HAVCR2* variants	Disinhibited T-cell–mediated immune response due to loss of function of HAVCR2 (TIM3) {1305}	Associated with HLH	Reported in > 50% of patients with SPTCL in predominantly Asian case series {2082, 3274}; can involve mesentery {4336}

AID, activation-induced cytidine deaminase; ALPS, autoimmune lymphoproliferative syndrome; ALPS-FAS, ALPS with germline *FAS* variants; AT, ataxia–telangiectasia; BL, Burkitt lymphoma; CAEBV, chronic active EBV; CHL, classic Hodgkin lymphoma; DLBCL, diffuse large B-cell lymphoma; EMZL, extranodal marginal zone lymphoma; HLH, haemophagocytic lymphohistiocytosis; HSV, herpes simplex virus; IM, infectious mononucleosis; IPEX, immunodysregulation, polyendocrinopathy, and enteropathy, X-linked; LPD, lymphoproliferative disorder; NBS, Nijmegen breakage syndrome; NLPHL, nodular lymphocyte-predominant Hodgkin lymphoma; PID, primary immunodeficiency disorder; PTCL, peripheral T-cell lymphoma; SCID, severe combined immunodeficiency; SPTCL, subcutaneous panniculitis-like T-cell lymphoma; T-LBL, T-lymphoblastic lymphoma; T-LGLL, T-large granular lymphocyte leukaemia; T-PLL, T-prolymphocytic leukaemia; XLP1, X-linked lymphoproliferative syndrome 1; XMEN, X-linked immunodeficiency with magnesium defect, EBV infection, and neoplasia.

characterized; recent prevalence estimates are in the range of 1:1000 to 1:5000 {3968}. Although the majority of patients present early in childhood {4183}, those with CVID may present in young or middle adulthood {4465}. The M:F ratio is 1.5:1, with a male predominance in X-linked entities. Predominantly antibody deficiencies are reported to be most common in Australia, eastern Asia, Egypt, Europe, Latin America, and North America, whereas combined immunodeficiencies are reported as more common in Middle Eastern countries and Tunisia {13}. Most IEI-associated lymphomas (57%) occur in patients with combined immunodeficiencies, particularly those associated with chromosomal instability and predisposition to malignancy (e.g. ataxia–telangiectasia, 29%), followed by B-cell deficiencies (including CVID) (29%) and innate immunodeficiency (14%) {1558}.

Etiology

Among patients with combined immunodeficiency with predisposition to malignancy, 20% of patients with ataxia–telangiectasia and 70% of patients with Nijmegen breakage syndrome develop lymphoma or (T-cell) leukaemia by the age of 20 years {3863, 3702}. Among patients with predominantly antibody deficiency, 4–28% develop lymphoma, often in young to middle adulthood {1066,818,4465,3767}. Biopsy-proven granulomatous disease occurs in about 10% of patients with CVID {4339,1599}. Patients with immune dysregulation with EBV susceptibility and B lymphoproliferation develop lymphoma in childhood or young adulthood; lymphoma develops in 43% of those with CD27/CD70 deficiency {1335}. In autoimmune lymphoproliferative syndrome (ALPS) with a heterozygous *FAS* mutation (ALPS-FAS), about 12% of patients develop LPDs and lymphoma across a broad

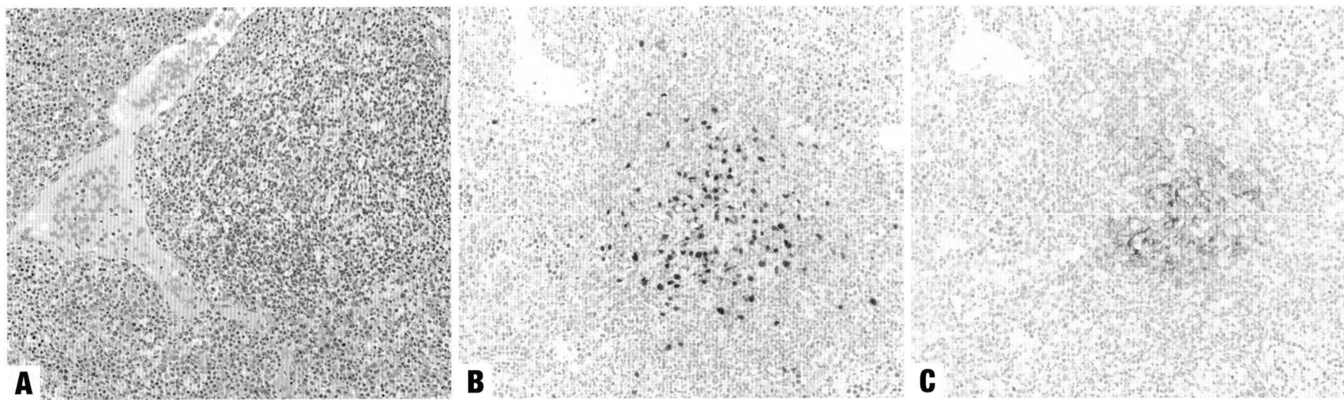

Fig. 4.257 Inborn error of immunity–associated lymphoid proliferations and lymphomas. **A** Bone marrow biopsy of a patient with common variable immunodeficiency reveals numerous well-formed lymphoid aggregates containing scattered larger cells. **B** The bone marrow germinal centre B cells are highlighted on PAX5 immunohistochemistry within a T-cell–rich background in common variable immunodeficiency. **C** CD21 immunohistochemistry demonstrates that the large B cells are reactive germinal centre B cells within poorly formed, T-cell–rich germinal centres.

Table 4.52 Nodal and extranodal lymphoproliferative manifestations of common variable immunodeficiency

Organ system	Common presentation	Histological findings
Lymph nodes	Lymphadenopathy	Enlarged and poorly defined germinal centres, decreased plasma cells, non-necrotizing granulomas {4124}
Gastrointestinal tract	Chronic diarrhoea	Increased intraepithelial lymphocytes with villous blunting; nodular lymphoid hyperplasia; decreased lamina propria plasma cells {865,4323,2500}
Liver	Hepatomegaly	Nodular regenerative hyperplasia with intrasinusoidal cytotoxic T-cell proliferation {3914,4592}; granulomatous disease {1599}
Respiratory tract	Pneumonia, infiltrates on imaging; bronchiectasis	Interstitial lung disease with variable organizing pneumonia, interstitial lymphoid infiltrates, granulomas, and lymphoid hyperplasia {2409,32235152}
Extrapulmonary granulomatous/ CD8+ T-cell–rich lesions {1599,4172}	Sometimes destructive lesions of skin, eye, lymph nodes, spleen, kidney, and other sites	Non-necrotizing granulomas with variable associated T-cell–rich infiltrate; rarely associated with clonal CD8+ lymphoproliferation {1280,2565}
Spleen	Splenomegaly	Reactive germinal centres, sometimes with marginal zone and periarteriolar lymphoid sheath hyperplasia; epithelioid granulomas in red pulp and around follicles {1263}
Peripheral blood	Cytopenias	Large granular lymphocytosis {1617}

age range {3298}. (See Chapter 7: *Genetic tumour syndromes associated with haematolymphoid tumours*.)

Pathogenesis

Defective T-cell–mediated immunosurveillance and an increased susceptibility to EBV infection are associated with both an overall increase in susceptibility to lymphoma, predominantly diffuse large B-cell lymphoma and classic Hodgkin lymphoma, and over-representation of EBV+ LPDs similar to those seen in secondary immunodeficiency/dysregulation settings. Ongoing uncontrolled EBV infection can trigger haemophagocytic lymphohistiocytosis {1747,2227}. A subset of syndromic IEIs, including ataxia–telangiectasia and Nijmegen breakage syndrome, have a direct predisposition to malignancy related to chromosomal instability with an impaired DNA damage response, resulting in predisposition to T-lymphoblastic leukaemia/lymphoma and peripheral T-cell lymphomas (see Table 4.51, p. 574, and Chapter 7: *Genetic tumour syndromes associated with haematolymphoid tumours*).

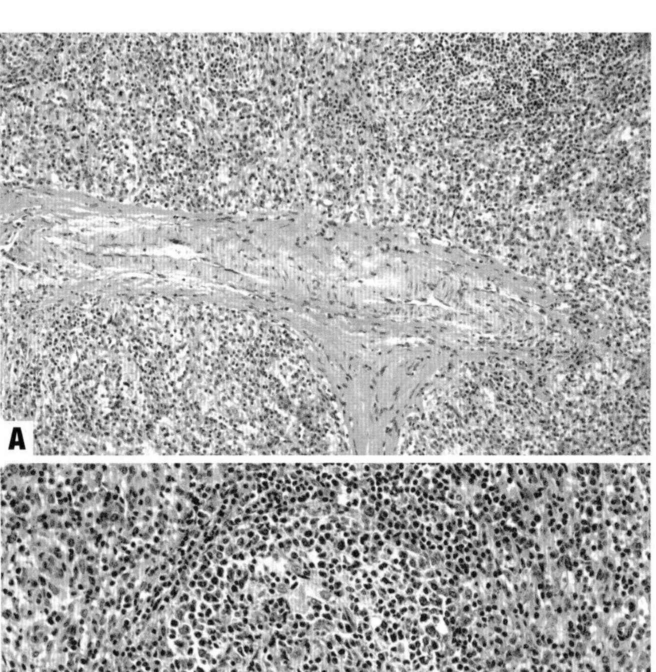

Fig. 4.258 Inborn error of immunity–associated lymphoid proliferations and lymphoma. **A** Splenectomy from a patient with Wiskott–Aldrich syndrome. Bare, thick-walled vessels signify the lack of normal periarteriolar lymphoid sheath T-cell zones. **B** Abnormal follicles show germinal centres with a characteristic lack of splenic marginal zones.

Macroscopic appearance

Firmer, fleshy or necrotic areas of specimens should be sampled to assess for lymphoma.

Histopathology

IEI-LPDs are highly heterogeneous because of the varied specific immune dysfunctions caused by the underlying IEI (see Table 4.51, p. 574); the subtypes below are broad conceptual headings that align with LPDs occurring across immune deficiency/dysregulation settings.

Hyperplasias, EBV-positive mucocutaneous ulcers, and polymorphic LPDs

EBV+ B-cell LPDs occurring in the context of IEIs resemble those seen across immunodeficiency settings {1397}. Histological features of hyperplasias vary according to the underlying IEI. Poorly formed germinal centres and decreased plasma cells are characteristic of CVID {4124}. T-zone hyperplasia with plasmacytosis is typical of ALPS (see *Autoimmune lymphoproliferative syndrome*, p. 646). Granulomatous/CD8+ T-cell–rich lesions are common extranodal features of CVID (see Table 4.52) but are also reported in other IEIs (see Table 4.51, p. 574).

Lymphomas

Predisposition to lymphoma varies according to the IEI (see Table 4.51, p. 574); diffuse large B-cell lymphoma, classic Hodgkin lymphoma, Burkitt lymphoma, and marginal zone lymphoma are common overall {3400}, whereas follicular lymphoma is seen in late-onset IEI {1558}.

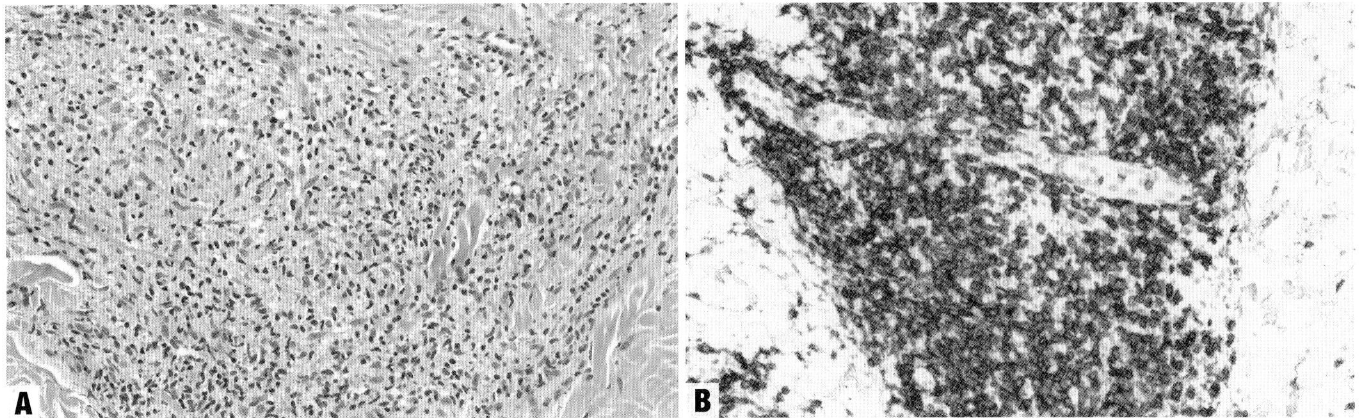

Fig. 4.259 Inborn error of immunity–associated lymphoid proliferations and lymphomas. **A** A cutaneous biopsy of progressive rash in a patient with common variable immunodeficiency reveals dense dermal lymphohistiocytic infiltrates. **B** The dense dermal lymphohistiocytic infiltrate is CD8+ T-cell–rich.

Immunophenotype

Flow cytometry is helpful in lymphoma diagnosis and may provide a clue to the underlying IEI.

Cytology

Cytological preparations are valuable in screening for lymphoma or infection; a diagnosis of lymphoma based on cytological smear preparations alone is not recommended {2134}. HRS-like cells on the cytological preparation raise a broad differential diagnosis similar to that in other immunodeficiency settings, from infectious mononucleosis to EBV+ mucocutaneous ulcer, polymorphic LPD, diffuse large B-cell lymphoma, and classic Hodgkin lymphoma.

Diagnostic molecular pathology

Molecular testing should be performed as indicated in the immunocompetent setting. Caution is indicated in interpreting clonality where expansion of restricted subsets of T and B cells

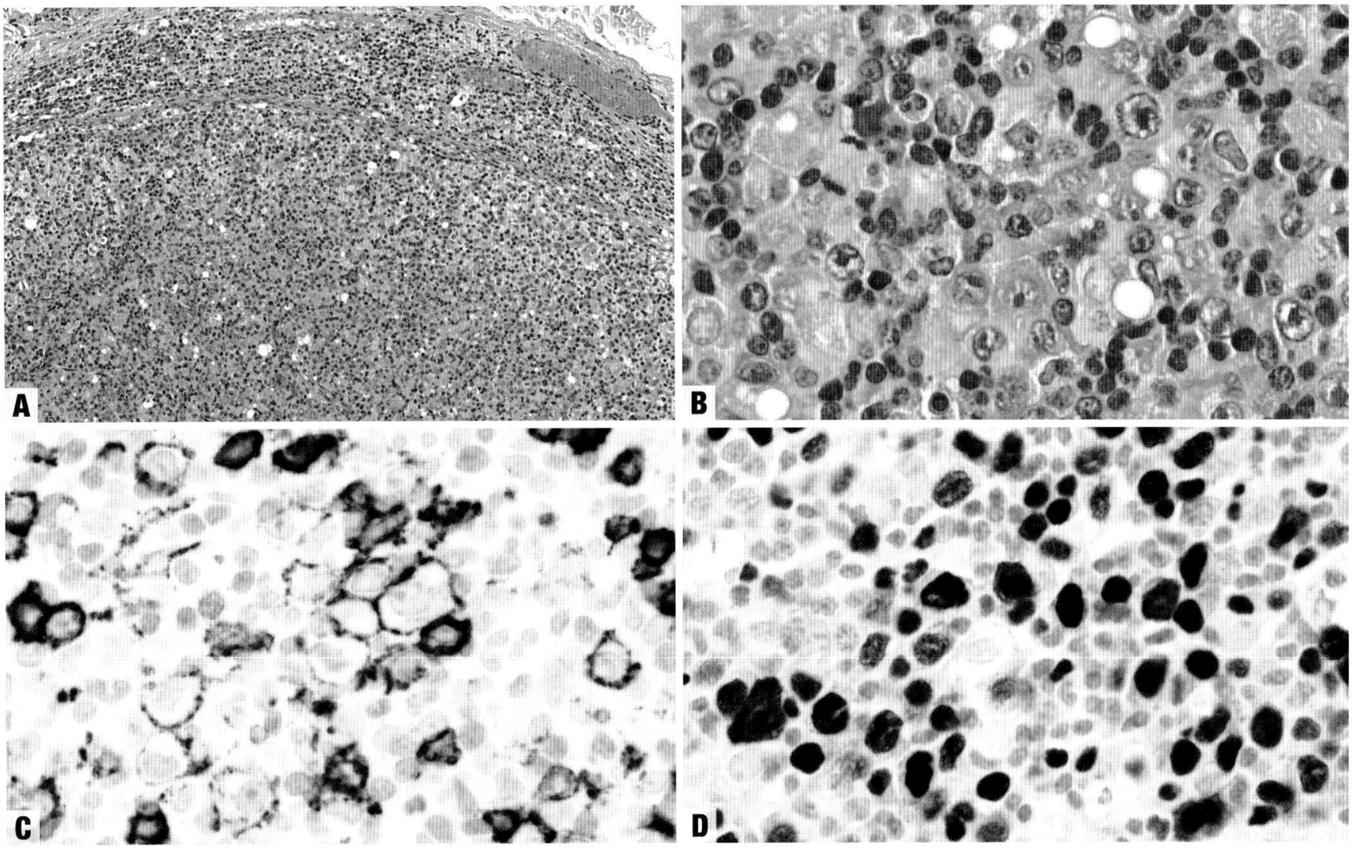

Fig. 4.260 Inborn error of immunity–associated lymphoid proliferations and lymphomas. Chronic active EBV disease in the setting of CD27 deficiency–associated immunodeficiency. **A** There are sheets of medium to large lymphoid cells with prominent nucleoli, which leave a rim of uninvolved lymph node and intact sinusoid. **B** At higher magnification, a proliferation of medium to large lymphoid cells with prominent nucleoli is visible. **C** The large atypical cells are variably CD20+ on immunohistochemistry. **D** Medium-sized to large atypical cells are EBV-positive by EBV-encoded small RNA (EBER) in situ hybridization.

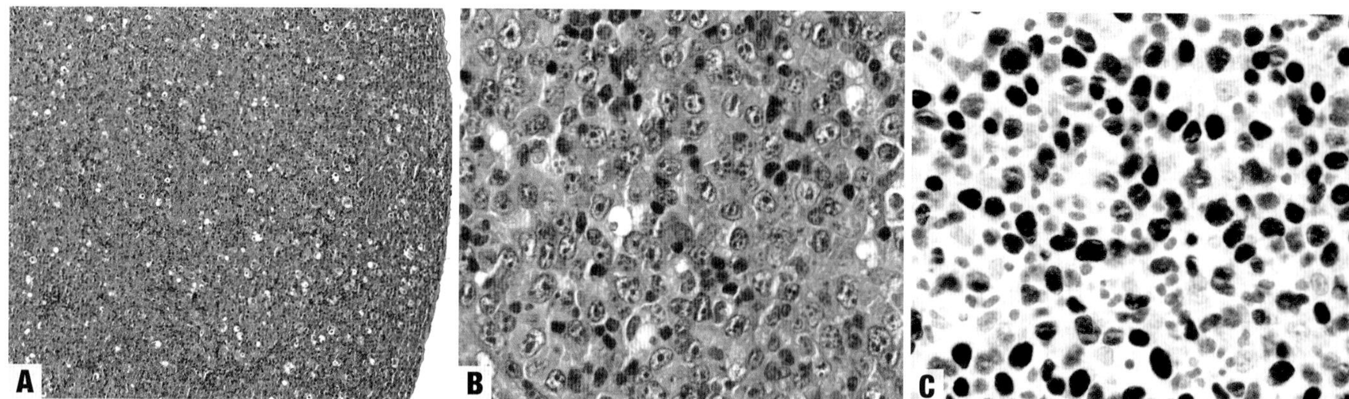

Fig. 4.261 Inborn error of immunity–associated lymphoid proliferations and lymphomas. Diffuse large B-cell lymphoma in the setting of CD27 deficiency–associated immunodeficiency. **A** Sheets of monomorphic atypical large cells efface lymph node architecture. **B** Sheets of large cells have prominent nucleoli and admixed apoptotic debris. **C** EBV-encoded small RNA (EBER) in situ hybridization highlighting sheets of large cells.

in IEI could potentially produce misleading results {3475,4191}. Germline testing is recommended in order to prove the diagnosis of the underlying IEI. It should be noted that IEI-associated mutations overlap with those seen in lymphomas and may be incidentally detected in tumour biopsy specimens tested for somatic mutations, and therefore germline testing should not be performed on tumour biopsy samples.

Essential and desirable diagnostic criteria

Essential: the diagnostic criteria for EBV+ B-cell LPD are the same as those listed in the section *Polymorphic lymphoproliferative disorders arising in immune deficiency/dysregulation* (p. 561); the diagnostic criteria for lymphoma are the same as those for sporadic lymphomas; EBV status must be assessed, and the immunodeficiency background (IEI) should be mentioned; a diagnosis of a granulomatous and/or CD8+ T-cell–rich lesion requires exclusion of an infectious etiology or occult malignancy, such as T-cell/histocyte–rich B-cell lymphoma or overt T-cell lymphoma.

Desirable: molecular classification, including germline genetic testing for the underlying IEI.

Staging

Lymphoma staging is performed and reported according to the diagnosis-appropriate staging system, such as the Lugano Classification (modified Ann Arbor staging system) or the revised International Pediatric Non-Hodgkin Lymphoma Staging System (IPNHLSS) {688,3476}.

Prognosis and predictionw

The prognosis varies markedly, both by diagnostic entity and by IEI background. Although chemotherapy with or without rituximab often achieves remission, morbidity and mortality due to infectious complications are high {1558}. When possible, allogeneic stem cell transplantation (alloSCT) can cure both the lymphoma and the underlying IEI {2797}, albeit with an increased risk of LPDs arising in the posttransplant setting and significant alloSCT-related morbidity and mortality rates {1856}.

Hodgkin lymphoma: Introduction

de Jong D
Gujral S

Hodgkin lymphoma (HL) has a venerable history and began as a "disease of the lymph glands and the spleen". The iconic Reed–Sternberg cells, in a milieu whose description was left appropriately vague, formed the definition of the disease. Over the decades, the Reed–Sternberg cells and their mononuclear variants were shown to be derived from germinal-centre B cells. Nodular lymphocyte-predominant HL (NLPHL) has been recognized as a separate clinicopathological entity since the third edition of the WHO classification of haematolymphoid tumours. Despite the similarities between classic HL (CHL), especially the lymphocyte-rich variant, and NLPHL, there is ample clinicopathological, etiological, and pathogenetic evidence that NLPHL is a different neoplasm from CHL. These differences may justify the consideration of removing NLPHL from the parent category of HL in favour of placing it under the category of mature B-cell neoplasms. However, in the short term, to avoid unnecessary confusion in clinical practice, including in clinical trials and protocols, and for clinical and epidemiological research purposes, the use of the original name of NLPHL is retained in the present fifth edition of the classification. The newly suggested name "nodular lymphocyte-predominant B-cell lymphoma" is accepted to be used as a synonym in the interim period, until new terminology can be introduced in future editions of the WHO classification.

Although the basic description of CHL has not changed much since the last century, knowledge about its etiology and pathogenesis has increased exponentially over the years. Biological insights have led to the recognition of an expanding spectrum of grey zones and mimics that lead to diagnostic pitfalls, which have been the subject of professional discussions in the pathology community. These insights have paved the way for redefining the boundaries surrounding CHL. They have also impacted its epidemiology, because cases previously diagnosed as CHL may be differently classified now. Therefore, previously reported information needs to be critically reassessed in the light of the changing diagnostic criteria. Moreover, it should be noted that on the basis of morphology alone, HL may seem by far to be the easiest subtype of lymphoma to diagnose, but it is equally the easiest to misdiagnose.

In the fourth-edition *WHO classification of tumours of haematopoietic and lymphoid tissues*, a group of lymphomas was considered to be formally unclassifiable, with overlapping features between diffuse large B-cell lymphoma and CHL. The term "mediastinal grey zone lymphoma" was introduced but not formally defined. Major efforts on genetic characterization together with clinicopathological studies have elucidated the concept of a continuous biological spectrum between CHL and primary mediastinal B-cell lymphoma, with mediastinal grey zone lymphoma straddling the two. This concept now justifies a definition of mediastinal grey zone lymphoma, a redefinition of CHL, and the boundary between the two. It should be understood, however, that the spectrum is a continuous one, with many shades of grey. The defining criteria are inevitably arbitrary and may be subject to change when novel, objective evidence becomes available.

Lymphoproliferative disorders arising in immune deficiency/dysregulation settings have emerged as another major source of diagnostic difficulty impacting EBV-positive CHL. Proliferations in immune deficiency/dysregulation settings, including HIV, posttransplantation, and iatrogenic immunosuppression settings, may be morphologically and immunophenotypically indistinguishable from CHL. The clinical context and presenting features (e.g. primary extranodal presentation) help to differentiate such proliferations from CHL. Multidisciplinary discussions and optimal communication between pathologists and clinicians are the key to a final interpretation of such cases.

Traditionally, four histological subtypes of CHL are distinguished: nodular sclerosis, mixed-cellularity, lymphocyte-rich, and lymphocyte-depleted. With modern treatment protocols, these subtypes have lost most of their prognostic relevance. However, there is still merit in describing these subtypes to support epidemiological and translational studies, since specific subtypes seem to differ in their underlying biology, as well as perhaps different geographical distributions. Moreover, the differential diagnosis of the various subtypes covers a diverse spectrum, which helps to alert the pathologist to differential diagnostic options and thereby avoid pitfalls in daily practice.

The definition of the entities that have been recognized for years as HL is in flux. This comes at a time when the clinical outcomes for these diseases are considered to be well established. Therefore, the refinement of diagnostic criteria is not due to uncertainty; on the contrary, it reflects a deeper and more complete understanding of CHL. The biological underpinnings of this fascinating group of lymphomas, in which the malignant cells are in the minority and where the myriad subsets of cells in the immune microenvironment play a crucial role in the modulation of the disease, pave the way for improved understanding and classification, as well as guiding diagnostic and therapeutic options for patients.

Classic Hodgkin lymphoma

Borges AM
Anagnostopoulos I
Borchmann P
d'Amore ESG
Delabie J
Diepstra A
Fromm JR
Garcia JF
Hebeda KM
Küppers R
Laskar S
Naresh KN
Nicolae A
Steidl C
Tamaru J
Vielh P

Definition

Classic Hodgkin lymphoma (CHL) is a neoplasm derived from germinal-centre B cells, characterized by a low fraction of tumour cells embedded in a reactive microenvironment rich in immune cells. The large neoplastic Hodgkin and Reed–Sternberg cells show a defective B-cell expression programme.

ICD-O coding

9650/3 Classic Hodgkin lymphoma
9663/3 Classic Hodgkin lymphoma, nodular sclerosis
9652/3 Classic Hodgkin lymphoma, mixed cellularity
9651/3 Classic Hodgkin lymphoma, lymphocyte-rich
9653/3 Classic Hodgkin lymphoma, lymphocyte-depleted

ICD-11 coding

2B30.1Z Classic Hodgkin lymphoma, unspecified
2B30.10 Nodular sclerosis classic Hodgkin lymphoma
2B30.12 Mixed-cellularity classic Hodgkin lymphoma
2B30.11 Lymphocyte-rich classic Hodgkin lymphoma
2B30.13 Lymphocyte-depleted classic Hodgkin lymphoma

Related terminology

Not recommended: Hodgkin disease.

Subtype(s)

Nodular sclerosis classic Hodgkin lymphoma; mixed-cellularity classic Hodgkin lymphoma; lymphocyte-rich classic Hodgkin lymphoma; lymphocyte-depleted classic Hodgkin lymphoma

Localization

CHL mainly involves lymph nodes, with a striking predilection for the supradiaphragmatic nodes. More than 70% of patients with early-stage CHL present with enlarged cervical or supraclavicular lymph nodes, and > 60% have mediastinal involvement. Fewer than 5% of patients present with exclusive infradiaphragmatic involvement of abdominopelvic lymph nodes and/or spleen; these sites are often involved in high-stage disease. Mediastinal and subdiaphragmatic sites are commonly encountered in the nodular sclerosis and mixed-cellularity subtypes, respectively. Extranodal sites of involvement in stage IV disease include the lung (21%), bone (15%), liver (10%), and bone marrow (9%) (German Hodgkin Study Group [GHSG] database) {3053}. Primary extranodal involvement, in sites such as the skin, gastrointestinal tract, Waldeyer ring, and CNS, is rare and should prompt consideration of alternative diagnoses and evaluation for an underlying immunodeficiency, especially HIV/AIDS, in which setting advanced-stage disease and extranodal

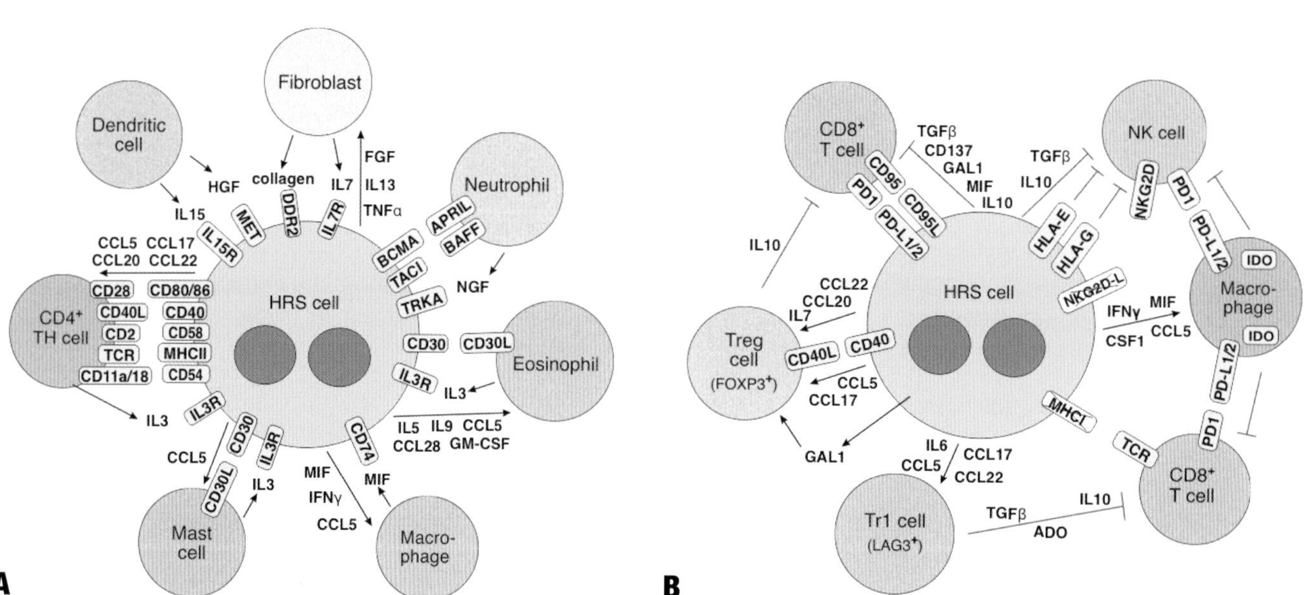

Fig. 4.262 Pathogenesis of classic Hodgkin lymphoma. **A** Cellular interactions in the classic Hodgkin lymphoma microenvironment supporting HRS cell survival and/or proliferation. HRS cells secrete a multitude of cytokines and chemokines to attract other immune cells into the lymphoma microenvironment. Some factors also support the survival, proliferation, and/or specific differentiation processes of the attracted cells {4356,2386}. **B** Main immune evasion strategies of HRS cells. Besides the attraction of T regulatory (Treg and Tr1) cells and macrophages, which have inhibitory effects on cytotoxic cells, HRS cells also directly suppress cytotoxic CD8+ T cells and NK cells by the expression of inhibitory surface receptors and the secretion of immunosuppressive factors {4356,2386}. ADO, adenosine; HGF, hepatocyte growth factor; IDO, indoleamine 2,3-dioxygenase; MIF, macrophage migration inhibitory factor.

involvement may be seen more frequently {2759,3056,3798} (see the sections on lymphoid proliferations and lymphomas associated with immune deficiency and dysregulation, p. 549).

Clinical features

Patients usually present with painless, firm peripheral lymphadenopathy, with characteristic contiguous nodal involvement. About 20% of patients with localized disease and 70% with advanced-stage disease have systemic B symptoms. Bulky mediastinal disease may cause persistent cough, shortness of breath, or even superior vena cava syndrome. Less frequently observed is pruritus. Alcohol-induced pain of affected lymph node regions is a rare but characteristic symptom in CHL. Paraneoplastic phenomena including autoimmune haemolysis, ichthyosis, neuropathy, and cerebellar degeneration have been infrequently described as the initial presentation. Anaemia, leukocytosis with neutrophilia, lymphocytopenia, and elevated C-reactive protein are the most frequently encountered laboratory findings.

Epidemiology

The incidence of CHL varies. Higher rates are observed in groups with a higher socioeconomic index {1162}. An incidence of 2.63 cases per 100 000 person-years {3711} has been reported in the US SEER data. CHL has a slight male predominance, with the exception of nodular sclerosis CHL (NSCHL), which has a slight female predominance. Incidence rates also vary with age; it is a rare disease in children and shows a first peak (~4 cases per 100 000 person-years) in young adults aged 25–35 years and a second peak starting at 60 years, in the USA (SEER incidence rates 2014–2018) {1040}. CHL displays this bimodal age distribution in White and Asian/Pacific Islander populations, but not in Black or Hispanic populations {1099}. The incidence of CHL increases with socioeconomic living standards in general and within a given population with a higher socioeconomic status {755}. There is a 2.55-fold increased risk of developing CHL after infectious mononucleosis in adolescence, which is most pronounced shortly after the infection but remains increased as long as 20 years later {1597}. Mixed-cellularity CHL (MCCHL) is seen in children mostly in low- and middle-income countries. In

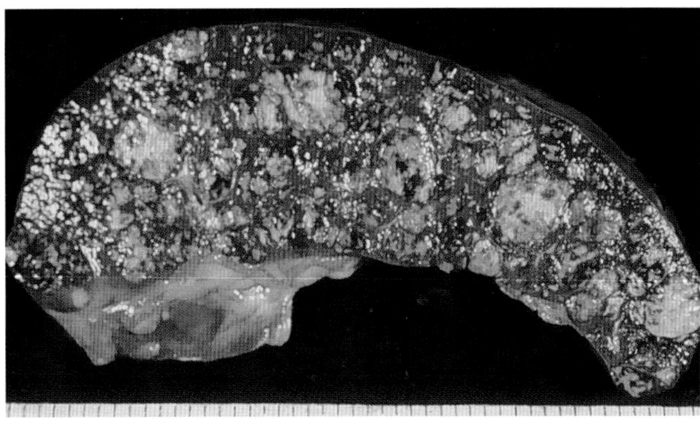

Fig. 4.263 Classic Hodgkin lymphoma, mixed cellularity. Splenectomy specimen of a patient with classic Hodgkin lymphoma, mixed cellularity, showing extensive tumour infiltration with confluent tumour nodules.

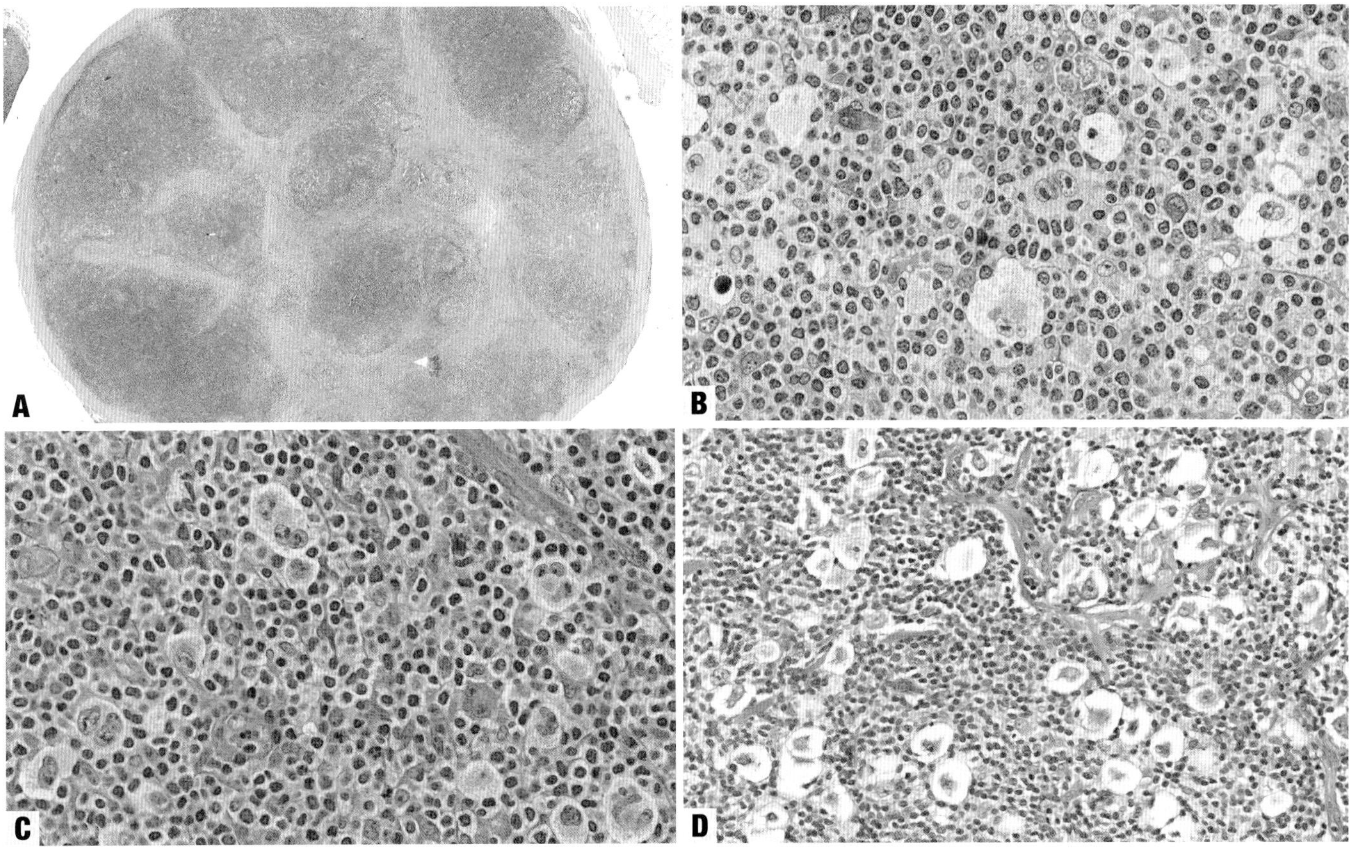

Fig. 4.264 Classic Hodgkin lymphoma, nodular sclerosis. **A** Low-power histology shows fibrous septa. **B** The infiltrate consists of typical HRS cells with conspicuous nucleoli and abundant cytoplasm admixed with reactive immune cells. **C** Polymorphic HRS cells. **D** Numerous lacunar cells show smaller nucleoli and retraction of the cytoplasm upon fixation.

general, the risk of MCCHL steadily increases with age. In a retrospective analysis of the US SEER database, of 21 372 patients with CHL reported between 1992 and 2011, the lymphocyte-rich, mixed-cellularity, lymphocyte-depleted, nodular sclerosis, and not-further-classified types of CHL accounted for 5.8%, 18.9%, 1.5%, 58.1%, and 15.7%, respectively {1040}. It should be noted that the defining criteria of CHL and its subtypes have been subject to change during and after the monitoring period of this study, impacting on epidemiological features. For specific epidemiological aspects of CHL in the setting of immunodeficiencies, including HIV/AIDS and immunosenescence, see *Lymphomas arising in immune deficiency/dysregulation*, p. 568).

Together, these observations indicate that environmental factors play a role in the development of CHL. In addition, both geographical clustering and familial aggregation have been described {2828}.

Etiology

The etiology of CHL remains elusive. However, there is strong evidence that latent EBV infection drives malignant transformation in EBV-positive CHL. In young individuals, primary EBV infection is associated with a higher incidence of EBV-positive CHL, usually 5–10 years later {1596}. In low- and middle-income countries, EBV is usually acquired at a young age and, accordingly, CHL presenting in childhood is often EBV-positive. The delay in primary EBV infection in countries with a higher socioeconomic status results in a small incidence peak in early adulthood. Apart from the peak in young people, the incidence of EBV-positive CHL steadily increases with age. As most adults carry EBV, a gradually declining immune system (immunosenescence) probably explains this phenomenon. EBV-positive CHL is also observed in patients with acquired immunodeficiency or those with solid-organ transplants, albeit that with the changing criteria for immunodeficiency-associated lymphoproliferative disorders, fewer cases are being diagnosed as CHL than in the past. In addition, EBV-positive CHL is strongly associated with HLA-A*01, an allele that cannot present EBV antigenic peptides, whereas HLA-A*02 is protective and can induce anti-EBV immune responses {953,2959,1598}. The mixed-cellularity and lymphocyte-depleted CHL subtypes are most frequently EBV-positive, although any of the subtypes may be positive.

Much less is known about the etiology of EBV-negative CHL. This group follows a different age distribution from that of EBV-positive CHL, with a steady increase until the peak in middle age and a gradual decline in older age. EBV-negative CHL is most frequently of the nodular sclerosis subtype. Genome-wide analyses have identified susceptibility loci in HLA that differ between EBV-positive and EBV-negative cases, as well as susceptibility variants in a variety of immune system–related gene loci {1075,4128,1227,3868}. Genetic susceptibility probably explains the observed familial clustering of CHL and the high concordance in monozygotic twins {1974,763}. Most data on etiology are derived from western Europe and North America.

Pathogenesis

The pathogenesis of CHL is complex and not fully understood. It involves genomic alterations intrinsic to the neoplastic HRS cells, an intense crosstalk of neoplastic HRS cells with the abundant tumour microenvironment, and latent EBV infection in a subset of cases. The binucleated or multinucleated Reed–Sternberg cells are generated from Hodgkin cells through a process of incomplete cytokinesis {3394}. The B-cell origin of HRS cells was elucidated by demonstration of monoclonal IG gene rearrangements in microdissected neoplastic cells, and the high load of somatic mutations in their rearranged IGHV genes, which indicated a germinal-centre B-cell derivation {1883}. Detection of destructive somatic IGHV mutations in 25% of cases led to the concept that HRS cells in general develop from germinal-centre B cells that have acquired deleterious mutations that would normally lead to apoptosis in the germinal centre, but that are rescued

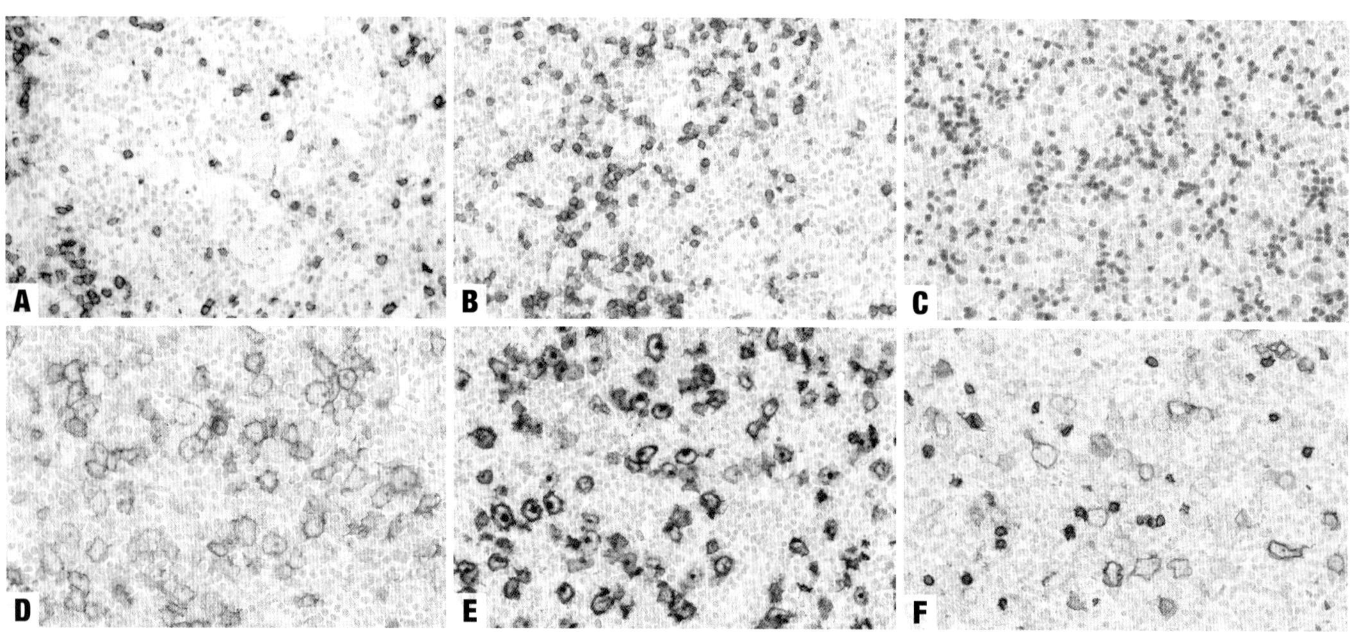

Fig. 4.265 Classic Hodgkin lymphoma, nodular sclerosis, typical immunophenotype. The neoplastic cells show a defective B-cell phenotype, with a lack of CD20 (**A**) and an absence of CD79a expression (**B**). **C** PAX5 shows typical weak expression. HRS cells are positive for CD30 (**D**) and CD15 with membrane and perinuclear dot-like staining (**E**). **F** A subset of HRS cells may express CD20 with variable and weak intensity.

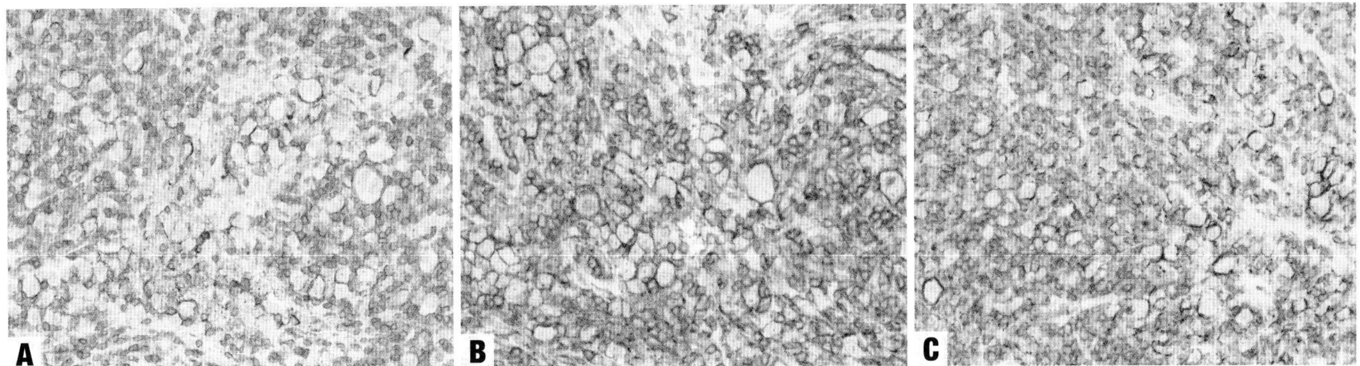

Fig. 4.266 Classic Hodgkin lymphoma, nodular sclerosis, aberrant immunophenotype. Nodular sclerosis classic Hodgkin lymphoma, with a subset of HRS cells showing aberrant expression of CD3 (**A**), CD4 (**B**), and CD2 (**C**) in a case rich in neoplastic cells. Staining for PAX5 (not shown) and the presence of monoclonal IGH and polyclonal TRG gene rearrangements further support the diagnosis.

by pathogenic survival signals such as those from EBV infection {1883}. At the time of diagnosis, HRS cells are remarkably aberrant at the genetic, metabolic, and morphological levels and have lost most of their B-cell phenotype {3651}. Recurrent chromosomal gains/losses and somatic mutations leading to constitutive activation of oncogenic signalling pathways (in particular NF-κB and JAK/STAT) and immune evasion are considered characteristic of CHL biology and essential for HRS cell survival and proliferation. Cytogenetically, besides aneuploidy and hypertetraploidy {4333}, HRS cells show recurrent chromosomal imbalances, including gains of 2p13 (*REL*), 9p24.1 (*CD274* [*PDL1*], *PDCD1LG2* [*PDL2*], *JAK2*), and 17q21 (*MAP3K14*), and loss of 6q23-q24 (*TNFAIP3*) {3628,1826,2562,3825,1404}. In addition, genetic studies have revealed recurrent somatic mutations in components of the NF-κB pathway (*TNFAIP3*, *NFKBIA*, *REL*), the JAK/STAT pathway (*SOCS1*, *PTPN1*, *STAT6*, *STAT3*, *CSF2RB*) {3628,4357,1451,3390,4014,2581,4356}, and regulators of immune escape (e.g. inactivating mutations in the gene encoding the MHC class I component B2M and the MHC class II transactivator gene *CIITA* [*C2TA*]) {3390,3824}. Other signalling pathways important in CHL pathogenesis include MAPK/ERK, AP-1, PI3K/AKT, and NOTCH1 {4356}.

HRS cells release a large array of chemokines (e.g. CCL17 [TARC], CCL5), cytokines (e.g. IL-5, IL-7, IL-13), and growth factors (macrophage colony–stimulating factor, FGF2) to attract and modulate CD4+ regulatory and helper T cells, myeloid cells (eosinophils, macrophages, mast cells), and stromal cells (fibroblasts, mesenchymal stromal cells) {2386,4356}. This milieu is not reactive to the neoplastic cells but rather is symbiotic, promoting HRS cell survival, angiogenesis, and host immune system evasion through cytokines and cell surface ligands. HRS cell immune escape is facilitated by the protective shield conferred by CD4+ T-cell rosettes surrounding the HRS cells, polarization of CD4+ T cells towards T regulatory (Treg) cells, monocyte differentiation into anti-inflammatory M2 macrophages, and secretion of immunosuppressive cytokines (IL-10, TGF-β) {2386,4356}. Of paramount importance is the expression of the immune checkpoint ligands, PDL1 and PDL2, by HRS cells {1404,3446}. Interference in the interaction between PD1 and PDL1/PDL2 is currently therapeutically exploited.

EBV-infected HRS cells show a type II latency programme, which includes expression of EBV-encoded small RNAs (EBERs), EBNA1, LMP1, and LMP2A {1884}. LMP1 is an oncogene and mimics an active CD40 receptor, whereas LMP2A mimics B-cell receptor signalling, i.e. these two viral proteins can replace two main survival signals for germinal-centre B cells {1995,2514}.

Macroscopic appearance

Involved lymph nodes are enlarged, usually discrete, and firm in consistency. The gross appearance varies with the histological subtype. The nodular sclerosis subtype may be grossly or subtly nodular, and involved lymph nodes are not uncommonly matted together. The mixed-cellularity and lymphocyte-rich subtypes may show no specific alteration, being homogeneous and fleshy in appearance. Areas of necrosis may be present. Splenic involvement usually shows scattered nodules, although large masses are sometimes seen. Rare cases can be confined to the thymus and can be associated with cystic change. After

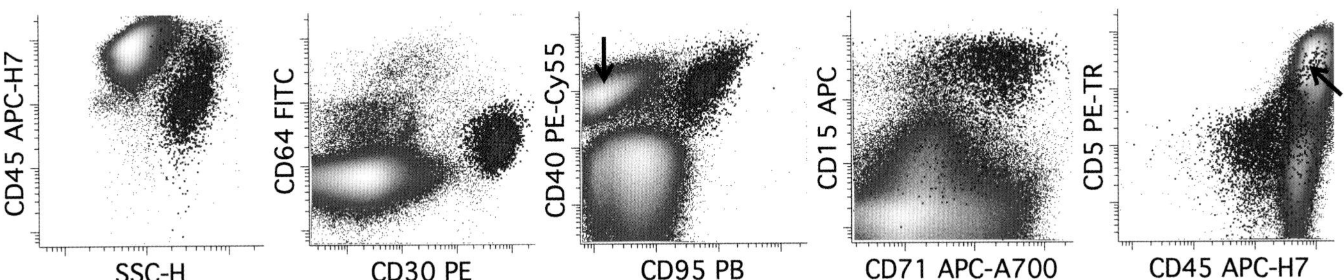

Fig. 4.267 Immunophenotyping of HRS cells in a case of classic Hodgkin lymphoma by flow cytometry. HRS cells (red) show expression of CD15, CD30, CD40 (at level of reactive B cells, vertical arrow), CD45 (weak), CD71, and FAS (CD95), without expression of CD20 (data not shown) or CD64 (apparent expression due to autofluorescence). The large population of HRS cells shows little to no CD5 expression. A small subset of HRS cells (oblique arrow) shows CD5 expression at the level of reactive T cells, indicative of HRS cells with bound T cells (T-cell rosetting).

therapy, it is not uncommon to find a persistent fibrotic mass that resembles the appearance of a lymph node treated for a chronic infection, such as tuberculosis.

Histopathology

The histopathological descriptions of CHL have essentially not changed since the nodular lymphocyte-predominant variant was defined and separately classified. CHL is defined by the presence of mononuclear Hodgkin cells and binucleated or multinucleated Reed–Sternberg cells within a characteristic cellular microenvironment. Lymph nodes may be totally, partially, or focally involved. When involvement is subtle, distinguishing genuine HRS cells in the appropriate milieu becomes important. CHL shows a paucity of the defining HRS cells in the affected lymph node, which may constitute 0.1–10% of the cells in the infiltrate. One may, therefore, have to search extensively to locate an HRS cell. It is possible to find the classic Reed–Sternberg cell in almost every case, but they are usually not as numerous as the mononuclear Hodgkin cells.

HRS cells display various forms. They are at least four to five times the size of background lymphocytes and have large nuclei with prominent eosinophilic nucleoli. The prototypical Reed–Sternberg cell, which has at least two nuclei with large, eosinophilic, centrally placed nucleoli surrounded by a perinuclear halo, giving it the classic owl-eye appearance, may represent a minority of the neoplastic population. A Hodgkin cell usually has a round nucleus with a prominent nucleolus. Lacunar cells are characteristic of NSCHL. A common finding is the presence of mummified cells with a dense cytoplasm and pyknotic nuclei; these represent apoptotic forms.

The cellular microenvironment surrounding the HRS cells is non-neoplastic and is increasingly being recognized as an important factor in the biology and progression of CHL, as well as in the prognosis and response to therapy. It varies with the subtype and EBV status. The background lymphocytes in most cases are T cells accompanied by variable numbers of eosinophils, histiocytes, neutrophils, and plasma cells. Epithelioid granulomas may be focal or may sometimes dominate the picture. The lymphocyte-rich subtype may include abundant reactive B cells of mantle cell type.

Core needle biopsy

Most descriptions of the histopathology have been made on the findings of whole-node biopsies. There is, however, an increasing trend to use core needle biopsies. This makes diagnosis challenging because of the scarcity and uneven distribution of HRS cells. It is also difficult to assess features, such as fibrosis, which are important for subtyping the nodular sclerosis variant. Epithelioid cell granulomas, when present, may lead to a mistaken diagnosis of mycobacterial disease, especially in FNA smears.

Subtypes

CHL has traditionally been subclassified into four groups: NSCHL, MCCHL, lymphocyte-rich CHL (LRCHL), and lymphocyte-depleted CHL (LDCHL). Typical examples of each subtype are readily identifiable on histology; however, there are some overlaps. Subtyping CHL may not be relevant for modern therapeutic management, but subtypes seem to reflect biological entities and should be recognized and reported whenever possible, with the provision that this may not be possible or even advisable on limited material.

NSCHL is characterized by sclerotic bands that surround one to several nodules containing HRS cells and the reactive infiltrate. It is usually also associated with capsular fibrosis {4291}. Lacunar cells are characteristic and result from retraction of the cytoplasm during fixation, resulting in the appearance of neoplastic cells residing in holes or lacunae {3258}. Typical HRS cells are common, and Hodgkin cells with pleomorphic morphology can be seen. The inflammatory infiltrate comprises eosinophils, histiocytes, small lymphocytes, and occasionally neutrophils. Remnant reactive lymphoid follicles and focal necrosis can also be observed in this variant {2517}. In rare instances, the cellular background resembles LRCHL. Cases of NSCHL with numerous neoplastic cells in sheets are called the syncytial variant. Necrosis is common in areas with numerous tumour cells. Although NSCHL was historically graded on the basis of the relative number of neoplastic cells {2517,2465}, this practice is now obsolete.

In MCCHL, the lymph node architecture is diffusely effaced. Compared with other CHL subtypes, binucleated or multinucleated Reed–Sternberg cells are relatively frequent. HRS cells are diffusely scattered in a mixed inflammatory infiltrate comprising small lymphocytes, histiocytes, eosinophils, and plasma cells. The abundance of these immune cells varies from case to case. Not infrequently, and especially in EBV-positive cases, epithelioid histiocytes or granulomas are seen. Fibrosis, when present, is finely reticular in nature and not prominent {2445}. Fibrous septa and capsular fibrosis are absent.

LRCHL is characterized by a nodular or, less commonly, diffuse infiltrate with abundant small lymphocytes, and it virtually

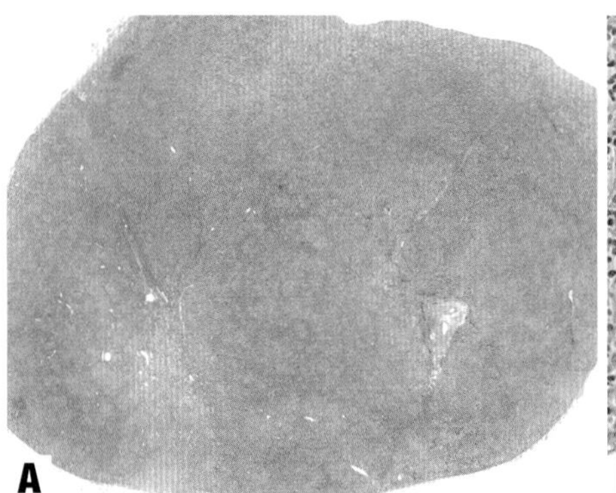

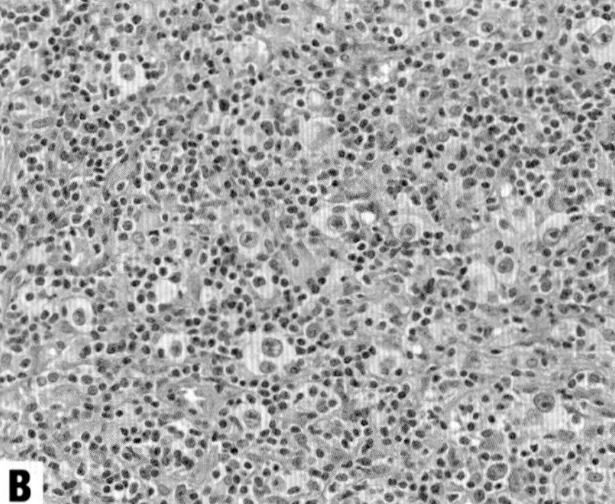

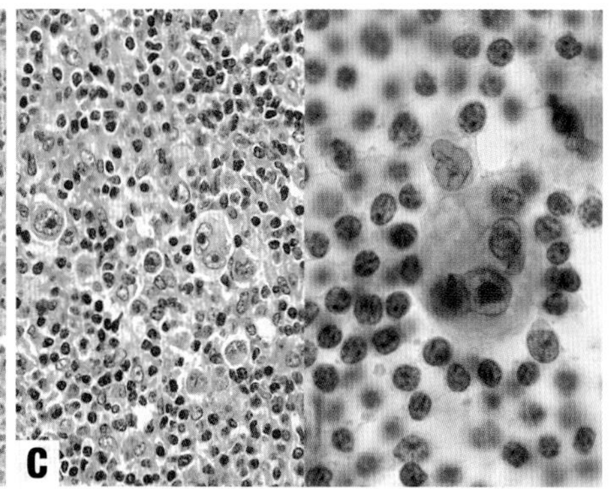

Fig. 4.268 Classic Hodgkin lymphoma, mixed cellularity. **A** Low-power histology showing a diffuse, vaguely nodular architecture. **B** Higher-power magnification showing an inflammatory microenvironment comprising small lymphocytes, histiocytes, eosinophils, and plasma cells. **C** HRS cell morphology in histology and cytology.

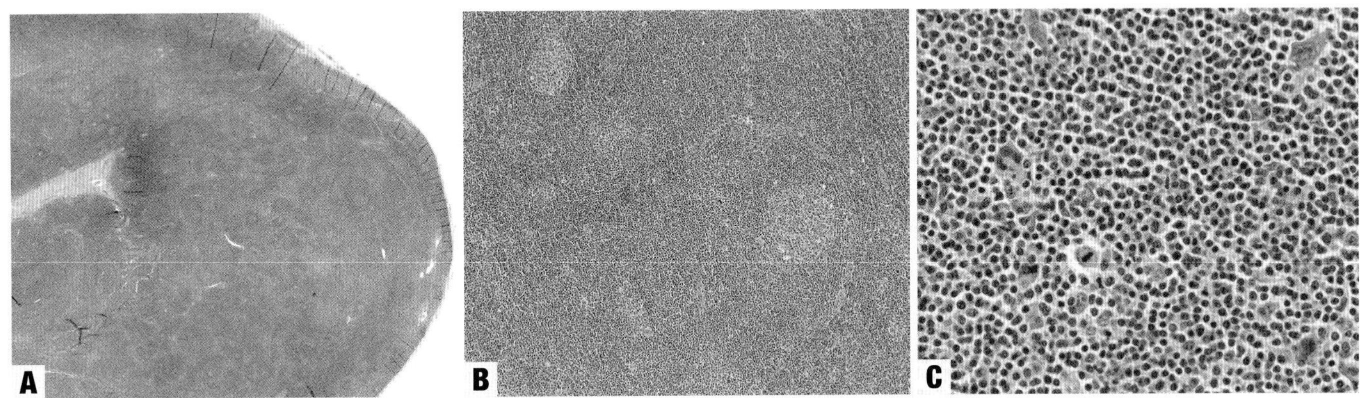

Fig. 4.269 Lymphocyte-rich classic Hodgkin lymphoma. **A** Histologically, the lymph node architecture is altered by a nodular lymphoid proliferation. **B** The nodules show expanded mantle zones and regressed germinal centres. **C** Scattered HRS cells are observed throughout the nodules, which are mainly composed of small lymphocytes; eosinophils and neutrophils are absent.

lacks neutrophils and eosinophils. In nodular cases, the nodules encompass most of the involved tissue so that the interfollicular zones are compressed. The nodules are composed of small B lymphocytes and may harbour germinal centres that are relatively small or regressed and usually eccentrically located. HRS cells are predominantly found within the nodules but consistently outside the germinal centres. A proportion of the HRS cells may resemble lymphocyte-predominant cells or mononuclear lacunar cells. Eosinophils and/or neutrophils are absent from the nodules; if present, they are located in the interfollicular zones in small numbers. In diffuse cases, the small lymphocytes of the cellular background may be admixed with histiocytes with or without epithelioid features. This subtype can easily be confused with nodular lymphocyte-predominant Hodgkin lymphoma. In the past, approximately 30% of cases initially diagnosed as nodular lymphocyte-predominant Hodgkin lymphoma were later found to be LRCHL {109}. The demonstration of an immunophenotype typical for classic HRS cells is essential in making this distinction. In rare cases, small lymphocytic lymphoma may show scattered classic HRS cells, mimicking LRCHL.

LDCHL is rare (≤ 2%) and is strongly associated with EBV. Like MCCHL, it has a diffuse growth pattern, pleomorphic HRS cell features, and frequent association with EBV {4291}. LDCHL and MCCHL may therefore represent two ends of the same spectrum {1036}. The defining features of LDCHL are a predominance of HRS cells and a scarcity of background lymphocytes. Eosinophils and plasma cells are equally scarce, and fibrous bands are absent. Two patterns can be observed, one with sheets of HRS cells and the other with diffuse fibrosis and abundant histiocytes {3758}.

Immunophenotype

The HRS cells of CHL express CD30 in almost all cases {3649, 3827,3829} and CD15 in the majority of cases {1652,3830}. Both CD30 and CD15 are typically present in a membranous pattern,

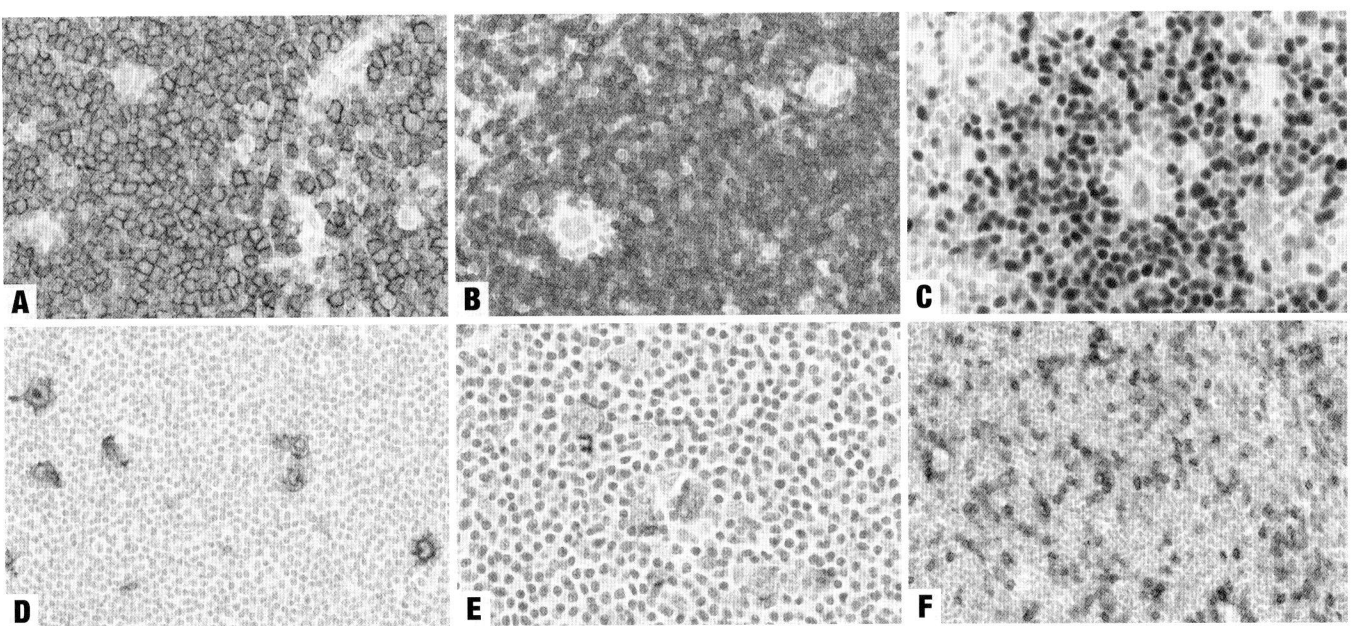

Fig. 4.270 Lymphocyte-rich classic Hodgkin lymphoma immunophenotype. Scattered HRS cells negative for CD20 (**A**) and CD79a (**B**), and weakly positive for PAX5, are noticed in a background rich in small mantle zone B cells (**C**). The neoplastic lymphocytes strongly express CD30 (**D**) and IRF4 (MUM1) (not shown) and are also highlighted with LMP1 (**E**). **F** HRS cells are encircled by rosettes of non-atypical PD1-positive T cells.

with accentuation in the Golgi area of the cytoplasm. However, CD15 may also be expressed in a cytoplasmic granular pattern. CD30 expression is generally uniform across all HRS cells, whereas CD15 expression can be focal. HRS cells are usually negative for CD45 and are consistently negative for immunoglobulin J chain, immunoglobulin heavy and light chains, and CD68R {718,1115}.

The B-cell nature of HRS cells is best demonstrated by PAX5, which is expressed in almost all cases (~95%). PAX5 expression is characteristically weaker than in reactive B cells. Most of the B-cell programme is downregulated in CHL. In 30–40% of cases, CD20 may be detectable but is usually of varied intensity and present only on a minority of the neoplastic cells {3617,4596}. Other B-cell–associated antigens, such as CD19 and CD79a, are less often expressed. The expression of B-cell transcription factors such as OCT2, BOB1, PU.1 and BCL6 is downregulated in most cases {2891}. OCT2 and BOB1 are both negative in nearly 90% of cases and PU.1 in almost all cases {2396,4048}. In rare cases, there is expression of either OCT2 or BOB1 (but usually not both) in HRS cells {3758}. In LRCHL, these B-cell transcription factors are more frequently expressed than in the other CHL subtypes {2891}. Immunoglobulin staining is typically negative in HRS cells. Occasionally, staining may be seen for both light chains in the same cell, related to absorption from free protein in the tissue extracellular matrix. In such cases, kappa or lambda mRNA cannot be demonstrated in HRS cells. The transcription factor IRF4 (MUM1) is consistently and strongly expressed in HRS cells, but the plasma cell–associated adhesion molecule CD138 is consistently negative {485}. Germinal-centre cell markers other than BCL6, which may be weakly positive, are rarely expressed in CHL.

The association with EBV demonstrated by in situ hybridization for EBER is variable. EBV-infected HRS cells express LMP1 and EBNA1 without EBNA2, a pattern characteristic of type II EBV latency {1559,1560,4133,4349,2695}.

Aberrant expression of one or more T-cell antigens is noted in the HRS cells in a minority (~5%) of cases. Expression may be seen in a membranous and/or cytoplasmic location {4111, 159,4211,859}. In these cases, CD4 and CD2 are the more frequently expressed, and CD3 is less common. Similarly, expression of cytotoxic molecules is rarely encountered. Most HRS cells express proliferation-associated nuclear antigens, such as PCNA or MIB1 {2902,1324}. Nuclear expression of GATA3 is present in about 80% of CHLs {1964}. HRS cells in most cases express fascin {3539}. Strong expression of PDL1 in a majority of HRS cells is seen in over 40% of cases {4249}. Furthermore, most cases of CHL are negative for CD23 {3539,59}. Immunohistochemistry showing nuclear expression of STAT6 with or without cytoplasmic staining in HRS cells is a useful marker seen in about 80% of cases {4171}. These additional immunohistochemical markers may be useful in diagnostically challenging cases.

The background small lymphoid cells in CHL include both B cells and T cells that vary in number among histological subtypes. B cells are most prominent in LRCHL and least prominent in LDCHL. The small B cells in LRCHL represent expanded mantle zones (positive for IgM and IgD). The follicular architecture of the B-cell nodules in LRCHL is highlighted by a dense meshwork of CD21+ follicular dendritic cells. The cells forming rosettes around the HRS cells are usually CD4+ T cells in all subtypes of CHL. Rosettes with PD1+ T cells (T follicular helper [TFH] cells) surround the neoplastic cells in nearly half of the cases of LRCHL {2891}. Background cells also include CD15-expressing eosinophils and neutrophils and CD163/CD68-positive macrophages {2042}.

Differential diagnosis

CHL must be distinguished from both nodular lymphocyte-predominant Hodgkin lymphoma and a variety of T- and B-cell proliferations, both reactive and neoplastic, that present with large cells that express CD30 and resemble HRS cells. Non-Hodgkin lymphomas with HRS cells should not be considered as composite lymphoma (see Table 4.53).

T-cell/histiocyte–rich large B-cell lymphoma (THRLBCL): Given its background rich in histiocytes and small lymphocytes, THRLBCL may show morphological overlap with either MCCHL or LRCHL. The large neoplastic cells, however, exhibit a full B-cell immunophenotype. Expression of BCL6 and a lack of CD15 and CD30 support THRLBCL, whereas EBV positivity argues against this diagnosis.

Infectious mononucleosis (IM): In IM, architectural distortion of the lymph node is more subtle, with paracortical expansion and many immunoblasts in a background of smaller lymphocytes and plasma cells. Although a proportion of immunoblasts may resemble HRS cells, most large cells have features of conventional immunoblasts. HRS-like cells in IM are usually CD45+, CD20+, CD30+, CD15−, EBER+. IM immunoblasts including the Reed–Sternberg–like cells show polytypic expression of kappa and lambda light chains. The smaller lymphoid cells in the background show a predominance of CD8+ T cells in IM, whereas CD4+ reactive T cells predominate in CHL. Smaller cells of a range of sizes are EBV+ in IM, whereas EBV is predominantly found in the HRS cells of EBV+ CHL, with only rare EBV+ small lymphocytes {2431}.

EBV-positive diffuse large B-cell lymphoma (DLBCL): EBV-positive DLBCL, particularly of the polymorphic subtype, may show morphological overlap with CHL, given the morphology of the tumour cells and the composition of the immune microenvironment. However, EBV+ DLBCL lacks the eosinophils and rosette formation by T cells usually found in CHL. Unlike in CHL, the neoplastic cells in EBV-positive DLBCL show a preserved B-cell expression programme, are CD45 positive, and usually lack CD15.

Mediastinal grey zone lymphoma (MGZL): One of the most difficult lines to draw is between NSCHL and MGZL when the

Table 4.53 Criteria for distinguishing nodular lymphocyte-predominant Hodgkin lymphoma (NLPHL) and T-cell/histiocyte–rich large B-cell lymphoma (THRLBCL) from classic Hodgkin lymphoma (CHL)

Entity	Distinguishing features vs CHL
NLPHL	Nodules lacking residual germinal centres Neoplastic lymphocyte-predominant cells robustly express B-cell lineage markers, variably express EMA and IgD, and typically lack CD30 and CD15
THRLBCL	Lack of nodules Inflammatory microenvironment lacking eosinophils and small B cells, as well as PD1+ T-cell infiltrates and rosettes surrounding neoplastic cells The large cells express pan–B-cell markers, BCL6, and MEF2B, and lack CD30, CD15, and EBV

latter exhibits CHL-like morphology. The difficulty has been compounded by a lack of consistent and universally accepted criteria thus far for MGZL {3578}. A diagnosis of MGZL is favoured over CHL in the mediastinum when preservation of the B-cell programme is seen in the large neoplastic cells, especially when the neoplastic cells are present in sheets (see Table 4.54).

Immune deficiency/dysregulation–associated lymphoproliferative disorders (IDD-LPDs): EBV-positive CHL shares overlapping features with several IDD-LPDs (see Table 4.55). Shared among these entities are the variable proportions and cytological features of immunoblasts, including multinucleated cells that may mimic the HRS cells of CHL. Localization of CHL to lymph nodes and the mediastinum allows the separation of CHL from some IDD-LPDs. Detailed clinical evaluation, staging, and information on medical history are important considerations in the separation of these entities from most cases of CHL.

Nodal TFH cell lymphoma, angioimmunoblastic type (nTFHL-AI), and other nodal TFH cell lymphomas: nTFHL-AI can show reactive immunoblasts or clonally expanded large B cells that may mimic HRS cells and express CD30. These may be variably EBV+. They show variable expression of CD20 but otherwise have a preserved B-cell programme, expressing CD79a, PAX5, OCT2, and BOB1, and frequently expressing light chains. In a minority of cases, the large cells not only have the morphological features of HRS cells, but they also show the typical immunophenotype of HRS cells (CD30+, CD15+/–, and EBV+/–). HRS-like cells in angioimmunoblastic T-cell lymphoma are rosetted by neoplastic T cells of TFH phenotype and are often accompanied by an increase in more typical B immunoblasts {412}. In contrast, reactive T cells in CHL are typically CD4+ T cells that do not have a TFH phenotype, except in LRCHL where TFH cells often rosette HRS cells (see above). In difficult cases, TR gene rearrangement studies would be required to make the distinction. Detection of characteristic mutations as described in nTFHL-AI, especially the hotspot *RHOA* (p.G17V) and *IDH2* (p.R172) mutations, favour a diagnosis of nTFHL-AI {174,2904} (see Table 4.56).

Peripheral T-cell lymphoma (PTCL) NOS and anaplastic large cell lymphoma: EBV-positive and (more rarely) EBV-negative

Table 4.54 Differential diagnosis between mediastinal grey zone lymphoma (MGZL) and classic Hodgkin lymphoma (CHL) expressing CD20 and/or strong PAX5 in HRS cells

Criterion	Consider CHL	Consider MGZL
CD30	Uniform in HRS cells	Mostly heterogeneous in HRS-like cells
CD15	Positive in at least some HRS cells	Usually negative
B-cell programme	Defective B-cell programme with lack of expression of other B-cell markers	Retained B-cell programme with uniform and strong expression of CD20 and PAX5 in combination with at least one additional B-cell marker (CD19 and CD79a or OCT2 and BOB1)
EBV (LMP or EBER)	Supports the diagnosis	Exceedingly rare in a mediastinal presentation Precludes the diagnosis in non-mediastinal sites

EBER, EBV-encoded small RNA.

Table 4.55 Differential diagnosis of classic Hodgkin lymphoma (CHL) versus lymphoid proliferations and lymphomas associated with immune deficiency and dysregulation (IDD-LPDs)

IDD-LPD type	Typical features of IDD-LPDs that allow separation from CHL
Infectious mononucleosis–like hyperplasia	Localization in tonsils and adenoids (but not lymph nodes) Absence of architectural destruction EBV+ cells range in size from small to large
Polymorphic LPDs	Localization in one or more extranodal sites (but not lymph nodes) EBV+ cells range in size from small to large, including B-cell differentiation stages (small B cells, plasmacytoid cells, plasma cells, and immunoblasts)
EBV-positive mucocutaneous ulcer	Localization of sharply circumscribed ulcers in cutaneous and mucosal sites including the gastrointestinal tract EBV+ cells range in size from small to large
EBV-positive diffuse large B-cell lymphoma	Localization in one or more extranodal sites Presence of sheets or scattered EBV+ large B cells in a T-cell and histiocyte–rich background Immunophenotype of intact B-cell programme in large cells Lack of an inflammatory microenvironment

Table 4.56 Differential diagnosis of classic Hodgkin lymphoma (CHL) versus nodal T follicular helper cell lymphoma, angioimmunoblastic type (nTFHL-AI); nodal T follicular helper cell lymphoma, follicular type (nTFHL-F); peripheral T-cell lymphoma (PTCL) NOS; and anaplastic large cell lymphoma (ALCL)

Entity	Features
nTFHL-AI with HRS cells	Characteristic clinical features and immune manifestations may provide a clue; a large mediastinal mass favours CHL No clear demarcation between areas with HRS-like cells and areas more of typical nTFHL-AI HRS-like cells exhibit a relatively intact B-cell programme (not always) HRS-like cells rosetted by neoplastic T cells with a TFH phenotype; CD10 in T cells is useful when expressed Often many B immunoblasts in addition to HRS cells Flow cytometry: dim sCD3 and CD4/CD10+ or CD4/PD1+ T cells help identify nTFHL-AI Detection of *RHOA* p.G17V or *IDH2* p.R172 variants
nTFHL-F with HRS cells (progressive transformation of germinal centres pattern)	Similar to nTFHL-AI Detection of *RHOA* p.G17V
PTCL-NOS with HRS cells	Atypical features of background cells T-cell immunophenotypic aberrations Often many B immunoblasts in addition to HRS-like cells HRS-like cells are usually CD15–, EBER+/– TR gene clonal rearrangement
ALCL	HRS-like cells and hallmark cells Cohesive or intrasinusoidal growth HRS-like cells are PAX5– and CD15– TR gene clonal rearrangement

EBER, EBV-encoded small RNA; TFH, T follicular helper.

HRS-like cells of B-cell lineage can sometimes be found in PTCL-NOS {3332,1057} and should not be mistaken for CHL or a composite lymphoma. In addition, the neoplastic T cells in some cases of PTCL may have morphological features similar to HRS cells {174}.

The differential diagnosis between ALK-negative anaplastic large cell lymphoma and CHL can be challenging, and the former differs from the latter in its T-cell nature, reflected (among other features) by the clonal TR gene rearrangement and absence of a B-cell immunophenotype, including negative PAX5 expression (with rare exceptions {1154}). HRS-like cells have also been described in lymph nodes of Hodgkin-like adult T-cell leukaemia/lymphoma and can be of B-cell lineage infected with EBV, or of T-cell lineage infected with HTLV-1 {3023,1899}. Most of the Hodgkin-like lymphoproliferations in draining lymph nodes of CD30-positive primary cutaneous lymphoproliferative diseases represent nodal dissemination rather than a second neoplasm. The history of cutaneous lesions is not always available, so establishing a diagnosis may be challenging. The lack of expression of PAX5 is a clue that the lymphoid proliferation does not represent CHL {174}.

The diagnosis of PAX5-negative CHL cases must always be made with caution {3952}. Helpful features for the differential diagnosis are the recognition of atypical features of the T-cell background, and the detection of immunophenotypic aberrations. Clonality analysis for TR gene rearrangements may be necessary in difficult cases {174}.

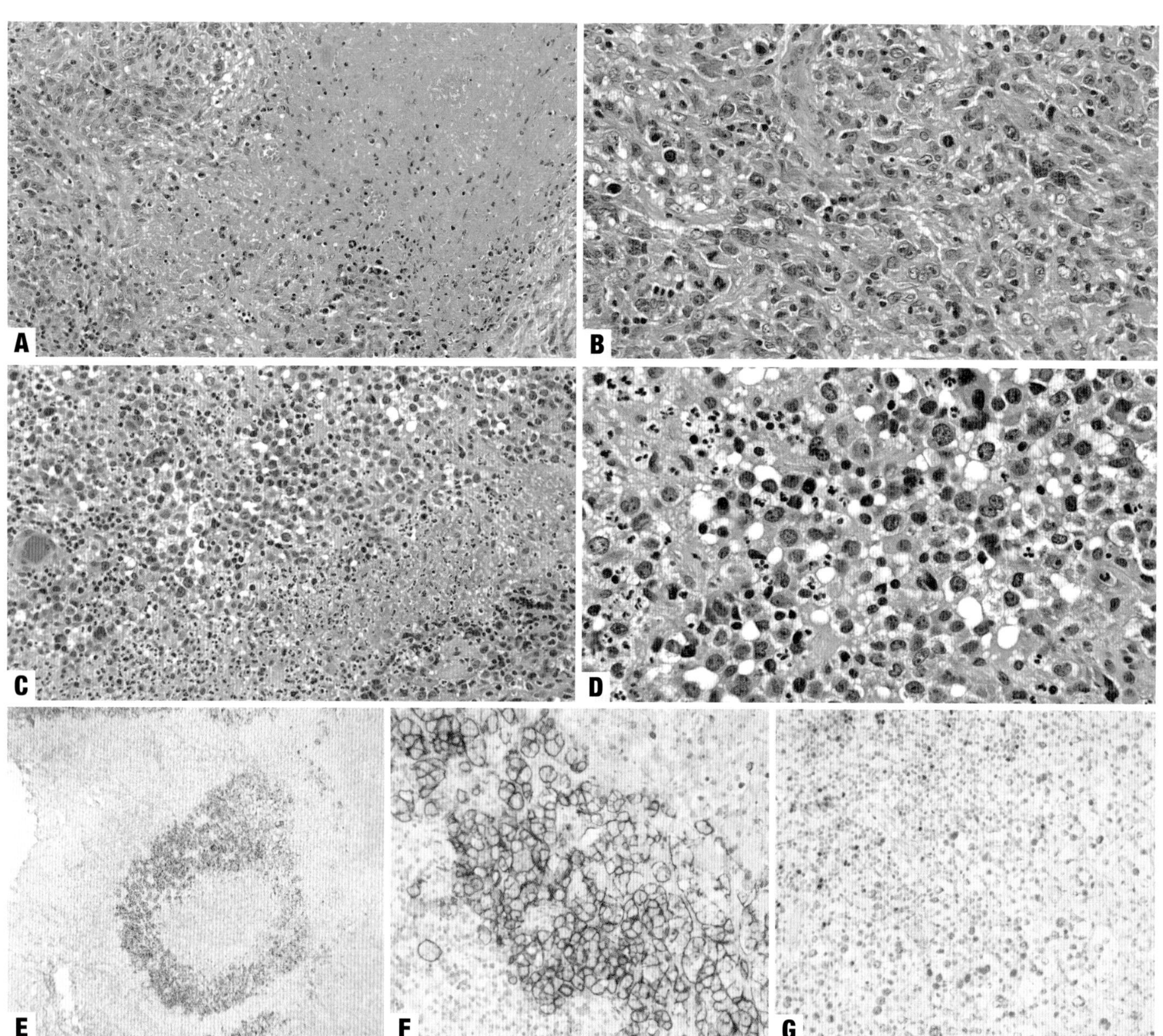

Fig. 4.271 Nodular sclerosis classic Hodgkin lymphoma, syncytial variant. **A** Numerous lacunar cells show smaller nucleoli and retraction of the cytoplasm upon fixation. **B** Sheets of pleomorphic, mitotically active neoplastic cells, some with an HRS cell–like appearance. **C** Necrosis is common in areas with numerous neoplastic cells. **D** High magnification shows sheets of polymorphic, mostly mononuclear HRS cells. **E** Immunohistochemistry shows CD30 expression in tumour cells surrounding an area of necrosis. **F** CD30 expression. **G** PAX5 is positive in HRS cells.

Cytology

For a primary diagnosis of CHL, cytology alone should not be advised as an alternative to a core needle or whole lymph node biopsy, because the differential diagnosis can be very complex. In recurrent disease, cytology can be of value and should be complemented by immunocytochemistry on corresponding cell blocks or by immunophenotyping by flow cytometry. Certain laboratories have demonstrated that the neoplastic cells of CHL can be characterized by flow cytometry and thereby show an immunophenotype similar to that seen in tissue sections {1242,611}. Flow cytometry characteristically demonstrates T cells bound (rosetting) to HRS cells, mediated by the adhesion macromolecules CD54 and CD58 {1240}. Routine clinical immunophenotyping of the reactive T-cell infiltrate typically shows increases in the CD4:CD8 ratio and Treg cells {1675,2541,2456}, and increased expression of CD7 and CD45 on CD4+ T cells {4422}.

Diagnostic molecular pathology

For the primary diagnosis of CHL and its differential diagnostic considerations, TR clonality assays can be helpful in excluding PTCL in selected cases. Because 9p24/*CD274*/*PDCD1LG2* copy-number status is predictive of response to immune checkpoint inhibition therapy, assessment of this locus may be considered when clinical protocols necessitate it {3447}.

Essential and desirable diagnostic criteria

Essential: primary nodal or mediastinal presentation; HRS cells and variants in a reactive microenvironment composed of varying proportions of small lymphocytes, eosinophils, histiocytes, plasma cells, and neutrophils; immunophenotype of HRS cells: CD30+, PAX5+ (weak to moderate), CD20–/weak/heterogeneous.

Desirable: immunophenotype of HRS cells: CD15+, CD45–, decreased expression of OCT2 and BOB1; EBV positivity (~40% of cases); histological subtyping (if possible); exclusion of mimics of CHL by appropriate workup.

Staging

The principles of staging and risk stratification in CHL have evolved along with the better understanding of the prognostic factors influencing treatment outcomes and the related changes in management. The Cotswold modification of the Ann Arbor Staging system still forms the basis for staging in Hodgkin lymphoma. This includes factors like the number of lymph nodal regions involved and their relationship relative to the diaphragm, nodal bulk, and sites of involvement, along with surrogate markers of disease burden like ESR and the presence or absence of B symptoms {2369}. Staging based on FDG PET-CT, when possible (according to the Lugano classification), is the most important predictor of outcome {688}. In the era of routine PET before treatment, a significantly higher proportion of focal bone marrow involvement is detected {4252}.

The presence or absence of the known risk factors is used to classify cases into early-stage favourable, early-stage unfavourable, and advanced-stage disease, for choosing the most appropriate therapy {2051}. The International Prognostic Score (IPS) classifies advanced disease into good-, fair-, and poor-risk groups on the basis of factors like albumin, haemoglobin, male sex, age, stage IV disease, leukocytosis, and lymphopenia {1528}. However, recent studies suggest that the IPS is

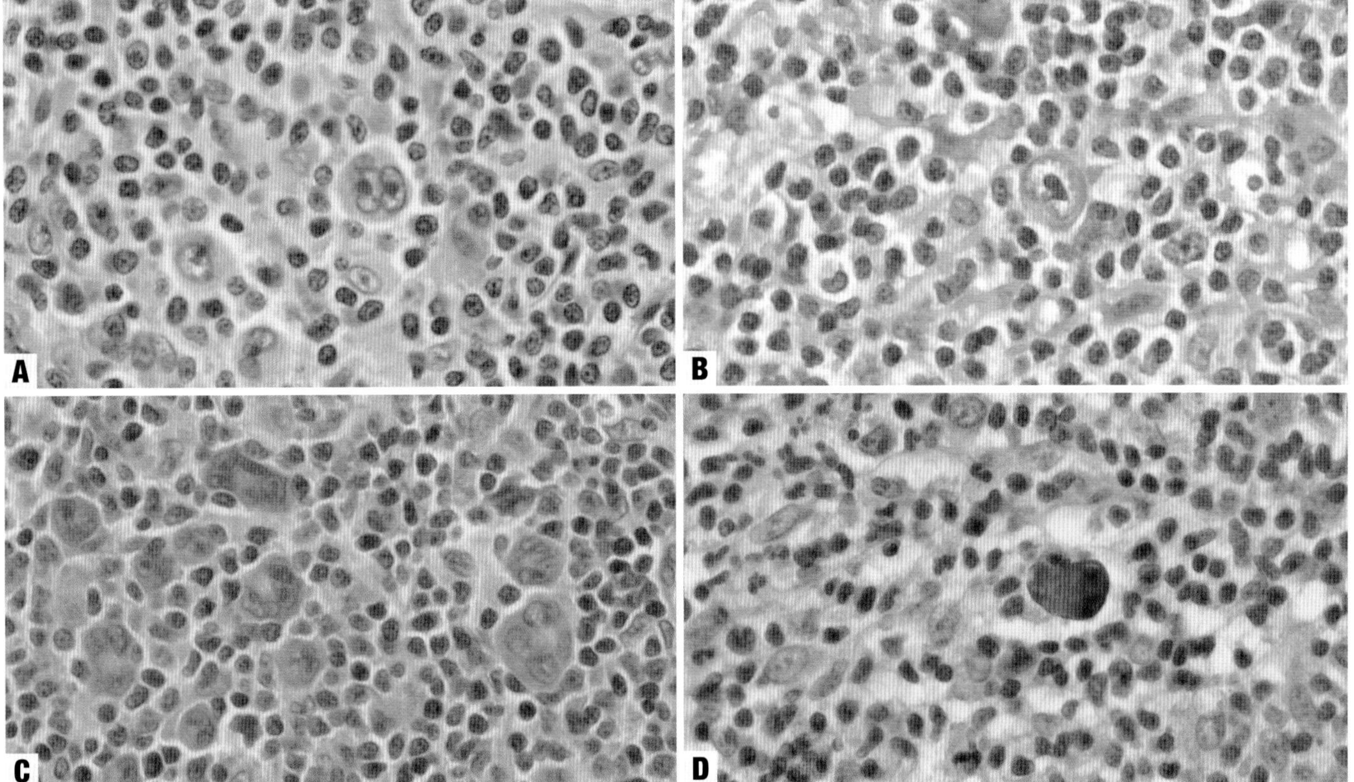

Fig. 4.272 Classic Hodgkin lymphoma, nodular sclerosis. Tumour cell types in classic Hodgkin lymphoma. **A** A binucleated Reed–Sternberg cell. **B** A mononuclear Hodgkin cell. **C** Multinucleated Reed–Sternberg cells. **D** A mummified (apoptotic) Hodgkin cell.

becoming less discriminating, owing to improved outcomes with currently used therapy and staging procedures {1441,2707, 952}. Current therapeutic strategies are not only based on these pretreatment prognostic factors but also tailored to the early response to chemotherapy.

Prognosis and prediction

More than 80% of patients with CHL can be cured with modern polychemotherapy, selectively combined with radiotherapy. To reduce long-term organ dysfunction and to increase efficacy, individual treatment is tailored to defined risk groups, based on Ann Arbor stage (with or without FDG PET), bulky (mediastinal) disease, extranodal localization, B symptoms, and the IPS {1528}. In addition, response to therapy is being evaluated by interim FDG PET imaging to allow intensification or reduction of therapy. Salvage polychemotherapy followed by high-dose chemotherapy and autologous stem cell transplantation, immune checkpoint inhibitors, and the CD30 antibody–drug conjugate brentuximab vedotin are considered acceptable options in relapsed or refractory CHL {2726}.

Multiple studies have used gene expression profiling to identify signatures that are associated with treatment outcomes {938,3560,3656}. In concordance, high numbers of macrophages and non-malignant B cells in the tumour microenvironment were validated as adverse and favourable prognostic factors, respectively {3823,614,1758}. However, neither gene expression profiling nor enumeration of cells have found their way into clinical practice. Many other tissue-based prognostic or predictive biomarkers in either HRS cells or the tumour microenvironment have suffered the same fate, owing to a lack of validation or limited utility for clinical decision-making. Therapy response monitoring in plasma, based on the detection of circulating tumour cell DNA or the tumour-derived chemokine CCL17 (TARC), may complement PET in the near future {753}.

Nodular lymphocyte-predominant Hodgkin lymphoma

Hartmann S
Borchmann P
Borges AM
Laskar S
Medeiros LJ
Naresh KN
Natkunam Y
Siebert R
Sohani AR
Tamaru J
Vielh P

Definition

Nodular lymphocyte-predominant Hodgkin lymphoma (NLPHL) is a germinal centre–derived B-cell neoplasm composed of scattered large neoplastic B cells with multilobated nuclei (lymphocyte-predominant [LP] cells) within nodules dominated by mantle zone B cells and follicular dendritic cells (FDCs). Variant histological growth patterns also occur, in which small B cells are few and/or nodules are infrequent.

ICD-O coding

9659/3 Nodular lymphocyte-predominant Hodgkin lymphoma

ICD-11 coding

2B30.0 Nodular lymphocyte-predominant Hodgkin lymphoma

Related terminology

Acceptable: nodular lymphocyte predominant B-cell lymphoma.
Not recommended: nodular paragranuloma.

Subtype(s)

Six different nodular and diffuse morphological patterns are recognized {1129}.

Localization

NLPHL is characterized by lymph node involvement. Early-stage disease (stage I and II) accounts for about 60% of all cases, and is even more frequent in children (80%) {3695}. In contrast to classic Hodgkin lymphoma (CHL), the sites of involvement are less focused on supradiaphragmatic lymph nodes, with about 40% of cases arising in the cervical or axillary regions and about 20% in the iliac and inguinal regions. Bulky disease (> 50 mm) occurs less frequently (up to 40%) than in CHL. Also, organ involvement is much less frequent (< 20%) than in CHL and includes bone (12%), liver (8%), and lung (4%), as reported from the German Hodgkin Study Group (GHSG) database {211}.

Clinical features

Most patients present with painless, localized lymphadenopathy at the time of initial diagnosis, sometimes present for years. Approximately 40% of patients present with advanced-stage (stage III or IV) disease {3732,3053}. About 15–20% of patients

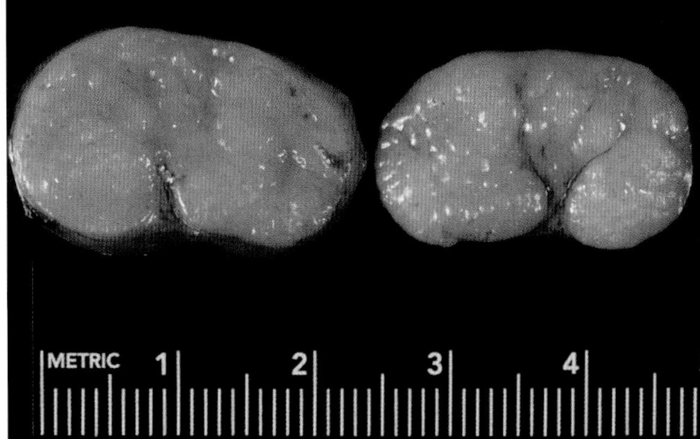

Fig. 4.273 Nodular lymphocyte-predominant Hodgkin lymphoma. The gross appearance of a lymph node involved by nodular lymphocyte-predominant Hodgkin lymphoma and progressive transformation of germinal centres demonstrating a nodular cut surface.

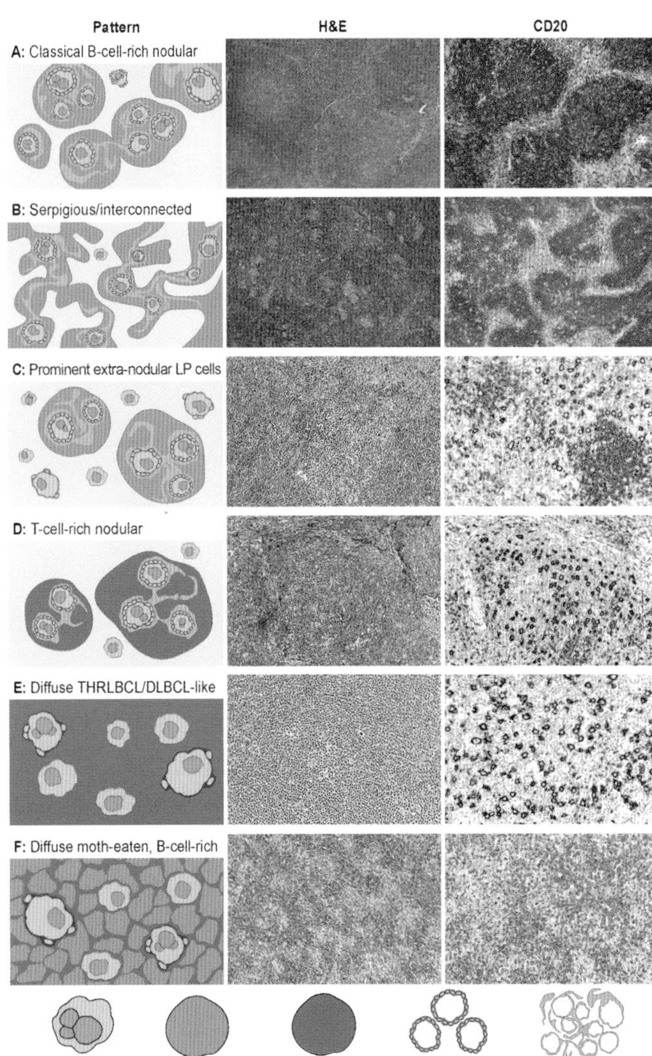

Fig. 4.274 Nodular lymphocyte-predominant (LP) Hodgkin lymphoma. Schematic representation of the six growth patterns of nodular lymphocyte-predominant Hodgkin lymphoma. The recognition of the growth patterns is supported by immunohistochemistry, especially CD20 to highlight the distribution of lymphocyte-predominant cells. DLBCL, diffuse large B-cell lymphoma; FDC, follicular dendritic cell; THRLBCL, T-cell/histiocyte–rich large B-cell lymphoma.

have B symptoms, including night sweats, fever, and significant weight loss (GHSG database {3053}). There are no characteristic laboratory findings.

Epidemiology

NLPHL has an incidence of 0.11 cases per 100 000 person-years {3711}. The incidence varies worldwide, with higher incidence rates in Europe, the USA, and the Middle East, and a lower incidence in Asia {3711,2235,2727,2251,2858,55}. US SEER data reflect a lower incidence in people of Asian descent, and a higher incidence in African Americans, than in White people {3711,3053}. Histological patterns in NLPHL do not vary by geographical region {4436}.

There is a male predominance (M:F ratio: 2.5–3:1) and a wide age distribution, from childhood to > 80 years, with most patients diagnosed between 30 and 60 years of age {3711,3854,2717,3732}. The median age at diagnosis is higher in women than men {2717,3732}. NLPHL with IgD-positive LP cells occurs more commonly in young men {3292}.

Etiology

The etiology is unknown. Genetic predisposition leading to rare familial NLPHL is noted, associated with germline *NPAT* variants or *TET2* haploinsufficiency {3511,2660,3513,1841}. NLPHL is associated with primary immunodeficiency syndromes, such as Hermansky–Pudlak syndrome type 2 and autoimmune lymphoproliferative syndrome (ALPS) {4143,2421}. IgD-positive NLPHL occurs preferentially in individuals with HLA haplotypes HLA-DRB1*04 and HLA-DRB1*07, indicating a role for cognate T-cell help {4011,291,1523}. In contrast to CHL, EBV plays no significant role in the genesis of NLPHL, which shows EBV positivity in only exceptional cases {1688}.

Pathogenesis

The pathogenesis of NLPHL involves genomic alterations in tumour cells of NLPHL (LP cells) and immunological interactions with the microenvironment. The tumour cells of NLPHL are clonal germinal-centre B cells exhibiting ongoing somatic hypermutation and intraclonal diversity in their rearranged IG genes {2159,444}. Aberrant somatic hypermutation affects *PIM1*, *RHOH* (*TTF*), *PAX5*, *MYC*, *SOCS1*, *JUNB*, *DUSP2*, and *SGK1*; the latter four are more frequently targeted in variant growth patterns {2368,2812,1524,3647}. *BCL6* translocations (46–48%) or amplifications (27%) are common genetic alterations {4392,3395,215}.

A subset of NLPHL is likely triggered by preceding bacterial infections, resulting in an extensive immune reaction in susceptible patients. The LP precursor cells may enter germinal centres and undergo clonal selection and malignant transformation due to aberrant somatic hypermutation events driven by the germinal-centre reaction. In IgD-positive NLPHL, additive stimulation by *Moraxella*-derived antigen and superantigen are important

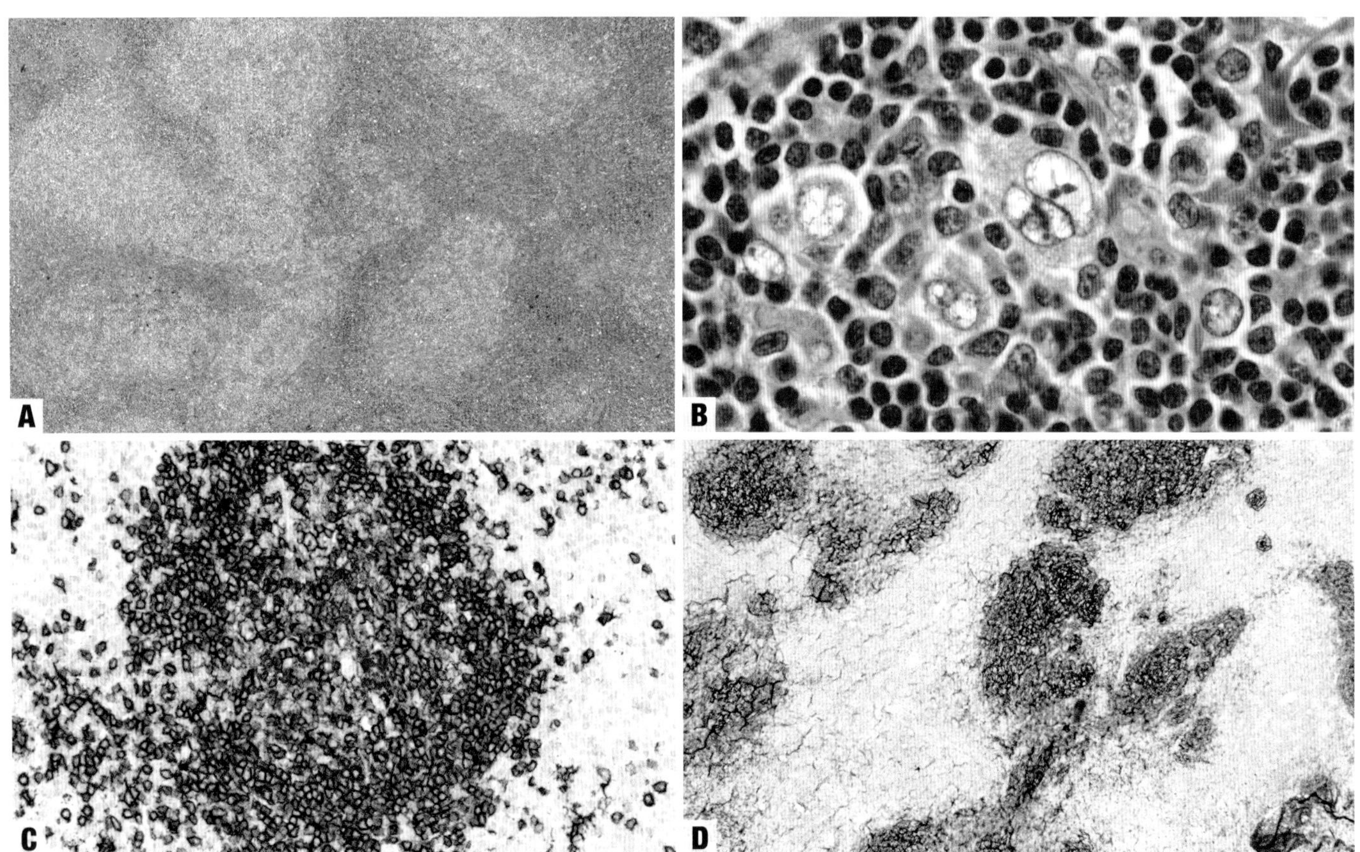

Fig. 4.275 Nodular lymphocyte-predominant Hodgkin lymphoma. **A** Pattern A is the most common presentation of nodular lymphocyte-predominant Hodgkin lymphoma and is characterized by large round or oval nodules. **B** High magnification of typical lymphocyte-predominant cells. **C** The majority of lymphocyte-predominant cells are contained within the nodule of small B cells as highlighted by CD20, which is strongly positive in the lymphocyte-predominant cells and the small B cells. **D** CD21 immunohistochemistry highlights the expanded meshworks of follicular dendritic cells in the nodules of the nodular lymphocyte-predominant Hodgkin lymphoma pattern.

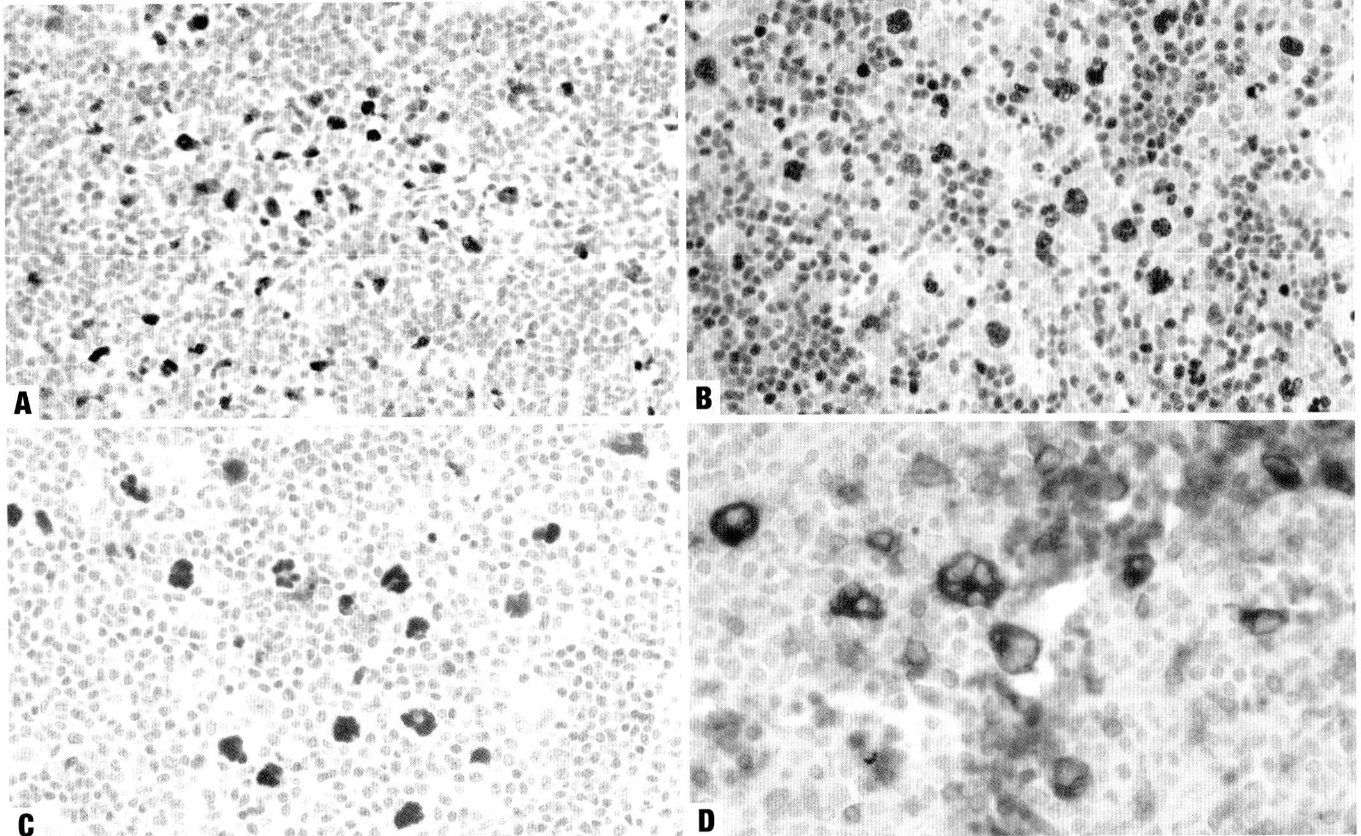

Fig. 4.276 Nodular lymphocyte-predominant Hodgkin lymphoma. **A** The lymphocyte-predominant tumour cells are typically positive for BCL6, as are the background T follicular helper (TFH) cells. **B** OCT2 is strongly positive in lymphocyte-predominant cells and moderately positive in background small B cells. **C** MEF2B is typically positive in nodular lymphocyte-predominant Hodgkin lymphoma, in contrast to classic Hodgkin lymphoma. **D** IgD is expressed in a subset of lymphocyte-predominant cells in nodular lymphocyte-predominant Hodgkin lymphoma.

factors for lymphoma development {4011}. A close interaction between LP cells and rosetting PD1-positive T cells via immunological synapses has been observed {291,1523}, suggesting a role for the microenvironment in lymphomagenesis.

Macroscopic appearance

Lymph nodes are usually enlarged, frequently > 30 mm, and firm. Cut surfaces are grey-tan and often nodular. Splenic involvement is characterized by large tumour nodules or selective involvement of the white pulp in a grossly normal spleen {631}.

Histopathology

Lymph nodes involved by NLPHL show partial or complete architectural effacement by a nodular proliferation with or without diffuse areas. Neoplastic LP cells are large, with multilobated nuclei with one or more nucleoli, and pale cytoplasm (often resembling popcorn) and represent 1–5% of the mass. LP cells usually occur singly, although rarely increased numbers or clusters of LP cells may be seen within nodules. The immune microenvironment is composed of many non-neoplastic B cells and T cells, often with activated morphological features, including clear cytoplasm and a more open chromatin structure {2916}, and histiocytes, including epithelioid histiocytes. Histiocytes may cluster or form granulomas around tumour nodules. Neutrophils and eosinophils are absent. Sclerosis is uncommon at diagnosis but often present at recurrence {1129}. A rim of normal lymph node may remain present in the periphery of the affected lymph node showing follicular hyperplasia and progressive transformation of germinal centres.

Immunohistochemistry

Most cases express a broad panel of B-related markers (CD20, CD79a, OCT2, BOB1, PU.1) (see Table 4.57, p. 594). Of these, OCT2 is the most reliable positive marker, and CD79a only rarely shows weaker expression {3983,2647}. CD20 and one or more of the B-cell transcription factors (BOB1, OCT2, PU.1) may be lost in rare cases {2647}. CD19 is frequently negative {2572, 3983,477}. Germinal-centre B-cell markers such as BCL6, LMO2 and HGAL are positive in the vast majority, but CD10 is negative. LP cells are usually negative for CD30 and rarely positive for CD15 {3367,1129,2891,3331,4209,1516,3672}. IgD is typically expressed in LP cells in a clinicopathological subtype often associated with extranodular tumour cells (pattern C) and mild cytological atypia of background T cells {3292,3774, 1516}. EBV is rarely positive in LP cells {759,2891,1688,4436}. In contrast to CHL, MEF2B is typically expressed in LP cells of NLPHL {2765}, whereas STAT6 is negative {4171}. These markers support the distinction of NLPHL from CHL.

Background small B cells have a mantle zone phenotype (positive for IgD, negative for germinal-centre markers) and are associated with expanded CD21+, CD23+ FDC meshworks.

T follicular helper (TFH) cells, which express CD3, PD1, CD57, BCL6, CXCL13, and ICOS, are typically abundant and typically form rosettes encircling LP cells {2892,1514,4241}. A CD4+/CD8-dim T-cell population is frequently detected by flow cytometry {3347,1241}, indicating T-cell activation.

Morphological patterns of NLPHL

Six growth patterns defined by histological and immunophenotypic features have been recognized (see Table 4.58) {1129}; 75% of cases show typical B-cell–rich patterns (patterns A and B) and 25% show variant patterns (patterns C–F). A mixture of growth patterns is commonly seen. Immunohistochemistry for CD20 to highlight the number and distribution of both tumour and reactive B cells is important for recognizing variant patterns {1129,424,1517,1514}. In cases with a predominantly diffuse

Table 4.57 Immunophenotype of the lymphocyte-predominant (LP) tumour cells of nodular lymphocyte-predominant Hodgkin lymphoma

Category	Markers	Expression profile of LP tumour cells
B-cell markers	CD20, CD79a, CD22	Positive; CD20 loss or downregulation reported in 2.8% of cases {2647}
B-cell transcription factors	PAX5, OCT2, BOB1	Positive; loss or downregulation in some cases; OCT2 staining often strong in comparison to mantle zone B cells {470,3828}
Immunoglobulins	J chain	Positive
	IgD	Positive in distinct subset {3292,1516}
Pan-leukocyte	CD45RB/LCA	Positive
Germinal-centre B-cell markers	BCL6, HGAL, LMO2	Positive
	CD10	Negative
Classic Hodgkin lymphoma markers	CD30, CD15	Infrequent; CD30 is positive in reactive immunoblasts {1129,3672,4209,2891, 3331,3367}
Immune checkpoint	PDL1	Diminished in LP cells; variably positive in background histiocytes {655,3127}
EBV	EBER	Positive in rare cases {1688,4301, 1516}
Miscellaneous	IRF4 (MUM1)	Variably positive
	EMA	Variably positive
	MEF2B	Positive {2765}
	STAT6	Weak cytoplasmic staining (nuclear staining in classic Hodgkin lymphoma) {4171}
	IgG4	Negative in LP cells; no positive plasma cells (unlike progressive transformation of germinal centres) {1988}
Category	**Markers**	**Expression in microenvironment**
Follicular dendritic cell markers	CD21, CD23	Positive in nodular growth patterns A, B, C, and D; loss in diffuse patterns E and F {1129,4126}
TFH cell markers	PD1, ICOS, CXCL13, BCL6, CD57	TFH-cell rosettes surround LP cells {2892}; loss or downregulation in variant growth patterns {746}; negative in LP cells

EBER, EBV-encoded small RNA; TFH, T follicular helper.

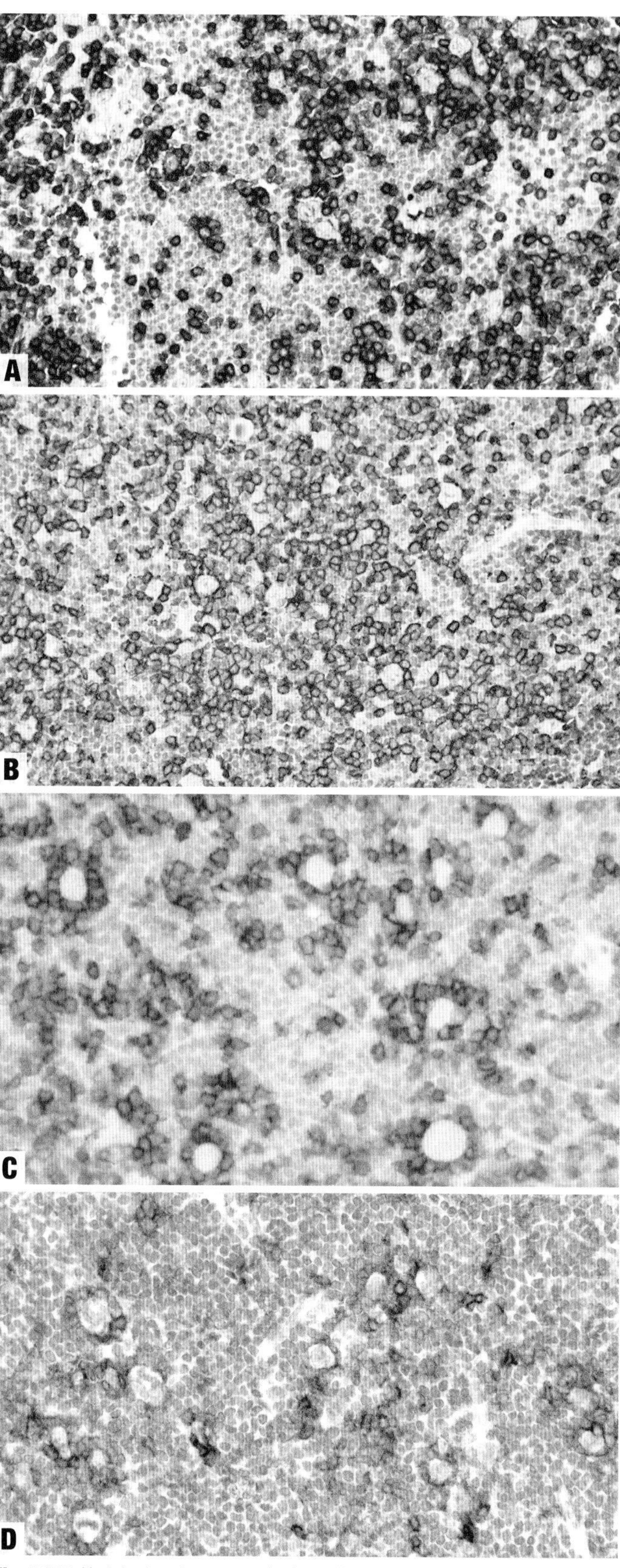

Fig. 4.277 Nodular lymphocyte-predominant Hodgkin lymphoma. T follicular helper (TFH) cells characteristically constitute a large component of the non-neoplastic infiltrate of nodular lymphocyte-predominant Hodgkin lymphoma. They form rosettes around lymphocyte-predominant cells and are positive for CD3 (**A**), CD57 (**B**), PD1 (**C**), and ICOS (**D**).

Table 4.58 Characteristic features of nodular lymphocyte-predominant Hodgkin lymphoma (NLPHL) growth patterns

Pattern	Descriptive pattern	Overall architecture	LP tumour cell distribution	Immune microenvironment
A	B-cell–rich nodular	Nodules have a classic circular or oval appearance; intact FDC meshworks are present	The majority of tumour cells are contained within nodules	Nodules contain a predominance of small mantle zone–type B cells; small CD4+ TFH cells and histiocytes are present; PD1+ T-cell rosettes are typically present
B	Serpiginous-interconnected	Irregularly shaped nodules in a serpiginous/interconnected pattern; FDC meshworks are present	The majority of tumour cells are contained within nodules	Nodules contain a predominance of small mantle zone–type B cells; small CD4+ TFH cells and histiocytes are present; PD1+ T-cell rosettes are typically present
C	Prominent extranodular tumour cells	Nodules are frequently condensed; FDC meshworks are present	A high proportion of tumour cells are outside and in between nodules	Nodules contain a predominance of small mantle zone–type B cells; small CD4+ TFH cells and histiocytes are present; tumour cells outside nodules are surrounded by small CD4+ TFH cells and histiocytes and are not associated with FDC meshworks; PD1+ T-cell rosettes are usually present but may be diminished
D	T-cell–rich nodular	Nodules typically have a classic appearance, with somewhat activated clear T cells; irregular shapes of nodules may also be present; FDC meshworks are present	The majority of tumour cells are contained within nodules	Nodules contain a predominance of TFH cells that are surrounded by a small rim of mantle zone–type B cells
E	Diffuse (T-cell/histiocyte–rich large B-cell lymphoma–like or diffuse large B-cell lymphoma–like)	Diffuse growth without nodules (other areas in the same biopsy must contain one or more of the other patterns to be classified as NLPHL); absence of FDC meshworks	Tumour cells are singly and diffusely scattered; confluence or sheets of tumour cells should raise consideration of diffuse large B-cell lymphoma	Diffuse background with a predominance of small T cells and histiocytes; CD4:CD8 ratio may be variable between cases {1417,1514}; PD1+ T-cell rosettes may be diminished or absent
F	Diffuse moth-eaten, B-cell–rich	Diffuse growth without distinct nodules in a mosaic or moth-eaten configuration; partial FDC meshworks are present	Tumour cells are singly and diffusely scattered with surrounding TFH rosettes	Diffuse with areas containing a predominance of small B cells alternating with areas dominated by small CD4+ TFH cells and histiocytes; the B-cell areas are usually associated with FDC meshworks

FDC, follicular dendritic cell; TFH cell, T follicular helper cell; LP, lymphocyte-predominant.

T-cell/histiocyte–rich large B-cell lymphoma (THRLBCL)-like pattern (pattern E), at least one unequivocal NLPHL nodule is required to distinguish this variant pattern from de novo THRLBCL. Partial nodal involvement with few affected nodules containing tumour cells has been postulated to represent an in situ phase of NLPHL {550,548}; however, further confirmatory studies are warranted.

Transformation to aggressive lymphoma

NLPHL can transform to large B-cell lymphoma with a heterogeneous appearance with respect to overall architecture, cell types in the immune microenvironment, and proportion of neoplastic cells. Transformation typically involves loss of nodular architecture, FDC meshworks, and non-neoplastic B cells with increased T cells and histiocytes and a variable proportion of neoplastic large B cells {1663,358,1760,1518,1492,3885}. Sometimes composite patterns of NLPHL, diffuse large B-cell lymphoma, and THRLBCL-like areas occur in the same lymph node. NLPHL with variant patterns, particularly pattern E (THRLBCL-like) areas, is also frequently observed when the liver, spleen, and bone marrow are involved, and it must be distinguished from transformation to large B-cell lymphoma. Transformation should be considered when there are either confluent sheets or scattered large B cells without any other typical or variant patterns of NLPHL. Individual cases, however, show a wide morphological spectrum, and reliable predictions of clinical behaviour based on histological features are challenging. As with de novo diagnosis, ample tissue sampling is critical: on core biopsies or small tissue samples, distinction between NLPHL with an extensive pattern E component and THRLBCL may not be possible. Rare NLPHL variants with increased TFH cells in the microenvironment and lacking FDC meshworks despite a nodular growth pattern have been associated with an aggressive clinical course {4070,3011}, and probably represent a continuum between NLPHL and THRLBCL.

Differential diagnosis

The differential diagnosis includes THRLBCL, the nodular variant of lymphocyte-rich CHL, progressive transformation of germinal centres, and (less commonly) peripheral T-cell lymphoma (see Table 4.59, p. 596).

Cytology

Smears show numerous small lymphocytes, histiocytes, and few LP cells. Because the diagnosis is largely based on immunoarchitectural features, and distinguishing NLPHL with an extensive pattern E component from THRLBCL requires ample tissue sampling, fine core needle biopsies should generally be avoided. Histological confirmation of incisional or excisional biopsies and exclusion of differential diagnoses is required.

Diagnostic molecular pathology

No single and particular molecular diagnostic assay is currently helpful in establishing the diagnosis. Although LP cells are clonal by single-cell PCR analyses, conventional clonality assays for IG gene loci on whole tissue sections are frequently unable to detect the tumour cell clone.

Essential and desirable diagnostic criteria

Essential: nodular architecture, at least focally; LP tumour cells: single scattered large cells with multilobated nuclei, vesicular chromatin, and one or more generally small nucleoli; immunophenotype: uniform positivity for several B-cell antigens (usually CD20-positive); immune microenvironment: many small lymphocytes, histiocytes, and follicular dendritic cells; no eosinophils.

Desirable: characteristic immunophenotype of LP cells (CD20, OCT2, BCL6) and of background TFH cells (PD1-positive) rosetting around tumour cells; defining growth patterns (A–F) – because this may be highly challenging on core needle biopsies, a lymph node excision is preferred.

Staging

The Lugano system adopted by the Union for International Cancer Control (UICC) TNM classification {688} is used for staging.

Prognosis and prediction

Patients with NLPHL have a 10-year overall survival rate of > 90% and a progression-free survival rate of > 75% {3854, 1051,2989}. Relapses occur more frequently in NLPHL than in CHL {109}. Variant histopathological growth patterns (patterns C–F), male sex, and a low serum albumin level are risk factors for relapse {1517}. Variant growth patterns correlate with shorter time to relapse {1517,1522}. Infradiaphragmatic

Table 4.59 Clinicopathological features of nodular lymphocyte-predominant Hodgkin lymphoma (NLPHL) and comparison with entities in the differential diagnosis

Feature	NLPHL	THRLBCL	LRCHL	nTFHL-AI	Progressive transformation of germinal centres
Age group, sex, and ethnic predilection	Children and young adults M:F ratio: 2.5–3:1 More common in Black people than White people in the USA	Middle age to elderly M > F	Children and young adults M:F ratio: 2:1 No ethnic predilection	Middle age to elderly M:F ratio: 1:1 No ethnic predilection	Children and young adults M:F ratio: 1:1 No ethnic predilection
Sites of involvement	Peripheral lymph nodes, typically single site; mediastinal involvement and bulky disease are uncommon	Systemic disease with B symptoms, splenomegaly, and/or hepatomegaly	Peripheral lymph nodes; mediastinal involvement and bulky disease are uncommon	Systemic disease with B symptoms, bulky lymphadenopathy, and cutaneous manifestations	Peripheral lymph nodes, typically single site; mediastinal involvement and bulky disease are uncommon
Lesional cells	Single scattered large B cells (LP cells) with multilobated nuclei, single prominent or multiple nucleoli, and scant pale cytoplasm	Single scattered large B cells with pleomorphic nuclei, variable nucleoli, and moderate cytoplasm	Single scattered large B cells with prominent eosinophilic nucleoli, binucleation or multinucleation, and abundant pale cytoplasm	Small to medium-sized lymphoid cells with clear or pale cytoplasm and moderate cytological atypia	No tumour cells; may be associated with NLPHL or, less commonly, CHL
Tissue architecture and immune microenvironment	Nodular growth with or without diffuse areas; predominance of mantle zone–type small B cells, admixed T cells, and histiocytes including epithelioid histiocytes; eosinophils are rare or absent; variant growth patterns with T-cell and histiocyte–rich background in subset	Diffuse growth with predominance of T cells and histiocytes	Nodular or rarely diffuse growth; predominance of mantle zone–type small B cells; small germinal centres may be seen within nodular areas; histiocytes are less common; eosinophils can be present at periphery of nodules	Diffuse growth with nodal effacement; polymorphous lymphoid infiltrate with prominent vasculature and inflammatory background including eosinophils; plasma cells may be abundant	Nodular growth with involution of mantle zone–type small B cells and progressive disruption of germinal centres
Immunophenotype	Positive for B-cell markers and transcription factors; CD30 and CD15 are rare; TFH rosettes; FDC markers show presence of at least partial nodularity	Positive for B-cell markers and transcription factors; no TFH rosettes; no FDC meshworks	Positive for CD30 and CD15 with minimal B-cell markers and diminished B-cell transcription factors; nuclear GATA3 expression and STAT6 (in contrast to weak cytoplasmic staining in LP cells)	Positive for TFH markers; CD30 positive in subset; CD15 usually absent; may show CD20+ B-cell lymphoproliferative disease with or without EBV	PTGC follicles show involution of BCL2+ and IgD+ mantle zone–type B cells within germinal centres
Genetic profile / pathogenesis	Rearranged IGH; *Moraxella* spp.; *SGK1, DUSP2, JUNB, SOCS1* mutations; *BCL6* rearrangements	Rearranged IGH; *SGK1, DUSP2, JUNB, SOCS1* mutations	None	Rearranged TR; *RHOA, TET2, IDH2, DNMT3A* mutations	None

CHL, classic Hodgkin lymphoma; FDC, follicular dendritic cell; LP, lymphocyte-predominant; LRCHL, lymphocyte-rich CHL; nTFHL-AI, nodal T follicular helper cell lymphoma, angioimmunoblastic type; PTGC, progressively transformed germinal centre; TFH, T follicular helper; THRLBCL, T-cell/histiocyte–rich large B-cell lymphoma.

and splenic involvement, as well as clonal IG rearrangement detected at initial diagnosis, are risk factors for transformation to large B-cell lymphoma {79,3150}. The 5-year overall survival rate is reportedly better in patients with late relapses (after > 12–24 months) than in those with early relapses (65.4% vs 94.9%) {1052,1051}.

Therapy protocols are highly varied, with excision, immunotherapy, chemotherapy and radiation therapy all applied. The choice of modality depends largely on the patient's age and disease stage. For children with limited-stage disease, watchful waiting after resection can be employed {2610,132,2049}. For adults with limited-stage disease, there is no consensus approach and either radiation therapy or chemotherapy may be used; rarely, patients are followed by active surveillance {414}. Patients with advanced-stage disease require systemic therapy {4444,224,1050}. Rituximab monotherapy results in good overall survival despite high relapse rates {1049,28}.

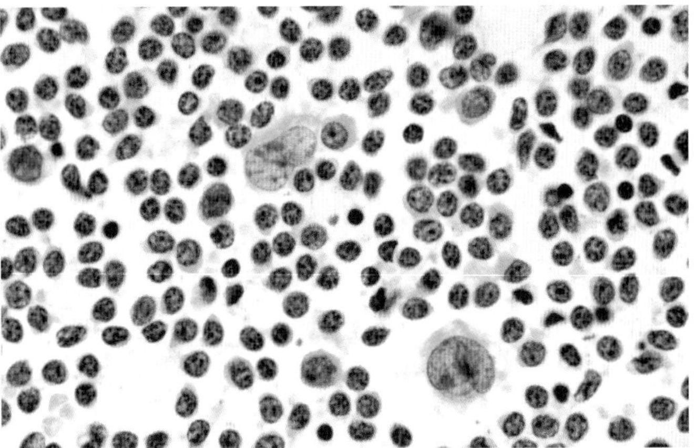

Fig. 4.278 Nodular lymphocyte-predominant Hodgkin lymphoma. Cytological smear showing lymphocyte-predominant cells with multilobated nuclei, fine pale chromatin, and prominent nucleoli.

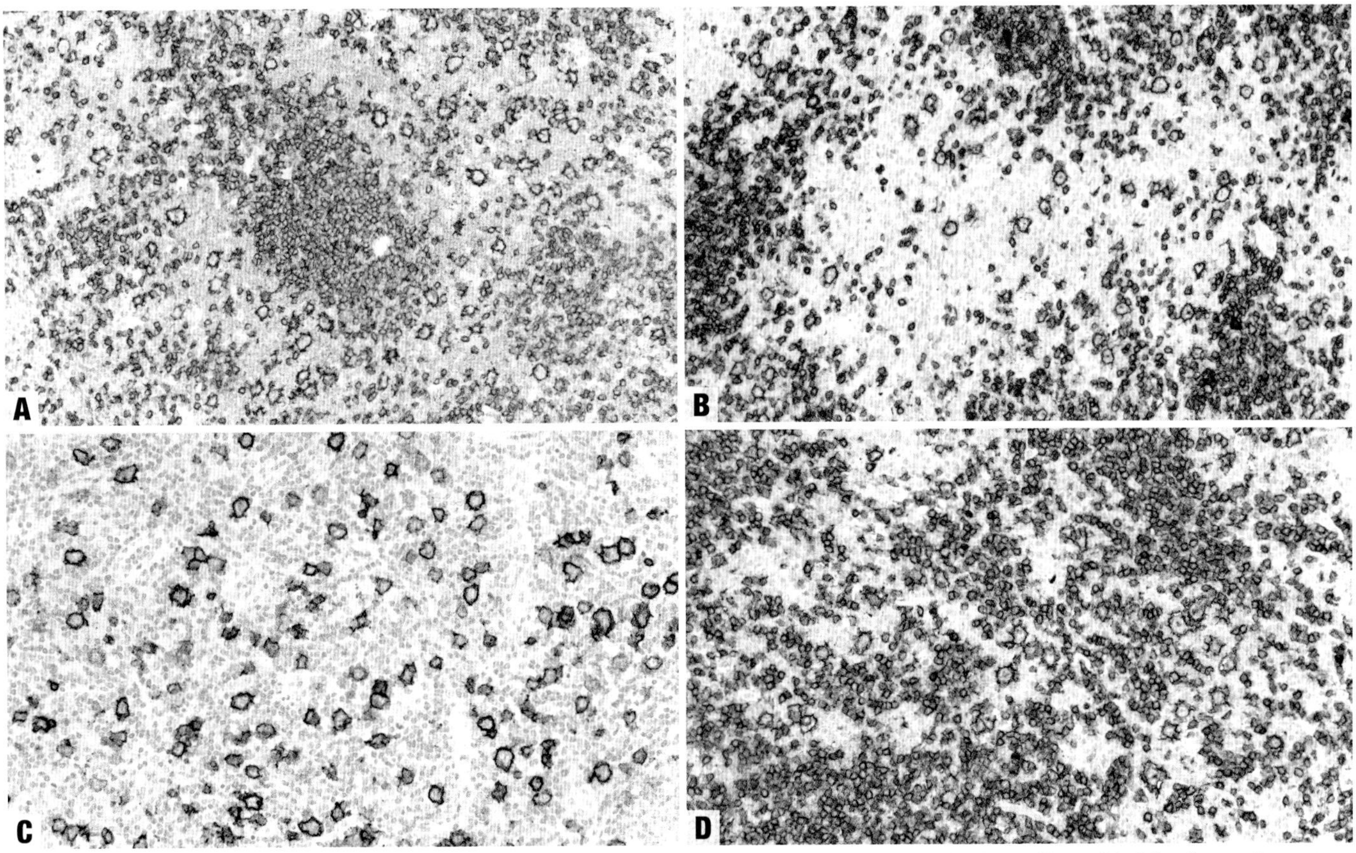

Fig. 4.279 Variant patterns of nodular lymphocyte-predominant Hodgkin lymphoma as highlighted by CD20 immunohistochemistry. **A** Pattern C is defined by prominent extranodular lymphocyte-predominant cells. Pattern D has a nodular architecture with a T-cell–rich non-neoplastic background infiltrate (**B**), whereas pattern E has a diffuse architecture and a dense T-cell infiltrate (**C**). **D** Pattern F also has a diffuse growth pattern, but the non-neoplastic background infiltrate consists of small B cells, and follicular dendritic cell meshworks are lacking.

Plasma cell neoplasms and other diseases with paraproteins: Introduction

Chng WJ

A number of conditions produce paraproteins or M proteins, which are either monoclonal intact immunoglobulins, light chains, or occasionally heavy chains or misfolded immunoglobulins that are deposited. The conditions range from mature B-cell neoplasms to plasma cell neoplasms. They range from asymptomatic precursor conditions (IgM and non-IgM monoclonal gammopathy of undetermined significance [MGUS]) to symptomatic conditions that require treatment. The paraproteins produced could be IgM or, rarely, heavy chain only, which tend to be associated with B-cell disorders such as lymphoplasmacytic lymphoma, chronic lymphocytic leukaemia / small lymphocytic lymphoma, or extranodal marginal zone lymphoma of mucosa-associated lymphoid tissue (EMZL) (these entities are described elsewhere in this volume), or non-IgM (IgG, IgA, IgD, IgE, or light chain only), which tend to be associated with plasma cell neoplasms and are further detailed in the following sections. In some of the conditions, such as immunoglobulin deposition diseases and immunoglobulin light chain amyloidosis, the paraproteins form abnormal deposits in the kidneys and other organs, which results in organ damage. There is also a group of conditions where the presence of monoclonal gammopathy is associated with renal disease; however, they may not fulfil the diagnostic criteria for B-cell or plasma cell neoplasms. These conditions are now recognized as monoclonal gammopathy of renal significance (MGRS). The differentiation of these conditions therefore requires a combination of clinical features, such as organ involvement and symptoms, as well as the characteristics of the paraproteins and the pathological changes in the affected tissues, and the clonal origin of the cells producing the paraproteins.

In this edition, compared with the fourth edition, some new conditions are introduced, including MGRS; TEMPI syndrome (telangiectases, elevated erythropoietin and erythrocytosis, monoclonal gammopathy, perinephric fluid collection, and intrapulmonary shunting), which was a provisional entity in the fourth edition; and AESOP syndrome (adenopathy and extensive skin patch overlying a plasmacytoma). The sections have been reorganized according to the types of paraproteins and the disease burden. IgM and non-IgM MGUS and MGRS are grouped as monoclonal gammopathies, and the diseases with abnormal monoclonal immunoglobulin deposits are grouped together.

Cold agglutinin disease

Naresh KN
Berentsen S
Chen X
Randen U
Rossi D

Definition

Cold agglutinin disease (CAD) is an autoimmune haemolytic anaemia mediated by monoclonal cold agglutinins (autoantibodies that agglutinate erythrocytes at an optimum temperature of 0–4 °C) in the absence of any infection or lymphoma. The process is driven by an underlying clonal B-cell proliferation; however, it does not fulfil criteria for a B-cell lymphoma.

ICD-O coding

9760/1 Cold agglutinin disease

ICD-11 coding

3A20.1 Autoimmune haemolytic anaemia, cold type

Related terminology

Acceptable: primary cold agglutinin–associated lymphoproliferative disease; primary cold agglutinin disease.

Subtype(s)

None

Localization

Clonal B cells are best identified in the bone marrow. There is no evidence of extramedullary lymphoma {3366}.

Clinical features

Anaemia due to complement-mediated extravascular haemolysis and cold-induced symptoms due to red blood cell agglutination (e.g. acrocyanosis, Raynaud phenomenon, livedo reticularis) are the primary manifestations {321,320}. A small serum monoclonal IgM paraprotein (mostly kappa) is detected in > 90% of cases {321}.

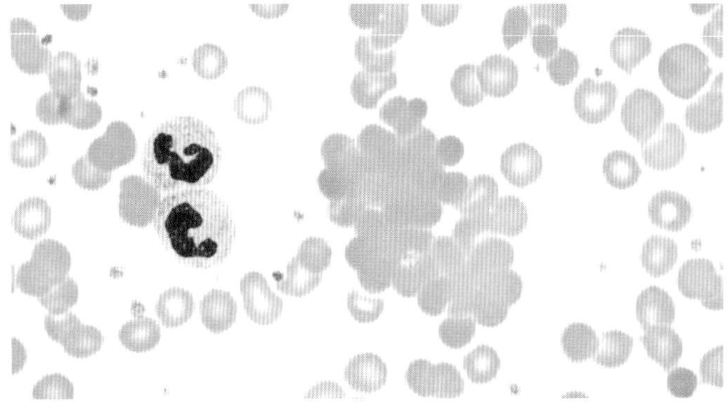

Fig. 4.281 Cold agglutinin disease. A peripheral blood smear shows red cell agglutination, anisocytosis, and polychromasia.

Epidemiology

CAD is rare: the incidence is estimated at 1–1.8 cases per 1 million person-years. As reported from Scandinavian populations, the prevalence is 4-fold higher in countries and areas with a colder climate as compared to more moderate or warm climates {321,510}. CAD is slightly more frequent in women, and the median age at diagnosis is in the late sixties {321,320}.

Etiology

Unknown

Pathogenesis

CAD harbours clonal rearrangements of immunoglobulin heavy and light chain genes. Somatic mutation of the IG genes occurs in all cases. The usage of the IG gene repertoire is significantly skewed, with the IGHV4-34 gene being used by about 80% of cases, mostly along with IGKV3-20 or IGKV3-15. Multiple regions

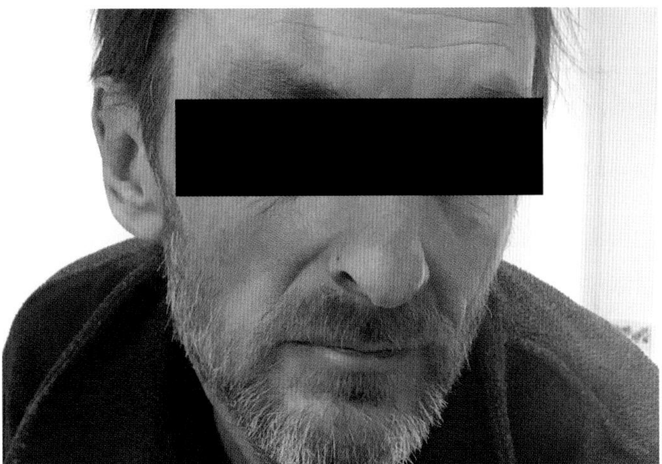

Fig. 4.280 Cold agglutinin disease. Typical facial acrocyanosis as can be seen in a patient with cold agglutinin disease.

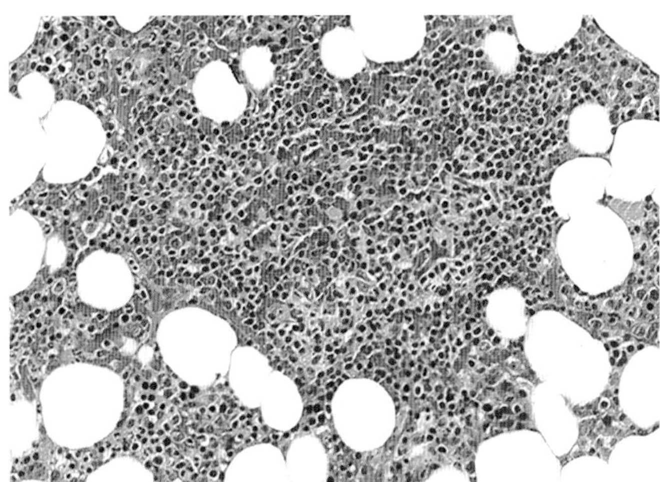

Fig. 4.282 Cold agglutinin disease. High-power view of a bone marrow biopsy showing a small aggregate of small lymphoid cells with round to oval nuclei and scant cytoplasm.

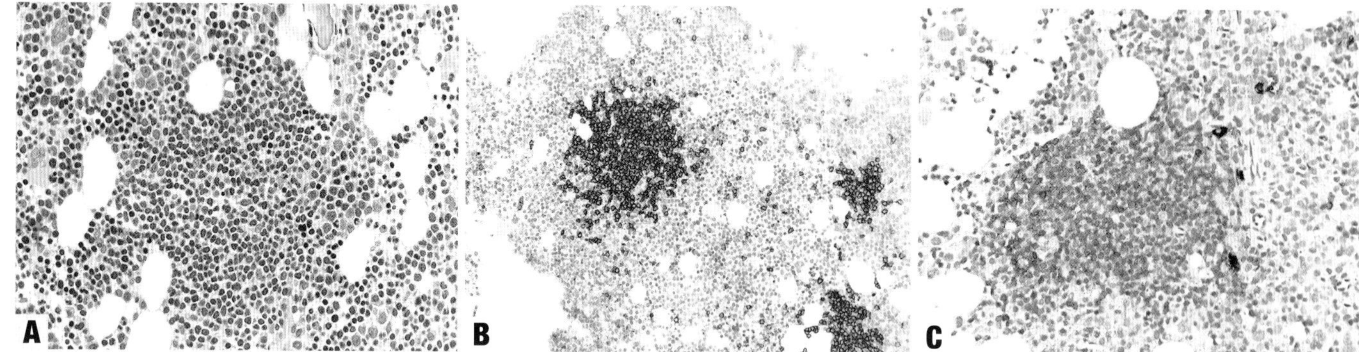

Fig. 4.283 Cold agglutinin disease. **A** Bone marrow core biopsy shows an intertrabecular lymphoid aggregate, typical of cold agglutinin disease. **B** CD20 immunostain highlights small nodules of B cells as well as scattered B cells in an interstitial distribution. **C** There are scattered and clustered IgM-positive B cells, as well as a few scattered IgM-positive plasma cells in the bone marrow outside the aggregate.

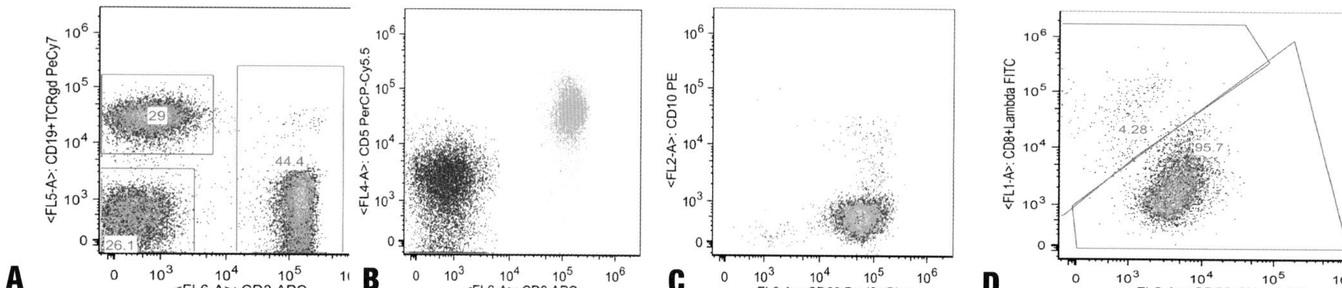

Fig. 4.284 Cold agglutinin disease. **A** Flow cytometry of lymphoid cells, CD3 versus CD19; B cells are in the upper-left quadrant (29% of the lymphoid cells). **B** Flow cytometry of B cells, CD3 versus CD5; B cells (blue, CD3–) are negative for CD5. CD3+, CD5+ T cells are the control (grey). **C** CD20 versus CD10; dot plot shows that the B cells are negative for CD10. **D** Flow cytometry of B cells, kappa versus lambda light chain; the B-cell population shows kappa light chain restriction.

within the IG genes contribute to I antigen–binding. Mutations at the N-glycosylation sites of the IGHV CDR2 are frequent and increase specific binding of the I antigen, translating into more severe anaemia {2506}. At the cytogenetic level, complete or partial gains of chromosome 3 occur in > 90%, and these often co-occur with a gain of chromosome 12 or 18 (70%) {2504}. These changes are similar to those seen in marginal zone lymphoma. Genes that are recurrently mutated in CAD include *KMT2D* (70%) and *CARD11* (30%) {2505}. The *MYD88* p.L265P mutation is not present in CAD {3366}.

The IgM monoclonal autoantibodies typically bind to the I antigen on the red blood cell surface at an optimum temperature of 0–4 °C {321,2506}. The binding of multiple red blood cells by one pentameric IgM molecule is the basis for agglutination. The bound IgM triggers the classic complement pathway and leads to extravascular haemolysis. Activation of the terminal complement cascade with intravascular haemolysis can occur to a variable extent.

Macroscopic appearance

Not relevant

Histopathology

Blood smear shows red blood cell agglutination, red cell anisocytosis, and polychromasia. Bone marrow aspirate morphology is usually unremarkable apart from an often-expanded erythropoiesis.

Bone marrow core biopsy shows small lymphoid cells mainly as nodular aggregates and as a sparse interstitial infiltrate; these cells have round to slightly oval nuclei with a homogeneous dark chromatin pattern and scant clear cytoplasm. Mature plasma cells (< 5% of the marrow cells) surround these lymphoid aggregates and are also seen singly scattered throughout the marrow. No paratrabecular growth pattern, lymphoplasmacytic morphology, increased mast cells, or fibrosis is seen {3366,1767,320}.

Immunophenotype

Lymphoid cells express B-cell markers (CD19, CD20, PAX5, CD79a, CD22, and CD79b), monotypic light chain (most often kappa), and IgM; CD5 is positive in 40% of the cases. They are negative for BCL6, IRF4 (MUM1), CD23, and cyclin D1. The plasma cells express IgM and monotypic light chain (most often kappa).

Differential diagnosis

The differential diagnosis includes secondary cold agglutinin syndromes associated with a clinically overt lymphoid malignancy, in particular lymphoplasmacytic lymphoma (see Table 4.60) or with an infection.

Table 4.60 Differential diagnosis based on bone marrow findings: cold agglutinin disease and lymphoplasmacytic lymphoma

Cold agglutinin disease	Lymphoplasmacytic lymphoma
Small nodules, no diffuse infiltrates or intrasinusoidal growth	Nodular and/or diffuse
Intertrabecular infiltrates	Paratrabecular/intertrabecular infiltrates
Small B cells and (usually) plasma cells	Small B cells, lymphoplasmacytoid cells, plasma cells
Plasma cells widely spread in the marrow, outside the aggregates	Plasma cells admixed in the infiltrates
No mast cell infiltration	Mast cell infiltration present

Cytology
FNAB is not sufficient to establish a diagnosis.

Diagnostic molecular pathology
An absence of *MYD88* p.L265P mutation aids in distinguishing CAD from lymphoplasmacytic lymphoma.

Essential and desirable diagnostic criteria
See Box 4.03.

Staging
Not relevant

Prognosis and prediction
Prognostic scores for CAD do not exist. Survival appears to be similar to or only slightly worse than in an age-matched healthy population {321,320,3910}. CAD does not progress to another indolent lymphoma and the frequency of transformation to an aggressive lymphoma is very low (< 5%) {321,320}.

Box 4.03 Diagnostic criteria for cold agglutinin disease {1767,3366,319,1585}

Essential:
- Chronic haemolysis – as assessed by high indirect bilirubin, low haptoglobin, high LDH, and (often) high absolute reticulocyte count
- Monospecific direct antiglobulin test (DAT) strongly positive for C3d; DAT is usually negative for IgG but occasionally is weakly positive
- Cold agglutinin titre > 64 at 4 °C; the specimen must be kept at 37–38 °C from sampling until plasma/serum has been removed from the cells/clot
- No overt malignant disease or relevant infection – clinical assessment for malignancy; radiology as required; exclude recent infection with *Mycoplasma* or EBV
- Evidence of a clonal B-cell disorder – as assessed by electrophoresis, flow cytometry, and/or bone marrow biopsy

Desirable:
- Monoclonal IgM/kappa in plasma/serum (or, rarely, IgG or lambda phenotype); the specimen must be kept at 37–38 °C from sampling until plasma/serum has been removed from the cells/clot
- B-cell kappa-to-lambda ratio > 3.5 (or, rarely, < 0.9) – as assessed by flow cytometry in bone marrow aspirate
- Cold agglutinin–associated lymphoproliferative disorder by histopathology (on bone marrow biopsy)
- *MYD88* p.L265P mutation not found – as assessed in bone marrow

IgM monoclonal gammopathy of undetermined significance

Rajkumar SV
Fernández de Larrea C
Kristinsson SY
Landgren OC

Definition

IgM monoclonal gammopathy of undetermined significance (MGUS) is defined by the presence of a serum monoclonal (M) protein of < 3 g/dL, < 10% bone marrow lymphoplasmacytic infiltration (clonal B cells and plasma cells together), and no evidence of anaemia, constitutional symptoms, hyperviscosity, lymphadenopathy, or hepatosplenomegaly that can be attributed to the underlying lymphoproliferative disorder.

ICD-O coding

9761/1 IgM monoclonal gammopathy of undetermined significance

ICD-11 coding

2A83.0 & XH16T1 Monoclonal gammopathy of undetermined significance & IgM monoclonal gammopathy of undetermined significance

Related terminology

None

Subtype(s)

None

Localization

The neoplastic cells reside in the bone marrow.

Clinical features

IgM MGUS is not associated with clinical manifestations. It is usually diagnosed incidentally on laboratory tests performed during workup for a wide variety of clinical symptoms and reasons. IgM MGUS carries a risk of progression to Waldenström macroglobulinaemia (lymphoplasmacytic lymphoma), although rarely patients can develop IgM plasma cell (multiple) myeloma, chronic lymphocytic leukaemia, or other lymphomas {4106, 2183}. It may progress to immunoglobulin light chain amyloidosis. The most important causally related disorders that occur in a small proportion of patients with IgM MGUS are IgM-related peripheral neuropathy and Schnitzler syndrome, a rare disorder characterized by chronic urticaria {3352}.

Epidemiology

IgM MGUS is a subset of MGUS, accounting for about 20% of all MGUS cases. Thus, the estimated prevalence in the general population aged ≥ 50 years is approximately 0.6% {2185}. The incidence of IgM MGUS increases with age. The age-adjusted incidence is higher in males than females, and higher in Black people than White people. First-degree relatives may have a higher risk of MGUS {2212}.

Etiology

See *Non-IgM monoclonal gammopathy of undetermined significance* (p. 603).

Pathogenesis

See *Non-IgM monoclonal gammopathy of undetermined significance* (p. 603).

Macroscopic appearance

Not relevant

Histopathology

Bone marrow is characterized by < 10% clonal involvement by neoplastic cells that are light chain–restricted on immunostaining or flow cytometry. The neoplastic cells exhibit lymphoplasmacytoid or plasma cell differentiation. They have a typical immunophenotype, including surface IgM+, CD5+/−, CD10−, CD19+, CD20+, and CD23−, that would satisfactorily exclude other lymphoproliferative disorders, including chronic lymphocytic leukaemia.

Cytology

Not relevant

Diagnostic molecular pathology

A recurrent mutation, *MYD88* p.L265P, that has been found in > 90% of patients with Waldenström macroglobulinaemia (lymphoplasmacytic lymphoma), can also be present at the MGUS stage.

Essential and desirable diagnostic criteria

Essential: serum M protein of < 3 g/dL; < 10% bone marrow infiltration by clonal neoplastic cells; no evidence of anaemia, constitutional symptoms, hyperviscosity, lymphadenopathy, or hepatosplenomegaly that can be attributed to the underlying lymphoproliferative disorder (see Box 4.04).

Staging

See *Non-IgM monoclonal gammopathy of undetermined significance* (p. 603).

Prognosis and prediction

The risk of progression of IgM MGUS to Waldenström macroglobulinaemia (lymphoplasmacytic lymphoma) or a related malignancy is approximately 1.5% per year. This risk persists indefinitely {2183}.

Box 4.04 Diagnostic criteria for IgM monoclonal gammopathy of undetermined significance

Essential:
- Serum IgM monoclonal protein < 3 g/dL
- Bone marrow lymphoplasmacytic infiltration < 10%
- No evidence of anaemia, constitutional symptoms, hyperviscosity, lymphadenopathy, or hepatosplenomegaly that can be attributed to the underlying lymphoproliferative disorder

Non-IgM monoclonal gammopathy of undetermined significance

Rajkumar SV
Fernández de Larrea C
Kristinsson SY
Landgren OC

Definition

Non-IgM monoclonal gammopathy of undetermined significance (MGUS) is defined by the presence of a non-IgM (mainly IgG or IgA; rarely IgE, IgD, and light chain only) serum monoclonal (M) protein of < 3 g/dL, clonal bone marrow plasma cells < 10%, and absence of end-organ damage, such as hypercalcaemia, renal insufficiency, anaemia, and bone lesions (CRAB), that can be attributed to the plasma cell proliferative disorder. Light chain MGUS is a subtype characterized by an abnormal serum free light chain ratio (< 0.26 or > 1.65), increased level of the involved light chain, no immunoglobulin heavy chain expression on immunofixation, and an absence of end-organ damage that can be attributed to the plasma cell proliferative disorder.

ICD-O coding

9765/1 Non-IgM monoclonal gammopathy of undetermined significance
9765/1 IgG monoclonal gammopathy of undetermined significance
9765/1 IgA monoclonal gammopathy of undetermined significance
9765/1 IgD monoclonal gammopathy of undetermined significance
9765/1 IgE monoclonal gammopathy of undetermined significance
9765/1 Light chain monoclonal gammopathy of undetermined significance

ICD-11 coding

2A83.0 Monoclonal gammopathy of undetermined significance

Related terminology

None

Subtype(s)

IgG MGUS; IgA MGUS; IgD MGUS; IgE MGUS; light chain MGUS

Localization

The neoplastic cells reside in the bone marrow.

Clinical features

Non-IgM MGUS is generally not associated with clinical symptoms, especially myeloma-associated clinical manifestations. It is usually diagnosed incidentally on laboratory tests done during the workup of a variety of unrelated medical conditions {3744}. Non-IgM MGUS carries a risk of progression to plasma cell (multiple) myeloma, plasmacytoma, or immunoglobulin light chain amyloidosis {4106,2183}. The most important causally related disorders that occur in a small proportion of patients with non-IgM MGUS are proliferative glomerulonephritis, dermatological diseases (e.g. lichen myxoedematosus, necrobiotic xanthogranuloma, scleromyxoedema, and pyoderma gangrenosum), and (rarely) peripheral neuropathy.

Epidemiology

Non-IgM MGUS is a subset of MGUS that accounts for about 80% of all MGUS cases. Thus, the estimated prevalence in the general population aged ≥ 50 years is approximately 3% {2185}. The incidence of non-IgM MGUS increases with age. The age-adjusted incidence is higher in males than females, and higher in Black people than White people. First-degree relatives may have a higher risk of MGUS {2212}.

Etiology

The etiology is unknown; however, a higher risk has been associated with a family history, obesity, exposure to pesticides, and immunosuppression.

Pathogenesis

MGUS probably originates when plasma cells divide in response to antigenic stimulation. During this period of antigenic stimulation, primary cytogenetic abnormalities occur. The two major types of primary cytogenetic abnormalities are hyperdiploidy and IGH translocations. IGH translocations involve the immunoglobulin heavy chain switch region on chromosome 14q32, and one of five common partner chromosomes loci: 11q13 (*CCND1*), 4p16.3 (*FGFR3* and *NSD2*), 6p21 (*CCND3*), 16q23 (*MAF*), and 20q11 (*MAFB*). The development of additional second-hit events and changes in the tumour microenvironment are thought to be responsible for the progression of MGUS to malignancy.

Macroscopic appearance

Not relevant

Histopathology

Bone marrow is characterized by infiltration with clonal mature plasma cells that are light chain–restricted on immunostaining or flow cytometry of < 10% of total nucleated cells in the bone marrow. Clonal neoplastic cells are typically CD38+, CD45 dim to negative, CD19-negative, and CD138-positive.

Cytology

Not relevant

Diagnostic molecular pathology

FISH studies will reveal the presence of primary cytogenetic abnormalities (t(11;14); t(4;14); t(14;16); hyperdiploidy with trisomies of chromosomes 7, 9, 11, 15, 19) in most patients with an adequate number of plasma cells for analysis.

Box 4.05 Diagnostic criteria for monoclonal gammopathy of undetermined significance (MGUS)

Non-IgM MGUS

Essential:

- Serum monoclonal protein (non-IgM type) < 3 g/dL
- Clonal bone marrow plasma cells < 10%[a]
- Absence of end-organ damage, such as CRAB, that can be attributed to the plasma cell proliferative disorder

Light chain MGUS

Essential:

- Abnormal FLC ratio (< 0.26 or > 1.65)
- Increased level of the appropriate involved light chain (increased kappa FLC in patients with ratio > 1.65 and increased lambda FLC in patients with ratio < 0.26)
- No immunoglobulin heavy chain expression on immunofixation
- Absence of end-organ damage that can be attributed to the plasma cell proliferative disorder
- Clonal bone marrow plasma cells < 10%
- Urinary monoclonal protein < 500 mg/24 h

CRAB, hypercalcaemia, renal insufficiency, anaemia, and bone lesions; FLC, free light chain.
[a]A bone marrow biopsy can be deferred in patients with low-risk MGUS (IgG type, M protein < 15 g/L, normal FLC ratio) in whom there are no clinical features concerning for myeloma.
Note: For each entity, all criteria must be met.

Essential and desirable diagnostic criteria

Essential: serum monoclonal (M) protein < 3 g/dL; clonal bone marrow plasma cells < 10% of total nucleated cells; absence of CRAB features that can be attributed to the plasma cell proliferative disorder (see Box 4.05).

Staging

Risk-stratification of MGUS (IgM MGUS and non-IgM MGUS) is based on the size and type of the M protein and the free light chain ratio (see Table 4.61) {3353}. The presence of all three risk factors (abnormal serum free light chain ratio, IgA-type or IgM-type MGUS, and serum M protein > 1.5 g/dL) is considered high risk, with approximately 50–60% risk of progression at 20 years, whereas the risk is only 5% when none of the risk factors are present.

Prognosis and prediction

The overall risk of progression of non-IgM MGUS to plasma cell (multiple) myeloma or a related malignancy is approximately 1% per year. This risk persists indefinitely {2183}.

Table 4.61 Risk stratification model to predict the progression of monoclonal gammopathy of undetermined significance (MGUS) to myeloma or a related disorder

Risk group based on the following risk factors: 1. serum M protein > 1.5 g/dL 2. IgA or IgM subtype 3. elevated free light chain ratio > 1.65	Relative risk	Absolute risk of progression at 20 years	Absolute risk of progression at 20 years accounting for death as a competing risk
Low risk (no risk factors present)	1	5%	2%
Low to intermediate risk (any one risk factor present)	5.4	21%	10%
High to intermediate risk (any two risk factors present)	10.1	37%	18%
High risk (all three risk factors present)	20.8	58%	27%

Monoclonal gammopathy of renal significance

Leung N
Fernández de Larrea C
Kristinsson SY
Landgren OC
Nasr SH
Rajkumar SV

Definition

Monoclonal gammopathy of renal significance (MGRS) is a plasma cell or B-cell neoplasm that does not meet the accepted criteria for malignancy or initiation of treatment but secretes a monoclonal immunoglobulin (Ig) or Ig fragment resulting in kidney injury. It is important to note that renal impairment secondary to light chain cast nephropathy in plasma cell neoplasm is a multiple myeloma / plasma cell myeloma–defining event.

ICD-O coding

9765/1 Monoclonal gammopathy of renal significance

ICD-11 coding

2A83.0 Monoclonal gammopathy of undetermined significance

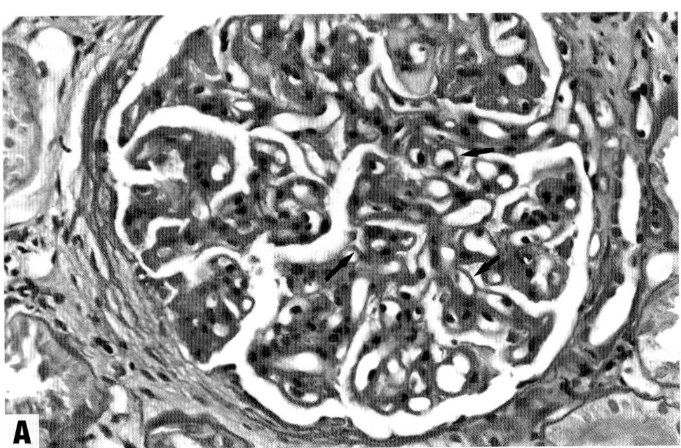

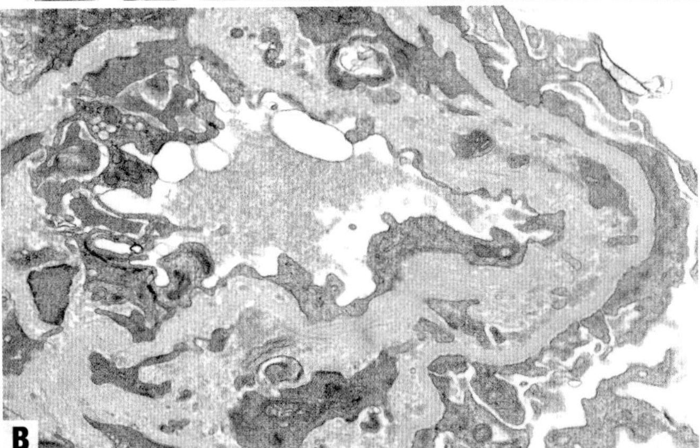

Fig. 4.285 Monoclonal gammopathy of renal significance. Chronic glomerular microangiopathy associated with monoclonal gammopathy. **A** A high-power light microscopy image showing glomerular basement membrane thickening and segmental narrow duplication (arrows) (PAS). **B** An electron microscopy image showing glomerular basement membrane duplication, cellular interposition, and widening of the subendothelial zone by electron-lucent fluffy-appearing material. No electron-dense deposits were seen, and immunofluorescence was negative.

Related terminology

None

Subtype(s)

See Table 4.62 (p. 607).

Localization

The kidney is always affected. The B-cell or plasma cell neoplasm in most cases involves the bone marrow or lymph nodes.

Clinical features

The clinical presentation of MGRS is broad and encompasses variable combinations of proteinuria, haematuria, acute or chronic renal insufficiency, hypertension, and hypocomplementaemia {457}. Microscopic haematuria and hypertension are common, but hypotension is common in patients with Ig-associated amyloidosis. The severity of proteinuria or renal impairment depends on the kidney lesion. Patients with Ig-associated amyloidosis, monoclonal Ig deposition disease, and cryoglobulinaemia often have extrarenal manifestations, including congestive heart failure, autonomic/peripheral neuropathy, liver failure, and skin rash/purpura {2285}.

Epidemiology

MGRS represents a subset of cases of monoclonal gammopathy of undetermined significance (MGUS), of smouldering (asymptomatic) myeloma, and of clonal B-cell proliferation that does not meet the diagnostic criteria for lymphoma {2180,2179,2285}. The true prevalence is unknown but may be close to 1.5% of patients with MGUS {3831,2054}. The median age at diagnosis is about 60 years, but the disease can occur in people in their late teens and early twenties {2909,2910,3843,3840,4256,1819,2825,2908}. There is a male predominance of 60–75%.

Etiology

A plasma cell neoplasm is the most common cause of Ig-associated amyloidosis, monoclonal Ig deposition disease, light chain proximal tubulopathy, crystal-storing histiocytosis, crystalglobulin induced nephropathy, C3 glomerulopathy with monoclonal gammopathy, and thrombotic microangiopathy. B-cell clones are the most common cause of cryoglobulinaemia secondary to monoclonal gammopathy. In proliferative glomerulonephritis with monoclonal Ig deposits, plasma cell neoplasm makes up 50% of the cases. CD20-positive B-cell lymphomas account for the other half, one third of which coexpress CD20 and CD38 {2285}.

Pathogenesis

Monoclonal Igs injure the kidney by deposition, vascular occlusion, or activation of complement.

Macroscopic appearance

Not relevant

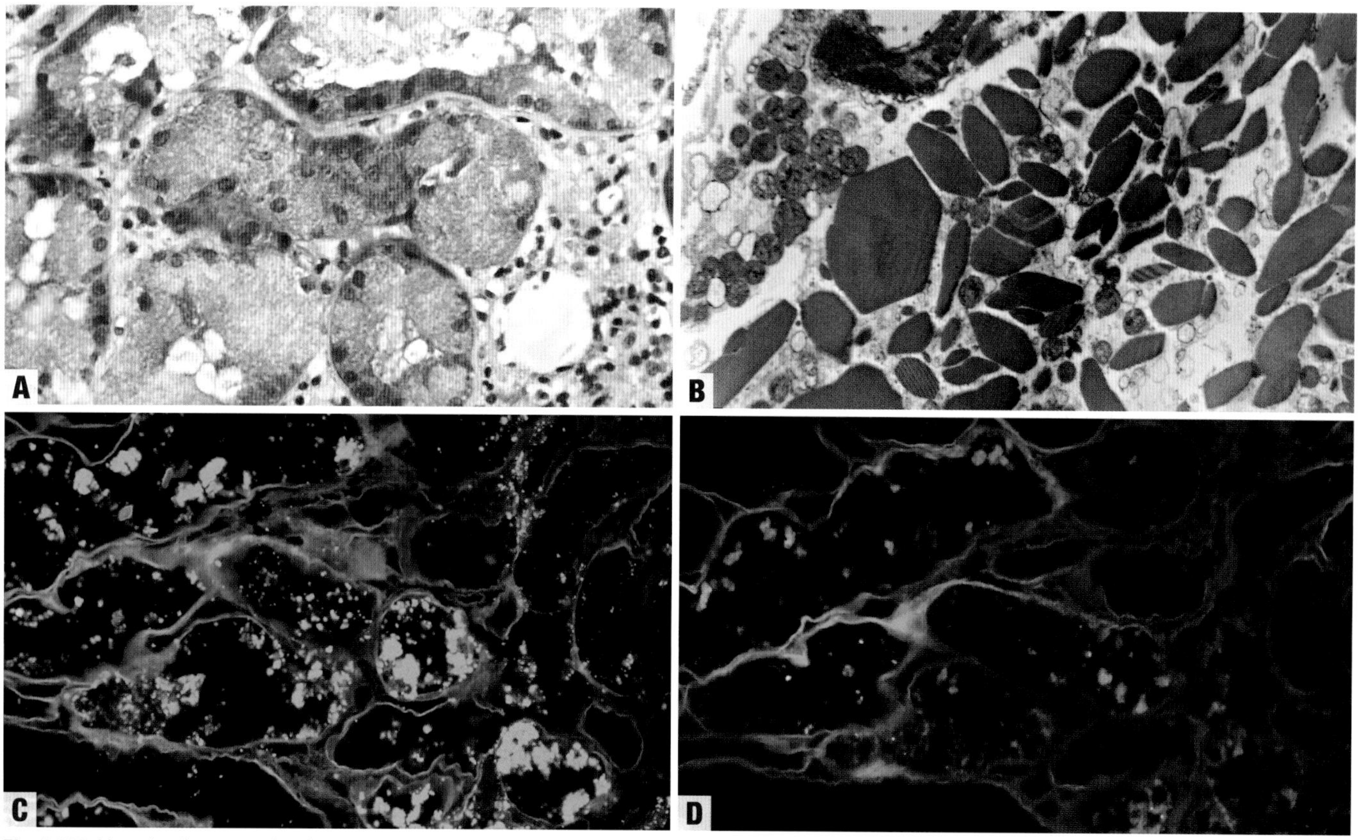

Fig. 4.286 Monoclonal gammopathy of renal significance. Light chain proximal tubulopathy. **A** Proximal tubular cells are variably extended by numerous light-blue inclusions (trichrome stain). **B** A high-power electron microscopy image of a proximal tubular cell shows intracytoplasmic crystalline inclusions with variable shapes (rhomboidal, polygonal, rod-shaped); the majority of crystals appear to lie free within the cytosol. **C,D** Immunofluorescence performed on Pronase-digested, paraffin-embedded tissue shows proximal tubular intracytoplasmic crystals staining positive for kappa light chain I (**C**) with negative staining for lambda light chain (**D**).

Histopathology

See *IgM monoclonal gammopathy of undetermined significance* (p. 602) and *Non-IgM monoclonal gammopathy of undetermined significance* (p. 603).

Cytology

See *IgM monoclonal gammopathy of undetermined significance* (p. 602) and *Non-IgM monoclonal gammopathy of undetermined significance* (p. 603).

Diagnostic molecular pathology

See *IgM monoclonal gammopathy of undetermined significance* (p. 602) and *Non-IgM monoclonal gammopathy of undetermined significance* (p. 603).

Essential and desirable diagnostic criteria

Essential: kidney biopsy demonstrating injury as a result of a monoclonal Ig; proteinuria > 1 g/day (mostly albuminuria); progressive acute or subacute kidney injury.

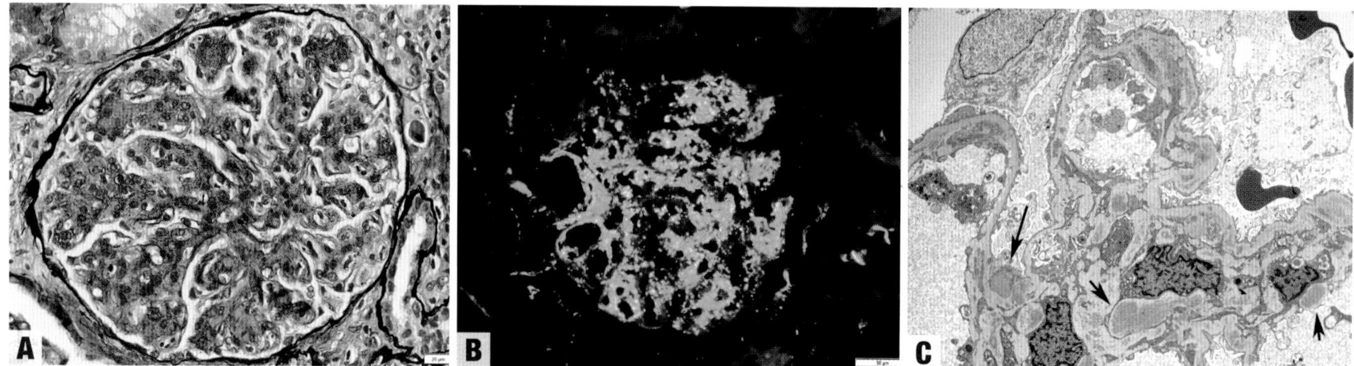

Fig. 4.287 Monoclonal gammopathy of renal significance. C3 glomerulonephritis associated with monoclonal gammopathy. **A** The glomerulus exhibits a membranoproliferative glomerulonephritis pattern of injury, with global mesangial expansion by an increase in mesangial cell number and abundant silver-negative glassy immune deposits, together with segmental duplication of the glomerular basement membrane (JMS stain). **B** On immunofluorescence, there is bright granular global glomerular staining for C3. Glomeruli were negative for IgG, IgA, kappa, and lambda (not shown). **C** An electron microscopy image showing mesangial electron-dense deposits (short arrows) as well as a hump-shaped subepithelial deposit at the mesangial waist (long arrow).

Table 4.62 Subtypes of monoclonal gammopathy of renal significance (MGRS)

Subtype	Most common clone	Ig deposits	Immunological and ultrastructural characteristics	Extrarenal manifestations
Always associated with MGRS				
Crystal-storing histiocytosis	Plasma cell	LC	Intracellular LC crystals in interstitial histiocytes (with or without crystals in tubular and glomerular cells)	Yes
Crystalglobulin-induced nephropathy	Plasma cell	Ig	Extracellular MIg crystals within glomerular and vessel lumina (with or without TMA)	Yes
Ig-related amyloidosis	Plasma cell	LC, Ig, HC	Extracellular deposition of congophilic randomly oriented fibrils	Yes
LC proximal tubulopathy	Plasma cell	LC	Crystalline or non-crystalline LC inclusions within proximal tubular cells	Yes
Monoclonal Ig deposition disease	Plasma cell	LC, Ig, HC	Finely granular, punctate MIg deposits in tubular and glomerular basement membranes and mesangium	Yes
Proliferative glomerulonephritis with monoclonal Ig deposits	Plasma cell and B cell	Ig, LC	Amorphous MIg deposits in mesangium and subendothelial zone (and occasionally in subepithelial zone)	No
Frequently associated with MGRS				
C3 glomerulopathy with MG	Plasma cell	C3 only	C3 deposits in mesangium and subendothelial and subepithelial zones (and the lamina densa of the glomerular basement membranes in dense deposit disease)	No
Cryoglobulinaemic glomerulonephritis (type I and [mostly] type II)	B cell	Ig	Short microtubular and annular deposits composed of MIg only or of MIg and polyclonal Igs	Yes
Monoclonal immunotactoid glomerulonephritis	B cell	Ig	Microtubular deposits composed of MIg	No
Thrombotic microangiopathy with MG	Plasma cell	None	Chronic endothelial cell injury, no MIg or C3 deposits	Yes
Rarely associated with MGRS				
Monotypic membranous nephropathy	Plasma cell	Ig	Subepithelial deposits of MIg	No
Monotypic anti-GBM disease	Plasma cell	Ig	Linear deposits of MIg along the glomerular basement membranes, no electron-dense deposits ultrastructurally	No
Monotypic IgA nephropathy / Henoch Schönlein purpura nephritis	Plasma cell	Ig	Monoclonal IgA deposits in the mesangium (and occasionally in subepithelial and/or subepithelial zones)	No/yes

GBM, glomerular basement membrane; HC, heavy chain; Ig, immunoglobulin; LC, light chain; MG, monoclonal gammopathy; MIg, monoclonal immunoglobulin; TMA, thrombotic microangiopathy.

Desirable: lack of lytic bone lesions; no extramedullary plasmacytoma; no hypercalcaemia secondary to bone lesions; no anaemia with haemoglobin < 10 g/dL; clonal bone marrow plasma cells < 10% of total nucleated cells; involved to uninvolved free light chain ratio < 100; no hyperviscosity; no bulky lymphadenopathy; no thrombocytopenia (< 100 × 10^9/L).

Staging

Staging is not required except in case of MGRS associated with Ig light chain amyloidosis (see *Immunoglobulin-related amyloidosis (AL amyloidosis)*, p. 608).

Prognosis and prediction

The treatment of MGRS is directed at the underlying B-cell or plasma cell clones and is based on a combination of various chemotherapy agents, aiming to preserve kidney function and prevent recurrence after kidney transplantation {1164}. No randomized controlled trials exist to guide the optimal approach to therapy, but bortezomib-based regimens are frequently used {94}. Anti-CD20 monoclonal antibodies such as rituximab are used for B-cell clones expressing CD20.

Immunoglobulin-related amyloidosis (AL amyloidosis)

Wechalekar AD
Gertz M
Naresh KN

Definition

Immunoglobulin light chain amyloidosis (AL amyloidosis) is defined as extracellular deposition of immunoglobulin light chain–derived linear non-branching fibrils (with a width of 9 nm) produced by clonal plasma cells or B cells causing progressive end-organ dysfunction.

ICD-O coding

9769/1 Immunoglobulin-related amyloidosis (AL amyloidosis)
9769/1 Systemic AL amyloidosis
9769/1 Localized AL amyloidosis
9769/1 Heavy chain AL amyloidosis

ICD-11 coding

5D00.0 AL amyloidosis

Related terminology

Acceptable: light chain amyloidosis; AL amyloidosis.

Subtype(s)

Systemic AL amyloidosis; localized AL amyloidosis; heavy chain AL amyloidosis

Localization

The heart, kidneys, liver, soft tissues (tongue, submandibular soft tissues, carpal tunnel, conjunctiva, cornea), gut, peripheral and autonomic nerves, skin, and lymph nodes can be involved.

Clinical features

AL amyloidosis should be considered in any patient with multisystem disease and a monoclonal protein in blood or urine. Heart failure with preserved ejection fraction associated with echocardiographic evidence of thickened ventricular walls, often confused with hypertrophic cardiomyopathy and left ventricular hypertrophy due to longstanding hypertension, is a common presentation {1119}. Amyloidosis is a differential diagnosis of any patient with non-diabetic proteinuria, peripheral neuropathy (particularly when associated with autonomic dysfunction), bilateral carpal tunnel syndrome, and hepatomegaly {2661}. The symptoms of amyloidosis are nonspecific and include fatigue, oedema, weight loss, and dyspnoea, which are seen with disorders that are far more common, leading patients to be misdiagnosed as having monoclonal gammopathy of undetermined significance (MGUS) and smouldering myeloma due to a failure to recognize the cardinal features of AL amyloidosis. Classic signs of amyloidosis, including macroglossia, submandibular swelling, and periorbital purpura, are highly characteristic but are found in only 15% of patients and are not specific. Most patients are seen primarily in cardiology and nephrology departments rather than haematology departments {2433}.

Epidemiology

AL amyloidosis occurs with an annual incidence of 1 case per 100 000 person-years, making it one sixth as common as plasma cell myeloma (PCM) {2182}. Cardiac amyloidosis

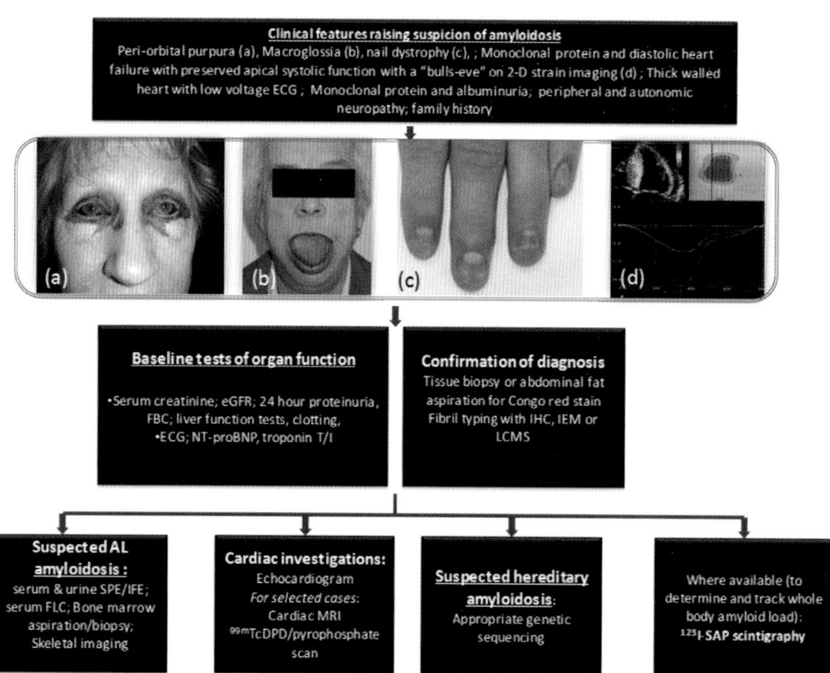

Fig. 4.288 Immunoglobulin-related amyloidosis (AL amyloidosis). Characteristic clinical features and a diagnostic algorithm for AL amyloidosis {4334}.

caused by wildtype transthyretin is common in elderly people, with a population prevalence as high as 1.1% of patients with heart failure {2362}. Differentiation from AL amyloidosis is important. Clues to the diagnosis of AL include multiple organ involvement, with two thirds of patients having more than one organ symptomatically involved with amyloid. The key to diagnostic recognition is obtaining immunofixation of the serum and urine and conducting an immunoglobulin free light chain (FLC) assay in patients with a symptom complex suggestive of AL.

Etiology

Unknown

Pathogenesis

In AL amyloidosis, an unstable immunoglobulin light chain (or fragments) interacts with the extracellular environment, leading to proteolytic cleavage, and binding to matrix components such as glycosaminoglycans, serum amyloid P, and collagen, which facilitate aggregation {2663}. The prefibrillar AL oligomers can be a cytotoxic species. Amyloid deposits are cleared by complement-mediated macrophages; the exact in vivo regulation remains unclear, but the process can be accelerated by antibodies directed to amyloid fibrils or fibrillar components {384}.

Macroscopic appearance

The macroscopic appearance varies between tissues. Affected organs may have a waxy appearance.

Histopathology

Bone marrow core biopsy

Bone marrow specimens vary, from revealing no pathological findings to showing involvement with amyloid, MGUS, PCM, or (rarely) lymphoplasmacytic lymphoma. The most common finding is a mildly increased infiltration with plasma cells (median: 9%), best demonstrated on CD138 immunohistochemistry, which may appear normal or may exhibit any of the changes found in PCM. Amyloid deposits are found in the bone marrow in about 60% of cases {2181,3215,3900,933}.

Biopsy of other tissues

Amyloid deposits may be present in many other tissues and organs, including parenchyma massively replaced by amyloid deposits. Macrophages and foreign body giant cells may be found around deposits. In localized AL, plasma cells may be increased in the adjacent tissues.

Amyloid demonstration and typing

On H&E-stained sections, amyloid is a pink, amorphous, waxy-looking substance with a characteristic cracking artefact. Typically, it is found focally in thickened blood vessel walls, on basement membranes, and in the interstitium of tissues such as fat and bone marrow {3900}. In bone marrow core biopsies, periosteal locations frequently show amyloid deposition. Congo red stains amyloid pink to red by standard light microscopy, and under polarized light it produces a characteristic apple-green birefringence. Congo red fluorescence microscopy is the more sensitive method for amyloid detection {2533}. Electron microscopic studies can differentiate light chain amyloidosis from non-amyloid immunoglobulin deposition diseases.

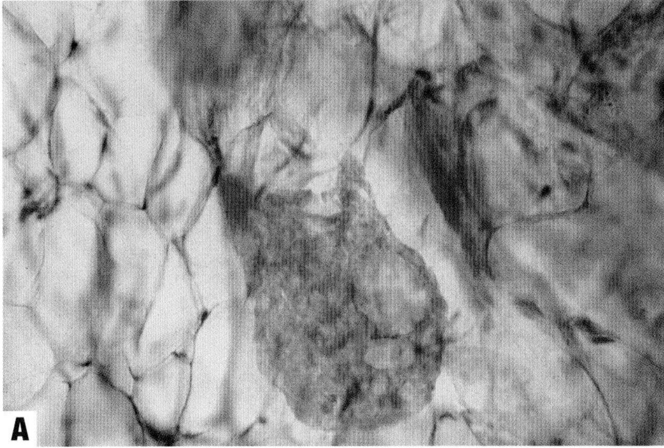

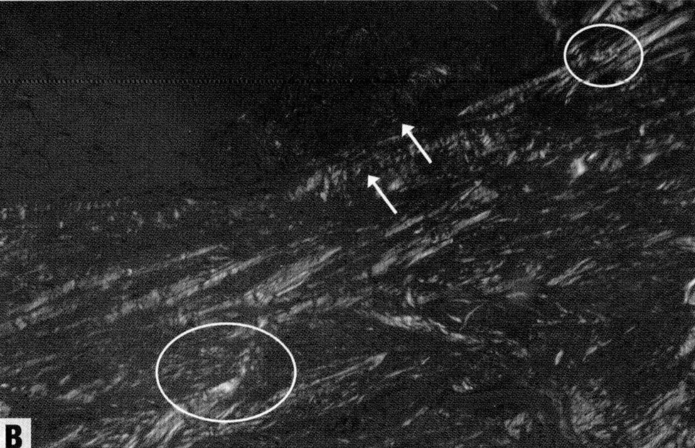

Fig. 4.289 Immunoglobulin-related amyloidosis (AL amyloidosis). **A** Amyloid deposition. Congo red staining of abdominal fat aspirate in a patient with AL amyloidosis (bright field). **B** Amyloid deposition in bone marrow biopsy that shows green birefringence under polarized light microscopy (circled in two places), with arrows pointing to blood vessels.

MGUS or another plasma cell proliferative disorder may be incidentally present in patients with secondary or familial amyloidosis {2190,787}. It is essential to characterize the amyloid fibril type. Laser microdissection of the amyloid in a biopsy specimen and analysis by mass spectrometry is the most effective method of characterizing amyloid type, with nearly 100% sensitivity and specificity {4258}.

Immunophenotype

The immunophenotypic features of the abnormal plasma cells in AL amyloidosis are like those of PCM, with aberrant expression of CD56 and/or cyclin D1 in 50% of cases and the majority showing light chain restriction. In a minority of cases with a smaller clone of neoplastic plasma cells admixed with normal plasma cells, light chain restriction is not demonstrable by immunohistochemistry. Neoplastic plasma cells express lambda light chains in > 80% of cases, and the rest are positive for kappa light chain {3900,4425, 933,4399}. Clonal abnormal plasma cells can also be detected using multiparameter flow cytometry in most cases of AL amyloidosis. Documentation of disease by multiparameter flow cytometry is useful assessing response to treatment {3109,2826}.

Cytology

The diagnosis cannot be made on the basis of FNAB.

Definition	Stage	HR for OS	Median OS, months	Ref. No.
Mayo Clinic, 2004 [10]				
One higher stage each for elevated troponin and elevated NT-proBNP[1]	I	Reference	130	35
	II	2.3	54	
	III	6.4	10	
Mayo Clinic, 2012 [15]				
One higher stage each for elevated troponin, elevated NT-proBNP, and elevated dFLC[2]	I	Reference	130	35
	II	1.8	72	
	III	3.7	24	
	IV	7.1	6	
European modification [26, 60]				
Derived from Mayo 2004: stage I–II correspond, stage III separated by additional NT-proBNP >8,500 ng/L	I	Reference	130	35
	II	2.4	54	
	IIIa	4.2	24	
	IIIb	11.3	4	

Thresholds for biomarkers are reported based on proposed modifications of the staging systems [29].
[1] cTnT >0.035 μg/L or cTnI >0.1 μg/L or hsTnT >54 pg/mL; NT-proBNP >332 ng/L.
[2] cTnT >0.025 μg/L or cTnI >0.1 μg/L or hsTnT >54 pg/mL; NT-proBNP >1,800 ng/L; dFLC >180 mg/L.

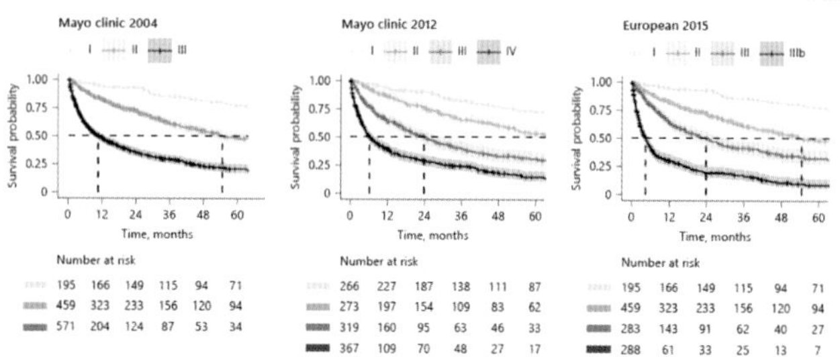

Fig. 4.290 Staging of immunoglobulin-related amyloidosis (AL amyloidosis). The shaded areas in these Kaplan–Meier overall survival (OS) plots indicate the 95% CI. cTnI, cardiac troponin I; cTnT, cardiac troponin T; dFLC, difference between involved and uninvolved free light chains; HR, hazard ratio; hsTnT, high-sensitivity troponin T; NT-proBNP, N-terminal pro–B-type natriuretic peptide. Reference citations per original publication {970B}: [10] Dispenzieri et al., 2004 {968A}; [15] Kumar et al., 2012 {2149A}; [26] Palladini et al., 2003 {3111A}; [29] Lilleness et al., 2019 {2341A}; [35] Dittrich et al., 2019 {970A}; [60] Sidana et al., 2020 {3739A}.

Diagnostic molecular pathology

There is no molecular diagnostic test for AL amyloidosis. Testing for mutations predisposing to familial amyloidosis in genes encoding transthyretin, Apo-A1/A2, fibrinogen, lysozyme and gelsolin is important to avoid misdiagnosis (mutations are listed on the Mutations in Hereditary Amyloidosis website, available at http://amyloidosismutations.com/ {3491}).

Essential and desirable diagnostic criteria

Essential: documentation of amyloid-related end-organ dysfunction by clinical examination (soft tissue deposition, polyneuropathy, autonomic neuropathy), supported by abnormality on tests for organ function in blood or urine; monoclonal protein in serum or urine or abnormal serum FLCs; demonstration of amyloid deposition on tissue biopsy (of abdominal fat, bone marrow, salivary gland, or the affected organ) by Congo red (or similar thioflavin) stain or typical fibrils on electron microscopy.

Desirable: typing of amyloid fibril protein by laser capture followed by mass spectrometry or immunohistochemistry / immunoelectron microscopy; confirmation of organ involvement by imaging (echocardiography or cardiac MRI for the heart); mutation of one or more genes associated with hereditary amyloidosis (especially when typing by mass spectrometry is unavailable or inconclusive).

Staging

Heart involvement is the most important determinant of survival in AL. The staging for AL is based on blood levels of cardiac biomarkers (N-terminal pro–B-type natriuretic peptide [NT-proBNP], B-type natriuretic peptide [BNP], and cardiac troponin T/I). The two widely used staging systems are the European modification of the Mayo 2004 staging system (stages I, II, IIIa, IIIb) {4335} and the Mayo 2012 staging system (stages I–IV), additionally incorporating serum FLCs as an indirect measure of plasma cell burden {2152}. Additional incorporation of cardiac global longitudinal strain by echocardiography may further refine the staging {778}.

Prognosis and prediction

The survival of patients with AL has substantially improved over the last decade, with a median survival time of 5 years in contemporary cohorts {2824,3374}. However, patients with advanced cardiac AL still have a high mortality rate after diagnosis (~30–40% at 6 months) {3374}.

Monitoring of the disease is done by assessing the haematological response using the difference between involved and uninvolved FLC. "Response" represents a 50% reduction, "very good partial response" (VGPR) a reduction to < 40 mg/L, and "complete response" represents normalization of the FLC with no detectable M protein in serum/urine {3113}. Patients achieving a rapid VGPR or better have a 58% predicted survival rate at 10 years {3373}. Organ response is defined as follows: for the heart, a reduction in the biomarker NT-proBNP by > 30% and by > 300 ng/L if baseline NT-proBNP is ≥ 650 ng/L; for kidneys, a reduction in urinary protein loss by 50%; and for the liver, a 50% reduction in serum alkaline phosphatase level {3112,3113}. Haematological response appears necessary but not sufficient for organ response; the latter translates into improved survival and reduced risk of developing end-stage renal disease.

Monoclonal immunoglobulin deposition disease

Leung N
Fernández de Larrea C
Kristinsson SY
Landgren OC
Rajkumar SV

Chapter 4

Definition

Monoclonal immunoglobulin (Ig) deposition disease results from non-amyloid deposition of monoclonal Ig in tissue secondary to a plasma cell neoplasm or (rarely) a B-cell neoplasm.

ICD-O coding

9769/1 Monoclonal immunoglobulin deposition disease
9769/1 Light chain deposition disease
9769/1 Light and heavy chain deposition disease
9762/3 Heavy chain deposition disease

ICD-11 coding

2A83.52 Light chain deposition disease
2A83.50 Heavy chain deposition disease

Related terminology

Acceptable: Randall-type monoclonal immunoglobulin deposition disease.

Subtype(s)

Light chain deposition disease; light and heavy chain deposition disease; heavy chain deposition disease

Localization

The kidney is nearly always involved in monoclonal Ig deposition disease {2910,1819}. Heart, liver, lung, gastrointestinal tract, autonomic and peripheral nervous system, and skin involvement has been also reported {781,344}. Extrarenal involvement seems to be more common in patients with plasma cell myeloma {2910,2713}.

Clinical features

Monoclonal Ig deposition disease has three subtypes based on the monoclonal Ig deposits. Light chain deposition disease is the most common and makes up 80% of cases, followed by heavy chain deposition disease and light and heavy chain deposition disease.

The most common monoclonal Ig detected in the serum is IgG, followed by monoclonal light chain, IgA, and IgM {2355,3291,3600,2713,1819}. The tissue Ig deposits can differ from the monoclonal Ig in the blood. In patients with light chain deposition disease, only the monoclonal Ig light chain is deposited, even if the entire Ig is detected in the serum. In heavy chain deposition disease, the serum will show the presence of the monoclonal light chain but the tissue deposits will only contain the monoclonal heavy chain. Proteinuria is often in the nephrotic range, with varying degrees of renal impairment {2910,1819}. Acute kidney injury and acute renal failure occur in patients with coexisting light chain cast nephropathy {2355}. Patients with heart involvement present with diastolic heart failure and atrial arrhythmias. Septal thickening can be seen on echocardiogram {508}. Troponin T, B-type natriuretic peptide (BNP), and N-terminal pro–B-type natriuretic peptide (NT-proBNP) are elevated in patients with heart involvement {2713}. Liver involvement is manifested by elevation of liver function tests, hepatomegaly, portal hypertension, and liver failure. Cough, oxygen desaturation, and dyspnoea are common in pulmonary involvement {344}. The monoclonal Ig deposition can be interstitial or nodular on imaging studies. Another pattern is pulmonary cystic disease resulting in emphysematous changes and obstructive lung disease {781}. Peripheral and autonomic neuropathy can be seen in patients with nerve involvement. A nerve biopsy is typically required to confirm nerve involvement {1819}.

Epidemiology

The median age at diagnosis is in the mid-fifties to mid-sixties, ranging from 20 to 91 years {2355,3291,3600,2713,1819,4570}. Nearly 60% of the patients are male. Plasma cell neoplasms make up > 95% of the associated neoplasms. Plasma cell (multiple) myeloma makes up 20–30% of cases of monoclonal Ig deposition disease, whereas monoclonal gammopathy of renal significance accounts for 65–75% of cases {2284,2285}. In patients with plasma cell myeloma, light chain deposition can coexist with light chain cast nephropathy {2355,4540}. B-cell neoplasms are associated with 2–3% of cases {3291,2910, 2284}. The B-cell neoplasms involved are most commonly IgM-expressing B-lymphoid neoplasms, such as lymphoplasmacytic lymphoma, chronic lymphocytic leukaemia, and marginal zone lymphomas {4084,3845,4256,1581}.

Etiology

Unknown

Pathogenesis

Various characteristics of the Ig protein determine the risk of developing monoclonal Ig deposition disease {1573}. Monoclonal light chains in the VκIV family are overrepresented in light chain deposition disease {4229}. CH1 deletion is required for the development of heavy chain deposition disease, but this abnormality is also present in patients with Ig heavy chain amyloidosis and heavy chain disease {772,456}. Somatic mutations that increase the hydrophobicity of the Ig contribute to the pathogenesis, but no single mutation has been identified as predictive of the disease.

Macroscopic appearance

The macroscopic appearance varies depending on the tissue affected.

Histopathology

For details of the histological presentation of the underlying lymphoid neoplasms, see the appropriate sections.

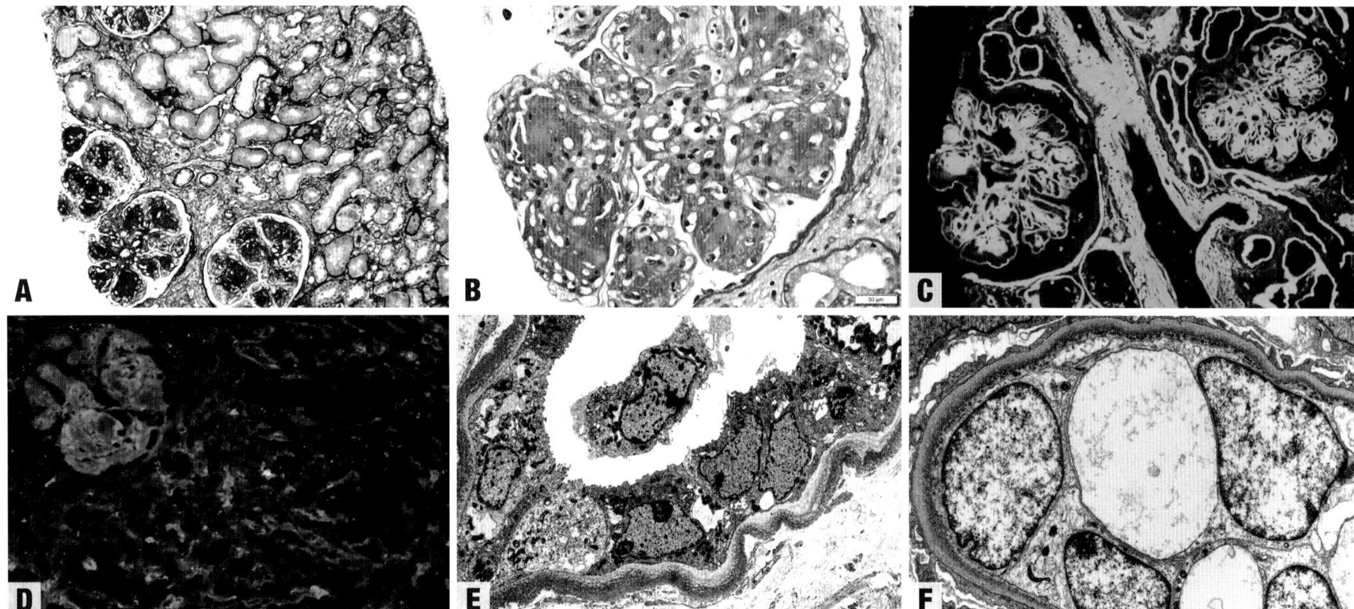

Fig. 4.291 Monoclonal immunoglobulin deposition disease. Light chain deposition disease. **A** Low-power view showing nodular glomerulosclerosis. The mesangial nodules stain black (JMS). **B** High-power image of a glomerulus showing nodular mesangial expansion by PAS-positive mesangial sclerosis and glassy immune deposits. The glomerular basement membrane is mildly thickened with segmental duplication (PAS). **C,D** On immunofluorescence, there is bright diffuse linear staining of the basement membranes of glomeruli, tubules, and vessel wall myocytes for kappa light chain (**C**), with negative staining for lambda light chain (**D**). **E,F** On electron microscopy, punctate, powdery, electron-dense deposits are present extensively along the outer aspect of the tubular basement membrane (**E**) and the inner aspect of the glomerular basement membrane (**F**).

The deposits are most frequently found in tubular basement membranes, glomerular basement membranes, vascular walls, and the interstitium of the kidney {2910}. Cardiac deposits involve the myocardial interstitium throughout the endocardium and epicardium as well as vascular walls, and deposits in the liver predominantly involve the perisinusoidal spaces {508,2639}. In the lung, nodular perivascular deposits are seen {1980,4415}. Ig deposits appear eosinophilic on H&E staining, are positive on PAS and silver stains, and are negative on Congo red staining.

Renal monoclonal Ig deposition disease on light microscopy exhibits nodular glomerulosclerosis in two thirds of cases. Immunofluorescence reveals diffuse linear deposits of one light chain (in light chain deposition disease), one light chain and one heavy chain (in light and heavy chain deposition disease), or one heavy chain (in heavy chain deposition disease) along the basement membranes of glomeruli, tubules, and vessels. The characteristic ultrastructural finding is punctate, powdery (non-fibrillar), electron-dense deposits along the basement membranes of tubules and glomeruli.

Inflammatory or lymphoplasmacytic involvement may occur outside the kidney but is characteristically absent in the kidney.

Cytology

FNA would not provide enough tissue for diagnosis.

Diagnostic molecular pathology

In nearly 50% of patients with monoclonal Ig deposition disease with an underlying plasma cell neoplasm, a t(11;14) is identified {2116}.

Essential and desirable diagnostic criteria

Essential: demonstration of monoclonal Ig deposition in tissue – in the kidney, this should be demonstrated by immunohistochemistry and electron microscopy; in cases where there is coexistence of light chain cast nephropathy, monoclonal Ig deposition disease may be demonstrated by immunohistochemistry only; diagnosis in other tissues relies on immunohistochemistry, as electron microscopy is not commonly used; besides light chain cast nephropathy, Ig light chain amyloidosis and light chain proximal tubulopathy have been found to coexist with monoclonal Ig deposition disease in the same kidney.

Staging

No staging system currently exists.

Prognosis and prediction

The overall median survival time is > 5 years, but it varies and is influenced by the presence of plasma cell myeloma, kidney function at the time of diagnosis, cardiac involvement, type of treatment received, and response to treatment {2355,3600, 2116,4591,2713,1819,123}. Patients who achieve a very good partial haematological response or better, and renal response, have the best outcomes {773,3600}.

Heavy chain diseases: Introduction

Chng WJ
Sohani AR

The heavy chain diseases (HCDs) are three rare B-cell neoplasms (alpha, gamma, and mu) each characterized by the production of a shortened monoclonal immunoglobulin heavy chain, with typically no light chain {4269,355}. The heavy chain is usually truncated because of deletions, insertions, and point mutations presumed to be acquired during somatic hypermutation, resulting in the absence of portions of the variable heavy chain (VH) domain and the first constant heavy chain (CH1) domain {4269}. The latter domain normally contains binding sites for light chain, and for heavy chain binding protein, which directs unassociated heavy chains to the proteasome for degradation {1551}. Therefore, in the absence of normal CH1, the mutant heavy chain neither associates with light chain to form a normal immunoglobulin molecule nor is it targeted for degradation. Variably sized proteins are produced, which may not yield a characteristic monoclonal peak by routine serum protein electrophoresis and require immunofixation to detect. Deletions affecting the genes encoding the VH domain may lead to false negative results on IGH PCR for B-cell clonality, requiring IGK PCR for this assessment {360}.

In some cases, HCD shows morphological features consistent with another well-defined histological entity. Some cases of gamma HCD have morphological features that resemble lymphoplasmacytic lymphoma, splenic marginal zone lymphoma, or extranodal marginal zone lymphoma of mucosa-associated lymphoid tissue (EMZL) {360}, whereas mu HCD typically resembles chronic lymphocytic leukaemia /

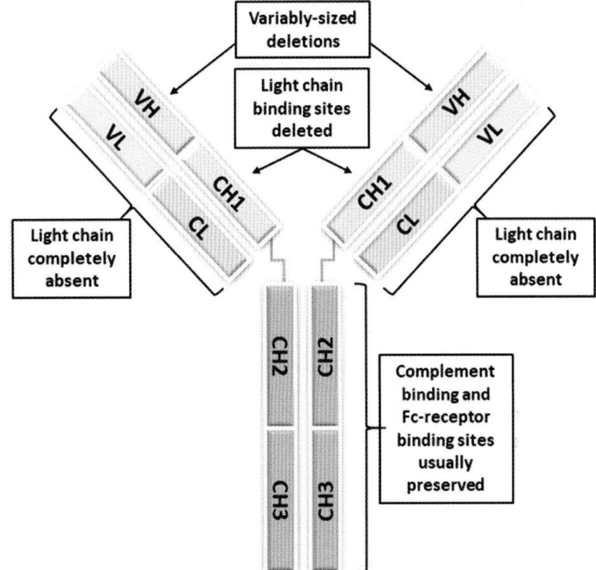

Fig. 4.292 Immunoglobulin molecule indicating abnormalities in heavy chain disease. In all forms of heavy chain disease, there is an abnormal heavy chain CH1 domain, including the region containing sites for binding to immunoglobulin light chains. Therefore, in heavy chain disease, free heavy chains are both structurally abnormal and abnormally secreted without light chains. Variably sized deletions are also present in the VH domain. The CH2 and CH3 domains are usually preserved, enabling the heavy chain to be detected by immunofixation.

Table 4.63 Essential clinicopathological and diagnostic features of heavy chain diseases (HCDs) (continued on next page)

Feature	Mu HCD	Gamma HCD	Alpha HCD
Epidemiology	Extremely rare Male predominance	Rare Female predominance	Higher incidence in Mediterranean and Middle East Association with low socioeconomic status
Median age at diagnosis	58 years	51–68 years	32 years
Associated lymphoma	Features resembling CLL with plasmacytic differentiation or, in some cases, lymphoplasmacytic lymphoma	Small B-cell lymphoma with plasmacytic differentiation resembling a polymorphous lymphoplasmacytic neoplasm (*MYD88* wildtype) or, in some cases, another well-defined entity such as marginal zone lymphoma (usually of nodal or splenic types) or a splenic B-cell leukaemia/lymphoma	MALT lymphoma with extensive plasmacytic differentiation (IPSID)
Other associated diseases	Case reports of SLE, amyloidosis, portal hypertension, myelodysplastic neoplasm, recurrent pulmonary infections, carpal tunnel syndrome	Underlying autoimmune disease in a subset of patients, most commonly RA, AIHA, or SLE; immune thrombocytopenia, various forms of vasculitis, Sjögren syndrome, myasthenia gravis, and thyroiditis also reported; autoimmune disease onset usually precedes diagnosis by several years Concurrent T- or NK-large granular lymphocytic disorders reported in some patients	Infection with *Helicobacter pylori*, *Vibrio cholerae*, *Campylobacter jejuni*, or intestinal parasites

AIHA, autoimmune haemolytic anaemia; CLL, chronic lymphocytic leukaemia; IFE, immunofixation electrophoresis; IPSID, immunoproliferative small intestinal disease; MALT, mucosa-associated lymphoid tissue; MGUS, monoclonal gammopathy of undetermined significance; PFT, pulmonary function test; RA, rheumatoid arthritis; SLE, systemic lupus erythematosus; SPEP, serum protein electrophoresis.

Table 4.63 Essential clinicopathological and diagnostic features of heavy chain diseases (HCDs) (continued)

Feature	Mu HCD	Gamma HCD	Alpha HCD
Clinical presentation	Splenomegaly, hepatomegaly, lymphadenopathy Renal complications rare, despite Bence Jones proteinuria	Disseminated disease (60%): fever, weight loss, malaise, generalized lymphadenopathy (50% of cases); splenomegaly and hepatomegaly less common Localized disease (25%): manifestations depend on involved organ, e.g. cytopenias in bone marrow disease, erythematous plaques in cutaneous disease; other reported sites: thyroid, salivary gland, oropharynx, and gastrointestinal tract Symptoms of autoimmune disease without overt lymphoma (15%): clinically resembles MGUS	Most common presenting symptoms and signs in gastrointestinal disease: chronic watery diarrhoea, weight loss, malabsorption, abdominal pain, finger clubbing, vomiting, and fever Respiratory disease: dyspnoea, hypoxaemia, diffuse pulmonary infiltrates, hilar lymphadenopathy, direct involvement of pharyngeal mucosa by IPSID, restrictive pattern on PFTs Advanced disease: generalized lymphadenopathy, hepatosplenomegaly, ascites
Additional findings on imaging and other modalities	Lytic bone lesions	Enlarged lymph nodes or other involved organs	X-ray / CT / abdominal ultrasound: small bowel wall thickening, enlarged mesenteric lymph nodes; small bowel dilation or strictures on contrast-enhanced imaging Upper gastrointestinal endoscopy: polypoid or nodular mucosa, erythematous or thickened mucosal folds, mucosal oedema
SPEP/IFE and related findings	SPEP may be normal (> 50% of cases) IFE shows anti-IgM heavy chain reactivity usually without associated light chain Free monoclonal light chains (usually kappa) also secreted, resulting in detection of serum free light chains and urine Bence Jones protein	Elevated serum IgG Monoclonal band in beta globulins fraction of SPEP that types as IgG heavy chain without associated kappa or lambda light chain Abnormal monoclonal IgG heavy chain also found in urine protein electrophoresis because of low molecular weight of IgG and existence as a dimer	Elevated serum IgA Broad monoclonal band in alpha-2 globulins or beta globulins fraction of SPEP that types as IgA heavy chain without associated kappa or lambda light chain Abnormal IgA heavy chain detectable in both serum and intestinal juice
Other laboratory findings	Hypoproliferative anaemia, mild lymphocytosis Thrombocytopenia less common *MYD88* p.L265P mutation in a subset of cases	Normocytic anaemia Cytopenias related to underlying autoimmune disease or bone marrow infiltration	Hypochromic anaemia, lymphocytosis, hypoalbuminaemia Electrolyte imbalances with hypokalaemia, hyponatraemia, hypocalcaemia Elevated alkaline phosphatase (gastrointestinal isozyme)
Histological/ cytological characteristics	Bone marrow aspirates and touch preparations show infiltration of small, mature-appearing lymphocytes resembling CLL cells admixed with plasma cells with a single prominent intracytoplasmic vacuole	Polymorphous infiltrate of small lymphocytes, plasmacytoid and plasma cells, immunoblasts, and histiocytes; some cases with increased eosinophils or high endothelial venules Diffuse or interfollicular infiltrates with sparing of follicles in nodal specimens, while extranodal tissues may show follicular colonization and lymphoepithelial lesions	Dense infiltrates composed of abundant plasma cells or lymphocytes with marked plasmacytic differentiation Marginal zone B cells and lymphoepithelial lesions may be present Infiltrate displaces intestinal crypts and is associated with villous atrophy Large-cell transformation shows sheets of immunoblasts or plasmablasts with surface ulceration and mucosal destruction
Immuno-phenotype	Positive for CD19, CD20, CD38, and IgM Light chain restriction in some cases, usually kappa Weak expression of CD5 reported in rare cases	Lymphocytes positive for CD19, CD20, PAX5, and CD79a, without expression of CD5, CD10, or CD23 Plasmacytic / plasma cell component positive for CD19, CD79a, CD38, CD138, and IRF4 (MUM1) Both components express monoclonal IgG typically without light chain staining, although monotypic kappa staining is reported in rare cases	Lymphocytes positive for CD19, CD20, PAX5, and CD79a and typically negative for CD5 and CD10 Plasma cells positive for CD138, CD79a, and IRF4 (MUM1) and negative for CD20 and PAX5 Both components express monoclonal IgA without light chain staining

AIHA, autoimmune haemolytic anaemia; CLL, chronic lymphocytic leukaemia; IFE, immunofixation electrophoresis; IPSID, immunoproliferative small intestinal disease; MALT, mucosa-associated lymphoid tissue; MGUS, monoclonal gammopathy of undetermined significance; PFT, pulmonary function test; RA, rheumatoid arthritis; SLE, systemic lupus erythematosus; SPEP, serum protein electrophoresis.

small lymphocytic lymphoma (CLL/SLL), or in some cases lymphoplasmacytic lymphoma, and alpha HCD is considered a variant of MALT lymphoma {4269,355}. However, each of these HCDs is sufficiently distinct to be considered a separate entity (see Table 4.63, p. 613). Establishing a diagnosis of HCD requires demonstration of the relevant free heavy chain by immunofixation. Of note, it is important to distinguish HCDs from heavy chain deposition diseases, which are described in a different section (see *Monoclonal immunoglobulin deposition disease*, p. 611).

Mu heavy chain disease

Sohani AR
Bianchi G
Geddie WR

Definition
Mu heavy chain disease (HCD) is a systemic B-cell neoplasm with hepatosplenic, nodal, and bone involvement characterized by vacuolated plasma cells and secretion of defective serum mu heavy chains that lack associated light chains; free serum and/or urine kappa light chains may also be present.

ICD-O coding
9762/3 Mu heavy chain disease

ICD-11 coding
2A84.2 Mu heavy chain disease

Related terminology
None

Subtype(s)
None

Localization
The spleen is almost universally involved, with hepatic involvement in 75% of patients, nodal disease in 40%, and bone marrow involvement in 20% {4270,355}.

Clinical features
Bone involvement is characterized by lytic bone lesions. When associated with systemic illnesses such as amyloidosis or systemic lupus erythematosus, features of the underlying disorders are present. Anaemia is commonly present, with or without lymphocytosis, typically secondary to bone marrow infiltration by neoplastic cells {355}. Lymphocytosis is typically milder than that seen in chronic lymphocytic leukaemia {227}.

Epidemiology
Mu HCD is the rarest form of HCD. It shows a male predominance and occurs in the sixth decade of life.

Etiology
A few reported cases with *MYD88* p.L265P mutation suggests that at least some cases are biologically related to lymphoplasmacytic lymphoma (LPL) {227,4218}.

Pathogenesis
Mu HCD arises from a clonal expansion of cells of B lineage producing truncated mu heavy chain that lacks light chain binding sites {4391,2485}.

Macroscopic appearance
Not relevant

Histopathology
Involved tissues are infiltrated by vacuolated plasma cells and small round lymphoid cells with mature chromatin, resembling cells of chronic lymphocytic leukaemia / small lymphocytic lymphoma (CLL/SLL) or LPL {355,822,227}.

Cytology
FNA may be used in association with core biopsy to sample splenic or liver lesions, acquire material for flow cytometry or other ancillary tests, and detect associated systemic amyloidosis.

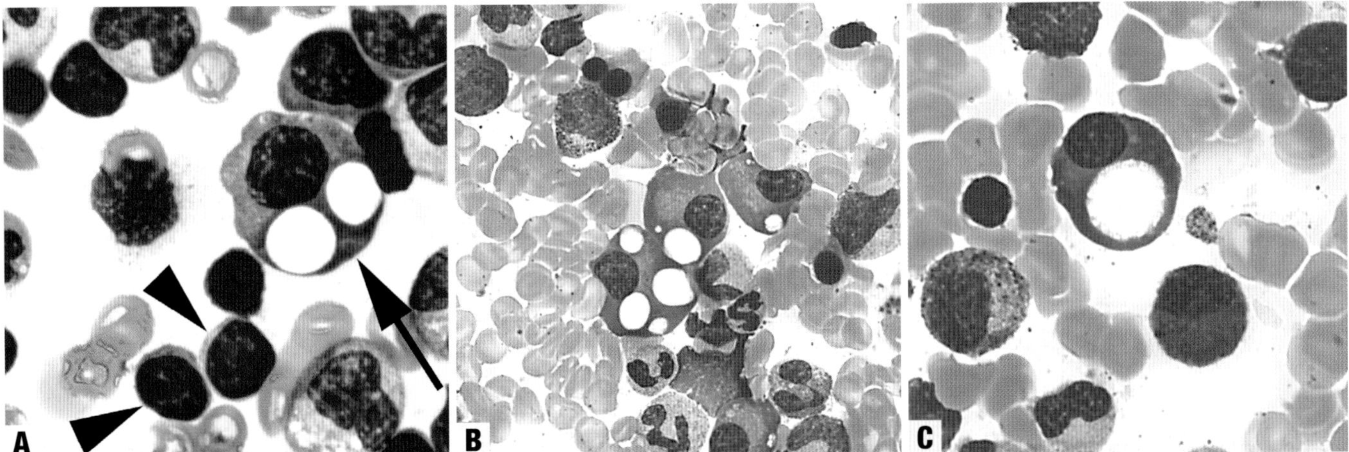

Fig. 4.293 Mu heavy chain disease. **A** The bone marrow aspirate smear (Wright–Giemsa) contains a spectrum of neoplastic cells including small, mature-appearing lymphocytes with scant cytoplasm (arrowheads) and plasma cells with prominent cytoplasmic vacuoles (arrow). Background bone marrow elements (erythroid and myeloid precursors) are also present. **B,C** In this case of mu heavy chain disease, the aspirate smear (MGG) shows plasma cells with eccentric nuclei, clumped chromatin, and prominent cytoplasmic vacuoles, including some with multiple vacuoles (**B**) and others with large single vacuoles (**C**). Background small lymphocytes and normal maturing myeloid and erythroid elements are also present.

Diagnostic molecular pathology

Clonal IG gene rearrangements may be present with high levels of somatic hypermutation. *MYD88* p.L265P mutation has recently been reported in a subset of cases {227,4218}.

Essential and desirable diagnostic criteria

Essential: bone marrow or tissue involvement by IgM-positive small round lymphocytes and vacuolated plasma cells; elevated serum free kappa light chains or kappa Bence Jones proteinuria.

Desirable: serum immunofixation or other modality demonstrating anti-mu reactivity without associated light chain.

Staging

The modified Lugano staging system for underlying lymphoma (e.g. CLL/SLL, LPL) applies.

Prognosis and prediction

The prognosis is highly variable, with reported overall survival times ranging from < 1 month to decades (median: 2 years). Delays in diagnosis negatively impact survival. Watchful waiting without therapy is recommended for indolent, asymptomatic cases. In cases of active, symptomatic lymphoma, CLL/SLL-directed therapy (or LPL-directed therapy if *MYD88*-mutated) is indicated {355,4218}.

Gamma heavy chain disease

Sohani AR
Bianchi G
Geddie WR

Definition

Gamma heavy chain disease (HCD) is a B-cell lymphoplasmacytic neoplasm exhibiting variable morphology with nodal, bone marrow, and extranodal involvement. All cases secrete an M protein characterized as gamma heavy chain, without associated light chains.

ICD-O coding

9762/3 Gamma heavy chain disease

ICD-11 coding

2A84.1 Gamma heavy chain disease

Related terminology

Not recommended: Franklin disease.

Subtype(s)

None

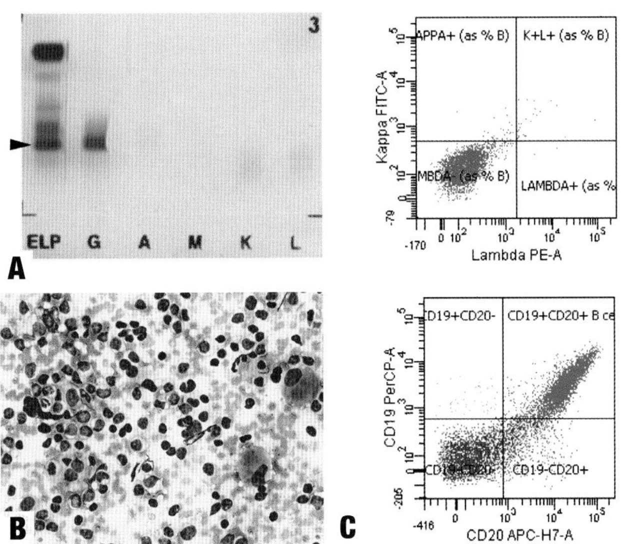

Fig. 4.294 Gamma heavy chain disease. **A** Serum protein electrophoresis and immunofixation in gamma heavy chain disease. The serum protein electrophoresis lane (ELP) shows a distinct broad band (arrowhead), consistent with an M component. There is a corresponding band in the gamma lane (G), indicating that the M component is composed of gamma heavy chain. However, no corresponding bands are seen in either the kappa (K) or lambda (L) light chain lanes, which show only faint polyclonal patterns. (Other lane labels: A, alpha; M, mu.) **B** FNA of a parotid mass (Giemsa) demonstrates a heterogeneous population of numerous small lymphocytes with round to slightly irregular nuclei, clumped chromatin, and moderate eccentric basophilic cytoplasm, indicative of plasmacytic differentiation. Also present are occasional epithelioid histiocytes with oval nuclei and abundant cytoplasm, seen on the right side of the image. **C** Concurrent flow cytometry demonstrated a population of CD19+, CD20+ B cells (blue, bottom) that were negative for both kappa and lambda immunoglobulin light chains (blue, top).

Localization

Most patients have disseminated nodal disease, with or without splenomegaly or marrow involvement. Localized extranodal disease may be limited to the bone marrow or another site, most commonly the skin.

Clinical features

Underlying autoimmune disease (present in a subset of patients) generally precedes the onset of HCD by several years {1165, 4271}. Cytopenias are related to underlying autoimmunity or bone marrow infiltration.

Epidemiology

HCD is a rare disease, with a female predominance; patients are in their sixth or seventh decade of life {1165,4271}.

Etiology

The association with an underlying autoimmune disease in many cases suggests an etiological link to lymphoma development, but further studies are needed {1165,4271}.

Pathogenesis

Gamma HCD arises from a clonal expansion of cells producing abnormal truncated gamma heavy chain that lacks light chain binding sites {2844}.

Macroscopic appearance

Enlarged lymph nodes and spleen

Histopathology

The morphological findings are heterogeneous. In lymph nodes, most cases contain an interfollicular or diffuse infiltrate of small lymphocytes, plasmacytoid lymphocytes, plasma cells, and admixed immunoblasts and histiocytes, resembling a polymorphous lymphoplasmacytic or (nodal and extranodal) marginal zone lymphoma. In biopsies with features of extranodal marginal zone lymphoma, lymphoepithelial lesions and follicular colonization may be present. Monocytoid differentiation is typically absent {360}. In some cases, increased eosinophils and hypervascularity raise the differential diagnosis of Hodgkin or peripheral T-cell lymphoma {2844}. Transformation to diffuse large B-cell lymphoma may occur {4269,355}.

Cytology

Cytological sampling may be used for primary diagnosis in conjunction with flow cytometry, immunofixation, or molecular testing {1600}.

Diagnostic molecular pathology

Clonal IG gene rearrangements are found. No known recurrent genetic mutations are known {360}. *MYD88* is wildtype {1476}.

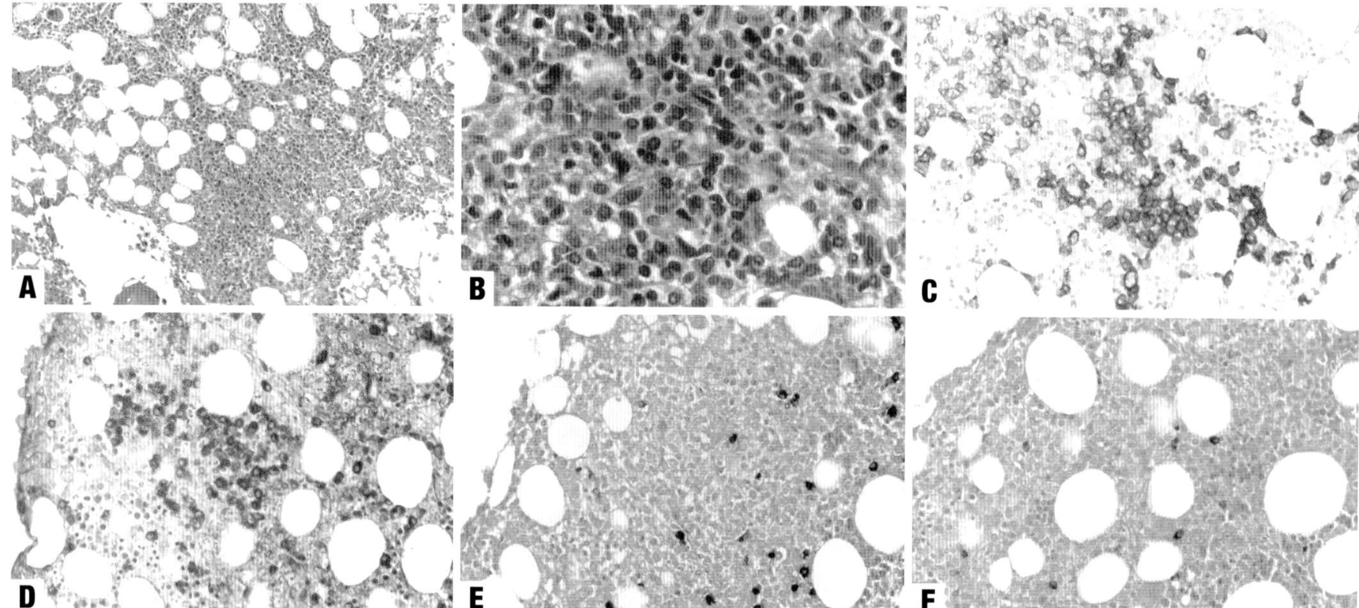

Fig. 4.295 Gamma heavy chain disease. **A,B** Bone marrow evaluation of a 46-year-old man with a history of rheumatoid arthritis shows loose lymphoid aggregates consisting of small lymphocytes, plasmacytoid lymphocytes, and plasma cells. The lymphoplasmacytic cells are positive for CD138 (**C**) and IgG heavy chain (**D**) by immunohistochemistry. In situ hybridization for kappa (**E**) and lambda (**F**) light chains highlights fewer plasma cells, in a different distribution from that of the IgG-expressing plasma cells.

Essential and desirable diagnostic criteria

Essential: serum or urine immunofixation electrophoresis demonstrating a gamma monoclonal band without an associated light chain (this may be the only manifestation in patients with autoimmune disease).

Desirable: FNA or tissue biopsy demonstrating atypical lymphoplasmacytic proliferation expressing IgG, typically without light chains.

Staging

Staging follows the Lugano modification of the Ann Arbor staging system for the underlying lymphoma.

Prognosis and prediction

Gamma HCD has a highly variable clinical course, with overall survival ranging from < 1 to 20 years. Disseminated or medullary disease requires systemic chemotherapy, whereas surgery or radiation is effective for localized extranodal disease {355}. Rituximab is recommended for CD20-positive disease, and durable responses have been reported with the use of novel agents, including bendamustine, lenalidomide, and bortezomib {3754}. Treatment of the underlying autoimmune disease is indicated.

Alpha heavy chain disease

Sohani AR
Bianchi G
Geddie WR

Definition

Alpha heavy chain disease (HCD) is a variant of extranodal marginal zone lymphoma of mucosa-associated lymphoid tissue (EMZL) that typically involves the gastrointestinal tract and secretes defective, truncated alpha heavy chains lacking light chains.

ICD-O coding

9762/3 Alpha heavy chain disease

ICD-11 coding

2A84.0 Alpha heavy chain disease

Related terminology

Acceptable: Mediterranean lymphoma; immunoproliferative small intestinal disease (IPSID).

Subtype(s)

None

Localization

The duodenum is most often involved (63% of cases), followed by the jejunum (17%) and ileum (8%). Involvement of the stomach, colon, mesenteric lymph nodes, respiratory tract, thyroid, or more than one anatomical site has been reported in rare cases {3205,357}.

Clinical features

The most common gastrointestinal manifestations are malabsorption with diarrhoea, abdominal pain, weight loss, hypoalbuminaemia, and electrolyte abnormalities {3205,357,1095}.

Epidemiology

Patients are predominantly young and male, and the incidence is higher in the Mediterranean, Middle East, and low- and middle-income countries than in other geographical areas {1095}. The overall incidence is declining following broader accessibility of antibiotics.

Etiology

Impaired localized immunity secondary to prior infection leads to diminished clearance of *Campylobacter jejuni*. Chronic *C. jejuni* infection and toxin exposure induce an IgA-secreting lymphoplasmacytic proliferation that acquires somatic hypermutation and double-stranded DNA breaks, ultimately resulting in clonal expansion {357}.

Pathogenesis

Alpha HCD arises from a clonal expansion of cells producing abnormal truncated alpha heavy chains with loss of light chain binding sites and B-cell receptor idiotype, allowing immune escape. Mutant heavy chains cluster with the B-cell receptor, resulting in activated signal transduction, antigen-independent proliferation, and tumour cell growth {357}.

Macroscopic appearance

Endoscopy shows polypoid or nodular lesions, erythematous mucosal thickening, or mucosal oedema {357,1095}.

Histopathology

Tissue biopsies contain a dense infiltrate composed of abundant plasma or lymphoplasmacytic cells with splaying of intestinal crypts and villous atrophy. Other features of EMZL may also be

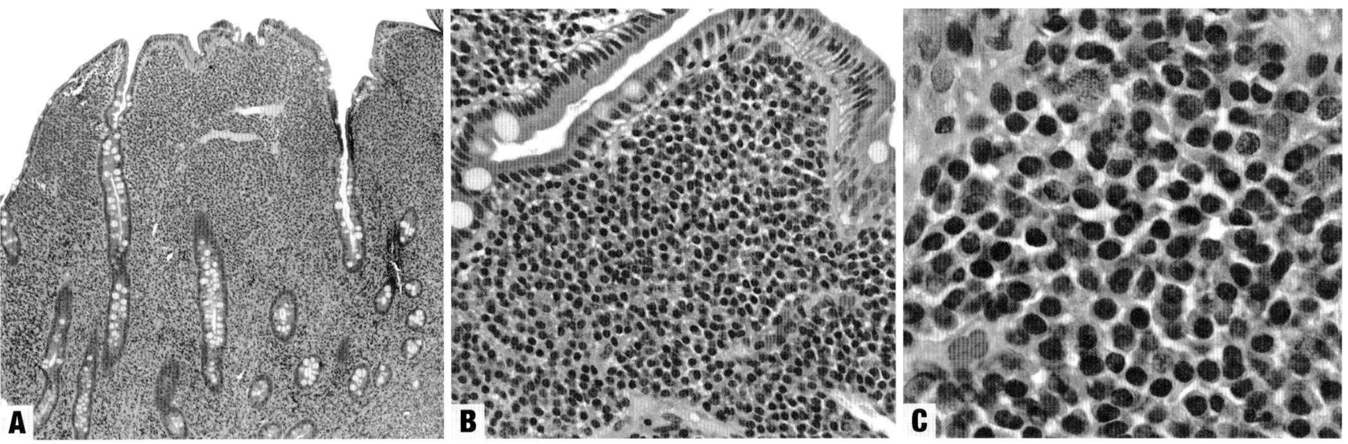

Fig. 4.296 Alpha heavy chain disease. **A** Duodenal biopsy demonstrates marked infiltration of the lamina propria by a dense lymphoid infiltrate with splaying of crypts and overlying villous blunting. **B** Details are shown at higher magnification. **C** High-power examination shows that the infiltrate consists of small cells with round, eccentric nuclei and moderate pink cytoplasm, histologically consistent with an extranodal marginal zone lymphoma of mucosa-associated lymphoid tissue (EMZL) with extensive plasmacytic differentiation. Immunohistochemical stains (not shown) demonstrated that the plasmacytic cells were positive for alpha heavy chain, with little to no staining for mu and gamma heavy chains or kappa and lambda light chains, supporting a diagnosis of alpha heavy chain disease or immunoproliferative small intestinal disease.

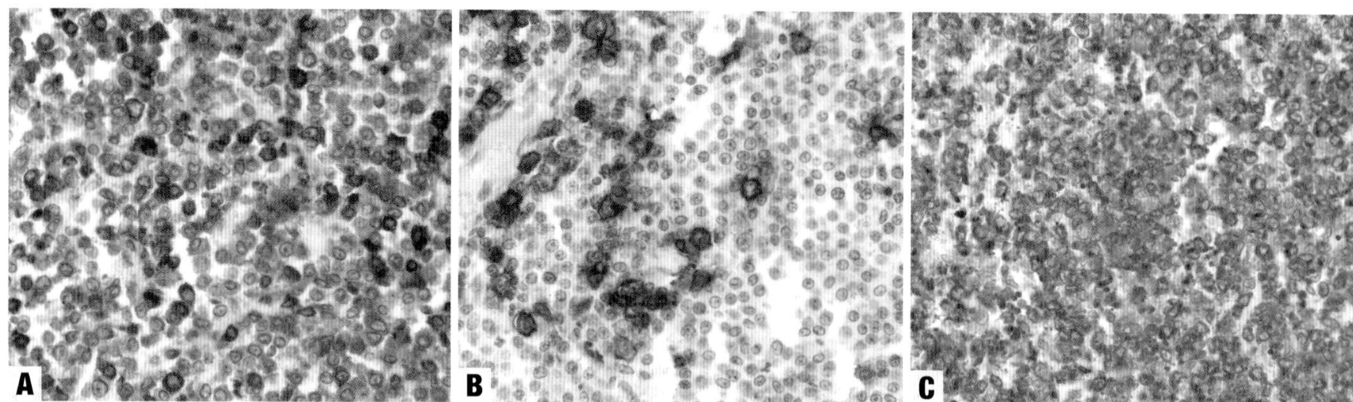

Fig. 4.297 Alpha heavy chain disease. **A** The neoplastic cells are diffusely positive for CD79a. **B** Only a small subset express CD20. **C** There is diffuse staining for IgA, but staining for kappa and lambda light chains was negative (not shown).

present (see *Histology* in *Extranodal marginal zone lymphoma of mucosa-associated lymphoid tissue*, p. 401). Large-cell transformation with sheets of immunoblasts or plasmablasts may occur.

Cytology

EUS-FNAB may be used to augment an endoscopic mucosal biopsy and collect material for ancillary testing.

Diagnostic molecular pathology

Clonal IG gene rearrangements are present. No known recurrent mutations or translocations are known, including, for example, rearrangements involving *MALT1* or other typical aberrations found in EMZL {357}.

Essential and desirable diagnostic criteria

Essential: tissue biopsy with features of EMZL with extensive plasmacytic differentiation expressing IgA without light chains.

Desirable: serum immunofixation demonstrating anti-alpha reactivity without associated light chain.

Staging

The disease is staged as localized (single-organ involvement) or systemic (nodal and multiorgan involvement) {357}.

Prognosis and prediction

The natural history is local progression followed by systemic spread. Complications of bowel obstruction or perforation, severe malnutrition, or infection may be fatal. In early disease, 6-month antimicrobial treatment leads to remission in 30–70% of cases, although recurrence is common {357}. Anthracycline-based chemotherapy and rituximab have been effective in treating systemic disease or large-cell transformation {1095}.

Plasma cell neoplasms: Introduction

Chng WJ

Plasma cell neoplasms arise from the monoclonal expansion of post–germinal-centre, class-switched, terminally differentiated B cells that secrete monoclonal immunoglobulins (Igs) called M proteins or paraproteins. The plasma cell neoplasms discussed in the following sections include plasma cell myeloma, plasmacytoma, and plasma cell neoplasms with an associated paraneoplastic syndrome (POEMS syndrome [polyneuropathy, organomegaly, endocrinopathy, myeloma protein, and skin changes], TEMPI syndrome [telangiectases, elevated erythropoietin and erythrocytosis, monoclonal gammopathy, perinephric fluid collection, and intrapulmonary shunting], and AESOP syndrome [adenopathy and extensive skin patch overlying plasmacytoma]) (see Box 4.06). Compared with the fourth edition of the WHO classification of haematolymphoid tumours, a few changes have been made. First, TEMPI syndrome, which was a provisional entry, is now confirmed as a subtype of plasma cell neoplasms with an associated paraneoplastic syndrome. In addition, AESOP syndrome has been added as a subtype. Second, following the hierarchical structure of the present edition of the WHO classification, non-IgM monoclonal gammopathy of undetermined significance (MGUS), a precursor lesion with the potential to evolve into a plasma cell neoplasm, has been omitted from the plasma cell neoplasms family/class and grouped with other monoclonal gammopathies. The third change is that diseases characterized by monoclonal Ig deposition, such as Ig light chain amyloidosis and monoclonal Ig deposition disease, previously classified as plasma cell neoplasms, have now also been grouped separately. Other Ig-secreting disorders that consist of both monoclonal lymphocytes and plasma cells, including lymphoplasmacytic lymphoma and the heavy chain diseases, are also discussed in other sections.

The uniform morphological and immunological features of plasma cell myeloma / multiple myeloma justify its classification as a single entity. It is a matter of ongoing discussion whether subclassification according to underlying primary cytogenetic abnormalities – as is done in various myelodysplastic neoplasms, acute myeloid leukaemias, and B-lymphoblastic leukaemias/lymphomas – would be timely. Arguments in favour are the mutually exclusive nature of cytogenetic alterations and the enrichment of major clinical characteristics in cytogenetically defined subtypes, although such associations are not unique. Moreover, some primary cytogenetic alterations are associated with more a favourable or unfavourable outcome. However, the current state of knowledge has not sufficiently elucidated the underlying biology and does not allow unique biology-based treatment decisions. Primary cytogenetic alterations currently rather serve as an important adjunct in risk-stratification systems that may also include serum markers, stage, and secondary genetic alterations. The impact of such risk-stratification methods thus far lacks strong, validated evidence; therefore, cytogenetic-based subtyping was deemed too early. Biology-based subclassification should be reconsidered in the future, however, as more data on genetic alterations – including cytogenetics, gene expression profiling, and mutation profiles – and their clinical correlations become available, especially in clinical trials involving new drugs such as immunomodulatory agents, proteasome inhibitors, and monoclonal antibodies.

Box 4.06 Plasma cell neoplasms

- Plasmacytoma
  - Solitary plasmacytoma of bone
  - Extramedullary plasmacytoma
- Plasma cell myeloma
  - Plasma cell myeloma
  - Clinical variants
    - Smouldering (asymptomatic) myeloma
    - Non-secretory myeloma
    - Plasma cell leukaemia
- Plasma cell neoplasms with associated paraneoplastic syndrome
  - POEMS syndrome (polyneuropathy, organomegaly, endocrinopathy, myeloma protein, and skin changes)
  - TEMPI syndrome (telangiectases, elevated erythropoietin and erythrocytosis, monoclonal gammopathy, perinephric fluid collection, and intrapulmonary shunting)
  - AESOP syndrome (adenopathy and extensive skin patch overlying plasmacytoma)

Plasmacytoma

Ferry JA
Coupland SE
Cowan AJ
Deshpande V
Gupta R
Karadimitris A
Leoncini L
Lim MS
Lorsbach RB
Medeiros LJ
Rajkumar SV
Siebert R
Walker BA

Definition

Plasmacytoma is a solitary neoplasm of clonal plasma cells without evidence of plasma cell (multiple) myeloma or end-organ damage due to plasma cell neoplasia.

ICD-O coding

9731/3 Solitary plasmacytoma of bone
9734/3 Extramedullary plasmacytoma

ICD-11 coding

2A83.2 & XH4BL1 Solitary plasmacytoma & Plasmacytoma, NOS

Related terminology

None

Subtype(s)

Solitary plasmacytoma of bone (SPB); extramedullary plasmacytoma (EMP)

Localization

SPB mainly arises in bones with active haematopoiesis, affecting the axial skeleton more often than the appendicular skeleton. The spine is most commonly involved, followed by pelvis, ribs, skull, and long bones {4321,3873,3709,70}.

EMP most commonly arises in the upper respiratory tract (nasal cavity, paranasal sinuses, nasopharynx, larynx) {69, 2125,38,70}. EMP rarely involves the lymph nodes {69,2646, 2125}, lungs, gastrointestinal tract {69,4010}, genitourinary tract {69,2125}, and skin {69,788}.

Clinical features

Patients present with localized pain, swelling, fracture, and/or spinal cord compression {3873}. Approximately half of patients have a serum paraprotein; IgG is most common, followed by IgA, and rarely light chain only {3873,2682,38}. Rare patients with plasmacytoma have a paraneoplastic syndrome, such as POEMS syndrome (polyneuropathy, organomegaly, endocrinopathy,

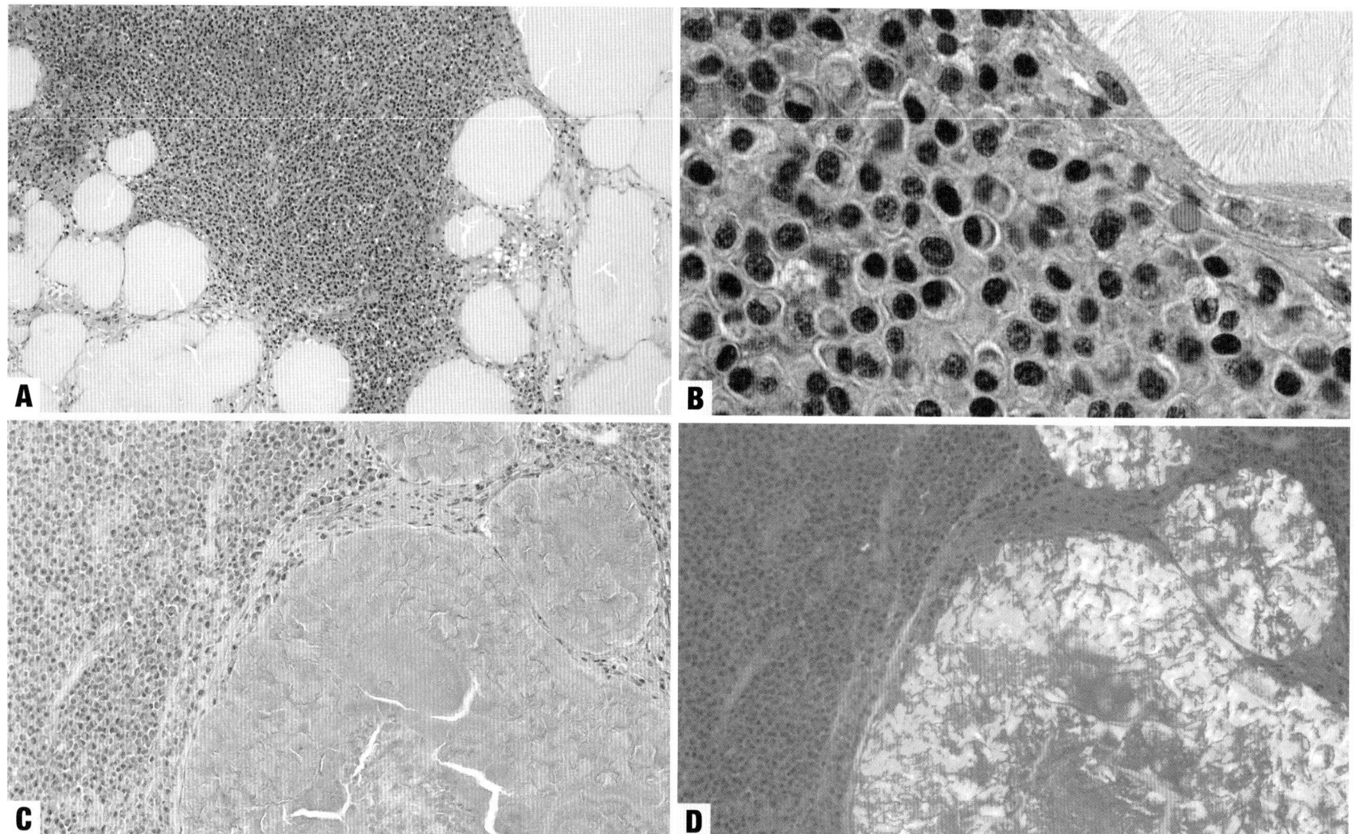

Fig. 4.298 Solitary plasmacytoma of bone with amyloid deposition. **A** A patient presented with pain and a lytic lesion in the femoral neck. The biopsy shows sheets of plasma cells and large aggregates of pale-pink amyloid. At 25 months, a second lytic lesion was found, but the marrow remained negative. There is no known systemic amyloidosis. **B** The lesion is composed of sheets of mature and slightly atypical plasma cells adjacent to amyloid with a fibrillar quality. **C,D** With Congo red stain, the amyloid is positive (**C**), and apple-green in polarized light (**D**).

myeloma protein, and skin changes) {2890,967}, TEMPI syndrome (telangiectases, elevated erythropoietin and erythrocytosis, monoclonal gammopathy, perinephric fluid collection, and intrapulmonary shunting), or AESOP syndrome (adenopathy and extensive skin patch overlying plasmacytoma) {554}.

Radiographically, SPB is a solitary lytic bone lesion {2640, 4332,4321,3752}.

Epidemiology

The incidence rates of SPB and EMP in the USA are 0.45 cases per 100 000 person-years and 0.09 cases per 100 000 person-years, respectively {1068}. About 2–5% of all plasma cell neoplasms are plasmacytomas {2063,961,3709}. EMP is less common than SPB {2341}, accounting for 20–30% of all plasmacytomas {38,70,1068}.

Plasmacytomas affect more men than women (M:F ratio: ~1.5–2:1 for SPB, ~2–3:1 for EMP) {4010,259,2682,1068}. Black people are at higher risk than White people for SPB, whereas Hispanic individuals have an intermediate risk {1994,1068}. Risk for EMP shows less difference among racial groups {1068}. Patients are mostly middle-aged and older adults (median age: 55–65 years) {4332,4321,1994,4010}. Incidence increases with age {1068}. Young adults are occasionally affected {2060,4321,1068}.

Etiology

EMP mainly arises in sites of ongoing antigen exposure. Rare posttransplantation plasmacytomas are related to immune dysregulation (see *Hyperplasias arising in immune deficiency/dysregulation*, p. 555).

Pathogenesis

Cytogenetic abnormalities in EMP overlap with those of plasma cell myeloma / multiple myeloma (see *Plasma cell myeloma / multiple myeloma*, p. 625) {366,788}.

Macroscopic appearance

SPB is a soft, gelatinous, haemorrhagic lesion.

Histopathology

Neoplastic plasma cells grow in sheets. In bone, these cells replace marrow and trabeculae, sometimes causing fracture. The cellular morphology varies among cases. Some are composed of normal-appearing plasma cells; others of enlarged, atypical plasma cells with distinct nucleoli; and a few of plasmablasts with large nuclei, vesicular chromatin, and prominent central nucleoli {69,2646,2890}. Rare cases have anaplastic morphology {2799} or amyloid deposition {1332}. Dutcher bodies may be seen.

Immunophenotype

The immunophenotype is similar to that of plasma cell myeloma / multiple myeloma, except that expression of cyclin D1 and CD56 is rare or absent in EMP {2125}. IgG is most commonly expressed, followed by IgA {69}. IgA+ EMP may have

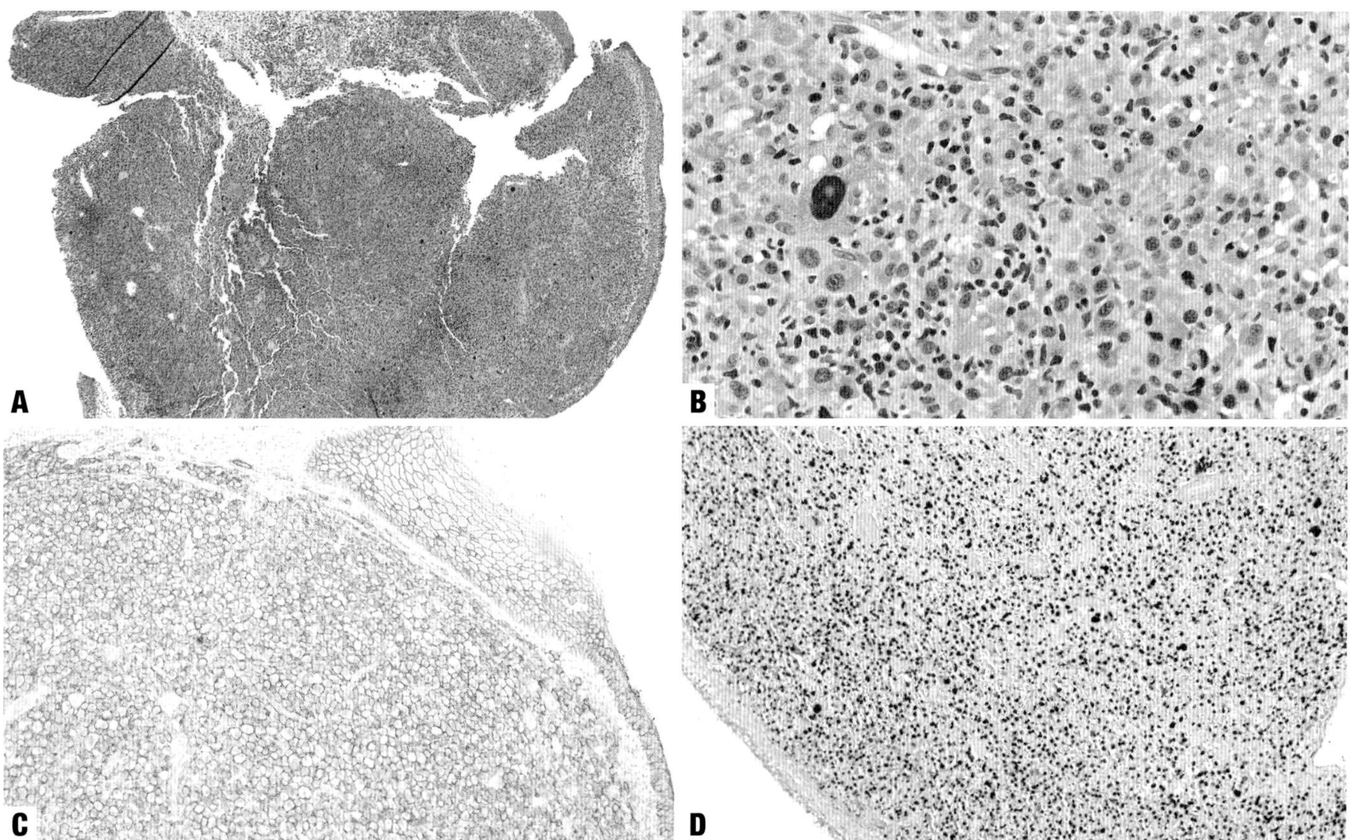

Fig. 4.299 EBV+ extramedullary plasmacytoma in an immunocompetent patient (EPIC). **A** Biopsy of a fleshy exophytic lesion in the nasal cavity. The cellular infiltrate extends under intact, pre-existing normal epithelium. **B** The lesion is composed of mature and slightly enlarged plasma cells, with rare large bizarre cells and admixed small lymphocytes. **C** CD138 is diffusely positive. Plasma cells also express monotypic IgA lambda (not shown). **D** Neoplastic plasma cells are positive for EBV (in situ hybridization for EBV-encoded small RNA [EBER]).

distinctive features, including frequent nodal as well as extranodal involvement, and a tendency to affect younger patients, some with immune dysregulation {3697}. Plasmacytomas are almost always negative for EBV. Rare cases of EBV+ EMP in immunocompetent patients (EPIC) have been reported {2398}. EPIC involves the nasal cavity and, less often, other head and neck sites or the gastrointestinal tract {4042,4478,3529}. The histological and immunophenotypic features are similar to those of other EMPs, except that EPIC often contains many CD8+ T cells {2398}. Rare EBV+ osseous plasmacytomas have been described {2869,2398}.

Differential diagnosis

The presence of B cells and/or IgM expression suggests B-cell lymphoma with marked plasmacytic differentiation.

Plasmablastic morphology, tingible-body macrophages, a high proliferation index, and *MYC* rearrangements in an immunosuppressed or older patient, particularly in the oral cavity, suggest plasmablastic lymphoma. Plasmablastic lymphoma is usually EBV+, in contrast to the vast majority of plasmacytomas. Plasmacytoma can mimic a neuroendocrine neoplasm on routinely stained sections, and CD138 stains epithelial cells as well as plasma cells. A panel of immunostains including keratins, neuroendocrine markers, IRF4 (MUM1), and kappa and lambda can help establish a diagnosis.

Cytology

On cytological preparations, SPB can show a spectrum of differentiation, from small bland plasma cells to plasma cells with atypia. Cases of EMP tend to be more differentiated.

Diagnostic molecular pathology

Clonal IG gene rearrangement may assist in cases with ambiguous clonality by light chain immunohistochemistry, in situ hybridization, or flow cytometry.

Essential and desirable diagnostic criteria

Essential: a biopsy-proven clonal plasma cell neoplasm of bone or an extramedullary site; no clonal B cells; no other (plasma cell) lesions on physical examination or radiographic studies; no end-organ damage (hypercalcaemia, renal insufficiency, anaemia, and bone lesions [CRAB]) due to plasma cell neoplasm; < 10% clonal plasma cells on non-targeted bone marrow sampling – plasmacytomas with no marrow involvement must be distinguished from those with minimal (< 10%) marrow involvement.

Staging

Patients should undergo thorough evaluation to exclude plasma cell myeloma / multiple myeloma, including complete blood count; serum creatinine, calcium, and free light chains; serum and urine protein electrophoresis and immunofixation; bone marrow aspiration and biopsy to investigate the presence of clonal plasma cells (including flow cytometry, FISH, and conventional cytogenetics); and highly sensitive imaging with whole-body CT, PET-CT, or MRI.

Prognosis and prediction

Standard management of EMP comprises involved field radiation therapy, typically at doses of 40–45 Gy {4086}. Local recurrences occur in 5–20% of cases {3095,1993,3389}. The risk of progression of EMP to plasma cell myeloma is lower than that for SPB, with 5-year progression-free survival rates of 70–93% and 38–44%, respectively {3389,908}. Cytogenetic abnormalities in EMP appear to lack the prognostic significance they have in plasma cell myeloma / multiple myeloma (PCM/MM) {366,788}.

Radiation is also standard therapy for SPB, providing effective local control in most cases. Without radiation-based treatment, the local recurrence rate is high {2060,1994,3873,4576}. SPB > 50 mm is associated with an increased risk of local recurrence {4332,851,38}. The risk of progression to PCM/MM increases with lesions > 50 mm {851}, older patient age, and persistent paraprotein > 1 year after therapy {4332,2060,1994, 38}. Surgical resection helps stabilize affected vertebra and may decrease the risk of progression {4441,3709}. Addition of systemic therapy may improve outcome {2682}. Patients with SPB with minimal bone marrow involvement are significantly more likely to develop PCM/MM than those with no clonal plasma cells on bone marrow aspirate by flow cytometry or on biopsy by immunohistochemistry {4321,1994,3105,1586,3352}; administering systemic, multiple myeloma–type therapy to such patients has been suggested {962}. Patients diagnosed more recently have a better prognosis, probably due to improved staging techniques and therapy {3709,1068}. Plasmablastic morphology is associated with aggressive behaviour {1332}. A subset of patients with SPB have a long survival (> 10 years) without progression to PCM/MM {1994}.

Plasma cell myeloma / multiple myeloma

Kumar S
Baughn LB
Cowan AJ
Gujral S
Gupta R
Karadimitris A
Lim MS
Malhotra P
Maruyama D
Medeiros LJ
Naresh KN
Paiva B
Rajkumar SV
Walker BA

Definition

Plasma cell myeloma is a bone marrow-based, multifocal neoplastic proliferation of plasma cells. Multiple myeloma is defined by the combination of plasma cell myeloma, usually associated with a serum and/or urine monoclonal immunoglobulin (Ig), and either evidence of organ damage related to the disease, or in the absence of organ damage, laboratory or imaging findings that suggest a high risk of developing end-organ damage within 2 years.

ICD-O coding

9732/3 Plasma cell myeloma
9732/3 Smouldering (asymptomatic) myeloma
9732/3 Non-secretory myeloma
9733/3 Plasma cell leukaemia

ICD-11 coding

2A83.1 Plasma cell myeloma

Related terminology

Acceptable: myeloma; multiple myeloma (plasma cell myeloma) NOS.

Subtype(s)

Smouldering (asymptomatic) myeloma; non-secretory myeloma; plasma cell leukaemia

Localization

Generalized or multifocal bone marrow involvement is typically present at diagnosis. Lytic bone lesions and focal tumoural masses of plasma cells also occur, most commonly in sites of active haematopoiesis. Extramedullary involvement in the form of soft tissue masses, diffuse organ infiltration, or circulating plasma cells is usually a manifestation of advanced disease, with a higher prevalence among patients with relapsed plasma cell myeloma / multiple myeloma (PCM/MM).

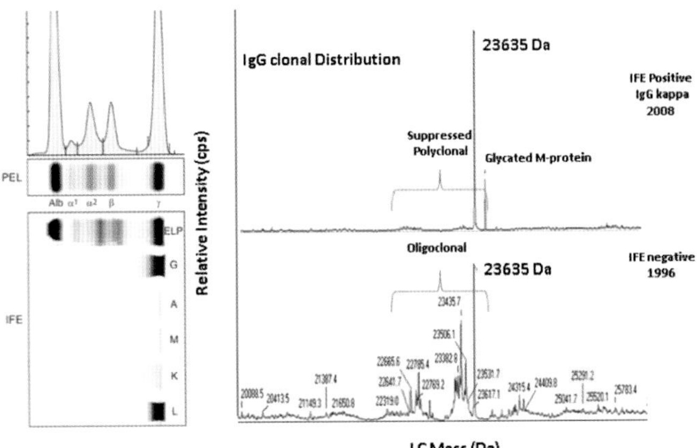

Fig. 4.300 Plasma cell myeloma / multiple myeloma. The upper-left panel demonstrates the electrophoretic pattern in a patient with a monoclonal protein that was confirmed to be IgG lambda by immunofixation (shown in the lower-left panel). The right panel demonstrates an IgG kappa monoclonal protein detected by mass spectrometry over two time points 12 years apart, highlighting the sensitivity of the technique and the ability to track the protein over time using the protein mass.

Clinical features

The clinical behaviour of PCM/MM is highly heterogeneous. All cases of PCM/MM evolve from an asymptomatic premalignant stage termed monoclonal gammopathy of undetermined significance (MGUS) {2213,4347} and are often preceded by smouldering myeloma {2184,2855}. Generally, most patients with PCM/MM have evidence of multiple myeloma–related damage to one or more end-organs, such as hypercalcaemia, renal insufficiency, anaemia, and bone lesions (CRAB). The International Myeloma Working Group (IMWG) updated the definition of multiple myeloma to include multiple myeloma–defining biomarkers: bone marrow plasma cells ≥ 60%, ratio of involved to uninvolved serum free light chain (FLC) ≥ 100, and more than one focal bone lesion ≥ 5 mm in size on whole-body MRI (SLiM), all indicators of imminent development of CRAB features {3352}.

Lytic bone lesion is the most frequent multiple myeloma–associated end-organ damage. Bone pain and hypercalcaemia can result from multiple myeloma–induced lytic lesions, osteoporosis, and pathological fractures. Nearly half of patients present with bone pain, mainly affecting the back {3665}. Renal impairment typically occurs due to tubular damage from multiple myeloma cast nephropathy, and anaemia from marrow replacement as well as renal damage. Other etiologies of renal dysfunction may include renal amyloidosis, light chain deposition disease, cryoglobulinaemia, or drug-induced kidney injury. In some patients, concurrent light chain amyloidosis can cause nephrotic syndrome (< 5%). Acquired Fanconi syndrome with glycosuria, phosphaturia, and aminoaciduria can also occur with multiple myeloma. Other presenting findings may include recurrent infections due to impaired lymphocyte function, suppression of normal plasma cell function, hypogammaglobulinaemia, and neurological manifestations due to spinal cord compression or peripheral neuropathy. Hyperviscosity syndrome due to high levels of M protein is uncommon. Soft tissue masses or organomegaly due to extramedullary plasmacytomas or amyloidosis is found in approximately 10% of patients. Physical findings are often absent or nonspecific. The presenting features can be altered by other concomitant plasma cell disorders such as Ig light chain amyloidosis or monoclonal Ig deposition disease.

An M protein is found in the serum or urine in about 97% of patients: IgG in 50%; IgA in 20%; light chain (Bence Jones protein) in 20%. IgD, IgE, IgM, or a biclonal M protein is found in < 10%. About 3% of patients have non-secretory disease. In 90%

of patients, there is a decrease in polyclonal Ig to < 50% of normal (immunoparesis). Other laboratory findings include hypercalcaemia in as many as 10% of patients, elevated creatinine in 20–30%, and hypoalbuminaemia in as many as 15%. Protein electrophoresis with immunofixation in the serum and 24-hour urine collection will allow for the detection, characterization, and quantitation of the monoclonal protein and is essential for diagnosis as well as assessment of treatment response. In as many as 20% of patients, an intact monoclonal Ig is not present, and the PCM/MM cells secrete only kappa or lambda FLC, which can be measured using a specific assay for the FLC. More recently, mass spectrometry–based assays for the detection and quantitation of monoclonal protein have been shown to be more sensitive than the conventional protein electrophoresis {2853}.

Epidemiology

PCM/MM was the 14th most common cancer diagnosed in the USA in 2021, representing about 1.8% of all new cancer cases {3742}. Globally, PCM/MM has increased in incidence since 1990 {829,4581}, with an age-standardized incidence rate of 1.92 cases per 100 000 persons in 2019 {4581}. PCM/MM is most common in high-income/high-sociodemographic-index regions, including Australasia, North America, and western Europe, although the largest increases in incidence since 1990 have been seen in low- and middle-income countries {829, 4581}. In the USA in 2021, there were an estimated 34 920 new diagnoses of PCM/MM, and an estimated 12 410 deaths due to PCM/MM {3742}. Among Black Americans, PCM/MM is diagnosed twice as frequently as in White Americans {3888}. The risk of developing PCM/MM is approximately 2- to 4-fold higher in individuals with a first-degree relative with PCM/MM. Although PCM/MM is uncommon in adults aged < 30 years, its incidence increases progressively with age. With a median age of diagnosis of 69 years in the USA, PCM/MM is predominantly a disease of the older population.

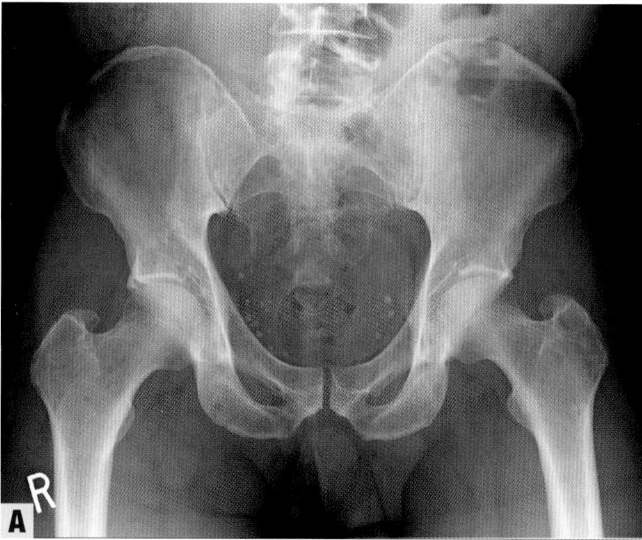

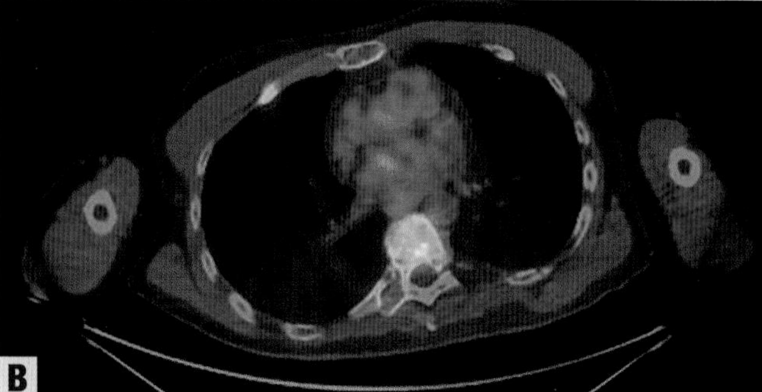

Fig. 4.301 Plasma cell myeloma / multiple myeloma. **A** A conventional radiograph showing lytic lesions involving the femur and iliac bones. **B** Increased FDG uptake is seen in areas of bone lesions on FDG PET.

Etiology

The cause of PCM/MM is unknown but is believed to represent a combined effect of genetic susceptibility and environmental exposures. First-degree relatives of patients with MGUS and PCM/MM have a higher risk of plasma cell dyscrasia {3202}, possibly linked to non-coding genetic variants which predispose to the disease. Twenty-three such variants account for 15% of PCM/MM heritability and are predicted to influence the expression of genes involved in B-cell and plasma cell differentiation and function, regulation of the cell cycle and genomic instability, chromatin remodelling, and autophagy {4358}. Although the reasons behind the higher incidence of MGUS and PCM/MM in people of African ancestry remain unknown, it may have a genetic basis. Conversely, persistent antigenic stimulation is thought to favour expansion of antigen-specific B-cell and plasma cell clones, providing the ground for random primary genetic events to initiate the malignant transformation of plasma cells. This is best exemplified in the case of Gaucher disease type I, a monogenic sphingolipid lysosomal storage disease characterized by accumulation of the sphingolipids lyso-glucosylsphingosine and beta-glucosylceramide. Presentation of these sphingolipids by CD1d activates type II natural killer T cells which provide help to sphingolipid-specific B cells, leading to their persistent activation and differentiation to oligoclonal plasma cells {2877}. As a result, paraproteins are found in as many as 35% of young and middle-aged patients with Gaucher disease {4132}, and the lifetime relative risk of patients with Gaucher disease developing PCM/MM is 5% {3467}. Obesity in mid-life has also been reported to increase the risk of progression of MGUS to plasma cell (multiple) myeloma, but it is not associated with a higher risk of MGUS {633,4006}.

Pathogenesis

The pathogenesis of PCM/MM is characterized by increasing numbers of plasma cells in bone marrow {3352}, which progressively displace normal cells {3106}. Bone marrow stromal cells and non-haematopoietic multipotent cells contribute to the development and progression of PCM/MM by regulating cell migration, homing {356}, and angiogenesis {4131,3268}. Accordingly, the development of PCM/MM is also characterized by progressively higher numbers of circulating plasma cells in the peripheral blood {3569}, which likely contribute to intramedullary and extramedullary disease dissemination {1290} and greater clonal heterogeneity {3369}. There is growing evidence that immune evasion {4546, 2292} and a progressively permissive tumour microenvironment {892} are involved in the pathogenesis of PCM/MM.

Genetic factors

There are two main initiating genetic events that occur early in the course of the disease: multiple trisomies of the odd-numbered

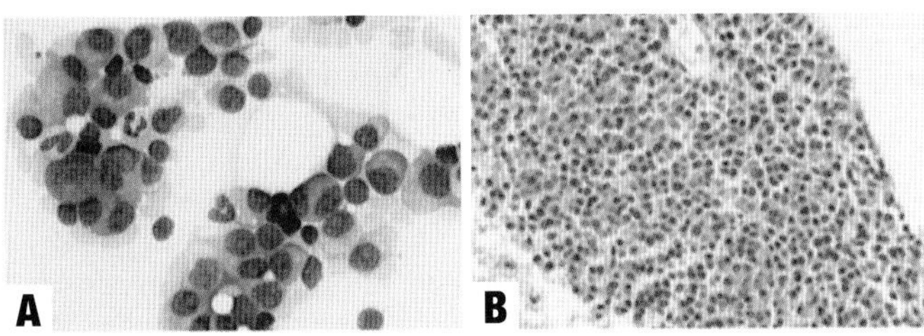

Fig. 4.302 Plasma cell myeloma / multiple myeloma. **A** Plasma cells on a bone marrow aspirate with distinct eccentric nuclei as well as binucleated forms. **B** Diffuse infiltration with plasma cells in a bone marrow biopsy.

chromosomes (i.e. hyperdiploid) and recurrent chromosomal translocations involving the IGH locus at 14q32.33 that result in overexpression of key oncogenes, including *CCND1*, *CCND2*, *CCND3*, *NSD2* (*MMSET*, *WHSC1*), *MAF*, *MAFA*, and *MAFB* {328,2153}. These are considered primary genetic events, present in nearly all tumour cells, and are detected at the MGUS stage {2412,2413}. IGH translocations and hyperdiploidy appear to be early events in the pathogenesis of PCM/MM, unified by an associated upregulation of one of the cyclin D genes (*CCND1*, *CCND2*, or *CCND3*) {328,2142}. Clonal heterogeneity occurs early and is present in MGUS and smouldering myeloma {4279}. Progression from precursor states to PCM/MM involves branching evolutionary patterns, novel mutations, biallelic hits in tumour suppressor genes, and segmental copy-number changes {396,505,441}. Although the first gain at 1q21 is often an early event, jumping translocations and additional amplifications of 1q21 emerge later in the course of PCM/MM {57,2606}. Recurrent mutations in driver genes impacting cellular signalling pathways, such as the RAS/MAPK and NF-κB pathways, are characteristic of PCM/MM {2518}. They include alterations of the MAPK pathway (*KRAS*, *NRAS*, *FGFR3*, and *BRAF* SNVs), a variety of mutations (SNVs, homozygous deletions, translocations) that activate the NF-κB pathway (*TRAF3*, *TRAF2*, *BIRC2*, *BIRC3*, *CYLD*, *MAP3K14*), the DNA repair pathway (deletion 17p, *TP53*, and *ATM* SNVs), and *MYC* (translocations or copy-number variations), which are most likely secondary or late events as they are infrequently observed in MGUS {2684} and smouldering myeloma {396,505,441}. Complex structural variant events (e.g. chromothripsis), and specific mutation signatures implicating enhanced activities of activation-induced cytidine deaminase (AID) and APOBEC deaminases {3950}, indicate higher genomic instability in PCM/MM {4278}.

Macroscopic appearance

The bone defects on gross examination are filled with a soft, gelatinous, fish-flesh and/or haemorrhagic tissue.

Histopathology

The morphology varies from mature-appearing plasma cells to immature, plasmablastic and pleomorphic variants (including multinucleated and multilobated forms). Mature plasma cells are oval-shaped, with an eccentric nucleus and spoke-wheel or clock-face chromatin and without a nucleolus. There is abundant basophilic cytoplasm, with a perinuclear hof. Immature forms have more-dispersed nuclear chromatin, a higher N:C ratio, and a prominent nucleolus {1410,255}. As nuclear immaturity and pleomorphism rarely occur in reactive plasma cells, these are reliable indicators of malignancy. The cytoplasm of PCM/MM cells has abundant endoplasmic reticulum, which may contain condensed or crystallized cytoplasmic Ig producing a variety of morphologically distinctive findings, including multiple pale bluish-white, grape-like accumulations (Mott cells, morula cells), cherry-red refractile round bodies (refractile bodies), vermilion-staining glycogen-rich IgA (flame cells), overstuffed fibrils (Gaucher-like cells, thesaurocytes), and crystalline rods. However, these changes are not pathognomonic of PCM/MM.

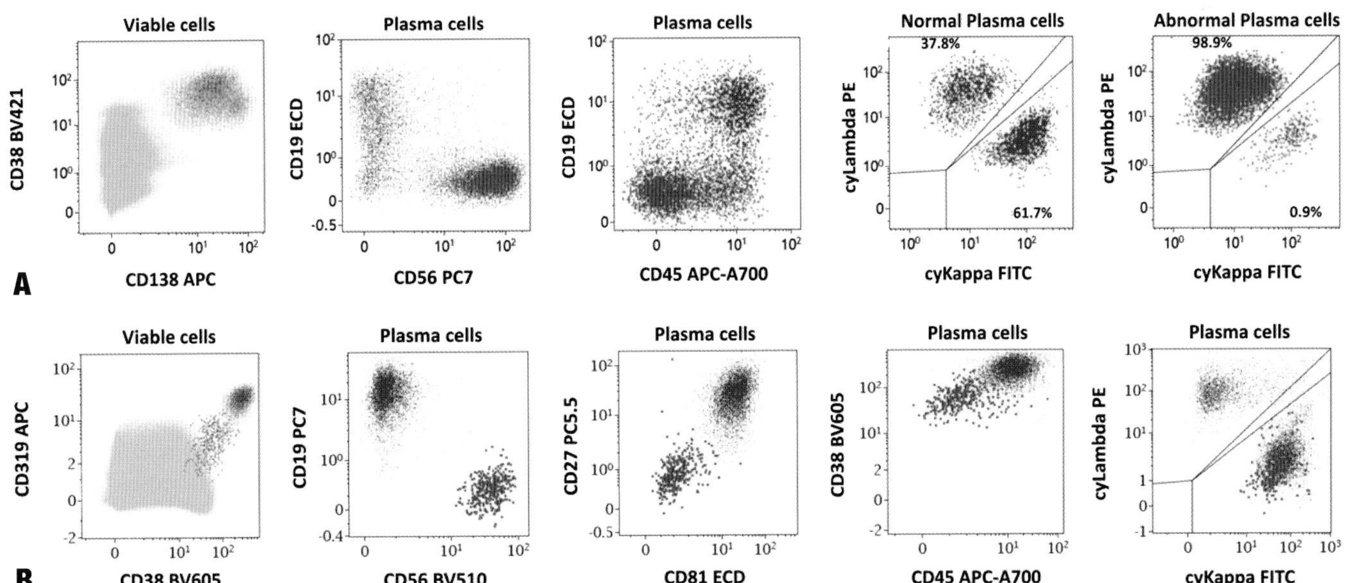

Fig. 4.303 Plasma cell myeloma / multiple myeloma. **A** A case of plasma cell neoplasm at baseline demonstrating the abnormal plasma cells (red dots) that express moderate CD38, bright CD138, and bright CD56, show negative expression of CD19 and CD45, and show cytoplasmic immunoglobulin lambda light chain restriction. The normal plasma cells (black dots) show a polytypic distribution of cytoplasmic immunoglobulin kappa and lambda light chains. **B** A typical example of measurable residual disease assessment using multicolour flow cytometry. The residual tumour cells (0.06%) are highlighted in red and express moderate CD38, dim CD319, and bright CD56, show negative expression of CD27, CD81, and CD45, and show cytoplasmic immunoglobulin kappa light chain restriction. The normal plasma cells present in the sample are shown in black.

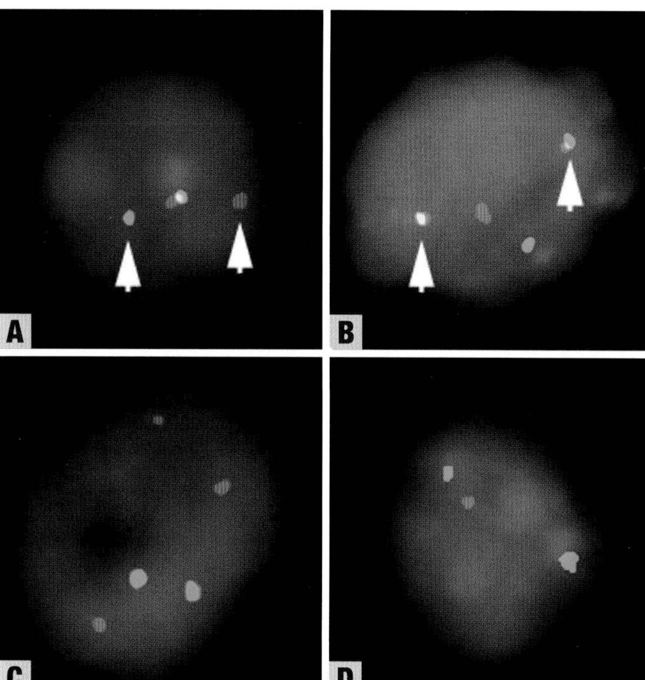

Fig. 4.304 Plasma cell myeloma / multiple myeloma. Interphase FISH analysis of recurrent abnormalities in multiple myeloma using purified plasma cells. **A** Break-apart signal pattern for IGH at 14q32 (3′ in green, 5′ in red). Split red and green signals are indicated by arrowheads, and intact 3′ and 5′ IGH is seen as the single fusion of red and green signals. **B** Fusion signals for t(11;14)(q13;q32). Probes for IGH are in green and probes for *CCND1* are in red. The two fusion signals (indicated by arrowheads) probably represent the der(11) and der(14). **C** An additional copy of 1q22 (red) and two copies of 1p36 (green) are seen. **D** Loss of *TP53* (red) at 17p13 and two copies of chromosome 17 (CEP17, green) are seen.

The number of plasma cells varies from barely increased to > 90%. Rare PCM/MM cases may show < 10% plasma cells in the aspirate smears, likely caused by a suboptimal bone marrow aspirate or focal distribution of PCM/MM in the marrow. In such instances, trephine biopsy sections may show more plasma cells with or without focal clusters / nodular aggregates or sheets of plasma cells. It is advisable to stain and examine all aspirate smears as well as touch imprints for a more reliable evaluation of plasma cell numbers. Rarely, they may be seen as bare nuclei (degenerating cells).

Normal plasma cells are found in trephine biopsy as small clusters around arterioles. PCM/MM plasma cells may occur as interstitial clusters, focal nodules, broad bands / diffuse sheets, and even packed marrow {255}. A nodule / tumoural mass of plasma cells within the trephine strongly favours a diagnosis of PCM/MM. It may vary from classic plasma cell morphology to lymphoid, immunoblastic, spindle/oval, or signet-ring cell. Normal haematopoiesis is generally preserved; however, in diffuse involvement it may be suppressed. Scattered osteoclasts may be seen. Fibrosis may be seen in a few cases {4180}. A trephine biopsy is useful in assessing suspected light chain–associated amyloidosis and may show vascular or interstitial amyloid deposition.

Peripheral blood

Rouleaux formation is the most striking feature on peripheral blood smears and is related to the quantity and type of M protein. A leukoerythroblastic picture may be seen in some cases. Circulating plasma cells can be found in a significant proportion of patients by sensitive flow cytometry approaches, usually in small numbers. Marked plasmacytosis accompanies plasma cell leukaemia (consensus threshold: > 5% {3352}).

Kidney

Bence Jones protein accumulates as aggregates of eosinophilic material in the lumina of the renal tubules. Renal tubular reabsorption of Bence Jones proteins is largely responsible for renal damage in multiple myeloma.

Immunohistochemistry

Immunohistochemistry is useful in highlighting and quantifying plasma cells (using CD138 and IRF4 [MUM1]), confirming monoclonal proliferation (by light chain restriction using kappa and lambda light chains), and distinguishing PCM/MM from other neoplasms. Sometimes, immunohistochemical staining may result in high background staining due to the presence of normal physiological interstitial immunoglobulins, resulting in interpretational challenges. It can be avoided using colorimetric in situ hybridization for kappa and lambda mRNA-based staining methods {3412}.

Flow cytometric immunophenotyping

Plasma cells express CD138, strong CD38, and strong SLAM-family proteins such as CD229 and CD319 {3270,2823,3987, 4292}. PCM/MM cells are characterized by negative expression of CD19 (> 95% of cases), weak or negative expression of CD45 (70–75% of cases), and moderate to strong expression of CD56 (60–80% of cases), with cytoplasmic kappa or lambda light chain restriction. Some cases also show loss of CD27 and/or CD81 expression. Abnormal expression of CD20, CD28, CD33, and KIT (CD117) can also be noted in approximately one third of cases; rarely, CD10 expression can be seen {270,3104,3989, 1203,648,1796}. Plasma cells with aberrant antigen expression showing light chain restriction should be considered neoplastic. The level of clonal plasma cells is prognostic in smouldering and active PCM/MM (e.g. MGUS-like profile), and specific immunophenotypes (e.g. CD19 and CD81 coexpression) are associated with a longer time to progression and favourable survival {3108,3110,3441,2484}.

Cytology

The typical morphology of PCM/MM cells described above is seen in aspirates from pleural effusion and cerebrospinal fluid when involved by extramedullary disease.

Diagnostic molecular pathology

Cytogenetic abnormalities in PCM/MM

Cytogenetic abnormalities can be detected by conventional chromosome studies in about one third of PCM/MM cases {1208,3599,2636}, whereas interphase FISH has greater sensitivity and abnormalities can be detected in > 90% of PCM/MM cases {1208,1209,2636}. CD138-positive selection should be used to optimize the yield of FISH studies {3308}. Cytogenetic abnormalities are both numerical and structural and include trisomies, whole or partial chromosomal deletions and gains, and chromosomal translocations {2153}. About half of PCM/MM tumours are hyperdiploid, with 48–75 chromosomes, and have gains of three or more of the odd-numbered chromosomes 3, 5, 7, 9, 11, 15, 19, and 21 {3790,3351,2153}. The other half of

PCM/MM tumours mostly have < 48 or > 75 chromosomes and usually have an IGH translocation at chromosome 14q32 {1210,3790,3351,2153}. Seven oncogenes are involved in recurrent IG gene translocations: *CCND1* on 11q13 (involved in 16% of cases); *NSD2*, often with *FGFR3*, on 4p16 (in 15%); *MAF* on 16q23 (in 5%); *CCND3* on 6p21 (in 3%); *MAFB* on 20q11 (in 3%); *MAFA* on 8q24 (in < 1%); and *CCND2* on 12p13 (in < 1%) (see Table 4.64) {3790,3351,2153}. Just over 90% of these translocations involve IGH on 14q32; the remaining ones involve primarily the Ig light chain loci, more commonly lambda at 22q11.2 and rarely kappa at 2p11.2, or other loci such as *TENT5C* (*FAM46C*) or *CXCR4*. Hyperdiploid PCM/MM tumours infrequently have one of the seven recurrent IGH translocations listed above {3790,3351,2153}.

Common secondary cytogenetic abnormalities in PCM/MM include deletion of chromosome 13q (or monosomy 13), found in about 50% of cases {194,1211,365}; deletion of chromosome 17p including *TP53* (or monosomy 17), found in about 10% {3998, 4277}; deletion of 1p, found in about 20% {1545}; and duplication or amplification of 1q, found in about 40% {1486,1212,3623, 6,3624}. In addition, *MYC* locus translocations are also present in about 40% of PCM/MM cases. These reposition *MYC* near a promiscuous array of plasma cell–specific super-enhancers (including IGH, IGK, IGL, and non-Ig enhancers) {258,3704,3507}. *MYC* translocations can contribute to the progression from MGUS to plasma cell (multiple) myeloma {723,2698}.

The consensus recommendations on testing by FISH on bone marrow are listed in Table 4.65 {2151}.

Essential and desirable diagnostic criteria

Plasma cell myeloma

Essential: demonstration of clonal plasma cells in the bone marrow using flow cytometry or immunohistochemistry (≥ 10%).

Multiple myeloma

Essential: diagnosis requires a combination of laboratory and clinical features (see Box 4.07); demonstration of plasma cell myeloma or biopsy-proven bony or extramedullary plasmacytoma; demonstration of one or more myeloma-defining criteria (SLiM-CRAB): MRI showing more than one focal lesion, and/or serum FLC ratio > 100, and/or bone marrow plasma cell percentage > 60%, and/or anaemia, and/or hypercalcaemia, and/or lytic lesions, and/or osteoporosis with compression fracture demonstrated by low dose CT or skeletal X-ray, and/or renal impairment.

Table 4.64 Primary cytogenetic abnormalities in plasma cell myeloma / multiple myeloma

Primary cytogenetic abnormality	Genes involved	Frequency
t(4;14)(p16;q32)	IGH::*NSD2*	15%
t(11;14)(q13;q32)	IGH::*CCND1*	16%
t(6;14)(p21;q32)	IGH::*CCND3*	3%
t(12;14)(p13;q32)	IGH::*CCND2*	< 1%
t(14;16)(q32;q23)	IGH::*MAF*	5%
t(14;20)(q32;q11)	IGH::*MAFB*	2%
t(8;14)(q24;q32)	IGH::*MAFA*	< 1%
Hyperdiploid (without above translocations)	n/a	50%
Unclassified (other)	n/a	10%

n/a, not applicable.

Table 4.65 Cytogenetic abnormalities in plasma cell myeloma / multiple myeloma detected by interphase FISH

Cytogenetic abnormality	Gene(s) involved	Frequency
t(4;14)(p16;q32)	*NSD2*/IGH	15%
t(11;14)(q13;q32)	*CCND1*/IGH	16%
t(14;16)(q32;q23)	IGH/*MAF*	5%
1q21 gain/amplification	*CKS1B*, *ADAR* (*ADAR1*)	40%
1p deletion	*CDKN2C*	20%
17p13 deletion	*TP53*	10%
13q deletion	*RB1*	50%

Staging

The Revised International Staging System (R-ISS) for multiple myeloma, based on pretreatment serum B2M, albumin, and LDH levels, as well as on interphase FISH–based chromosomal

Box 4.07 International Myeloma Working Group (IMWG) diagnostic criteria for multiple myeloma and related plasma cell disorders (modified from Rajkumar et al., 2014 {3352})

Smouldering multiple myeloma

Essential:
Serum monoclonal protein (IgG or IgA) ≥ 3 g/dL, or urinary monoclonal protein ≥ 500 mg per 24 h and/or clonal bone marrow plasma cells 10–60%
AND
Absence of myeloma-defining events or amyloidosis

Multiple myeloma

Essential:
Clonal bone marrow plasma cells ≥ 10% or biopsy-proven bony or extramedullary plasmacytoma
AND
Any one or more of the following myeloma-defining events:
Evidence of end-organ damage that can be attributed to the underlying plasma cell proliferative disorder, specifically:
- Hypercalcaemia: serum calcium > 0.25 mmol/L (> 1 mg/dL) higher than the upper limit of normal or > 2.75 mmol/L (> 11 mg/dL)
- Renal insufficiency: creatinine clearance < 40 mL per minute or serum creatinine > 177 μmol/L (> 2 mg/dL)
- Anaemia: haemoglobin value > 2 g/dL below the lower limit of normal, or a haemoglobin value of < 10 g/dL
- Bone lesions: one or more osteolytic lesions on skeletal radiography, CT, or PET-CT

OR
Clonal bone marrow plasma cell percentage ≥ 60%
OR
Involved: uninvolved serum free light chain ratio ≥ 100 (involved free light chain level must be ≥ 100 mg/L)
OR
More than one focal lesion (≥ 5 mm in size) on MRI studies

Plasma cell leukaemia {1166}

Essential:
Presence of ≥ 5% circulating plasma cells in peripheral blood smears in patients otherwise diagnosed with plasma cell myeloma

Table 4.66 Risk stratification in plasma cell myeloma / multiple myeloma

Risk model	Low	Standard	High
ISS {1411}	I: Serum B2M < 3.5 mg/L, serum albumin ≥ 3.5 g/dL	II: Not stage I or III	III: Serum B2M ≥ 5.5 mg/L
IMWG {722}	ISS I/II, age < 55 years, and absence of all of t(4;14), del(17p13), and 1q21+	Not low or high risk	ISS II/III and t(4;14) or del(17p13)
R-ISS {3116}	I: ISS I and absence of all of del(17p13), t(4;14), and t(14;16)	II: Not R-ISS I or III	III: ISS III with either high serum LDH or presence of any of del(17p13), t(4;14), or t(14;16)

IMWG, International Myeloma Working Group; ISS, International Staging System; R-ISS, Revised International Staging System.

abnormalities, provides a strong predictor of survival (see Table 4.66). For R-ISS stage I, II, and III disease, overall survival rates of 82%, 62%, and 40%, respectively, and 5-year progression-free survival rates of 55%, 36%, and 24%, respectively, are reported {3116}. The R-ISS combines elements of tumour burden and disease biology (presence of high-risk cytogenetic abnormalities or elevated LDH level) to create a unified prognostic index that helps in clinical care as well as in comparisons of clinical trial data.

Prognosis and prediction

Multiple myeloma is considered incurable for most patients, with an average 5-year survival rate of 55.6%, but new therapies have significantly extended progression-free and overall survival. Patients aged > 70 years and those with comorbidities have a less favourable prognosis. The prognosis of multiple myeloma is determined by a combination of clinical, biochemical, and molecular features, assessed at diagnosis and after treatment.

Prognosis at diagnosis has been established through the International Staging System (ISS) {1411} and further refined by the addition of high-risk genomic abnormalities into the R-ISS {3116} and the IMWG risk-stratification methods {722}. The genomic abnormalities considered by the IMWG as high-risk are t(4;14)(p16;q32), t(14;16)(q32;q23), del(17p13), and gain/amplification of 1q21 (see Table 4.65, p. 629, and Table 4.66, above); therefore, at the minimum, these abnormalities should be analysed to identify high-risk cases. For del(17p), the proportion of CD138+ cells with the deletion has an impact on outcome: cases with ≥ 55–60% of cells with del(17p) are associated with a worse outcome {3998,3997}. Del(1p32) is an emerging poor-prognostic marker that identifies a subgroup of patients with a dismal outcome {4276,4277}. Patients with t(4;14)(p16;q32) were historically a high-risk group, but the introduction of proteasome inhibitors has improved outcomes for this group {3792, 3791,3842}. Similarly, the use of BCL2 inhibitors has increased overall response rates in patients with t(11;14)(q13;q32) from 6% with standard therapy to 40% using BCL2 inhibitors {2150}.

There are ongoing efforts to transition interphase FISH into next-generation sequencing that could additionally assess patients' mutation status, although its impact on prognosis requires further cross-validation. One exception is the genetic status of *TP53*, where biallelic alterations drive the poor outcome of these patients {4277,3997}. Gene expression profiles are prognostic in newly diagnosed multiple myeloma, but they are not routinely assessed {4553,2143}. Similarly, the presence of extramedullary disease identified with PET-CT {4535,4129} and circulating plasma cells {3569,1365} is prognostic, but it is not incorporated in current risk models.

Minimal/measurable residual disease assessment, using next-generation flow cytometry or next-generation sequencing of Ig rearrangements as well as PET-CT {4534}, is used to assess response after treatment {3196,3107,580}. Undetectable measurable residual disease is associated with improved progression-free and overall survival {2843,2195}. The combination of diagnostic and measurable residual disease biomarkers improves risk-stratification {3107,1357}.

Plasma cell neoplasms with associated paraneoplastic syndrome

Lim MS
Baughn LB
Gupta R

Definition
This is a group of rare paraneoplastic syndromes associated with plasma cell neoplasms: POEMS syndrome (polyneuropathy, organomegaly, endocrinopathy, M protein, and skin changes), TEMPI syndrome (telangiectases, elevated erythropoietin and erythrocytosis, monoclonal gammopathy, perinephric fluid collection, and intrapulmonary shunting), and AESOP syndrome (adenopathy and extensive skin patch overlying plasmacytoma).

ICD-O coding
Code as tumour type.

ICD-11 coding
Code as affected site, e.g.
8E4A.1 Paraneoplastic or autoimmune disorders of the peripheral or autonomic nervous system
EL10 Paraneoplastic syndromes involving skin

Related terminology
Acceptable: for POEMS syndrome: osteosclerotic myeloma.

Subtype(s)
POEMS syndrome; TEMPI syndrome; AESOP syndrome

Localization
The plasma cell neoplasm typically involves the bone marrow as single or multiple osteosclerotic lesions. In AESOP syndrome, the skin overlying a solitary plasmacytoma involving the bone is affected by violaceous patches.

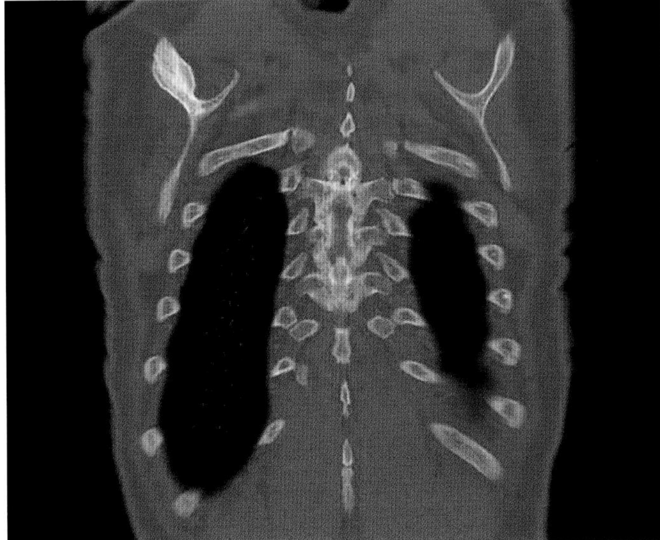

Fig. 4.305 POEMS syndrome (polyneuropathy, organomegaly, endocrinopathy, myeloma protein, and skin changes). Radiological studies demonstrate osteosclerotic lesions.

Clinical features
Patients with POEMS syndrome classically present with a subacute, distal, symmetrical, sensorimotor neuropathy {2913}. The paraproteinaemia is IgA or IgG with lambda light chain restriction {969}. The quantity of M protein in the serum and/or urine is typically below plasma cell myeloma / multiple myeloma levels {969, 12}. Osteosclerotic bone lesions are seen in most patients {3718}, involving the pelvis, thoracic and lumbar vertebrae, and ribs, and (less commonly) the scapula, clavicle, sternum, skull, and long bones {3117}. N-terminal propeptide of type I collagen (P1NP), a marker for osteosclerotic metastasis, is markedly elevated {4286}. VEGF levels are markedly elevated in plasma {1001} and serum {4286} and correlate with disease severity {2697}. Organomegaly, involving the liver or spleen, and lymphadenopathy are common {3717}. Skin changes with hyperpigmentation and haemangiomas {241,2681}, as well as nail changes and rubor, are common. Other common features include papilloedema, hypogonadotropic hypogonadism, volume overload, acrocyanosis, weight loss, clubbing, hyperhidrosis, pulmonary hypertension / restrictive lung disease, thrombotic diatheses, diarrhoea, and low vitamin B12 values. Approximately 15% of patients with POEMS syndrome also have KSHV/HHV8-negative multicentric Castleman disease {969,2863}.

TEMPI syndrome is associated with unexplained erythrocytosis, monoclonal gammopathy, and perinephric fluid collections {1969,2712,3149}. Telangiectases are seen on the face, upper back, and chest, with frequent involvement of the hands, whereas the lower extremities are spared. Erythrocytosis progresses to secondary polycythaemia. Serum erythropoietin levels exceed most other causes of erythrocytosis. There is a characteristic absence of *JAK2* mutations. The progressive increase in erythropoietin levels precedes the development of intrapulmonary shunting and perinephric fluid collections. The monoclonal paraprotein is IgG kappa in most cases {4231, 3913,2169}. Unlike in POEMS syndrome, VEGF levels are not elevated in TEMPI syndrome {2662}.

AESOP syndrome can be the presentation in rare cases of solitary plasmacytoma {3458}. Patients develop slow-growing red, brown, or violaceous skin patches with visible blood vessels on the thorax. The skin lesions are variable in size, with fine desquamation especially at the edge; smaller satellite lesions may be observed {1138}. Polyneuropathy and lymphadenopathy, which are unilateral or bilateral, typically become apparent after the development of skin lesions. There may be overlap with POEMS syndrome as some patients develop organomegaly and endocrinopathy {3535}.

Epidemiology
All of these syndromes are rare. The exact prevalence of POEMS syndrome is unknown, but it may be more common in Asia. The prevalence of POEMS syndrome is estimated to be 0.3 per 100 000 individuals in Japan {3874}. The median age at

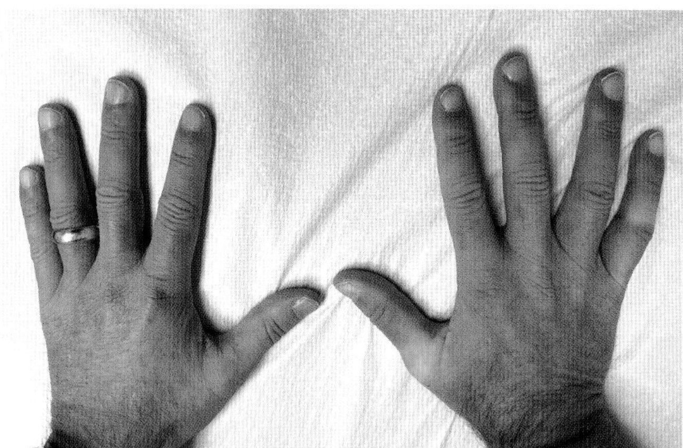

Fig. 4.306 POEMS syndrome (polyneuropathy, organomegaly, endocrinopathy, myeloma protein, and skin changes). Skin changes, including general rubor and whitening of nails, in a patient with POEMS syndrome.

presentation is about 50 years, and the M:F ratio is 1.5:1 {969}. TEMPI syndrome occurs in the fourth or fifth decade of life and affects both men and women, without a specific geographical predisposition {3913,3912}.

Etiology

The etiology and pathogenesis are not well characterized {966}. Levels of VEGF correlate with disease activity but may not be a driving force of the disease in POEMS syndrome. No known single chemokine or cytokine abnormality has been identified in TEMPI syndrome {3912}.

Pathogenesis

The constellation of features seen in POEMS syndrome and TEMPI syndrome is secondary to cytokines (e.g. IL-1β, TNF-α, IL-6) and inflammatory and vascular growth factors (e.g. VEGF) secreted from the plasma cells and platelets {1330}.

The cytogenetic abnormalities in POEMS syndrome are similar to those in other plasma cell neoplasms, but with different prevalence rates {481,1874}. IGH translocations and deletion of chromosome 13 have been reported. Sequencing studies identified variants in *KLHL6*, *LTB*, *EHD1*, *EML4*, *HEPHL1*, *HIPK2*, and *PCDH10* {2870}. Restricted usage of certain IGLV and IGLJ genes has been identified {308}. There are currently no known molecular or genetic risk factors that predict overall survival {966}. FISH analysis of 37 POEMS syndrome cases identified monosomy 13 in 14 cases (38%); 1 case had trisomy 3 and trisomy 7, and 3 cases had IGH translocation t(11;14)(q13;q32). No 17p deletions were found. There is a low prevalence of hyperdiploidy and 14q32 rearrangements. No recurrent underlying genetic abnormalities have been identified in TEMPI syndrome {3912}. Duplication of 22q11.23 and an elevated level of macrophage migration inhibitory factor (MIF) have been reported {3877}.

Macroscopic appearance

The macroscopic appearance varies according to the syndrome and the tissues affected.

Histopathology

POEMS syndrome

The majority of patients with POEMS syndrome show bone marrow involvement by clonal plasma cells. However, one third of patients presenting with solitary or multiple plasmacytomas show no bone marrow involvement. The median percentage of plasma cells identified in the bone marrow is < 5% {869}. Within osteosclerotic lesions, atypical plasma cells infiltrate normal marrow with sclerosis of the bony lamellae {2147}. Reactive lymphoid aggregates containing admixed B and T cells are seen, with plasma cells rimming the aggregates {869}. Other findings include megakaryocyte hyperplasia and clustering, as well as atypia with small monolobated and hypolobated nuclei, hyperchromatic nuclei, nuclear segmentation, and/or larger forms. Peripheral blood smears are essentially normal. The histological findings in the lymph node are consistent with the plasma cell variant of Castleman disease.

The immunophenotypic profile of neoplastic plasma cells in POEMS syndrome is similar to that of clonal plasma cells in other plasma cell neoplasms except that the vast majority of cases are lambda-restricted {3349,966,1712}.

TEMPI syndrome

There are no specific morphological findings of TEMPI syndrome, and the bone marrow is unremarkable in the majority of cases {4231,2169,2712}. Erythroid hyperplasia with mild atypia in erythroid cells and megakaryocytes is reported. Bone marrow shows few monoclonal plasma cells (< 5%), with an increase in clonal plasma cells reaching the levels seen in smouldering myeloma reported in only 1 case {3460}. Non-paratrabecular lymphoid aggregates with small, normal-appearing lymphocytes are noted in a few cases. Features observed in myeloproliferative neoplasms, including megakaryocyte clusters and fibrosis, are not identified in patients with TEMPI syndrome. The monoclonal paraprotein component seen in most cases of TEMPI syndrome is IgG kappa, although IgG lambda and IgA lambda have also been reported.

AESOP syndrome

Skin biopsies of patients with AESOP syndrome show diffuse reactive vascular hyperplasia within the dermis and may be associated with surrounding dermal mucin. The subcutis is typically uninvolved. Excised lymph nodes reveal nonspecific findings, including sinusoidal lymphoplasmacytic infiltrates with variable degrees of endothelial proliferation, and may mimic features seen in Castleman disease. The underlying plasmacytoma / plasma cell neoplasm exhibits features consistent with a clonal plasma cell neoplasm and demonstrates light chain restriction and expression of CD138.

Cytology

Not relevant

Diagnostic molecular pathology

Not applicable

Box 4.08 Diagnostic criteria for POEMS syndrome (polyneuropathy, organomegaly, endocrinopathy, myeloma protein, and skin changes), adapted from Dispenzieri et al., 2019 {966}

Mandatory major criteria:
- Polyneuropathy (typically demyelinating)
- Monoclonal plasma cell proliferative disorder (almost always lambda)

Major criteria (one required):
- Castleman disease
- Sclerotic bone lesions
- VEGF elevation

Minor criteria:
- Organomegaly (splenomegaly, hepatomegaly, or lymphadenopathy)
- Extravascular volume overload (oedema, pleural effusion, or ascites)
- Endocrinopathy (adrenal, thyroid, pituitary, gonadal, parathyroid, pancreatic)
- Skin changes
- Papilloedema
- Thrombocytosis/polycythaemia

For the diagnosis of POEMS syndrome, one major criterion and one or more minor criteria must be met, in addition to both mandatory criteria.

Essential and desirable diagnostic criteria

For the diagnosis of POEMS syndrome, one major criterion and one or more minor criteria must be met, in addition to the two mandatory criteria (see Box 4.08). For the diagnosis of TEMPI syndrome, all the major criteria and one or more minor criteria must be met (see Box 4.09).

Staging

Not applicable

Box 4.09 Diagnostic criteria for TEMPI syndrome (telangiectasias, elevated erythropoietin and erythrocytosis, monoclonal gammopathy, perinephric fluid collection, and intrapulmonary shunting), adapted from Sykes et al., 2020 {3912}

Major criteria:
- Telangiectases
- Elevated erythropoietin and erythrocytosis
- Monoclonal gammopathy (IgG kappa)

Minor criteria:
- Perinephric fluid
- Intrapulmonary shunting

Other:
- Venous thrombosis

For the diagnosis of TEMPI syndrome, all three major criteria and one or more minor criteria must be met. Venous thrombosis has been described in a subset of patients and supports the diagnosis.

Prognosis and prediction

In most cases of POEMS syndrome, the disease is chronic and progressive. Patients with localized plasma cell tumours (one to three isolated bone lesions) treated with radiation have a good clinical outcome, with a 4-year overall survival rate of 97% and a 4-year failure-free survival rate of 52% {2115}. Patients with widespread bone lesions or with extensive bone marrow involvement are treated as patients with plasma cell myeloma / multiple myeloma, with either conventional chemotherapy and/or consolidation of conventional chemotherapy with high-dose melphalan and autologous haematopoietic stem cell transplantation, which is associated with excellent long-term survival {1002}. An insufficient number of TEMPI syndrome and AESOP syndrome cases have been evaluated to make statements regarding prognosis and prediction.

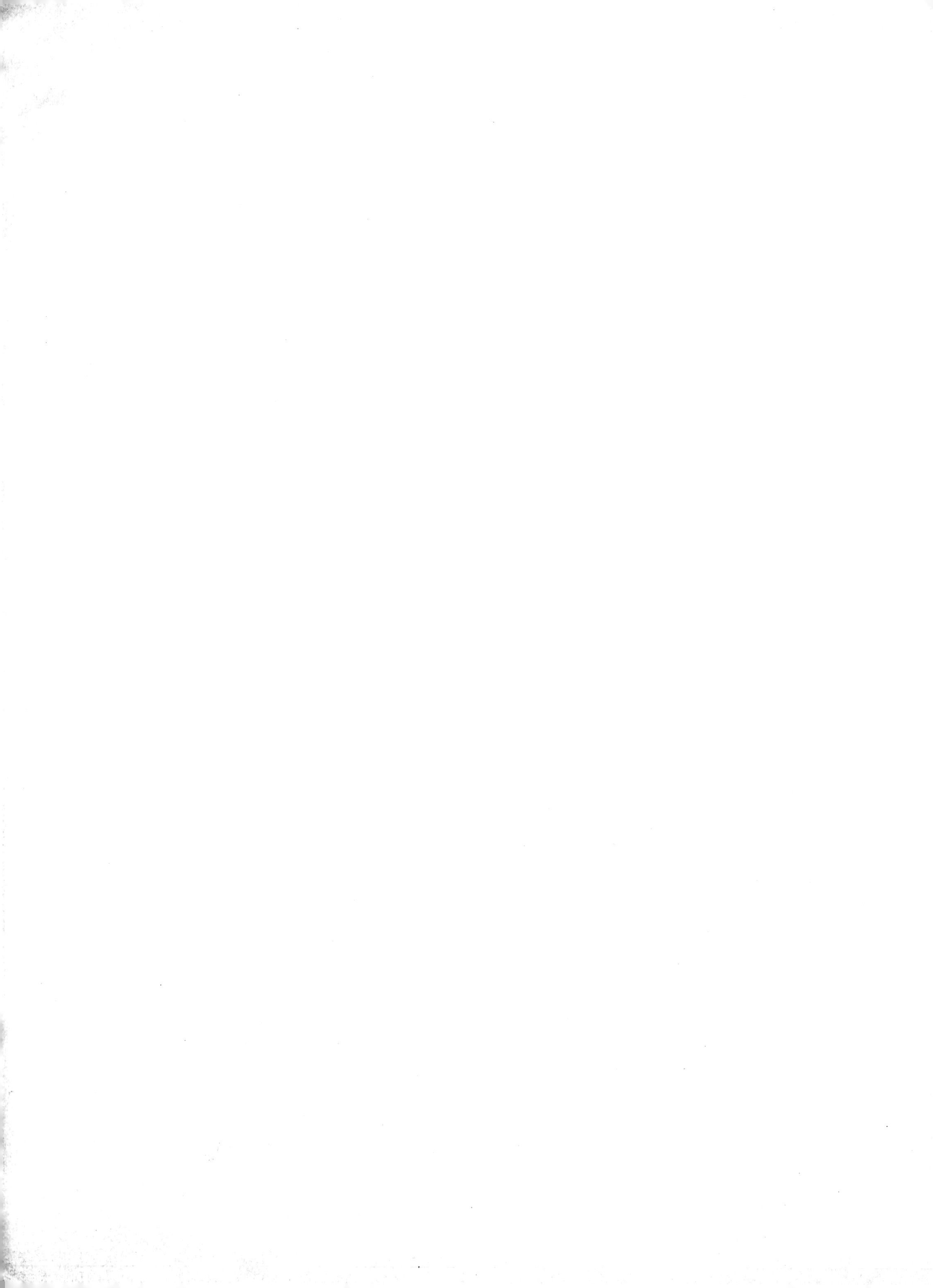

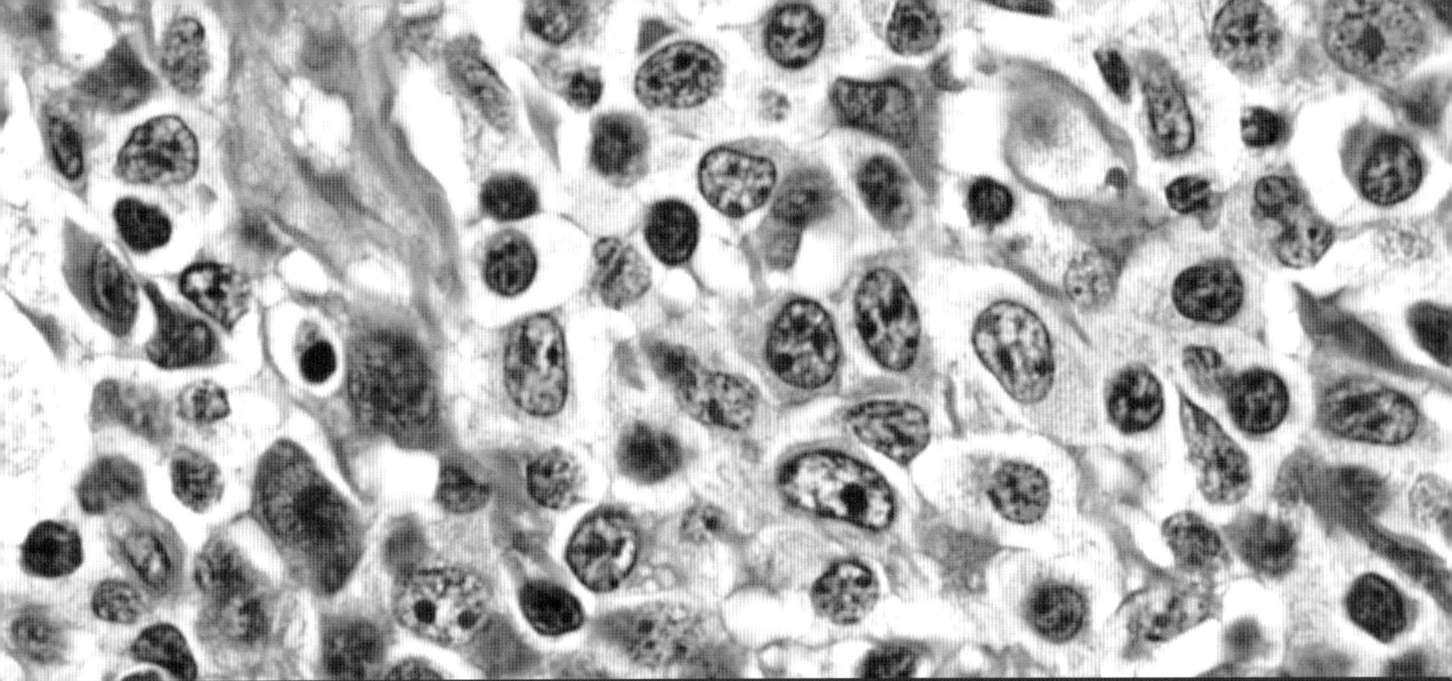

5

T-cell and NK-cell lymphoid proliferations and lymphomas

Edited by: Akkari Y, Alaggio R, Chan JKC, Chng WJ, Coupland SE, Dave SS, de Jong D, Du MQ, Khoury JD, Lazar AJ, Lim MS, Nagai H, Pulitzer M, Sewell WA, Tan PH, Washington MK, Wood BL

(Continued on next page)

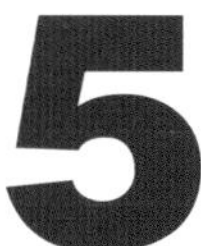

T-cell and NK-cell lymphoid proliferations and lymphomas (continued)

Nodal T follicular helper cell lymphoma
- Nodal T follicular helper cell lymphoma, angioimmunoblastic type
- Nodal T follicular helper cell lymphoma, follicular type
- Nodal T follicular helper cell lymphoma NOS

Other peripheral T-cell lymphomas
- Peripheral T-cell lymphoma NOS

EBV-positive T-cell and NK-cell lymphomas
- EBV-positive nodal T- and NK-cell lymphoma
- Extranodal NK/T-cell lymphoma

EBV-positive T-cell and NK-cell lymphoid proliferations and lymphomas of childhood
- Severe mosquito bite allergy
- Hydroa vacciniforme lymphoproliferative disorder
- Systemic chronic active EBV disease
- Systemic EBV-positive T-cell lymphoma of childhood

T-cell and NK-cell lymphoid proliferations and lymphomas: Introduction

Lim MS
Chan JKC
de Jong D
Elenitoba-Johnson KSJ
Ferry JA
Ott G

T-cell and NK-cell lymphoid proliferations and lymphomas represent a broad spectrum of entities that range from non-clonal proliferations to highly aggressive lymphomas. They can arise in a variety of anatomical locations, including lymph nodes, blood and bone marrow, and organ sites such as the intestine, liver, spleen, and skin. Thirty-six distinct T-cell and NK-cell lymphoma entities are recognized in this edition, and the changes from the previous (revised fourth) edition of the WHO classification of haematolymphoid tumours are shown in Box 5.01 and Box 5.02. Although the entities are hierarchically ordered in families/classes largely on the basis of their site of presentation (blood / bone marrow, skin, gastrointestinal tract, liver, spleen), some are grouped into families/classes according to the current understanding of well-defined T-cell subsets as the cell of origin (e.g. nodal T follicular helper cell lymphoma), or by shared morphological and immunophenotypic features (e.g. anaplastic large cell lymphoma). In addition, there is increasing recognition of exuberant non-clonal proliferations of mature and precursor T cells that mimic neoplastic conditions and arise as abnormal immune responses to infection, inflammation, or genetic dysregulation of T-cell homeostasis, and these are included in this fifth-edition volume. Two entities are included that represent clonal T-cell or NK-cell lymphoproliferative disorders arising primarily in the intestine: indolent T-cell lymphoma of the gastrointestinal tract and indolent NK-cell lymphoproliferative disorder of the gastrointestinal tract. These low-grade neoplasms must be distinguished from inflammatory conditions as well as from the highly aggressive lymphomas that they may mimic, including enteropathy-associated T-cell lymphoma and extranodal NK/T-cell lymphoma, which have a more aggressive clinical course. Thereby, this edition now covers the full spectrum of lymphoid proliferations, from reactive disorders mimicking malignancy to the most aggressive T- and NK-cell proliferations.

Box 5.01 T-cell and NK-cell entities added since the previous edition

Non-neoplastic entities
- Kikuchi–Fujimoto disease
- Indolent T-lymphoblastic proliferation
- Autoimmune lymphoproliferative syndrome (ALPS)

Lymphomas
- Primary cutaneous peripheral T-cell lymphoma NOS
- Indolent NK-cell lymphoproliferative disorder of the gastrointestinal tract
- EBV-positive nodal T- and NK-cell lymphoma

Box 5.02 Lymphoma/leukaemia entities with minor changes in terminology compared with the previous edition[a]

- T-lymphoblastic leukaemia/lymphoma *NOS*
- Early *T-precursor* lymphoblastic leukaemia/lymphoma
- T-large granular lymphocytic leukaemia (*"cell" dropped*)
- NK-large granular lymphocytic leukaemia (*"cell" dropped*)
- Primary cutaneous acral CD8-positive T-cell *lymphoproliferative disorder*
- Indolent T-cell *lymphoma* of the gastrointestinal tract
- *ALK-positive* anaplastic large cell lymphoma
- *ALK-negative* anaplastic large cell lymphoma
- *Nodal T follicular helper cell lymphoma*, angioimmunoblastic type
- *Nodal T follicular helper cell lymphoma*, follicular type
- *Nodal T follicular helper cell lymphoma* NOS
- Extranodal NK/T-cell lymphoma (*qualifier "nasal-type" dropped*)
- *Hydroa vacciniforme* lymphoproliferative disorder
- *Systemic* chronic active EBV *disease*

[a]Key changes are shown in *italics*.

T cells and NK cells in the immune system

T cells and NK cells play important roles in the immune system. T cells recognize foreign antigens derived from pathogens, which are typically displayed on the surface of the body's own cells. NK cells, NK-like T cells, and $\gamma\delta$ T cells play important roles in mucosal and skin defence where a rapid response of the innate immune system is required. The innate immune system is independent of antigen presentation and does not require encounters with antigens in the context of MHC molecules to initiate the immune response. The adaptive immune system, in contrast, represents a more sophisticated response, requiring antigen specificity through antigen-presenting cells in the context of MHC molecules as well as immunological memory. Although conventional $\alpha\beta$ CD4+ and CD8+ T cells are the best characterized of the T-cell subsets, recent studies have identified other, unconventional forms of T cells, such as mucosa-associated invariant T (MAIT) cells {3183} with limited T-cell receptor (TCR) diversity, which function as a bridge between the innate and adaptive immune responses. Distinct subtypes of mature T- and NK-cell neoplasms are thought to arise from cells within the innate and adaptive immune systems.

T-cell and NK-cell differentiation and function

T-cell differentiation is a highly regulated process that originates from multipotent progenitors in the bone marrow that undergo subsequent maturation and selection into antigen-specific T cells in the thymic cortex. Thymic T-cell precursors embedded in a network of thymic stroma provide critical cues for T-cell development via the microenvironment. The thymus is fully developed at birth, and the rate of T-cell production is greatest before puberty, declining in adults. Once the T-cell repertoire is established, the pool of peripheral T cells is

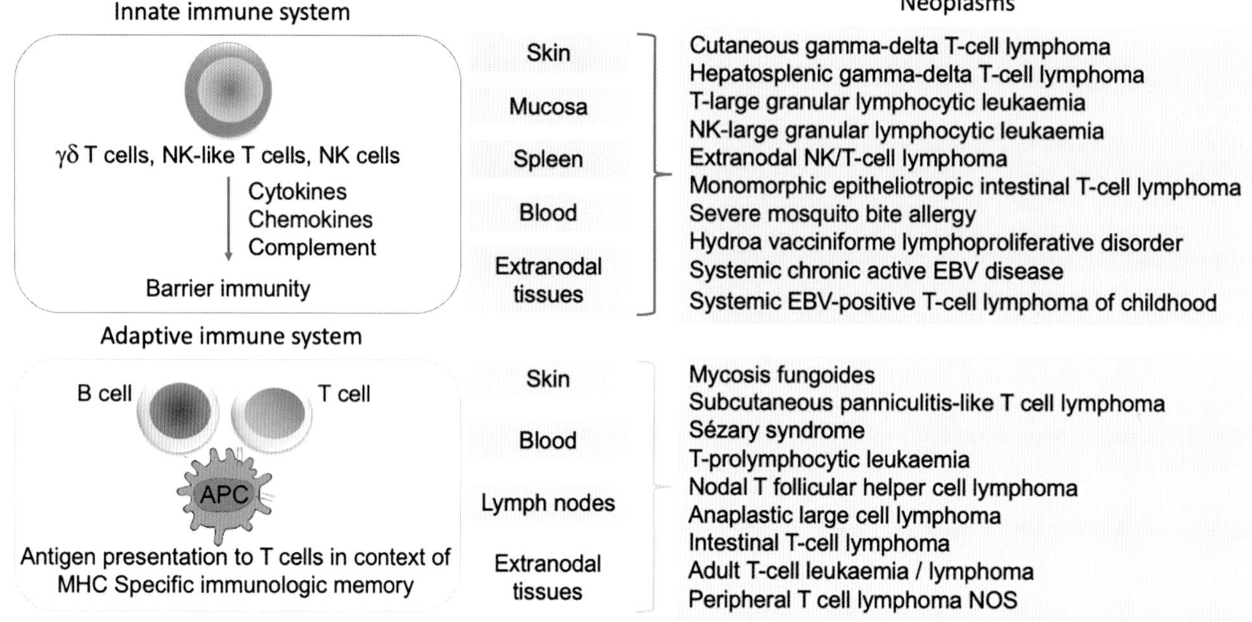

Fig. 5.01 T-cell and NK-cell lymphoid proliferations and lymphomas. T and NK cells of the innate and adaptive immune systems. The innate immune system functions to recognize foreign antigens and involve NK cells, NK-like T cells, and γδ T cells. It is independent of antigen presentation, and effector functions are mediated by the release of cytokines, chemokines, and complement. The adaptive immune system is more sophisticated, requiring antigen specificity through interactions with B cells and antigen-presenting cells (APCs), which through MHC class molecules confers immunological memory and allows for the generation of effector/memory T cells and T regulatory (Treg) cells. Neoplasms of T and NK cells are thought to arise from distinct T-cell subsets representative of both the innate and the adaptive immune systems.

further maintained by the division of mature T cells in peripheral lymphoid organs.

Cortical thymocytes exhibit an immature phenotype, with expression of TdT, BCL6, CD99, CD1a, CD3, CD5, and CD7. They are initially double-negative for CD4 and CD8 and acquire their expression during maturation into double-positive (CD4+, CD8+) T cells before differentiating into single-positive CD4+ or CD8+ T cells. CD4 and CD8 are co-receptors for TCR, and they associate on the T-cell surface with TCR and bind to the MHC. Precursor T-cell neoplasms have an immunophenotype similar to that of cortical thymocytes, except for the more recently characterized early T-precursor lymphoblastic leukaemia/lymphoma {826}. Because of the deregulated nature of the tumour cells, loss or aberrant expression of markers may occur.

T cells within the medullary thymus have phenotypes similar to those of mature T cells within the peripheral lymphoid organs, including the spleen and lymph nodes. There are two major types of T cells: αβ T cells and γδ T cells, defined by the TCR expressed. The αβ and γδ chains of TCR are each composed of a variable region and a constant region. They are both associated with the CD3 complex, which contains γ, δ, and ε chains. αβ and γδ T cells diverge early in T-cell development in the thymus. TR (TCR) genes are assembled and expressed from the V, D, and J gene segments, which generate rearranged V genes encoding the antigen receptor variable region. Successful rearrangement of both α and β (or γ and δ) chain genes of TCR is required (productive rearrangement) for the expression of the protein product, which represents the signal for progression to the next stage of development. Of note, αβ T cells exhibit rearrangements of the TRD and TRG genes, which precede productive rearrangements of the TRB and TRA genes. Cells that do not make productive rearrangements die by in situ apoptosis.

In the peripheral lymphoid organs, T cells and NK cells function in innate and adaptive immune responses.

γδ T cells account for < 5% of normal T cells and have a restricted anatomical distribution, being found mainly in the splenic red pulp, intestinal epithelium, some mucosal sites, and the skin. γδ T cells have a restricted range of antigen recognition and serve as the first line of defence in mucosal immunity and bacterial infections. Lymphomas of γδ T cells are more common in these sites and are rare in lymph nodes.

NK cells function in cell-mediated cytotoxicity, through antibody-dependent mechanisms in addition to killer activation receptors and inhibitory killer cell immunoglobulin receptors (KIRs). NK cells do not rearrange TR (TCR) genes and do not express the complete TCR complex. Activated NK cells express the ε and ζ chains of CD3 in the cytoplasm and express CD2, CD7, and variably CD8, but not sCD3. They express CD16, CD56, variably CD57, and cytoplasmic cytotoxic granules. NK-cell clonality can be assessed using antibodies to various KIRs.

T cells and NK cells within the adaptive immune system are highly heterogeneous and functionally complex. Multiple T-cell subsets are characterized by their specialized functions and differential expression of surface antigens, cytokines, and transcription factors. Numerous subsets of naïve, effector (regulatory and cytotoxic), and memory T cells are known, and additional subsets are being recognized with multidimensional omics technologies.

The highly coordinated expression of transcription factors and chromatin-based epigenetic programmes regulate T-cell lineage commitment and stage-specific differentiation. Such transcription factors include the basic helix-loop-helix (bHLH) factors E2A and HEB, as well as PU.1, GATA3, TCF1, BCL11B, RUNX-family factors, and Ikaros-family factors {4529}. Importantly, many of these transcription factors and chromatin-remodelling genes such as *ARID1A*, *ARID1B*, *KMT2D*, and *SETD2* are affected by genetic alterations in many forms of T-cell and NK-cell lymphomas.

Lineage-specific transcription factors and cytokine expression profiles can be used for the functional categorization of T cells. TBX21 is a regulator of T helper 1 (Th1) and cytotoxic T-cell differentiation. Th1 cells provide functional help to other T cells and macrophages; they express TBX21 and secrete IL-2 and interferon-γ. T helper 2 (Th2) cells provide support for B cells in the production of antibodies; they express GATA3 and secrete IL-4, IL-5, IL-6, and IL-10. GATA3 promotes CD4+ lineage over CD8+ lineage and promotes Th2 cell differentiation over Th1 or T helper 17 (Th17) cell differentiation. T regulatory (Treg) cells express FOXP3 and have diverse functions in suppressing the immune response to cancer and limiting inflammatory responses in tissues. Th17 cells have an effector function and express IL-17 and RORγt, as well as playing a role in immune-mediated inflammatory disease. T follicular helper (TFH) cells help in B-cell maturation within the germinal-centre reaction and express BCL6, CD10, PD1, CXCL13, and CXCR5. CXCL13 induces the proliferation of follicular dendritic cells and facilitates the migration of B and T cells into the germinal centre. The TFH cell phenotype is characteristic of several types of T-cell lymphomas; these include, among others, nodal TFH cell lymphomas, which are now grouped within one family/class.

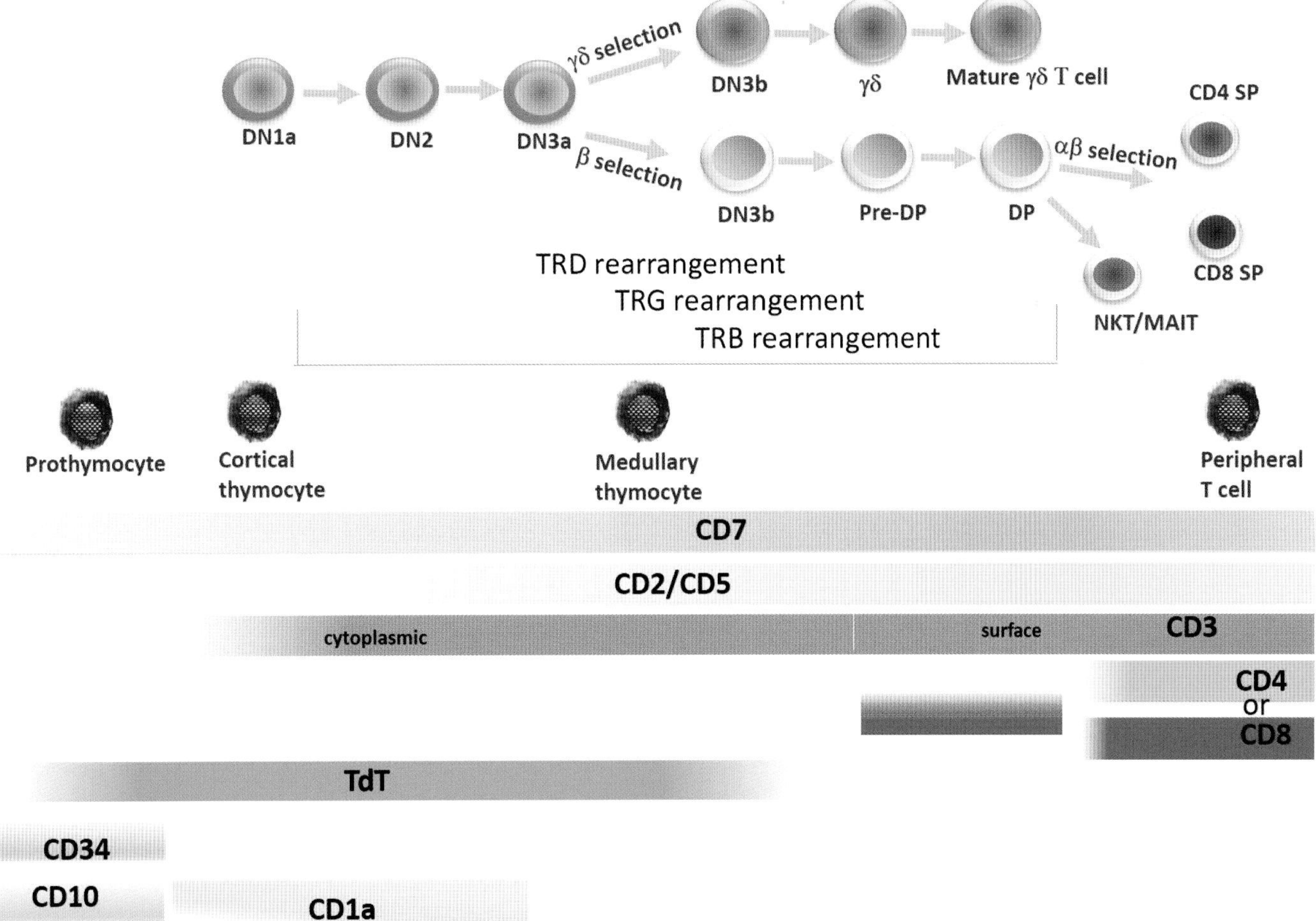

Fig. 5.02 T-cell and NK-cell lymphoid proliferations and lymphomas. T-cell maturation occurs in the thymus, and stages of T-cell differentiation exhibit characteristic antigen expression. Cortical thymocytes exhibit an immature T-cell phenotype and express CD34, CD10, CD1a, and TdT. T-cell lineage commitment follows the rearrangement of the TR (TCR) genes TRD and TRG as they progress through the double-negative stages (DN1a, DN2, DN3a). Those that undergo γδ selection or bypass the β-selection checkpoint differentiate into γδ T cells. Productive TRB rearrangements occurring in the medullary thymus give rise to αβ T cells, which are CD3+, CD4+, CD8+ double-positive (DP) cells, and subsequently to CD4+ and CD8+ single-positive (SP) T cells. A subset of mature T cells differentiate into natural killer T (NKT) / mucosa-associated invariant T (MAIT) cells.

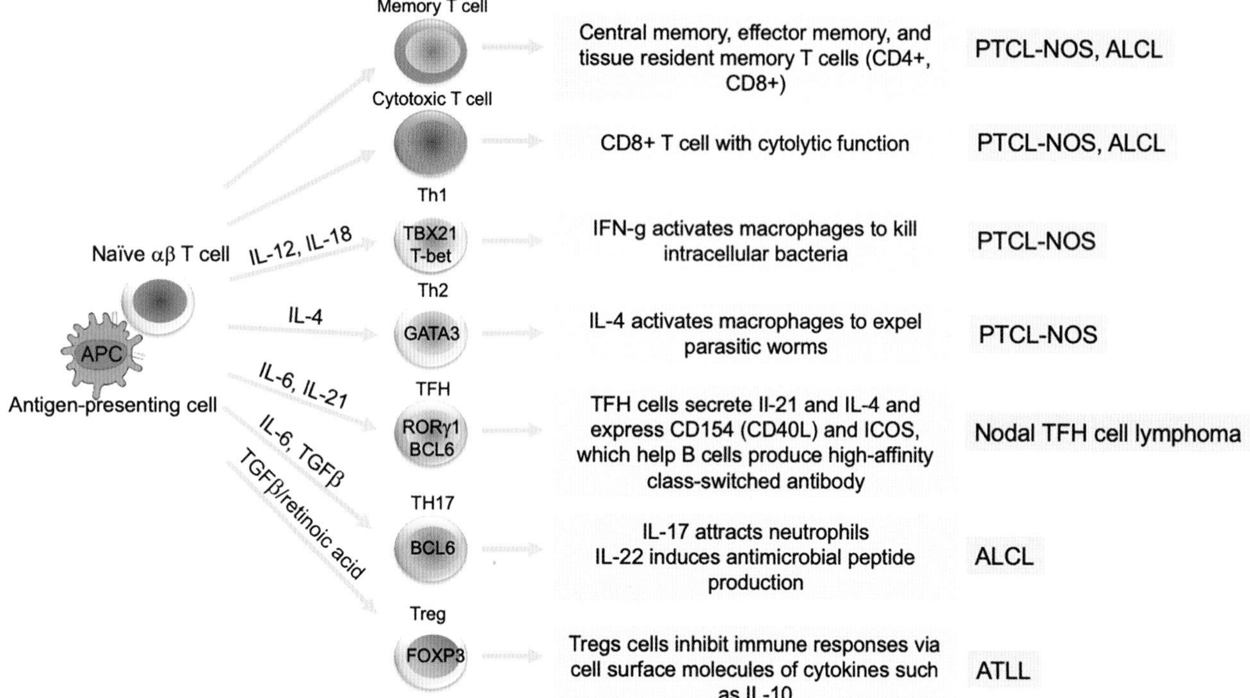

Fig. 5.03 T-cell and NK-cell lymphoid proliferations and lymphomas. Differentiation of effector T-cell subsets. Effector T-cell subsets are derived from the interaction of naïve CD4+ or CD8+ T cells with antigen-presenting cells through antigen-specific MHC-dependent interaction. Antigen-specific memory T cells can be found in central, effector, or tissue resident subsets, which can be either CD4+ or CD8+. Polarizing cytokines that are present during T-cell activation lead to epigenetic modifications and expression of transcription factors that contribute to the differentiation of naïve helper T cells into T helper cell subsets (TH1, TH2, T follicular helper [TFH], TH17, and T regulatory [Treg] cells). The expression of transcription factors, cell surface molecules, and cytokines is helpful in the characterization of T-cell subsets. Examples of putative neoplastic counterparts of T-cell subsets are listed. ALCL, anaplastic large cell lymphoma; ATLL, adult T-cell leukaemia/lymphoma; PTCL, peripheral T-cell lymphoma.

Impact of ontogeny on the classification of T-cell and NK-cell neoplasms

Lymphomas are related to all the lymphoid cell types of the innate and adaptive immune systems. Traditional classification systems for T-cell and NK-cell neoplasms primarily incorporated the dif- ferential expression of cellular proteins for the assess- ment of dif- ferentiation stages, lineages, and limited aspects of T-cell func- tion such as cytotoxicity or activation status (CD30 and CD25). Conceptually, T cells within these functional compartments are thought to acquire genetic aberrations that contribute to the biol- ogy of T-cell malignancies that are characteristic of lymphomas. The diagnostic utility of chemokines, immune checkpoint pro- teins, and transcription factors allows for the recognition of dis- tinct T-cell subsets that may be incorporated into clinical practice.

Neoplasms that are derived from the innate immune system include aggressive NK-cell leukaemias, systemic EBV-positive T-cell lymphoma of childhood, hepatosplenic gamma-delta T-cell lymphoma, and gamma-delta T-cell lymphomas arising from cutaneous and mucosal sites. Gene expression profiling studies have identified molecular subtypes of peripheral T-cell lymphoma NOS based on their expression of proteins in major T-cell subsets. However, the current status of knowledge on the clinicopathological context and prognostic implications is still considered insufficient for including these variants as formal subtypes at this stage.

Genetics of T-cell and NK-cell lymphoid proliferations and lymphomas

Advances in molecular techniques, including the use of next-generation sequencing, have led to an enhanced understanding of the genetic basis of many T-cell and NK-cell lymphoma subtypes. In addition to providing insights into pathogenetic mechanisms, they have enabled the identification of molecular features that are critical for establishing the diagnosis (as essential and/or desirable diagnostic criteria), that have prognostic significance, and that may serve as therapeutic targets {3561,4176,4193}.

The *NPM1* (*NPM*)::*ALK* fusion was identified in 1995 as the predominant genetic alteration in ALK-positive ALCL {2800}; however, recurrent gene fusions (involving *DUSP22*, *TP63*, *ROS1*, and *TYK2*) {837} have only recently emerged as important pathogenetic events and prognostic indicators in certain subtypes, such as ALK-negative ALCL. The vast majority of oncogenic alterations in mature T-cell lymphomas are represented by point mutations, indels, and copy-number changes. T-cell lymphomas frequently carry mutations leading to the constitutive activation of pathways downstream of TCR (including JAK/STAT, PI3K/AKT, and NF-κB), of costimulatory proteins, and/or of cytokine receptors and their downstream pathways. Highly recurrent mutations of various classes of epigenetic modulators are identified in most forms of T-cell lymphoma. The numerous alterations in the DNA methylation and histone posttranslational modification machinery that result from mutations in epigenetic regulators are only beginning to be understood, but they are likely to be early events in oncogenesis {3561,4176,4193}.

Genes that regulate chromatin and histones are not only involved in tumorigenesis but may also be critical for T-cell differentiation. For example, mutations of *SETD2*, a lysine methyltransferase responsible for H3 p.K36 methylation, are highly recurrent in T-cell lymphomas of γδ T cells, such as hepatosplenic T-cell lymphoma {2619}, cutaneous gamma-delta T-cell lymphoma {864}, and monomorphic epitheliotropic intestinal T-cell lymphoma {2709}. Significantly, transgenic mouse models with a loss of function of *SETD2* develop an expansion of γδ T cells, suggesting a role for *SETD2* in T-cell development. Genetic subversion of mechanisms exploiting immune evasion is also observed in various types of T-cell lymphomas {1910,2081,1912}.

Specific molecular alterations in a variety of T-cell and NK-cell neoplasms are associated with morphological or immunophenotypic correlates. ALCLs with *DUSP22* rearrangement are characterized by neoplastic cells with a doughnut-cell appearance {2025}, sheet-like growth pattern, and reduced numbers of pleomorphic cells. A subset of ALCLs with Hodgkin-like morphology have aberrant expression of ERBB4 {3603}, whereas more anaplastic cells are seen in ALCLs with

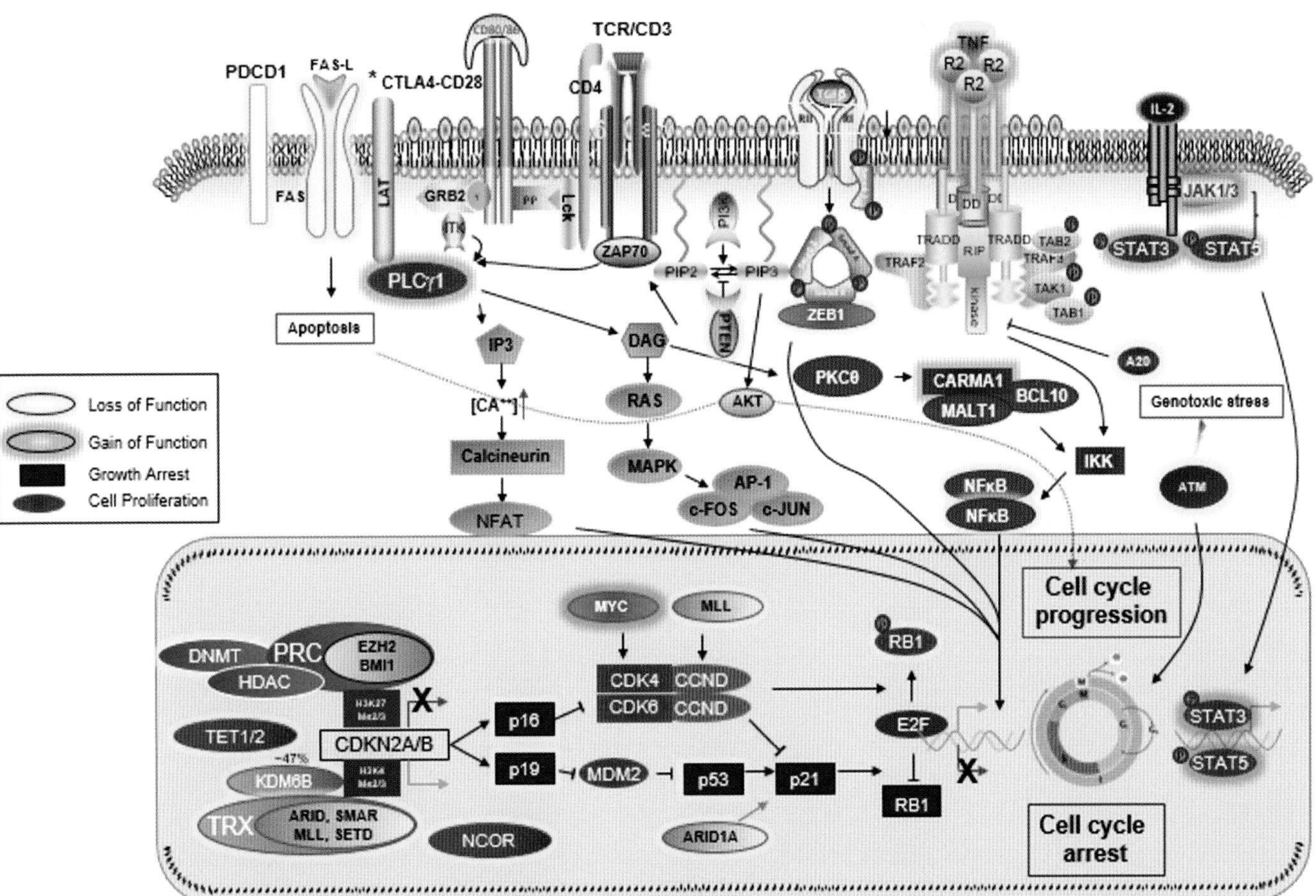

Fig. 5.04 Genetics of T-cell and NK-cell lymphoid proliferations and lymphomas. The vast majority of oncogenic alterations in mature T-cell lymphomas are represented by point mutations, indels, and copy-number changes. T-cell lymphomas frequently carry mutations leading to the constitutive activation of pathways downstream of the T-cell receptor (TCR), costimulatory proteins, and/or cytokine receptors. Highly recurrent mutations of many classes of epigenetic modulators are identified in most forms of T-cell lymphoma {1063}.

JAK2 rearrangement {1199}. There is emerging evidence to support the clinical and phenotypic significance of specific mutations in T-large granular lymphocytic leukaemia and NK-large granular lymphocytic leukaemia. *STAT3* mutations are enriched in CD8+ T-large granular lymphocytic leukaemia with CD16 expression {3991,3714} and are associated with neutropenia and poorer overall survival {3568,242,3320}.

Summary

The current edition of the WHO classification of T-cell and NK-cell lymphoproliferative disorders and neoplasms represents an ongoing refinement of previously used paradigms that integrate the clinical, immunophenotypic, and genetic features of these heterogeneous neoplasms. It also recognizes the presence of T-cell and NK-cell proliferations with indolent clinical behaviour, as well as a spectrum of mature and immature non-clonal T-cell proliferations that may arise secondary to dysregulated T-cell homeostasis in a variety of conditions such as inflammation, infection, and autoimmunity. The current understanding will serve as a basis for further research using novel technology such as multimodal analytical platforms (including linear and 3D genomics) and epigenetic and proteomic analyses at the single-cell level. Answers to open questions on the cellular origins of T- and NK-cell proliferations and neoplasms, their clonal evolution, and their genetic and phenotypic heterogeneity will help to drive future editions of the WHO classification of haematolymphoid tumours towards an increasingly biologically meaningful basis.

Kikuchi–Fujimoto disease

Ng S-B
Chan JKC
Gratzinger D
Lim MS
Medeiros LJ
Sukswai N

Definition

Kikuchi–Fujimoto disease (KFD) is a self-limiting disorder characterized by lymphadenopathy with paracortical proliferation of immunoblasts, infiltration by histiocytes with characteristic nuclear features, and apoptosis or necrosis with abundant nuclear debris.

ICD-O coding

None

ICD-11 coding

4B2Y Other specified disorders involving the immune system

Related terminology

Acceptable: histiocytic necrotizing lymphadenitis; Kikuchi disease; Kikuchi lymphadenitis.

Subtype(s)

None

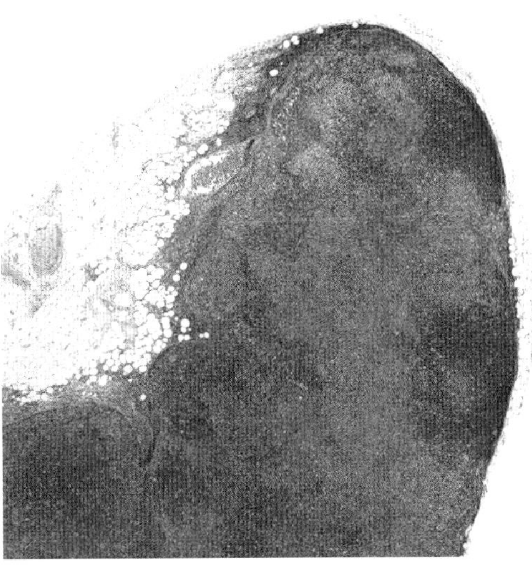

Fig. 5.05 Kikuchi–Fujimoto disease. The lesional foci in the lymph node are typically non-expansile, pale-staining, and well demarcated from the surrounding parenchyma.

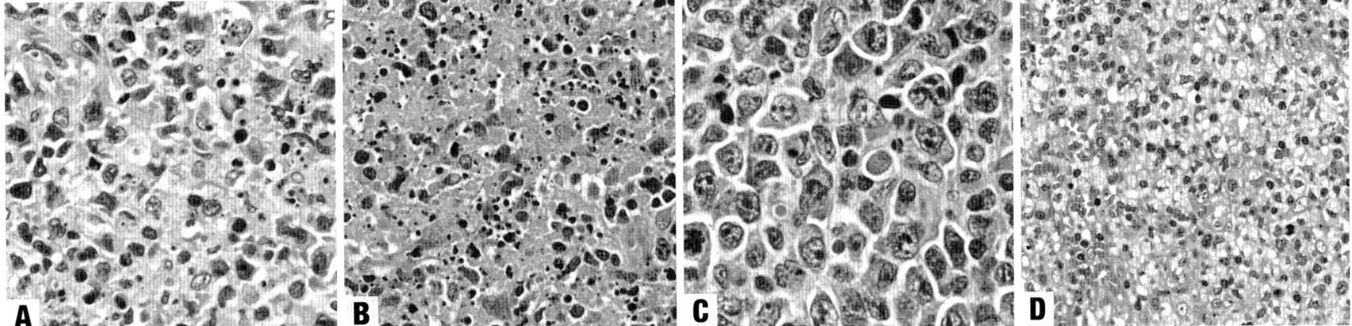

Fig. 5.06 Kikuchi–Fujimoto disease: cellular composition of karyorrhectic foci. **A** The foci can be composed predominantly of histiocytes. The histiocytes show irregular twisted nuclei. Some have crescentic nuclei and contain ingested nuclear debris. **B** Overt necrosis can be present. **C** A focus with numerous large lymphoid cells, some of which exhibit atypia in the form of irregular nuclear folds. Nuclear debris is found among the lymphoid cells. **D** In late lesions, there can be accumulation of foamy histiocytes.

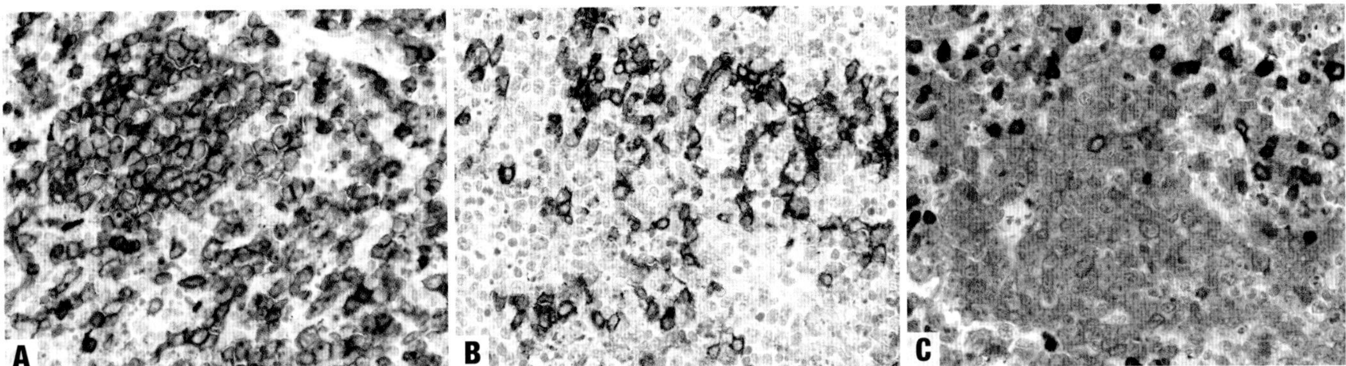

Fig. 5.07 Kikuchi–Fujimoto disease: immunohistochemistry. **A** Almost all the T cells are CD8-positive. **B** The plasmacytoid dendritic cells within the karyorrhectic foci are highlighted by CD123 staining. **C** An aberrant immunophenotype is common in the large lymphoid cells within the karyorrhectic foci. Double immunostaining for CD8 (red) and CD5 (brown) shows that most large lymphoid cells show red cell-membrane staining without a brownish hue, indicating a loss of CD5 expression.

Localization

Lymph nodes are involved, with rare concurrent skin lesions {2002,3806}.

Clinical features

KFD is an acute or subacute disorder involving unilateral cervical lymph nodes in the majority of patients. Less frequently, the disease is bilateral and involves other lymph nodes. Clinical manifestations may include fever (which can be prolonged), asthenia, weight loss, rash, and arthromyalgia {1257,1991,2257,1018}. Anaemia (occurring in 55% of cases) and leukopenia (in 9–58%) can be present, and the erythrocyte sedimentation rate (in 32–56%), LDH level (in 32–81%), and/or aminotransferase level (in 24–27%) can be elevated {1990,3234,4107,996,4090,2157, 4522,3782,681,1018,3186}. Rare cases are associated with autoimmune diseases, such as systemic lupus erythematosus and Graves disease {681,3794,1018,3186}, or with other conditions such as meningoencephalitis, myocarditis, and haemophagocytic lymphohistiocytosis {624,1018,511,3671}. High FDG uptake may be observed on PET-CT, mimicking lymphoma {4098,2098, 2001}, and this correlates with disease severity {3682}.

Epidemiology

KFD has a high prevalence among Asian populations but occurs worldwide. It affects young adults (median age: 23–30 years) and shows a female predominance {1990,3234,4107,996,4090,2157, 4522,3782,681,1018}. In paediatric patients, KFD is more common in boys {2011,277,3674}. The geographical predominance of KFD in the Republic of Korea and in Japan is related to the presence of the HLA class II alleles HLA-DPA1 and HLA-DPB1 {3960}; however, this disorder is seen in patients of any ethnicity {1018}.

Etiology

The etiology is unclear, although infection and autoimmune diseases are postulated to be triggers of the disease {1716,420}. A causal relationship with viruses, including EBV, parvovirus B19, and human herpesviruses, has not been demonstrated {4568, 1676,3461,733,1018}.

Pathogenesis

KFD is characterized by an exuberant T cell–mediated immune response to a variety of stimuli in genetically susceptible individuals {1716,645,420}. Apoptosis, a prominent feature of KFD, is induced by CD8+ cytotoxic T cells via the FAS and perforin pathways {3931,1156,3022,3020}. Plasmacytoid dendritic cells (pDCs) play a role in promoting the cytotoxic reaction by producing type I interferon, and elevated levels of cytokines and chemokines, such as interferon-γ, IL-6, and IL-18, have been demonstrated in patients with KFD {1104,2136,1914,3018,4259, 3875}. An IgD+/CD38+ small B-cell population has been identified in KFD and systemic lupus erythematosus, suggesting a possible pathological role for anergic/autoreactive B cells {3659}.

Macroscopic appearance

Not relevant

Histopathology

The lymph node shows single or multiple non-expansile, circumscribed, sometimes wedge-shaped, light-staining karyorrhectic foci in the paracortex. The cellular composition of the karyorrhectic foci evolves through three phases {2157}. The proliferative phase is characterized by abundant karyorrhectic debris admixed with a variable number of histiocytes with twisted or

Table 5.01 Differential diagnosis of Kikuchi–Fujimoto disease (KFD)

Disorder	Overlapping features with KFD	Distinguishing features from KFD
Systemic lupus erythematosus–associated lymphadenopathy	Non-granulomatous histiocytic infiltrates with necrosis and lacking granulocytes	Histological features may or may not simulate KFD; clinical and serological criteria for the diagnosis of systemic lupus erythematosus, including elevated anti-dsDNA antibodies {3212}, haematoxylin bodies (not invariably present), vasculitis, deposits of nuclear material in the vessel walls (Azzopardi effect), presence of many plasma cells
Infectious mononucleosis	Necrosis, presence of immunoblasts	Prominent proliferation of immunoblasts, often showing a spectrum of maturation; lacks discrete karyorrhectic foci; Reed–Sternberg–like cells may be present; presence of many EBV-encoded small RNA (EBER)-positive cells
Infectious necrotizing granulomatous lymphadenitis (e.g. mycobacterial and fungal infections, cat scratch disease)	Necrosis, clusters of plasmacytoid dendritic cells, histiocytes	Granulomas with epithelioid histiocytes and multinucleated giant cells; evidence of infective agents by special stains, cultures, serology, and/or molecular techniques
Kawasaki disease	Necrosis	Usually in patients aged < 5 years; despite prominence of apoptotic debris, the main histological change is geographical necrosis rather than cellular proliferation; fibrin thrombi in non-necrotic areas; granulocytic infiltration
Herpes simplex lymphadenitis	Necrosis	Viral inclusions and multinucleated giant cells; abundant granulocytes in necrotic areas; viral antigens detected by immunohistochemistry
Lymph node infarction	Necrosis	Coagulative necrosis without karyorrhexis; ghost cells may retain expression of pan–B- or T-cell markers
Drug-induced necrosis (e.g. phenytoin)	Necrosis	Necrosis associated with eosinophils, history of medication
Peripheral T-cell lymphoma	Proliferative and slightly atypical T-cell infiltrates; CD30 expression; aberrant loss of CD5, CD7, or CD2 {4340}; rarely clonal by TR gene rearrangement studies	Effacement of architecture, malignant lymphoid cells with atypia, monoclonal T-cell proliferation

dsDNA, double-stranded DNA.

crescentic nuclei (often accompanied by phagocytosed debris), immunoblasts, and pDCs. Abundant immunoblasts with irregular nuclear folds may mimic lymphoma. The necrotizing phase is characterized by discrete to confluent areas of coagulative necrosis among the proliferating cells and karyorrhectic debris, whereas the xanthomatous phase is characterized by the accumulation of foamy macrophages. Granulocytes and eosinophils are notably absent, and plasma cells are scarce {4090}.

Immunohistochemistry

The karyorrhectic foci typically comprise a mixture of cell types. (1) The histiocytes express CD68, CD163, and CD4, and they also characteristically express myeloperoxidase {3235}. (2) pDCs express pDC markers (e.g. CD123, TCL1, and TCF4), CD4, and CD68, and they tend to cluster around proliferative or necrotic areas {2529,3875}. Although characteristic, pDCs are not specific to KFD and can be present in other reactive settings {3452}. (3) The lymphocytes are predominantly CD8+ cytotoxic T cells and may express CD30 {3917}. The majority express TCRβ and a minority express TCRγ {3875}. Aberrant immunophenotypes, in the form of partial or complete loss of expression of CD5, CD7, or CD2, are not uncommon {4340} and may lead to misdiagnosis as T-cell lymphoma.

Differential diagnosis

See Table 5.01.

Cytology

Characteristic cytological features include the presence of karyorrhectic debris, phagocytic histiocytes with crescentic nuclei, and pDCs {4088}.

Diagnostic molecular pathology

Uncommonly, monoclonal or oligoclonal TR gene rearrangements are identified in KFD, and care should be taken not to overdiagnose T-cell lymphoma {2353}.

Essential and desirable diagnostic criteria

Essential: lymphadenopathy; discrete paracortical karyorrhectic foci with proliferation of histiocytes, pDCs, and immunoblasts; no granulocytes and few plasma cells; exclusion of mimics of KFD – in particular, relevant infections, lymphomas, and autoimmune diseases should be ruled out whenever possible (see Table 5.01).

Desirable: histiocytes with crescentic nuclei and phagocytosed debris.

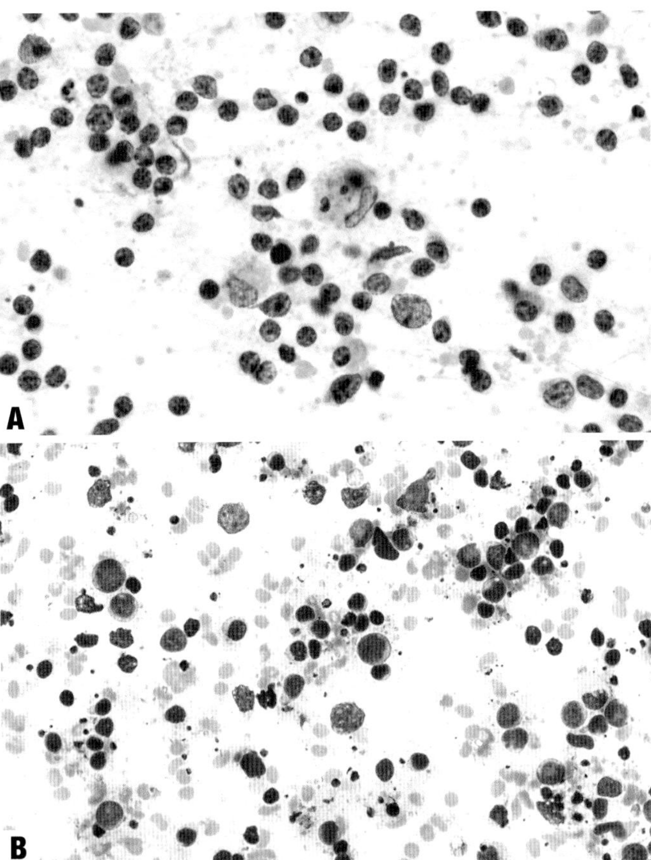

Fig. 5.08 Kikuchi–Fujimoto disease: FNAC. Lymph node fine-needle aspirate smear shows histiocytes (some with crescentic morphology and ingested debris), small lymphoid cells, large lymphoid cells, and karyorrhectic debris in Pap staining (**A**) and in Giemsa staining (**B**).

Staging

None

Prognosis and prediction

KFD resolves spontaneously in most patients, but 3–21% of patients develop recurrent disease {3782,1018,3186}, and rare fatalities from pulmonary haemorrhage, haemophagocytic syndrome, and heart failure can occur {624,4402,1860,236}. When recurrent, there is involvement in multiple nodal sites (in 73% of cases) and an association with underlying autoimmune diseases (in 32%) {390}.

Autoimmune lymphoproliferative syndrome

Gratzinger D
Allende LM
Chan JKC
Ott G
Yang DT

Definition

Autoimmune lymphoproliferative syndrome (ALPS) is an inborn or acquired error of immunity characterized by lymphadenopathy, hepatosplenomegaly, autoimmune cytopenias, and an increased risk of lymphoma. It is associated with germline or somatic defects in the FAS-mediated apoptosis pathway and the accumulation of αβ CD4/CD8 double-negative T (DNT) cells.

ICD-O coding

None

ICD-11 coding

4A01.22 Immune dysregulation syndromes presenting primarily with lymphoproliferation

Related terminology

Not recommended: Canale–Smith syndrome.

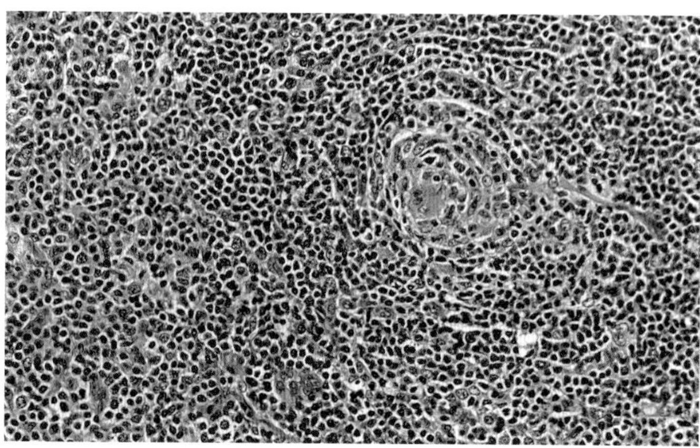

Fig. 5.09 Autoimmune lymphoproliferative syndrome (ALPS) lymph node with Castleman disease–like changes. Typical Castleman disease–like follicles with regressed germinal centres, onion-skinning, and penetrating small-calibre vessels.

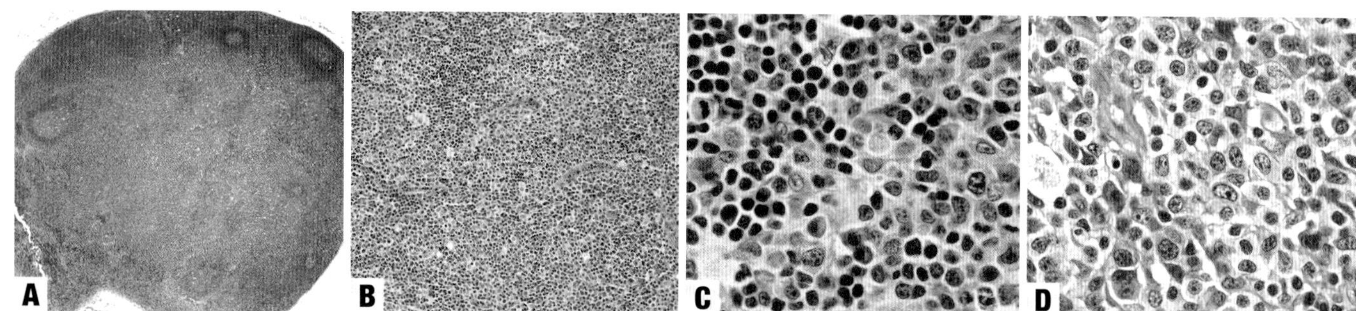

Fig. 5.10 Typical lymph node histology in autoimmune lymphoproliferative syndrome (ALPS). **A** Low-power magnification shows reactive follicles with visible germinal centres and well-formed mantle zones; the paracortex is expanded by a pale-staining lymphoid infiltrate, but the overall lymph node architecture is intact. **B** The interfollicular infiltrate is composed of sheets of pale-staining medium-sized lymphocytes with admixed small lymphocytes, plasma cells, and high endothelial venules. **C** The medium-sized lymphocytes have irregular nuclear contours and prominent nucleoli; mitotic figures are frequent. **D** The paracortex is expanded by sheets of cytologically atypical lymphocytes with open chromatin, slightly irregular nuclear contours, and visible nucleoli.

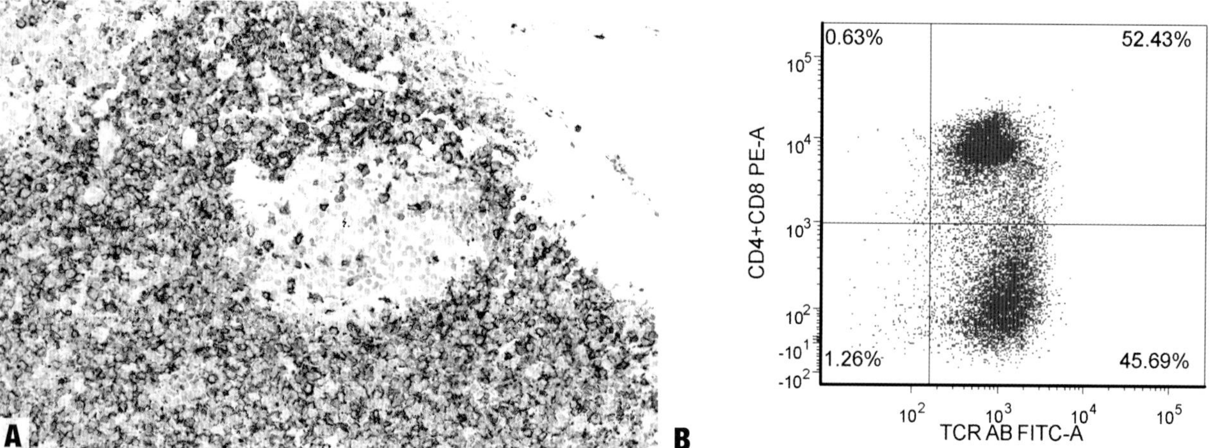

Fig. 5.11 Typical immunohistochemical findings in autoimmune lymphoproliferative syndrome (ALPS). **A** The paracortical expansion is composed of T cells that coexpress CD57 by immunohistochemistry. **B** Flow immunophenotyping shows a large population of TCRαβ+, CD4−, CD8− T-cell events.

Subtype(s)

ALPS with germline *FAS* mutation (ALPS-FAS), either homozygous (autosomal recessive) or heterozygous (autosomal dominant); ALPS with somatic *FAS* mutation (ALPS-sFAS); ALPS with other specified FAS-pathway germline mutation (*FASLG, CASP10, CASP8, FADD*); ALPS with unknown underlying mutation (ALPS-U) {3052,3967}

Localization

The lymph nodes and spleen are the main sites of involvement; less commonly, extranodal sites {1397}, including the bone marrow {4443}, are involved.

Clinical features

Clinical features include lymphadenopathy, hepatosplenomegaly, autoimmune cytopenias, an increased risk of lymphoma, and a high risk of sepsis after splenectomy {3768,3848,2937, 3298}. ALPS-FAS is usually diagnosed in early childhood, whereas ALPS-sFAS is diagnosed across a broad age range {997,1621}. Coexisting IgG4-related disease may occur {4142}.

Radiological features

The PET imaging features of ALPS overlap with those of lymphoma {562}.

Epidemiology

The global prevalence of ALPS is unknown; a recent systematic review relied on data predominantly from the USA, Italy, and France {1464}. *FAS* mutations accounted for 85% of cases of ALPS; 87% of these mutations were germline.

Box 5.03 Characteristic histological findings and pitfalls of autoimmune lymphoproliferative syndrome (ALPS)

Characteristic histological findings
- Pale-staining proliferative paracortical DNT cell hyperplasia with plasmacytosis and foci of RDD
- B-cell follicles with a range of features, from reactive follicular hyperplasia to progressive transformation of germinal centres to Castleman disease–like findings
- Extranodal sites with mixed lymphoid infiltrates including proliferative DNT cells

Pitfalls
- Misdiagnosis as peripheral T-cell lymphoma due to cytological atypia, DNT cell phenotype, high Ki-67 index, cytotoxic markers, extranodal infiltrates, occasional $\gamma\delta$ T-cell phenotype
- Masking of underlying ALPS by associated Castleman disease–like findings, RDD, or superimposed IgG4-related disease
- Increased risk of lymphoma, including some types that may be obscured by a prominent non-neoplastic T-cell component, such as T-cell/histiocyte–rich large B-cell lymphoma and nodular lymphocyte-predominant Hodgkin lymphoma

DNT, CD4/CD8 double-negative T; RDD, Rosai–Dorfman disease.

Etiology

Genetic factors are characterized by germline or somatic mutations in *FAS* or genes encoding the FAS pathway {3052}.

Pathogenesis

FAS pathway gene mutations lead to a failure of lymphocyte apoptosis {3768,1198} and increased proliferation {2583,4251}, resulting in the persistence of physiological CD38+, CD45RA+, IL-10+ CD4+, CD8+, and DNT cell populations {2458}. Failure of FAS-dependent T-cell immune surveillance {31} and

Table 5.02 Clinical, laboratory, histological, and genetic features suggestive of autoimmune lymphoproliferative syndrome (ALPS) and ALPS-like disorders

Features	ALPS	Overlap	ALPS-like disorders
Clinical	Lymphadenopathy, hepatosplenomegaly Autoimmune cytopenia Risk of malignancy	Lymphadenopathy, hepatosplenomegaly Autoimmune cytopenia Risk of malignancy	Frequent: recurrent infections, enteropathy, skin lesions Infrequent: HLH, arthritis, neurological symptoms, endocrinopathy, and cardiomyopathy
Laboratory	Increased: CD3+, TCRαβ+, CD4−, CD8− (DNT) cells; vitamin B12, sFASL, IL-10; IgG Normal: IgG antibody responses Decreased: FAS-induced apoptosis; anti-polysaccharide IgM response in active disease	Memory B-cell lymphopenia	Variable levels of DNT cells, vitamin B12, sFASL, IL-10 Variable levels of IgG, IgM Specific alteration of T, B, and/or NK cells Normal FAS-induced apoptosis except in cases with *STAT3* gain of function or deficiencies of LRBA or TET2
Histological	Infiltration of DNT cells in lymph nodes (paracortical), spleen, and (occasionally) extranodal sites	Lymphoid infiltrates at extranodal sites	Lymphocytic infiltration of non-lymphoid organs including gut, lung, or brain (especially in cases with LRBA and CTLA-4 defects)
Genetic	Germline mutations: *FAS, FASLG, FADD, CASP10*, and *CASP8* Somatic mutations: *FAS*	None	Immune dysregulation (EBV susceptibility): *PRKCD, MAGT1, XIAP, SH2D1A, RASGRP1, TNFRSF9* Immune dysregulation (Treg cell defect): *STAT3, CTLA4, LRBA, IL2RA, IL2RB, DEF6* Antibody deficiencies: *PIK3CD* and *CARD11* gain of function, *PIK3R1* loss of function Combined immunodeficiency: *ITK, STK4* Defects in innate immunity: *STAT1* gain of function, *IL12RB1* Autoinflammatory disorders: *ADA2, TNFAIP3, TET2* Phenocopies of IEIs: somatic mutations in *NRAS, KRAS* {3967,3969}

DNT, CD4/CD8 double-negative T; HLH, haemophagocytic lymphohistiocytosis; IEI, inborn error of immunity; sFASL, serum FASL; Treg, T regulatory.

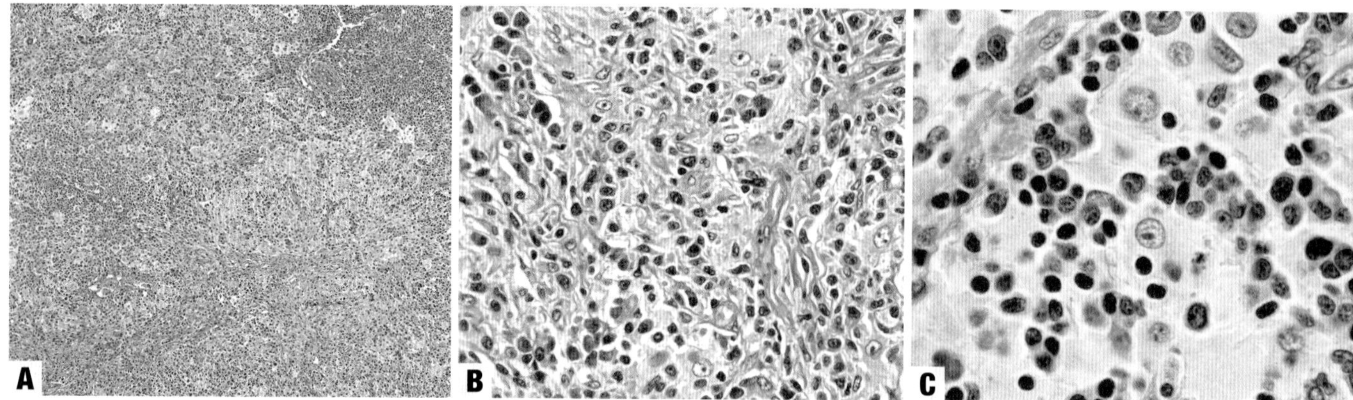

Fig. 5.12 Autoimmune lymphoproliferative syndrome (ALPS) lymph node with Rosai–Dorfman disease. **A** Low-power view of the lymph node reveals irregular eosinophilic foci that stand out against the characteristic paracortical expansion. **B** The characteristic eosinophilic histiocytes of Rosai–Dorfman disease, notable for their round nuclei and prominent central nucleoli, are admixed with numerous plasma cells. **C** Emperipolesis, with engulfed lymphocytes and plasma cells within the histiocyte cytoplasm, is evident at high magnification.

FAS-deficient germinal-centre B cells {3382} may contribute to the predisposition to lymphoma.

Macroscopic appearance

The lymph nodes and spleen are enlarged and homogeneous in appearance. Firm, fleshy, or necrotic areas should be sampled to exclude lymphoma.

Histopathology

Lymph nodes are enlarged by reactive follicular hyperplasia and pronounced pale-staining paracortical hyperplasia, with admixed proliferations of DNT cells and polytypic plasma cells. Progressive transformation of germinal centres, Castleman disease–like histology, or superimposed plasmacytosis {2347} may mask histological findings {446}. Rosai–Dorfman disease is found in about a quarter of ALPS lymph nodes {3298,2537A}. Similar infiltrates occur at extranodal sites, including the spleen and bone marrow {1397,4443,2347}.

Immunohistochemistry

The DNT cell population is positive for CD45RA, negative for CD45RO, and positive for cytotoxic markers, including perforin, TIA1, and CD57 (see Box 5.03, p. 647) {2347,4144,4191}.

Differential diagnosis

The differential diagnosis includes RAS-associated leukoproliferative disease; unicentric Castleman disease (UCD), especially the mixed/plasmacytic subtype, and idiopathic multicentric Castleman disease (iMCD); IgG4-related disease; Rosai–Dorfman disease; and lymphoma. Although IgG4-related disease and Rosai–Dorfman disease can co-occur with ALPS, the diagnosis of KSHV/HHV8-negative multicentric Castleman disease is definitionally excluded in the setting of ALPS {1110}. ALPS may mimic T-cell lymphoma by its high proliferation index, unusual immunophenotype, and extranodal involvement (including the bone marrow) {3348}.

Bone marrow involvement by benign lymphoproliferation must not be overinterpreted as lymphoma {4443}.

Numerous ALPS-like primary immune regulation disorders share an autoimmune lymphoproliferative phenotype (see Table 5.02, p. 647).

Cytology

Not relevant

Diagnostic molecular pathology

Germline and acquired mutations should be assessed according to diagnostic guidelines {3052,566,2416,2553}. Similar *FAS* death domain mutations are also found in lymphoma {2608}. ALPS DNT cells have a restricted TCRVβ repertoire {460}, raising the concern for possible false positive T-cell clonality results.

Essential and desirable diagnostic criteria

Essential: > 6 months of benign, non-infectious adenopathy and/or splenomegaly, peripheral blood flow cytometry showing normal or increased lymphocyte count; αβ DNT cells > 1.5% of total or > 2.5% of CD3+ lymphocytes; detection of *FAS*, *FASLG*, *CASP8*, *FADD*, or *CASP10* mutation.

Desirable: a probable diagnosis can be made if typical lymph node findings are also present – however, expanded lymph node αβ DNT cells do not substitute for peripheral blood flow; elevated plasma vitamin B12, serum FASL, and IL-10; autoimmune cytopenias with polyclonal hypergammaglobulinaemia; a compatible family history can support a probable ALPS diagnosis.

Staging

Not relevant

Prognosis and prediction

ALPS is associated with an increased risk of B-cell lymphomas, including classic Hodgkin lymphoma, nodular lymphocyte-predominant Hodgkin lymphoma, diffuse large B-cell lymphoma, Burkitt lymphoma, follicular lymphoma, and (rarely) T-cell lymphoma and histiocytic sarcoma {3848,2937,3298,4208}.

Indolent T-lymphoblastic proliferation

Parrens M
Ohgami RS
Ott G

Definition

Indolent T-lymphoblastic proliferation (iT-LBP) is an extrathymic non-clonal expansion of T lymphoblasts occurring alone or in association with other disorders, such as Castleman disease.

ICD-O coding

None

ICD-11 coding

2B0Y Other specified primary cutaneous mature T-cell or NK-cell lymphomas and lymphoproliferative disorders

Related terminology

None

Subtype(s)

None

Localization

iT-LBP is most frequently identified in mandibular, cervical, supraclavicular, abdominal, retroperitoneal, or oropharyngeal lymph nodes {3846,3010} and in upper aerodigestive tract lymphoid tissues {4202,4482}. It has also been reported in association with tissues involved by myasthenia gravis {3846,2012}; Castleman disease {3317,3012,4404,1881,651,1239}; hepatocellular carcinoma {4319,1094,2099}; follicular dendritic cell sarcoma {2012,3012,4284,664}; nodal T follicular helper cell lymphoma (nTFHL), angioimmunoblastic type {3012}; and acinic cell carcinoma {3012,4488}. iT-LBP has not been identified in the bone marrow.

Clinical features

The clinical presentation is typically indolent and varies according to the features of associated disorders. However, in many cases, it consists of isolated lymphadenopathy or an isolated

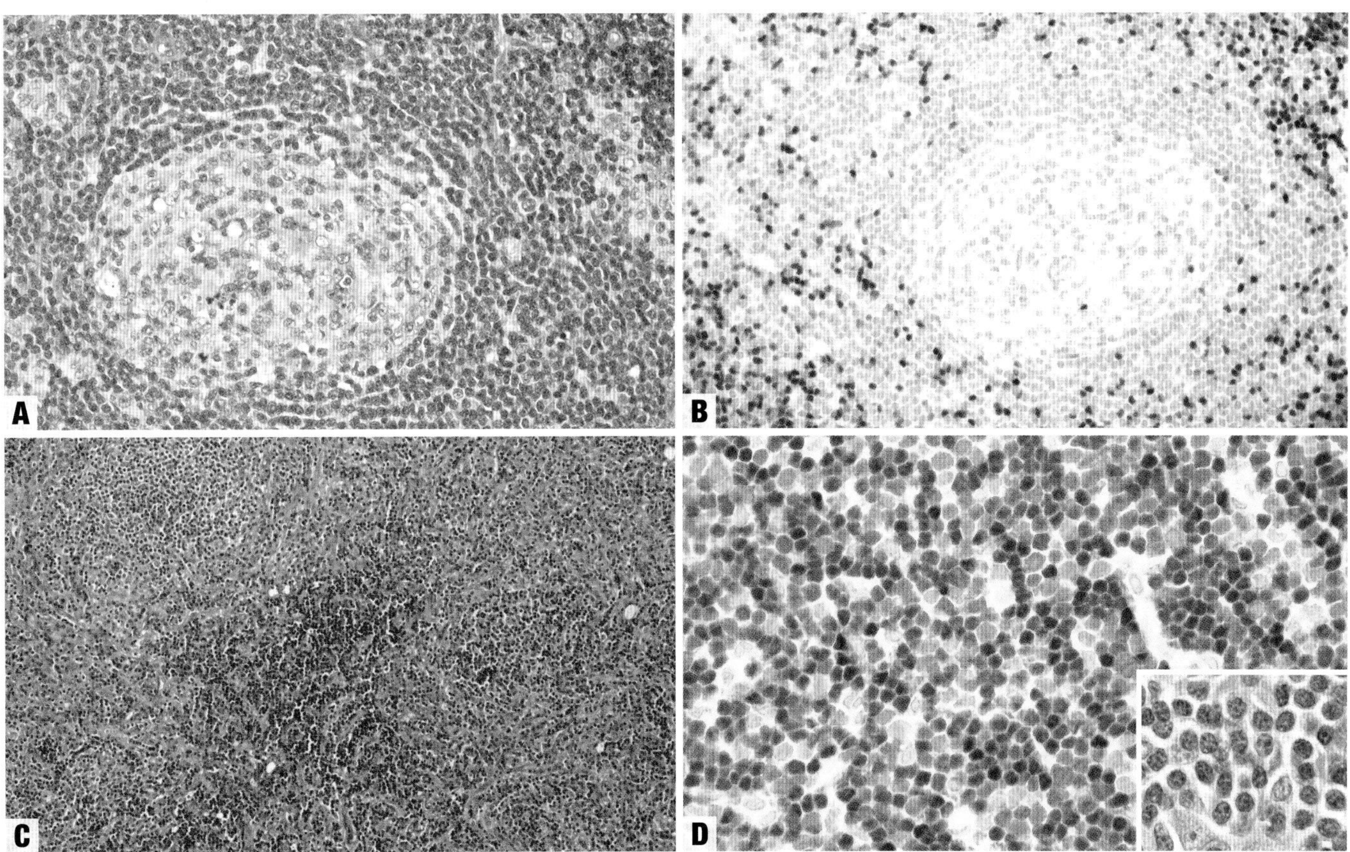

Fig. 5.13 Indolent T-lymphoblastic proliferation. **A** Sheets of small immature lymphocytes are seen surrounding a reactive follicle but with preservation of normal lymphoid architecture and without invasion into the germinal centre. Note the absence of morphological atypia in the small cells. These lymphoblasts resemble haematogones as seen in a marrow biopsy. **B** Small TdT-positive T cells ringing reactive follicles. **C** An interfollicular expansion of small to medium-sized lymphoid cells with immature blastic chromatin and inconspicuous nucleoli, lacking significant atypia. **D** Nuclear TdT immunostaining highlights the small lymphocytes, which are present in sheets and lack nuclear atypia. **Inset:** High magnification shows small to medium-sized lymphoid cells with immature blastic chromatin and inconspicuous nucleoli without significant atypia.

tumour mass in an otherwise healthy individual. Cases of diffuse lymphadenopathy have been described {3010}. Lymphadenopathy or a mass lesion may persist for years or spontaneously resolve. In follicular dendritic cell sarcoma, iT-LBP may be more frequent in patients who also have paraneoplastic autoimmune multiorgan syndrome {4284}.

Epidemiology

Cases have been reported with increasing frequency in recent years, indicating that the entity is not as rare as originally thought. There may be a slight male predominance, and most cases described have been in individuals in their fourth or fifth decade of life, although paediatric cases have been reported {1881}.

Etiology

The etiology is unknown. Some studies suggest that T lymphoblasts are perpetually released from the thymus, although this has not yet been established {1239,445}.

Pathogenesis

The pathogenesis of iT-LBP is unclear, although several studies have shown that small numbers of TdT-positive T lymphoblasts may be present normally in reactive secondary lymphoid organs in paediatric and adult populations {1239,3265,3847, 3061,2616,371}. One hypothesis is that iT-LBP originates from T lymphoblasts that have been released from the thymus and have homed to extrathymic sites with a favourable local microenvironment {3012,1094,3846,4319}. An alternative hypothesis is that an altered cytokine milieu (e.g. IL-6, IL-7) in tissues may stimulate local rare TdT+ T cells to proliferate, which may result in iT-LBPs {664,3012}. These hypotheses have not been confirmed.

Macroscopic appearance

The macroscopic aspect is related to the associated diseases or tumours but frequently consists of a mass composed of pink-tan, firm, fleshy tissue. Areas of necrosis have been reported when associated with hepatocellular carcinoma {3012}.

Histopathology

In lymph nodes, the overall architecture is preserved. T lymphoblasts form clusters or confluent sheets, preferentially in interfollicular and paracortical regions. Lymphoblasts are small to medium in size, lack atypia, and have open immature chromatin with inconspicuous nucleoli. Mitoses are frequent, as are scattered histiocytes. When associated with Castleman disease, the T lymphoblasts are located in the interfollicular regions. When associated with carcinoma, the T lymphoblasts are interspersed or clustered between malignant epithelial cells {3008,3523, 3012}.

Immunophenotype

The immunophenotype of iT-LBP is consistent with that of immature thymocytes expressing CD3 and TdT. Most cases are double-positive for CD4/CD8; however, a double-negative phenotype can be seen {1239}. Other T-cell markers (including CD2, CD5, and CD7) are positive, but their expression level may be decreased. CD10, CD99, and CD1a are variably expressed. CD34 is frequently negative. B-cell markers are not expressed. LMO2 is negative in iT-LBP but positive in most cases of T-lymphoblastic leukaemia {445}. The Ki-67 index is high, ranging from 40% to 90%. CD33 is rarely positive {3010}. Cytokeratin is negative, unlike in ectopic thymic epithelial cells.

Differential diagnosis

In contrast to iT-LBP, T-lymphoblastic leukaemia exhibits cellular atypia, frequently shows aberrant antigen expression (CD34, CD33, CD79a) and/or loss of the usual T-cell markers, exhibits clonal TR gene rearrangement, and progresses rapidly (often with bone marrow involvement).

Cytology

Not applicable

Diagnostic molecular pathology

Molecular testing for TR gene rearrangements shows a polyclonal population.

Essential and desirable diagnostic criteria

Essential: clinically indolent disease; no evidence of disease related to precursor T-cell neoplasia; confluent groups of TdT-positive T cells without atypia or tissue destruction; immunophenotype of developmentally normal precursor thymocytes, most often (but not always) of the cortical type (CD4+/CD8+); absence of clonal TR gene rearrangements

Desirable: absence of bone marrow involvement.

Staging

Not applicable

Prognosis and prediction

iT-LBP is an indolent process that does not require specific treatment. It must be distinguished from T-lymphoblastic leukaemia to avoid unnecessary aggressive therapy.

T-lymphoblastic leukaemia/lymphoma NOS

Czader M
Chandy M
Choi JK
Leventaki V
Lin P
Miles RR
Molina TJ
Saha V
Tembhare PR

Definition

T-lymphoblastic leukaemia/lymphoma (T-ALL/LBL) NOS is a neoplasm of haematopoietic progenitors committed to T-lineage differentiation.

ICD-O coding

9837/3 T-lymphoblastic leukaemia/lymphoma, NOS

ICD-11 coding

2A71 & XH50W7 Precursor T-lymphoblastic neoplasms & Precursor T-cell lymphoblastic neoplasms

Related terminology

Acceptable: precursor T-lymphoblastic leukaemia/lymphoma; T-cell acute lymphoblastic leukaemia.

Subtype(s)

None

Localization

By convention, the term "T-lymphoblastic leukaemia" (T-ALL) is used when the peripheral blood and bone marrow are the primary sites of involvement, and the term "T-lymphoblastic lymphoma" (T-LBL) is used when the primary sites of involvement are lymph node, mediastinum (thymus), or other extranodal sites including the skin, tonsils, liver, spleen, CNS, and testes. Presentation at these extramedullary sites without nodal or mediastinal involvement is uncommon {2370}. Unlike in B-lymphoblastic leukaemia (B-ALL), aleukaemic presentations in the setting of significant bone marrow involvement are uncommon. The distinction between T-ALL and T-LBL becomes arbitrary when both marrow and non-marrow sites are involved, although many treatment protocols use > 25% marrow blasts to define leukaemia. Unlike for myeloid neoplasms, however, a defined number of blasts in the blood or marrow is not required for the diagnosis of T-ALL/LBL, although in practice, the diagnosis should be made with care when blasts are < 20%, because there is no convincing evidence to suggest that outcome is adversely affected by deferring therapy until blasts reach 20%.

Clinical features

T-ALL typically manifests with a high leukocyte count, and often with a concurrent large mediastinal or other tissue mass. Lymphadenopathy and hepatosplenomegaly are common. For a given leukocyte count and tumour burden, T-ALL often shows relative sparing of normal bone marrow haematopoiesis compared with B-ALL. T-LBL frequently presents with a mass in the anterior mediastinum, often exhibiting rapid growth and sometimes presenting as a respiratory emergency. Pleural and/or pericardial effusions are reported {2300}.

Epidemiology

T-ALL accounts for about 15% of childhood cases of acute lymphoblastic leukaemia (ALL); it is more common in adolescents than in younger children, and it has a male predilection. T-ALL accounts for approximately 25% of cases of adult ALL. T-LBL accounts for approximately 85–90% of all lymphoblastic lymphomas; like its leukaemic counterpart, it is most frequent in adolescent boys, but it can occur in any age group {2370, 3344,1455}.

Etiology

Unknown

Pathogenesis

The pathogenesis of T-ALL/LBL involves the multistep accumulation of genetic/epigenetic alterations in oncogenic and tumour suppressor pathways, as well as ribosomal dysfunction and deregulated expression of oncogenic microRNAs or long ncRNAs related to T-cell development. These alterations affect genes responsible for cell growth, survival, and differentiation. The most common are mutations affecting the NOTCH pathway, translocations of transcription factors to chromosomal regions of TR loci, and mutations in epigenetic regulators (*EZH2*, *SUZ12*, and *EED*) and chromatin modifiers (*PHF6*, *KDM6A*, and *USP7*). Other genetic abnormalities include alterations of genes involved in the JAK/STAT (*IL7R*, *JAK1*, *JAK3*, and *STAT5B*), PI3K/AKT (*PIK3CA* and *PTEN*), and RAS/MAPK (*HRAS*, *KRAS*, and *PTPN11*) signalling pathways, as well as deletions in cell-cycle regulatory genes (*CDKN2A*, *CDKN2B*, *CDKN1B*, *RB1*, *CCND2*, *CCND3*, *CTCF*, and *MYB*) {1143,1469,2821,3954,810}.

One study described T-ALL cases in a pair of monozygotic twins that shared the same TR gene rearrangement {1219}, suggesting an in utero origin of the earliest genetic lesions.

Macroscopic appearance

Not relevant

Histopathology

Microscopy

The lymphoblasts in T-ALL/LBL are morphologically indistinguishable from those of B-ALL/LBL. On smears or touch preparations, the blasts have scant basophilic agranular or (rarely) vacuolated cytoplasm and round to irregular or convoluted nuclei. They range from blasts that are small or medium in size and have a high N:C ratio, condensed chromatin, and no evident nucleoli, to larger blasts with finely dispersed chromatin and relatively prominent nucleoli. Occasionally, the blasts in T-ALL may resemble more mature lymphocytes, and immunophenotypic studies are then required to distinguish this disease from a mature (peripheral) T-cell leukaemia/lymphoma {1301,4511}.

In bone marrow trephine sections, the blasts infiltrate between and displace normal marrow elements, and they have high N:C ratios, thin nuclear membranes, finely stippled chromatin, and inconspicuous nucleoli. The lymph node generally shows complete effacement of the architecture and involvement of the capsule, although partial involvement of the paracortex with sparing of germinal centres may be seen. A starry-sky pattern mimicking Burkitt lymphoma may be present, although the nucleoli and cytoplasm are typically less prominent in T-LBL {2574}. In the thymus, there is extensive disruption and replacement of the thymic epithelial cell network, with loss of the cortical/medullary architecture and permeative infiltration of the surrounding adipose tissue.

Cytological smears from fine-needle aspirates or effusions are hypercellular with a monotonous population of individually scattered immature lymphoid cells whose cytomorphology is similar to that described above. Cytoplasmic pseudopods (hand-mirror cells) can be observed in some cases. Lymphoglandular bodies, apoptosis, frequent mitoses, and tingible-body macrophages are often observed {4274}.

Cytochemical stains are still often performed for the subtyping of acute leukaemia, particularly in resource-limited settings, but immunophenotyping is required for definitive lineage assignment. Lymphoblasts are invariably negative for myeloperoxidase but may stain light grey and weakly with Sudan Black B when granules are present. Nonspecific esterase may show multifocal punctate or Golgi staining that is variably inhibited by sodium fluoride. PAS shows coarse, chunky cytoplasmic staining in some cases.

Immunophenotype

Lymphoblasts in T-ALL/LBL express the T lineage–associated antigens cCD3, CD7, and CD5 in 84–97% of cases {3157}. Of these, cCD3 is the most lineage-specific and defines T-lineage differentiation, as does sCD3, which is expressed less frequently and usually at a lower level than in mature T cells. CD7 expression is often uniform and higher than in mature T cells, but it may be lower or (very rarely) even absent. CD5 expression is usually lower than in mature T cells and may be very low or absent. CD2 is expressed in a majority of cases.

Patterns of antigen expression associated with T-cell immaturity are commonly present and imperfectly recapitulate stages of early T-cell maturation. This includes CD45 expression, which is invariably lower than in mature lymphocytes, although not as low as it commonly is in B-ALL/LBL. The progenitor nature of T lymphoblasts is demonstrated by the expression of CD1a, CD34 (in one third of cases), KIT (CD117), and/or CD99, in addition to TdT, which is present in most cases {3985,3157,3430, 4511}. T-ALL/LBL has previously been stratified into four immunophenotypic subtypes corresponding to the stages of normal intrathymic T-cell differentiation {309}: (1) pro-T/T-I, (2) pre-T/T-II, (3) cortical T / T-III, and (4) medullary T / T-IV. Many cases

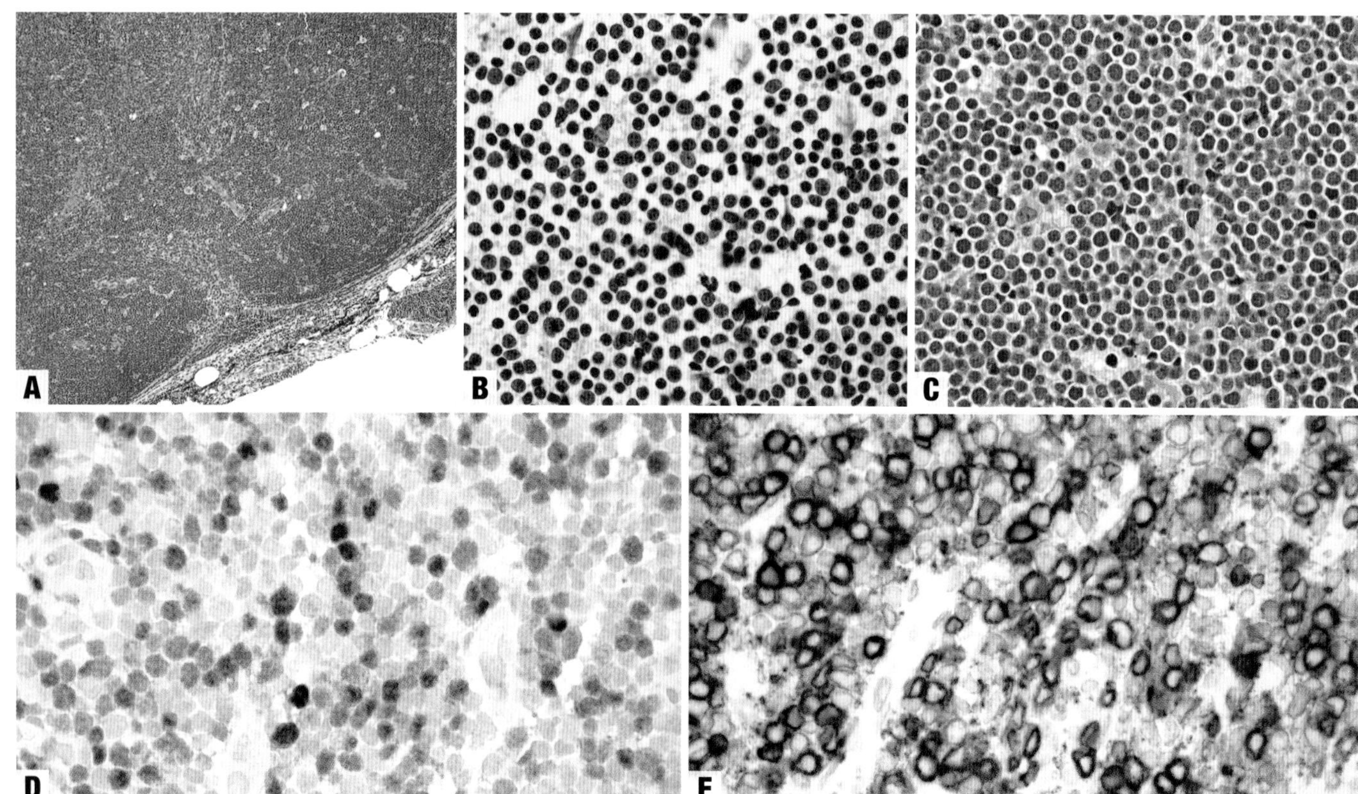

Fig. 5.14 T-lymphoblastic leukaemia: lymph node biopsy. **A** The lymph node architecture is effaced by diffuse sheets of mononuclear cells that extend into perinodal soft tissue. More limited lymph node involvement by acute lymphoblastic leukaemia may show infiltration confined to the subcapsular sinus with inconspicuous spread into the underlying lymph node. **B** Touch imprint at triage of the fresh lymph node highlights the monotonous morphology and fine chromatin of the lymphoblasts. **C** The neoplastic cells are small to intermediate-sized lymphoid cells with finely stippled nuclear chromatin, scant cytoplasm, and conspicuous associated mitoses. **D** Immunohistochemistry shows that the neoplastic cells express TdT (nuclear localization). **E** Immunohistochemistry shows neoplastic cells expressing CD3 (cytoplasmic localization, weak expression) among non-neoplastic T cells expressing both cytoplasmic and membranous CD3 (strong expression).

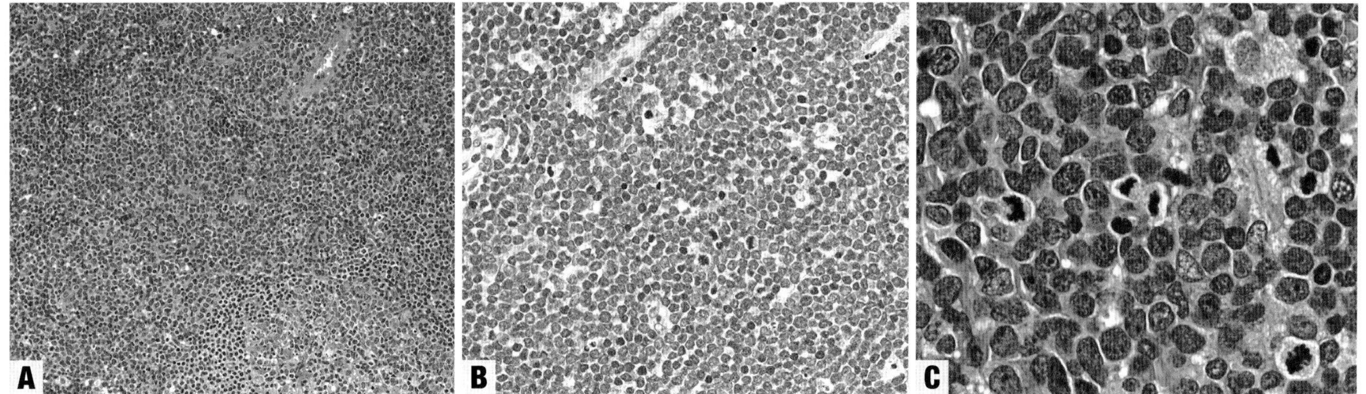

Fig. 5.15 T-lymphoblastic leukaemia/lymphoma: mediastinal biopsy. **A** This biopsy shows a diffuse infiltrate of atypical lymphoid cells. **B** Giemsa illustrates medium-sized cells with scant cytoplasm and round to irregular nuclear contours. **C** Medium-sized atypical lymphoid cells display irregular nuclear contours, small nucleoli, and finely dispersed chromatin. Note the presence of several mitotic figures.

previously classified as pro-T or pre-T now meet the criteria for early T-precursor ALL (ETP-ALL) and should be classified as such (see next section). CD4 and CD8 are frequently coexpressed (~46% of T-ALL/LBL cases), often with CD1a, and CD10 may be positive in as many as 40% of cases {3985,3157}.

Components of these immunophenotypes are not entirely specific for T-ALL, as coexpression of CD4 and CD8 can also be seen in T-prolymphocytic leukaemia and CD10 positivity can be seen in peripheral T-cell lymphomas, most commonly in nodal T follicular helper (TFH) cell lymphoma. In 29–48% of cases there is nuclear staining for TAL1, but this does not necessarily correlate with the presence of *TAL1* gene alteration {691,921}. LMO2 is expressed in the majority of cases, in contrast to non-neoplastic thymocytes, which are LMO2-negative. CD56 is expressed in a subset of cases and does not by itself suggest NK-cell differentiation {3985,1247}.

Heterogeneous, usually dim, expression of CD79a is observed in at least 10% of cases, and CD19 expression can be seen occasionally {3245,3985,3157}, hence neither of these define B-lineage differentiation in isolation. Expression of one or more of the myeloid-associated antigens (e.g. CD13 or CD33) is seen in 19–32% of cases {1966,4113,3157}, and KIT (CD117) expression is seen in a subset of cases and may be associated with activating mutations of *FLT3* {3100}, so their expression alone does not suggest myeloid lineage differentiation. HLA-DR is negative in the majority of cases.

Differential diagnosis

The main differential diagnoses for T-ALL/LBL include thymoma and other subtypes of acute leukaemia, including their extramedullary presentations.

In lymphocyte-rich thymoma, larger epithelial cells with low mitotic activity and more vesicular chromatin are present. In particular, immunohistochemical staining highlights the keratin-positive epithelial cells in an interlocking pattern reminiscent of normal thymic architecture, something absent in T-LBL. When analysed by flow cytometry, lymphoid cells demonstrate normal thymocyte maturational patterns, albeit often skewed towards the common thymocyte maturation stage, which along with polyclonal TR gene rearrangements can be helpful in diagnosis {2309}. Thymic hyperplasia and ectopic thymus are rare but can be distinguished from T-ALL/LBL using similar criteria.

The distinction of T-ALL/LBL from other subtypes of acute leukaemia is greatly facilitated by flow cytometry. ETP-ALL is a distinct entity of T-ALL/LBL with a primitive immunophenotype defined by the expression of one or more of the myeloid / stem cell markers (e.g. CD13, CD33, CD34, KIT [CD117], or HLA-DR), an absence of CD1a and CD8, and decreased to absent CD5. T-ALL/LBL is distinguished from T/myeloid mixed-phenotype acute leukaemia by an absence of cytoplasmic myeloperoxidase and a lack of monocytic differentiation. Acute undifferentiated leukaemia differs from T-ALL by a lack of cCD3 expression, but it must be borne in mind that a subset of T-ALL/LBL cases, mostly of the ETP-ALL type, show dim cCD3.

Cases of T-LBL with a significant eosinophilic component or associated myeloproliferative features may represent one of the entities/types within the family of myeloid/lymphoid neoplasms with eosinophilia and tyrosine kinase gene fusions (see the dedicated sections) {17,1723,3290}. Molecular testing is required to establish the diagnosis.

A subset of T-ALL/LBL cases show sCD3 expression, and the distinction from a mature T-cell lymphoma or leukaemia such as T-prolymphocytic leukaemia or angioimmunoblastic T-cell lymphoma is based on a combination of morphology, immunophenotypic profile, and molecular genetics. Mature T-cell lymphoma/leukaemia lacks immature antigens (e.g. CD34, TdT, or CD1a) and typically shows dimmer CD7 expression than the bright CD7 seen in T-ALL/LBL. Detection of *NOTCH1* mutation favours T-ALL/LBL, whereas TCL1 expression or rearrangement supports T-prolymphocytic leukaemia.

NK-lymphoblastic lymphoma/leukaemia is rare and problematic to define. Normal NK cells lack sCD3 by definition and commonly express CD2 and CD7, and immature subsets can express CD5 and cCD3 (ζ and ε chains) {2783}, an immunophenotype that overlaps with that of T-ALL/LBL. CD56 expression, although characteristic of NK cells, is also present in a subset of T-ALL/LBL cases with features resembling ETP-ALL {3985, 1247}. The absence of clonal TR gene rearrangement is seen in both NK cells and in a subset of T-ALL/LBL cases, particularly of the early T-precursor type. Other NK cell–associated antigens such as CD94 and CD161 are not sufficiently well studied to use for this purpose. Consequently, it is unclear at present if NK-lymphoblastic lymphoma/leukaemia exists or how it could

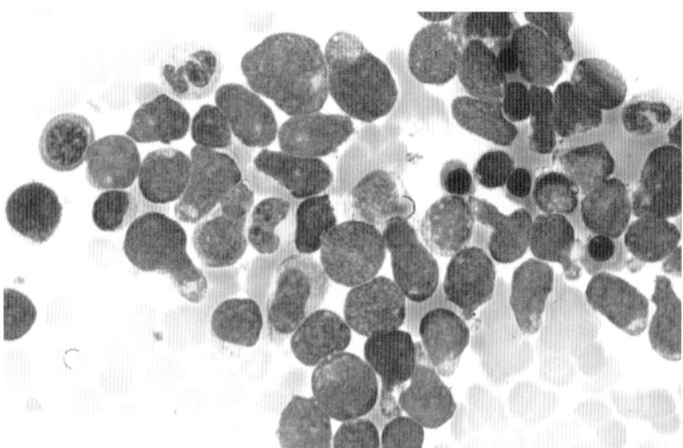

Fig. 5.16 Histopathology of T-lymphoblastic leukaemia at diagnosis. Bone marrow aspirate smear (Wright–Giemsa staining). The lymphoblasts may vary slightly in size, particularly on air-dried smears. The morphology of T-lymphoblastic leukaemia is indistinguishable from that of B-lymphoblastic leukaemia. Both may show eccentric orientation of scant cytoplasm (hand-mirror cells).

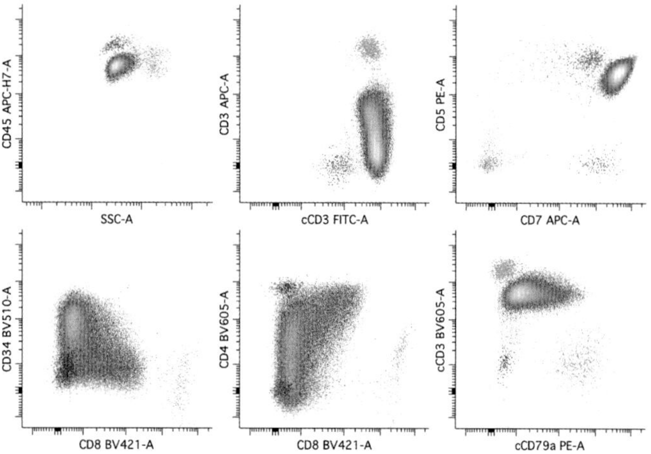

Fig. 5.17 T-lymphoblastic leukaemia/lymphoma NOS. Flow cytometry of T-lymphoblastic leukaemia/lymphoma at diagnosis. Leukaemic blasts (red) show an immature T-lineage immunophenotype with expression of cCD3, dim to absent sCD3, and variable CD34. Compared with normal mature T cells (green and magenta), the leukaemia shows abnormal expression of increased CD7, decreased CD5, decreased CD45, and variable CD4 and CD8 in a pattern reminiscent of that of thymic T cells. The immunophenotype also differs from that of NK cells (dark blue) and B cells (cyan). Note the presence of variable cCD79a, a relatively common finding in T-lymphoblastic leukaemia/lymphoma and not indicative of B lineage.

be distinguished from T-ALL/LBL, particularly of the early T-precursor type.

Indolent T-lymphoblastic proliferations are benign polyclonal proliferations of T lymphoblasts in extrathymic sites, primarily in lymph nodes {3008}. The majority of cases represent focal aggregates of T lymphoblasts without effacement of nodal architecture. Extensive nodal involvement has been reported, however. Such cases may be challenging to differentiate from T-LBL, especially on core needle biopsies. Flow cytometric immunophenotyping of indolent T-lymphoblastic proliferations demonstrates a variety of normal T-cell maturation stages, which together with polyclonal TR gene rearrangements and a lack of LMO2 expression by immunohistochemistry help to differentiate it from T-ALL/LBL {1239,445}.

Cytology

See above.

Diagnostic molecular pathology

Antigen receptor genes

T-ALL/LBL shows clonal rearrangements of the genes TRB and/or TRG in > 90% of cases, and there are simultaneous IGH gene rearrangements in approximately 20% of cases {3244,3915}. The subset of cases lacking an identifiable clonal TR gene rearrangement are largely immunophenotypically primitive, corresponding to ETP-ALL. Of note, TR gene rearrangements can also be found in B-ALL and acute myeloid leukaemia (AML), so they are not reliable for lineage assignment in acute leukaemia. Clonal TR-rearranged sequences may be used to monitor residual disease after therapy {4421,475}.

Cytogenetic abnormalities and oncogenes

An abnormal karyotype is found in 50–70% of cases {1398, 1484}. The most common recurrent cytogenetic abnormalities are rearrangements of TRA and TRD at 14q11.2, TRB at 7q34, and TRG at 7p14.1, with a variety of partner genes. In most cases, these translocations lead to the transcriptional dysregulation of the partner gene by juxtaposition with the regulatory region of one of the TR loci. The most commonly involved genes include the T-lineage transcription factor genes *TLX1*, *TLX3*, *TAL1*, *TAL2*, *LMO1*, *LMO2*, *LYL1*, *NKX2-1*, *NKX2-2*, *NKX2-5*, *OLIG2*, and HOXA family genes {917,1398,1718,1704,2383}. Other transcription factor genes that may be involved in translocations include *MYC* and *MYB*, and the cytoplasmic tyrosine kinase gene *LCK*.

In many cases, translocations are not detected by karyotyping but only by molecular genetic studies. For example, the*TAL1* locus is deregulated in about 20–30% of cases of T-ALL, but a t(1;14)(p33;q11.2) translocation can be detected by karyotyping in only about 3% of cases. More often, cryptic insertion or deletion events upstream of *TAL1* lead to deregulation {467,1544, 1784,1718}. Other important rearrangements in T-ALL involve *MLLT10*, *KMT2A*, *ABL1*, and *NUP98* {1398,2630,2383}.

It has been proposed that T-ALL be divided into four distinct, non-overlapping genetic subgroups on the basis of specific translocations that lead to the aberrant expression of (1) TAL or LMO genes, (2) *TLX1*, (3) *TLX3*, and (4) HOXA genes, resulting in the arrest of T-cell maturation at distinct stages of thymocyte development {2630,4173}. The *TLX1* subgroup appears to have a relatively favourable prognosis {1170}. Another group, characterized by the overexpression of *LYL1*, may correspond more closely to ETP-ALL {2630}. More recently, eight subgroups of T-ALL were proposed, based on genetic alterations and gene expression: *TAL1*, *TAL2*, *TLX1*, *TLX3*, HOXA genes, *LMO1*/*LMO2*, *LMO2*/*LYL1*, and *NKX2-1* {2383}. In that study, the ETP-ALL cases commonly fitted in the *LMO2*/*LYL1* group.

Deletions also occur in T-ALL. The most important is del(9p) with loss of the tumour suppressor gene *CDKN2A*, which is detected at a frequency of about 30% by classic karyotyping, and at a higher frequency by molecular testing, and results in cell-cycle deregulation at the G1 checkpoint. Other tumour suppressors deleted or inactivated in T-ALL include BCL11B, LEF1, WT1, neurofibromin (NF1), ETV6, RUNX1, and GATA3, but the last three are associated with the ETP-ALL phenotype {305}.

Signalling pathway deregulation in T-ALL occurs in the NOTCH, PI3K/AKT, JAK/STAT, RAS/MAPK, and ABL kinase pathways {1718,1465}. More than 75% of cases show NOTCH1 pathway activation, which can be caused by activating mutations involving the extracellular heterodimerization domain and/or the C-terminal PEST domain of *NOTCH1* (50% of cases) and/or by loss-of-function mutations in *FBXW7*, a negative regulator of *NOTCH1* (30% of cases) {4353,2510,1718,1704,2383,3068}. The direct downstream target of *NOTCH1* appears to be *MYC*, which contributes to the growth of the neoplastic cells {4354}.

Epigenetic dysregulation occurs via mutations in *PHF6*, *SUZ12*, *EZH2*, *TET2*, *H3-3A* (*H3F3A*), *KDM6A*, *EED*, *SETD2*, and *DNMT3A* {1704,305}.

Although most studies have focused on T-ALL, T-LBL cases show overall similar genetic findings and pathway dysregulation {1970}.

NOTCH1 and/or *FBXW7* mutations have been associated with better clinical outcomes, whereas loss of heterozygosity at 6q, *PTEN* mutations, and *KMT2D* mutations have been associated with worse outcomes {1970}.

Essential and desirable diagnostic criteria

Essential: the presence of haematopoietic progenitors of T lineage (defined largely by the expression of surface and/or cytoplasmic CD3) that have an aberrant immunophenotype; the diagnostic criteria for ETP-ALL are not met.

Desirable: the percentage of abnormal T progenitors or blasts exceeds 20% in the peripheral blood or bone marrow, or an extramedullary site is involved; however, unlike in myeloid neoplasms, a defined number of blasts in the blood or marrow is not required for the diagnosis of T-ALL/LBL – in practice, the diagnosis should be made with caution when blasts are < 20%, because there is no convincing evidence to suggest outcome is adversely affected by deferring therapy until blasts reach 20%.

Staging

None

Prognosis and prediction

Long-term response rates approach 85% in children and adolescents, and 60% in adults {1023,2791,3163,502}. Age, genetics, presenting white blood cell count, and measurable residual disease at the end of induction are less prognostic than in B-ALL. The most significant predictor of outcome is measurable residual disease at the end of consolidation {4375,3643}. Along with multiagent chemotherapy, dexamethasone {3163, 2791}, nelarabine {1023}, and escalating intravenous methotrexate with asparaginase {1023} are associated with improved outcomes. Prophylactic CNS radiotherapy does not appear to be required. Outcomes of relapsed T-ALL remain poor, at least partially because of limited therapeutic options {1041}. In adult protocols, T-ALL is treated similarly to other types of ALL. The prognosis of T-ALL may be better than that of B-ALL in adults, although this may reflect the lower incidence of adverse cytogenetic abnormalities. The prognosis of T-LBL, like that of other lymphomas, depends on patient age, disease stage, and LDH levels {2780}.

Early T-precursor lymphoblastic leukaemia/lymphoma

Czader M
Chandy M
Choi JK
Jain N
Lin P
Miles RR
Molina TJ
Saha V
Tembhare PR

Definition

Early T-precursor lymphoblastic leukaemia/lymphoma (ETP-ALL) is a neoplasm composed of blasts committed to the T-cell lineage with a unique immunophenotype that includes the expression of stem cell markers and/or myeloid lineage markers.

ICD-O coding

9837/3 Early T-precursor lymphoblastic leukaemia/lymphoma

ICD-11 coding

2A71 & XH8F29 Precursor T-lymphoblastic neoplasms & Early T-cell precursor acute lymphoblastic leukaemia

Related terminology

None

Subtype(s)

None

Localization

Patients typically present with bone marrow and peripheral blood involvement. Some patients may present with lymphoblastic lymphoma {4454,1773,3157}. Lymph node and hepatosplenic involvement is common. Mediastinal involvement is detected in 10–40% of patients {1773,2935,4571,1315}. CNS involvement is reported in as many as 18% of patients {1773, 2935,1315}.

Clinical features

Symptoms and signs at presentation are related to cytopenias or manifestations of extramedullary disease. The white blood cell count may or may not be elevated, and in some studies, patients with ETP-ALL tend to have a lower white blood cell count than those with non-ETP ALL {502}.

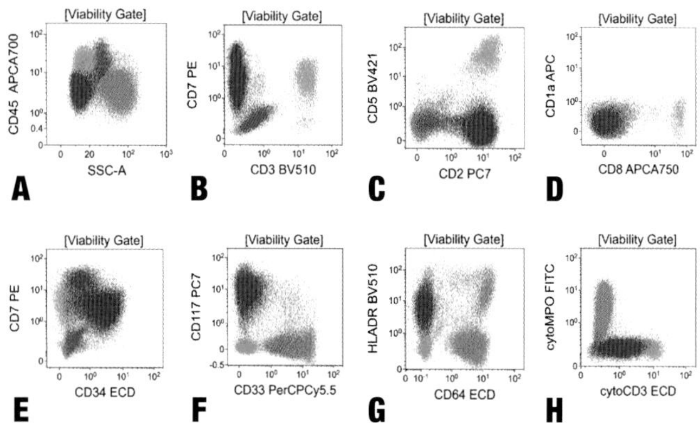

Fig. 5.18 Early T-cell precursor lymphoblastic leukaemia: flow cytometry scattergrams. Blasts (red) show low side scatter and dim CD45 (**A**), bright to dim CD7 and negative sCD3 (**B**), positive CD2 and negative CD5 (**C**), negative CD1a and CD8 (**D**), partial CD34 (**E**), moderate KIT (CD117) and negative CD33 (**F**), moderate HLA-DR with negative CD64 (**G**), and moderate to dim cCD3 and negative cytoplasmic myeloperoxidase (**H**) expression.

Epidemiology

ETP-ALL represents 12–17% of paediatric T-lymphoblastic leukaemia (T-ALL) cases {794,826,1136} and 22–40% of adult cases {400,2935,1976}. In the adult population, patients with ETP-ALL tend to be older than those with non-ETP ALL {1976, 2935,3014}.

Etiology

The etiology is unknown in most cases. Genome-wide association studies previously demonstrated several susceptibility loci for T-ALL. In a recent study, germline *RUNX1* variants were enriched in ETP-ALL; and in a mouse model, *RUNX1* variants cooperated with mutated *JAK3* to induce ETP-ALL {2327}.

Pathogenesis

ETP-ALL was initially recognized as a distinct type of T-ALL on the basis of a gene expression signature that overlaps with that of normal early T-precursors {826}. Physiologically, these precursors are the earliest recognizable stage in T-cell ontogeny and represent recent immigrants from the bone marrow to the thymus. They are characterized by multilineage differentiation potential and the expression of lymphoid, myeloid, and stem cell markers {298,4261}. In an analogous manner, ETP-ALL is characterized by a specific transcriptional signature close to that of haematopoietic stem cells and myeloid progenitors {4557}. Single-cell RNA sequencing also showed that leukaemic cells express plasticity, with both stem cell and T-cell signatures, and can differentiate to stimulate an immunosuppressive microenvironment through the expression of the checkpoint molecule LGALS9 and the support of dysfunctional CD8+ T cells {110}. The expression profile of ETP-ALL is characterized by increased expression of MEF2C {1622} and decreased expression of BCL11B {942,1133} and GATA3 {1639,2934}.

A recent murine molecular pathogenesis model postulates concurrent *EZH2* and *RUNX1* inactivating mutations as initiating events leading to the expansion of early thymic progenitors with an ETP-ALL gene expression signature whose leukaemic potential is further promoted by the acquisition of mutations (e.g. *FLT3*), resulting in the constitutive activation of the RAS signalling pathway {413}. This model recapitulates the distinctive mutation profile of ETP-ALL, which resembles that of myeloid neoplasms and is characterized by activating mutations in genes regulating cytokine receptor and RAS signalling (*FLT3*, *NRAS*, *KRAS*, *IL7R*, *JAK3*, *JAK1*, *SH2B3*, *BRAF*), haematopoietic development (*GATA3*, *ETV6*, *RUNX1*, *IKZF1*), and histone modifications (*EZH2*, *EED*, *SUZ12*, *SETD2*, *EP300*) {4557,2936, 2934}. *NOTCH1* mutations are uncommon in ETP-ALL, in contrast to other types of T-ALL {2934}.

The frequency of *CDKN2A/CDKN2B* deletion is low in patients with ETP-ALL {1315,4290,4454}.

The majority of ETP-ALL cases do not have TRG gene rearrangements, and they frequently lack biallelic deletion of the TRG locus, in contrast to non-ETP ALL, supporting an early maturation stage {2934,4599,1315}.

Macroscopic appearance

Not relevant

Histopathology

In smears, lymphoblasts are small to medium in size and have round to convoluted nuclei, finely dispersed chromatin, small or absent nucleoli, and mildly to moderately basophilic cytoplasm {826}.

Histological sections show sheets of lymphoblasts with high N:C ratios, finely stippled chromatin, and inconspicuous nucleoli.

Immunophenotype

The ETP-ALL immunophenotype is defined as follows: (1) expression of cCD3, (2) absent CD1a and CD8 expression (< 5% positive blasts); (3) absent or dim CD5 expression (< 75% positive blasts); and (4) expression of one or more myeloid (CD11b, CD13, CD33, CD65, KIT [CD117]) and/or stem cell (CD34, HLA-DR) markers (≥ 25% positive blasts) {826, 1773} (see Box 5.04). The expression of CD123 has also been reported {125}. The ETP-ALL immunophenotype may be established by immunohistochemistry.

A proportion of ETP-ALL cases show heterogeneous expression of cCD3, with a subset of blasts being negative {3985}. sCD3 is usually absent {1976,826}. CD7 is consistently positive, a feature that, when combined with the expression of stem cell or myeloid markers, provides a distinct phenotype for measurable residual disease evaluation by flow cytometry.

It has been suggested that defining ETP-ALL by immunophenotyping may lead to an underestimation of the number of cases of true ETP-ALL, relative to gene expression profiling {4599, 1457}. This may be due in part to the challenges of using a percentage threshold for CD5 expression. Proposed alternative approaches include using the absence of expression of CD4 instead of CD5, which in some studies allowed for a closer correlation between immunophenotype-based and gene expression profile–based designations {4599,1315}. Other approaches incorporating scoring systems have also been proposed {1976, 1729}. T-ALL cases with an immunophenotype similar to that of ETP-ALL but with CD5 expression (in ≥ 75% of blasts) have been designated as near–ETP-ALL, but at present the clinical implications of such a designation remain unclear {2794,1773}.

An initial diagnosis of ETP-ALL should not be based on flow cytometry on a peripheral blood sample, because of the potential immunophenotypic overlap with T/myeloid mixed-phenotype acute leukaemia (MPAL) and occasional immunophenotypic discordance between the circulating and medullary components of some acute leukaemia types {682}.

Differential diagnosis

Exclusion of MPAL as defined in this volume of the WHO classification requires particular attention, given the close biological relationship of ETP-ALL to T/myeloid MPAL. The initial definition of ETP-ALL incorporated a conservative threshold of < 3% to define negative myeloperoxidase expression by cytochemistry and flow cytometry {826}. This threshold may not be optimal for defining myeloperoxidase positivity for MPAL diagnosis, and further studies are needed to define the boundary between these neoplasms. Until further data are available, the original threshold of < 3% to define negative myeloperoxidase in ETP-ALL is retained.

Box 5.04 Immunophenotype of early T-precursor lymphoblastic leukaemia/lymphoma (ETP-ALL) {826}

ETP-ALL

Must meet all five criteria for antigen expression:

1. CD3 (cytoplasmic+; surface−)[a]
2. Absent myeloperoxidase (< 10% by flow cytometry, < 3% by cytochemistry)
3. Absent CD1a and CD8
4. ≥ 25% of blasts with at least one of the following stem cell or myeloid markers: CD34, KIT (CD117), CD13, CD33, CD65, CD11b, HLA-DR
5. Dim to negative CD5 (< 75% of blasts positive)[b]

Near–ETP-ALL

Criteria 1–4 met but ≥ 75% blasts are CD5+

[a]Expression of sCD3 is rare. [b]Dim CD5 can be also defined as mean fluorescence intensity (MFI) that is at least 1 log less than that of normal T cells; with this approach, the MFI of T cells should be at least 2 log greater than that of the negative control.

Cytology

See above.

Diagnostic molecular pathology

Not relevant for diagnostic evaluation

Essential and desirable diagnostic criteria

Essential: lymphoblastic leukaemia/lymphoma features by morphology; blasts must express an early T-precursor immunophenotype, characterized by the following (see Box 5.04): positive for cCD3, absent CD1a and CD8 expression (< 5% positive blasts), absent or dim CD5 expression (< 75% positive blasts), expression of one or more myeloid (CD11b, CD13, CD33, CD65, KIT [CD117]) and/or stem cell (CD34, HLA-DR) markers (≥ 25% positive blasts), and negative myeloperoxidase (< 3%).

Staging

Not relevant

Prognosis and prediction

Clinical outcomes for children with ETP-ALL were initially reported to be poor when compared with non-ETP ALL, and similar outcomes were observed in adults {826,1729,2454,1773, 1315,502}. In subsequent years, several studies showed that long-term outcomes of paediatric and adult patients with ETP-ALL were comparable to those of patients with other T-ALLs {3163,794,1453,400,1247,1794,1023}. Such favourable outcomes were reported despite higher rates of measurable residual disease after induction among patients with ETP-ALL. This could be due to treatment intensification for ETP-ALL patients with measurable residual disease and the increased rate of allogeneic stem cell transplantation after the first remission.

Because BCL2 is overexpressed in ETP-ALL, ongoing clinical trials are exploring BCL2 inhibition as a potential targeted therapy {734,3314}.

Mature T-cell and NK-cell leukaemias: Introduction

Lim MS
Dave SS
Lazar AJ
Pulitzer M
Willemze R
Wood BL

The category of mature T-cell and NK-cell leukaemias includes six entities representative of T- and NK-cell proliferations that primarily present as leukaemic disease. They are T-prolymphocytic leukaemia, T-large granular lymphocytic leukaemia (T-LGLL), NK-large granular lymphocytic leukaemia (NK-LGLL), adult T-cell leukaemia/lymphoma, Sézary syndrome, and aggressive NK-cell leukaemia. The respective sections provide updates on these diseases, especially on our enhanced molecular understanding of them. These updates are now incorporated into the essential or desirable diagnostic criteria and will have an impact on clinical practice.

Rare cases of mature T-cell leukaemias that meet the clinical and immunophenotypic criteria for T-prolymphocytic leukaemia (T-PLL) but do not exhibit defining genetic features such as juxtaposition of *TCL1A* or *MTCP1* to T-cell receptor loci are being recognized and referred to as "TCL1 family–negative T-PLL" by some investigators {1458,1936}. The relationship of TCL1 family–negative T-PLL to T-PLL is currently not clear, and in the present classification such cases should be classified as peripheral T-cell lymphoma NOS (with leukaemic involvement) after exclusion of other specific leukaemic T-cell entities.

Emerging evidence indicates that genetic mutations in T-LGLL and NK-LGLL have clinical and phenotypic significance. *STAT3* mutations are enriched in CD8+ T-LGLL and are associated with CD16 expression {3991,3714}, neutropenia, and poorer overall survival {3568,242,3320}. In contrast, recurrent *STAT5B* mutations are present in approximately 30% of CD4+ T-LGLL cases and are rare in CD8+ T-LGLL and gamma-delta T-LGLL, but they confer an aggressive disease course only in CD8+ T-LGLL.

Genetic analyses of adult T-cell leukaemia/lymphoma have revealed novel events that highlight the importance of immune evasion, including *CTLA4*::*CD28* and *ICOS*::*CD28* fusions, *REL* C-terminal truncations {1910,2081}, recurrent alterations in *HLA-A* and *HLA-B*, and structural variations disrupting the 3′ untranslated region of *CD274* (*PDL1*) {1912}. Furthermore, the frequency and pattern of somatic alterations are correlated with clinical behaviour. Specifically, aggressive subtypes show more genetic alterations, whereas *STAT3* mutations are more common in indolent subtypes. Prognostic subtypes of adult T-cell leukaemia/lymphoma {1908} have been better characterized and are now implemented in the current edition.

Notable changes have been made in the terminology associated with NK-cell proliferations. Chronic lymphoproliferative disorder of NK cells has been renamed NK-LGLL. Recent studies show that NK-LGLLs are clonal or oligoclonal expansions, providing a rationale for renaming and recognition as the NK-cell counterpart of T-LGLLs. Genome-wide sequencing studies provide novel insights into the pathogenetic events in aggressive NK-cell leukaemia and implicate the role of genetic alterations of the JAK/STAT and RAS/MAPK pathways, histone modifiers (*TET2*, *CREBBP*, KMT2 [*MLL2*], *DDX3X*), and immune checkpoint molecules PDL1/PDL2 {3966,1016,1665,1056} in their pathogenesis.

Although Sézary syndrome is closely related to mycosis fungoides at the clinical and biological level, it is included in these sections on mature T-cell and NK-cell leukaemias to highlight its primary site of clinical presentation and the importance of its inclusion in the diagnostic workup of mature T-cell leukaemias. Comprehensive analyses of genomic signatures {1821} highlight the contribution of cellular ageing and ultraviolet (UV) radiation exposure in Sézary syndrome.

T-prolymphocytic leukaemia

Elenitoba-Johnson KSJ
Chen X
Herling M

Definition

T-prolymphocytic leukaemia (T-PLL) is a clonal proliferation of small to medium-sized prolymphocytes with a mature post-thymic T-cell phenotype characterized by the juxtaposition of *TCL1A* or *MTCP1* to a TR locus, most often the TRA/TRD locus.

ICD-O coding

9834/3 T-prolymphocytic leukaemia

ICD-11 coding

2A90.0 T-cell prolymphocytic leukaemia

Related terminology

None

Subtype(s)

None

Localization

Peripheral blood, bone marrow, spleen, liver, lymph node, and (sometimes) skin and serosa involvement is observed.

Clinical features

The most frequent presentation is a marked lymphocytosis of > 100 × 10^9/L, seen in 75% of cases. Patients exhibit anaemia and thrombocytopenia due to bone marrow infiltration. Frequently, hepatosplenomegaly and generalized lymphadenopathy with only slightly enlarged lymph nodes are observed. Cutaneous involvement is seen in approximately 20% of cases, and malignant effusions are seen in approximately 15% {2596}. About 30% of cases may present at an asymptomatic and indolent phase, but these eventually progress to active disease with exponentially rising blood lymphocytosis. Serum immunoglobulins are normal.

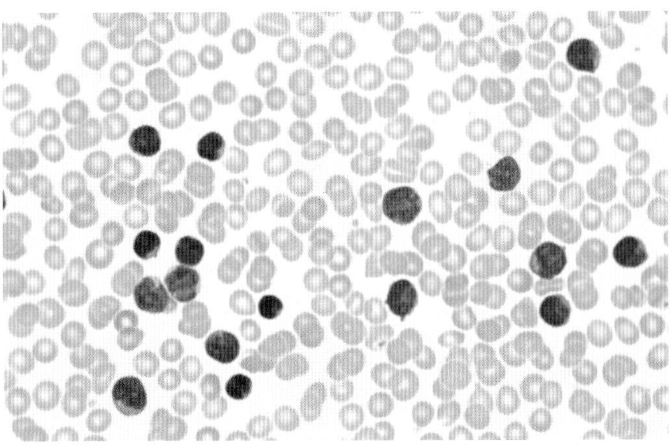

Fig. 5.19 T-prolymphocytic leukaemia. Peripheral blood smear. The neoplastic cells are small to medium-sized with irregular nuclear contours, prominent round to oval nucleoli, basophilic cytoplasm, and cytoplasmic blebs. Normal small lymphocytes are also present.

Epidemiology

T-PLL is rare and accounts for approximately 2% of cases of mature lymphoid leukaemias in adults aged > 30 years {2596}. The disease predominates in the elderly (median age: 65 years, range: 30–94 years). There is a slight male predominance (M:F ratio: 1.33:1).

Etiology

The etiology is unknown. A subset may arise in the context of ataxia–telangiectasia, characterized by germline mutations in *ATM* {3982,3863} (see *Ataxia–telangiectasia*, p. 810).

Pathogenesis

The chromosomal rearrangements inv(14)(q11q32) and t(14;14)(q11;q32) juxtapose *TCL1A* to the TR gene enhancer loci of

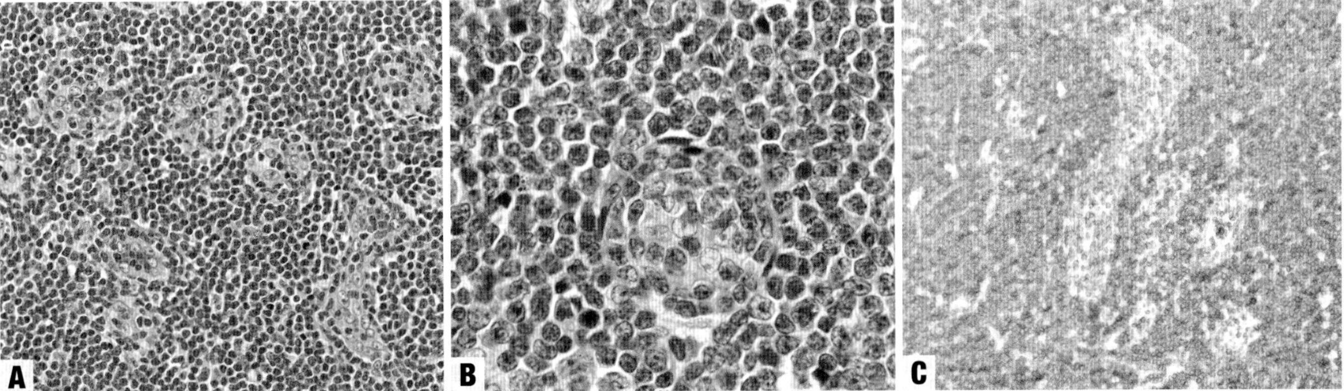

Fig. 5.20 T-prolymphocytic leukaemia involving lymph node. **A** Much of the lymph node is replaced by atypical small lymphoid cells that infiltrate multiple high endothelial venules. **B** A small blood vessel engulfed by small lymphoid cells with oval to irregular nuclei and small but distinct nucleoli. **C** CD3 stains the atypical cells, including those invading blood vessels.

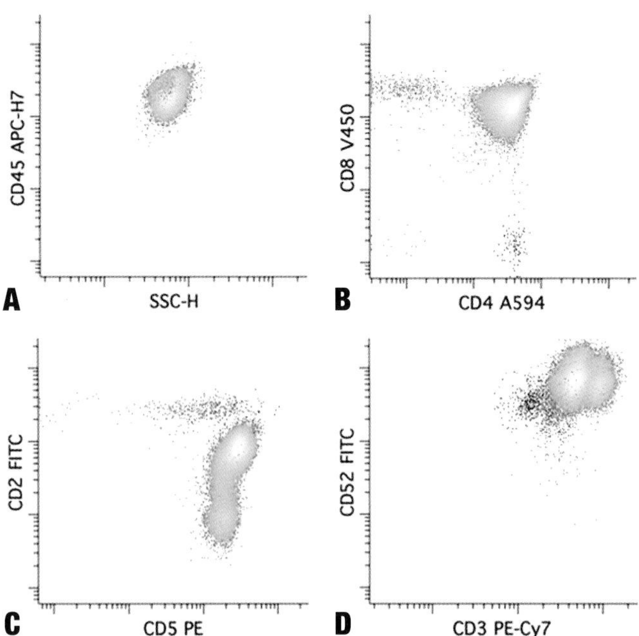

Fig. 5.21 T-prolymphocytic leukaemia. Flow cytometry of T-prolymphocytic leukaemia. All plots show CD3+ T cells. Neoplastic cells are coloured aqua; normal CD4+ T cells are red, and CD8+ T cells are green. The neoplastic cells are positive for CD45 (**A**) and coexpress CD4 and CD8 (**B**) in addition to CD2 (variably decreased) (**C**), CD3, CD5, CD45, and CD52 (**D**).

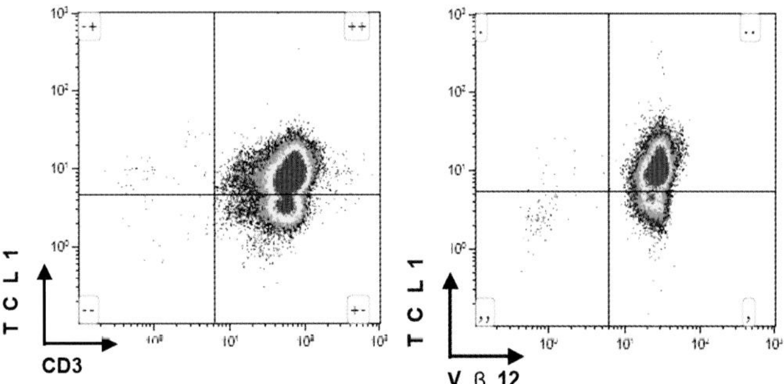

Fig. 5.22 T-prolymphocytic leukaemia. Flow cytometric assessment of TCL1A expression in clonal CD3+ T cells characteristic of T-prolymphocytic leukaemia.

TRA/TRD (rarely TRB). In approximately 5% of cases, a t(X;14)(q28;q11.2) translocation places the homologous *MTCP1* under in-trans regulation of T-cell receptor regulatory sequences. The resulting constitutive expression of these TCL1 oncogene family members is considered an initiating event in leukaemogenesis {461,2507,2596,3161}. These structural variants or chromosomal alterations result in dysregulated expression of members of the TCL1 oncoprotein family, which enhance T-cell receptor signalling and inhibit activation-induced death {2993}. Aberrant expression of TCL1 results in enhanced AKT signalling and increased cell proliferation and survival. Mouse models that overexpress human TCL1A or MTCP1 recapitulate human T-PLL {1419,4237}. Hypomorphic (reduced function) ATM resulting from mutations and/or deletions leads to impaired DNA damage repair and cooperates with TCL1 deregulation to accumulate DNA lesions, hence contributing to leukaemogenesis {3637}. Activating mutations of *IL2RG*, *JAK1*, *JAK3*, and *STAT5B* leading to constitutive STAT5 signalling are recurrent, with a total frequency as high as 75% of T-PLL {300,1982,2410, 4272}. Mutations in *EZH2*, *FBXW10*, and *CHEK2* may further contribute to the pathogenesis of T-PLL, putatively through their respective functions in epigenetic regulation, proteasome degradation, and DNA repair pathways {1982,3637}. Complex karyotypes are observed in 70–80% of cases. Abnormalities of chromosome 8, including idic(8)(p11.2), t(8;8)(p11.2;q12), and trisomy 8q, are seen in 70–80% of cases {3180}. Deletions in 12p13 {1577} and 22q {486}, gains in 8q24 (*MYC*) {1649}, and abnormalities of chromosomes 5p, 6, and 17 {461,817,2984} have also been described. Some studies have shown that the minimally amplified region of the chromosome 8 events includes not only *MYC*, but rather *AGO2* with or without *MYC* alterations {3637,448}.

Macroscopic appearance

Not relevant

Histopathology

Peripheral blood and bone marrow

Blood smears display anaemia, thrombocytopenia, and leukocytosis that comprises mainly atypical lymphocytes. The most commonly observed morphology (75% of cases) is a predominance of small to medium-sized cells with nongranular basophilic cytoplasm and round, oval, or markedly irregular nuclei with visible nucleoli. A less common morphology, named the small cell variant (25% of cases) exhibits cells that are relatively small in size with scant cytoplasm and small nuclei containing condensed chromatin and inconspicuous nucleoli. In the least frequently observed cytology (5% of cases), the neoplastic cells are small to medium-sized with irregular nuclear contours resembling cerebriform cells of Sézary syndrome. Regardless of nuclear morphology, a characteristic feature is basophilic cytoplasm with protrusions or blebs. Bone marrow aspirates show aggregates of neoplastic lymphoid cells, and core biopsies demonstrate diffuse and interstitial infiltrates {1564}.

Other tissues

Splenic involvement is characterized by red pulp expansion and white pulp attenuation by neoplastic cells {3082}. Lymph nodes show diffuse paracortical infiltration and attenuation of germinal centres. Cutaneous involvement consists of dense perivascular and periadnexal infiltrates without epidermotropism {2596, 2508}.

Immunophenotype

T-prolymphocytes exhibit a mature T-cell immunophenotype of mostly central memory–like differentiation {2993}. They are characteristically positive for CD2, CD3 (may be weak), CD5, and CD7, and negative for TdT and CD1a {2596,1564,672}. The neoplastic cells are commonly positive for CD4, with CD4+/CD8– in 40–60%, CD4+/CD8+ in 25–41%, and CD4–/CD8+ in about 15% of cases {1565}. Coexpression of CD4 and CD8 is a distinct feature of T-PLL that is rarely seen in other postthymic T-cell neoplasms. CD52 is usually expressed at a high level and often targeted therapeutically in T-PLL {2596,672}. Overexpression of the oncoprotein TCL1A can be detected by immunohistochemistry in tissues and by flow cytometry {1564,1565}.

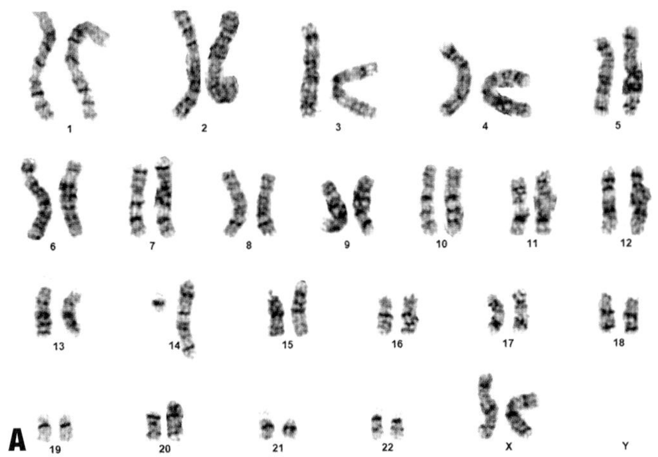

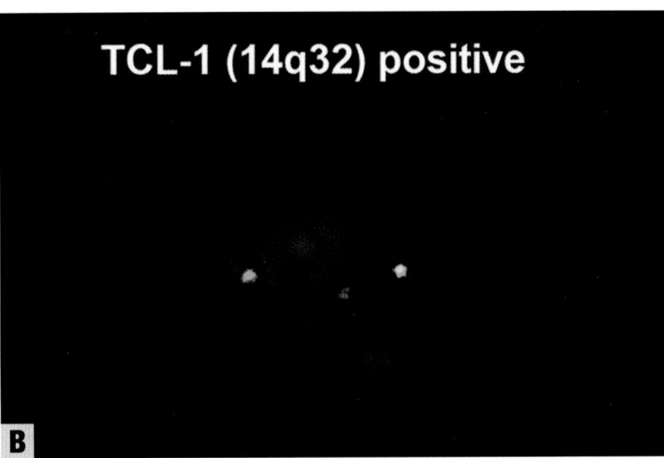

Fig. 5.23 T-prolymphocytic leukaemia. **A** An abnormal female karyotype 46,XX,t(14;14)(q11.2;q32)[10]/46,XX[21] was observed in a patient with bone marrow involvement by T-prolymphocytic leukaemia. A reciprocal translocation between the long arms of the two copies of chromosome 14 at bands 14q11.2 and 14q32 was observed. **B** Interphase FISH study using the *TCL1A* (14q32.13) dual-colour break-apart probe set was positive in 20 (10%) of 200 cells examined. The positive cells displayed one colocalized fusion signal, representing the intact *TCL1A* locus, and one red and one green signal representing the disrupted region around the *TCL1A* locus due to a chromosomal translocation/rearrangement.

Differential diagnosis

The differential diagnosis of T-PLL includes mature T-cell neoplasms with leukaemic presentation, such as adult T-cell leukaemia/lymphoma, Sézary syndrome, and T-large granular lymphocytic leukaemia {1564}. Other considerations include lymphoid neoplasms with leukaemic presentation, such as T- or B-lymphoblastic leukaemia, hepatosplenic T-cell lymphoma, chronic lymphocytic leukaemia / small lymphocytic lymphoma, and mantle cell lymphoma. Some investigators recognize rare cases of TCL1 family–negative T-PLL {1458,1131,1936}. In these cases, deletions and/or mutations of *ATM*, which are found in 80–90% of all T-PLL cases but are usually absent in other mature T-cell malignancies, are considered to best aid in establishing the diagnosis of presumed TCL1 family–negative T-PLL {3637}. However, given the insufficient clinicopathological and molecular data, the relationship of TCL1 family–negative T-PLL to T-PLL is currently not clear, and such cases should preferably be classified as peripheral T-cell lymphoma NOS (with leukaemic involvement) after exclusion of other specific leukaemic T-cell entities.

Cytology

See above.

Diagnostic molecular pathology

Clonal TR gene rearrangements (in TRB or TRG) are detected, but without prominent clonotypic biases {2113}. Rearrangements involving TCL1 genes (*TCL1A*, *MTCP1*) and the TRA/TRD loci are present in all cases of T-PLL.

Essential and desirable diagnostic criteria

See Box 5.05.

Staging

About 30% of cases are in the inactive stage at diagnosis, and approximately 70% of patients present with active disease {3812}.

Box 5.05 Diagnostic criteria for T-prolymphocytic leukaemia (T-PLL) according to consensus guidelines {3812}

Essential (major) diagnostic criteria

- Peripheral blood lymphocytosis > 5×10^9/L or bone marrow infiltrate with T-PLL immunophenotype
- Evidence of T-cell monoclonality
- Demonstration of *TCL1A* (14q32) or *MTCP1* (Xq28) rearrangement (desirable identification of juxtaposed TR locus, most frequently TRD) or TCL1A protein expression[a]

Minor diagnostic criteria (at least one required)

- Abnormalities involving chromosome 11 (11q22.3, *ATM*)
- Abnormalities in chromosome 8: idic(8)(p11), t(8;8), trisomy 8q
- Abnormalities in chromosome 5, 12, 13, or 22, or complex karyotype
- Involvement of specific sites (e.g. splenomegaly, effusions)

[a]In 90–95% of cases, the diagnosis is established by all three major criteria being met. For discussion of (and diagnostic criteria for) TCL1-negative T-PLL, see the text {1131}.

Prognosis and prediction

Although the disease course is characteristically aggressive in most cases {2596,4137}, as many as 20–30% of patients demonstrate initially stable or slowly progressive disease {1288,627, 3812}. However, nearly all cases of inactive T-PLL progress to active disease within 1–2 years {3812}. The median overall survival time is approximately 21 months {627}. Adverse prognostic factors vary between series; they include age > 65 years, presence of serous effusions, hepatic or CNS involvement, bulky lymphadenopathy, very high absolute lymphocyte counts, complex karyotype, very high TCL1A protein, bone marrow suppression, or organ dysfunction {910,1565,1775,447}. Initiation of treatment is dependent on the presence of active disease, defined by clinical and relatively simple laboratory parameters such as haemoglobin and platelet counts, and progressive lymphocytosis {3812}. Response rates and prognosis have significantly improved after introduction of the anti-CD52 monoclonal antibody alemtuzumab in the first-line treatment of T-PLL {627}. However, cure is only observed in a small fraction of patients who undergo allogeneic stem cell transplantation.

T-large granular lymphocytic leukaemia

Morice WG
Cheng CL
Gujral S
Lamy T
Loughran TP Jr
Naresh KN
Semenzato GC

Definition

T-large granular lymphocytic leukaemia (T-LGLL) is a neoplastic proliferation of cytotoxic large granular T cells presenting with persistent absolute lymphocytosis (> 2×10^9/L).

ICD-O coding

9831/3 T-large granular lymphocytic leukaemia

ICD-11 coding

2A90.1 T-cell large granular lymphocytic leukaemia

Related terminology

Acceptable: T-cell lymphoproliferative disease of granular lymphocytes; T-cell large granular lymphocytic leukaemia.

Not recommended: T-cell large granular lymphocytosis; T-gamma lymphoproliferative disease.

Subtype(s)

None

Localization

T-LGLL involves the peripheral blood, bone marrow, and spleen. Liver involvement may be present, whereas lymph node involvement is exceedingly rare.

Clinical features

One third of T-LGLL cases are asymptomatic. When symptomatic, the clinical features are typically attributable to disease-associated cytopenias; fatigue and B symptoms are not common {940,240}. Neutropenia (absolute neutrophil count < 1.5×10^9/L) is present in as many as 80% of cases and severe neutropenia (absolute neutrophil count < 0.5×10^9/L) in 20–25%. Neutropenia may be complicated by aphthous ulcers of the oral mucosa and ulceration or recurrent bacterial infections of the skin, oropharynx, or perirectum {2207,2926}. T-LGLL–associated anaemia may be transfusion-dependent; pure red blood cell aplasia is seen in a minority of cases {1488, 3714}. Thrombocytopenia and/or associated bleeding complications are uncommon.

T-LGLL is frequently associated with autoimmune disorders. Rheumatoid arthritis is present in as many as 20% of cases, and other autoimmune diseases such as systemic lupus erythematosus and Sjögren syndrome are also described {1235}. More than 30% of patients with T-LGLL have abnormal serological findings indicative of immune activation, such as polyclonal hypergammaglobulinaemia or positive antinuclear antibodies {2382}. Monoclonal B-cell lymphocytosis can be identified in as many as 25% of T-LGLL cases; 5% are associated with haematological malignancies, which are most often B-cell lymphomas {1384,1645,4235}. Splenomegaly is described in 15–50% of T-LGLL cases; it is usually modest and often only identified by radiological examination {2207,3082}. Lymphadenopathy and hepatomegaly are rare.

Epidemiology

T-LGLL is rare, accounting for < 5% of lymphoproliferative disorders overall, although it appears to have a slightly higher prevalence in Asia (5–6%) {3689,2428,2171}. The age-adjusted incidence of T-LGLL is 0.02 cases per 100 000 person-years based on the SEER Program database and the US National Cancer Database (NCDB) {3689}. T-LGLL is a disease of adults (median age: 60 years); the majority of cases occur in people aged 45–75 years. It is rare in individuals aged < 25 years. There is no sex predilection.

Etiology

The frequent association of T-LGLL with autoimmunity and haematolymphoid malignancies, as well as the frequent seroreactivity to HTLV-1–related proteins, suggest that chronic antigenic stimulation plays a central role {2429,3776,2990}.

Pathogenesis

Chronic antigenic stimulation leading to oligoclonal or clonal expansion of memory effector T cells and acquired resistance to

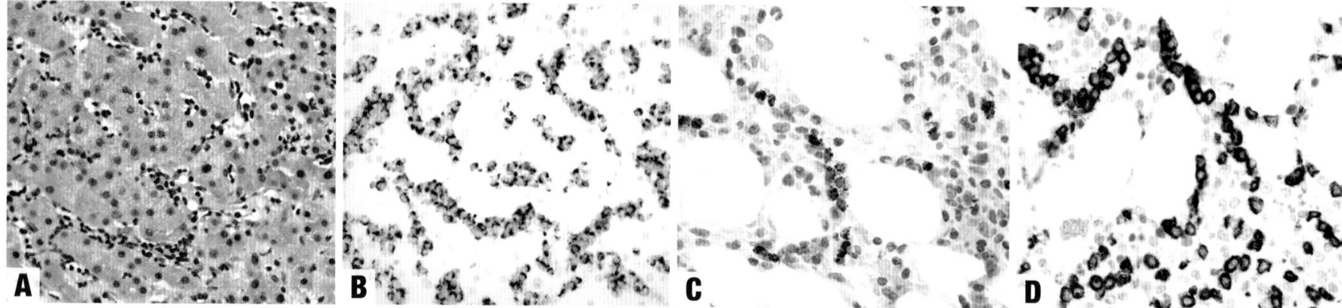

Fig. 5.24 T-large granular lymphocytic leukaemia. **A** Liver biopsy reveals sinusoidal infiltration by small lymphocytes. **B** The small lymphocytes in the liver sinusoids are strongly TIA1-positive by immunohistochemistry. **C** Immunohistochemistry of a bone marrow biopsy reveals intrasinusoidal infiltrates by granzyme B–positive cells. **D** Immunohistochemistry of a bone marrow biopsy reveals intrasinusoidal infiltrates and interstitial clusters of CD8-positive cells.

activation-induced cell death are key events in the development of T-LGLL. T-LGLL expansion can be stimulated by IL-15 and autocrine PDGF stimulation, and the cells are resistant to FAS/FASL-mediated apoptosis {2206,665,4483}. Abnormalities in cell signalling are also key. Constitutive activation of STAT3, with or without mutation, appears to play a central role in promoting cellular survival {1798,1089}. Recurrent *STAT5B* mutations (most often p.N642H and p.Y665F; NP_036580.2) are disproportionately present in indolent CD4+ T-LGLL (30%); these mutations are rare in CD8+ T-LGLL or gamma-delta T-LGLL. In CD8+ cases they are associated with an aggressive disease course {4476,118}. In addition, perturbations in the PI3K/AKT and NF-κB signalling pathways have been implicated in the pathogenesis of T-LGLL {2244, 3606,1853}. Other genes recurrently mutated in T-LGLL are *TET2*, *TNFAIP3*, *BCL11B*, *FLT3*, and *PTPN23* {685,3990}.

Macroscopic appearance

Not relevant

Histopathology

In the peripheral blood, T-LGLL usually shows small and minimally irregular nuclei, condensed chromatin, and abundant pale-staining cytoplasm containing variably abundant azurophilic granules. The cytological features of T-LGLL are difficult to identify in bone marrow aspirate specimens.

Bone marrow examination is not required but can aid in confirmation of the diagnosis and the exclusion of other potential causes of cytopenias, such as myelodysplasia {2208}. The bone marrow is slightly hypercellular in approximately half of the cases, and the remainder are normocellular or hypocellular {2789,3081}. In most cases, bone marrow shows a mixed interstitial and intrasinusoidal infiltrate of small lymphoid cells without significant atypia. The volume/density of the infiltrate is variable, and it can be subtle, making morphological assessment difficult. The interstitial infiltrates are frequently accompanied by nodular aggregates of small lymphocytes.

Splenic involvement by T-LGLL is characterized by red pulp sinusoidal and cordal infiltration, frequently associated with white pulp hyperplasia {3082,2382}.

Immunophenotype

Most cases of T-LGLL are of CD8+ αβ T-cell lineage (CD8+ T-LGLL) with a mature effector memory phenotype (CD3+, CD8+, CD57+, CD45RA+, CD62L−). A minority of cases express CD4 either alone or in association with CD8^{dim} (CD4+ T-LGLL) {2350}. Fewer than 10% of T-LGLL cases are of γδ T-cell lineage; these cases fully express CD57 and CD16, partially express CD8, and preferentially display the Vγ9/Vδ2 profile {429,3992}.

By immunohistochemistry, the lymphoid cells usually express CD2, CD3, CD8, TCRβ, CD7, and the cytotoxic granule proteins TIA1, perforin, granzyme B, and granzyme M. They rarely express CD56 and are often negative for CD5 {2787,4462}. Interstitial lymphoid aggregates composed of mixed T cells and B cells are frequent. Expression of the NK cell–associated antigens CD16 and CD57 is frequent (80% and 90%, respectively), although this feature is not disease-specific {3009,2788,2448,512}.

By flow cytometric analysis of TCRβ constant region (TRBC1) or TCRVβ expression, the dominant clone typically exceeds 70%, and this finding is helpful for explaining difficult-to-interpret TR gene PCR results {1635}. The NK cell–associated receptors killer cell immunoglobulin-like receptor (KIR) and CD94/NKG2 are expressed in more than one-third of cases of T-LGLL, and the cells expressing these receptors represent late-stage, fully differentiated cytotoxic T lymphocytes {1611,2788,1090,3148}. Abnormal uniform expression of a single KIR isoform (CD158a, CD158b, or CD158e) is indicative of clonality.

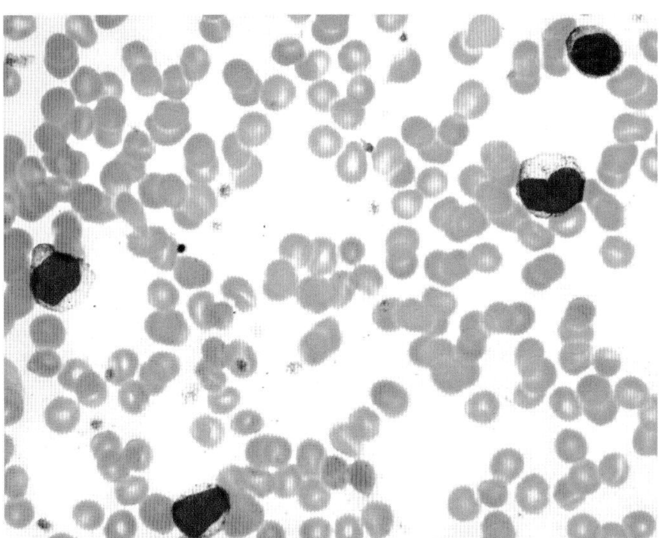

Fig. 5.25 T-large granular lymphocytic leukaemia. Peripheral smear. Small, minimally irregular nuclei with condensed chromatin and abundant pale-staining cytoplasm containing azurophilic granules (Giemsa).

Differential diagnosis

The differential diagnosis for T-LGLL includes reactive CD8+ T-cell expansions/infiltrates (T-cell clonopathy of undetermined significance), NK-large granular lymphocytic leukaemia, and mature T-cell neoplasms with leukaemic presentation such as T-prolymphocytic leukaemia, adult T-cell leukaemia/lymphoma, and Sézary syndrome. CD8+ T-lymphocytosis with features of large granular lymphocytes can be seen in the context of autoimmune disorders and chronic infectious states (e.g. HTLV-1). In such cases, the levels of lymphocytosis are usually low but are occasionally higher. Features to differentiate reactive CD8+

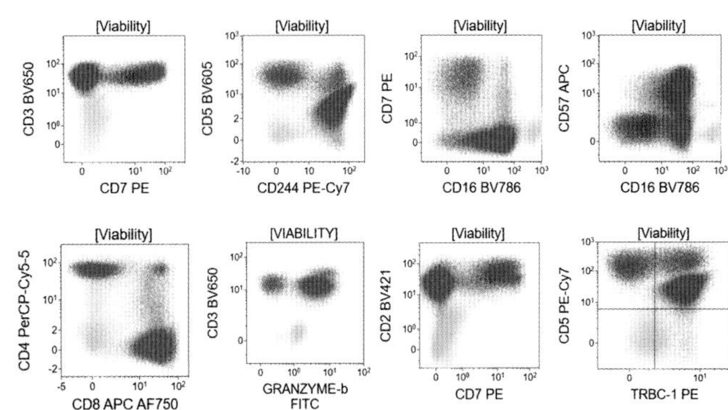

Fig. 5.26 T-large granular lymphocytic leukaemia. Flow cytometry. The abnormal T cells (red dots) show moderate expression of CD3 and CD2, as well as multiple immunophenotypic aberrations such as loss of CD7 and CD5; expression of the T/NK markers CD16, CD244, and CD57; expression of the cytotoxic marker granzyme B; CD8 restriction; and restricted TRBC1 expression indicating clonality. The normal T cells are shown in blue. All other cells present in the sample are shown in light grey.

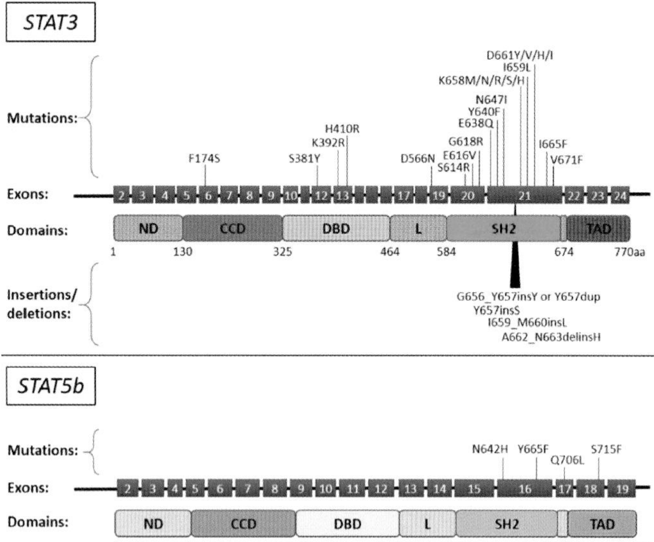

Fig. 5.27 T-large granular lymphocytic leukaemia. The *STAT3* and *STAT5B* mutations are indicated at their position in the exon upstream of the corresponding protein domain. The point mutations and the insertions/deletions are reported above and below the schematic representation of the gene, respectively. CCD, coiled-coil domain; DBD, DNA-binding domain; L, linker; ND, N-terminal domain; TAD, transactivation domain.

T-lymphocytosis from neoplastic T-LGLL include the absence of tissue infiltrates (other than bone marrow localization) and absence of significant cytopenias. A neoplastic nature of the proliferation is supported by T-cell receptor monoclonality and/or *STAT3*/*STAT5B* mutation analysis {3715}.

Cytology

See *Histopathology* for blood results.

Diagnostic molecular pathology

T-LGLLs show monoclonal or oligoclonal TR gene rearrangement, although the predominant clone may change over time {762}. *STAT3* and *STAT5B* mutations are the most commonly recognized gain-of-function genetic lesions in T-LGLL {1798,2108,3350}.

Essential and desirable diagnostic criteria

Note: The presence of all three essential criteria or of two essential criteria plus one of the two desirable criteria is sufficient for a diagnosis of T-LGLL.

Essential: (1) an increase in circulating cytotoxic T cells (often 2×10^9/L but may be lower); (2) a T-cell population with an aberrant phenotype, usually CD8-positive and with downregulation of CD5 and/or CD7 and/or abnormal expression of CD16 and NK cell–associated receptors; (3) evidence of T-cell monoclonality.

Desirable: demonstration of intrasinusoidal cytotoxic lymphocyte infiltrates in the bone marrow by immunohistochemistry; demonstration of *STAT3* or *STAT5B* mutation.

Staging

None

Prognosis and prediction

The majority of patients with T-LGLL develop disease-associated cytopenias requiring treatment. Single-agent therapy with methotrexate, cyclophosphamide, or ciclosporin is often employed as first-line therapy, with or without corticosteroids {4586,3124,2208}. The prognosis is generally good, with most patients exhibiting long survival. Neutropenia, transfusion-dependent anaemia, and *STAT3* mutation are associated with a worse prognosis. Rare cases of progression to aggressive T-cell lymphoma have been described {2604}.

NK-large granular lymphocytic leukaemia

Morice WG
Cheng CL
Gujral S
Lamy T
Loughran TP Jr
Naresh KN
Semenzato GC

Definition

NK-large granular lymphocytic leukaemia (NK-LGLL) is a neoplasm characterized by a persistent increase in peripheral blood NK cells (usually > 2×10^9/L) and a chronic indolent clinical course.

ICD-O coding

9831/3 NK-large granular lymphocytic leukaemia

ICD-11 coding

2A90.2 Chronic lymphoproliferative disorders of NK cells

Related terminology

Acceptable: chronic lymphoproliferative disorder of NK cells; chronic NK-large granular lymphocyte lymphoproliferative disorder.

Not recommended: chronic NK-cell lymphocytosis; indolent leukaemia of NK cells.

Subtype(s)

None

Localization

NK-LGLL typically involves the peripheral blood and bone marrow. Splenomegaly is uncommon, and hepatomegaly, lymphadenopathy, and skin involvement are not typical {3286}.

Clinical features

Most patients are asymptomatic. Some may present with neutropenia and/or anaemia or these may develop over the course of the disease. NK-LGLL may occur in association with other diseases such as autoimmune disorders, solid tumours, haematological neoplasms, and neuropathy {990}. However, these associations might not be as frequent as in T-large granular lymphocytic leukaemia (T-LGLL) {3678}.

Epidemiology

NK-LGLL is predominantly a disease of adults (median age: 60 years). It has no sex predilection. Unlike aggressive NK-cell leukaemia, NK-LGLL does not show a racial, geographical, or genetic predisposition.

Etiology

The etiology is unknown. Stimulation of innate immunity, possibly due to viral infection, is postulated to play a role in the development of NK-LGLL {343}. However, direct viral infection of NK cells does not appear to be a factor in the development of the disease.

Pathogenesis

Activating mutations of *STAT3* affecting the SH2 domain {1798} are present in approximately one third of NK-LGLL cases. About 25–30% of NK-LGLL cases have mutations in *TET2*, and some may have mutations of both *TET2* and *STAT3* {3156,1300}. Mutations of *CCL22* are found in 21.5% of cases of NK-LGLL; these are mutually exclusive of *STAT3* and *STAT5B* mutations and are not found in T-LGLL {208}, suggesting that such mutations may define a distinct subgroup of NK-LGLL. Mutations in *TNFAIP3* and PI3K pathway genes are also found in a minority of cases {2243}. *STAT5B* mutations are exceedingly rare {3990, 3350}. Interplay between killer cell immunoglobulin-like receptors (KIRs) expressed by the NK cells and their ability to recognize self–MHC class I may also be a contributing factor to leukaemogenesis {4537}.

Macroscopic appearance

Not relevant

Histopathology

The abnormal cells in the blood are usually intermediate to large in size, with abundant pale-staining cytoplasm and variably abundant azurophilic granules. The granules may be fine to coarse but can be difficult to visualize in some cases. The nuclei are typically small and round, with condensed chromatin and minimally irregular nuclear contours {2428}. NK-LGLL cannot be distinguished from T-LGLL by cytological features.

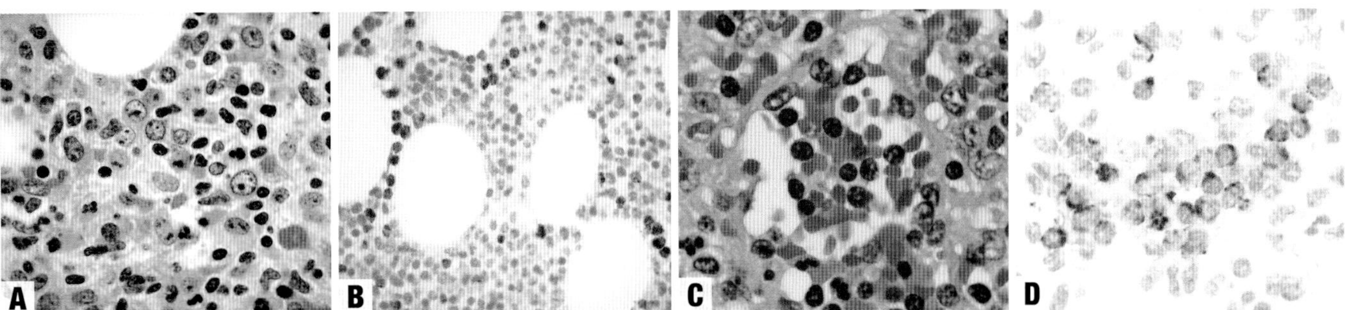

Fig. 5.28 NK-large granular lymphocytic leukaemia. **A** Bone marrow biopsy reveals a subtle increase in interstitial small lymphocytes. **B** Bone marrow. Immunohistochemistry reveals granzyme B–positive intrasinusoidal infiltrates. **C** Splenic involvement characterized by increased sinusoidal small lymphocytes. **D** Immunohistochemistry for TIA1 highlights the splenic sinusoidal infiltrates.

Chapter 5

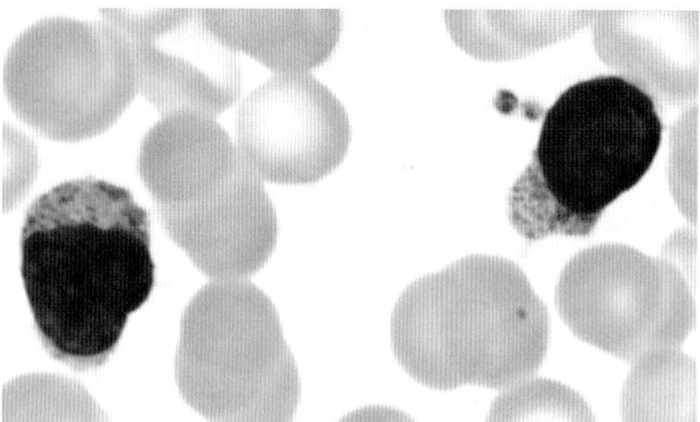

Fig. 5.29 NK-large granular lymphocytic leukaemia. Peripheral blood cytology. Peripheral blood smear examination reveals lymphocytes with small, bland nuclei and abundant cytoplasm containing visible granules (Giemsa). In this instance the cytoplasm contains numerous granules, but this feature varies both between and within cases. There are no cytological features that reliably distinguish between NK-large granular lymphocytic leukaemia and normal cytotoxic lymphocytes.

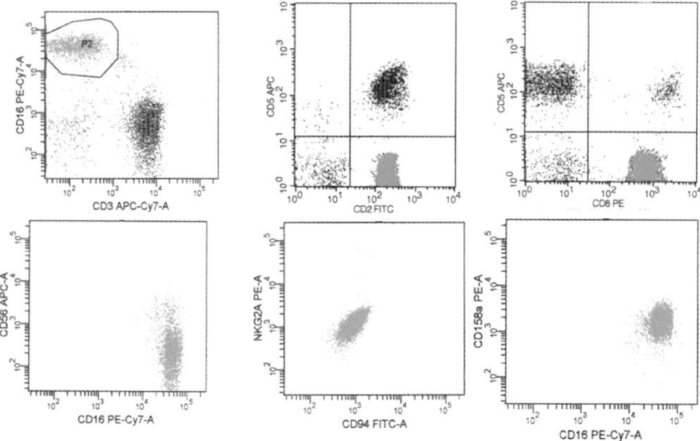

Fig. 5.30 NK-large granular lymphocytic leukaemia. Flow cytometric immunophenotyping in NK-large granular lymphocytic leukaemia reveals CD16+, CD3− NK cells (upper left; NK cells shown in green, normal T cells shown in red) that are CD2-positive (upper middle) and have uniform expression of CD8 (upper right). Selective gating on the NK cells reveals loss of CD56 (lower left), uniform expression of the CD94/NKG2A heterodimer (lower middle), and restricted expression of the killer cell immunoglobulin-like receptor (KIR) CD158a (lower right).

Lymphocytes may be increased in bone marrow aspirate smears, but the lymphocyte cytoplasm is often difficult to visualize in these preparations and therefore the distinctive features of NK-LGLL are not readily appreciated {2790}. Bone marrow involvement is common, usually displaying an intrasinusoidal pattern although interstitial infiltrates may also be seen {2788}. The infiltrating cells typically have small, minimally irregular nuclei and lack distinctive cytological features. In the spleen, intrasinusoidal infiltration of the red pulp may also be seen {2428}.

Immunophenotype

Flow cytometry shows that NK-LGLL cells are CD16-positive and sCD3-negative; cCD3ε expression may be present. CD56 is often positive, but approximately 50% of cases show weak or absent expression {542,902}. Diminished expression of CD2 and CD7 may also be present. Expression of CD8 is variably reported {3677,2162}. Abnormalities in NK-cell receptor expression are a hallmark of NK-LGLL {4536,1088,3148,2786}. All cases have abnormal expression of KIR: either a complete lack of detectable KIR or restricted KIR isoform expression is seen, the latter more often in CD56-negative cases. Other abnormalities of NK-cell receptors are uniform, bright CD94/NKG2A heterodimer expression and weak or absent expression of CD161.

Expression of cytotoxic granule proteins (TIA1, granzyme B, granzyme M) is detectable by flow cytometric immunophenotyping and immunohistochemistry {2787}. The latter typically illustrates the presence of intrasinusoidal infiltrates in the bone marrow and spleen, which is otherwise difficult to detect by histological examination {2788}. NK-LGLL and T-LGLL are indistinguishable by immunohistochemical analysis alone.

Differential diagnosis

The differential diagnosis of NK-LGLL includes mature T-cell neoplasms with a leukaemic presentation, in particular T-LGLL, a disorder with considerable clinical and pathological overlap. When lymphocytosis is prominent, aggressive NK-cell leukaemia may be considered; NK-LGLL is distinguished by the indolent clinical presentation and lack of nuclear EBV positivity.

Cytology

See *Histopathology* for blood results.

Diagnostic molecular pathology

Mutations of *STAT3* (in 30% of cases) {1798} and *TET2* (in 25–30%) are seen in NK-LGLL, with a subset having both gene alterations {3156}. TR gene rearrangement studies show an absence of clonal T-cell populations.

Essential and desirable diagnostic criteria

Essential: (1) increase in circulating NK cells, typically > 2 × 10^9/L, persisting for > 6 months; (2) flow cytometric evidence of peripheral blood or bone marrow involvement by a uniform population of sCD3−, CD16+ NK cells; (3) demonstration of a restricted pattern of KIR expression (either dominant expression of a relevant KIR or a lack of KIRs) by flow cytometry (this is accepted as a surrogate marker of clonal expansion).

Note: If essential criteria 2 and 3 are both present, a diagnosis of NK-LGLL can be made in the absence of documented persistence of an absolute peripheral blood NK-cell count of > 2 × 10^9/L.

Desirable: bone marrow involved by intrasinusoidal NK cells; demonstration of *STAT3* and/or *TET2* mutations with NK-cell lineage (confirmed by flow cytometry).

Staging

Not relevant

Prognosis and prediction

In over half of all NK-LGLL cases, the clinical course is indolent and no therapy is required; some cases may even show spontaneous regression. Overall, the management of NK-LGLL is similar to that of T-LGLL, with the need for treatment usually determined by the presence or absence of associated cytopenias. Cytopenias and recurrent infections may be harbingers of a worse prognosis.

Adult T-cell leukaemia/lymphoma

Karube K
Cook LB
Ishitsuka K
Iwatsuki K
Kataoka K
Miyoshi H
Naresh KN
Tokura Y
Tsukasaki K

Definition

Adult T-cell leukaemia/lymphoma (ATLL) is a mature T-cell neoplasm associated with HTLV-1.

ICD-O coding

9827/3 Adult T-cell leukaemia/lymphoma
9827/3 Smouldering adult T-cell leukaemia/lymphoma
9827/3 Chronic adult T-cell leukaemia/lymphoma
9827/3 Lymphoma adult T-cell leukaemia/lymphoma
9827/3 Acute adult T-cell leukaemia/lymphoma

ICD-11 coding

2A90.5 Adult T-cell lymphoma or leukaemia, human T-cell lymphotropic virus type 1–associated

Related terminology

Acceptable: adult T-cell leukaemia/lymphoma, HTLV-1 associated.

Subtype(s)

Smouldering ATLL; chronic ATLL; lymphoma ATLL; acute ATLL

Localization

The peripheral blood, bone marrow, lymph node, skin, spleen, liver, gastrointestinal tract, bone, lung, CNS, and other organs may be involved {488}.

Clinical features

Patients with ATLL exhibit diverse clinical features, including generalized lymphadenopathy, cutaneous lesions, hepatosplenomegaly, and features related to the infiltration of various organs, particularly the CNS, gastrointestinal tract, bone, and lung {3996}. Many patients have an associated immunodeficiency, with frequent opportunistic infections caused by *Pneumocystis jirovecii*, *Candida* spp., CMV, or *Strongyloides stercoralis* {3899}. Some patients with indolent ATLL show leukaemic manifestation alone, without symptoms or signs.

Approximately half of all patients present with skin lesions, some of which are clinically indistinguishable from those of mycosis fungoides or Sézary syndrome {3598}. The cutaneous lesions can be of patch (6.7%), plaque (26.9%), multipapular (19.3%), nodulotumoural (38.7%), erythrodermic (4.2%), or purpuric (4.2%) type {3598}. Among them, the nodulotumoural type shows a poor prognosis, comparable to that of lymphoma ATLL.

Laboratory investigations frequently reveal leukocytosis with increased abnormal lymphocytes showing cerebriform or flower-like nuclei, elevation of serum LDH and soluble IL-2R, hypercalcaemia, and paraneoplastic neutrophilia/eosinophilia. Leukaemic manifestation, hypercalcaemia, and infiltration of the skin and gastrointestinal tract are the distinctive features of ATLL versus other lymphomas and leukaemias. Seropositivity of HTLV-1 is confirmatory, particularly if patients are not from an endemic area for HTLV-1 or do not show the typical presentation of ATLL {4123,536,3048}.

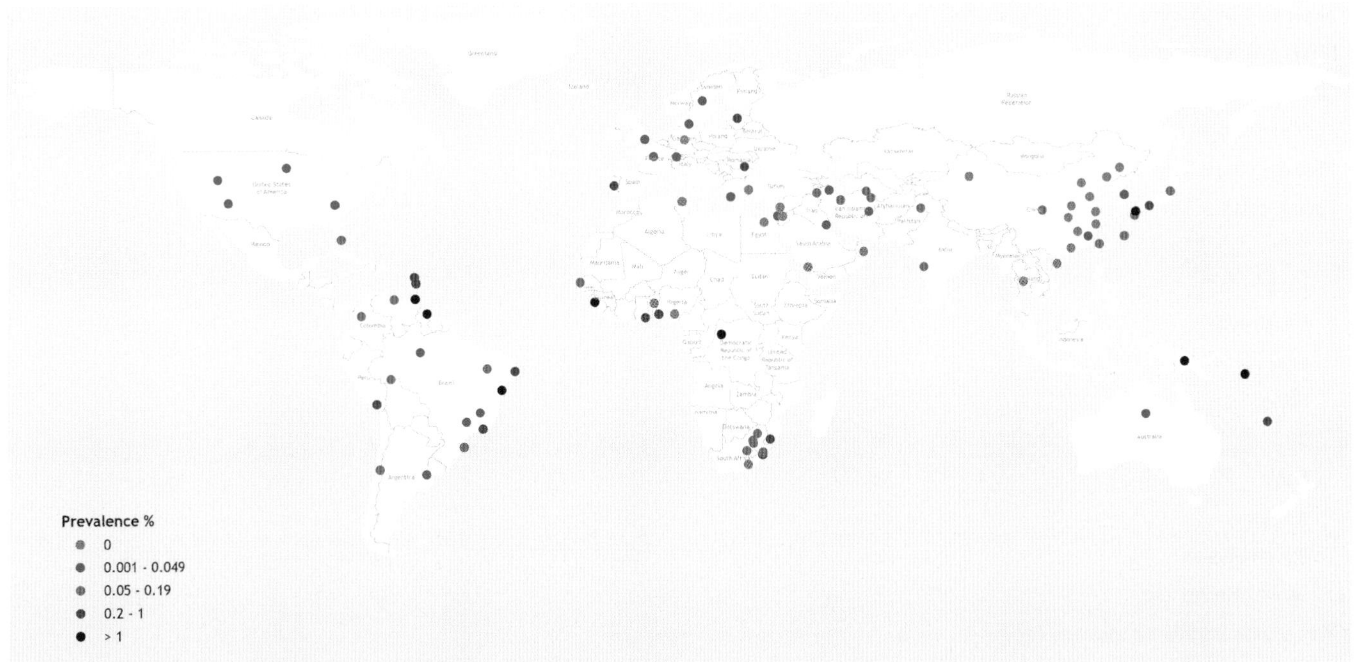

Fig. 5.31 Distribution and results of studies examining HTLV-1 seroprevalence among blood donors.

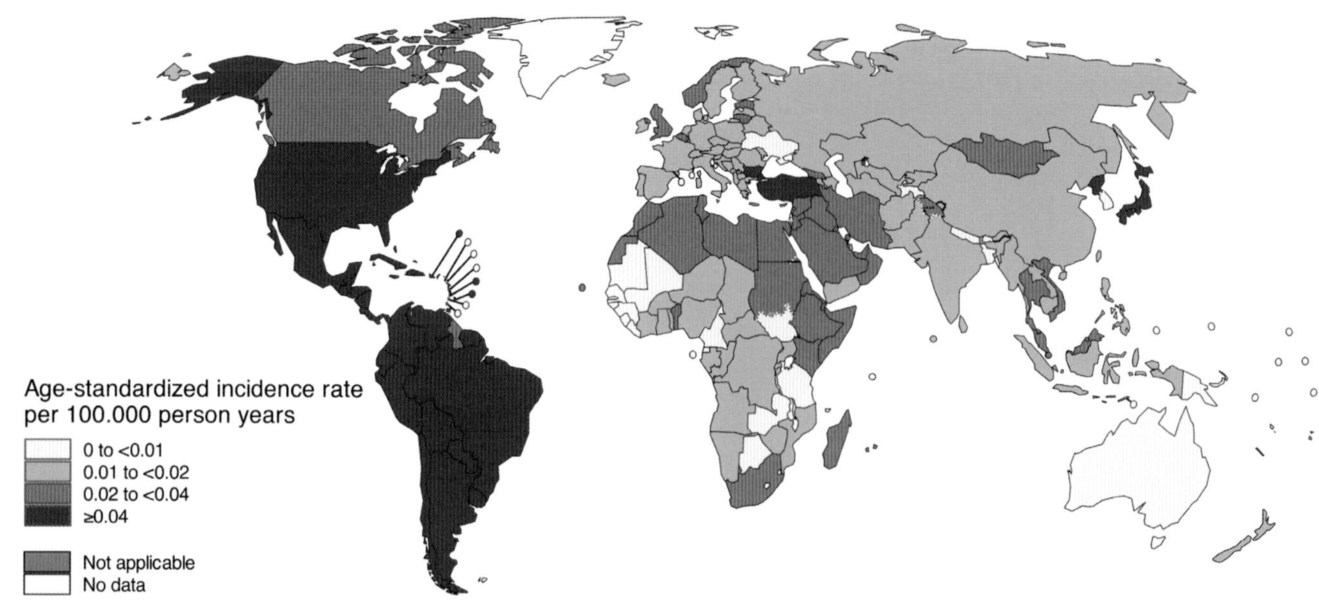

Fig. 5.32 Country-specific age-standardized incidence rates of cancer attributable to HTLV-1, 2020. Incidence rates of adult T-cell leukaemia/lymphoma.

The clinical presentation and course of ATLL are highly variable. Four clinical subtypes have been identified: acute, lymphoma, chronic, and smouldering, defined by the pattern of organ involvement, LDH/calcium values, and degree of leukaemic manifestation (see Table 5.03) {1918}. The acute subtype is diagnosed by the exclusion of the other three subtypes. Chronic-type ATLL is further divided into unfavourable and favourable subtypes according to the presence of LDH or blood urea nitrogen (BUN) levels above the normal upper limits or an albumin level below the normal lower limit {1918}. The acute, lymphoma, and unfavourable chronic subtypes of ATLL, which have a similar prognosis, are grouped as aggressive

Table 5.03 Shimoyama classification: diagnostic criteria for the clinical subtypes of adult T-cell leukaemia/lymphoma (modified from {3728})

Diagnostic criteria	Smouldering	Chronic	Lymphoma	Acute
Anti-HTLV-1 antibody	+	+	+	+
Lymphocytes (× 10^9/L)	< 4	≥ 4	< 4	n/a[a]
Abnormal T lymphocytes	≥ 5%	+[b]	≤ 1%	+
Flower cells with T-cell marker	Occasionally	Occasionally	No	Yes
LDH	≤ 1.5 × N	≤ 2 × N	n/a[a]	n/a[a]
Corrected calcium (mmol/L)	< 2.74	< 2.74	n/a[a]	n/a[a]
Histology-proven lymphadenopathy	No	n/a[a]	Yes	n/a[a]
Tumour lesion				
Skin	n/a[c]	n/a[a]	n/a[a]	n/a[a]
Lung	n/a[c]	n/a[a]	n/a[a]	n/a[a]
Lymph node	No	n/a[a]	Yes	n/a[a]
Liver	No	n/a[a]	n/a[a]	n/a[a]
Spleen	No	n/a[a]	n/a[a]	n/a[a]
CNS	No	No	n/a[a]	n/a[a]
Bone	No	No	n/a[a]	n/a[a]
Ascites	No	No	n/a[a]	n/a[a]
Pleural effusion	No	No	n/a[a]	n/a[a]
Gastrointestinal tract	No	No	n/a[a]	n/a[a]

N, normal upper limit; n/a, not applicable.
[a]No essential quantification except terms required for other subtype(s). [b]In cases with < 5% abnormal T lymphocytes in the peripheral blood, a histology-proven tumour lesion is required. [c]No essential quantification if other terms are fulfilled, but a histology-proven malignant lesion is required in cases with < 5% abnormal T lymphocytes in the peripheral blood.

ATLL, whereas the favourable chronic and smouldering subtypes are grouped as indolent ATLL {4100}. About half of all cases of indolent ATLL will transform into aggressive ATLL within 5 years.

Epidemiology

ATLL is endemic in several regions of the world, in particular south-western Japan, the Caribbean, intertropical Africa, the Middle East, South America, and Papua New Guinea. The distribution of the disease is closely linked to the prevalence of HTLV-1 in the population. Three major routes of infection by HTLV-1 have been recognized: breastfeeding, sexual intercourse, and blood transfusion. Individuals infected by HTLV-1 early in life, mainly by breastfeeding, are at (low-level) risk of developing ATLL after a long latency period. The development of ATLL after HTLV-1 infection via blood transfusion or sexual intercourse is very rare, in contrast to the development of HTLV-1–associated myelopathy / tropical spastic paraparesis {4374,1754}.

The median age of onset varies by geographical location. In Jamaica, the USA, and Latin America, the median ages are 43, 47, and 57 years, respectively {1487,3226,2509}. According to recent epidemiological studies in Japan, ATLL is currently diagnosed only in adults, with a median age of 68 years, which is 10 years older than that reported in the 1980s, probably because of the decline of HTLV-1–infected individuals in the younger population in Japan {1750,2096}. The cumulative incidence of ATLL is estimated to be 3–5% among HTLV-1 carriers in Japan {2096,1754,1885}.

Etiology

Only a small fraction (3–5%) of patients with HTLV-1 infection develop ATLL, and the estimated incidence is 46–710 cases per 100 000 person-years, with higher incidence rates in endemic regions. A variety of risk factors and determinants for developing ATLL among people with HTLV-1 infection have been reported, including male sex, older age, higher HTLV-1 proviral load (≥ 40 copies per 1000 peripheral blood mononuclear cells), longer duration of infection (> 20 years), and younger age at acquisition (infancy or childhood) {4367}. Although chronic infection with HTLV-1 is the cause of ATLL, this alone is not sufficient for neoplastic transformation. In asymptomatic carriers, low-abundance HTLV-1–infected CD4+ T-cell clones make up most of the HTLV-1 PVL (the proportion of infected mononuclear cells detected by PCR) in the peripheral blood. When one or more clones have started to undergo malignant transformation, they constitute a disproportionately high fraction of the PVL and may be detected in the peripheral blood years before the development of ATLL. High PVL (> 4%) carriers are those at greatest risk of future ATLL, and they are more likely to carry ATLL-like clonal expansions {2980,2096}. However, full transformation of expanded clones probably requires additional genetic and/or epigenetic events.

Pathogenesis

The HTLV-1 genome encodes two crucial proteins, Tax and HBZ, that regulate the persistence, expression, and pathogenesis of HTLV-1, although neither are directly oncogenic. Tax is a transcriptional transactivator that can drive viral replication and activate cellular pathways involved in T-cell proliferation, mainly via the NF-κB and AP-1 pathways. HBZ, a bZIP protein, also drives cell proliferation, inhibits apoptosis, and induces TIGIT and CCR4 expression on the cell surface, which is implicated in the proliferation and trafficking of malignant cells {229}. Expression of HTLV-1 proteins exposes infected cells to virus-specific cytotoxic T lymphocytes, and the quality of the cytotoxic T lymphocyte response is a key determinant of the host PVL {228}. Cytotoxic T lymphocyte escape is evident in ATLL, with immunodominant viral epitopes and host genes involved in antigen presentation frequently altered.

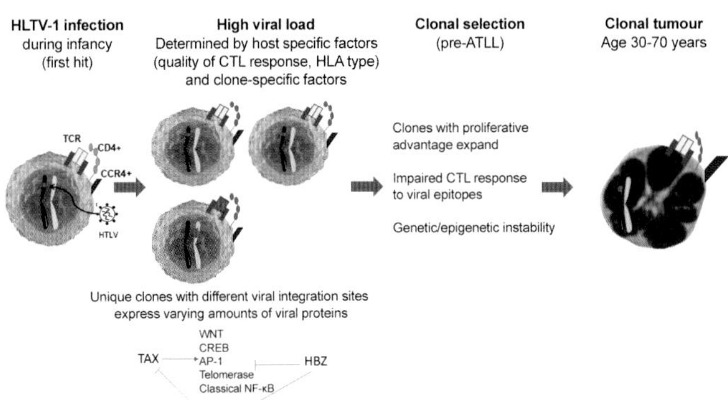

Fig. 5.33 Pathogenesis overview in adult T-cell leukaemia/lymphoma (ATLL). ATLL typically arises in HTLV-1 carriers infected by cell-to-cell transmission that occurs during birth or via breastfeeding. Infected cells are typically CD3+, CD4+, CD26−, CCR4+. During chronic infection, the blood of healthy carriers will contain > 10 000 distinct infected T-cell clones, each with a unique integration site and T-cell receptor. Each distinct clone is under different selection forces (different viral protein expression counterbalanced by cytotoxic T lymphocyte [CTL] killing), and some clones will have a proliferative advantage over others. ATLL-like clones harbouring driver mutations may be detected in the peripheral blood years before clinical ATLL development.

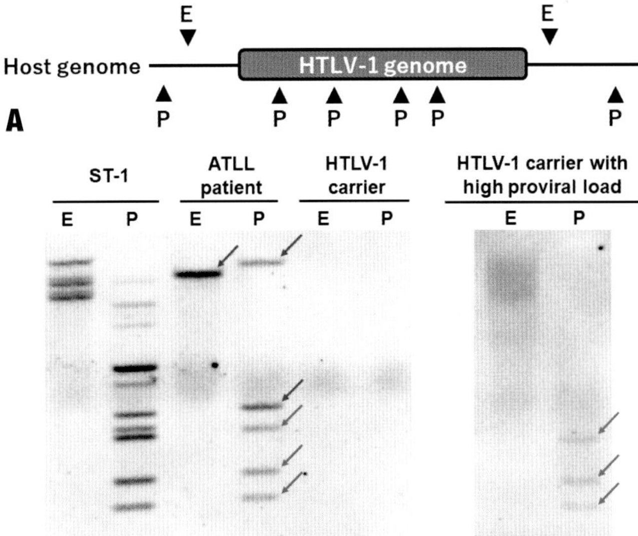

Fig. 5.34 Adult T-cell leukaemia/lymphoma. Southern blot analysis using HTLV-1 probes. Extracted DNA samples from peripheral blood or fresh tissue specimens are digested by two restriction enzymes, *Eco*RI (E) and *Pst*I (P), and electrophoresed. **A** Restriction enzyme recognition sites for each enzyme are shown. **B** Positive bands (red arrows) indicating monoclonal HTLV-1 integrations are recognized in a sample from a patient with adult T-cell leukaemia/lymphoma, like in ST-1 cells (positive control), whereas no bands or only internal fragments (blue arrows) are observed in an HTLV-1 carrier sample. In an HTLV-1 carrier with a high proviral load, smears and internal fragments are detected.

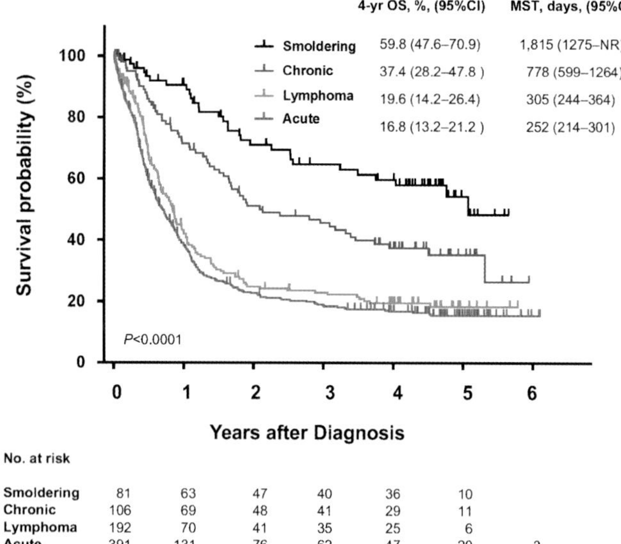

Fig. 5.35 Adult T-cell leukaemia/lymphoma. Overall survival of patients with adult T-cell leukaemia/lymphoma according to each clinical subtype. MST, median survival time; NR, not reached; OS, overall survival.

ATLL harbours clonally rearranged TR genes and one or a few HTLV-1 integrations. It is characterized by frequent gain-of-function alterations in T-cell receptor / NF-κB signalling, including activating mutations in *PLCG1*, *PRKCB*, and *CARD11*; *CTLA4*::*CD28* and *ICOS*::*CD28* fusions; and *REL* C-terminal truncational changes {1910,2081}. Other genetic targets include transcription factors (including alterations in the genes encoding the CIC-ATXN1 complex, and intragenic deletions in *IKZF2*), transcriptional co-regulators (*TBL1XR1* alterations), chemokine receptors (*CCR4* and *CCR7* C-terminal truncating mutations), epigenetic regulators (*ARID2* and *EP300* alterations), and tumour suppressors (*TP53* and *CDKN2A* alterations) {1910,2880,3691,2081}. Immune evasion–related molecules, such as *HLA-A* and *HLA-B*, are recurrently altered. Significantly, one quarter of ATLL cases harbour structural variations disrupting the 3′ untranslated region of *CD274* (*PDL1*), leading to its overexpression {1912}. Many ATLL cases show widespread accumulation of repressive epigenetic changes (H3 p.K27me3 and CpG island DNA hypermethylation), which modulate multiple pathways, including NF-κB signalling, MHC class I molecules, and Cys2-His2 zinc finger genes involved in retroelement silencing {1910, 4469}. The frequency and pattern of somatic alterations differ among clinical subtypes. Aggressive subtypes show more genetic alterations, whereas *STAT3* mutations are more common in indolent subtypes {1908}. The subtypes are further stratified into different subsets with different prognoses by their genetic alterations (see Table 5.04).

Macroscopic appearance

The macroscopic appearance corresponds to the clinical features.

Histopathology

The morphological features depend on the organ of involvement. Involved lymph node can show a diffuse or paracortical pattern of infiltration, or rarely a leukaemic pattern, characterized by preserved or dilated nodal sinuses containing malignant cells {3728}. The skin often shows epidermal infiltration with Pautrier-like microabscesses, along with a dermal infiltrate in perivascular locations. Some patients with cutaneous lesions have tumour nodules with extension to the subcutaneous fat {3017}.

The cytomorphological features of ATLL are highly variable. Tumour cells vary in size, nuclear shape, and extent of pleomorphism within an infiltrate. The morphological patterns include pleomorphic small, medium, and large cells, as well as anaplastic cells. Generally, the neoplastic lymphoid cells are medium to large in size, with nuclear pleomorphism and prominent convolutions and lobulation. The cells have coarsely clumped chromatin and prominent nucleoli {3017}. Lymphoid cells in the chronic and smouldering forms are generally smaller and show less atypia {3728,1764}. Cases of T-cell lymphoma with a prominence of cells showing striking nuclear lobulation should raise the suspicion of ATLL.

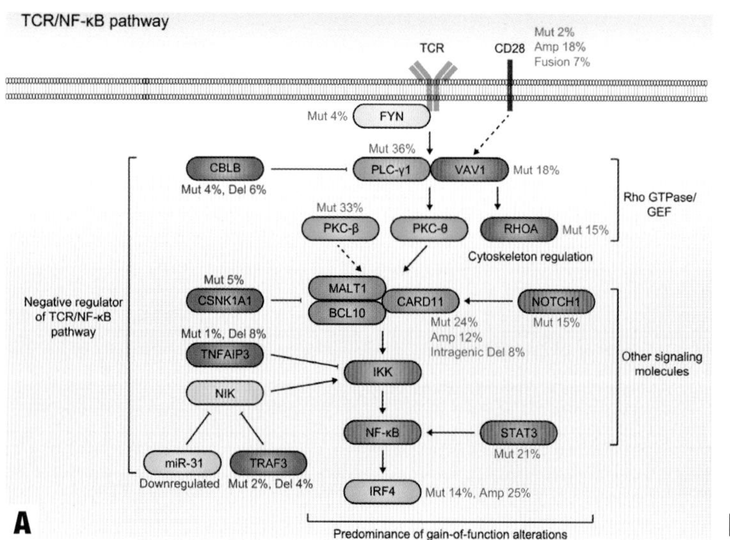

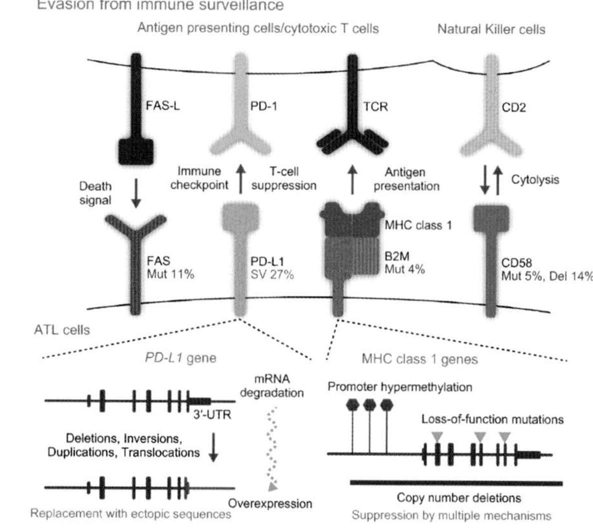

Fig. 5.36 Adult T-cell leukaemia/lymphoma. Molecular pathways frequently affected by somatic alterations. T-cell receptor (TCR) / NF-κB pathway (**A**) and evasion from immunosurveillance (**B**). Amp, amplification; Del, deletion; Mut, mutation; SV, structural variation.

Table 5.04 Clinical prognostic indexes and genetic prognostic markers for adult T-cell leukaemia/lymphoma

<table>
<tr><th></th><th>Acute subtype</th><th>Lymphoma subtype</th><th>Unfavourable chronic subtype</th><th>Favourable chronic subtype</th><th>Smouldering subtype</th></tr>
<tr><td colspan="6">Clinical prognostic indexes</td></tr>
<tr><td>ATL-PI {1920}</td><td colspan="2">Stage, PS, age, albumin, sIL2-R</td><td></td><td></td><td></td></tr>
<tr><td>iATL-PI {1919}</td><td></td><td></td><td colspan="3">sIL-2R</td></tr>
<tr><td>JCOG-PI {1261}</td><td colspan="3">Corrected calcium, PS</td><td></td><td></td></tr>
<tr><td>Modified ATL-PI {1248}</td><td colspan="2">Clinical subtype, PS, corrected calcium, sIL-2R</td><td></td><td></td><td></td></tr>
<tr><td>New Prognostic Score for ATL from North America {3226}</td><td colspan="5">PS, stage, calcium, age</td></tr>
<tr><td colspan="6">Genetic prognostic markers</td></tr>
<tr><td>Kataoka et al., 2018 {1908}</td><td colspan="2">CD274 (PDL1) amplification, PRKCB mutations</td><td colspan="3">IRF4 mutations, CD274 (PDL1) amplification, CDKN2A deletions</td></tr>
</table>

ATL-PI, adult T-cell leukaemia prognostic index; iATL-PI, indolent adult T-cell leukaemia prognostic index; JCOG-PI, Japan Clinical Oncology Group prognostic index; PS, Eastern Cooperative Oncology Group (ECOG) performance status; sIL-2R, soluble IL-2R.

Early in the course of ATLL, lymph nodes can show large EBV+ Hodgkin-like B lymphocytes in a background of small to medium-sized ATLL cells, which may result from the underlying immunodeficiency in patients with ATLL {3023}.

Immunohistochemistry and flow cytometry

On immunohistochemistry, the tumour cells express some pan–T-cell antigens (CD2, CD3, CD5) but usually lack CD7. Most cases are CD4+ and CD8–, but some are CD4– CD8+, double-positive, or double-negative. CD25 is expressed in most cases. Cytotoxic markers are negative. Especially in larger cells, CD30 may be variably positive. Tumour cells frequently express CCR4, and a proportion of cells express FOXP3 {3943,1896,3455}.

Flow cytometric evaluation may be helpful for the evaluation of disease progression. In addition to the immunophenotypic profile described above, the expression pattern of CD26, CD7, CCR7, CD127, and CADM1 can predict disease status including HTLV-1 carrier, indolent ATLL, and aggressive ATLL. In particular, the downregulation of CD7 and upregulation of CCR7 and CADM1 are more frequently observed in aggressive ATLL than in indolent ATLL {1849,2070}.

Differential diagnosis

The differential diagnosis may include almost any type of T-cell lymphoma or leukaemia, such as Sézary syndrome and T-prolymphocytic leukaemia in the peripheral blood; mycosis fungoides and primary cutaneous anaplastic large cell lymphoma

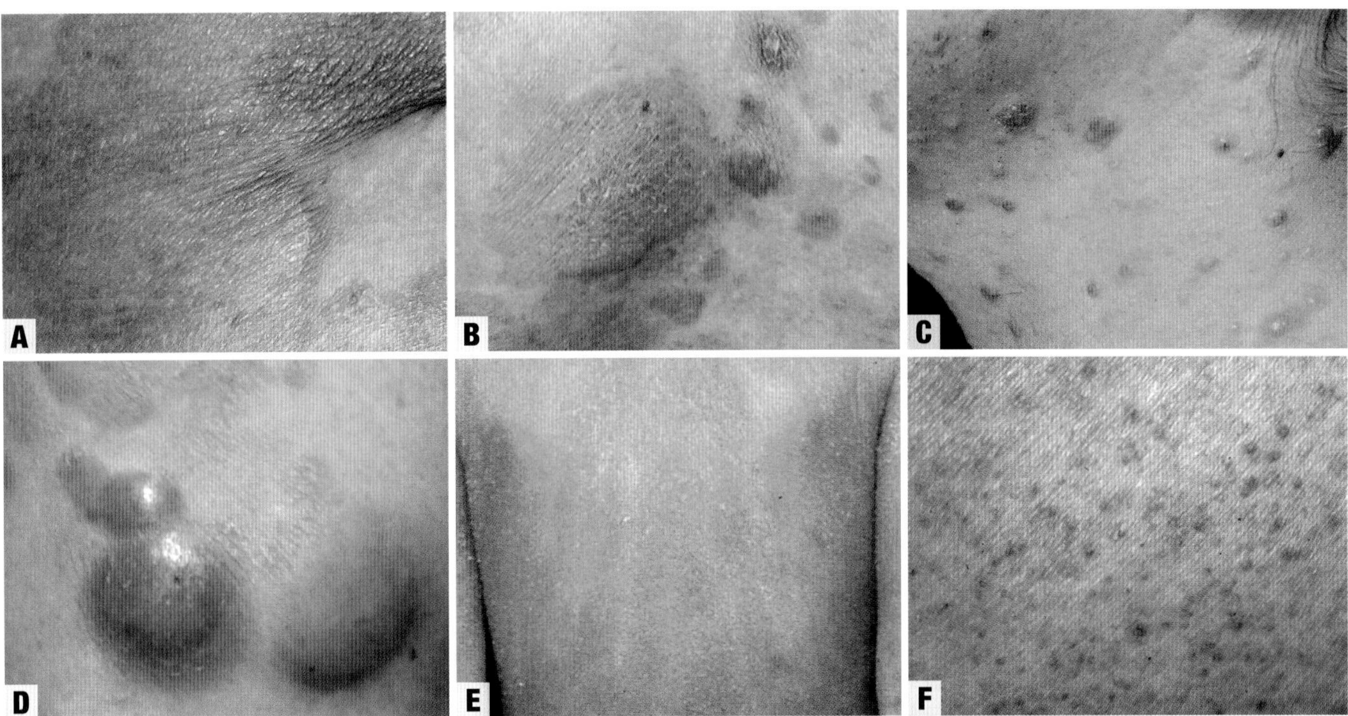

Fig. 5.37 Adult T-cell leukaemia/lymphoma: cutaneous manifestations. **A** Patch-type. The patches/plaques and erythrodermic lesions are similar to those of mycosis fungoides and Sézary syndrome, respectively. **B** Plaque type. **C** Multipapular type. **D** Nodulotumoural type. **E** Erythrodermic type. **F** Purpuric type.

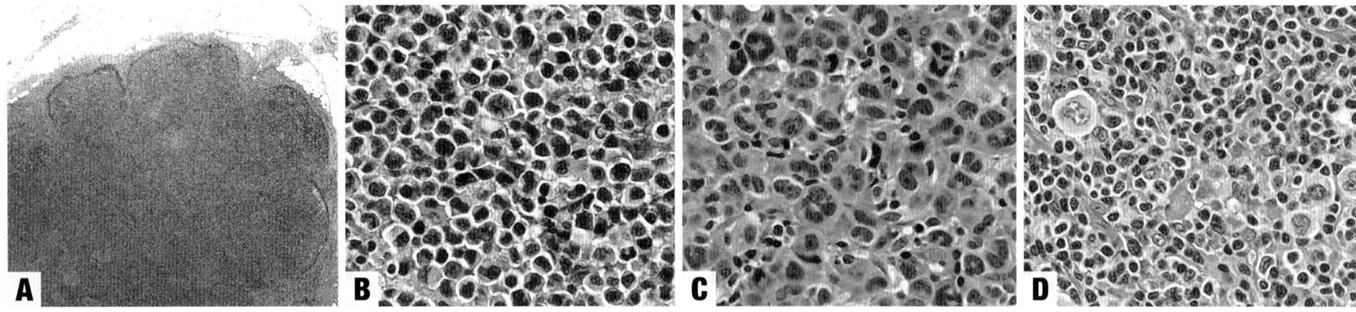

Fig. 5.38 Adult T-cell leukaemia/lymphoma involving a lymph node. **A** Low magnification shows diffuse infiltration with complete effacement of architecture. **B** The neoplastic cells typically show significant nuclear pleomorphism and irregular nuclear folds. **C** An example with anaplastic large cell lymphoma–like morphology. **D** An example with Hodgkin disease–like morphology.

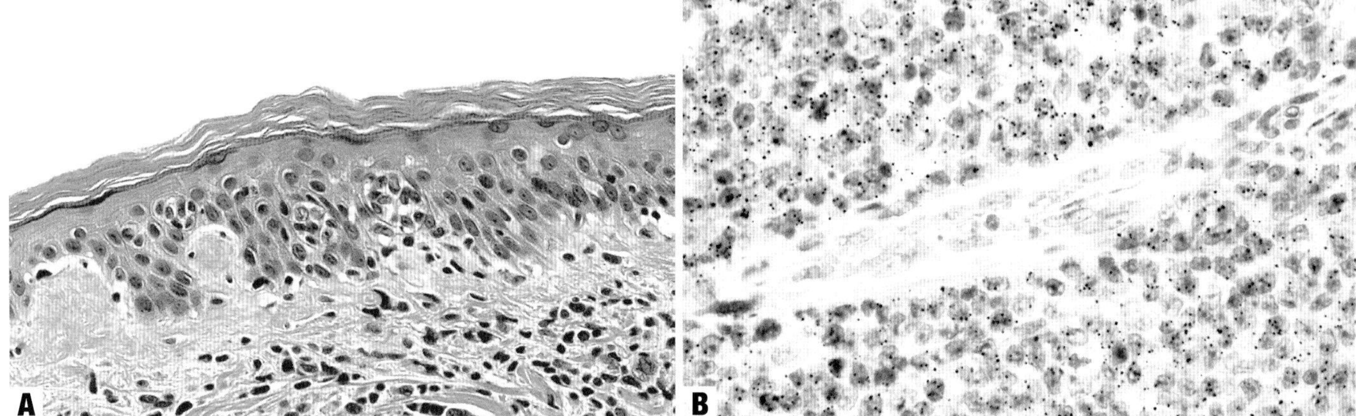

Fig. 5.39 Adult T-cell leukaemia/lymphoma involving skin. **A** The epidermis and dermis show infiltration by atypical lymphoid cells with irregularly folded nuclei. **B** In situ hybridization for HBZ, an HTLV-1–specific viral transcript. Numerous positive signals (brown dots) are observed in the neoplastic cells, whereas no signals are seen in the endothelial cells located in the centre of the figure.

in skin lesions; and peripheral T-cell lymphoma NOS, angioimmunoblastic-type nodal T follicular helper cell lymphoma, and systemic anaplastic large cell lymphoma in lymph nodes. The diagnosis of ATLL is confirmed by the detection of HTLV-1 antibody, or by demonstration of monoclonal integration of proviral HTLV-1 DNA. Nodal T follicular helper cell lymphoma, angioimmunoblastic type, can mimic ATLL cases because both can have a similar inflammatory background including eosinophilia. Regarding the distinction from classic Hodgkin lymphoma, atypia in the lymphoid cells surrounding HRS-like cells could be a clue to identifying Hodgkin like ATLL. The anaplastic variant of ATLL could be considered in the differential diagnosis

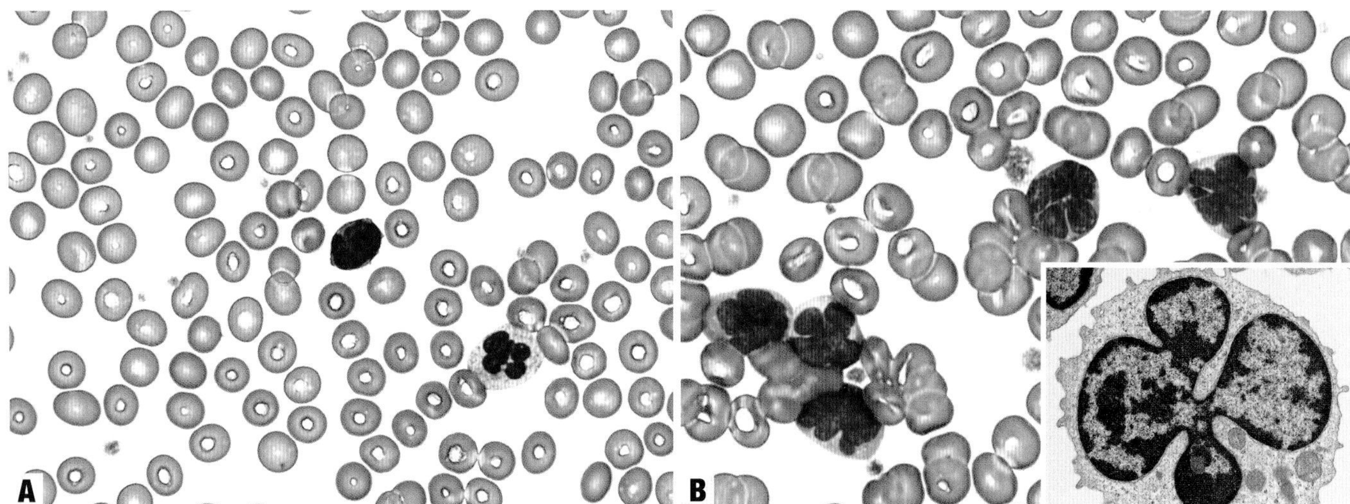

Fig. 5.40 Adult T-cell leukaemia/lymphoma: cytological findings of leukaemic cells. **A** In the smouldering subtype, small lymphoid cells with slight nuclear atypia are observed (Giemsa). **B** In the acute subtype, larger atypical cells with lobulated nuclei, namely flower cells, are usually seen (Giemsa). **Inset:** Electron microscopy shows a leukaemic cell with a characteristic flower-shaped nucleus.

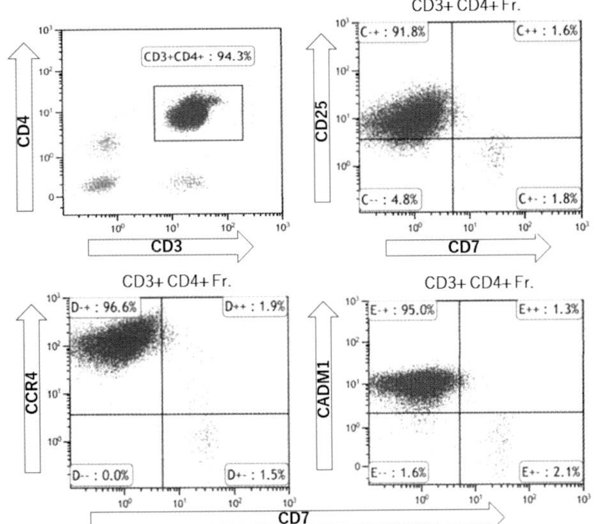

Fig. 5.41 Adult T-cell leukaemia/lymphoma. Flow cytometric analysis. Abnormal cells are detected as CD3+ and CD4+ (upper left). Those cells are CD25+ and CD7− (upper right), CCR4+ (lower left), and CADM1+ (lower right). This pattern could suggest aggressive adult T-cell leukaemia/lymphoma.

in the cases with cytotoxic molecule–negative ALK-negative anaplastic large cell lymphoma. In summary, it is crucial to test for HTLV-1 infection in all cases of T-cell lymphoma showing features of ATLL and in those with features of classic Hodgkin lymphoma where the background lymphoid cells (other than the HRS-like cells) appear atypical.

Cytology

The neoplastic cells in the peripheral blood and body cavity fluid are agranular, medium-sized to large lymphoid cells with irregular nuclei and basophilic cytoplasm, called flower cells in the acute variant. The cells in the smouldering or chronic variant are generally small, with a normal or less atypical appearance {4101}.

Diagnostic molecular pathology

Monoclonal integration of HTLV-1 can be demonstrated in neoplastic T cells using various molecular techniques on fresh; fresh-frozen; and formalin-fixed, paraffin-embedded material {3939,4466}.

Essential and desirable diagnostic criteria

Essential: neoplastic lymphoid cell proliferation with mature T-cell phenotype; proven HTLV-1 carriership.

Desirable: lymphoid cells with prominent convolutions and lobulation; identification of monoclonal integration of HTLV-1.

Staging

The Lugano classification (a modification of Ann Arbor staging) can be used.

Prognosis and prediction

Several clinicomolecular prognostic indexes have been proposed (see Table 5.04, p. 671) {3226,1908,1919,1920,1261,1248}. The prognosis of patients with stage I or II disease according to the Lugano classification is better than that of patients with advanced-stage disease; however, the clinical outcome is more closely correlated with the clinical subtype. The median survival times of patients with ATLL diagnosed in Japan in the 2000s were reported to be 8.3, 10.6, 31.5, and 55.0 months for the acute, lymphoma, chronic, and smouldering subtypes, respectively {1918}.

Sézary syndrome

Elenitoba-Johnson KSJ
Geddie WR
Ortonne N
Vermeer MH
Whittaker SJ
Willemze R

Definition

Sézary syndrome (SS) is a neoplasm of T lymphocytes, defined by the triad of erythroderma; generalized lymphadenopathy; and the presence of clonally related neoplastic T cells with cerebriform nuclei (Sézary cells) in the skin, lymph nodes, and peripheral blood.

ICD-O coding

9701/3 Sézary syndrome

ICD-11 coding

2B02 Sézary syndrome

Related terminology

None

Subtype(s)

None

Localization

SS is a generalized disease with a leukaemic presentation and characteristic involvement of the skin, with redness over most of the body (erythroderma). Lymphadenopathy and the involvement of any visceral organ can be observed at advanced stages, but the most common sites are the oropharynx, lungs, and CNS.

Clinical features

SS and mycosis fungoides share overlapping clinical and pathological features but are considered separate entities on the basis of differences in clinical behaviour and cell of origin {4379}.

Patients present with erythroderma and generalized lymphadenopathy. Other features are pruritus, alopecia, ectropion, palmar or plantar hyperkeratosis, lichenification, and onychodystrophy. Plaques (in the early stages) and generalized pruritus without erythroderma are rare {1554}. An increased prevalence of secondary cutaneous and systemic malignancies has been reported in SS and attributed to the immune dysregulation associated with skewing of the normal T-cell repertoire and loss of normal circulating CD4+ cells {1664}.

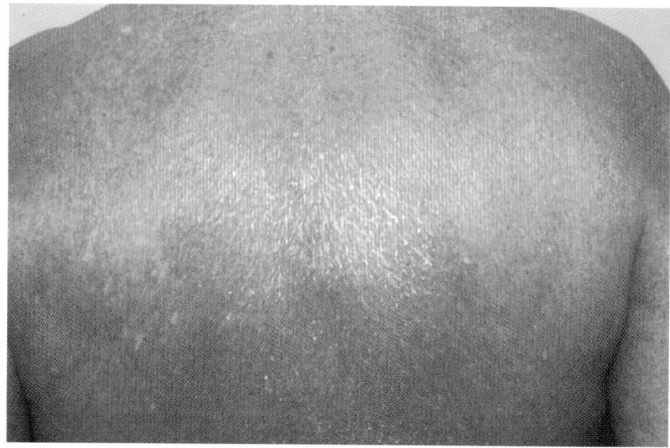

Fig. 5.42 Erythroderma in Sézary syndrome. A generalized erythrodermic rash with patchy reddening and scaling of skin.

Epidemiology

SS is rare, with a reported incidence of 0.36 cases per 100 000 person-years {1963}, accounting for 2–3% of all cutaneous T-cell lymphomas {4379,4377}. It occurs in adults, characteristically presenting in patients aged > 60 years, and shows a male predominance {3054,4379}.

Etiology

Computational studies of large genomic datasets have identified two mutation signatures in treatment-naïve SS: signature 1, associated with cellular ageing due to spontaneous deamination of methylated cytosines; and signature 7, characteristic of ultraviolet (UV) irradiation {1821}. This UV radiation signature is present in circulating tumour cells in SS and has also

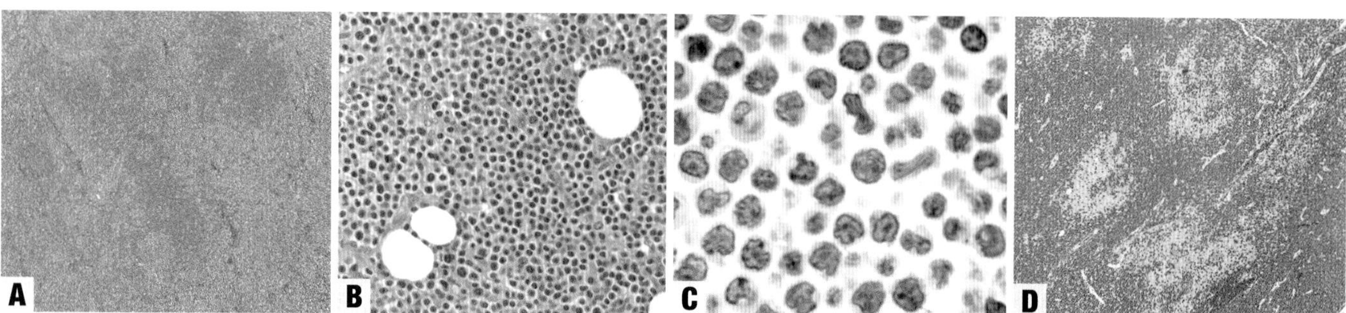

Fig. 5.43 Sézary syndrome involving lymph node. **A** There is paracortical expansion by an atypical lymphoid population composed of medium-sized lymphocytes. **B** The atypical lymphocytes have abundant clear cytoplasm and irregular nuclear features. **C** Neoplastic cells of Sézary syndrome demonstrate highly irregular, convoluted nuclei with clefts. **D** CD3 immunohistochemistry highlights the neoplastic cells of Sézary syndrome within the paracortical regions of the lymph node.

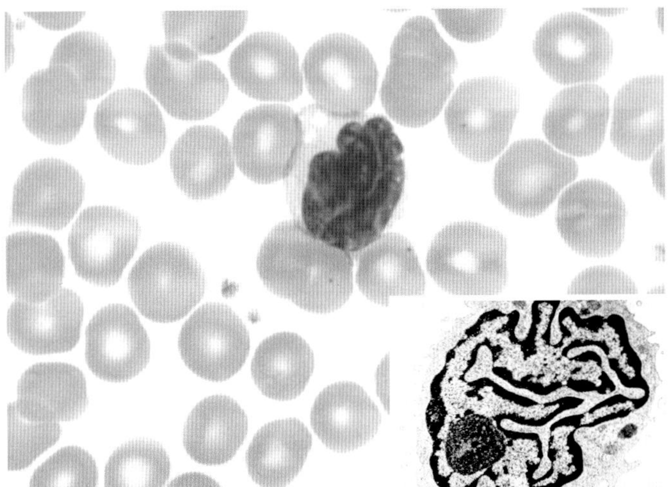

Fig. 5.44 Sézary syndrome. An atypical lymphocyte characteristic of Sézary syndrome (Giemsa). **Inset:** An electron micrograph of a Sézary cell showing a nucleus with invaginated nuclear membranes and deep nuclear clefting.

been found in mycosis fungoides but not in other mature T-cell lymphomas/leukaemias. This indicates that environmental UV radiation exposure is a key causal factor in the transformation of T cells that are either circulating through or resident in skin.

Pathogenesis

SS cells express markers indicative of a mature T-cell neoplasm, and the putative normal counterparts are circulating central memory T cells (CD27+, CD45RA–, CD45RO+) or skin-homing CD4+ T cells expressing CD45 (LCA), CCR4, and CCR7 contrasting with skin-resident memory T cells for mycosis fungoides {532}. Patients with SS are immunosuppressed because of the production of type 2 cytokines (T helper 2 [Th2]), which suppress T helper 1 (Th1) immunity. Genomic analyses of SS have revealed complex numerical and structural alterations similar to those in mycosis fungoides {273,2525,546}. SS is characterized by a high mutation burden reflecting causative UV radiation–induced mutations {1821}. Recurrent gain-of-function mutations (*PLCG1*, *CARD11*, *CD28*, *CARMIL2*[*RLTPR*]) {3137} affect T-cell receptor signalling pathways and upregulate NF-κB activity. Additionally, driver mutations are also found in DNA damage response pathways (*TP53*, *POT1*, *ATM*), JAK/STAT signalling (*STAT5B*; *JAK3*), and chromatin modifiers (*ARID1A*, *TRRAP*, *DNMT3A*, *TET2*) {3605,4184,729,4125,1981,4408,854,4298,3293,3160,3138,3137}. Recurrent balanced chromosomal translocations have not been detected, but isochromosome 17q is a recurrent feature of SS {4225}.

Macroscopic appearance

The macroscopic appearance corresponds to the clinical features.

Histopathology

Peripheral blood

Peripheral blood smears reveal characteristic Sézary cells, which are large atypical lymphocytes containing an abnormally shaped, deeply grooved nucleus with nuclear convolutions (cerebriform nucleus).

Lymph nodes and tissues

Involved lymph nodes show partial or complete effacement of the architecture by a dense, monotonous infiltrate of Sézary cells {3609}. The neoplastic cells are medium in size with irregular contours and deep clefts, and they show CD3 expression.

The cellular infiltrates involving skin tend to be monotonous, and epidermotropism is not invariably present. The dermal lymphocytic infiltrate is often perivascular. In as many as one third of biopsies from patients with otherwise classic SS, the histological picture may be nonspecific {4078}. Bone marrow may be involved, but infiltrates are often sparse and mainly interstitial {3737}.

Immunophenotype

The neoplastic T cells typically show a CD3+, CD4+, CD8– phenotype with frequent aberrant loss of pan–T-cell antigens such as CD2, CD5, CD7, and/or CD26 {2050}. PD1 (CD279) is expressed by neoplastic cells in skin and blood in almost all cases {598}. Sézary cells express cutaneous lymphocyte antigen (CLA) and the skin-homing receptor CCR4, as well as CCR7 {1190}. Sézary cells also typically express TCRαβ, CD25, and ICOS, and they sometimes express CXCL13. The natural killer cell markers CD158k (KIR3DL2) and NKp46 may also be expressed {3072,3073}.

Differential diagnosis

SS should be distinguished from inflammatory erythrodermic dermatoses and other haematological malignancies presenting with erythroderma. Additionally, SS should be distinguished from adult T-cell leukaemia/lymphoma. Benign conditions such as drug reactions, psoriasis, chronic eczema, pityriasis rubra pilaris, scabies, dermatomyositis, lupus, pemphigus foliaceus, and erythematous dermatitis should be excluded.

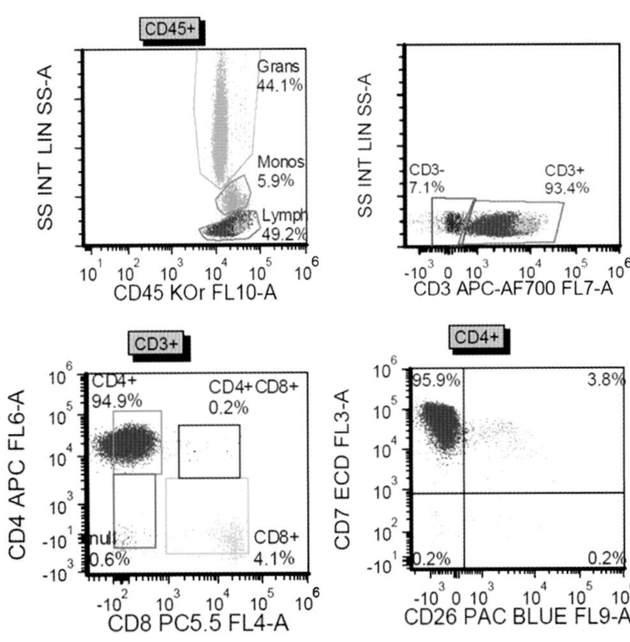

Fig. 5.45 Sézary syndrome. Flow cytometry demonstrating immunophenotypic features of Sézary syndrome. There is a large population of CD3^{dim}, CD4+ T cells with expression of CD7 but a total absence of CD26.

Cytology

See above

Diagnostic molecular pathology

The tumour cells are clonal by TR gene rearrangement analysis {3276,4365,4366}.

Essential and desirable diagnostic criteria

Essential: (1) erythroderma involving > 80% of the body surface area; (2) evidence of blood involvement by a neoplastic T-cell population defined by clonal TR gene rearrangements; (3) an absolute Sézary cell count ≥ 1000/µL, OR an expanded CD4+ T-cell population with a CD4:CD8 ratio > 10, OR an expanded CD4+ T-cell population with an abnormal phenotype (CD4+/CD7− T cells ≥ 40% or CD4+/CD26− T cells ≥ 30%).

Staging

Staging for SS involves evaluating the skin (T), lymph nodes (N), visceral organs (M), and blood (B). Given the systemic nature of the disease at presentation, patients with SS are considered to have stage IVA1, IVA2, or IVB disease depending on the presence of nodal and visceral involvement {3054} (see Table 5.08, p. 691, in *Mycosis fungoides*).

Prognosis and prediction

SS is an aggressive disease, with a median survival time of 32 months and a 5-year overall survival rate of 10–30%, depending on stage {4379}. Most patients die of opportunistic infections. The degree of peripheral blood involvement at diagnosis may have an impact on prognosis {4253}, but the prognostic relevance of bone marrow involvement is unknown.

Aggressive NK-cell leukaemia

Suzuki R
Cheng CL
Khoury JD
Kwong YL
Loughran TP Jr
Ng S-B
Ott G
Takeuchi K
Yamaguchi M

Definition

Aggressive NK-cell leukaemia (ANKL) is a systemic malignant proliferation of NK cells, with an acute presentation, highly aggressive clinical course, and frequent association with EBV.

ICD-O coding

9948/3 Aggressive NK-cell leukaemia

ICD-11 coding

2A90.3 Aggressive NK-cell leukaemia

Related terminology

Acceptable: aggressive NK-cell leukaemia/lymphoma.

Not recommended: NK-large granular lymphocyte leukaemia; aggressive large granular lymphocyte leukaemia.

Subtype(s)

None

Localization

The most commonly involved sites are the peripheral blood, bone marrow, liver, and spleen, but any organ can be involved {615,3894}.

Clinical features

Patients usually present with fever, constitutional symptoms, a leukaemic blood picture, and manifestations of haemophagocytic syndrome {3894,1742,2295}. The number of circulating leukaemic cells ranges from low to high and is < 20% in one third of patients. Hepatosplenomegaly is common and is sometimes accompanied by abnormal liver function tests and jaundice,

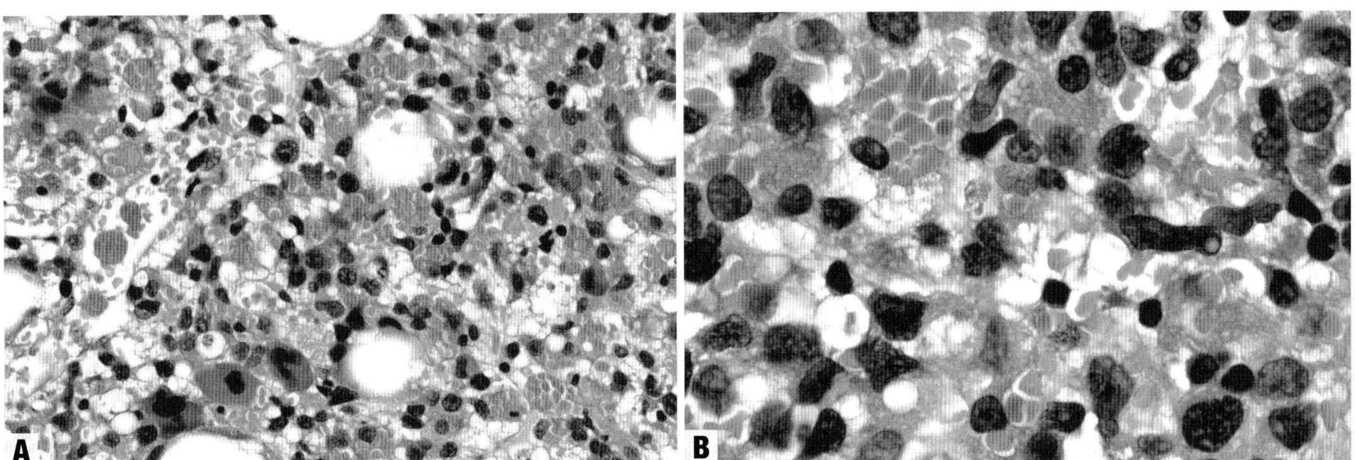

Fig. 5.46 Aggressive NK-cell leukaemia, bone marrow biopsy. **A** Extensive involvement by a monotonous population of uniform-appearing leukaemic cells. There are admixed histiocytes with phagocytosed red blood cells. **B** The leukaemic cells show nuclear pleomorphism and irregular folds.

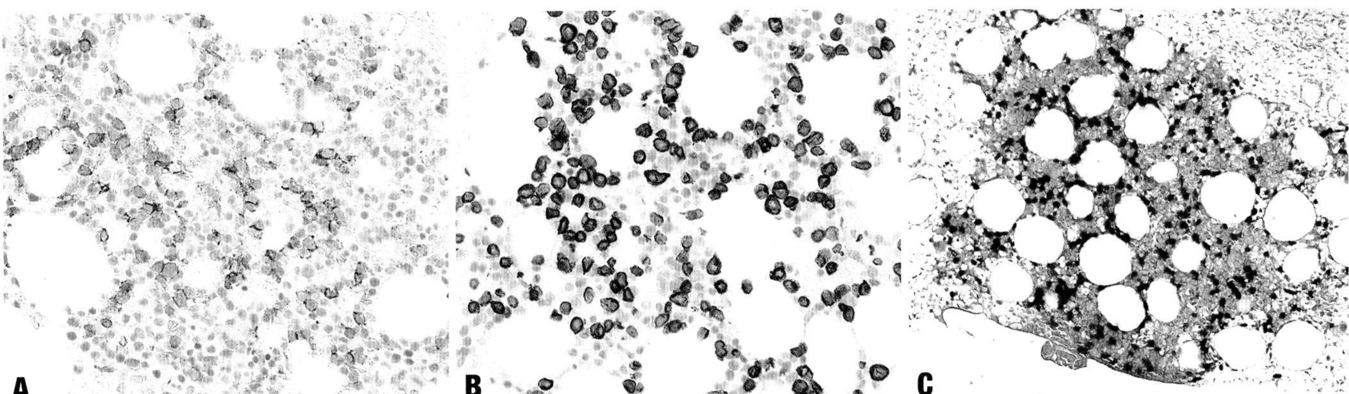

Fig. 5.47 Aggressive NK-cell leukaemia, bone marrow biopsy. **A** The leukaemic cells show positive staining for CD56 on the cell surface. **B** Immunostaining for CD3 highlights the leukaemic population and further accentuates the nuclear irregularities. **C** In situ hybridization for EBV-encoded small RNA (EBER) highlights the positive leukaemic cells in bone marrow.

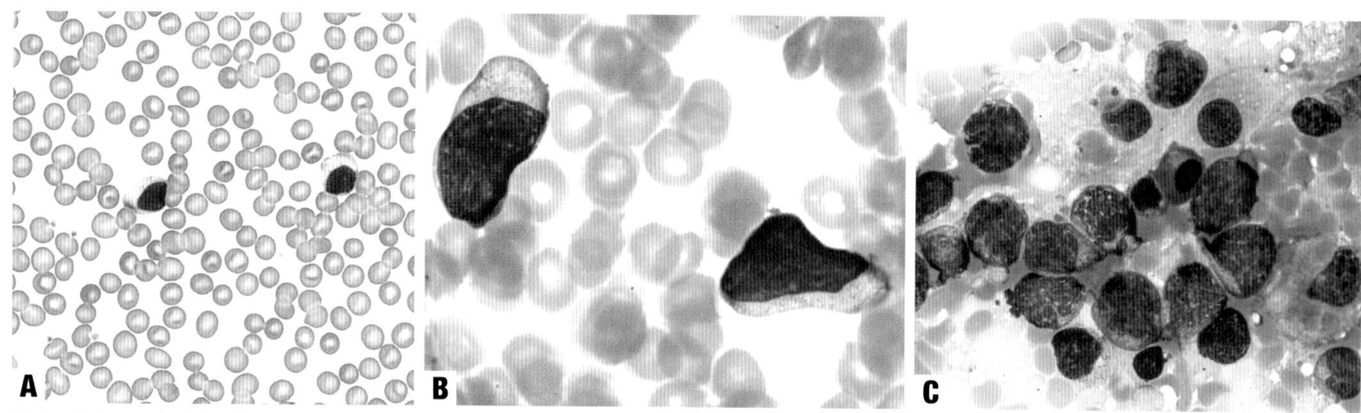

Fig. 5.48 Aggressive NK-cell leukaemia. **A** In a peripheral blood smear, the leukaemic cells are very similar to normal large granular lymphocytes in this case (Giemsa). **B** The leukaemic cells in the bone marrow show basophilic cytoplasm, and nuclei with more condensed chromatin and distinct nucleoli. Azurophilic granules can be observed in the cytoplasm (Giemsa). **C** Nuclear pleomorphism and haemophagocytosis are apparent (Giemsa).

mimicking hepatitis. Lymphadenopathy may be present, but skin and nasal lesions are uncommon. ANKL may be complicated by coagulopathy and multiorgan failure {3046,2785}.

Epidemiology

ANKL is a rare form of leukaemia that is more prevalent in Asian populations {3787,3894,2295}. Patients are most commonly young to middle-aged adults (median age: 40 years) {3787, 3894,1742,2295,3966}, and there is no sex predilection {3787, 3894,1742,2295,3966,1717,2178,620}.

Etiology

The etiology is unknown. A strong association with EBV (in ~90% of cases) suggests the virus has a pathogenetic role, but the overall low prevalence of ANKL implies the involvement of other (unknown) factors. In younger patients, ANKL may evolve from chronic active EBV disease {1745,3141,2021}. Exceptional cases may evolve from NK-large granular lymphocytic leukaemia (NK-LGLL) {3015,3016}.

Pathogenesis

EBV is reported to be positive in 85–100% of cases, and EBV is present in a clonal episomal form {620,1510,1932}. EBV-negative ANKLs occur de novo or evolve from NK-LGLL; they show clinicopathological features similar to those of EBV-positive cases, but it is currently unclear whether the clinical outcomes are similar {3894,1742,2068,2953,1283,1734}.

A variety of clonal cytogenetic abnormalities have been reported, such as del(6)(q21q25), i(7)(q10), and 11q deletion {3894,3509}. An array-based comparative genomic hybridization study has shown some differences in genetic changes between ANKL and extranodal NK/T-cell lymphoma (ENKTL): losses in 7p and 17p and gains in 1q are frequent in ANKL but not in ENKTL, whereas loss in 6q is more common in ENKTL {2888}. Genome-wide sequencing identified mutations in genes encoding components of the JAK/STAT and RAS/MAPK pathways, histone modifying molecules (*TET2*, *CREBBP*, *KMT2D*, *DDX3X*), and immune checkpoint molecules *CD274* (*PDL1*) / *PDCD1LG2* (*PDL2*) {3966, 1016,1665,1056}. *TP53* is mutated in one third of cases.

Macroscopic appearance

Not relevant

Histopathology

Circulating leukaemic cells vary in appearance from cells indistinguishable from normal large granular lymphocytes to cells with atypical nuclei featuring enlargement, irregular folds, open chromatin, or distinct nucleoli {615,1742}. They have ample pale or lightly basophilic cytoplasm containing fine or coarse azurophilic granules. Bone marrow smears show scant to abundant leukaemic cells, and there are commonly reactive histiocytes in the background showing haemophagocytosis.

The leukaemic infiltrates in organ sites (skin, liver, spleen, mucosal sites, bone marrow) are diffuse or patchy and destructive. The morphology is similar to that of the leukaemic populations, with round or irregularly folded nuclei, condensed chromatin, and small nucleoli, but significant nuclear pleomorphism can be present. Apoptosis of tumour cells is frequently seen.

Immunophenotype

The leukaemic cells are typically CD2+, sCD3−, CD3ε+, CD5−, CD7+, CD16+, CD56+, and positive for cytotoxic molecules (granzyme B, perforin, and/or TIA1) {3894,2295,3966}. CD8 and CD11b may be expressed, whereas CD57 is usually negative {3079,620}. There is a lack of T-cell receptor protein expression. The neoplastic cells express FASL, and high levels of FASL can be found in the serum of affected patients {1915,2492,3958}. The majority of cases show positive labelling for EBV-encoded small RNA (EBER) in leukaemic cells on in situ hybridization.

Differential diagnosis

The main differential diagnoses include disseminated ENKTL, NK-LGLL, T-large granular lymphocytic leukaemia (T-LGLL), and hepatosplenic T-cell lymphoma. All these diseases share the presence of neoplastic lymphoid cells that have azurophilic granules, but the clinical presentations, disease localizations, immunophenotypes, and genotypes are different. ANKL shows clinicopathological overlap with disseminated ENKTL, but it is differentiated by its acute fulminant systemic clinical presentation and lack of nasal involvement {615,3894}. The two indolent leukaemic neoplasms, NK-LGLL and T-LGLL, are associated with mild or no symptoms at presentation, lack of morphological atypia in the circulating large granular lymphocytes, and absence of EBV; furthermore, T-LGLL is of T rather than NK lineage. Hepatosplenic T-cell lymphoma may present similarly to

ANKL, but circulating leukaemic cells are uncommon, the neoplastic cells are of T lineage (often with TCRγδ expression), EBV is negative, and isochromosome 7q is frequently found.

Intravascular NK/T-cell lymphoma

With current limited data, intravascular NK/T-cell lymphoma is provisionally included under the category of ANKL {3575,2158, 592,2387,66,4541,1250}. In contrast to extranodal NK/T-cell lymphoma, intravascular NK/T-cell lymphoma does not present with mass lesions and shows a predilection for the skin and CNS. It is a highly aggressive neoplasm with a poor prognosis, especially in cases with multisystem involvement. The pathobiology has been linked to a tumorigenic role of EBV in most cases {354}. Somatic mutations in epigenetic regulators (*DDX3X*, *ARID1A*, histone genes) have been identified {1249}.

Cytology

See *Histopathology*.

Diagnostic molecular pathology

Germline configuration of TR genes supports an NK-cell lineage.

Essential and desirable diagnostic criteria

Essential: presentation with fever, constitutional symptoms, and a leukaemic blood picture; systemic (multiorgan) involvement by neoplastic lymphoid cells with an NK-cell immunophenotype; absence of T-cell receptor protein expression and/or clonal TR rearrangement.

Desirable: EBER positivity (positive in ~90% of cases); haemophagocytic lymphohistiocytosis.

Staging

None

Prognosis and prediction

Most cases pursue a fulminant clinical course, often complicated by coagulopathy, multiorgan failure, and/or haemophagocytic syndrome. The median survival time is measured in months {3787,3894,1742,2295,3966}. Response to conventional chemotherapy is poor, but L-asparaginase–containing regimens can be effective in some patients {1742,3893,3927}. Allogeneic haematopoietic stem cell transplantation performed in patients who achieve a response may potentially be curative {1475,1252}.

Introduction to primary cutaneous T-cell neoplasms

Kempf W
Pulitzer M
Willemze R

Primary cutaneous lymphomas constitute the second most common group of extranodal lymphomas. Cutaneous T-cell lymphomas (CTCLs) represent the majority of cutaneous lymphomas. They comprise a heterogeneous group of lymphoma entities with diverse clinical features (papules, patches, plaques, nodules, erythroderma) and histology (intraepidermal, dermal, and/

Table 5.05 Cutaneous T-cell lymphomas: epidemiological, clinicopathological, and prognostic features (adapted from {4377})

Type and subtypes	Frequency[a]	Clinical features	Histological features (predominant growth pattern and cytomorphology)	Course	5-year disease-specific survival rate[a]
Mycosis fungoides	39%	Patches, plaques, tumours	Epidermotropic infiltrate in all stages; nodular infiltrate with variable epidermotropism in tumour stage Small LCs in early-stage disease (patch) Admixture of medium-sized and large LCs in advanced stages (thick plaques, tumours)	Indolent	88%
Folliculotropic mycosis fungoides	5%			Variable	75%
Pagetoid reticulosis	1%			Indolent	100%
Granulomatous slack skin	1%			Indolent	100%
Sézary syndrome	2%	Erythroderma	Epidermotropic infiltrate Blood involvement	Aggressive	36%
Primary cutaneous CD30-positive lymphoproliferative disorders					
Lymphomatoid papulosis	12%	Papules and small nodules	Epidermotropic or dermal infiltrates Atypical CD30+ LCs of variable size	Indolent	99%
Cutaneous anaplastic large cell lymphoma	8%	Tumour(s)	Nodular infiltrate of CD30+ large LCs with severe nuclear atypia	Indolent	95%
Subcutaneous panniculitis-like T-cell lymphoma	1%	Deep-seated plaques or nodules	Subcutaneous infiltrates Medium-sized LCs	Indolent	80%
Primary cutaneous gamma-delta T-cell lymphoma	< 1%	Plaques and nodules	Epidermotropic or dermal nodular infiltrates Medium-sized to large LCs	Aggressive	11%
Cutaneous CD8+ aggressive epidermotropic T-cell lymphoma	< 1%	Erosive or ulcerated plaques and nodules	Epidermotropic infiltrate Medium-sized to large LCs	Aggressive	31%
Primary cutaneous CD4+ small/medium T-cell lymphoproliferative disorder	6%	Solitary nodule	Dermal nodular infiltrate Small LCs and intermingled medium-sized LCs	Indolent	100%
Primary cutaneous acral CD8+ T-cell lymphoma	< 1%	Solitary nodule	Dermal nodular infiltrate Small to medium-sized LCs	Indolent	100%
Primary cutaneous peripheral T-cell lymphoma NOS	< 1%	Nodule(s), rarely papules and plaques No patches	Nodular infiltrate Medium-sized to large LCs	Aggressive	15%
Adult T-cell lymphoma/leukaemia[b]	1%	Erythema, papules, plaques, tumours, erythroderma	Epidermotropic or dermal nodular infiltrates Medium-sized to large cells	Indolent/aggressive	Variable
Systemic chronic active EBV disease[b]	< 1%	Papulovesicular eruption	Dermal, often angiodestructive infiltrates Small to medium-sized LCs	Indolent	Variable

LC, lymphoid cell.
[a]Frequency and survival rates among cutaneous lymphomas, based on data included in Dutch and Austrian cutaneous lymphoma registries between 2002 and 2017. [b]Adult T-cell leukaemia/lymphoma and systemic chronic active EBV disease both also involve extracutaneous organs and are covered in separate sections.

or subcutaneous infiltrates of lymphocytes of variable size and morphology). Likewise, they exhibit differing phenotypes (cytotoxic and/or γδ T, T follicular helper [TFH]) and genetic features (see Table 5.05).

Primary cutaneous lymphomas are initially present in the skin, without extracutaneous disease. They often remain limited to the skin over long periods of disease evolution. Progression with extracutaneous spread usually occurs in the advanced stages.

Because the various forms of CTCL have overlapping histological and phenotypic features, correlation of the clinical features with the histological and immunophenotypic findings is an essential element of the diagnostic workup and implies that clinical photos and dermatological examination and discussion in multidisciplinary tumour boards are indispensable for diagnosis and management of CTCLs {4377,1955}.

The prognosis and treatment algorithms for CTCLs differ significantly among the various entities within this group {768}. In addition, despite identical histological, phenotypic, and genetic alterations being shared by some CTCL entities with nodal or other extranodal T-cell lymphomas, their diagnostic and prognostic significance and therapeutic implications may differ markedly {3322}. Mycosis fungoides and cutaneous CD30+ lymphoproliferative disorders (LPDs) account for 80% of all CTCLs, and although geographical differences exist in the prevalence of CTCL and its subtypes, mycosis fungoides is the most common form of CTCL worldwide. Certain subtypes (folliculotropic mycosis fungoides, pagetoid reticulosis) differ in their course and prognosis from classic patch/plaque mycosis fungoides and are identifiable by their distinct clinical and/or histological features {4376}.

CD30+ LPDs are the second most common CTCL group and represent a disease spectrum including primary cutaneous anaplastic large cell lymphoma (ALCL), lymphomatoid papulosis, and borderline cases {1953}. Primary cutaneous ALCL generally lacks t(2;5)(p23;q35)/*NPM1::ALK* and ALK expression and differs biologically from systemic ALCL by its good prognosis. Primary cutaneous ALCL and lymphomatoid papulosis show overlapping histological and phenotypic features not only with each other but also with other cutaneous or systemic T-cell lymphomas. As a consequence, knowledge of the clinical presentation and evolution of tumoural lesions is crucial for a definitive diagnosis. Although the pleomorphic cytomorphology of the neoplastic CD30+ cells suggests a highly malignant behaviour, the primary cutaneous CD30+ LPDs exhibit a favourable prognosis with absent or low mortality. Therefore, overtreatment in CD30+ LPD should be avoided.

Remarkably, primary mucosal and mucocutaneous CD30+ LPDs of the head and neck area share many clinicopathological features with primary cutaneous CD30+ LPDs, including indolent clinical behaviour {3655}. Therefore, they are probably closer to primary cutaneous CD30+ LPD than to systemic ALK− ALCL.

The other forms of CTCL included here are rare, with each entity accounting for < 1% of all CTCLs {4377}. This group encompasses subcutaneous panniculitis-like T-cell lymphoma, primary cutaneous CD8+ aggressive epidermotropic cytotoxic T-cell lymphoma, primary cutaneous gamma-delta T-cell lymphoma, primary cutaneous CD4+ small or medium T-cell LPD, and primary cutaneous acral CD8+ T-cell LPD {3841}. In the previous (revised fourth) edition of the WHO classification of haematolymphoid tumours, these lymphomas were grouped together, under "cutaneous peripheral T-cell lymphoma, rare subtypes". In the current edition they are listed as separate entities within the overarching hierarchical structure. The term "primary cutaneous peripheral T-cell lymphoma NOS" is used only for the very rare cases that do not fit into any of the other specified CTCL entities {4377}.

Primary cutaneous CD4-positive small or medium T-cell lymphoproliferative disorder

Vergier B
Jansen PM
Mitteldorf C
Ortonne N
Pulitzer M
Willemze R

Definition

Primary cutaneous CD4-positive small or medium T-cell lymphoproliferative disorder (PCSM-LPD) is characterized by a predominance of small to medium-sized CD4-positive pleomorphic T cells within a solitary skin lesion, without evidence of the plaques typical of mycosis fungoides.

ICD-O coding

9709/1 Primary cutaneous CD4-positive small or medium T-cell lymphoproliferative disorder

ICD-11 coding

2B0Y & XH3QE7 Other specified primary cutaneous mature T-cell or NK-cell lymphomas and lymphoproliferative disorders & Primary cutaneous CD4-positive small/medium T-cell lymphoproliferative disorder

Related terminology

Not recommended: primary cutaneous CD4+ small/medium pleomorphic T-cell lymphoma; pseudolymphomatous folliculitis.

Subtype(s)

None

Localization

The head and neck are most commonly involved (50% of cases), followed by the trunk and the upper and lower extremities.

Clinical features

The clinical presentation of PCSM-LPD is most frequently an asymptomatic erythematous solitary nodule, or less frequently a tumour, papule, macule, or plaque. The size ranges from 4 to 60 mm. PCSM-LPD affects men in the majority of cases {973}, and paediatric cases have been described {1421,301,304,280, 1782,62}.

PCSM-LPD has a benign clinical course, similar to that of cutaneous lymphoid hyperplasia. Because of this, the term "lymphoproliferative disorder" is preferred over "lymphoma".

Because multifocal presentation is exceedingly rare in PCSM-LPD, in patients with multifocal lesions a diagnosis of systemic T-cell lymphoma with secondary cutaneous involvement – especially peripheral T-cell lymphoma NOS and nodal T follicular helper (TFH) cell lymphomas – should be excluded.

Epidemiology

PCSM-LPD is the second most common cutaneous T-cell lymphoproliferative disorder after mycosis fungoides, accounting for 6% {4377} to 7.5% of primary cutaneous lymphomas {973}.

Etiology

Unknown

Pathogenesis

The pathogenesis is unknown. PCSM-LPD may reflect a response to an antigen stimulus with recruitment of both B cells and T cells, including a significant TFH-cell population {216}.

Macroscopic appearance

The macroscopic appearance corresponds to the clinical findings.

Histopathology

There are two common architectural patterns (see Table 5.06, p. 684). Most commonly (in 78% of cases) a nodular and/or diffuse lymphoproliferation infiltrating the entire dermis is seen, sometimes expanding into the subcutis. Less frequently, a subepidermal band-like infiltrate filling the superficial dermis is

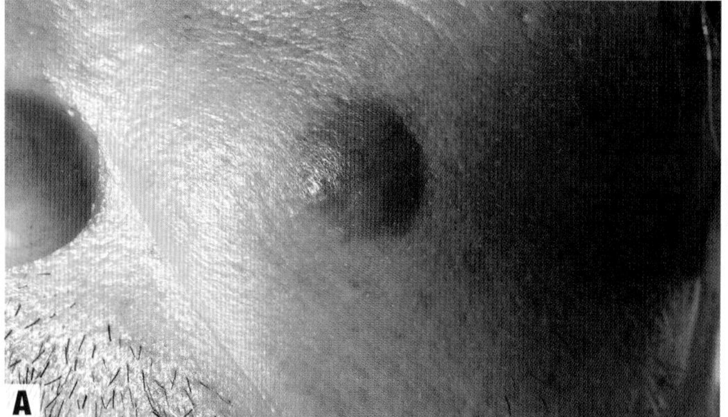

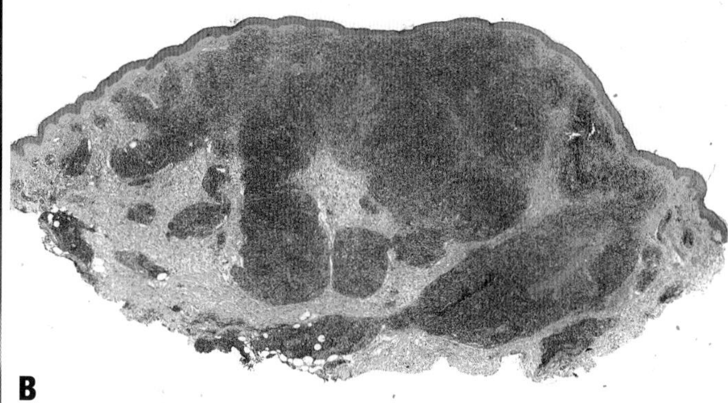

Fig. 5.49 Primary cutaneous CD4-positive small or medium T-cell lymphoproliferative disorder. **A** Clinical presentation with an erythematous solitary nodule on the face. **B** The histological architecture correlates with the clinical presentation. The nodular lymphoproliferation infiltrates the entire dermis (pattern 1).

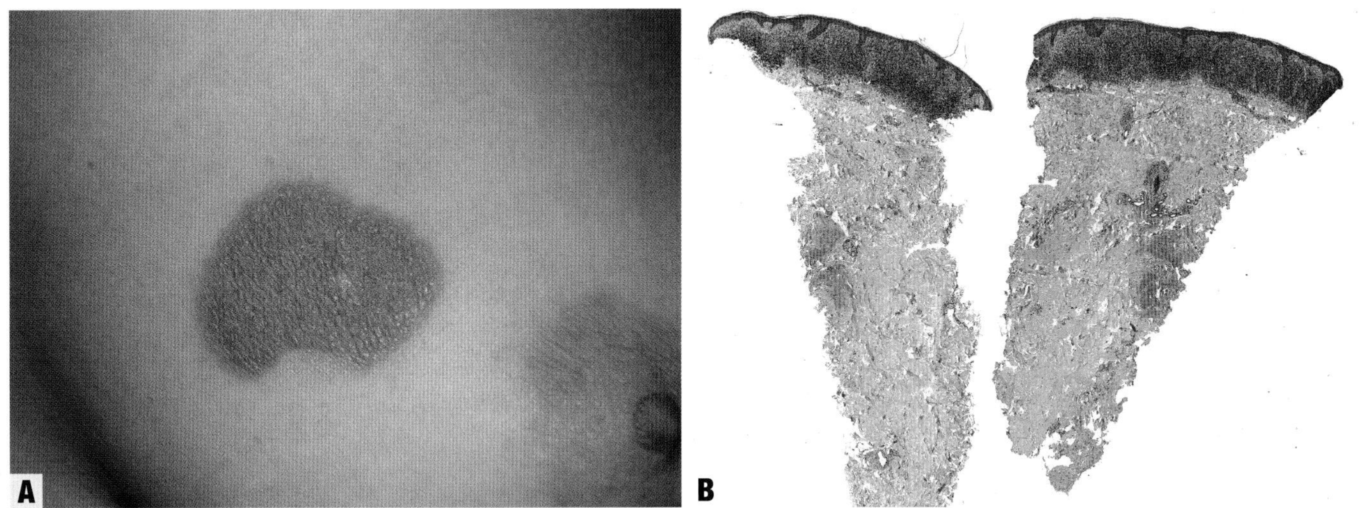

Fig. 5.50 Primary cutaneous CD4-positive small or medium T-cell lymphoproliferative disorder. **A** Clinical presentation with an erythematous macule/plaque. **B** The histological architecture correlates with the clinical presentation. The subepidermal band-like infiltrate fills the superficial dermis (pattern 2).

encountered, often associated with a periadnexal distribution and often resembling mycosis fungoides {304,599}. Epidermotropism may be present focally, but if it is particularly conspicuous, the diagnosis of mycosis fungoides should be considered. Adnexotropism accompanied by follicular destruction is very characteristic {301,304,3188}.

A predominance of small/medium-sized pleomorphic T cells with no more than 40% of large cells is characteristic {217,304, 2480}. Lymphoid follicles are uncommon.

Immunohistochemistry

The tumour cells of PCSM-LPD have a CD3+, CD4+, CD8−, CD30− phenotype. The infiltrate is admixed with a B-cell component, which can account for as many as 60% of the cells, sometimes with immunoblasts {217,2480}. The loss of pan–T-cell antigens (except for CD7) is uncommon. Cytotoxic proteins are not expressed {1421,301,599,3438}. Atypical CD4+ T cells express TFH-cell markers: PD1 (expressed by medium-sized to large cells that form clusters or rosettes {3438}, ICOS, CXCL13

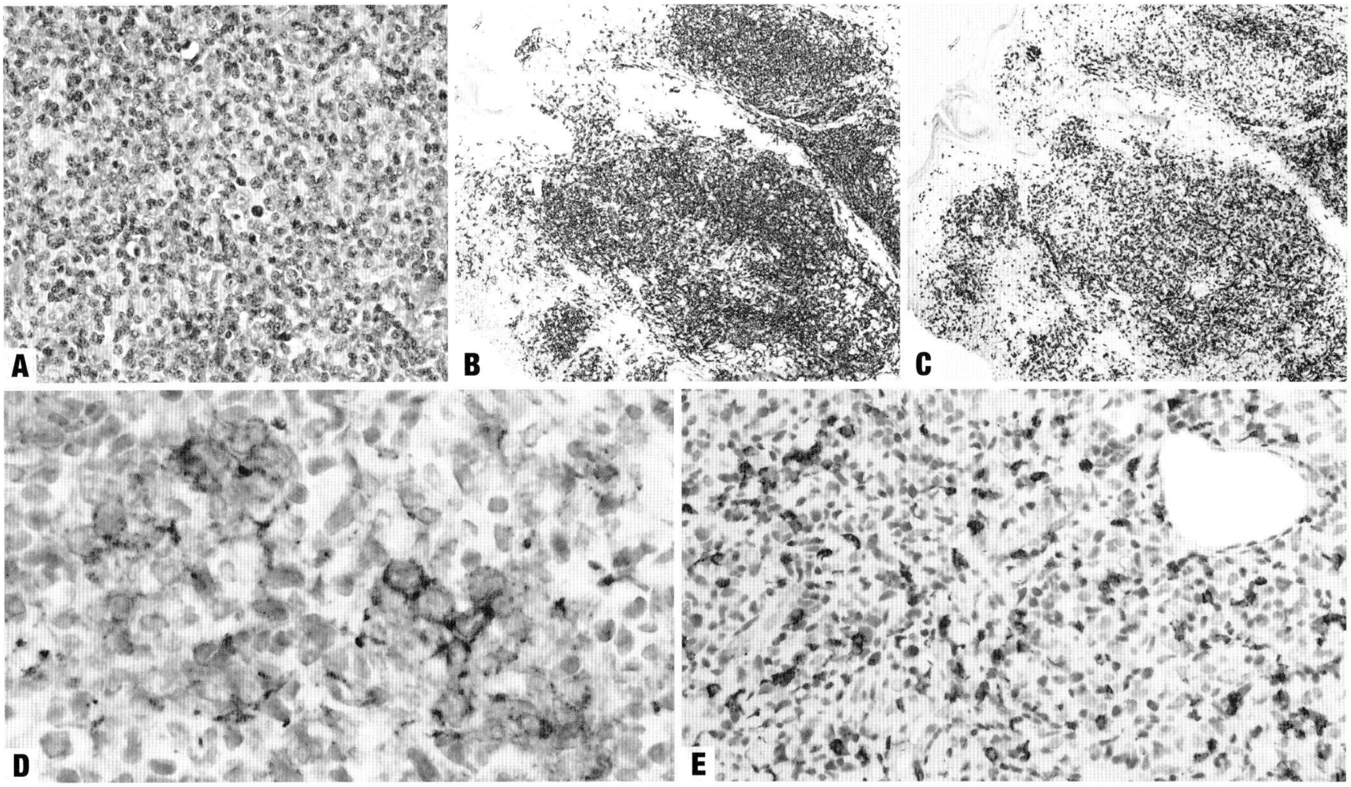

Fig. 5.51 Primary cutaneous CD4-positive small or medium T-cell lymphoproliferative disorder. **A** Infiltrate with a predominance of small/medium-sized pleomorphic cells. **B** CD4 immunostain revealing a CD4-positive lymphoproliferation. **C** CD20 immunostaining showing a prominent B-cell component. **D** Expression of PD1 by medium to large cells forming rosettes. **E** CD8 immunostaining showing sprinkling of small reactive CD8+ lymphocytes.

Table 5.06 Main features of the two patterns observed in primary cutaneous CD4-positive small or medium T-cell lymphoproliferative disorder

Features	Pattern 1 (75%)	Pattern 2 (25%)
Clinical	Reddish symmetrical papule/nodule Head and neck / upper trunk	Papule/macule/plaque Trunk and limbs
Infiltrate	Deep dermis +/− hypodermis Nodular and diffuse	Superficial dermis Band-like
Epidermotropism	Rare	Frequent
PD1	Clusters/rosettes	Clusters/rosettes
ICOS	Sparse	Clusters/rosettes
CXCL13	Rare positive cells	Often positive
Differential diagnosis	Cutaneous lymphoid hyperplasia, marginal zone lymphoma	Cutaneous lymphoid hyperplasia, mycosis fungoides

(a few positive cells), and BCL6 (expressed by sparse medium-sized to large lymphocytes), but not CD10 {304}. The Ki-67 proliferation index is often low (~25%) but in rare cases can reach 40% {3941}. Small reactive CD8+ T cells arranged in a starry-sky pattern {304}, sparse CD30+ T or B cells {217,3438,2480}, plasma cells, eosinophils, and histiocytes (including multinucleated giant cells) may be present {301,304,599}. Plasma cells can be light chain–restricted.

Differential diagnosis

The main differential diagnoses are cutaneous lymphoid hyperplasia (although this and PCSM-LPD exist on a spectrum), mycosis fungoides, CD30+ lymphomatoid papulosis (characterized by multiple skin lesions), and cutaneous marginal zone lymphoma {216}. Rare cases with widespread skin lesions, > 40% large pleomorphic T cells, and/or a high proliferative fraction are better classified, after multidisciplinary discussion, as primary cutaneous peripheral T-cell lymphoma NOS.

Cytology

Fine core needle biopsy is not recommended for the diagnosis of PCSM-LPD.

Diagnostic molecular pathology

TR genes are clonally rearranged in the majority (70%) of cases 21989349; 18987541; 33915243}, with no impact on the prognosis {304}. A coexisting B-cell clone can occur (26% of cases) {217,304}.

Essential and desirable diagnostic criteria

Essential: an asymptomatic solitary skin lesion; one of the two architectural patterns (nodular and/or diffuse vs band-like; see Table 5.06); predominance of CD4+ small or medium-sized pleomorphic T cells admixed with a B-cell component; TFH-cell phenotype: strong PD1 expression by atypical cells +/− ICOS, BCL6, and CXCL13 expression, but CD10 is negative.

Desirable: localization: head and neck > trunk > extremities; adnexotropism; absence of lymphoid follicles; scattered reactive cells: CD8+ T cells, CD30+ cells, plasma cells, eosinophils, and histiocytes.

Staging

Not relevant

Prognosis and prediction

Patients have an excellent prognosis with uncommon local or distant recurrences and no long-term risk of secondary lymphoma {3887,338}. Intralesional steroids, surgical excision, and radiotherapy are the preferred modes of treatment. Spontaneous regression after biopsy is frequent (reported in 32% of cases) {1421,304,1782,599}.

Primary cutaneous acral CD8-positive T-cell lymphoproliferative disorder

Kempf W
Mitteldorf C
Pulitzer M
Robson A

Definition

Primary cutaneous acral CD8-positive T-cell lymphoproliferative disorder is characterized by dermal, non-epidermotropic infiltrates of clonal medium-sized CD8+ cytotoxic lymphocytes, preferentially located at acral sites.

ICD-O coding

9709/3 Primary cutaneous acral CD8-positive T-cell lymphoproliferative disorder

ICD-11 coding

2B0Y & XH7S84 Other specified primary cutaneous mature T-cell or NK-cell lymphomas and lymphoproliferative disorders & Primary cutaneous acral CD8-positive T-cell lymphoma

Related terminology

Not recommended: indolent CD8+ lymphoid proliferation of the ear; primary cutaneous acral CD8-positive T-cell lymphoma.

Subtype(s)

None

Localization

There is a predilection for acral sites, especially the ears (the most common site), nose, hands, and feet {302,1407,3909,2303, 2058,4025}. Rare cases in other sites, such as the eyelids, trunk, genitals, and leg, have been reported {1968,1407,1466,1950}.

Clinical features

Primary cutaneous acral CD8-positive T-cell lymphoproliferative disorder manifests usually as an asymptomatic solitary, reddish, non-ulcerated papule or nodule, and less frequently as a plaque, measuring as large as 40 mm in size, that grows slowly over weeks or months. Rarely the lesions are multiple {1407} or bilateral, particularly on the ears and feet {302,506, 3211,4393}.

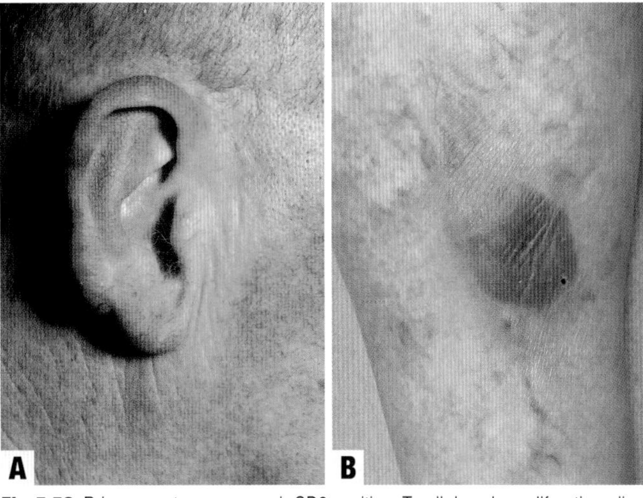

Fig. 5.52 Primary cutaneous acral CD8-positive T-cell lymphoproliferative disorder. **A** Presentation with a slightly reddish nodule on the lower half of the ear helix. **B** An erythematous, non-scaling plaque on the leg.

Epidemiology

The disease is rare, accounting for < 1% of all primary cutaneous lymphomas {4378}. It affects adults (median age: 56 years) with an M:F ratio of 2:1 {2058,4025}. Paediatric cases have not been reported.

Etiology

The etiology is unknown, and no infectious or causative agents have yet been identified.

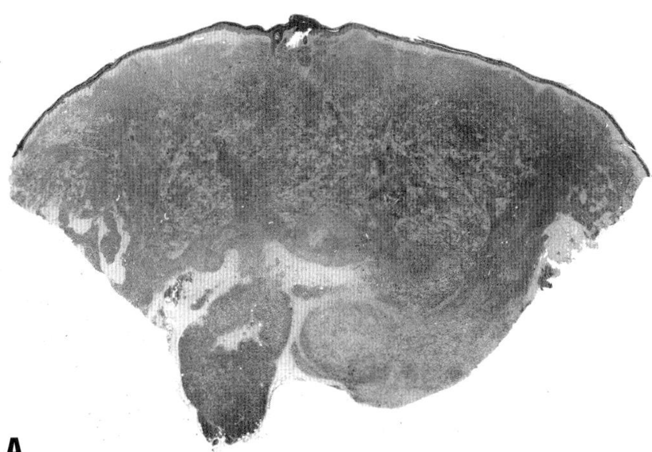

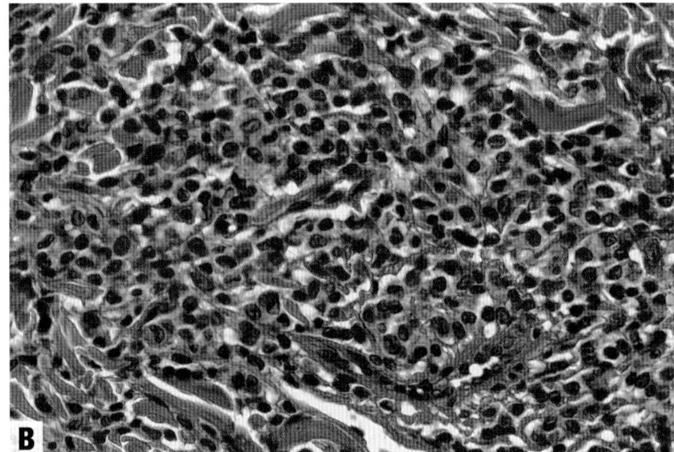

Fig. 5.53 Primary cutaneous acral CD8-positive T-cell lymphoproliferative disorder. **A** Low-power magnification shows a dense dermal monotonous infiltrate separated from the overlying epidermis by a grenz zone. **B** Higher-power magnification shows medium-sized tumour cells with moderate nuclear atypia, fine chromatin, and small nucleoli.

Table 5.07 Differential diagnosis of primary cutaneous acral CD8-positive T-cell lymphoproliferative disorder

Entity	Clinical features	Histological features	Phenotype	Course
CD8+ acral T-cell lymphoproliferative disorder	Solitary nodule at acral site	Dense monotonous infiltrate of mostly medium-sized tumour cells, moderate nuclear atypia, grenz zone, no epidermotropism	CD3+, CD4–, CD8+, CD30– TIA1+, granzyme B–, perforin– CD68 dot-like expression by tumour cells (disease-specific) Low proliferation (Ki-67/MIB1) EBV–	Indolent
Primary cutaneous peripheral T-cell lymphoma NOS (CD8+)	Rapidly growing solitary, multiple, or disseminated nodules	Dense infiltrates of mostly medium-sized to large tumour cells with prominent nuclear pleomorphism and mitotic activity Angioinvasive growth possible No epidermotropism	CD3+, CD4–, CD8+, CD30– TIA1+, granzyme B+/–, perforin+/– Moderate to high proliferation (Ki-67/MIB1) EBV–	Variable
CD8+ mycosis fungoides, tumour stage	Often ulcerated large tumour in a patient with preceding or concurrent patches and plaques	Tumour cells of variable size, moderate to severe nuclear pleomorphism Epidermotropism often present	CD3+, CD4–, CD8+, CD30+/– High proliferation (Ki-67/MIB1)	Aggressive
Primary cutaneous CD8+ aggressive epidermotropic cytotoxic T-cell lymphoma	Rapidly growing erosive or ulcerated multiple or disseminated plaques and nodules	Prominent epidermotropism of medium-sized atypical lymphocytes, apoptotic keratinocytes, ulceration	CD3+, CD4–, CD8+, CD30–, CD45RA+ TIA1+, granzyme B+/–, perforin+/– High proliferation (Ki-67/MIB1)	Aggressive
Lymphomatoid papulosis (subtype D)	Grouped papules and small nodules, with spontaneous regression of individual lesions within a few weeks	Prominent epidermotropism and dermal infiltrate of medium-sized atypical lymphocytes	CD3+, CD4–, CD8+, CD30+ TIA1+ High proliferation (Ki-67/MIB1)	Indolent
Lymphoproliferations in congenital immunodeficiency (inborn error of immunity)	Mostly multiple brownish papules and plaques	Dermal infiltrates of small lymphocytes with chromatin-dense nuclei and subtle or absent nuclear atypia, numerous histiocytes, and small granulomas No epidermotropism	CD3+, CD4–, CD8+, CD30– Numerous CD68+ histiocytes without dot-like staining Low proliferation (Ki-67/MIB1)	Indolent
Primary cutaneous gamma-delta T-cell lymphoma	Rapidly evolving ulcerated plaques and deep-seated nodules	Variable with epidermotropic, dermal, and/or subcutaneous infiltrates of medium-sized atypical lymphocytes Necrosis and angioinvasion may be present	TCRγ+ and TCRδ+ TCRβ– CD3+, CD2+, CD4–, CD5– CD7+/–, rarely CD8+ CD56+ (most cases) Expression of at least one cytotoxic protein: TIA1, granzyme B, perforin	Aggressive

Pathogenesis

No genetic or epigenetic factors contributing to tumour formation have yet been described.

Macroscopic appearance

The lesions appear as nodules (see *Clinical features*).

Histopathology

The tumour is composed of a dense and monotonous dermal proliferation of atypical medium-sized lymphocytes with irregular and frequently folded nuclei with fine chromatin and moderate nuclear pleomorphism {3211}. Less commonly, a perivascular pattern is observed. Mitotic activity is low (< 1%) or absent. The epidermis is mostly spared, but focal minimal epidermotropism and focal folliculotropism may be seen {506, 1407}. In one third of the cases, the epidermis is separated from the dermal infiltrate by a grenz zone. Plasma cells, histiocytes, neutrophils, and eosinophils are absent or few. The proliferation frequently extends into the underlying subcutis.

Immunohistochemistry

The tumour cells display a CD3+, CD4–, CD8+, CD30–, βF1+, and cytotoxic phenotype, with expression of TIA1, whereas granzyme B and perforin are usually negative. There has been 1 reported case with an exceptional CD4+, CD8+ phenotype {4027}. Loss or weak expression of one or more T-cell markers (CD2, CD5, CD7) is found in 85% of cases {4238}. The tumour cells express CD99 but are negative for CD56 and PD1 {2303}. CD57, CD30, TdT, and T follicular helper (TFH) cell markers are always negative {1407}. CD68 displays a characteristic Golgi dot-like staining pattern in the tumour cells, which is almost unique to this entity {4394}. The proliferation index (Ki-67/MIB1) is typically low (< 10%), although a few cases with a high proliferation index have been reported {3909}. There may be reactive B-cell aggregates or (rarely) secondary follicles. EBV is always negative.

Differential diagnosis

The differential diagnosis includes other non-epidermotropic dermal CD8-positive lymphoproliferations (see Table 5.07).

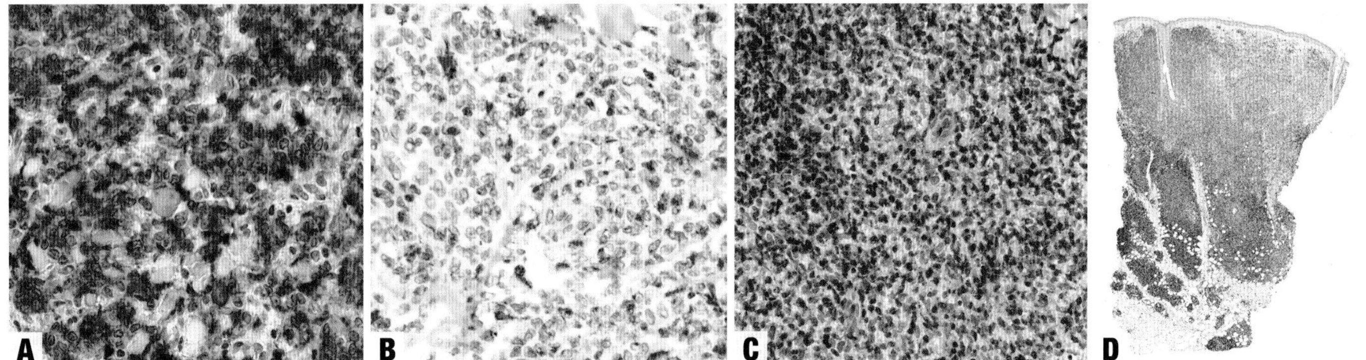

Fig. 5.54 Primary cutaneous acral CD8-positive T-cell lymphoproliferative disorder. Immunohistochemistry shows expression of CD8 by tumour cells (**A**), characteristic dot-like staining for CD68 in tumour cells (**B**), expression of TIA1 (**C**), and partial loss of CD5 (**D**).

Cytology

The cytology is not clinically relevant, because FNAB is not recommended for making this diagnosis.

Diagnostic molecular pathology

The neoplastic T cells show clonal rearrangements of TR (TCR) genes in nearly all cases {1958}.

Essential and desirable diagnostic criteria

Essential: a dense, predominantly dermal, non-epidermotropic infiltrate of atypical small to medium-sized CD8+ cytotoxic T cells; typical clinical presentation, most commonly as a solitary nodule at an acral site; no extracutaneous involvement at diagnosis.

Desirable: characteristic Golgi dot-like expression of CD68 by tumour cells; monoclonal rearrangement of TR genes; absence of immunodeficiency, EBV always negative.

Staging

The TNM classification system for primary cutaneous lymphomas other than mycosis fungoides is applied {2015}. Radiological staging is not mandatory if typical clinical and histopathological findings are present and in the absence of immunodeficiency {4377,4378}.

Prognosis and prediction

The tumour has an excellent prognosis {2058,1958}. Fatal outcomes have not been reported. Complete remission after surgical excision or local radiation therapy is the rule {4377, 1958}. Recurrence after treatment is possible; it may be more frequent in younger patients, and it can occasionally occur at other cutaneous sites {61,1407,4394,2303,2605}. Dissemination to extracutaneous sites has been reported in only 1 case {61}.

Mycosis fungoides

Pulitzer M
Berti E
Geddie WR
Guitart J
Kim JE
Pimpinelli N
Sander CA
Vermeer MH
Willemze R

Definition

Mycosis fungoides (MF) is a primary cutaneous T-cell lymphoma clinically characterized by the sequential evolution of patches, plaques, and tumours, and pathologically comprising infiltrates of clonal small to medium-sized mature T cells with hyperconvoluted nuclei, which are epitheliotropic in most cases.

ICD-O coding

9700/3 Mycosis fungoides
9700/3 Folliculotropic mycosis fungoides
9700/3 Pagetoid reticulosis
9700/3 Granulomatous slack skin disease

ICD-11 coding

2B01 Mycosis fungoides

Related terminology

Not recommended: classic mycosis fungoides (type Alibert–Bazin); Woringer–Kolopp disease.

Subtype(s)

Folliculotropic mycosis fungoides; pagetoid reticulosis; granulomatous slack skin disease

Localization

Skin lesions of MF can be one or few, localized or multiple and widespread, and sometimes even confluent. When localized, the lesions often occur in sun-protected areas, like skin flexures (axillae, groins) and the lower trunk / buttocks (bathing-trunk distribution). Extracutaneous dissemination occurs exclusively in the latest stages of disease, initially involving the draining lymph nodes, and occasionally spreading more extensively to the viscera and blood {1091}.

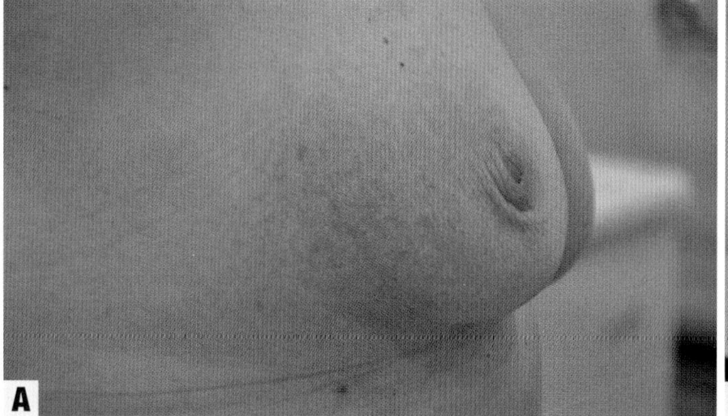

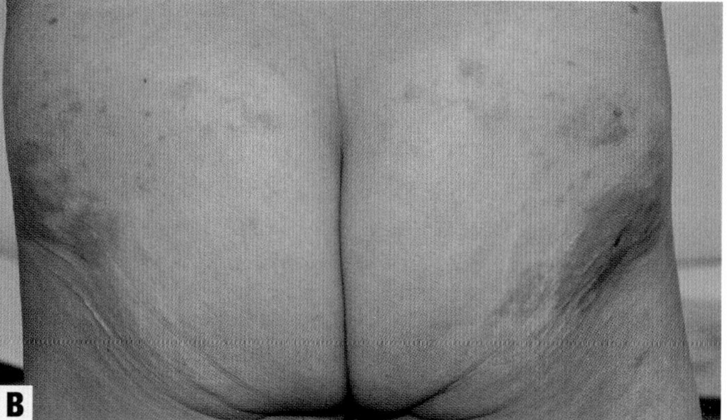

Fig. 5.55 Mycosis fungoides, stage IA. **A** Presentation with a poikilodermatous patch of the breast. **B** Patches localized in the bathing-trunk area.

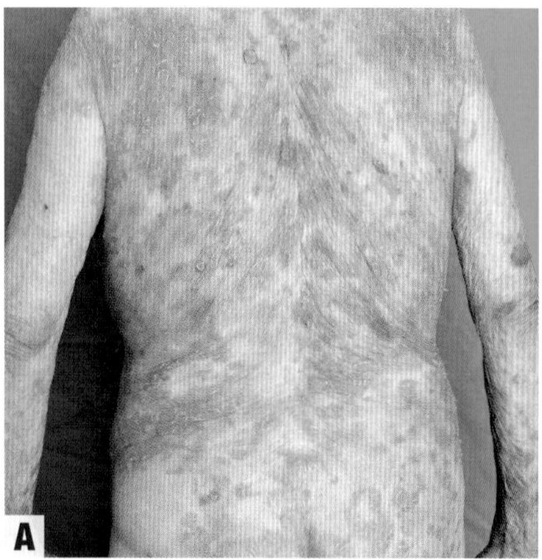

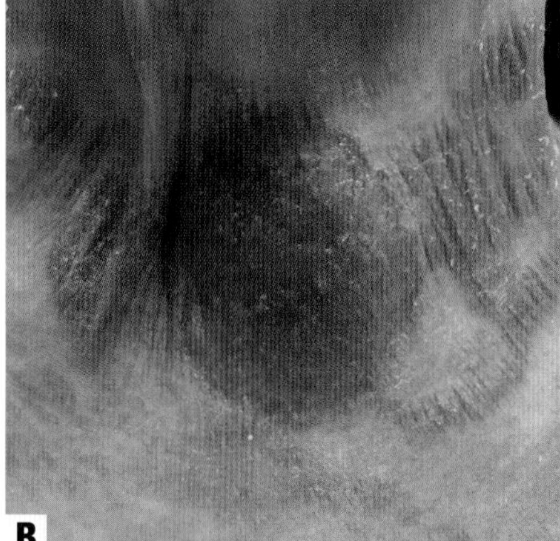

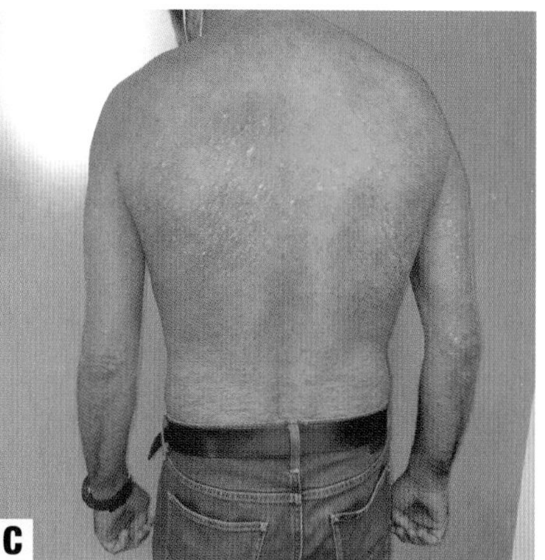

Fig. 5.56 Mycosis fungoides. **A** Stage IB, presenting with disseminated patches and thin plaques on the trunk. **B** Stage IIB, presenting as a confluent plaque on the neck. **C** Stage III, presenting as a diffuse erythroderma.

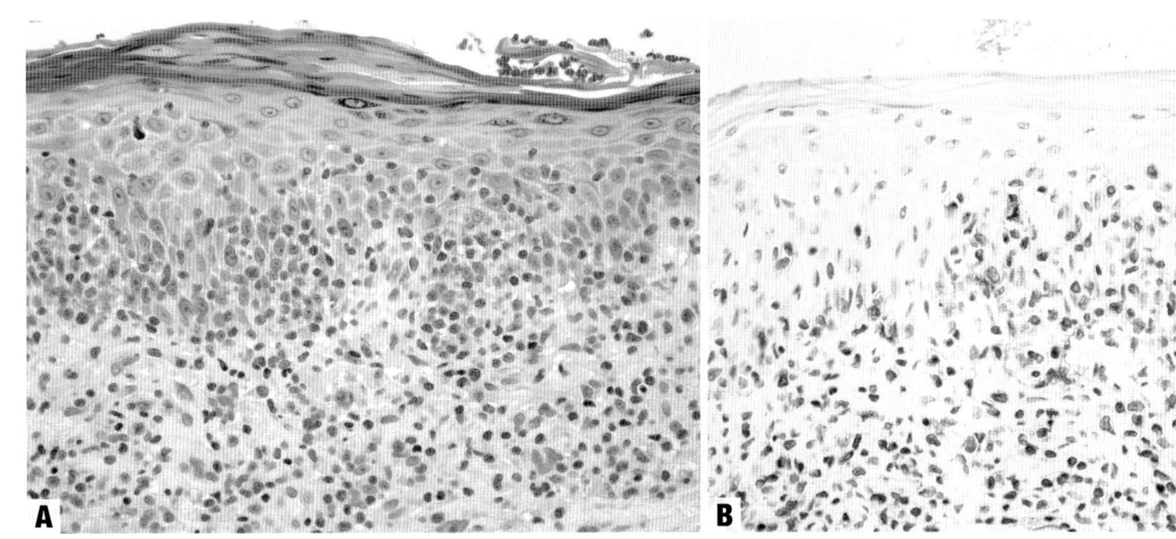

Fig. 5.57 Mycosis fungoides, patch/plaque stage. **A** Patch lesion. Small atypical lymphocytes migrate into the lower to middle layers of the epidermis and are present in the superficial papillary dermis. **B** TCRβ immunostaining shows atypical epidermotropic lymphocytes, with weak cytoplasmic TCRα/β heterodimer spotlighting cerebriform nuclei.

Clinical features

MF is characterized by an indolent clinical course over years or decades, with persistent, slowly growing lesions. Early-stage MF presents with patches and plaques {3246}, whereas advanced-stage MF characteristically shows progression to nodules/tumours or erythroderma.

MF patches are erythematous and scaling. The skin may look finely wrinkled and thinner than normal. MF plaques are variably infiltrated and scaling, with a red to brown hue. Patches and plaques are sharply demarcated, annular to arciform and polycyclic, and they might occur separately or simultaneously in the same patient. In dark skin, the lesions show dyschromia and are often hypopigmented rather than erythematous, although occasionally they are hyperpigmented {1313}. Tumours generally arise in advanced disease, typically occurring in patients with a long history of patches and plaques. Tumours may become eroded and ulcerate.

Bacterial superinfection is common in the advanced stages of the disease and is much rarer in the early stages. Skin and soft tissue infections and pneumonia are frequent causes of sepsis in these patients and a major cause of hospitalization and death {372}.

Subtypes of MF deviate from the classic clinical course. The clinical and histological features of these subtypes are described in *Histopathology*.

Epidemiology

MF is the most common type of cutaneous T-cell lymphoma, accounting for > 50% of cases, with an incidence of 5.8 cases per 1 million person-years {1792,1926}. MF can present at any age, with a peak incidence in patients in their late fifties {2815}. MF can also present in children and adolescents (4–11% of MF cases) {4424,1835}. The M:F ratio is 2:1 {1792}. The disease is reported in more White people (77.7%) than Black, Hispanic, or Asian people. However, the number of cases of MF is disproportionately high in Black populations {3859}, where MF seems to have a female predilection, an earlier onset, and a worse prognosis {3859,1659,931}.

Etiology

No clear etiological factor has been identified {3228}. Aggressive, transient antibiotic treatment is associated with decreases in the fraction of neoplastic T cells, cell proliferation, and STAT3 signalling, suggesting that the microbiome may be involved in the evolution of a malignant clone {2361}. Early MF is thought to be mediated by contact with immature antigen-presenting cells, leading to constitutive T-cell receptor activation, which along with defects in the apoptosis pathway may lead to early clonal expansion of T cells, contributing to the evolution of the disease {2124,323}.

Pathogenesis

Recent next-generation sequencing data have identified genetic aberrations in signalling pathways and epigenetic processes that may contribute to the pathogenesis of MF, i.e. in the context of chronic antigenic stimulation of skin-resident T lymphocytes {2124,323}. Alteration of tumour suppressor pathways {4125, 729,854}, and/or constitutive T-cell activation, chromatin modification, cell-cycle regulation, and alterations of NF-κB signalling

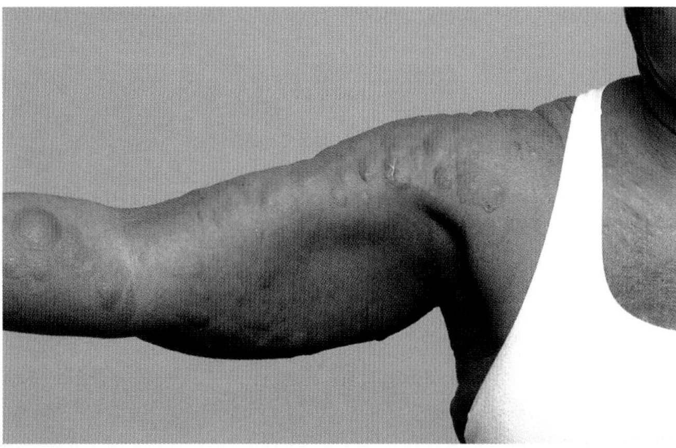

Fig. 5.58 Mycosis fungoides with large-cell transformation and erythroderma. Numerous skin nodules amenable to sampling by FNA are present on the arm.

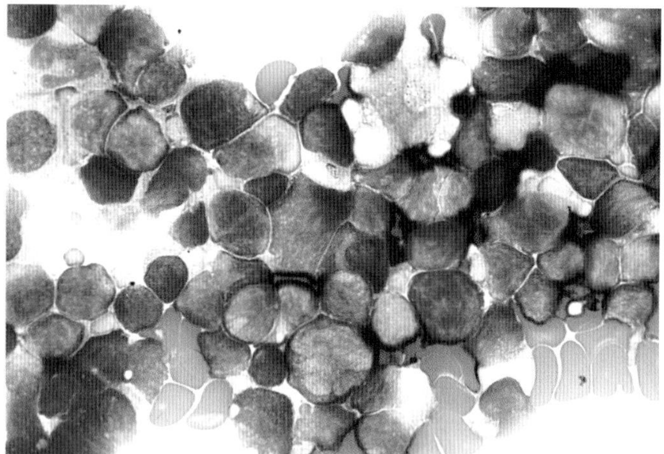

Fig. 5.59 Mycosis fungoides, large-cell transformation. FNAB of a skin nodule (Giemsa). Smears show large pleomorphic cells with convoluted nuclei.

downstream of the T-cell receptor may be involved in regulating T-cell survival and proliferation {632,3138}. Alterations of the JAK-3/STAT3 and MAPK signal transduction pathways may contribute to the survival and proliferation of malignant T cells in MF {210,4221,3781,3187,4275,1987}. Hypomethylation and hypermethylation signatures have been observed in MF; for example, *DNMT3A*, a gene encoding a methyltransferase, is often mutated or deleted in MF, signifying that genetic aberrations may underlie epigenetic dysregulation {3228,632}.

Macroscopic appearance

See *Clinical features*.

Histopathology

Histological features differ with disease stage. Early-stage (patch) lesions are characterized by subtle epidermotropic infiltrates of small to medium-sized haloed lymphocytes with hyperchromatic hyperconvoluted (cerebriform) nuclei, lining up along the basal and lower-middle layers of the epidermis, often associated with a mild to dense band of reactive small lymphocytes and admixed histiocytes. As the lesions transition to plaque-stage disease, lymphocytes may more prominently colonize both upper layers of the epidermis, in a pagetoid pattern or forming clusters or collections (Pautrier microabscesses) tightly associated with Langerhans cell scaffolding {2579}. MF tumours often fail to display the hallmark feature of epidermotropism, instead filling the dermis as diffuse sheets of small, medium-sized, and large atypical cells.

Large-cell transformation (LCT) is defined by the presence either of > 25% large lymphoid cells or of aggregates of large cells in dermal infiltrates. It should be noted that the designation of LCT

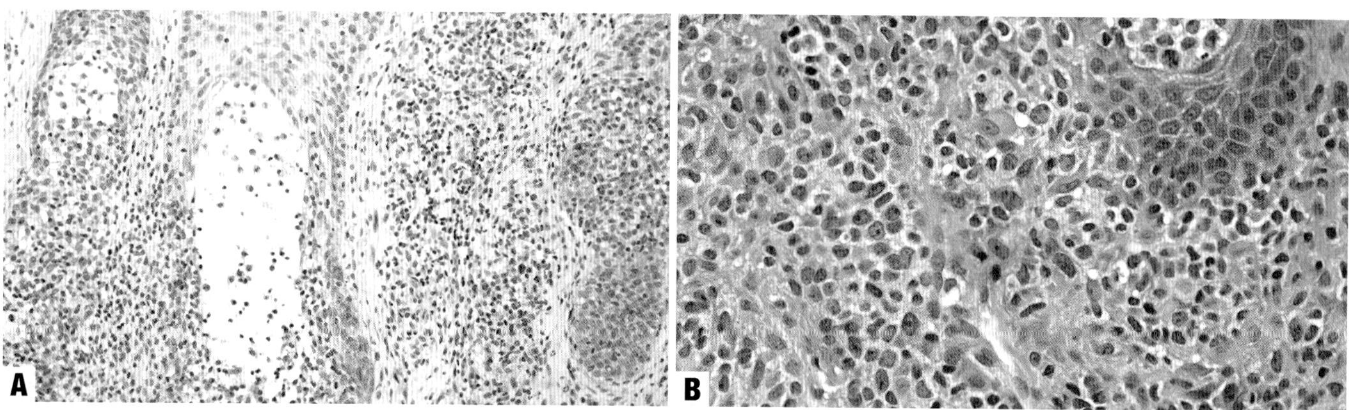

Fig. 5.60 Mycosis fungoides. **A** Folliculotropic mycosis fungoides, early lesion, with follicular mucin. Small to medium-sized atypical lymphocytes, epitheliotropic to follicular epithelium, and sebaceous gland structures. Mucin pools are present. **B** Plaque lesion. Medium-sized atypical lymphocytes with Pautrier microabscess formation and diffuse, band-like involvement of the papillary dermis.

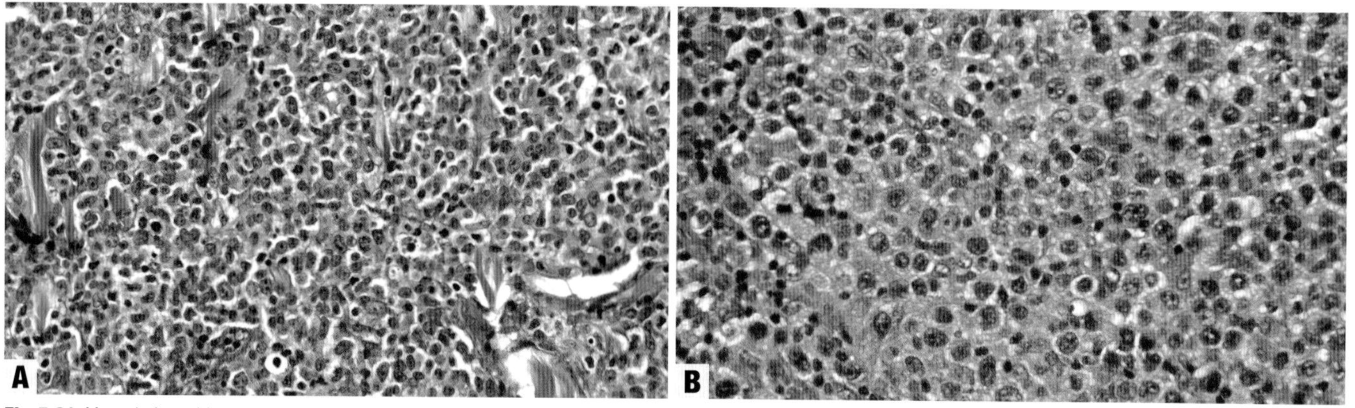

Fig. 5.61 Mycosis fungoides, tumour stage. **A** Tumour lesion showing diffuse sheets of medium-sized atypical lymphocytes with hyperchromatic convoluted nuclei. **B** At high magnification, the cytonuclear features of large transformed cells are appreciated.

has relatively poor interobserver reproducibility, however {1427}. It is commonly associated with or may herald disease progression.

Biopsy of enlarged lymph nodes is often performed for staging purposes. Enlarged lymph nodes from patients with MF frequently show dermatopathic lymphadenopathy with paracortical expansion due to the large number of histiocytes, some containing melanin pigment, and also Langerhans and interdigitating cells with abundant pale cytoplasm. Early involvement by MF cells may be difficult to identify in nodal tissue, requiring flow cytometric evaluation and molecular studies for TCR clonality; however, in higher N-stage disease, the normal architecture of the nodes becomes effaced by malignant cells, which are clearly recognizable {3054}.

Table 5.08 TNMB staging of mycosis fungoides and Sézary syndrome according to the International Society for Cutaneous Lymphomas (ISCL) and the European Organisation for Research and Treatment of Cancer (EORTC) {3054}

Category	T/N/M/B stage					Substage (if applicable)	
Skin	T1	Limited patches, papules, and/or plaques covering < 10% of the skin surface				T1a T1b	Patch only Plaque ± patch
	T2	Patches, papules, and/or plaques covering ≥ 10% of the skin surface				T2a T2b	Patch only Plaque ± patch
	T3	One or more tumours (≥ 10 mm diameter)					
	T4	Confluence of erythema covering ≥ 80% of the body surface area					
Node	N0	No clinically abnormal peripheral lymph nodes; biopsy not required					
	N1	Clinically abnormal peripheral lymph nodes; histopathology Dutch grade 1 or NCI LN 0–2				N1a N1b	Clone-negative Clone-positive
	N2	Clinically abnormal peripheral lymph nodes; histopathology Dutch grade 2 or NCI LN 3				N2a N2b	Clone-negative Clone-positive
	N3	Clinically abnormal peripheral lymph nodes; histopathology Dutch grade 3–4 or NCI LN 4; clone-positive or clone-negative					
	Nx	Clinically abnormal peripheral lymph nodes; no histological confirmation					
Viscera	M0	No visceral organ involvement					
	M1	Visceral organ involvement (must have pathology confirmation); the organ involved should be specified					
Blood	B0	Absence of significant blood involvement: ≤ 5% of peripheral blood lymphocytes are atypical (Sézary) cells				B0a B0b	Clone-negative Clone-positive
	B1	Low blood tumour burden: > 5% of peripheral blood lymphocytes are atypical (Sézary) cells, but the criteria for B2 are not met				B1a B1b	Clone-negative Clone-positive
	B2	High blood tumour burden, Sézary cell count of ≥ 1000/μL; clone-positive					
Stage	IA	T1	N0	M0	B0–1		
	IB	T2	N0	M0	B0–1		
	IIA	T1–2	N1–2	M0	B0–1		
	IIB	T3	N0–2	M0	B0–1		
	III	T4	N0–2	M0	B0–1		
	IIIA	T4	N0–2	M0	B0		
	IIIB	T4	N0–2	M0	B1		
	IVA1	T1–4	N0–2	M0	B0		
	IVA2	T1–4	N3	M0	B0–2		
	IVB	T1–4	N0–3	M1	B0–3		

Notes:

- For skin, "patch" means a skin lesion of any size with no significant elevation or induration; the presence or absence of hypopigmentation, hyperpigmentation, scale, crusting, and/or poikiloderma should be noted.
- For skin, "plaque" means a skin lesion of any size with elevation or induration; the presence or absence of ulceration, scale, crusting, and/or poikiloderma should be noted; histological features such as folliculotropism, large-cell transformation, and CD30 expression should be noted.
- For skin, "tumour" means a solid or nodular lesion ≥ 10 mm in diameter with evidence of depth and/or vertical growth; the total number and volume of lesions, largest lesion size, and body region involved should be noted; also note whether there is histological evidence of large-cell transformation; phenotyping for CD30 is encouraged.
- For node, "abnormal peripheral lymph node" means a palpable lymph node that is firm, irregular, clustered, fixed, and/or ≥ 15 mm in diameter.
- Node groups examined: cervical, supraclavicular, epitrochlear, axillary, and inguinal; central nodes are not assessed unless used to establish N3 histopathologically.
- Visceral involvement of spleen and liver can be assessed by radiological imaging.
- For blood, Sézary cells are defined as lymphocytes with hyperconvoluted/cerebriform nuclei; if Sézary cells cannot be used to determine tumour burden for B2, then a positive monoclonal rearrangement of the TR gene can be used instead: (1) expanded CD4+ or CD3+ cells with a CD4:CD8 ratio of ≥ 10, or (2) expanded CD4+ cells with abnormal immunophenotype including loss of CD7 or CD26.
- T-cell clones are identified by PCR or Southern blot analysis of the TR gene.

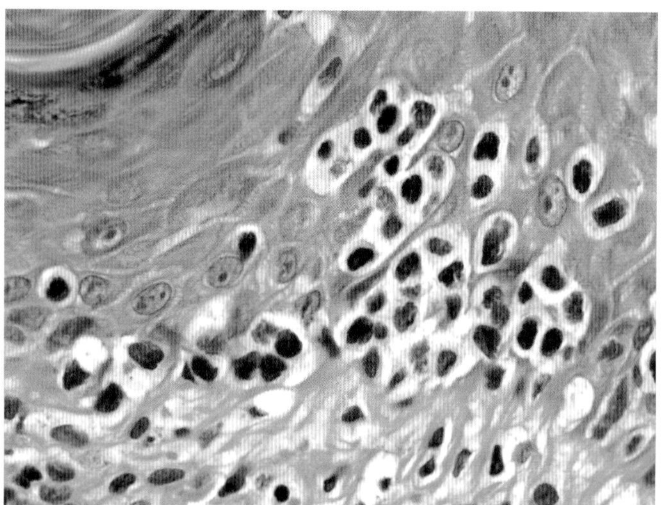

Fig. 5.62 Mycosis fungoides. Infiltrating cells show cerebriform nuclei.

Immunophenotype

Classic MF demonstrates a CD2+, CD3+, TCRβ+, CD5+, CD4+, CD8− phenotype. CD7 is often dimly expressed or partially lost, particularly in advanced disease. CD30 may be positive or negative, and, like other pan–T-cell antigens, may show varied levels of expression in contemporaneous biopsies. CD45 and CCR4 {1854}, both associated with lymphocyte homing to the skin, are expressed in most cases. Antigens suggestive of immune exhaustion (PD1), also common to T follicular helper (TFH) cells, are frequent in MF; however, other markers of TFH phenotype are rare. TOX may be an adjunct marker distinguishing early-stage MF {4573}. Advanced-stage MF may show numerous immunophenotypic aberrancies, including loss of the pan–T-cell antigens CD2 and CD5, diminution of CD4, or loss of TCRβ expression, as well as partial expression of CD30. Aggregates of B cells may be identified within these tumoural infiltrates, and Ki-67 labels a higher percentage of neoplastic cells than in early-stage MF.

Clinically, classic MF with a cytotoxic phenotype (CD8+ and/or TCRγδ) is well recognized. Of note, CD8+ paediatric MF and CD8+ hypopigmented MF, common in Black and Asian populations, may be associated with a more indolent course {7,1532, 2552,1313,2449}.

Nuclear expression of phosphorylated STAT3 can be found in a high proportion of MF / Sézary syndrome cases regardless of JAK mutation {2618}.

Subtypes

Folliculotropic mycosis fungoides

This refers to cases of MF with or without adnexal involvement beyond the hair follicles, which may occasionally present as predominantly syringotropic MF. It arises most commonly on the head and neck, upper extremities, and thorax. Alopecia, pruritus, and palmar/plantar lesions are characteristic {1318}. Folliculotropic MF may have a worse disease course than classic MF, especially in more advanced, tumour-like disease. Early-stage patients have an excellent prognosis on standard treatment, however {646,2699,1604,4169,4170}. Infiltrated plaques, acneiform lesions (comedo-like), and follicular keratosis pilaris–like lesions have been noted to be prominent features in folliculotropic MF {2840}.

In folliculotropic MF, atypical lymphocytes infiltrate the follicular epithelium, typically with sparing of the interfollicular epidermis. Cystic dilation or cornified plugging of hair follicles may be present. Follicular mucinosis and hyperplastic eccrine structures are common, with mucinous degeneration of the follicular epithelium occurring in 60% of cases {372}, ranging from widened intercellular spaces to large mucin lakes. Immunophenotypically, folliculotropic MF is CD4+.

Staging of the infiltrates enables prognostic and therapeutic stratification. Specifically, folliculotropic MF should be distinguished as either mild (early stage) or exuberant (advanced stage). Advanced-stage infiltrates show dense dermal interfollicular involvement {646,2699,1604,4169,4170}. An intermediate plaque-stage subset of folliculotropic MF can be stratified into better- or worse-outcome groups, with large cell size, higher Ki-67 proliferation index, interfollicular epidermotropism, and absent follicular mucinosis being associated with a worse outcome {4168}.

Pagetoid reticulosis (Woringer–Kolopp disease)

This is a slowly growing, well-circumscribed solitary psoriasiform or keratotic plaque (or plaques) affecting the distal extremities or trunk, occurring in all ages. Only exceptional cases show disease progression {78}, but such cases do not eventuate in death or extracutaneous disease. Histologically, pagetoid reticulosis shows sponge-like disaggregation of the epidermis by small to medium-sized lymphocytes, with additional epidermal changes (hyperplasia, acanthosis, hyperkeratosis). These intraepidermally located lymphocytes display atypical medium-sized to large cerebriform nuclei. They characteristically contrast with an underlying infiltrate of small lymphocytes at the dermoepidermal junction, which lack cytological atypia.

The florid scatter of CD8+ atypical lymphocytes in all levels of the epidermis (pagetosis) {78} is typical. CD4−/CD8− or CD4+ cases are rarely identified {1467}. CD30 may be expressed.

Granulomatous slack skin

This is exceedingly rare and arises predominantly in young adult patients, who present with pendulous skin in the axillae, groin, and gluteal folds, with pruritis, erythema, and patches and plaques in skin segments {275,1957,3688}, sometimes in the context of another lymphoma. Atypically, a few cases involve the blood, lymph nodes, or viscera. Treatment is challenging, and although the disease is mostly indolent, patients occasionally succumb to it {1835,275}. Granulomatous slack skin is characterized by a CD3+, CD4+, CD45RO+ atypical lymphocytic infiltrate; however the hallmark features are of a granulomatous infiltrate with loss of elastic fibres and numerous multinucleated CD14+, CD68+ histiocytes with many nuclei arranged in a wreath-like pattern. Elastophagocytosis can be seen, and elastic stain can highlight the destruction of elastic fibres throughout the dermis {4045,3688}.

Cytology

FNAB does not play a role in the initial diagnosis of MF. Later in the course of the disease, FNA may be used to sample skin nodules or parenchymal lesions to obtain material for ancillary testing, to look for morphological evidence of large-cell transformation {3099,4230,3864}, or to guide site selection for excisional lymph node biopsy {1276,3054}.

Table 5.09 Histopathological staging for abnormal lymph nodes[a] in mycosis fungoides and Sézary syndrome

ISCL/EORTC {3054}	**Dutch system** {3610}	**NCI classification** {3591}
N1	Category I: DL, no atypical CMCs	LN 0: No atypical lymphocytes LN 1: Occasional isolated atypical lymphocytes LN 2: Clusters (3–6 cells) of atypical lymphocytes
N2[b]	Category II: DL with early involvement and scattered atypical CMCs	LN 3: Aggregates of atypical lymphocytes, but architecture preserved
N3	Category III: Partial effacement of architecture, with many CMCs Category IV: Complete effacement of architecture	LN 4: Partial or complete effacement of architecture, with many atypical lymphocytes

CMC, cerebriform mononuclear cell with nucleus > 7.5 µm; DL, dermatopathic lymphadenopathy; EORTC, European Organisation for Research and Treatment of Cancer; ISCL, International Society for Cutaneous Lymphomas; NCI, US National Cancer Institute.
[a]Dimension ≥ 15 mm. [b]N2 is divided into two categories: N2a (without monoclonal TR gene rearrangement) and N2b (with monoclonal TR gene rearrangement).

Diagnostic molecular pathology

Like in other T-cell lymphomas, demonstration of a clonal TR gene rearrangement can be crucial in the diagnosis of MF {2034,2219,3383,3837,3870}. However, clonality results should be carefully interpreted in the proper clinicopathological context, because monoclonal TR gene rearrangement can be detected in some elderly individuals or in those with autoimmune diseases or chronic dermatoses {1444,2260,3284}. In contrast, early MF may yield false negative results {2034,1172}.

Essential and desirable diagnostic criteria

Essential (in early-stage MF): presence of persistent and/or progressive patches and plaques, especially in sun-protected areas; presence of small to medium-sized atypical T cells with hyperchromatic, hyperconvoluted (cerebriform) nuclei, preferentially in the epidermis.

Essential (in tumour stage MF): evidence of concurrent or preceding patches and plaques with histological features characteristic of MF.

Desirable: loss of pan–T-cell antigens; demonstration of clonal TR gene rearrangements in skin biopsy in difficult cases.

Staging

Staging of MF and Sézary syndrome is performed according to the International Society for Cutaneous Lymphomas (ISCL) / European Organisation for Research and Treatment of Cancer (EORTC) system, which stratifies cases into 10 overall clinical stages with consideration of the tumour, node, metastasis, and blood (TNMB) stage (Table 5.08, p. 691) {3054}. For the classification of blood or lymph node stage, T-cell clonality testing is necessary {3054}. Nodal status should be estimated only from clinically abnormal peripheral lymph nodes, defined as nodes ≥ 15 mm or as firm, clustered, or fixed palpable nodes regardless of size {3054,165,3591,3610}. Histopathological staging for clinically abnormal lymph nodes is specified in Table 5.09 {3054,165,3591,3610}.

Prognosis and prediction

Clinical stage, as assessed by TNMB classification, is the key prognostic factor for both disease progression and survival, with tumour-stage disease and blood, lymph node, and visceral involvement correlating with a poor prognosis. Patients with limited disease generally have an excellent prognosis, with a similar survival rate to that of the general population. Imaging is usually not recommended in early-stage MF {3054}. In the advanced stages of the disease, CT or PET-CT with or without contrast medium may be indicated at time of disease progression, before starting chemotherapy, and to evaluate visceral response or progression after a full treatment course. Ultrasound scan may be of help in the interpretation of lymph nodal enlargement. The presence of a circulating clone in the absence of phenotypic evidence of blood involvement, older age (> 60 years) at diagnosis, elevated LDH, and folliculotropism correlate with worse survival {32,931,317,3604}.

Primary cutaneous CD30-positive T-cell lymphoproliferative disorder: Lymphomatoid papulosis

Kempf W
Gujral S
Jansen PM
Kadin ME
Paulli M
Pulitzer M
Willemze R

Definition

Lymphomatoid papulosis (LyP) belongs to the spectrum of primary cutaneous CD30-positive T-cell lymphoproliferative disorders. It is characterized by self-healing but recurrent papulonodular skin lesions, atypical CD30-positive T cells by histology, and an excellent prognosis.

ICD-O coding

9718/1 Primary cutaneous CD30-positive T-cell lymphoproliferative disorder, lymphomatoid papulosis
9718/1 Primary mucosal CD30-positive T-cell lymphoproliferative disorder
9718/1 Lymphomatoid papulosis subtypes A, B, C, D, E
9718/1 Lymphomatoid papulosis with *DUSP22* locus rearrangement

ICD-11 coding

2B03.1 Lymphomatoid papulosis

Related terminology

None

Subtype(s)

Primary mucosal CD30-positive T-cell lymphoproliferative disorder; lymphomatoid papulosis subtypes A, B, C, D, and E; lymphomatoid papulosis with *DUSP22* locus rearrangement

Localization

LyP most frequently involves the trunk and extremities {292}. The disease may have primary mucosal involvement or, rarely, can concurrently involve various mucosal and cutaneous sites {3312,3655}.

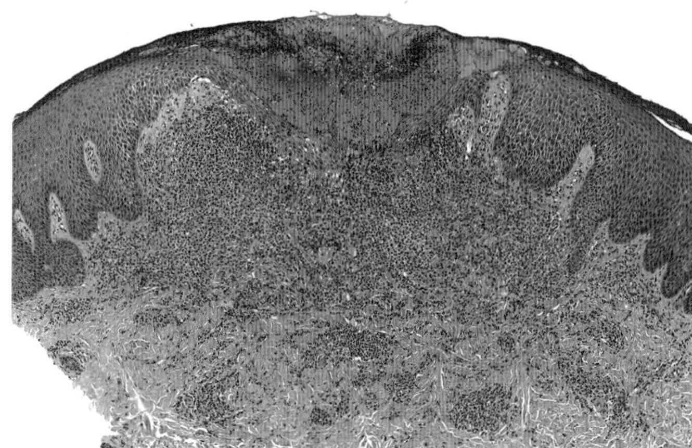

Fig. 5.64 Primary cutaneous CD30-positive T-cell lymphoproliferative disorder: Lymphomatoid papulosis. Wedge-shaped infiltrate of atypical lymphoid cells beneath an ulcer.

Clinical features

LyP manifests with recurrent eruptions with a waxing and waning course of papulonodular skin lesions that may ulcerate {2457}. The number of lesions may vary from a few to more than a hundred. Occasionally, larger (up to 20 mm) and longer-persisting nodular lesions can develop. Characteristically, skin lesions in different stages of evolution coexist {292,906}. The individual skin lesions spontaneously regress within 3–12 weeks, leaving scars and/or hypopigmentation or hyperpigmentation {2457}

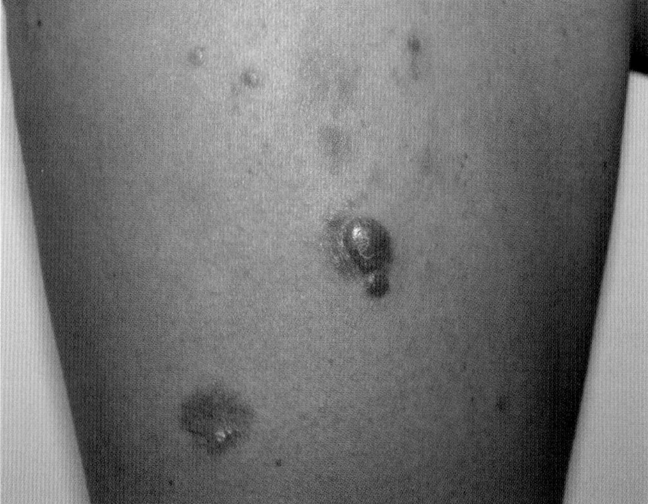

Fig. 5.63 Primary cutaneous CD30-positive T-cell lymphoproliferative disorder: Lymphomatoid papulosis. Papules and small nodules in various evolutionary stages, as well as hyperpigmented macules representing residuals of regressed lesions.

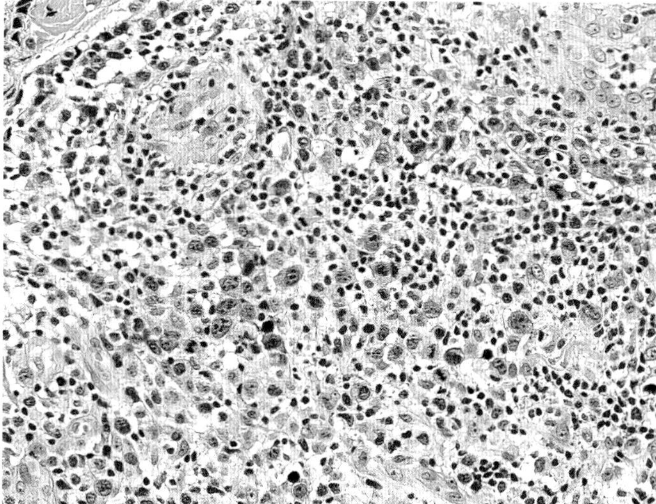

Fig. 5.65 Primary cutaneous CD30-positive T-cell lymphoproliferative disorder: Lymphomatoid papulosis. Type A. Mixed infiltrate of scattered medium-sized to large lymphoid cells within a background of small lymphocytes and histiocytes.

LyP may persist for several months, or occasionally for years or decades {2379,906}.

Epidemiology

The incidence is 1.2–1.9 cases per 1 million person-years, and the M:F ratio is 2–3:1 {4382,292,906,2379}. LyP most often affects adults (median age at onset: 35–45 years), but children may also be affected {4164,905,1317,4371}.

Etiology

The cause of LyP is largely unknown. Atopy and staphylococcal superantigens have been pathogenetically linked to LyP {1843}. A viral etiology has been suggested, but not proved {455,1846,1947}. Endogenous retroviral elements (i.e. inherited genomic elements with structural features of integrated retroviruses) have been detected, but their etiological role is unclear {1946,2229}.

Pathogenesis

The translocation t(2;5)(p23;q35), resulting in ALK expression, is not detected in LyP {914}. Identical T-cell clones have been demonstrated in some LyP lesions and associated lymphomas {738,894,884}. Rearrangements of the *DUSP22* locus on chromosome 6p25.3 are found in a small subset of LyP cases {1887,

Table 5.10 Diagnostic criteria and differential diagnosis for lymphomatoid papulosis (LyP) {1953}

Subtype (proportion of LyP cases)	Phenotype	Diagnostic histopathological and genetic criteria	Differential diagnosis	Discriminating features
A (80%)	CD4+, CD8−, CD30+	Wedge-shaped infiltrate with scattered or small clusters of large pleomorphic CD30+ cells (sometimes multinucleated or Reed–Sternberg–like) and numerous inflammatory cells, i.e. small lymphocytes, neutrophils, and/or eosinophils {4383,292,1070}	Mycosis fungoides, tumour stage	Clinical evolution with preceding patches and plaques
			Hodgkin lymphoma (almost always secondary cutaneous involvement)	Staging: nodal involvement
			C-ALCL	Clinical presentation: rapidly growing large tumour or multifocal nodules; cohesive sheets of large CD30+ T cells
B (< 5%)	CD4+, CD8−, CD30+/−	Epidermotropic infiltrate of small atypical CD30+ or CD30− cells with cerebriform nuclei {4383,292,1070}	Mycosis fungoides, patch/plaque stage	Clinical presentation with patches and plaques
C (10%)	CD4+, CD8−, CD30+	Monotonous infiltrate with cohesive sheets of large CD30+ T cells; few admixed inflammatory cells {4383,292,1070}	C-ALCL	Clinical presentation: rapidly growing large tumour or multifocal nodules
			Mycosis fungoides, tumour stage with large-cell transformation	Clinical evolution with preceding patches and plaques; variable expression of CD30
			Adult T-cell leukaemia/lymphoma	Detection of HTLV-1/2, geographical clustering
D (< 5%)	CD4−, CD8+, CD30+	Strongly epidermotropic, sometimes pagetoid infiltrate of atypical small to medium-sized CD8+, CD30+ pleomorphic T cells {3522}	Primary cutaneous CD8+ aggressive epidermotropic cytotoxic T-cell lymphoma	Clinical presentation: rapidly evolving erosive or ulcerated plaques and nodules CD8+, CD30− (rarely CD30+) CD45RA+ (70%)
			Pagetoid reticulosis (mycosis fungoides subtype)	Clinical presentation: solitary erythematous and scaly lesion Various phenotypes including expression of CD8 and CD30
E (< 5%)	CD4−, CD8+, CD30+	Angioinvasive infiltrates of mostly medium-sized CD8+, CD30+ pleomorphic cells Vascular occlusion, haemorrhages, extensive necrosis, and ulceration {1952} *Note:* Clinically, patients present with a few papulonodular lesions that rapidly ulcerate and evolve into large, necrotic, eschar-like lesions {1952}	Extranodal NK/T-cell lymphoma	Staging: systemic involvement Association with EBV (LMP, EBER+)
			Cutaneous gamma-delta T-cell lymphoma	Clinical presentation: rapidly evolving erosive or ulcerated plaques and nodules Often CD56+ CD30− (occasionally CD30+) TCRγδ+, TCRαβ−
			C-ALCL (angioinvasive form)	Clinical presentation: rapidly growing large tumour with ulceration CD4+ or CD8+, CD30+
LyP with *DUSP22* locus rearrangement (< 5%)	CD8+ or CD4/CD8 double-negative, CD30+	Biphasic pattern: epidermotropic, small to medium-sized, weakly CD30+ T cells with cerebriform nuclei, and a dense dermal infiltrate of strongly CD30+ medium-sized to large atypical cells {1887} Defining criterion: chromosomal rearrangements involving the *DUSP22-IRF4* locus on 6p25.3 {948}	Mycosis fungoides, tumour stage with large-cell transformation	Clinical evolution with preceding patches and plaques; variable expression of CD30

C-ALCL, primary cutaneous anaplastic large cell lymphoma; EBER, EBV-encoded small RNA.

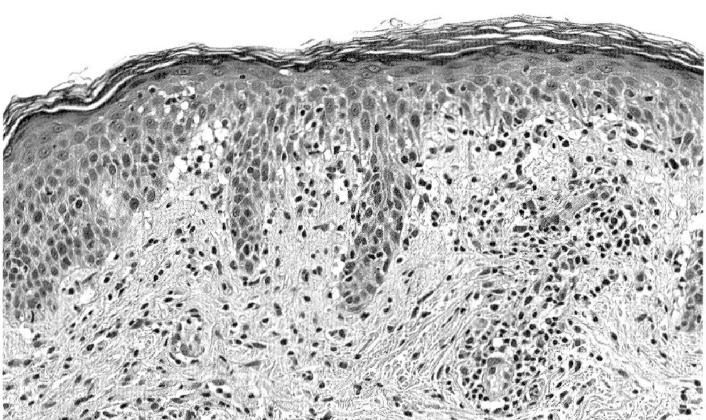

Fig. 5.66 Primary cutaneous CD30-positive T-cell lymphoproliferative disorder: Lymphomatoid papulosis. Type B. Epidermotropic infiltrate of small, slightly atypical lymphocytes that express CD4 and CD30.

4260}. *NPM1::TYK2* translocation, STAT mutations, and oncogenic fusion transcripts activating the JAK/STAT pathway have been identified {4205,2609}. SATB1 is expressed in the vast majority of LyP cases {3881}.

Macroscopic appearance

The lesions present as papules and small nodules (see *Clinical features*).

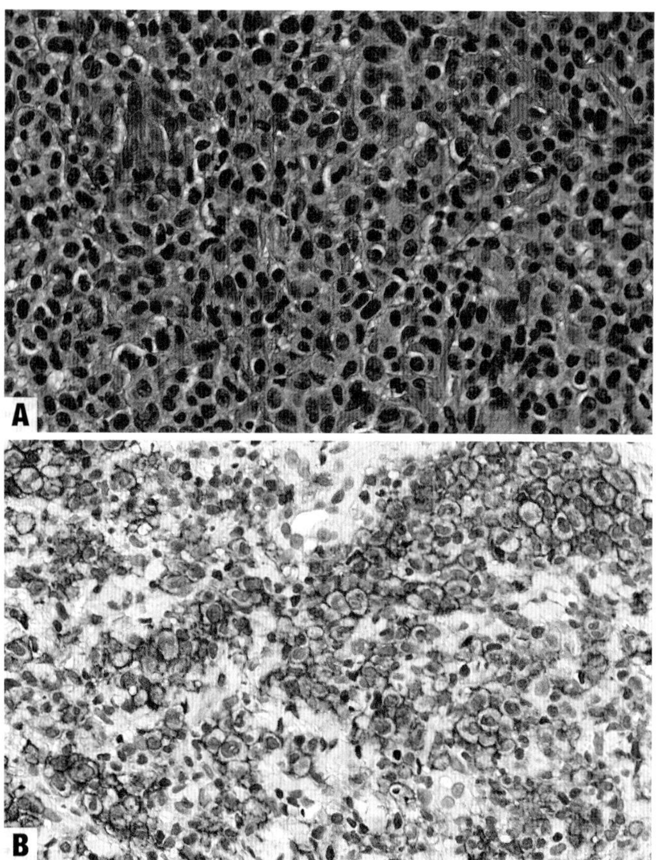

Fig. 5.67 Primary cutaneous CD30-positive T-cell lymphoproliferative disorder: Lymphomatoid papulosis. Type C. **A** Cohesive infiltrates of medium-sized to large lymphoid cells. **B** Expression of CD30 by all atypical cells.

Histopathology

The histological spectrum of LyP is extremely broad and in part depends on the evolution of the biopsied lesion {4383,4382, 1070,1953}. Six main subtypes (A–E and with 6p25.3 rearrangements involving the *DUSP22* locus) with distinct histological and/or genetic features are delineated (see Table 5.10, p. 695) {4383,292,1070,3522,1952,1887}. They may occur in different but concurrent lesions, and a single LyP lesion may show overlapping histological features of the different subtypes of LyP {1070,4382,1953}. Other rare subtypes have been described, including folliculotropic, syringotropic, and granulomatous LyP {1948,3444,843}. Mucosal lesions show a similar spectrum of findings {3312,3655}.

Immunohistochemistry

The atypical lymphoid cells express CD30, often with a Golgi dot-like pattern. They predominantly express CD4 in LyP subtypes A, B, and C; express CD8 in LyP subtypes D and E; and either express CD8 or are double-negative for CD4/CD8 in LyP with *DUSP22* locus rearrangement. Atypical cells may express TIA1 {2154}. Rare cases expressing CD56, TCRγδ, or a T follicular helper (TFH) cell phenotype have been reported {4056, 293,1201}.

Differential diagnosis

Although the LyP subtypes do not have any prognostic or therapeutic implications, recognition of these subtypes is important to avoid misdiagnosis of other, more aggressive lymphomas. Clinicopathological correlation is essential for differentiating LyP not only from these lymphomas but also from a wide variety of infectious and inflammatory skin diseases that can contain a substantial number of CD30+ cells {1446,1945, 4361}.

Cytology

Fine core needle biopsy is not recommended for making this diagnosis.

Diagnostic molecular pathology

Monoclonal rearrangements of TR (TCR) genes can be detected in 22–80% of LyP cases {738,1058,3833,1412}.

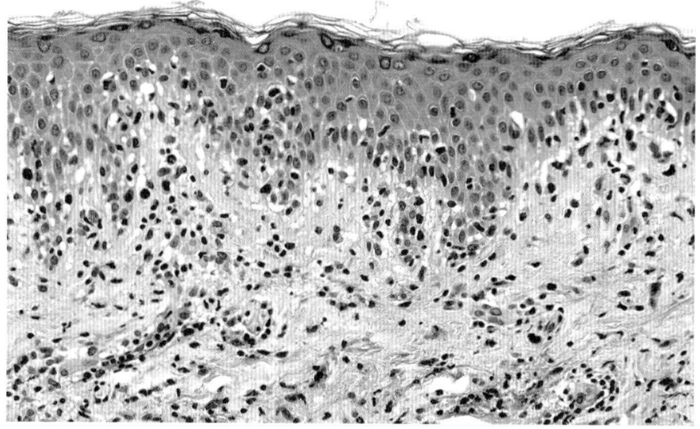

Fig. 5.68 Primary cutaneous CD30-positive T-cell lymphoproliferative disorder: Lymphomatoid papulosis. Type D. Epidermotropic infiltrate of small to medium-sized atypical lymphocytes.

Essential and desirable diagnostic criteria

Essential: infiltrates of mostly medium-sized atypical lymphoid cells with expression of CD30 and T-cell markers, and a variable inflammatory background; clinical presentation with waxing and waning papulonodular skin lesions; spontaneous regression within weeks to a few months; exclusion of other lymphomas by clinicopathological correlation.

Desirable: detection of monoclonal rearrangement of TR genes may be helpful in selected cases (especially in LyP subtype A).

Staging

In patients with the typical clinical presentation and no indication of extracutaneous disease by physical examination or blood tests, there is no need for further staging {1959,314}.

Prognosis and prediction

LyP has an excellent prognosis. However, patients are at increased risk for being diagnosed with a secondary cutaneous lymphoma (mycosis fungoides, primary cutaneous anaplastic large cell lymphoma), which may precede, be associated with, or follow LyP {4370,292,906,4289,807,2379,884,18,2633}. An increased risk for various non-haematological malignancies, such as cutaneous squamous cell carcinoma, melanoma, and organ-based malignancies, has also been suggested {2633, 4289}. Demonstration of fascin expression by CD30-positive cells and clonal TR gene rearrangement in LyP were suggested as risk factors for the development of LyP-associated lymphomas, pending confirmation in larger studies {906,1954}. Because of the increased risk of associated lymphomas, long-term follow-up is advised {1959,4382}.

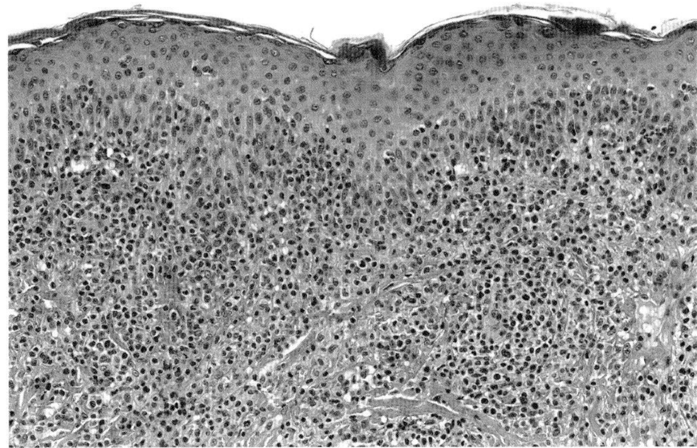

Fig. 5.69 Primary cutaneous CD30-positive T-cell lymphoproliferative disorder: Lymphomatoid papulosis with *DUSP22-IRF4* rearrangement. Epidermotropic infiltrate of small atypical lymphocytes and dermal small to medium-sized atypical lymphocytes.

Primary cutaneous CD30-positive T-cell lymphoproliferative disorder: Primary cutaneous anaplastic large cell lymphoma

Jansen PM
Gujral S
Kadin ME
Kempf W
Paulli M
Pulitzer M
Willemze R

Definition

Primary cutaneous anaplastic large cell lymphoma (C-ALCL) belongs to the spectrum of primary cutaneous CD30-positive T-cell lymphoproliferative disorders. C-ALCL is composed of large cells with an anaplastic, pleomorphic, or immunoblastic cytomorphology; > 75% of the tumour cells express CD30.

ICD-O coding

9718/3 Primary cutaneous CD30-positive T-cell lymphoproliferative disorder, primary cutaneous anaplastic large cell lymphoma

ICD-11 coding

2B03.0 & XH40C0 Primary cutaneous CD30-positive anaplastic large cell lymphoma & Primary cutaneous CD30-positive T-cell lymphoproliferative disorder

Related terminology

None

Subtype(s)

None

Localization

C-ALCL is a primary cutaneous disease that can involve the skin in any location {314,4405}. The disease may have primary mucosal involvement or, rarely, can concurrently involve mucosal and cutaneous sites {3312,3655}.

Clinical features

Most patients present with solitary or localized skin or mucosal plaques, nodules, tumours, or (rarely) papules, often with ulceration {292,2379}. Multifocal lesions are seen in about 20% of patients. Lesions may show partial or complete regression. Relapse in skin is common. Extracutaneous dissemination occurs in approximately 10% of cases, mainly in regional lymph nodes {292}.

Epidemiology

C-ALCL is the second most common cutaneous T-cell lymphoma {4377}. The median age is 60 years, and children can also be affected. The M:F ratio is 2–3:1 {292}.

Etiology

Unknown

Pathogenesis

The postulated normal counterpart is an activated skin-homing T lymphocyte. The vast majority of C-ALCLs do not carry translocations involving the *ALK* gene at 2p23 {914}. Exceptional cases of ALK-positive C-ALCL, including cases with t(2;5)(p23;q35)/*NPM1*::*ALK* and with other *ALK* fusion partners, have been reported in both children and adults, usually with excellent outcomes {174,1845,3076,3334,2634}.

Rearrangement of the *DUSP22* locus at 6p25.3 occurs in 20–25% of C-ALCLs {3222,4260}. Rearrangements of *TP63* on

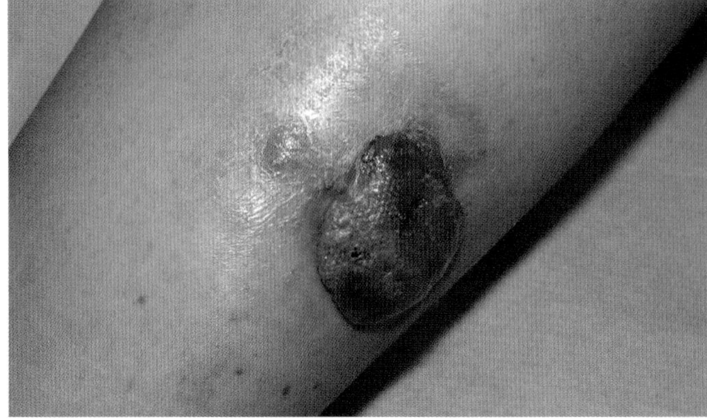

Fig. 5.70 Primary cutaneous anaplastic large cell lymphoma. Large polypoid tumour on the leg.

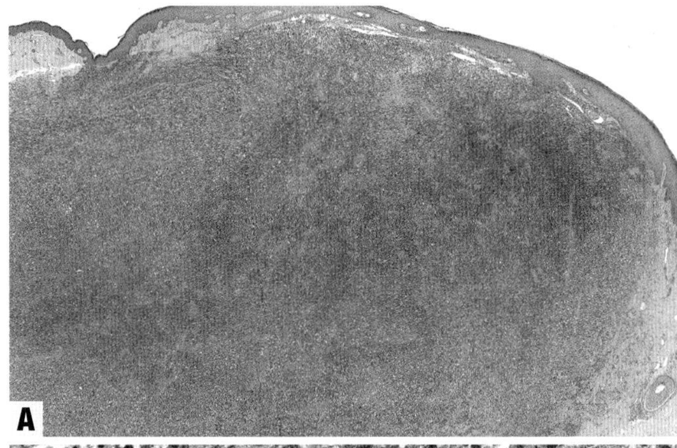

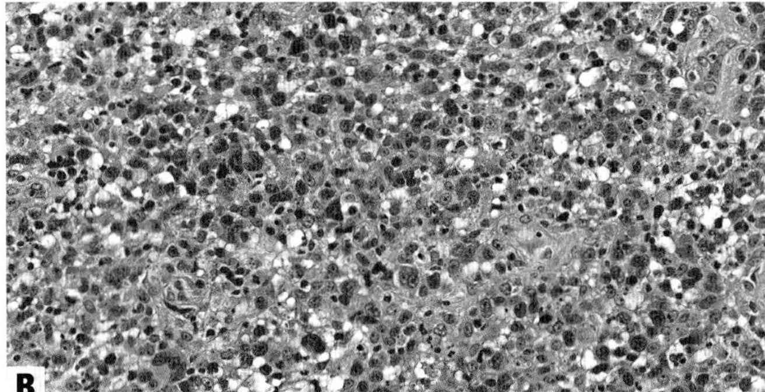

Fig. 5.71 Primary cutaneous anaplastic large cell lymphoma. **A** Low-power magnification shows a nodular infiltrate in the dermis and subcutis, with an absence of epidermotropism. **B** High-power magnification shows a confluent infiltrate of large anaplastic lymphoid cells.

chromosome 3q28, which are associated with poor survival in ALK-negative systemic anaplastic large cell lymphoma, are rare in C-ALCL {3638,4189}. Frequent chromosomal aberrations are gains of 7q31 and losses at 6q16-21 and 13q34 {2194,4160}.

The *NPM1::TYK2* gene fusion, resulting in constitutive STAT signalling, has been described in sporadic cases of C-ALCL {4205}. *TYK2* rearrangements have been found in 15% of cases. Upregulation of signal transduction associated with the PI3K, MAPK, and G-protein pathways has been revealed by transcriptome analysis {268}. Gene expression profiling has revealed high expression of the skin-homing chemokine receptors CCR10 and CCR8, possibly explaining skin tropism and infrequent extracutaneous dissemination {4160,4189,3638}. Recent genomic studies (albeit in only a small cohort of C-ALCL cases) demonstrated recurrent mutations in histone modifier genes (*KMT2D*, *KMT2A*, *SETD2*, *CREBBP*), as well as mutations in *STAT3* and *EOMES*, which encodes a transcription factor involved in lymphocyte development {9}.

Macroscopic appearance

See *Clinical features*.

Histopathology

The affected skin or mucosa shows diffuse infiltrates of large CD30+ tumour cells. Epidermotropism may be present, particularly in cases with *DUSP22* locus rearrangement {3063}. In most cases, the tumour cells have an anaplastic morphology, with round, oval, or irregularly shaped nuclei; prominent nucleoli; and abundant cytoplasm {4377}. Less commonly, lymphoma cells have a pleomorphic or immunoblastic appearance {292,2576, 3168}. Ulcerating lesions may show lymphomatoid papulosis–like histology, with an abundance of reactive T cells (mostly at lesion borders); admixed histiocytes, eosinophils, and neutrophils; and relatively few CD30+ cells. In such cases, epidermal hyperplasia may be prominent. The inflammatory background is prominent in the rare neutrophil-rich (pyogenic) and eosinophil-rich variants {490}. Rare cases of intralymphatic and intravascular C-ALCL have been reported {3556,4297}. Mucosal lesions show a similar spectrum of findings {3312,3655}.

Immunohistochemistry

The neoplastic cells have an activated CD4+ T-cell phenotype, with variable loss of CD2, CD3, CD5, and CD7, and frequent expression of cytotoxic proteins {292,427,2154}. Some cases may have a CD4−/CD8+ or CD4+/CD8+ T-cell phenotype {2575}. CD30 is expressed by > 75% of tumour cells {4377}. CD15 is expressed in approximately 40% of cases {313,4322}. Coexpression of CD56 is rarely observed and is not associated with a worse outcome {2921}.

Differential diagnosis

The term "primary cutaneous CD30-positive T-cell lymphoproliferative disorder, borderline lesion" refers to cases in which, despite careful clinicopathological correlation, a definitive distinction between C-ALCL and lymphomatoid papulosis cannot be made at diagnosis; a more precise diagnosis of C-ALCL or lymphomatoid papulosis may be evident, at least in some cases, on follow-up {292,4382,4377,3168}.

Cytology

Fine core needle biopsies are not recommended for establishing this diagnosis.

Diagnostic molecular pathology

Clonal rearrangements of TR (TCR) genes are detected in most cases {2459}.

Essential and desirable diagnostic criteria

Essential: lymphoma involvement limited to skin and/or mucosa; tumour cells with anaplastic, pleomorphic, or immunoblastic morphology; CD30 expression in > 75% of tumour cells; no clinical history or evidence of mycosis fungoides (exclude mycosis fungoides with CD30+ large-cell transformation); no history of lesions waxing and waning (exclude lymphomatoid papulosis).

Staging

The TNM classification system for primary cutaneous lymphomas other than mycosis fungoides is applied {2015}.

Prognosis and prediction

The prognosis is favourable, with a 10-year disease-related survival rate of approximately 90% {292,2379}. Presentation with multifocal skin lesions or regional lymph node involvement does not influence the prognosis. Worse outcomes have been associated with extensive skin lesions on the legs, or age > 60 years {314,2379,3662,4405,3576}.

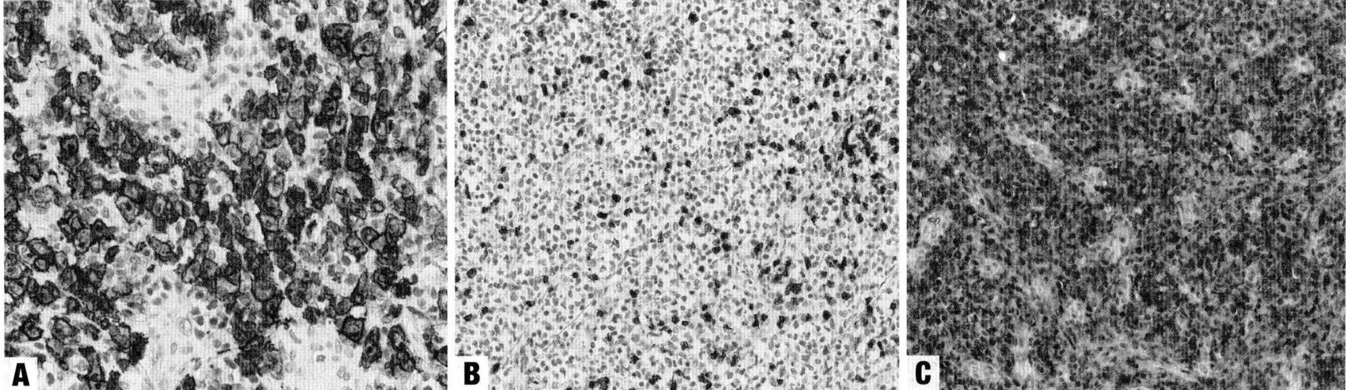

Fig. 5.72 Primary cutaneous anaplastic large cell lymphoma. **A** Expression of CD30 by the tumour cells, with a membranous and Golgi pattern. **B** Expression of CD3 by small reactive T cells and lack of expression of CD3 by the tumour cells. **C** Expression of CD4 by the tumour cells.

Subcutaneous panniculitis-like T-cell lymphoma

Guitart J
Jeon YK
Pulitzer M
Willemze R

Definition

Subcutaneous panniculitis-like T-cell lymphoma (SPTCL) is a lymphoproliferative disorder with adipotropism that mostly involves the subcutaneous tissue, but occasionally other sites. It is predominantly composed of activated cytotoxic medium-sized CD8+ lymphocytes expressing the TCRαβ heterodimer.

ICD-O coding

9708/3 Subcutaneous panniculitis-like T-cell lymphoma

ICD-11 coding

2B00 Subcutaneous panniculitis-like T-cell lymphoma

Related terminology

None

Subtype(s)

None

Localization

SPTCL primarily involves subcutaneous tissue, with a predilection for the lower extremities, followed by the upper extremities and trunk {4380}. Rarely, other sites rich in adipose tissue, such as the mesentery, perinodal fat, and bone marrow, can be involved {1351,1284}.

Clinical features

Patients present with tender non-ulcerated nodules ranging from 10 to > 200 mm in diameter and involving any anatomical site. A sequela of lipoatrophy is occasionally observed {2415}. Constitutional symptoms, including fever and malaise, are commonly observed, and approximately 20–30% of cases may evolve to haemophagocytic lymphohistiocytosis {2680,4380}. A minority of cases present with a single nodule that can trigger similar systemic symptoms {1351,1284}.

Epidemiology

SPTCL is exceedingly rare, with an incidence of approximately 1.5 cases per 10 million person-years in the USA {1382}, but it is more common in Asia {1474,2253,3139,3304}. It has a female predilection (M:F ratio: 1:2–3). Although the overall age range of presentation is broad, the median age is approximately 35 years, with a significant number of paediatric and adolescent cases {1690}. Autoimmune comorbidities are observed in at least 25%

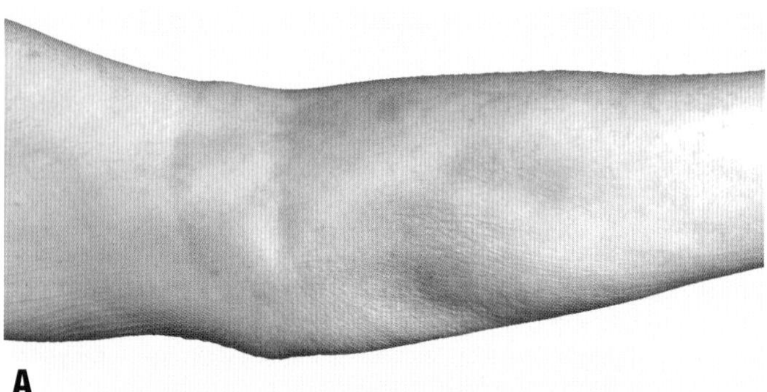

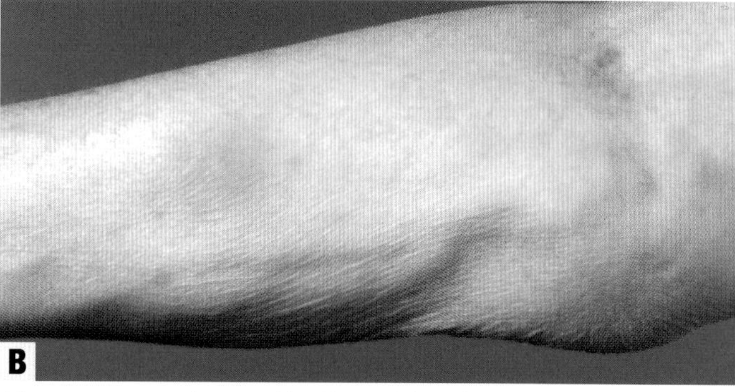

Fig. 5.73 Subcutaneous panniculitis-like T-cell lymphoma. **A** Multiple subcutaneous nodules are common on the extremities. The overlying epidermis may show mild to moderate erythema. **B** Subcutaneous nodules and lipoatrophy.

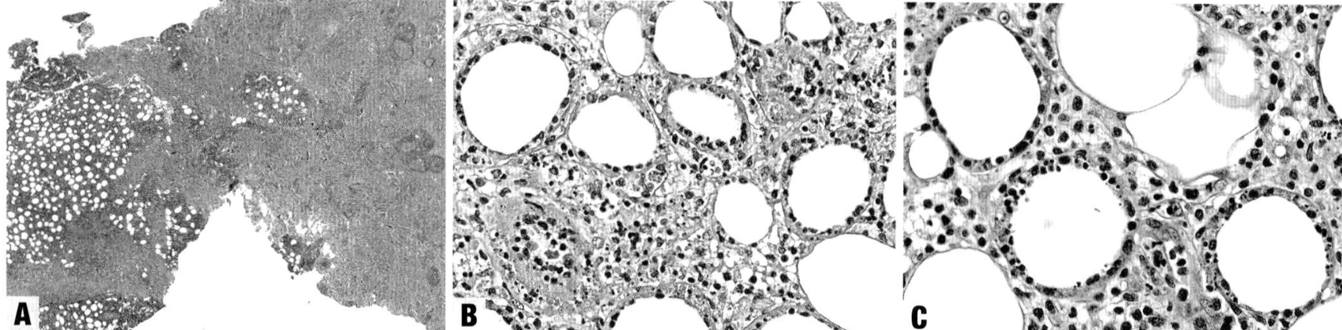

Fig. 5.74 Subcutaneous panniculitis-like T-cell lymphoma. **A** The infiltrate involves the subcutaneous tissue and spares the overlying dermis and epidermis. **B** Atypical cells rim fat spaces; macrophages are increased in number and contain apoptotic debris. **C** High magnification shows atypical medium-sized lymphocytes with karyorrhectic debris rimming the subcutaneous fat lobules.

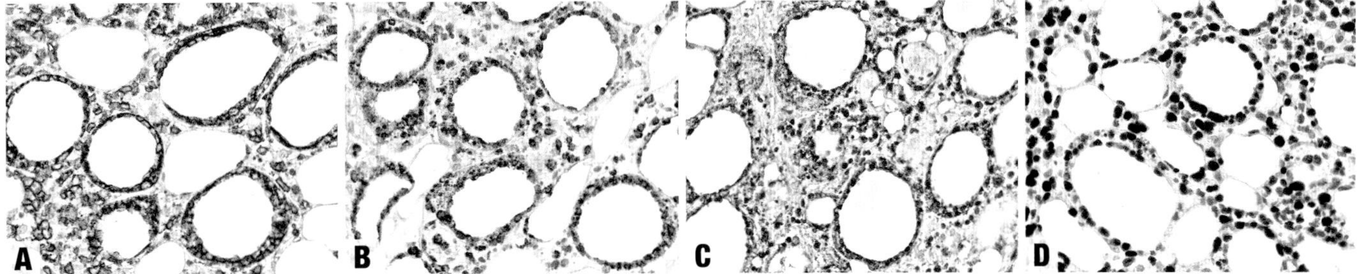

Fig. 5.75 Subcutaneous panniculitis-like T-cell lymphoma. **A** Atypical cells, which are positive for CD8, rim fat spaces. **B** The cells are positive for TIA1. **C** TCRβ with βF1 immunohistochemistry is also positive. **D** Ki-67 (MIB1) staining reveals high proliferation in the atypical cells.

of cases {4380,2680}. In particular, lupus erythematosus is a common comorbidity, which may cause difficulties in differentiating SPTCL from an associated lupus panniculitis {2460}.

Etiology

The etiology is unknown. Autoimmunity and immune dysregulation may play a role in many cases. Autoantibodies have been identified in approximately two thirds of cases {2680}. The constellation of findings may overlap with those of lupus erythematosus, raising the differential diagnosis of lupus panniculitis in cases presenting with lymphocyte-rich lobular infiltrates with adipotropic features {3251}.

Pathogenesis

Germline variants of *HAVCR2* (MIM number: 606652), encoding a negative membrane modulator of immune response (HAVCR2 [TIM3]), have been identified in at least 25% and as many as 85% of patients, with higher frequencies in Asian populations {3789,2082,3274}. Although whole-exome sequencing data have revealed a spectrum of somatic mutations involving genes encoding epigenetic modifiers, the PI3K/AKT/mTOR pathway, and the JAK/STAT pathway {1169,2330}, no pathognomonic driver mutation for SPTCL has been identified. Mutations resulting in protein misfolding abrogate expression of this negative immune checkpoint that regulates peripheral tolerance {1305}. Low levels of T regulatory (Treg) cells (FOXP3+, CCR4+) may lead to immune activation {1312}. Various triggers have been proposed for cases without germline mutations, including viral infections and autoimmunity {3274}.

Macroscopic appearance

See *Clinical features*.

Histopathology

The infiltrate is typically composed of medium-sized lymphocytes with irregular and hyperchromatic nuclei infiltrating the subcutaneous lobules and often extending into the periadnexal fat pad. The atypical cells may display a rimming pattern around adipocytes, accompanied by variable fat necrosis, karyorrhectic debris, and haemorrhage. Lipid-laden macrophages are abundant and may show haemophagocytosis. Plasma cells, granulocytes, and plasmacytoid dendritic cells are inconspicuous. Tumoural large-cell transformation is typically not observed {4380}.

Immunohistochemistry

Immunohistochemistry shows CD8+ mature αβ T cells (βF1+) and retention of pan–T-cell markers (CD2+, CD5+, CD7+). The cells typically express the cytotoxic markers TIA1, perforin, and granzyme B. CD30 and EBV-encoded small RNA (EBER) are negative. Markers for Treg cells (FOXP3, CCR4) are typically low or absent {1312}. Ki-67 shows foci of high proliferative activity. A variable subset of histiocytes and small subset of reactive T cells expressing TCRγδ may be observed.

Differential diagnosis

The differential diagnosis includes lupus erythematosus panniculitis and poorly categorized cases of lymphocyte-rich panniculitic infiltrates not meeting the criteria for SPTCL diagnosis. Primary cutaneous gamma-delta lymphomas and extranodal NK/T-cell lymphomas may also involve the subcutaneous tissue, with a similar cytotoxic pattern. Primary cutaneous gamma-delta lymphoma is excluded by the lack of TCRγδ expression, and extranodal NK/T-cell lymphoma is excluded by the absence of EBV {4380}.

Cytology

FNABs are not recommended for establishing this diagnosis.

Diagnostic molecular pathology

TRB and/or TRG gene rearrangement is mostly clonal. EBV in situ hybridization is negative {4380}.

Essential and desirable diagnostic criteria

Essential: a lobular subcutaneous infiltrate composed of atypical lymphocytes with rimming of adipocytes and expression of TCRαβ and CD8; absence of TCRγδ expression and absence of EBV/EBER within atypical cells.

Desirable: demonstration of clonal TR (TCR) gene rearrangement.

Staging

SPTCL is staged according to the TNM classification system for primary cutaneous lymphomas other than mycosis fungoides and Sézary syndrome {3054}.

Prognosis and prediction

SPTCL carries a good prognosis, often responding to a variety of therapies ranging from systemic steroids to immunosuppressive drugs like ciclosporin or methotrexate. Various single-agent or multiagent chemotherapies are also effective, tending to be used when immunomodulatory agents fail {2415,2680}. Approximately 20–30% of patients, especially those with *HAVCR2* germline mutations, will develop life-threatening haemophagocytic lymphohistiocytosis {2680}, which may require chemoablative therapy followed by stem cell transplantation {3789}.

Primary cutaneous gamma-delta T-cell lymphoma

Pulitzer M
Berti E
Guitart J
Nardi V
Willemze R

Definition

Primary cutaneous gamma-delta T-cell lymphoma (PCGD-TCL) is a clonal proliferation of mature, activated γδ T cells of the Vδ1 or Vδ2 subset, arising within the skin and subcutaneous tissues.

ICD-O coding

9726/3 Primary cutaneous gamma-delta T-cell lymphoma

ICD-11 coding

2B0Y & XH84A5 Other specified primary cutaneous mature T-cell or NK-cell lymphomas and lymphoproliferative disorders & Primary cutaneous gamma/delta T-cell lymphoma

Related terminology

None

Subtype(s)

None

Localization

PCGD-TCL manifests as single or generalized skin and subcutaneous lesions, occasionally with mucosal involvement, without preferential sites of involvement {1447}.

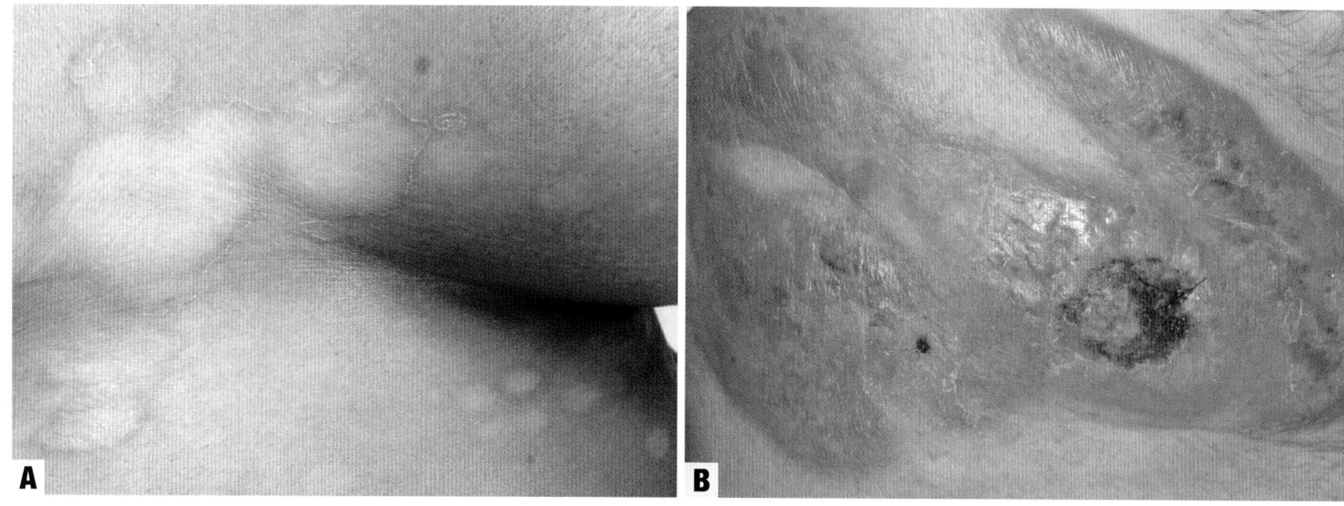

Fig. 5.76 Primary cutaneous gamma-delta T-cell lymphoma. **A** Polycyclic dyschromic patches and plaques with small, peripheral scaling in early-stage disease. **B** Presentation with an ulcerated tumour in more advanced disease.

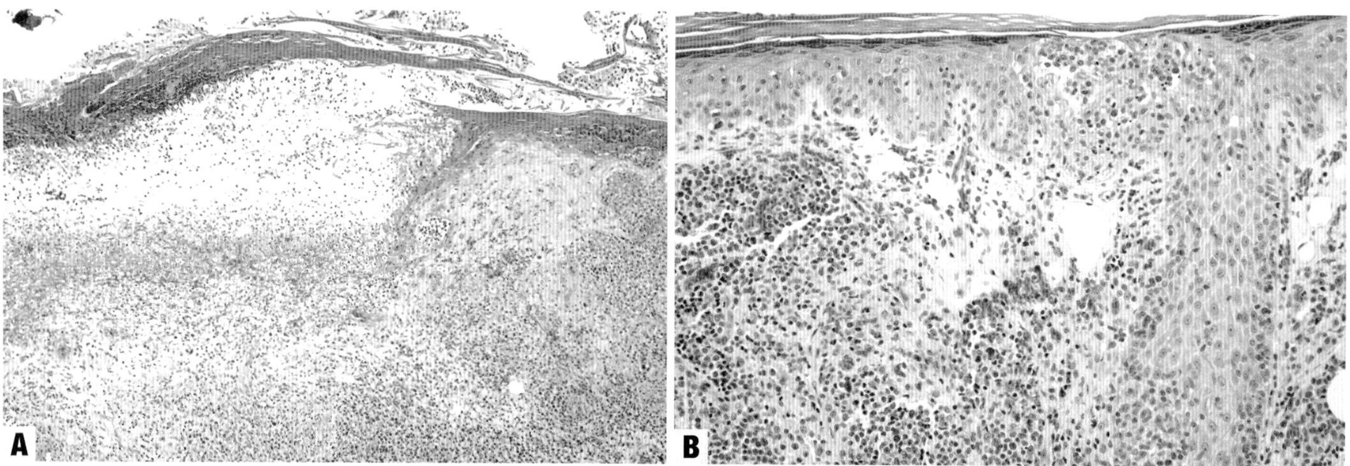

Fig. 5.77 Primary cutaneous gamma-delta T-cell lymphoma. **A** Ulcerated plaque of gamma-delta T-cell lymphoma showing a diffuse superficial and dermal infiltrate, with sheets of large atypical lymphocytes, cytotoxic tissue damage, and a large ulcer. **B** The intraepidermal and dermal component shows an epidermotropic and superficial dermal infiltration with cytotoxic tissue changes, haemorrhage, and Pautrier-like microabscesses.

Clinical features

The clinical presentation and disease course of patients with PCGD-TCL are variable, so a definitive diagnosis may not be achieved on the initial biopsy. Some patients present with generalized scaly patches and plaques suggestive of mycosis fungoides, whereas others present with deep dermal and/or subcutaneous nodules or tumours {4050,1447}. Ulceration and rapid evolution can be seen in either presentation. Both patterns may be present in the same patient. Haemophagocytic syndrome {4380,3548} and spread to extracutaneous (visceral) sites cause significant morbidity. Involvement of lymph nodes or bone marrow is uncommon {1468,37,1338}. B symptoms, including fever, night sweats, and weight loss, occur frequently.

Imaging findings on CT and PET-CT commonly signal cutaneous and extracutaneous sites of involvement {4380,1447,2515}.

Epidemiology

PCGD-TCL accounts for < 1% of primary cutaneous lymphomas. SEER Program data from 2006–2015 and 2000–2018 {1382,515} show a cumulative incidence of 0.05/million person-years, a median age of 63 years, and a male predominance.

Etiology

The etiology is unknown. Immune dysfunction associated with chronic antigenic stimulation may play a role in the origin of PCGD-TCL {149}. TR gene usage is non-random, suggesting common antigenic drivers {864}.

Pathogenesis

Studies show a heterogeneous genomic landscape with recurrent mutations of putative driver genes within the JAK/STAT {2141}, MAPK, MYC, and chromatin modification pathways, as well as mutations in consensus cancer genes and in tumour suppressor genes. Heterogeneity of PCGD-TCL may be related to different cells of origin with distinct roles in the immunity of their originating skin compartments: Vδ1 expression is associated with the superficial cutaneous or mucosal epitheliotropic lymphomas, and Vδ2 expression with the subcutaneous lymphomas {3306,864}. Ultraviolet (UV) light–associated mutation signatures are more common in Vδ1 cases, whereas senescence-related mutagenesis is noted in subcutaneous cases. Patients with deep dermal and subcutaneous lesions show enrichment in interferon-γ and other inflammatory cytokines, which probably drives the haemophagocytic syndrome {864}.

Macroscopic appearance

See *Clinical features*.

Histopathology

Malignant cells are predominantly medium-sized but can range from small to large, with elongated nuclei and coarse chromatin {4280}. Each skin compartment (epidermis, dermis, and subcutis), or any combination thereof, may be involved by PCGD-TCL, and sequential and contemporaneous biopsies may show different compartmental infiltration {4051}. Epidermal and intraepithelial (adnexal {4280}) infiltrates can be subtle or exuberant and pagetoid {333}. Angiotropism is occasionally observed. Dermal involvement may be nodular/perivascular or diffuse. Subcutaneous extension involves lobular and septal sites with rimming of adipocytes, apoptosis, and karyorrhexis.

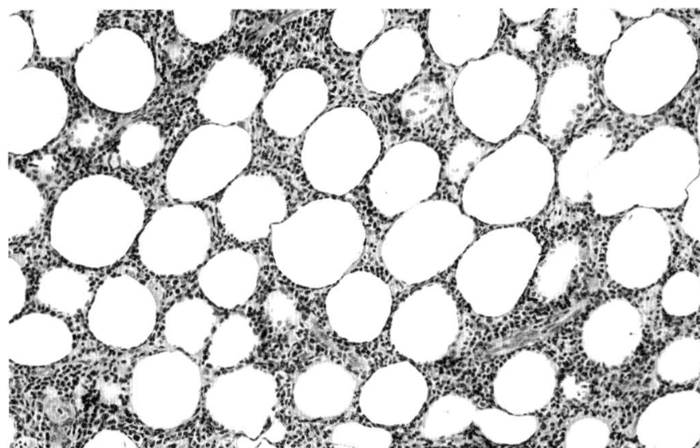

Fig. 5.78 Primary cutaneous gamma-delta T-cell lymphoma. Extension in the subcutis shows a panniculitis-like pattern with medium to large atypical cells that infiltrate the fat lobules and rim adipocytes.

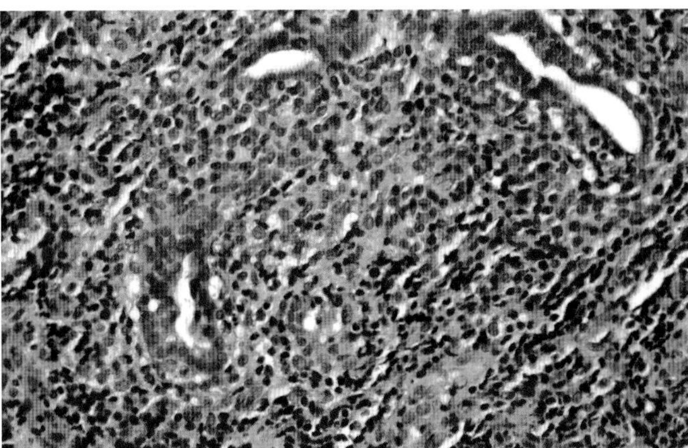

Fig. 5.79 Primary cutaneous gamma-delta T-cell lymphoma. Eccrine involvement in gamma-delta T-cell lymphoma. Deep dermal/panniculitic infiltrates encase and are tropic to the adnexal epithelium.

Additional cytotoxic tissue alteration includes vacuolar interface alteration at the dermoepidermal junction, coagulative necrosis, and angioinvasion.

Immunophenotype

Tumour cells are TCRγ+, TCRδ+, and TCRβ−. A CD3+, CD2+, CD7+/−, CD5− immunophenotype {4380,1857} with expression of at least one cytotoxic protein, including granzyme B, perforin, and/or TIA1, is typical. The majority of cases are negative for both CD4 and CD8, although CD8 positivity may be seen. CD56 expression is present in almost half of the cases {4380}. CD30 is expressed in a minority of cases. EBV is negative.

Differential diagnosis

The differential diagnosis includes, in particular, gamma-delta lymphoproliferative cutaneous disorders, such as gamma-delta subtypes of mycosis fungoides and lymphomatoid papulosis.

Cytology

FNAB is not recommended for establishing this diagnosis.

Diagnostic molecular pathology

Demonstration of clonal TR gene rearrangement can be helpful.

Essential and desirable diagnostic criteria

Essential: a monoclonal proliferation of CD3+, TCRγδ+ T cells in the skin or subcutis; exclusion of other lymphomas such as lymphomatoid papulosis and/or classic mycosis fungoides; EBV negative.

Desirable: CD4–/CD8– or CD4–/CD8+ phenotype; expression of at least one cytotoxic marker (TIA1, granzyme B, perforin); no extracutaneous disease at diagnosis (but this may develop during the course of the disease).

Staging

PCGD-TCL is staged according to the TNM classification system for primary cutaneous lymphomas other than mycosis fungoides and Sézary syndrome {3054}.

Prognosis and prediction

PCGD-TCLs are generally aggressive lymphomas with a median survival time of < 2 years. Decreased survival is described in patients with histological evidence of panniculitic rather than superficial involvement {4051,2665,864}. Haemophagocytic lymphohistiocytosis, metastatic disease, and infections are associated with poor survival {1447}. PCGD-TCLs respond poorly to chemotherapies. Allogeneic transplantation may provide the best option for prolonged remission {1338,1749,1222}.

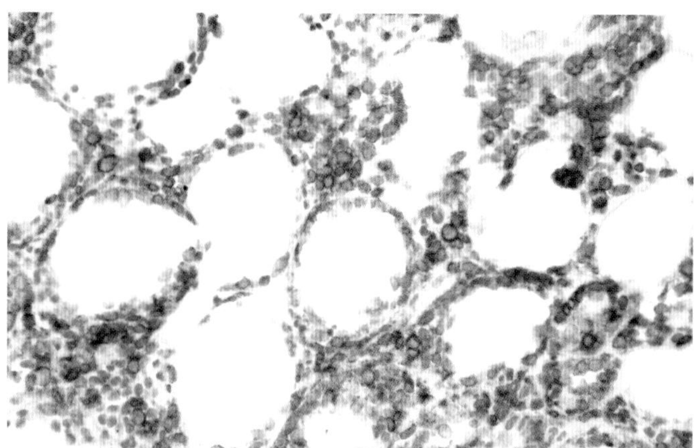

Fig. 5.80 Primary cutaneous gamma-delta T-cell lymphoma. TCRδ immunohistochemistry shows uniform staining of tumour cells.

Primary cutaneous CD8-positive aggressive epidermotropic cytotoxic T-cell lymphoma

Berti E
Guitart J
Nardi V
Pulitzer M
Robson A
Willemze R

Definition

Primary cutaneous CD8-positive aggressive epidermotropic cytotoxic T-cell lymphoma (PCAETL) is a neoplastic proliferation of T lymphocytes often expressing CD8 along with cytotoxic molecules, characterized by epidermal necrosis, a high proliferation index, and aggressive clinical behaviour.

ICD-O coding

9709/3 Primary cutaneous CD8-positive aggressive epidermotropic cytotoxic T-cell lymphoma

ICD-11 coding

2B0Y & XH2513 Other specified primary cutaneous mature T-cell or NK-cell lymphomas and lymphoproliferative disorders & Primary cutaneous CD8-positive aggressive epidermotropic cytotoxic T-cell lymphoma

Related terminology

Not recommended: Berti lymphoma; Ketron–Goodman / disseminated pagetoid reticulosis.

Subtype(s)

None

Localization

Patients present with generalized or localized skin lesions. The oral mucosa may be involved {1445,4060}.

Clinical features

PCAETL is characterized by localized or (more commonly) diffusely distributed papules, ulcerated nodules, tumours, and plaques, showing erosion or central necrosis {334,3432,1445}. In some patients these lesions may be preceded by chronic poorly defined patches {1445}. PCAETL may disseminate to visceral sites (lung, testes, CNS); lymph nodes are usually spared {1445}. Typically, PCAETL is not associated with immunosuppression.

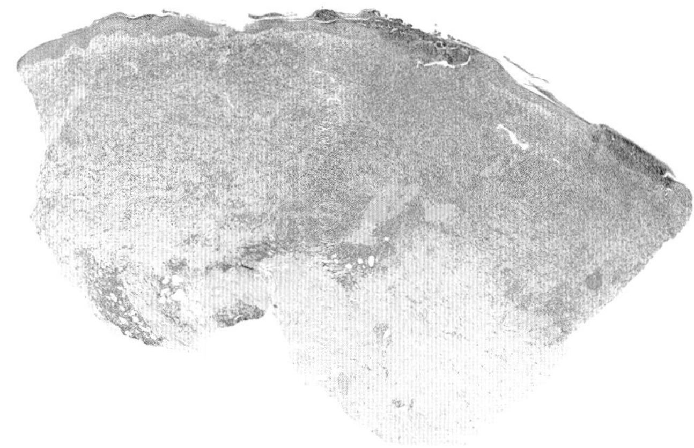

Fig. 5.81 Primary cutaneous CD8-positive aggressive epidermotropic cytotoxic T-cell lymphoma. Low magnification shows a dense nodular and diffuse epidermotropic infiltrate occupying the full dermis and leading to epidermal necrosis.

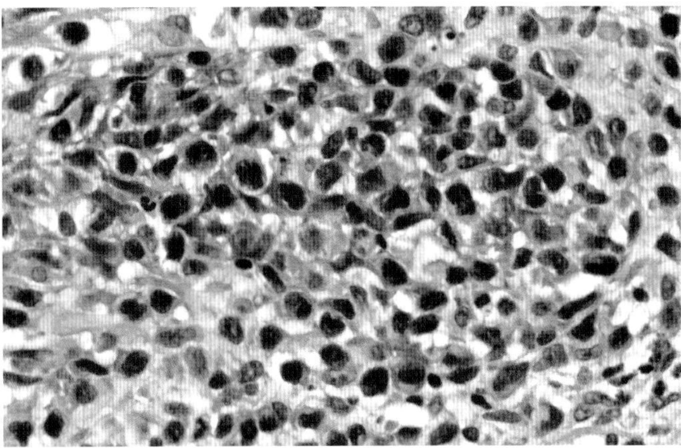

Fig. 5.82 Primary cutaneous CD8-positive aggressive epidermotropic cytotoxic T-cell lymphoma. High magnification revealing the presence of a large number of atypical pleomorphic lymphoid cells.

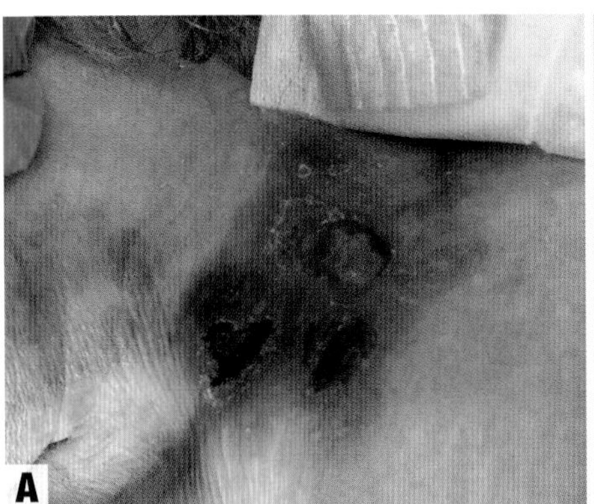

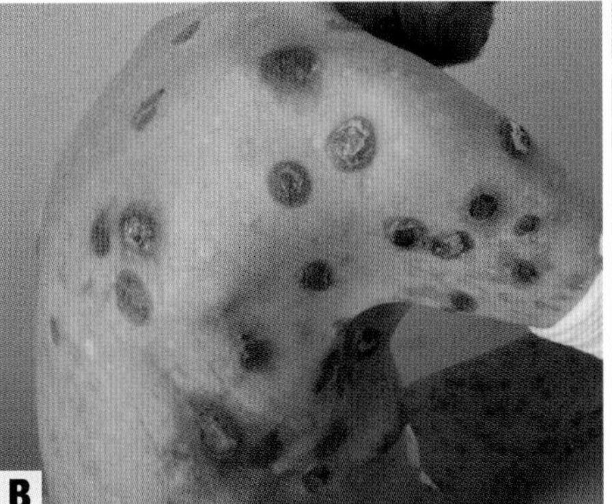

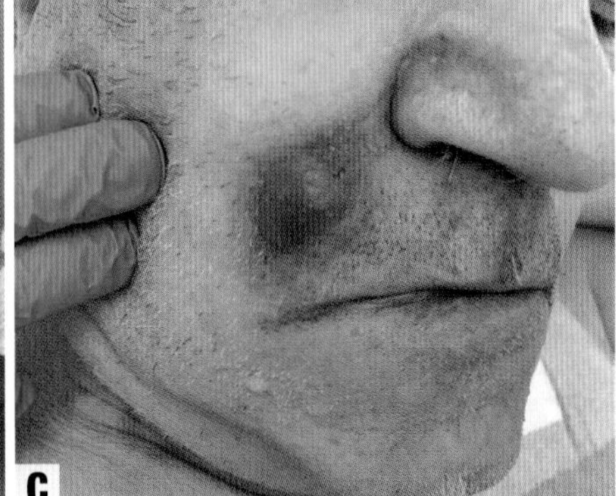

Fig. 5.83 Primary cutaneous CD8-positive aggressive epidermotropic cytotoxic T-cell lymphoma. Examples of the clinical presentation include ulcerating large plaques (**A**), diffuse roundish plaques with central necrotic evolution (**B**), and solitary large nodular lesions (**C**).

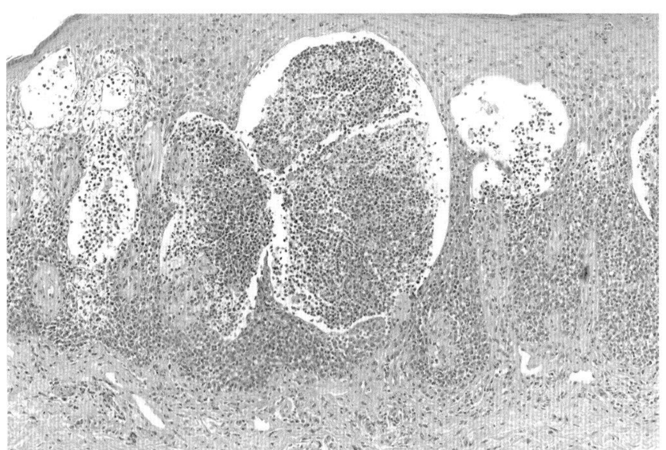

Fig. 5.84 Primary cutaneous CD8-positive aggressive epidermotropic cytotoxic T-cell lymphoma. The atypical lymphocytes extend towards the epidermis in a pagetoid fashion and form blisters.

Epidemiology

PCAETL is rare, accounting for < 1% of all cutaneous T-cell lymphomas. It occurs in adults and has a male predilection {334, 4377,3432,1445}.

Etiology

Unknown

Pathogenesis

Genomic events that recurrently impact genes with roles in the cell cycle, chromatin regulation, and the JAK/STAT pathway have been described in PCAETL, including complex genomic rearrangements and various *JAK2* fusions {267}. Upregulated JAK-2 signalling is observed in virtually all cases, whereas this feature is not detected in other cytotoxic cutaneous T-cell lymphomas. In fusion-negative cases, gain-of-function mutations in *JAK2*, *STAT3*, and *STAT5B*, and loss of negative regulators of the JAK/STAT pathway, particularly *SH2B3*, can be observed {267}.

Macroscopic appearance

PCAETL appears as roundish lesions showing erosive or ulcerative features (see *Clinical features*).

Histopathology

Although the infiltrate can involve the entire dermis, pagetoid epithelial involvement (epidermal and adnexal) is typically observed {3432,3581}. Spongiosis can lead to blister formation. The dermal infiltrates are monomorphic to pleomorphic. Rimming of subcutaneous fat spaces has been reported {2973}. Tumour cells are usually atypical small to large lymphocytes with indented nuclei, scant cytoplasm, and occasional immunoblastic features {334,1445}. Histological evidence of cytotoxicity, including epidermal necrosis/ulceration, dermal necrosis, karyorrhexis, and rare angiocentric destruction, is present {334,2973,3432,1445}. Ulceration may mimic pyoderma gangrenosum {4312,915}. Atypical CD8+ cytotoxic T cells show striking pagetoid epidermotropism {4379,334, 3432,1445}, especially in cases with diffuse lesions. The clinicopathological features are summarized in Table 5.11 {3432, 2973}.

Immunohistochemistry

The usual markers are listed in Table 5.11. Immunohistochemistry for phosphorylated STAT3 and phosphorylated STAT5 can also be used to detect activation of the JAK/STAT pathway {1135,267,2256}.

Table 5.11 Diagnostic features of aggressive epidermotropic CD8+ cutaneous T-cell lymphoma

Clinical features	Histological features	Immunophenotype
Generalized ulcerated papules, nodules, plaques, and/or tumours +/− Mucosal involvement	Pagetoid reticulosis pattern; epidermotropism and necrotic keratinocytes; cytological atypia	βF1+, TCRγδ−, TCRδ−, CD8+ or CD8−/CD4−, TIA1+, granzyme B+, perforin+, CCR4+, CD2− and/or CD5−, CD45RA+, pSTAT3+, pSTAT5+, Ki-67+
Solitary tumorous lesions	Diffuse or nodular dermal infiltrates	As above

Table 5.12 Histological differential diagnosis of primary cutaneous CD8+ aggressive epidermotropic cytotoxic T-cell lymphoma

Differential diagnosis	Clinical features	Immunophenotype			
		Positive	Negative	Variable	Ki-67
Lymphomatoid papulosis subtype D	Recurrent, self-healing, skin-limited papules and nodules	CD3, CD5, CD8, CCR4, βF1, TIA1, TBX21 (T-bet)	CD4, CD45RA, GATA3	CD2+/−, CD30+/−, granzyme B+/−, perforin+/−, CD7−/+, CD56−/+, TCRδ−/+	High in atypical cells
CD8+ mycosis fungoides	Chronic indolent patches and plaques or tumours	CD2, CD3, CD8, TIA1, CCR4, TBX21 (T-bet)	CD4, CD30, CD45RA, GATA3	CD5+/−, granzyme B+/−, perforin+/−, CD7−/+, CD56−/+	Low (high in transformed cases)
TCRγδ+ mycosis fungoides (epidermotropic)	Diffuse patches and plaques	CD2, CD3, TCRδ, TIA1, granzyme B, perforin, TBX21 (T-bet)	CD4, CD8, CCR4, CD56, βF1, GATA3	CD7+/−, CD45RA+/−, CD5−/+, CD30−/+	Intermediate
Primary cutaneous T-cell lymphoma NOS (cytotoxic pattern)	Rapidly diffused patches, plaques, or tumours; less often, solitary lesions	CD2, CD3, CD8, βF1, TIA1, TBX21 (T-bet)	CD5, CD7, CD4, CD30, CD45RA, TCRδ, GATA3	CCR4+/−, granzyme B+/−, perforin+/−, CD56−/+	High

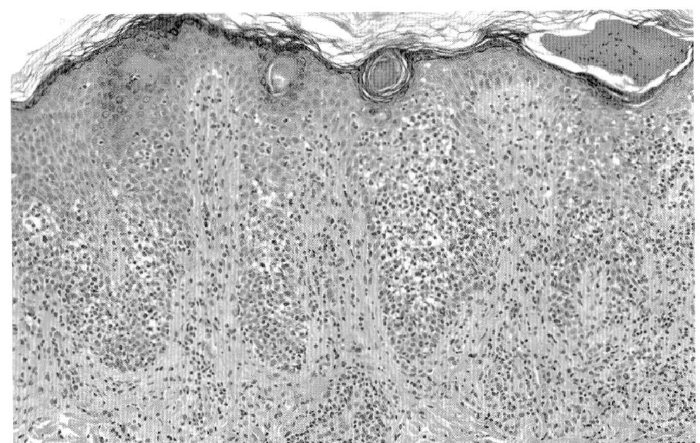

Fig. 5.85 Primary cutaneous CD8-positive aggressive epidermotropic cytotoxic T-cell lymphoma. The atypical lymphocytes infiltrate the upper dermis and extend towards the epidermis in a pagetoid fashion, accompanied by mild spongiosis.

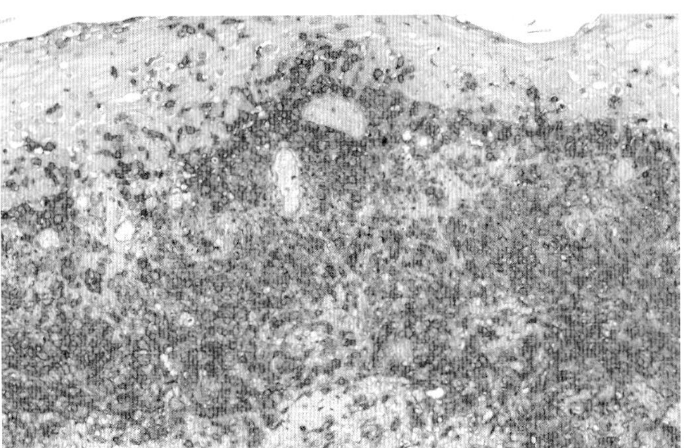

Fig. 5.86 Primary cutaneous CD8-positive aggressive epidermotropic cytotoxic T-cell lymphoma. Immunohistochemistry: CD8 stain highlights the neoplastic lymphocytes infiltrating the epidermis.

Differential diagnosis

This includes rare epidermotropic subtypes of cutaneous gamma-delta T-cell lymphomas (e.g. gamma-delta mycosis fungoides), CD8+ mycosis fungoides, localized pagetoid reticulosis, and type D lymphomatoid papulosis (Table 5.12).

Cytology

The use of FNAB is not recommended for the diagnosis of this entity.

Diagnostic molecular pathology

Evidence of clonal TR gene rearrangements supports the diagnosis.

Essential and desirable diagnostic criteria

Essential: an epidermotropic and adnexotropic cutaneous diffuse infiltrate composed of pleomorphic cytotoxic TCRαβ-expressing T lymphocytes; ulcerated or erosive plaques and tumours without spontaneous resolution.

Desirable: demonstration of activating mutations or fusions of JAK-2 pathway genes.

Staging

PCAETL is staged according to the TNM classification system for cutaneous T-cell lymphomas other than mycosis fungoides and Sézary syndrome {3054}.

Prognosis and prediction

PCAETL have an aggressive course (median survival time: 12 months). There are no differences between cases with small or large cell morphology or localized or diffuse lesions {1445}.

Primary cutaneous peripheral T-cell lymphoma NOS

Mitteldorf C
Berti E
Pulitzer M
Willemze R

Definition

Primary cutaneous peripheral T-cell lymphoma (pcPTCL) NOS is a poorly characterized group of T-cell lymphomas not meeting the criteria for any specifically defined primary cutaneous T-cell lymphoma entity; i.e. it is a diagnosis of exclusion.

ICD-O coding

9709/3 Primary cutaneous peripheral T-cell lymphoma, NOS

ICD-11 coding

2B0Z Primary cutaneous T-cell lymphoma of undetermined or unspecified type

Related terminology

Acceptable: primary cutaneous peripheral T-cell lymphoma, unspecified.

Subtype(s)

None

Localization

Disseminated skin lesions are predominantly located on the trunk and limbs {3233,1956}, whereas solitary tumours are more commonly found on the skin of the legs, arms, and (occasionally) head and neck {3233,1956}.

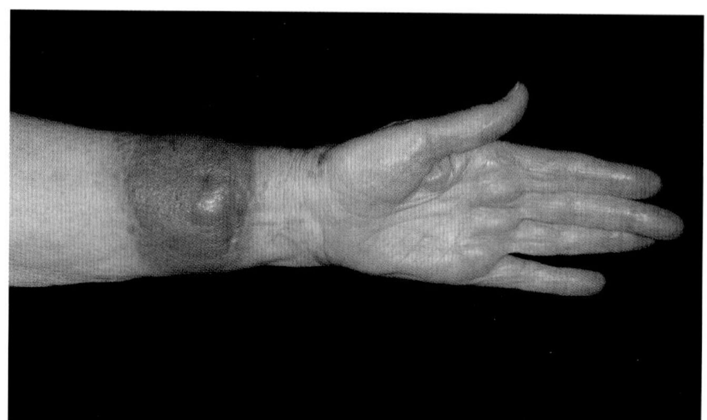

Fig. 5.87 Primary cutaneous peripheral T-cell lymphoma NOS. A large red tumour on the left forearm.

Clinical features

Most patients present with disseminated plaques, papules, or tumours {1956,3233,294}. About one third present with solitary lesions {1956,3233}.

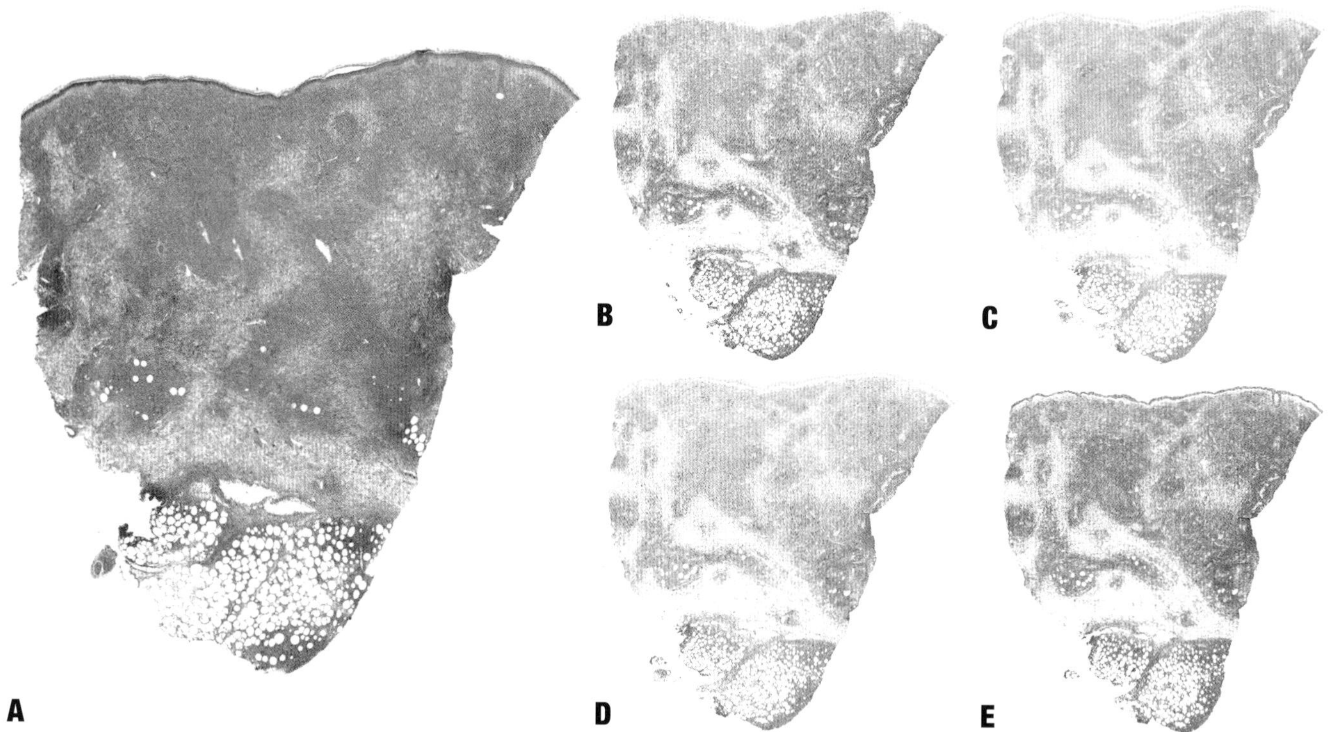

Fig. 5.88 Primary cutaneous peripheral T-cell lymphoma NOS. A diffuse infiltrate of cohesive sheets of lymphocytes extends into the dermis and involves the subcutis; the epidermis is spared (**A**). The tumour cells are positive for CD3 (**B**) and CD4 (**C**). The tumour cells are negative for CD8 (**D**). In this case, uniform GATA3 expression is seen (**E**).

The skin lesions can show ulceration (~15% of cases) {1956}. Although pcPTCL-NOS is limited to the skin at the time of diagnosis, systemic involvement commonly develops later during the course of the disease.

Epidemiology

pcPTCL-NOS is exceedingly rare, and it mostly arises in adults in their sixth decade of life. Presentation in the paediatric age group has also been described {1956,3233,294}. There is a male predilection (M:F ratio: 3:1) {294,3233,1956}.

Etiology

Unknown

Pathogenesis

Pathogenesis is largely unknown, although gains of chromosomes 7q, 8, and 17q and loss of chromosome 9p21 have been reported {4160}.

Macroscopic appearance

See *Clinical features*.

Histopathology

Because pcPTCL-NOS is a diagnosis of exclusion, distinct and characteristic histopathological and immunophenotypic features are lacking; however, features of any other cutaneous T-cell lymphoma entity can be observed, albeit outside the typical context. The skin shows diffuse or nodular dermal infiltration of cohesive sheets of mostly medium-sized to large lymphoid cells {294,4038,2258,1956}. The subcutis is commonly involved {1956}. A mild and focal epidermotropism is found in approximately one third of cases {1956}. Angiocentric/angiodestructive features and folliculotropism are rare {294,2258,1956}.

Immunophenotype

The tumour cells are positive for CD2 and CD3 {1956}. The most common phenotype is CD4+/CD8− {294,1956}. About one third show a CD4−/CD8− phenotype, and approximately 10% are CD4+/CD8+ {1956}. Cytotoxic markers (TIA1 and granzyme B) are mostly negative (75%) {1956}. Aberrant expression of CD20 can occur {1956}. The proliferative activity is moderate to high (30–90%). PD1 expression (> 40%) can be found {1956}. EBV is negative {1956}.

Very rare cases of primary cutaneous T-cell lymphoma with a T follicular helper (TFH) cell phenotype have been described {276, 3571}. Further data are needed to better characterize this entity. Therefore, primary cutaneous T-cell lymphomas with a TFH-cell phenotype (defined by the expression of at least two TFH-cell markers: PD1, ICOS, CD10, BCL6, CXCL13) should currently be placed in this group, i.e. pcPTCL-NOS with a TFH phenotype.

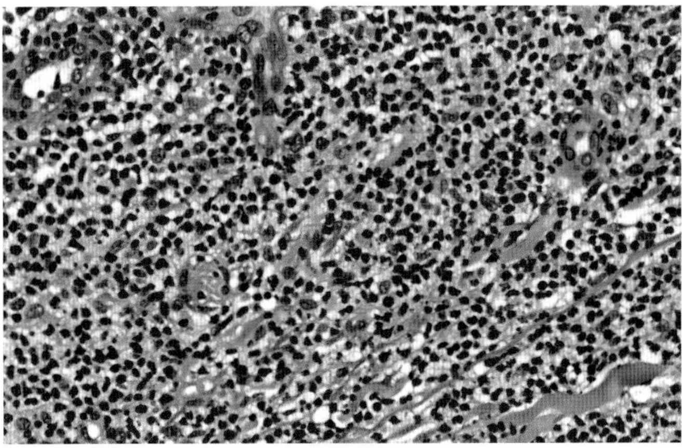

Fig. 5.89 Primary cutaneous peripheral T-cell lymphoma NOS. Sheets of pleomorphic small, medium-sized, and large tumour cells.

Cytology

Fine core needle biopsy usually does not provide sufficient material to make this diagnosis.

Diagnostic molecular pathology

Not generally relevant. TR gene rearrangements can be informative but are not specific.

Essential and desirable diagnostic criteria

Essential: diffuse or nodular dermal infiltrates of atypical T lymphocytes; no extracutaneous involvement of the lymphoma at time of diagnosis; a diagnosis of exclusion – does not meet the diagnostic criteria for defined cutaneous T-cell lymphoma entities.

Desirable: molecular studies to exclude other specific entities in selected cases.

Staging

pcPTCL-NOS is staged according to the International Society for Cutaneous Lymphomas (ISCL) / Cutaneous Lymphoma Task Force of the European Organization of Research and Treatment of Cancer (EORTC) system {2015}.

Prognosis and prediction

The prognosis of pcPTCL-NOS is poor, with mean overall survival times between 27 months {3233} and 5.6 years {4038}. Some studies showed a better prognosis in solitary lesions {3233}; this might provide a rationale for radiotherapy in such cases {294,3233,1956}. B symptoms, multifocal lesions, and systemic involvement are unfavourable prognostic factors {4038}. In disseminated lesions, multiagent chemotherapy is used, although it may not be effective {294,1956}.

Intestinal T-cell and NK-cell lymphoid proliferations and lymphomas: Introduction

Chan JKC
Alaggio R

In this edition, the following entities are listed under the category of intestinal T-cell and NK-cell lymphoid proliferations and lymphomas:

- Indolent T-cell lymphoma of the gastrointestinal tract
- Indolent NK-cell lymphoproliferative disorder of the gastrointestinal tract
- Enteropathy-associated T-cell lymphoma
- Monomorphic epitheliotropic intestinal T-cell lymphoma
- Intestinal T-cell lymphoma NOS

Compared with the previous edition, there is a change in nomenclature from "indolent T-cell lymphoproliferative disorder of the gastrointestinal tract" to "indolent T-cell lymphoma of the

Table 5.13 Comparison of different types of T-cell and NK-cell lymphoid proliferations and lymphomas involving the gastrointestinal tract[a]

Diagnostic criteria	Indolent T-cell lymphoma of the gastrointestinal tract	Indolent NK-cell lymphoproliferative disorder of the gastrointestinal tract	Enteropathy-associated T-cell lymphoma	Monomorphic epitheliotropic intestinal T-cell lymphoma	Extranodal NK/T-cell lymphoma[b]
Major clinical presentation	Abdominal symptoms (such as chronic diarrhoea, pain, vomiting, dyspepsia)	Asymptomatic or nonspecific gastrointestinal symptoms	Abdominal symptoms (such as pain, diarrhoea) and weight loss; common bowel perforation or obstruction	Abdominal symptoms (such as pain, bleeding) and weight loss; common bowel perforation or obstruction	Abdominal symptoms (such as pain, bleeding) and fever; common bowel perforation
Association with coeliac disease	–	–	+	–	–
Clinical course	Indolent, often chronic persistent or relapsing	Spontaneous regression, but recurrent new lesions may develop	Aggressive	Aggressive	Aggressive
Commonest localization in gastrointestinal tract	Small bowel or colon	Stomach, small and large intestines	Small intestine	Small intestine	Small and large intestines
Lesional involvement of gastrointestinal tract	Superficial (mucosal +/– submucosal)	Superficial (mucosal)	Deep	Deep	Deep
Cytomorphology	Small lymphoid cells with minimal nuclear atypia	Atypical medium-sized lymphoid cells with pale cytoplasm and eosinophilic granules	Pleomorphic large or medium-sized lymphoid cells, commonly with prominent inflammatory background	Monomorphic small to medium-sized lymphoid cells	Variable cytomorphology, from small to medium-sized to large cells
Epitheliotropism	–/focal	–/minimal	+	+	–
Necrosis	–	–	+/–	Usually –	+
EBV association	–	–	–	–	+
Lineage	T cell, CD4+ > CD8+	NK cell (cCD3+, sCD3–)	T cell, most often CD4–, CD8–	T cell, most often CD8+	NK cell (more common) or T cell
T-cell receptor expression	TCRαβ+	Negative	Usually negative	Usually TCRγδ+ or TCRαβ+	Usually negative
TR (TCR) gene rearrangements	Clonal	Negative	Clonal	Clonal	Usually negative
Molecular genetics	*JAK2::STAT3* fusion; mutations of JAK/STAT pathway genes and epigenetic modifier genes	*JAK3* mutation	Gains of 9q34; loss of 16q12; mutations of JAK/STAT pathway genes (commonly *JAK1*, *STAT3*)	Gains of 9q34; loss of 16q12; mutations of JAK/STAT pathway genes (commonly *JAK3*, *STAT5B*) and *SETD2*	6q21-25 deletion; mutations of JAK/STAT pathway genes, epigenetic regulators (*BCOR*, KMT2 [*MLL2*], *ARID1A*), tumour suppressor genes (*TP53*, *MGA*), and RNA helicase (*DDX3X*)

[a]Other differential diagnoses include intestinal T-cell lymphoma NOS and secondary involvement of the gastrointestinal tract by other mature T-cell lymphomas and leukaemias, such as adult T-cell leukaemia/lymphoma and peripheral T-cell lymphoma NOS. [b]This tumour is covered in the sections on EBV-positive T-cell and NK-cell lymphomas (p. 762).

gastrointestinal tract". The change from the more conservative designation of "lymphoproliferative disorder" to "lymphoma" is justified by the significant morbidities related to the tumour and the ability of the disease to disseminate, but the qualifier "indolent" remains to indicate the protracted clinical course {2537, 3703,3197,3773}.

The newly introduced entity indolent NK-cell lymphoproliferative disorder of the gastrointestinal tract is actually not new. Formerly known as lymphomatoid gastropathy or NK-cell enteropathy, this entity was first characterized more than a decade ago. It was not included as a lymphoma in previous editions of the WHO classification of haematolymphoid tumours because it was believed to be a reactive lesion mimicking malignancy. The recent finding of frequent mutations, particularly in *JAK3*, supports the notion that this disease has a neoplastic nature, hence its inclusion in the present edition {4439}. Nonetheless, the disease is practically benign in its clinical behaviour, with spontaneous regression of the individual lesions and only occasional development of new lesions over the years, without progression to more aggressive disease or dissemination {2522, 4439,3946}. Therefore, the entity is called a lymphoproliferative disorder instead of a lymphoma, and it is further qualified with the term "indolent" to indicate the excellent outcome. The most important differential diagnosis is extranodal NK/T-cell lymphoma, which often shows an identical immunophenotype but is highly aggressive (see Table 5.13).

The delineation of monomorphic epitheliotropic intestinal T-cell lymphoma as an entity separate from enteropathy-associated T-cell lymphoma, implemented in the revised fourth edition of the WHO classification of haematolymphoid tumours, remains highly valid, because these two entities show different epidemiological, etiological, pathological, immunophenotypic, and genetic features.

Intestinal T-cell lymphoma NOS remains a waste-basket entity; it is a heterogeneous category encompassing different types of primary T-cell lymphomas of the gastrointestinal tract, which are related to various classes of normal T cells resident in the mucosa of the intestine {2453}. Extranodal NK/T-cell lymphoma may also present as a primary gastrointestinal lymphoma. This lymphoma type is listed separately under the category of EBV-positive T-cell and NK-cell lymphomas because its primary localization is highly variable, with the upper respiratory tract being the most common site of involvement.

Indolent T-cell lymphoma of the gastrointestinal tract

Bhagat G
Dave SS
Naresh KN
Takeuchi K

Definition

Indolent T-cell lymphoma of the gastrointestinal tract (iTCL-GI) is a clonal T-cell proliferation characterized by the infiltration of the lamina propria by small mature lymphocytes lacking significant epitheliotropism, and typically a protracted clinical course.

ICD-O coding

9702/1 Indolent T-cell lymphoma of the gastrointestinal tract

ICD-11 coding

2B2Y & XH2LK2 Other specified mature T-cell or NK-cell neoplasms & Lymphoproliferative disorder, NOS

Related terminology

Acceptable: indolent T-cell lymphoproliferative disorder of the gastrointestinal tract; indolent clonal T-cell lymphoproliferative disorder of the gastrointestinal tract.

Subtype(s)

None

Localization

Most patients present with disease affecting the small intestine or colon {3201,2537,3703,3773,2499}. However, any site in the gastrointestinal tract can be involved, including the oral cavity and oesophagus {1046}. Dissemination to extragastrointestinal locations (e.g. bone marrow, tonsil, peripheral blood) is uncommon at diagnosis {3773} but can occur at disease progression or transformation {553,2499,2537,3197}.

Clinical features

Presenting symptoms include chronic diarrhoea, abdominal pain, vomiting, dyspepsia, and weight loss, mimicking inflammatory intestinal diseases (e.g. coeliac disease and inflammatory bowel disease) {3201,553,2537,3773,2499}. Peripheral lymphadenopathy is absent, but mesenteric lymphadenopathy may be observed {2584,2537,3773,2499}.

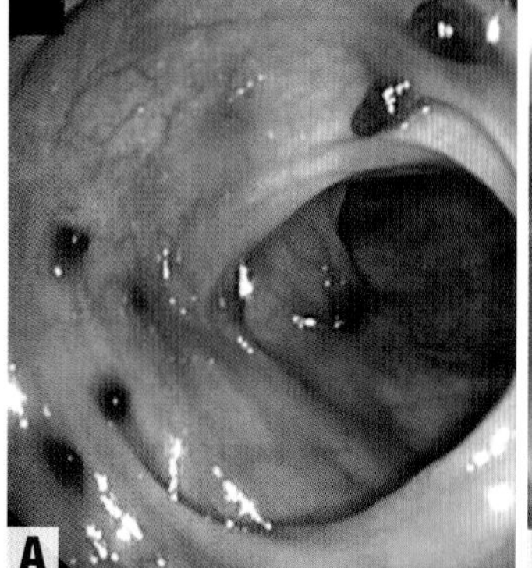

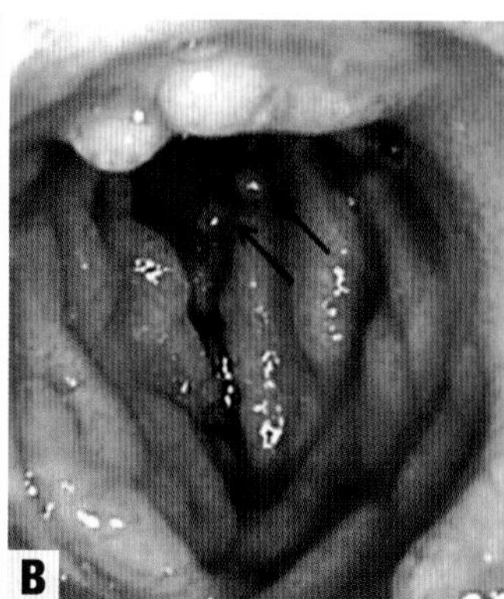

Fig. 5.90 Indolent T-cell lymphoproliferative disorder of the gastrointestinal tract. **A** Presentation with small polypoid hyperaemic lesions. **B** Presentation with multiple small, hyperaemic mucosal polyps (arrows).

Epidemiology

The geographical distribution of iTCL-GI is wide. It arises in adulthood (median ages: 51 years and 45 years for CD4+ and CD8+ diseases, respectively), more frequently in men than women (M:F ratio: 1.5–2:1), and rarely in adolescents {2584}.

Etiology

The etiology is unknown. Some patients have a history of inflammatory bowel disease or intestinal immune disorders {3201, 2499,3773}, but the relationship of these disorders with iTCL-GI is unclear.

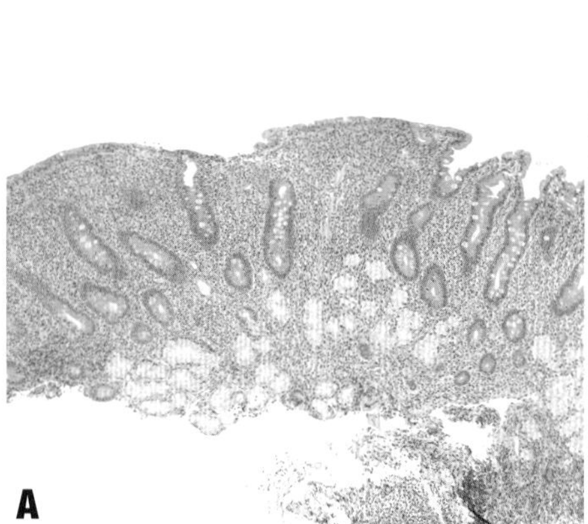

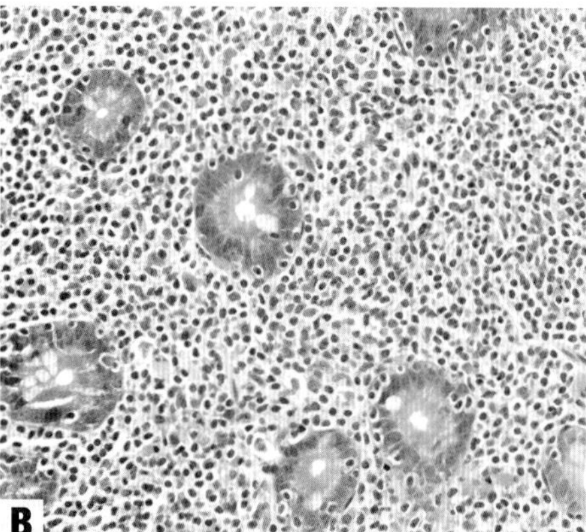

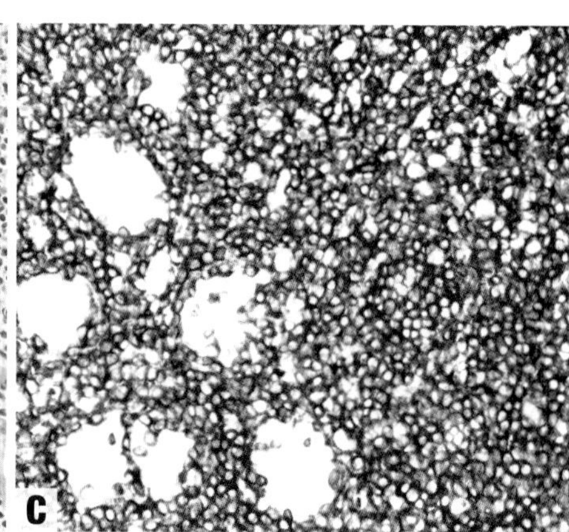

Fig. 5.91 Indolent T-cell lymphoma of the gastrointestinal tract, CD4 immunophenotype. **A** The duodenal biopsy shows villus atrophy, crypt hyperplasia, and expansion of the lamina propria by an infiltrate of small lymphocytes. Intraepithelial lymphocytes are not increased. **B** The lamina propria has a dense infiltrate of small lymphocytes exhibiting mature morphology. Focal infiltration of the crypt epithelium is present. **C** The lymphocytes are CD4-positive.

Pathogenesis

Clonal TRB and/or TRG rearrangements are detected in all cases {3201,2537,3703,3773}. Non-recurrent DNA copy-number variants have been reported in many CD4+ cases {2537, 2499}. However, mutations and structural variants appear to differ in distinct immunophenotypic subsets {3773,3703}. JAK/STAT pathway gene alterations, as well as mutations in epigenetic modifier genes (e.g. *TET2*, *KMT2D*), are present in CD4+, CD4+/CD8+, and CD4−/CD8− disorders, with CD4+ cases displaying recurrent *STAT3::JAK2* fusions, whereas some CD8+ cases have been shown to harbour structural alterations involving the 3′ untranslated region of *IL2* {3703, 3773}. The mutation profiles remain stable over long periods, and accrual of mutations may presage disease progression or transformation.

Macroscopic appearance

The mucosa of affected sites can be thickened, with prominent folds, nodules, fissures, or ulcers {1046,2584}. In some cases, the infiltrate produces intestinal polyps resembling lymphomatous polyposis {1592,1748}.

Histopathology

The lamina propria is usually expanded by a dense, non-destructive infiltrate of small lymphocytes; some biopsies show only patchy involvement {2584}. Infiltration of the muscularis mucosae and submucosa is seen at times. In small intestinal disease, the villous architecture is generally preserved, but crypt hyperplasia is not uncommon {3773}. Intraepithelial lymphocytes are not increased in most cases; however, epithelial infiltration of the crypts or lower portions of the villi may be present {2537,3773,2584}. The lymphocytes have round, ovoid, or slightly irregular nuclei; fine chromatin; indistinct nucleoli; and scant or moderate cytoplasm {2584}. Rare admixed chronic inflammatory cells and occasional lymphoid aggregates are seen {2584}. Epithelioid granulomas, similar to those observed in Crohn disease, can be focally present {3201,553,2537}.

Immunohistochemistry

The lymphocytes exhibit a mature T-cell phenotype. All cases express CD3, but downregulation/loss of CD5 or CD7 can be seen in a subset {2584}. CD4+ cases appear more common than CD8+ cases {553,2537,2499,3703,3201,3773}, and some might display CD4+/CD8+ or CD4−/CD8− immunophenotypes {3773,3703,3201}. CD4+ cases do not express FOXP3 or PD1 {2537}, and the CD8+ cases are TIA1+, but granzyme B expression is infrequent {3201,3773}. All published cases have documented TCRαβ expression. A small subset of cases are CD103+ and, rarely, focal/weak CD56 expression may be observed {1592,2499,3773}. CD30 is negative, except in transformed lymphomas {2537}. The neoplastic cells are negative for EBV-encoded small RNA (EBER). The Ki-67 proliferation index is extremely low (< 10%).

Differential diagnosis

Although iTCL-GI might resemble inflammatory intestinal diseases clinically, the presence of a relatively dense infiltrate of small mature lymphocytes in the lamina propria, sparse chronic inflammation, and dominant expression of CD4 or CD8, are supportive of iTCL-GI. The cytological attributes of indolent NK-cell lymphoproliferative disorder of the gastrointestinal tract (medium-sized cells, irregular nuclei, and pale pink cytoplasm) differ from those of iTCL-GI. Among primary aggressive intestinal T-cell lymphomas, monomorphic epitheliotropic intestinal T-cell lymphoma can show overlapping morphological and immunophenotypic features with CD8+ iTCL-GI; however, an absence of epitheliotropism and CD56 expression and a low Ki-67 proliferation index can aid in excluding monomorphic epitheliotropic intestinal T-cell lymphoma (see Table 5.13, p. 710). Secondary gastrointestinal involvement by peripheral or cutaneous T-cell lymphomas should be ruled out by clinical examination and imaging studies before diagnosing iTCL-GI.

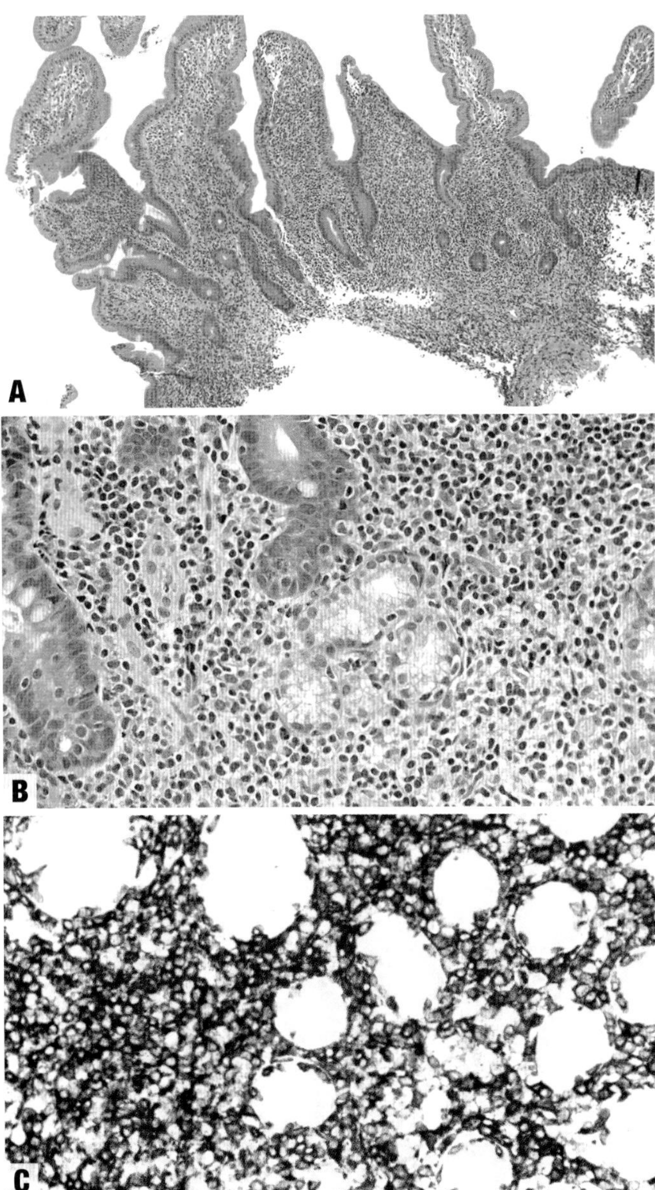

Fig. 5.92 Indolent T-cell lymphoma of the gastrointestinal tract, CD8 immunophenotype. **A** Some of the villi are broadened and the lamina propria is variably expanded by an infiltrate of small lymphocytes. **B** The lamina propria is infiltrated by small lymphocytes that have round or oval nuclei, inconspicuous nucleoli, and scant cytoplasm. **C** The lymphocytes are CD8-positive.

Cytology
Not clinically relevant

Diagnostic molecular pathology
In selected circumstances, demonstration of clonal TR rearrangement (or somatic mutations) can assist in the distinction from an inflammatory disorder.

Essential and desirable diagnostic criteria
Essential: a non-destructive, predominantly non-epitheliotropic infiltrate of small mature lymphocytes confined to the gastrointestinal mucosa +/− submucosa; T lineage (CD4+, CD8+, CD4+/CD8+, or CD4−/CD8−), with TCRαβ expression; low proliferation index (Ki-67 < 10%).

Desirable: detection of clonal TR rearrangement (or somatic mutations) can assist in the distinction from an inflammatory disorder.

Staging
Staging is performed according to the Lugano classification, which has been adopted by the eighth-edition Union for International Cancer Control (UICC) TNM classification {688}.

Prognosis and prediction
Multiple sites in the gastrointestinal tract are often involved, with chronic persistence of disease or a relapsing clinical course. Response to conventional chemotherapy is poor, but patients typically have prolonged survival with conservative management (e.g. steroid therapy). Disease progression with extragastrointestinal spread or transformation to aggressive lymphoma can occur, usually decades after diagnosis {553,2537,3703, 3197,3773}.

Indolent NK-cell lymphoproliferative disorder of the gastrointestinal tract

Xiao W
Cheng CL
Ferry JA
Takeuchi K

Definition
Indolent NK-cell lymphoproliferative disorder (iNK-LPD) of the gastrointestinal tract is an indolent but recurring EBV-negative NK-cell proliferation that predominantly involves the gastrointestinal tract but occasionally may affect other anatomical sites.

ICD-O coding
9702/1 Indolent NK-cell lymphoproliferative disorder of the gastrointestinal tract

ICD-11 coding
2B2Y & XH2LK2 Other specified mature T-cell or NK-cell neoplasms & Lymphoproliferative disorder, NOS

Related terminology
Acceptable: atypical NK-cell proliferation of the gastrointestinal tract; lymphomatoid gastropathy; NK-cell enteropathy.

Subtype(s)
None

Localization
iNK-LPD involves the stomach (in ~70% of cases) and the small/large intestine (in ~30%) {4195,2522,4439,3946}. Similar lesions have been rarely reported in the gallbladder {4435} and vagina {2132}, and (rarely) in adjacent lymph nodes {872}.

Clinical features
Patients are asymptomatic or have vague gastrointestinal symptoms including abdominal pain, with lesions identified on endoscopy. There is no history of coeliac disease or inflammatory bowel disease, and no systemic lymphadenopathy or organomegaly {2522,4439,3946}.

Epidemiology
iNK-LPD is rare. Patients are usually men and women in their third to eighth decade of life {2522,4439,3946}.

Etiology
Unknown

Pathogenesis
The proliferation in iNK-LPD may be an immune response to antigen(s) encountered in the gastrointestinal mucosa {2522, 3946}. A high prevalence of *Helicobacter pylori* infection has been reported in the gastric cases {3946}, and an anecdotal report of regression of chronic recurrent disease after anti-*Helicobacter* therapy {2881} suggests a possible etiological role of *Helicobacter*.

In one reported series, a molecular study identified somatic mutations in 7 of 10 patients, including mutations in *JAK3* (in 3 patients) and other genes, such as *RUNX1T1*, *CIC*, *ERBB4*, and *SETD5* {4439}. Strong immunostaining for phosphorylated STAT5 in all studied cases suggests that JAK-3/STAT5 pathway hyperactivation plays a role in pathogenesis {4439}. These findings further suggest that iNK-LPD is neoplastic.

Macroscopic appearance
Endoscopy reveals single or multiple superficial small lesions, approximately 10–20 mm, manifesting as elevated lesions, often with haemorrhage and oedema (blood blister–like lesion), erosion, or ulcer, involving single or multiple sites along the gastrointestinal tract {2522,3946}.

Histopathology
The lamina propria in iNK-LPD shows expansion by a relatively well circumscribed but confluent infiltrate of medium-sized cells with irregular nuclei (occasionally with small, distinct nucleoli),

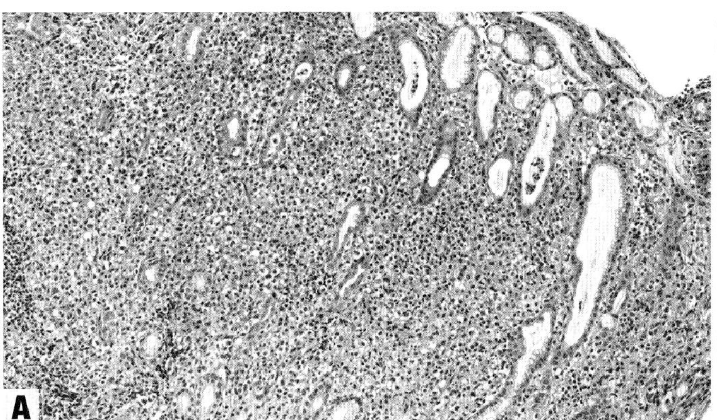

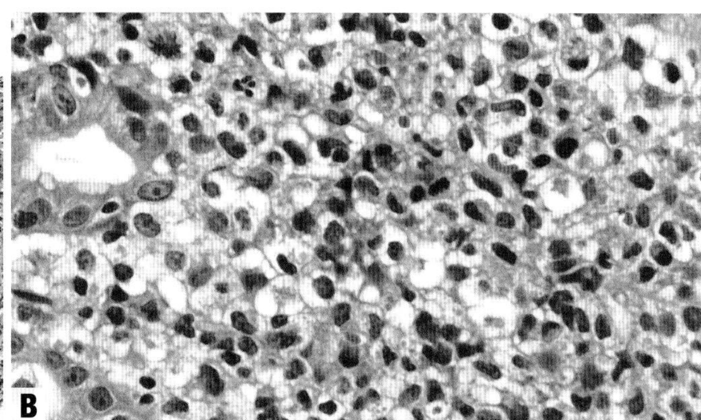

Fig. 5.93 Indolent NK-cell lymphoproliferative disorder of the gastrointestinal tract, involving the stomach. **A** The gastric mucosa shows expansion of the lamina propria by an atypical lymphoid infiltrate. **B** The lymphoid cells are medium-sized and usually have indented nuclei. Brightly eosinophilic granules can often be appreciated in the pale-staining cytoplasm.

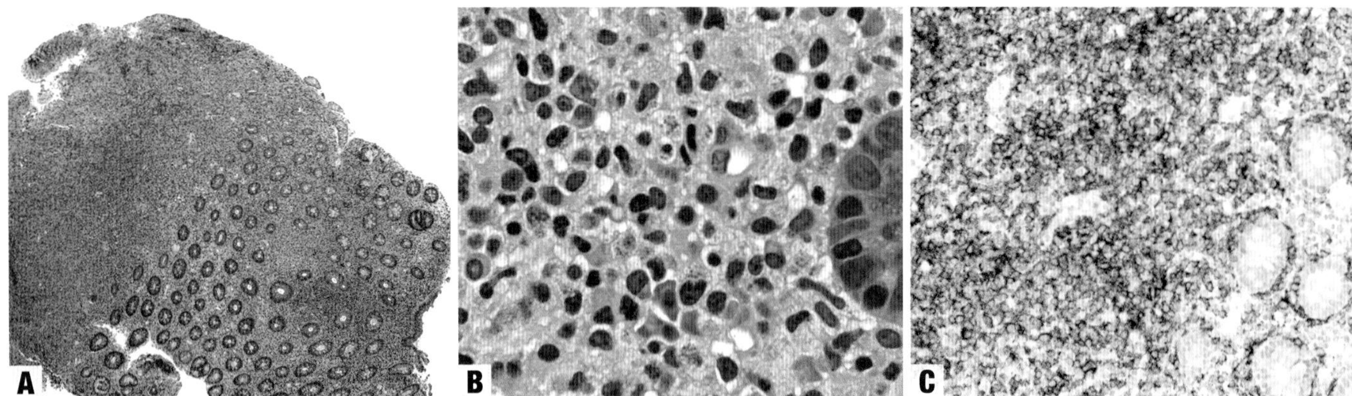

Fig. 5.94 Indolent NK-cell lymphoproliferative disorder of the gastrointestinal tract, involving the colon. **A** The mucosa shows a patchy dense infiltrate of atypical lymphoid cells. **B** The atypical lymphoid cells have indented nuclei and brightly eosinophilic granules. **C** Atypical lymphoid cells are positive for CD56.

finely clumped chromatin, and a moderate amount of pale cytoplasm {2522,4439,3946}, often with paranuclear eosinophilic cytoplasmic granules {3946}. Glands are displaced or destroyed. Epithelial invasion can be seen {3946}. Necrosis is occasionally seen, usually with mucosal ulceration. Other inflammatory cells (plasma cells, neutrophils, eosinophils) are often present. The muscularis mucosae remains intact. There is no angiocentric-angiodestructive growth, villous atrophy, or crypt hyperplasia.

Immunohistochemistry and in situ hybridization

Lesional cells express CD2, CD56, CD7, cCD3, TIA1, and granzyme B, but they do not express sCD3, TCRαβ, TCRγδ, CD5, CD4, CD10, CD20, PAX5, CD138, or CD68. CD8 is rarely positive {3935}. The Ki-67 proliferation index is usually low but can be as high as 40–50%. In situ hybridization for EBV-encoded small RNA (EBER) is negative.

Differential diagnosis

There is significant morphological and immunophenotypic overlap between iNK-LPD and extranodal NK/T-cell lymphoma, so their distinction is important to avoid unnecessary therapy. NK-large granular lymphocytic leukaemia differs from iNK-LPD by showing systemic (peripheral blood and marrow) involvement. See Table 5.13 (p. 710) for differential diagnostic features.

Cytology

Not relevant

Diagnostic molecular pathology

In situ hybridization for EBER is negative. No clonal TR gene rearrangements have been identified {2522,4439,3946}.

Essential and desirable diagnostic criteria

Essential: an infiltrate of atypical small lymphoid cells with an NK-cell immunophenotype, confined to the superficial mucosa of the gastrointestinal tract and rarely presenting at other anatomical sites, including lymph nodes; EBV negative.
Desirable: absence of clonal TR gene rearrangements.

Staging

None

Prognosis and prediction

Individual lesions usually regress spontaneously in a few months, but some patients may have persistent lesions or recurrent new lesions. Patients with iNK-LPD usually do not show a prolonged response to chemotherapy {2522,4439, 3946}. Progression to more aggressive disease has not been reported.

Enteropathy-associated T-cell lymphoma

Bhagat G
Cerf-Bensussan N
Dave SS
Naresh KN

Definition

Enteropathy-associated T-cell lymphoma (EATL) is an aggressive primary intestinal T-cell lymphoma of intraepithelial lymphocytes (IELs), which exhibits variable cellular pleomorphism and usually occurs in individuals with coeliac disease (CD).

ICD-O coding

9717/3 Enteropathy-associated T-cell lymphoma

ICD-11 coding

2A90.7 Enteropathy-associated T-cell lymphoma

Related terminology

Not recommended: type I enteropathy-associated T-cell lymphoma.

Subtype(s)

None

Localization

The small intestine is involved in about 90% of cases: most frequently the jejunum, but other segments of the small bowel, and less commonly the stomach and colon, may be affected {922, 1274,3743,2496}. Multifocal lesions are present in 32–54% of cases {1274,2496}. As many as one third of EATLs evolving from refractory coeliac disease (RCD) type 2 (RCD2) may initially manifest at extraintestinal locations (e.g. skin, lymph nodes, spleen) {2496}. Dissemination to extragastrointestinal sites is most often to mesenteric and abdominal lymph nodes, but other organs, including the bone marrow, lung, or liver, may also be involved {1045,2496,922}. Widespread disease (Lugano stage II2–IV) is observed in 43–70% of patients at diagnosis {922, 2496,3743}.

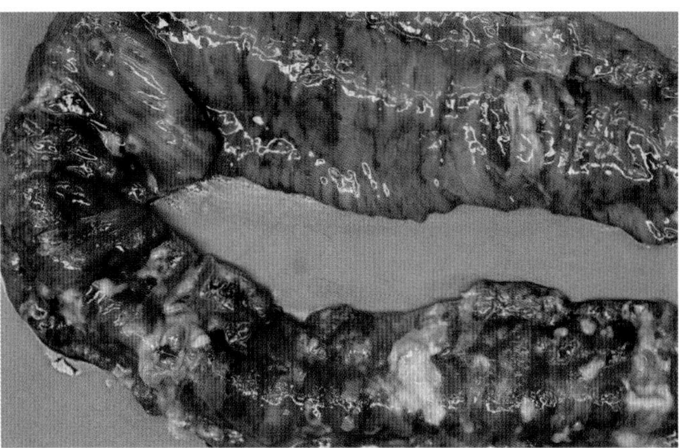

Fig. 5.95 Small intestinal resection for enteropathy-associated T-cell lymphoma. Multiple circumferential ulcers are seen with central exudates.

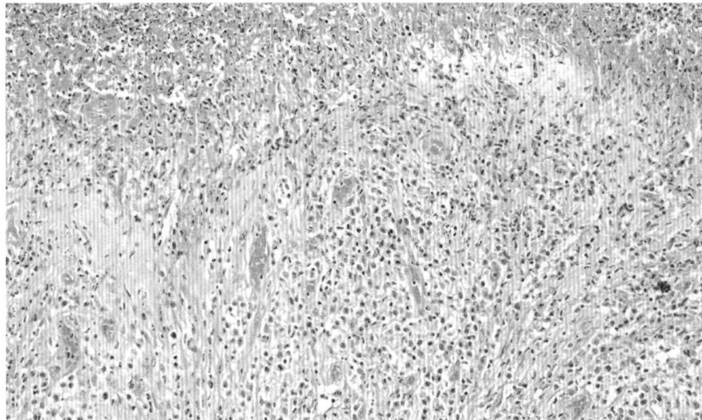

Fig. 5.96 Enteropathy-associated T-cell lymphoma with ulceration. Mucosal ulceration is present, overlying an infiltrate of lymphoma.

Clinical features

Abdominal pain, diarrhoea (due to malabsorption), and weight loss are the most common symptoms and signs. Almost half of the patients present with an acute abdominal emergency due to small bowel perforation or obstruction. Many patients are known to have adult (or childhood)-onset CD, but CD is frequently diagnosed only at the time of EATL diagnosis. The duration of symptoms before diagnosis of EATL varies widely (from weeks to years) {1274} but is < 3 months in most cases {3743}. About 50% of patients have a prodromal phase of unresponsiveness to a gluten-free diet before the development of EATL, referred to as RCD {2496}, which is sometimes associated with small-intestinal ulceration (ulcerative jejunitis) {164,209}. Such patients usually present with anorexia, severe malnutrition, and hypoalbuminaemia. B symptoms (other than weight loss) are present in a third of patients with EATL, and a significant proportion have anaemia, elevated LDH or hypercalcaemia {3743,922,2496}. A haemophagocytic syndrome has been reported in 16–40% of cases {108,2496}.

Refractory coeliac disease

Approximately 0.3–1% of adults with CD have persistent villous atrophy and fail to improve clinically or develop recurrent malabsorptive symptoms and signs despite adhering to a strict gluten-free diet for > 12 months. Upon exclusion of other gastrointestinal disorders and CD-related malignancies, these patients are considered to have RCD {91,1715,2444}. Two subtypes of RCD are recognized, according to the absence (type 1, RCD1) or presence (type 2, RCD2) of abnormal IELs {3770}.

RCD1

The majority of IELs are of TCRαβ lineage and express sCD3 and CD8 (i.e. a normal immunophenotype). TR gene rearrangement analysis usually shows polyclonal populations; monoclonality

Chapter 5

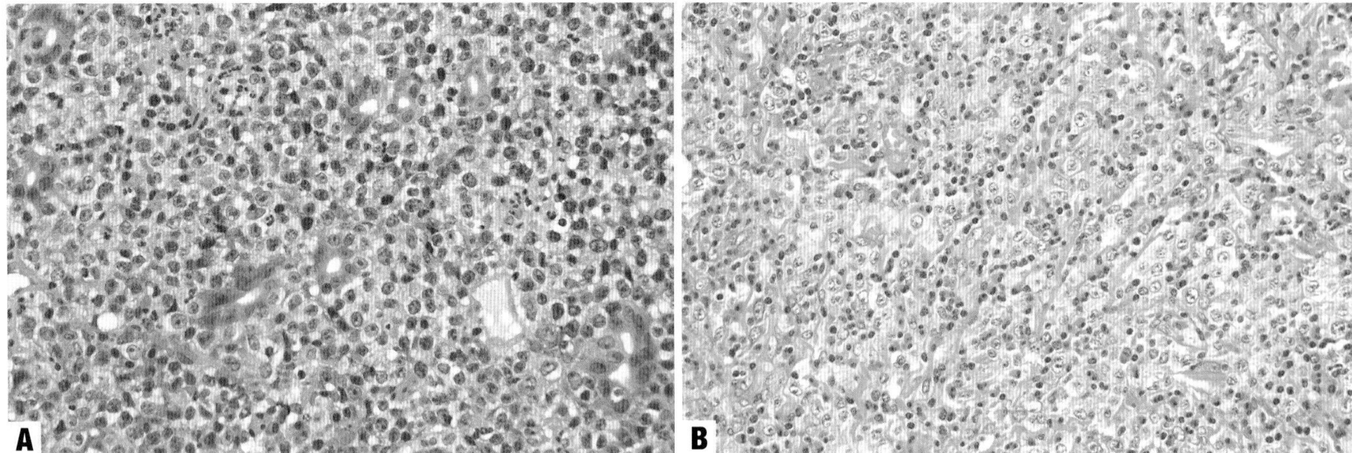

Fig. 5.97 Enteropathy-associated T-cell lymphoma. **A** An infiltrate of large lymphocytes with immunoblastic morphology is seen surrounding and infiltrating small intestinal epithelium. **B** Clusters of large atypical lymphocytes are seen amid numerous eosinophils and histiocytes.

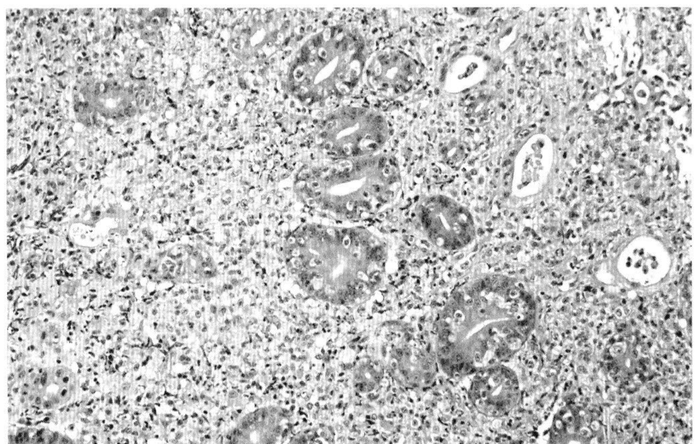

Fig. 5.98 Infiltration of small intestinal epithelium by enteropathy-associated T-cell lymphoma. Atypical lymphocytes infiltrate the small intestinal epithelium.

may be detected in a small proportion of RCD1 cases, but it is often transient. The etiology of this condition is not known, but surreptitious gluten ingestion is suspected in a subset of patients. No genetic alterations have been identified thus far. Mucosal pathological changes are the same as in uncomplicated CD. The symptoms are milder than in RCD2 {2495}, and the course is generally benign (5-year survival rate: 80–96%), with a low risk of EATL development (3–14%) {2495,91,1715, 3499}.

RCD2

The IELs usually express cCD3 and NK antigens, especially NKp46 (NCR1), but lack sCD3, CD8, and T-cell receptor {209, 654,584}. Other immunophenotypes (CD8+, sCD3+, and/or TCRαβ+ or TCRγδ+) can occasionally be seen {901,1140,3772}. The immunophenotypic and molecular profiles of the majority of RCD2 cases suggest an origin from an innate lymphoid cell subset with variable commitment to a T-cell lineage, which resides in the small intestinal epithelium {3918,3626,1093}. CD30 expression is considered an indicator of transformation to EATL {1140}. Flow cytometry is the best modality to assess IEL phenotype, and a cut-off point of > 20% abnormal cells has been shown to have high sensitivity in discriminating between RCD2 and RCD1 {4214}. For immunohistochemistry, a threshold of > 50% CD8− IELs (of all CD3ε+ IELs) is recommended for classification as RCD2, because the increased CD8− TCRγδ IELs in CD (and RCD1), which often comprise > 20% of all IELs, can be mistaken for aberrant IELs {4175,2498}. A threshold of > 25 NKp46+ IELs per 100 epithelial cells has been reported to be a reliable indicator of RCD2 {654}. Clonal TR gene rearrangements can be demonstrated in the majority of cases. However, about 70% of cases with clonal rearrangements have incomplete or non-functional TR rearrangements, and 25% lack clonal TR rearrangements {3918,1692,1093}. The majority of cases have somatic genetic alterations that overlap with EATL (see below). Villous atrophy is usually severe in RCD2. The abnormal IELs lack significant cytological atypia, and they can disseminate along the entire gastrointestinal tract (or to extragastrointestinal sites), with frequent infiltration of the lamina propria {4219,4216}. Mucosal ulcers are observed in some cases (ulcerative jejunitis). RCD2 is considered a cryptic lymphoma of IELs or EATL in situ and is associated with increased morbidity and mortality (5-year survival rate: 44–58%) and a high propensity to transform to EATL (30–52% within ~5 years) {2495,91, 1715,3499}.

Epidemiology

EATL constitutes about 3% of peripheral T-cell lymphomas and accounts for two thirds of all primary intestinal T-cell lymphomas reported in Europe and the USA; it is extremely rare in Asia {922}. It usually occurs in the sixth and seventh decades of life (median age: 61 years), with a slight male predominance (M:F ratio: 1.04–2.8:1) {922,1274,2496,3743,4215}. All patients have the genetic background of CD. Therefore, EATL is more common in regions with a high seroprevalence of CD, particularly Europe (0.05–0.14 cases per 100 000 population) {576, 3743,4215} and the USA (0.016 cases per 100 000 population) {3701}.

Etiology

EATL is strongly associated with CD. Evidence for an association between CD and EATL comes from the following: identical HLA-DQ2 haplotypes of patients with CD and EATL, the presence of gluten sensitivity in patients with EATL, the

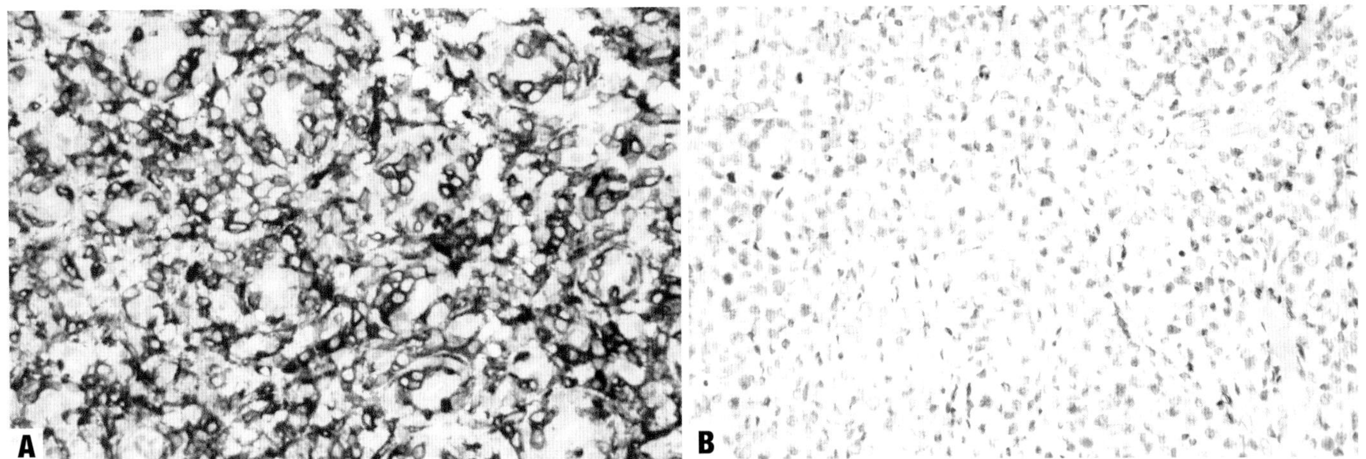

Fig. 5.99 Enteropathy-associated T-cell lymphoma. **A** The neoplastic cells express cCD3 by immunohistochemistry (no sCD3 expression was detected by flow cytometry). **B** The tumour cells are negative for CD8.

protective effect of a gluten-free diet, and case series showing progression from CD through RCD to EATL with clonal identity {1647,2998,1619,2375}. Homozygosity for HLA-DQ2 alleles, observed in 53–56% of patients with EATL (compared with 21% of patients with uncomplicated CD), and older age, both connoting increased exposure to gluten (gliadin peptides), are risk factors for the development of EATL {90,2496}.

Pathogenesis

Small-intestinal IELs are the postulated normal counterparts of EATL, based on immunophenotypic identity {3805,209,2496}. The lymphomas were thought to originate from TCRαβ IELs, but recent studies have suggested derivation from multiple IEL subsets. Virtually all cases harbour clonal TR gene rearrangements, which are identical to those in antecedent RCD2 when present {164,2852,876}. Besides developing in a stepwise manner with an intermediate RCD2 phase, EATL can also arise de novo {2496,876}. Similarities in the genomic landscapes of RCD2 and EATL indicate shared oncogenic mechanisms, initiated by highly prevalent mutations in members of the JAK-1/STAT3 signalling axis (80% of RCD2 and 90% of EATL cases) {3772,809, 3425,2709}. Epigenetic regulators (*TET2*, *KMT2D*) and *DDX3X*, as well as NF-κB (*TNFAIP3* [*A20*], *TNIP3*), DNA damage/repair (*POT1*, *TP53*), and immune escape (*CD58*, *FAS*, *B2M*) pathway genes, are also recurrently mutated in RCD2 and EATL {809, 3772,2709}.

The mutation spectrum of RCD2-related EATL overlaps with that of de novo EATL, but *TNFAIP3* mutations have so far only been observed in the former type. The genetic features of EATL and monomorphic epitheliotropic intestinal T-cell lymphoma (MEITL) overlap, although some alterations are differentially enriched in these two diseases (e.g. *JAK1* and *STAT3* in EATL; and *JAK3*, *STAT5B*, and *SETD2* in MEITL) {3425,809,2879, 2709}.

The identification of recurrent gain-of-function *JAK1* and *STAT3* mutations highlights the role of chronic inflammation in CD-associated lymphomagenesis. These mutations provide transformed IELs with a selective growth advantage and enhance cytotoxicity in the inflamed coeliac mucosa, which has an abundance of JAK/STAT-activating cytokines (IL-15 produced by stressed enterocytes and lamina propria macrophages; and IL-2, IL-21, and IFN-γ released by gliadin-responsive CD4+ T cells) {2655,1093,3626,2104}. Loss-of-function *TNFAIP3* mutations, resulting in NF-κB activation, may sensitize

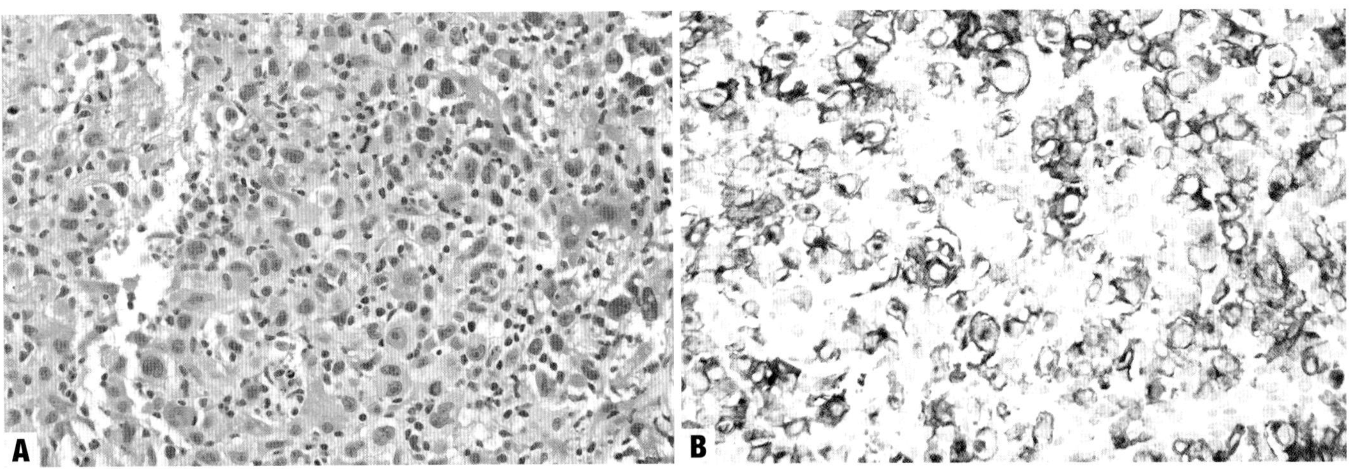

Fig. 5.100 Enteropathy-associated T-cell lymphoma exhibiting anaplastic morphology. **A** Numerous large anaplastic-appearing lymphocytes are seen, including occasional binucleated cells. **B** The neoplastic cells express CD30.

clonal IELs to the activating and pro-survival signals provided by cytokines released by CD4+ T cells {2104}. Protracted inflammation could lead to DNA damage and the acquisition of genomic alterations, further fuelling EATL progression {1093, 2497,3918,2104}.

Comparative genomic hybridization analysis has revealed a variety of chromosome aberrations in EATL, including segmental amplifications of chromosome 9q34 or deletions at 16q12.1 in > 80% of cases, and gains at 1q and 5q34-q35.2; some of these changes have also been observed in RCD2 {924,4220, 2495,809}. These abnormalities, however, are not specific to EATL, as they can be present in other types of intestinal T-cell lymphomas, including MEITL.

Macroscopic appearance

The intestinal tumour can manifest as circumferentially oriented ulcers, ulcerated nodules, plaques, or strictures, and less commonly as an exophytic mass. The uninvolved mucosa can be thin, with loss of mucosal folds.

Histopathology

EATLs can display different patterns of intestinal involvement, ranging from scattered single or variably sized clusters of atypical cells in the lamina propria and/or submucosa to transmural infiltrates of pleomorphic medium-sized and large lymphoid cells exhibiting immunoblastic or anaplastic morphology. The tumours may have a pronounced inflammatory background consisting of histiocytes, eosinophils, small lymphocytes, and plasma cells, obscuring the tumour cells. Intraepithelial spread may be striking. Angioinvasion and angiodestruction are commonly seen. Mucosa adjacent to the tumour usually shows villous atrophy, crypt hyperplasia, and intraepithelial lymphocytosis – histopathological features of CD. These CD-associated alterations are variable: more pronounced in the upper jejunum and less so in the distal small intestinal segments {1737,2496}.

Immunophenotype

The most common immunophenotypic profile is CD3+, CD5−, CD7+, CD4−, CD8−, CD56−, and CD103+; CD2 expression can vary. Cytotoxic granule proteins (TIA1, granzyme B, perforin) are generally expressed. T-cell receptor expression is mostly absent {4026}. Approximately 25% of EATLs are CD8+ (primarily de novo tumours), and rare cases express TCRγδ {2852,2496,4174}. Lymphomas with large cell or anaplastic morphology are often CD30+ and at times EMA+; ALK expression is extremely rare {737,2496,2706}. The Ki-67 labelling index is usually > 50% {2852}. In situ hybridization for EBV-encoded small RNA (EBER) is negative in the neoplastic cells.

Differential diagnosis

Differentiating EATL from MEITL can be challenging, because the lymphoma cells in some cases of MEITL may be pleomorphic

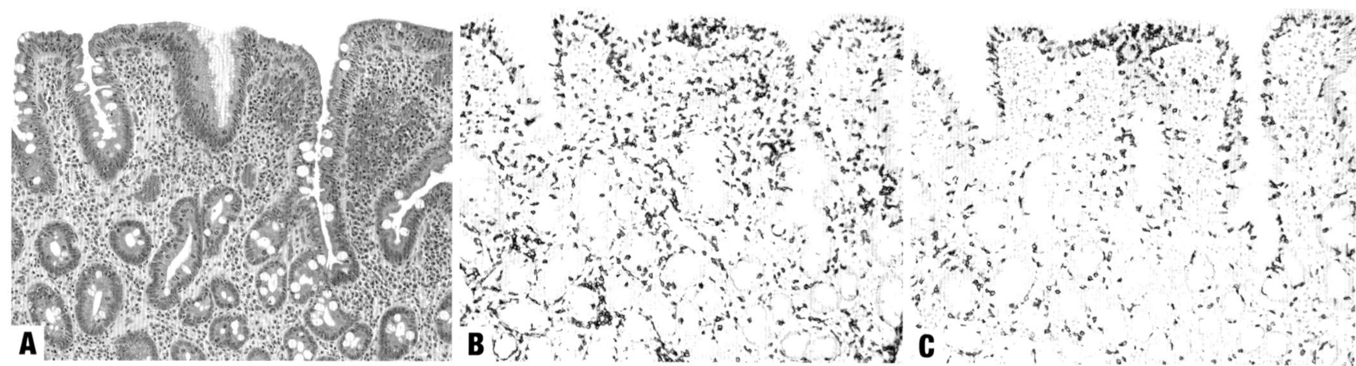

Fig. 5.101 Refractory coeliac disease type 1. **A** Duodenal biopsy showing partial villus atrophy, crypt hyperplasia, and increased intraepithelial lymphocytes. The intraepithelial lymphocytes express CD3 (**B**) and CD8 (**C**). By flow cytometry, sCD3 and TCRαβ expression was demonstrated, and TR rearrangement analysis showed polyclonal products.

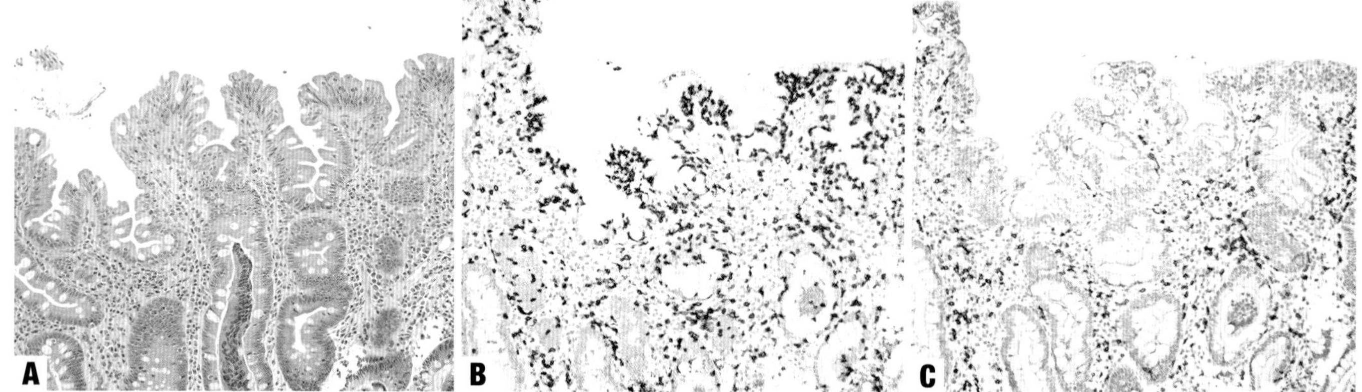

Fig. 5.102 Refractory coeliac disease type 2. **A** Duodenal biopsy showing subtotal villus atrophy, crypt hyperplasia, and increased intraepithelial lymphocytes lacking cytological atypia. **B** The intraepithelial lymphocytes are CD3-positive. Flow cytometry showed cCD3 expression and absence of sCD3 expression. **C** The intraepithelial lymphocytes are CD8-negative. Flow cytometry showed an absence of surface T-cell receptor expression, and TR rearrangement analysis revealed a clonal product.

or exhibit an atypical immunophenotype (CD8− and/or CD56−), and the villi at a distance from the tumour can be broad and show increased small IELs. The clinical features (no malabsorption and negative coeliac serologies), usually monomorphic lymphomatous infiltrate with few admixed inflammatory cells, lack of villous atrophy in the uninvolved small intestinal mucosa, and MATK expression can help support the diagnosis of MEITL. Similarly, intestinal T-cell lymphoma NOS and secondary intestinal involvement by peripheral T-cell lymphomas can be distinguished from EATL by the clinical presentation, an absence of epitheliotropism, and differences in immunophenotype. Adult T-cell leukaemia/lymphoma can involve or be localized to the gastrointestinal tract, display anaplastic cytomorphology, and express CD103 {1740}, so the evaluation of demographic information and HTLV-1 serology is paramount in excluding this possibility.

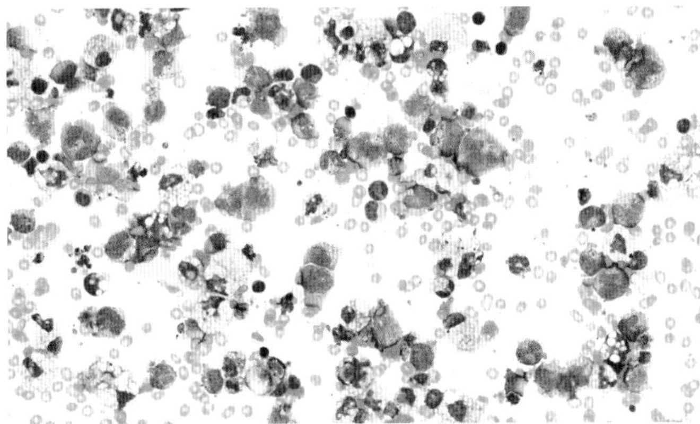

Fig. 5.103 Enteropathy-associated T-cell lymphoma presenting as pleural effusion. Large atypical cells are seen in a cytospin preparation of a pleural fluid sample. Many cells have azurophilic granules within the cytoplasm (Giemsa).

Cytology

In cytological preparations (such as from an effusion), the neoplastic cells are pleomorphic and medium to large in size, with round or oval vesicular nuclei, invariably prominent nucleoli, and moderate to abundant pale-staining cytoplasm. The cytoplasm may show azurophilic granules with Giemsa.

Diagnostic molecular pathology

Not clinically relevant

Essential and desirable diagnostic criteria

Essential: a lymphoma with the bulk of disease localized to the gastrointestinal tract; infiltration by pleomorphic medium-sized to large lymphoid cells; a variable inflammatory background, often including many eosinophils and histiocytes; uninvolved intestinal mucosa showing features of CD (villous atrophy, crypt hyperplasia, intraepithelial lymphocytosis); T-cell lineage, often with a CD4−/CD8− phenotype and expression of cytotoxic markers (TIA1, granzyme B, perforin).

Desirable: CD30 positivity (predominantly in cases of large cell or anaplastic morphology); in problematic cases, the presence of *JAK1* and/or *STAT3* SH2 domain hotspot mutations is helpful in differentiating EATL from MEITL.

Staging

EATL is staged according to the Lugano classification, which has been adopted by the eighth-edition Union for International Cancer Control (UICC) TNM classification system {688}.

Prognosis and prediction

The prognosis of EATL is very poor because of the frequent multifocal nature of the disease, high rate of intestinal (or extraintestinal) recurrence, and poor nutritional condition of patients, especially those with preceding RCD2. The median overall survival time is < 10 months. Patients with de novo EATL have better outcomes than those with RCD2-related EATL (5-year overall survival rate: 50% vs 0–8%) {2496,91}. The use of a novel aggressive chemotherapy regimen followed by autologous stem cell transplantation has been shown to enhance survival {3743,1785}, and patients with CD30+ EATLs have shown promising responses to CD30-targeted therapies {1965,4255}.

Prognostic factors are not well established. Recently, the EATL Prognostic Index (EPI) was introduced, which reportedly performs better than the International Prognostic Index (IPI) and another prognostic model for T-cell lymphomas (the Prognostic Index for Peripheral T-cell Lymphoma [PIT]) {885}.

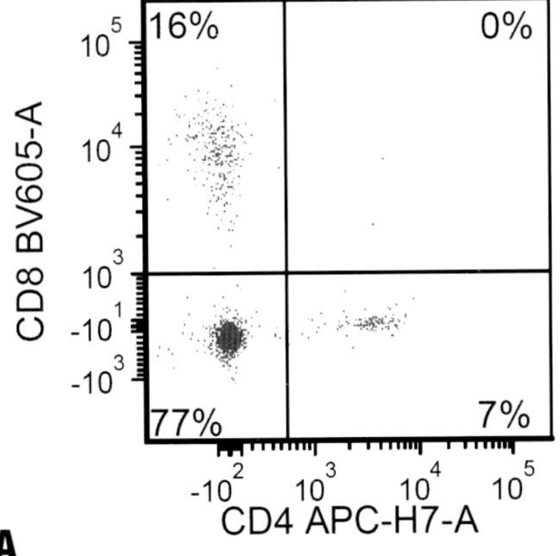

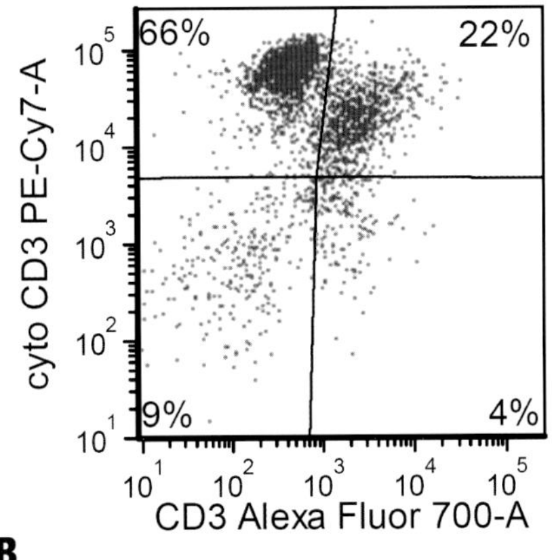

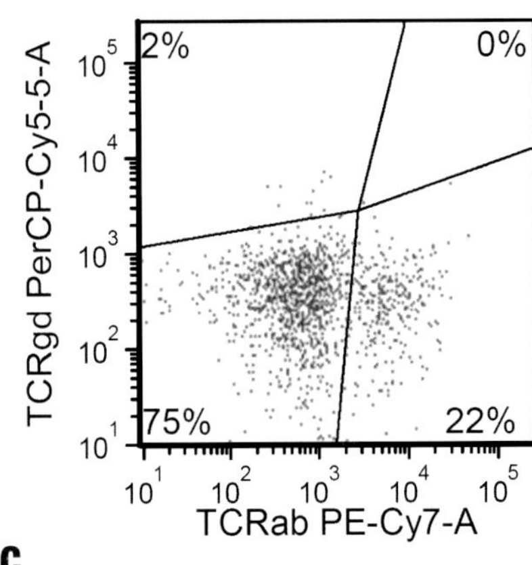

Fig. 5.104 Refractory coeliac disease type 2. **A** Flow cytometry shows no CD4 or CD8 expression by the intraepithelial lymphocytes (lower-left quadrant). **B** The intraepithelial lymphocytes show cCD3 expression and absent sCD3 expression (upper-left quadrant). **C** The intraepithelial lymphocytes lack surface T-cell receptor expression for both TCRαβ and TCRγδ (lower-left quadrant).

Monomorphic epitheliotropic intestinal T-cell lymphoma

Chan JKC
Bhagat G
Chuang S-S
Dave SS
Kato S
Nakamura N
Naresh KN
Tan SY

Definition

Monomorphic epitheliotropic intestinal T-cell lymphoma (MEITL) is an aggressive primary intestinal T-cell lymphoma of intraepithelial T lymphocytes, characterized by monomorphic cytomorphology and epitheliotropism, typically lacking association with coeliac disease.

ICD-O coding

9717/3 Monomorphic epitheliotropic intestinal T-cell lymphoma

ICD-11 coding

2A90.7 & XH1AG7 Enteropathy-associated T-cell lymphoma & Monomorphic epitheliotropic intestinal T-cell lymphoma

Related terminology

Not recommended: type II enteropathy-associated T-cell lymphoma.

Subtype(s)

None

Localization

MEITL arises most commonly in the small intestine, and less commonly in the colon, duodenum, or stomach; 20–35% of cases may show multifocal gastrointestinal tumours {3955, 4094,1741,616,4497}. Tumour may disseminate to mesenteric

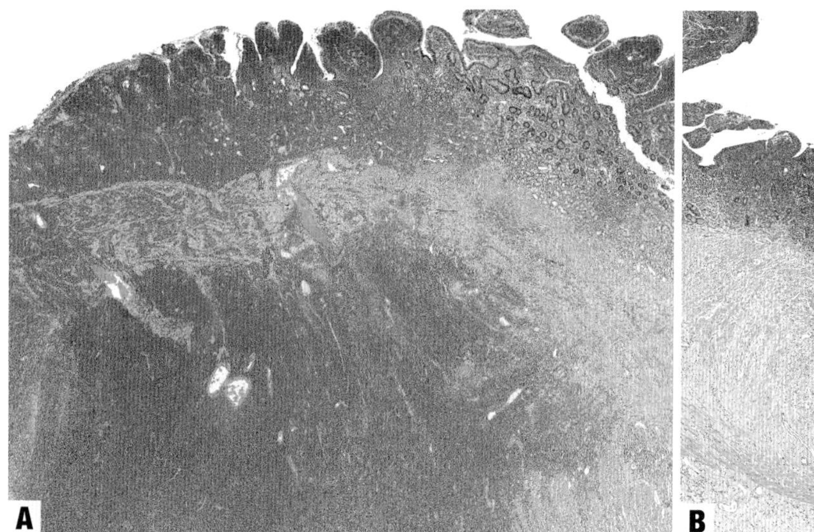

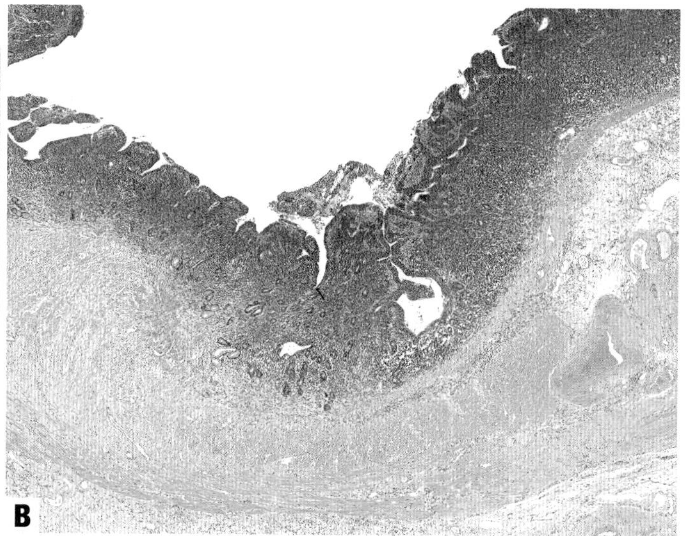

Fig. 5.105 Monomorphic epitheliotropic intestinal T-cell lymphoma involving small intestine: growth patterns. **A** The central portion of the tumour shows dense transmural infiltration by lymphoma, with no overt necrosis. The mucosa shows loss or reduction of villi. **B** Extensive horizontal mucosal spread of lymphoma is present in the peripheral zone.

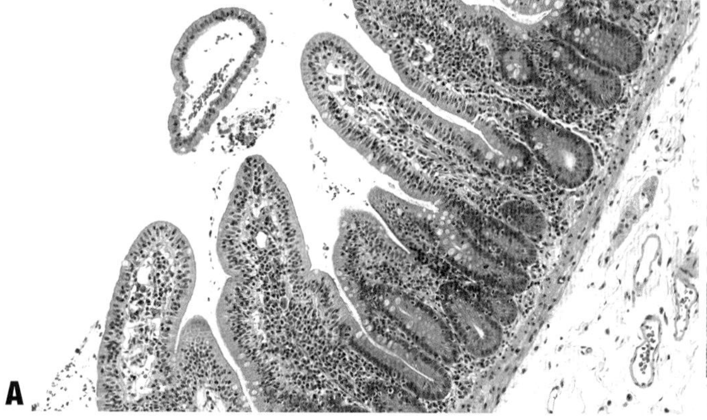

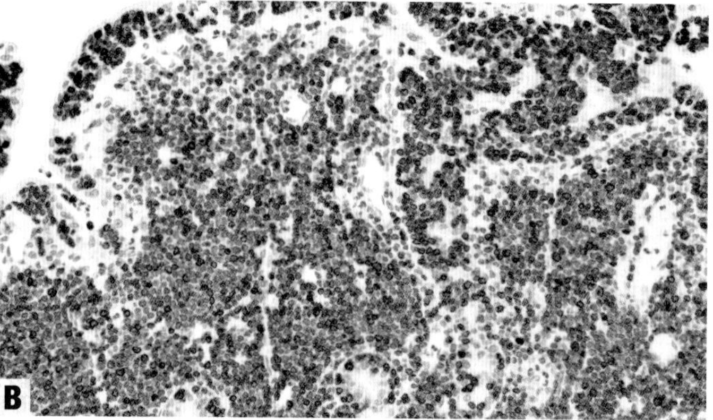

Fig. 5.106 Monomorphic epitheliotropic intestinal T-cell lymphoma involving small intestine: characteristic epitheliotropism. **A** The villi show prominent intraepithelial lymphocytosis in the mucosa distant from the tumour. Unlike in coeliac disease, villi are not atrophic, crypt hyperplasia is not seen, and there is no increase in plasma cells. **B** The lymphoma cells show positive immunostaining for CD3, which highlights the marked epitheliotropism.

lymph nodes, as well as to the lung, liver, brain, and skin {54, 2792,3898,922,2138,2922}.

Clinical features

Most patients present with abdominal pain; gastrointestinal bleeding, obstruction, or perforation; diarrhoea; and weight loss {3955,4094,616}.

Epidemiology

MEITL has a worldwide distribution {616,1295,3879}. Enteropathy-associated T-cell lymphoma (EATL) and MEITL together represent 2%, 6%, and 9% of all peripheral T-cell lymphomas in Asia, North America, and Europe, respectively {922}. MEITL cases greatly outnumber EATL cases in Asia; the reverse is true in Europe; and the incidence rates are approximately equal in North America. MEITL predominantly occurs in adults, with a reported median age of 54–67 years and a male predominance (M:F ratio: 2:1) {3955,616,3425,3944,4094, 658,4497,2859}.

Etiology

There is no association with coeliac disease, because studies have shown an absence of coeliac serologies {3955}. The rare reports of MEITL occurring in patients with coeliac disease may be coincidental events {2276,922,2859}.

Pathogenesis

MEITL classically originates from resident intestinal γδ T-cell populations involved in mucosal immunity, although some cases may be of an αβ T-cell nature or phenotypically T-cell receptor–silent. There is clonal TR gene rearrangement, even in T-cell receptor–silent cases {4041,1661}. In contrast to EATL, MEITL is not associated with coeliac disease. The genomic landscape of the two diseases bears some similarities. As with EATL, MEITL shows gains of 9q34.3-qter {2067,2879,4039, 657} and losses at 16q12.1 {2879,4039}, whereas alterations of 1q32.2-q41 and 5q34-q35.5 have been reported in MEITL by some {4041} but not others {2879,924}. Alterations such as gains of 9q22.31, 4p15.1, 7q34, 8p11.23, and 12p13.31, as well as loss of 7p14.1 {4039}, are more specific to MEITL. MEITL typically shows gains (and rarely translocations) of *MYC* {3049, 3955,1661}. The mutation spectrum of MEITL includes *SETD2* mutation and JAK/STAT deregulation as the pivotal pathways in oncogenesis {2879,2709,3425,4040,1489,4203}. *SETD2* is almost ubiquitously affected by nonsense mutations, frameshift insertions, or deletions, resulting in loss of function of this gene. SETD2 is an H3 p.K36–specific methyltransferase and interacts with RNA polymerase II. SETD2 expression is a key regulator of the transition from early double-negative to double-positive T cells in early T-cell development and probably directs the choice between αβ and γδ T-cell development {2317}. This notion is supported by the finding of increased intestinal γδ T cells in *SETD2*-knockout mice. Similar *SETD2* alterations are found in hepatosplenic T-cell lymphoma that is also prototypically of γδ T-cell derivation {2141}. SETD2 deficiency most likely contributes to lymphomagenesis. JAK/STAT activation, through mutations predominantly in *STAT5B*, *STAT3*, *JAK1*, and *JAK3*, and to a lesser extent in *SOCS3*, indicates constitutive cytokine-mediated drive as another major driver of oncogenesis in MEITL, like in EATL and various other T- and NK-cell lymphomas.

Macroscopic appearance

The tumour often appears as a large ulcerated mass showing full-thickness involvement of the intestinal wall, with or without perforation. Some tumours show coarse, cobble stone–like thickening of the mucosa.

Histopathology

In the majority of cases, the neoplastic cells are monotonous and small to medium-sized, with round nuclei, dispersed chromatin, and moderate amount of pale to clear cytoplasm. At times, the neoplastic cells may appear high-grade with a starry-sky appearance or, rarely, the lymphoma may show larger, pleomorphic cells with open chromatin and conspicuous nucleoli {1489}. Necrosis and an inflammatory background are uncommon. In the peripheral zone, the tumour invades the mucosa, inducing distortion, destruction, or expansion of villi, accompanied by epitheliotropic lymphoma cells.

The distant intestinal mucosa displays a normal architecture and may show an increase in morphologically bland, small intraepithelial lymphocytes, mimicking coeliac disease or lymphocytic colitis {3955,616,1741}.

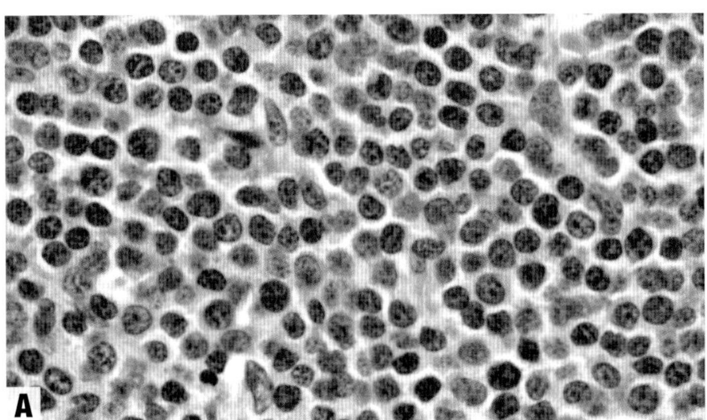

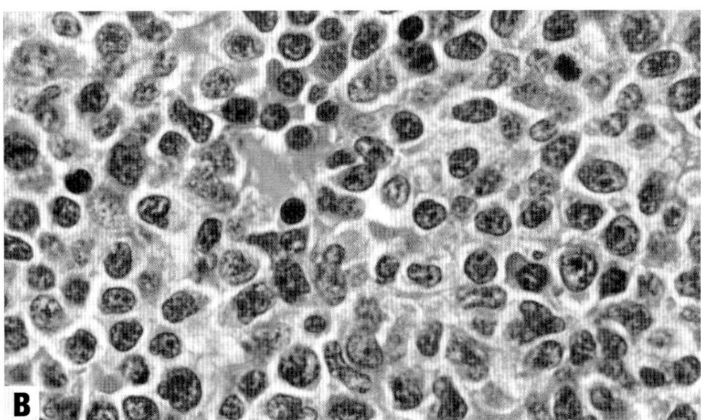

Fig. 5.107 Monomorphic epitheliotropic intestinal T-cell lymphoma: cytological spectrum. **A** Most frequently encountered are small to medium-sized cells with round or slightly irregular nuclei and dense chromatin. **B** Less frequently, medium-sized cells are admixed with occasional larger cells.

Chapter 5

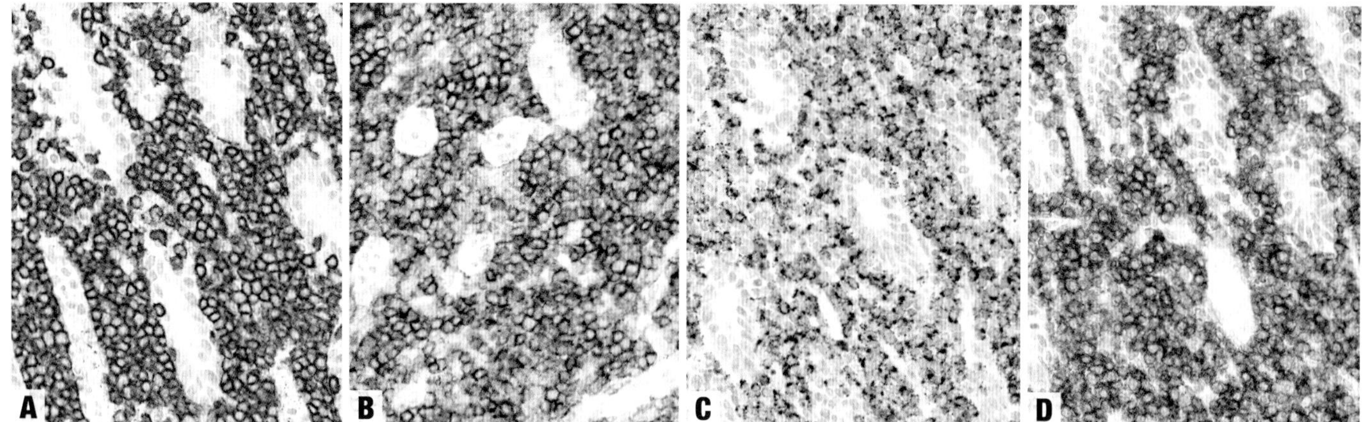

Fig. 5.108 Monomorphic epitheliotropic intestinal T-cell lymphoma: immunohistochemical profile. The tumour cells are positive for CD8 (**A**), CD56 (**B**), and TIA1 (**C**). They are usually also positive for TCRγ (**D**), although rare cases express TCRβ instead, express both TCRγ and TCRβ, or express neither.

Immunohistochemistry

The most common immunophenotypic profile is: CD2+, CD3+, CD4−, CD5−, CD7+, CD8+, CD56+ {3955,616}. However, CD8 and CD56 may be negative in 10–20% and 5–6% of cases, respectively {4497,616,1489}. Pooled data from several series show that 47% of cases express TCRγ and 35% express TCRβ, with occasional cases showing dual or negative T-cell receptor expression {3955,616,3425,4094,4040,2859}. The cytotoxic marker TIA1 is expressed in almost all cases, whereas positivity for granzyme B or perforin is less consistent {4039,3955, 658,3425}. A high frequency of CD103 and CD8a homodimer expression has been reported {3955,3425}, whereas CD30 expression is very rare {4497}. Extensive nuclear expression of MATK and cytoplasmic expression of Syk are seen in practically all MEITLs, whereas these are negative in EATLs {3957,2859}. Aberrant expression of CD20 is reported in 20% of cases {3955}.

The intraepithelial lymphocytes in the distant zone usually express CD3, CD8, and TIA1, but they can be positive or negative for CD56 {3955,1741,616}. These cells may represent precursors of MEITL.

Differential diagnosis

See Table 5.13 (p. 710).

Cytology

Pleural or peritoneal fluid cytological specimens show noncohesive atypical lymphoid cells with cytoplasmic azurophilic granules seen with Giemsa {3119,127}.

Diagnostic molecular pathology

In situ hybridization for EBV-encoded small RNA (EBER) is negative {3955,616,4497}. The report of EBV positivity in 3 of 38 cases in one series has raised controversy; it is unclear whether these cases might represent extranodal NK/T-cell lymphoma {4094,3956}. TR clonality assays may support the diagnosis in equivocal cases.

Essential and desirable diagnostic criteria

Essential: a lymphoma with the bulk of disease localized to the gastrointestinal tract; dense infiltration by relatively monotonous medium-sized or (occasionally) large lymphoma cells; typically lacking necrosis and an inflammatory background; epitheliotropism is common; no histological evidence of coeliac disease in uninvolved mucosa; proven T lineage, with expression of cytotoxic markers, and often CD5−, CD4−, CD8+, CD56+; EBV negative.

Desirable: in problematic cases, demonstration of *JAK3* and/or STAT5 mutations and/or of SETD2 inactivation are helpful in differentiating MEITL from EATL.

Staging

The lymphoma is staged according to the Lugano classification, which has been adopted by the eighth-edition Union for International Cancer Control (UICC) TNM classification {688}.

Prognosis and prediction

The clinical outcome is poor, with a median overall survival time of 7 months, 1-year overall survival rate of 36–57%, and 3-year overall survival rate of 13–26% {4094,3955,4497,4203}. The poor survival is attributable to intestinal perforation, the propensity of lymphoma to recur locally and to spread to various sites, and primary resistance to CHOP-like polychemotherapy {4497}.

Intestinal T-cell lymphoma NOS

Bhagat G
Dave SS
Kato S
Tan SY

Definition
Intestinal T-cell lymphoma NOS (ITCL-NOS) is an aggressive primary gastrointestinal T-cell lymphoma that lacks the clinicopathological features of defined lymphoma entities arising within the gastrointestinal tract.

ICD-O coding
9717/3 Intestinal T-cell lymphoma, NOS

ICD-11 coding
2A90.7 & XH9FT0 Enteropathy associated T-cell lymphoma & Intestinal T-cell lymphoma

Related terminology
None

Subtype(s)
None

Localization
ITCL-NOS can be confined to a single organ or involve multiple gastrointestinal sites, with the colon and small intestine being the most common {174,2003}. Dissemination to regional lymph nodes and extragastrointestinal sites may be seen {174,1937, 2003}.

Clinical features
The symptoms and signs depend on the anatomical site and extent of involvement. The presentation of patients with intestinal disease is similar to that of patients with enteropathy-associated T-cell lymphoma (EATL) and monomorphic epitheliotropic intestinal T-cell lymphoma (MEITL), although malabsorption is infrequent. Epigastric pain and haematemesis are common in individuals with primary gastric lymphomas {3879,1937}.

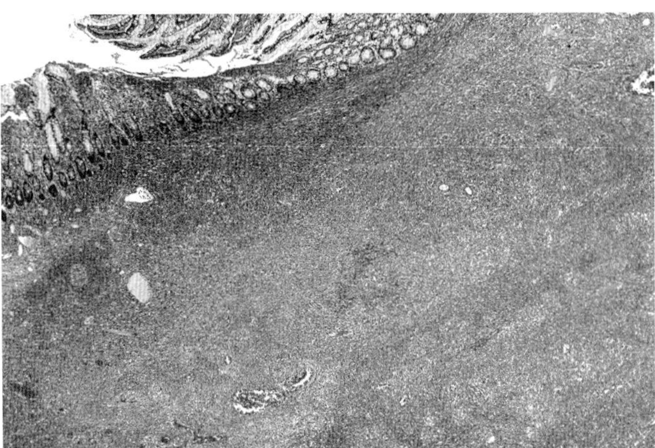

Fig. 5.109 Intestinal T-cell lymphoma NOS in the colon. Transmural infiltration by lymphoma.

Approximately 50% of patients present with stage III/IV disease {3879,2003}. Comprehensive clinical and laboratory evaluation and imaging studies are required, to exclude secondary gastrointestinal involvement by other types of peripheral T-cell lymphomas.

Epidemiology
The geographical distribution of ITCL-NOS is wide. In the USA and Europe, the frequency of ITCL-NOS is presumed to be low, because EATL and MEITL represent the vast majority of primary intestinal T- and NK-cell lymphomas {922}, whereas the proportion of intestinal T-cell lymphomas classified as ITCL-NOS in Asia ranges from 18% to 63% {1998,2003,3879}. The patient age (median: 49 years, range: 15–78 years) is similar to or slightly lower than that of MEITL (or EATL), and there is a male predilection (M:F ratio: 2:1) {3879,2003}.

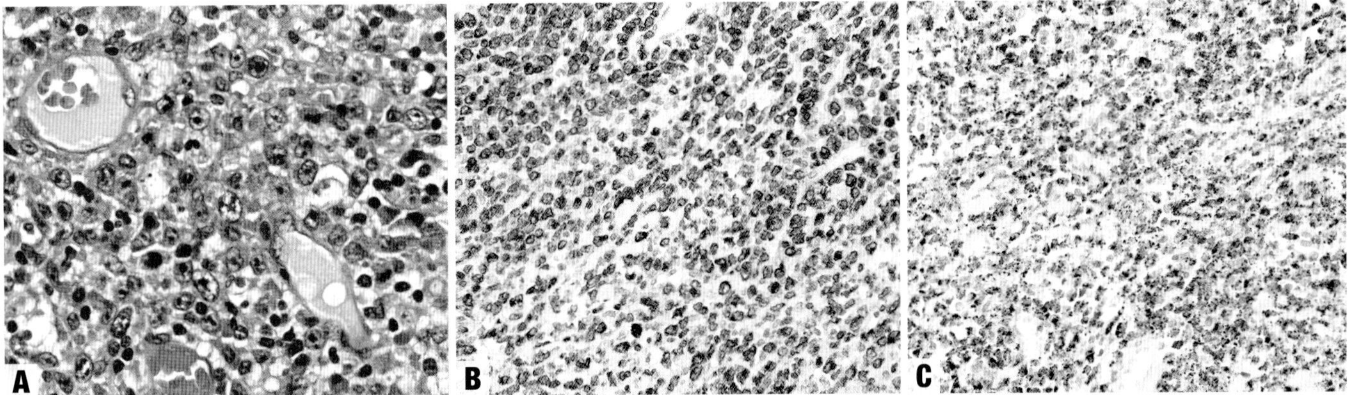

Fig. 5.110 Intestinal T-cell lymphoma NOS in the colon. Large pleomorphic lymphocytes with vesicular nuclei, prominent nucleoli, and scant or moderate cytoplasm (**A**). The tumour cells express CD3 (**B**) and are TIA1-positive (**C**).

Etiology

The etiology is unknown. Rare cases have been reported in individuals with inflammatory bowel disease and autoimmune enteropathy {1396,174,747}.

Pathogenesis

ITCL-NOS is probably a heterogeneous group. Insufficient information is available regarding the genetic landscape. JAK/STAT and MAPK pathway mutations have been identified in the few evaluated cases {2956}. There is a lower frequency of mutations in *SETD2*, STAT5 genes, and *JAK3* than there is in MEITL {1489}.

Macroscopic appearance

ITCL-NOS usually has an ulcerated, plaque-like appearance; protruding luminal masses can be seen in some cases {3879}.

Histopathology

The lymphoma shows mucosal and often transmural infiltration, commonly accompanied by ulceration. The neoplastic infiltrate can be patchy or diffuse. The lymphoma cells vary in size from medium to large, and they often show pleomorphism, with vesicular nuclei, prominent nucleoli, and scant or moderate cytoplasm. Epitheliotropism is only present in a minority (~20%) of cases {3879,1937}.

Immunophenotype

The neoplastic cells express CD3 and are usually CD4+ or CD4−/CD8−. Most cases express TCRαβ and a subset are T-cell receptor–silent {1937,3879,174}. The possibility of lymphoma derivation from a TCRγδ-positive T cell or another type of mucosal innate lymphoid cell in rare instances cannot be ruled out at present. The cytotoxic granule protein (TIA1) is frequently expressed, but granzyme B and CD30 expression is variable {1937,174}. Unlike in MEITL and extranodal NK/T-cell lymphoma, CD56 is negative. The Ki-67 labelling index tends to be high. EBV-encoded small RNA (EBER) positivity has been reported in rare cases, and it is presently unclear if these should be classified as ITCL-NOS or extranodal NK/T-cell lymphoma {3879}.

Differential diagnosis

ITCL-NOS should be diagnosed only after excluding well-defined primary gastrointestinal T- and NK-cell lymphoid proliferations and lymphomas (e.g. EATL, MEITL, extranodal NK/T-cell lymphoma, indolent T-cell lymphoma of the gastrointestinal tract, indolent NK-cell lymphoproliferative disorder of the gastrointestinal tract; see Table 5.13, p. 710) {3771}. This diagnosis should therefore be avoided when biopsies are limited, because cytoarchitectural features characteristic of the specific lymphoma types may not be evident.

Cytology

Not clinically relevant

Diagnostic molecular pathology

Studies of TR gene rearrangement may be helpful in excluding inflammatory disorders in selected circumstances.

Essential and desirable diagnostic criteria

Essential: a lymphoma with the bulk of disease localized to the gastrointestinal tract; infiltration with medium-sized to large lymphoma cells; proven T-cell lineage; exclusion of defined types of primary gastrointestinal T- and NK-cell lymphomas / lymphoproliferative disorders.

Staging

ITCL-NOS is staged according to the Lugano classification, which has been adopted by the eighth-edition Union for International Cancer Control (UICC) TNM classification {688}.

Prognosis and prediction

ITCL-NOS is associated with a poor prognosis, but some studies report better outcomes (median survival time: 35 months; 5-year overall survival rate: 23%) than for EATL and MEITL {2003,3879}. High stage and large cell morphology are associated with worse 5-year survival rates {1937,2003}.

Hepatosplenic T-cell lymphoma

Medeiros LJ
Behdad A
Miranda RN

Definition

Hepatosplenic T-cell lymphoma is an aggressive mature T-cell lymphoma characterized by a proliferation of cytotoxic T cells within the spleen, liver, and bone marrow.

ICD-O coding

9716/3 Hepatosplenic T-cell lymphoma

ICD-11 coding

2A90.8 Hepatosplenic T-cell lymphoma

Related terminology

Not recommended: erythrophagocytic Tγ lymphoma.

Subtype(s)

None

Localization

Hepatosplenic T-cell lymphoma involves the liver, spleen, and bone marrow {295,4461}. Peripheral lymph nodes are uncommonly involved {4461,4462}. A leukaemic phase is uncommon at initial diagnosis but can occur, particularly late in the clinical course {3266}.

Clinical features

Patients often present with marked hepatomegaly, splenomegaly, and B symptoms (see Table 5.14) {4341,295,1112,4461}. This neoplasm can (rarely) involve the skin, most often at the time of relapse {1892}. Laboratory abnormalities are common, particularly cytopenias and elevated serum levels of B2M and LDH (see Table 5.14) {295,4461}. Virtually all patients have advanced-stage disease, shown by pathological evaluation and/or radiological imaging studies {295,4461,393}.

Table 5.14 Clinical findings and laboratory abnormalities in patients with hepatosplenic T-cell lymphoma

Finding/abnormality	Frequency
Clinical findings	
Splenomegaly	80–95%
B-type symptoms	70–80%
Hepatomegaly	60–80%
Jaundice	30–50%
History of immunosuppression	15–25%
Lymphadenopathy	10–20%
Haematological abnormalities	
Thrombocytopenia	50–95%
Anaemia	60–80%
Neutropenia	50–80%
Lymphoma cells in blood	30–50%
Absolute monocytosis	10–20%
Absolute lymphocytosis	< 10%
Serological abnormalities	
Elevated B2M	80–90%
Elevated LDH	50–60%
Elevated bilirubin	50–60%
Elevated liver function enzymes	40–50%

Epidemiology

Hepatosplenic T-cell lymphoma is rare, representing 1.4–2% of peripheral T-cell lymphomas and far less than 1% of all non-Hodgkin lymphomas {4257,1222}. Early studies showed that most patients are adolescents or young adults, with a median age in the fourth decade of life {4463,3302}, but a recent study showed that 51% of patients were aged > 60 years {1222}. The gamma-delta subtype shows a male predominance {4463, 3302}. By contrast, patients with the alpha-beta subtype are more often women and tend to be older {2467}.

Etiology

Unknown

Pathogenesis

About 20% of hepatosplenic T-cell lymphoma cases arise in the context of immunosuppression or autoimmune disease, most often in transplant recipients or patients with Crohn disease treated with azathioprine and infliximab {3445,4463,4459}. Chronic antigenic stimulation and/or impaired immunosurveillance may therefore be involved in pathogenesis.

Isochromosome 7q is common and thought to be an early event in pathogenesis {4287,84}. Loss of 7p22.1-p14.1 and gain of 7q22.11-q31.1 are associated with overexpression of CHN2, ABCB1, RUNDC3B, and PPP1R9A {1191}. Mutations involving genes in the JAK/STAT pathway and/or chromatin epigenetic modification also occur (see Table 5.15, p. 728) {2141,2619}. Gene expression profiling has shown that the alpha-beta and gamma-delta subtypes have a similar profile, with overexpression of NK cell–associated molecules, FOS, VAV3, Syk, and S1PR5 {4068}.

Macroscopic appearance

The spleen is markedly enlarged, typically > 1000 g or > 200 mm in diameter by radiological imaging {4461}. The cut surface has a homogeneous appearance without nodules, reflecting diffuse red pulp involvement and atrophy of the white pulp. The liver is also diffusely enlarged.

Table 5.15 Cytogenetic abnormalities and gene mutations in hepatosplenic T-cell lymphoma

Abnormality/mutation	Frequency
Cytogenetic abnormality	
Isochromosome 7q	40–70%
Trisomy 8	10–50%
Y chromosome loss	20–25%
Chromosome 10q loss	10–20%
Chromosome 1q gain	10–15%
Ring chromosome 7	10%
Gene mutation	
STAT5B	30–40%
SETD2	25%
INO80	21%
TET3	15%
SMARCA2	10%
STAT3	5–10%

Histopathology

Hepatosplenic T-cell lymphoma involves cords and sinuses of the splenic red pulp {4341,295,4198}. The liver and bone marrow also show prominent sinusoidal involvement {4197,4462}. The neoplastic cells in the bone marrow usually expand sinusoids {4461,4462}. The bone marrow may also show mild to moderate haematopoietic cell dyspoiesis, but these features do not appear to have clinical importance {4460}. Erythrophagocytosis can be present, and uncommonly haemophagocytic lymphohistiocytosis can develop {2437}. The neoplastic cells are small to intermediate in size, with irregular nuclear contours, dense chromatin, inconspicuous nucleoli, and pale cytoplasm {295, 4198}. The lymphoma cells do not have cytoplasmic granules as shown by Giemsa {4462}. Occasionally, the neoplastic cells can resemble blasts, or they may exhibit substantial atypia and pleomorphism {4197,295}. Blastoid or pleomorphic cytological features can be detected at time of initial presentation or at time of progression {4197,295}.

Immunophenotype

The neoplastic cells are of cytotoxic T-cell lineage and have a distinctive immunophenotype {4198,4463} (see Table 5.16). They are usually positive for CD2 and CD3, they express

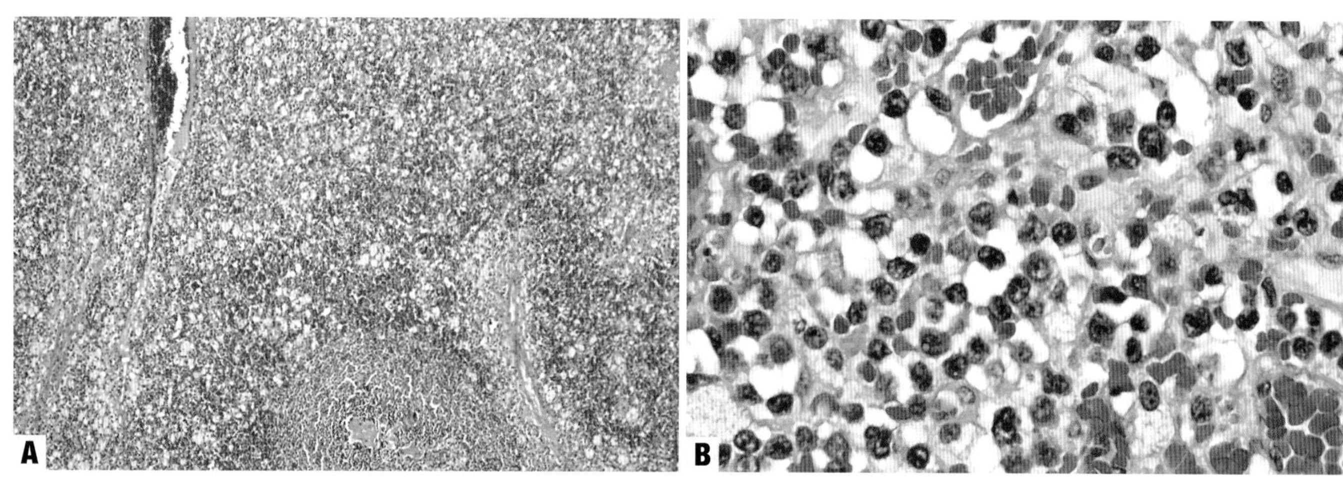

Fig. 5.111 Hepatosplenic T-cell lymphoma. **A** At low magnification, the splenic red pulp is expanded and appears hypercellular. The white pulp is atrophic. **B** High magnification of the splenic red pulp showing numerous lymphoma cells.

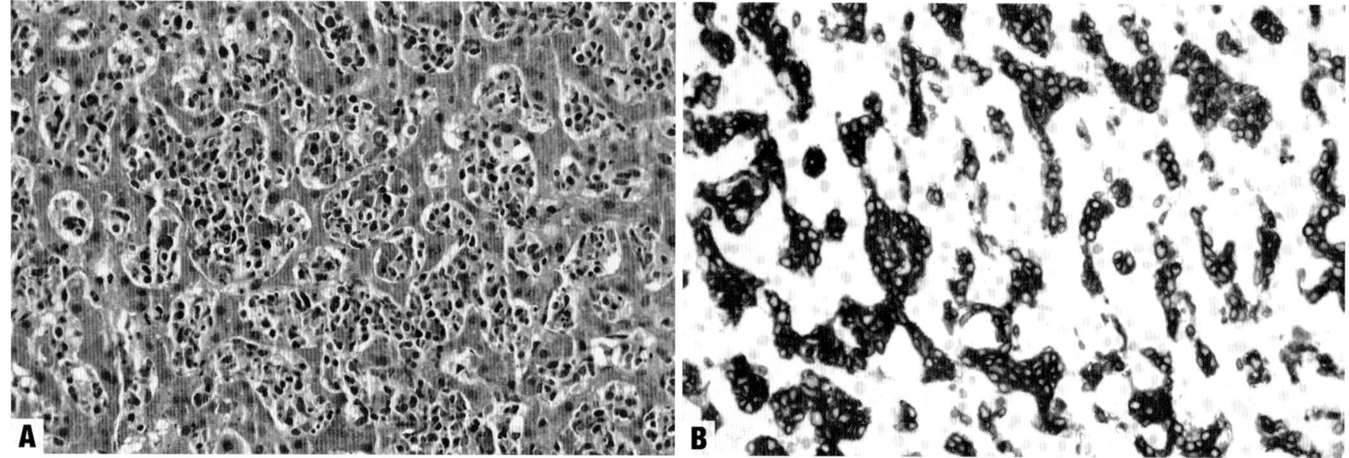

Fig. 5.112 Hepatosplenic T-cell lymphoma. **A** The sinusoids of the liver are extensively involved and expanded by lymphoma cells. **B** The lymphoma cells are positive for CD3, supporting a T-cell lineage.

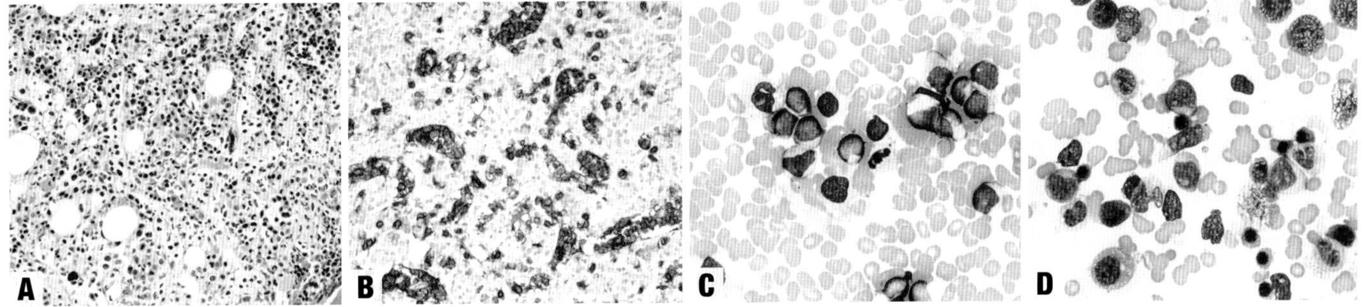

Fig. 5.113 Hepatosplenic T-cell lymphoma. **A** A trephine biopsy shows hypercellularity, and sinusoids are distended by many intermediate-sized lymphoma cells. **B** The tumour cells are positive for CD3. **C** A bone marrow aspirate smear shows many intermediate-sized lymphoma cells with agranular cytoplasm and inconspicuous nucleoli (Giemsa). **D** Morphology can be intermediate to large with prominent nucleoli imparting a blastoid appearance (Giemsa).

cytotoxic markers such as TIA1, perforin, granzyme M, and granzyme B (in 30–40% of cases), and they are usually negative for CD4, CD5 (~15% dim positive), and CD8 (~20% positive). Approximately 75% of cases are positive for TCRγδ, about 20% are positive for TCRαβ, and 5% lack T-cell receptors (silent or null). TCRVδ expression seems to be restricted to the Vδ1 chain {3306}. The NK cell–associated markers CD56 (~70%) and CD16 (~60%) are often positive. In situ hybridization analysis for EBV-encoded small RNA (EBER) is negative.

Differential diagnosis

Other mature T-cell lymphoma subtypes may involve the liver and spleen, and an extensive panel of immunohistochemical markers should be used {4192}.

Cytology

The diagnosis is most often established by bone marrow examination (described above) and there is a limited role for FNAB of the spleen or liver.

Diagnostic molecular pathology

Hepatosplenic T-cell lymphoma carries clonal TR rearrangements. Isochromosome 7q and/or trisomy 8, present in as many as two thirds and half of all cases, respectively, can help in establishing the diagnosis {4462,3302}.

Essential and desirable diagnostic criteria

Essential: characteristic pattern of extranodal disease with sinusoidal involvement of the liver, spleen, and bone marrow; small to intermediate-sized lymphoma cells without intracytoplasmic granules; demonstrated cytotoxic T-cell lineage.

Desirable: characteristic immunophenotype: CD4–, CD5–/+, CD8–/+, CD56+/–; isochromosome 7q; trisomy 8.

Staging

The Lugano system is used to stage lymphomas and has been adopted by the Union for International Cancer Control (UICC) TNM classification {688}.

Table 5.16 Immunophenotype of hepatosplenic T-cell lymphoma

Marker / T-cell receptor usage	Frequency
Marker	
CD2	> 95%
CD3	> 95%
TIA1	85–95%
Granzyme M	85–95%
CD7	70–85%
CD56	65–85%
CD16	50–60%
Granzyme B	30–40%
CD5 (often dim)	15–30%
CD8	10–20%
CD57	~10%
CD30	< 5%
EBV-encoded small RNA (EBER)	< 5%
CD4	0%
CD1a	0%
CD10	0%
Pan B-cell antigens	0%
T-cell receptor usage	
γδ	70–80%
αβ	15–20%
Silent (neither receptor)	~5%

Prognosis and prediction

Patients have a poor prognosis, with a median survival time of < 2 years {4257,393}. Patients with the TCRαβ subtype may have a poorer prognosis {2467}. Chemotherapy using highly aggressive regimens and/or allogeneic stem cell transplantation may improve long-term survival {3961}.

Anaplastic large cell lymphoma: Introduction

Lim MS

Anaplastic large cell lymphomas (ALCLs) are a group of mature T-cell lymphomas that share common cytomorphological and immunophenotypic features but are clinically, pathologically, and genetically heterogeneous. Both ALK+ and ALK− ALCL display large neoplastic lymphoid cells with abundant cytoplasm and pleomorphic features with horseshoe-shaped and reniform nuclei that show uniform strong expression of CD30 {3826}. ALK+ ALCL was considered a definite entity in the fourth edition of the WHO classification of haematolymphoid tumours, in 2008. ALK immunostaining has helped broaden the morphological spectrum of ALK+ ALCLs with the recognition of uncommon cytological variants {2031,1971}. ALK+ ALCLs have a characteristic epidemiology and pathogenetic origin {311,3261} that are distinct from those of ALK− ALCL and primary cutaneous ALCL (C-ALCL), which both have their own typical clinical and pathogenetic features {96}. ALK− ALCL, considered a provisional entity in the fourth edition of the WHO classification of haematolymphoid tumours, was recognized as a distinct entity in the revised fourth edition in 2016 {3146}. Although ALK− ALCLs represent a heterogeneous group of neoplasms, recent genomic analyses have led to significant enhancements of our understanding that are starting to impact the paradigm of classification of these neoplasms {837,4205}. Newly recognized cytogenetic groups are characterized by rearrangements of the *DUSP22-IRF4* locus on chromosome 6p25 and the *TP63* locus on chromosome 3q28 {3146,948}. Currently, there is insufficient consistent evidence on the biological and prognostic implications of these genetic alterations to allow their inclusion as formal subtypes of ALK− ALCL. Breast implant–associated ALCL is now recognized as a new entity within the ALCL family. It has a distinctive pathogenesis arising in response to textured-surface breast implants, a typical presentation as generally non-invasive disease, and a generally excellent outcome without need for chemotherapy or radiotherapy in low-stage disease {2690A,1097}.

ALK-positive anaplastic large cell lymphoma

Elenitoba-Johnson KSJ
Cozzolino I
d'Amore ESG
Klapper W
Lamant-Rochaix L
Mori T
Nagai H
Nakazawa A
Ott G
Takeuchi K

Definition

ALK-positive anaplastic large cell lymphoma (ALCL) is a CD30-positive mature T-cell lymphoma with aberrant expression of ALK secondary to rearrangements of the *ALK* gene.

ICD-O coding

9714/3 ALK-positive anaplastic large cell lymphoma

ICD-11 coding

2A90.A Anaplastic large cell lymphoma, ALK-positive

Related terminology

Acceptable: anaplastic large cell lymphoma, ALK-positive.

Subtype(s)

None

Localization

Lymph nodes are commonly involved (90%), and extranodal involvement is frequent (60%), most commonly the skin (26%), bone (14%), soft tissue (15%) and lung (14%) {3826,1101}. Bone marrow involvement is detected in 10–14% of patients when assessed by morphological examination alone, but this frequency is higher when immunostaining is used {1225}. CNS involvement is rare at diagnosis {1415}.

Clinical features

Patients usually present with advanced-stage disease (stage III or IV) and systemic symptoms (75%) {1101}.

Epidemiology

ALK+ ALCL is rare, accounting for 10–15% of paediatric and adolescent non-Hodgkin lymphoma cases and approximately 3% of adult non-Hodgkin lymphoma cases {3252}. There is a male predominance (M:F ratio: 3:1), and the median age is 30 years {3593}.

Etiology

Unknown

Pathogenesis

The aberrant expression of ALK is a consequence of chromosomal rearrangements that fuse the 3′ portion of ALK on chromosome 2p23 and the 5′ portion of a partner gene that provides the promoter and leads to constitutive expression of the chimeric oncoprotein, as well as to constitutive activation of the kinase function. There are more than 20 partner genes involved in ALK rearrangements {2286}. The predominant fusion partner is *NPM1*, which is involved in the t(2;5)(p23;q35) translocation, resulting in aberrant expression of the *NPM1::ALK* fusion protein (Table 5.17, p. 732). The *NPM1::ALK* oncogenic tyrosine kinase is constitutively active, triggering numerous cellular signalling pathways including the PLCγ {213}, PI3K/AKT {3765,214}, CDC42/RAC1 {739}, JNK/JUN (c-Jun) {2287}, RAS/ERK/MAPK, mTOR {2346}, JAK/STAT3 {4565}, and STAT5B {2957} pathways. Activation of these pathways promotes various aspects of oncogenesis to enhance cell survival, inhibit apoptosis {2346}, promote tumour dissemination, and evade the immune surveillance mechanisms. STAT3 also upregulates the transcription factor C/EBPβ, which is overexpressed in ALK+ ALCL and is critical for tumour cell survival through transcriptional activation of its target genes, *BCL2A1* and *DDX21* {406}. C/EBPβ contributes to the aberrant expression of the myeloid/histiocytic antigens CD13 and CD33, as well as clusterin. Transcription factors such as IRF and MYC are essential for the survival of ALCL {4344}. *NPM1::ALK* has also been reported to control T-cell identity by the epigenetic silencing of many T cell–associated antigens {99}.

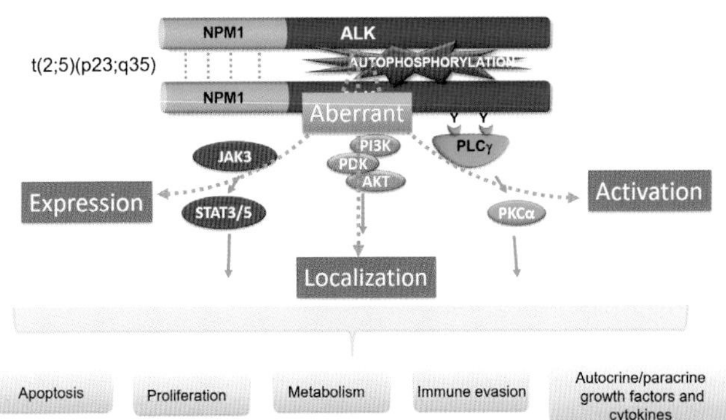

Fig. 5.114 ALK-positive anaplastic large cell lymphoma (ALCL). Pathogenesis. The oncogenic NPM1 (NPM)::ALK fusion protein is expressed as a consequence of the chromosomal translocation involving *NPM1* and *ALK*. Constitutively activated NPM1 (NPM)::ALK leads to the activation of numerous downstream oncogenic pathways that result in lymphoma.

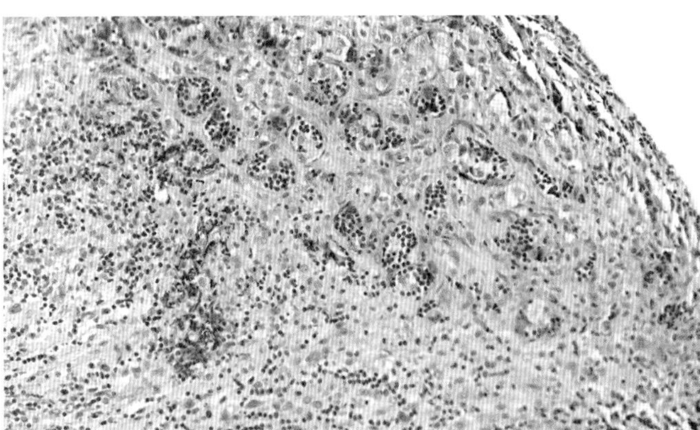

Fig. 5.115 ALK-positive anaplastic large cell lymphoma. Involvement of the sinusoids of the lymph node.

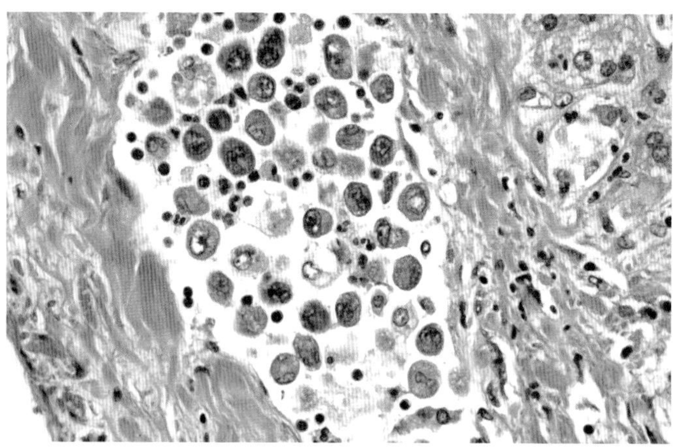

Fig. 5.116 ALK-positive anaplastic large cell lymphoma. Involvement of an intravascular space.

Macroscopic appearance

Not relevant

Histopathology

Lymph nodes show highly variable patterns of involvement, including paracortical, sinusoidal, perifollicular, intravascular, and diffuse. In extranodal sites the tumour cells show an infiltrative, diffuse proliferation that can be associated with tumour necrosis. Cases with classic morphology demonstrate variable numbers of characteristic (hallmark) cells with eccentrically placed large horseshoe-shaped nuclei, multiple nucleoli, and abundant amphophilic cytoplasm. The neoplastic cells may be distributed in sheets or in isolated clusters. The morphological spectrum is broad and includes small cell, lymphohistiocytic, and monomorphic patterns, as well as rare cases with a classic Hodgkin lymphoma (CHL)-like pattern, a neutrophil-rich background or with a sarcomatoid appearance. Small cell patterns tend to show a perivascular pattern of growth.

Bone marrow involvement is variable and typically shows small clusters of neoplastic cells in an interstitial pattern, which may be missed on casual examination. Immunostaining for CD30 may aid in highlighting the tumour cells {1225}.

Neoplastic cells circulating in the blood show variably sized (medium to large) atypical lymphoid cells with irregular multilobated nuclei and multiple nucleoli.

Immunophenotype

The neoplastic cells exhibit strong, uniform expression of CD30 highlighting the cell membrane and Golgi area. Immunohistochemistry for ALK highlights the neoplastic cells and is reflective of the aberrant expression of ALK secondary to *ALK* rearrangements. The presence of the *NPM1*::*ALK* translocation results in a nuclear and cytoplasmic pattern of ALK expression {3261}. *ALK* translocations with variant translocation partners result in cytoplasmic or membranous expression of ALK, which is seen in approximately 15% of ALK+ ALCL cases. There is frequent loss of T cell–associated antigens {1223}. CD2 and CD4 are most commonly expressed (40–70%), whereas CD3 is negative in > 75% of the cases. CD43 and CD45RO expression is commonly observed {1223,863,3498}. The tumour cells express cytotoxic markers, including TIA1, granzyme B, and perforin, even when they lack T-cell antigens, including CD8. They typically express CD25, clusterin, and BCL6 {4351}. CD15 and PAX5 are almost always absent but may be positive in rare cases. The tumour cells generally lack CD45 and the T-cell receptor molecules βF1 and TCRδ. EMA is positive in the vast majority of cases, whereas occasional cases aberrantly express epithelial markers such as cytokeratins. Myeloid

Table 5.17 Chromosomal rearrangements, partner genes and their functions, and patterns of ALK expression found in ALK-positive anaplastic large cell lymphoma

Chromosomal abnormality	*ALK* partner		ALK staining pattern	% of cases	References
	Gene	Function			
t(2;5)(p23;q35)	*NPM1*	Nuclear protein that shuttles between the nucleus and the cytoplasm	Nuclear and cytoplasmic	84%	{2800}
t(1;2)(q25;p23)	*TPM3*	Cytoskeletal protein	Strong cytoplasmic and membranous	13%	{2200}
Inv(2)(p23q53)	*ATIC*	Purine biosynthesis pathway	Diffuse cytoplasmic	1%	{779}
t(2;3)(p23;q21)	*TFGxl* *TFGl* *TFGs*	Associated with endoplasmic reticulum and microtubules	Diffuse cytoplasmic Diffuse cytoplasmic Diffuse cytoplasmic	< 1%	{1567}
t(2;17)(p23;q23)	*CLTC*	Component of the cytoplasmic face of intracellular organelles	Granular cytoplasmic	< 1%	{796}
t(2;X)(p23;q11.12)	*MSN*	Submembranous cytoskeletal protein	Membranous	< 1%	{796}
t(2;19)(p23;p13.1)	*TPM4*	Cytoskeletal protein	Diffuse cytoplasmic	< 1%	{2626}
t(2;22)(p23;q11.2)	*MYH9*	Cytoskeletal (major contractile protein)	Diffuse cytoplasmic	< 1%	{2201}
t(2;9)(p23;q33-34)	*TRAF1*	TNF signalling, signalling adaptor	Diffuse cytoplasmic	< 1%	{1155}
t(2;11)(2p23;11q12.3)	*EEF1G*	Translation elongation factor activity; subunit of elongation factor 1	Diffuse cytoplasmic	< 1%	{3111}
t(2;17)(p23;q25)	*RNF213* (*ALO17*)	E3 ubiquitin ligase	Diffuse cytoplasmic	< 1%	{796,4148}

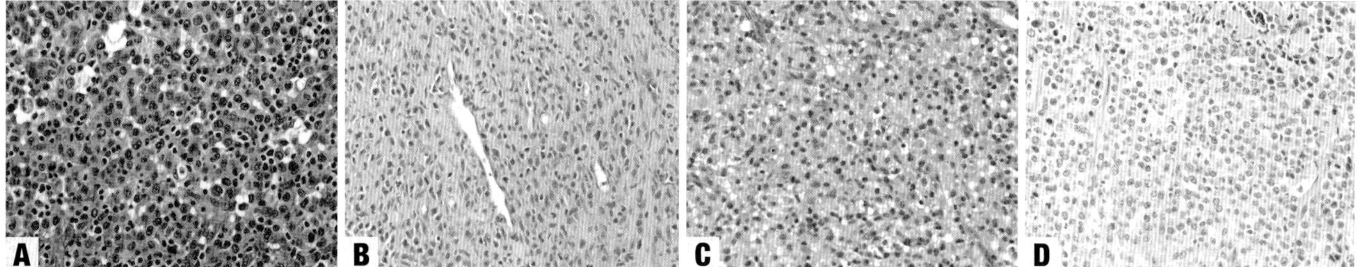

Fig. 5.117 ALK-positive anaplastic large cell lymphoma. **A** Classic morphology, characterized by a variable number of characteristic hallmark cells with abundant cytoplasm and large horseshoe-shaped nuclei and multiple nucleoli. **B** Small cell pattern, demonstrating depletion of background lymphoid cells. The neoplastic cells are predominantly small in size, with eosinophilic cytoplasm. **C** Lymphohistiocytic pattern, characterized by numerous histiocytes admixed with atypical lymphoid cells, some showing vacuolated cytoplasm. **D** Monomorphic pattern, comprising uniform large to medium-sized cells.

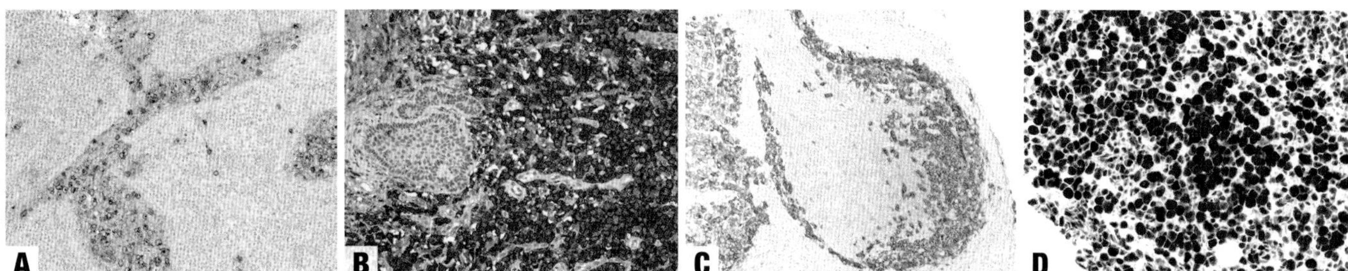

Fig. 5.118 ALK-positive anaplastic large cell lymphoma (ALCL). **A** Neoplastic cells demonstrating a sinusoidal growth pattern highlighted by strong, uniform expression of CD30. **B** Infiltration in the skin shows uniform and strong expression of CD30 in the perifollicular region. The hair follicle epithelium and endothelial cells are negative for CD30. **C** Tumour cell infiltration in the lymph node demonstrates strong and uniform expression of CD30 and highlights sheets and intrasinusoidal extension. **D** Strong nuclear and cytoplasmic expression of ALK is observed in ALCL with *NPM1::ALK* rearrangement.

antigens (CD13 and CD33), NK-cell markers (CD56), and stem cell transcriptional factors (including SOX2) are occasionally expressed {1311}. EBV is characteristically negative.

Differential diagnosis

Cases with a prominent sinusoidal growth pattern and large cohesive tumour cells may simulate metastatic carcinoma. Some ALK+ ALCLs show neoplastic cells that mimic Reed–Sternberg cells and should be distinguished from classic Hodgkin lymphoma. Plasmablastic lymphoma and primary effusion lymphoma (solid) may show cohesive sheets of large pleomorphic cells resembling the tumour cells of ALK+ ALCL. Other neoplasms that express ALK, such as ALK+ large B-cell lymphoma, inflammatory myofibroblastic tumour, histiocytic neoplasm, and carcinoma, must be excluded {2750,1722, 3826}.

Cytology

The large lymphoma cells show abundant basophilic cytoplasm with occasional vacuoles, and large pleomorphic nuclei with prominent nucleoli. Some may show a plasmacytoid appearance with a prominent perinuclear hof and cytoplasmic vacuoles.

Diagnostic molecular pathology

Most cases are diagnosed on the basis of the aberrant expression of ALK protein by immunohistochemistry. Genetic testing is not required, but it may be useful in selected cases to assess variant translocations. For cases that show downregulation or deletion of most T cell–associated antigens, demonstration of clonal T-cell populations by TR gene rearrangement may confirm the neoplastic process {404}.

Essential and desirable diagnostic criteria

Essential: complete or partial infiltration of lymph node or extranodal tissue by large pleomorphic cells with lobated nuclei and distinct nucleoli, including hallmark cells (other morphologies are acceptable); uniform strong expression of CD30 and ALK in lymphoma cells; negative for EBV.

Desirable: expression of T-cell markers and cytotoxic markers, albeit with frequent losses; clonal TR gene rearrangement.

Staging

The Cotswold modification {2369} of the Ann Arbor staging system is the standard anatomical staging system used for patients with ALK+ ALCL.

Prognosis and prediction

Long-term survival rates are about 80% {3739} and therefore significantly better than the vast majority of ALK− ALCL {3593}. The treatment failure rate for ALK+ ALCL patients is approximately 30%, regardless of first-line treatment strategy. Progression during chemotherapy portends a poor prognosis. Only 25% of patients who experience disease progression are expected to survive, even with aggressive salvage therapy including allogeneic transplantation. CNS involvement and a leukaemic component at presentation are adverse prognostic factors {2240, 4384,1415}. A small-cell and/or lymphohistiocytic component indicates a high risk of treatment failure in children {2202}. Detection of minimal disseminated disease by *NPM::ALK* RT-PCR analysis in bone marrow or peripheral blood at diagnosis or during treatment identifies patients at risk for relapse in the paediatric population {862,2436}. Targeted treatment, including small-molecule ALK inhibitors, may improve prognosis and modify the impact of prognostic factors {2810}.

ALK-negative anaplastic large cell lymphoma

Miranda RN
Cozzolino I
Ott G

Definition

ALK-negative anaplastic large cell lymphoma (ALCL) is a mature T-cell lymphoma with uniform strong expression of CD30, without ALK expression or *ALK* rearrangement.

ICD-O coding

9715/3 ALK-negative anaplastic large cell lymphoma

ICD-11 coding

2A90.B Anaplastic large cell lymphoma, ALK-negative

Related terminology

Acceptable: anaplastic large cell lymphoma, ALK-negative.

Subtype(s)

None

Localization

Lymph nodes and extranodal sites are affected in a 1:1 ratio {3593}, with single extranodal sites involved in about 50% of

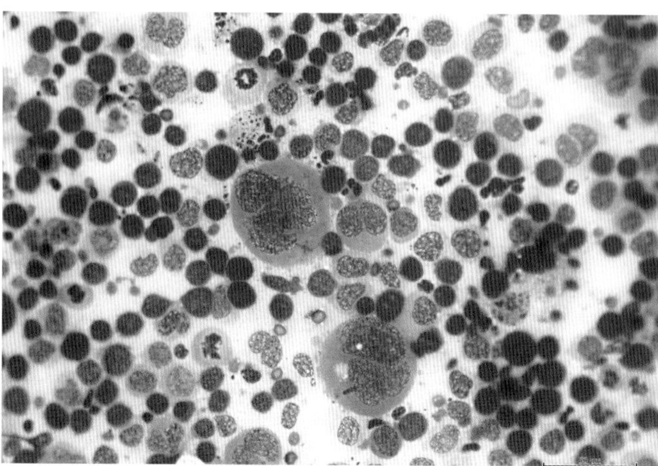

Fig. 5.119 ALK-negative anaplastic large cell lymphoma. Large tumour cells with abundant bluish and vacuolated cytoplasm. Nuclei are central and lobated, with multiple conspicuous nucleoli (Giemsa).

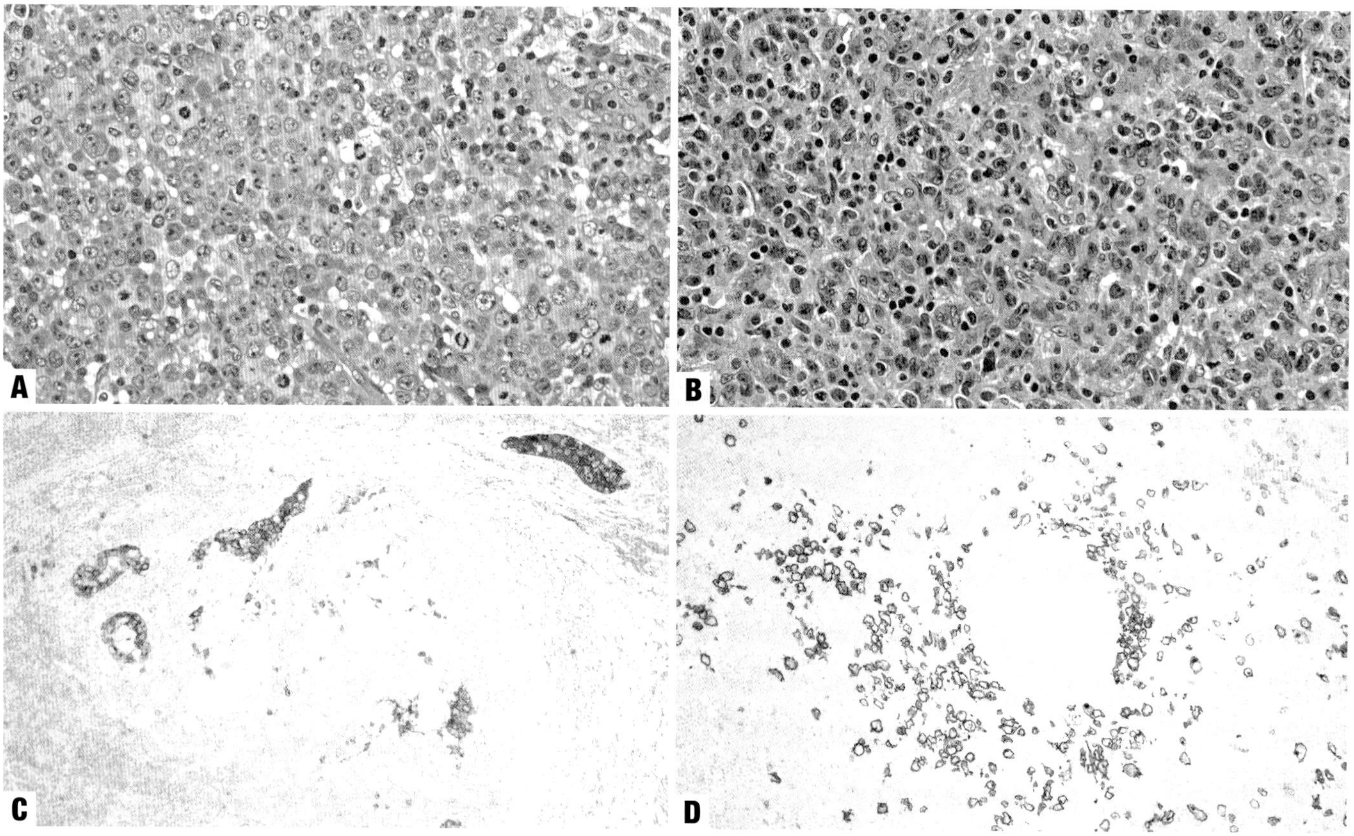

Fig. 5.120 ALK-negative anaplastic large cell lymphoma. **A** Diffuse infiltration of large oval cells and scattered hallmark cells; there are frequent mitoses. **B** Pleomorphic cells are admixed with reactive lymphocytes in the background. FISH for *DUSP22* rearrangement was negative. **C** CD30 highlights clusters of lymphoma cells with a sinusoidal pattern. **D** CD30 highlights lymphoma cells in a paracortical/perifollicular pattern.

cases and multiple extranodal sites in 26% of cases {4508,3736}. Sites include soft tissue, mediastinum, bone marrow, liver, spleen, gastrointestinal tract, and breast {3627,3738,3593}.

Clinical features

Patients usually present with stage III or IV disease, associated with B symptoms {3736}.

Epidemiology

ALK– ALCL represents 5.5–15% of mature T-cell neoplasms {3736,4508}, with some geographical variation {3736}. Most cases occur in adults (median age: 54 years, range: 18–89 years) {3736,1113,3826}, with an M:F ratio of 1.6:1 {3736}.

Etiology

Unknown

Pathogenesis

The tumour cells are CD4+ lymphocytes with features of an innate cytotoxic immune cell {4108}. Most cases show clonal rearrangement of TR genes. Activating mutations of *JAK1* and *STAT3* lead to constitutive activation of the JAK/STAT3 pathway {837}. Oncogenic fusions involving tyrosine kinase genes other than *ALK* also lead to STAT3 activation {837,4205}. Rearrangements of the *DUSP22* locus at 6p25.3 occur in about 20–30% of cases {3146}, and these cases appear distinct from other ALK– ALCL cases in that they lack STAT3 activation and result in a DNA hypomethylation state leading to enhanced immunogenicity through reduced expression of PDL1 and overexpression of CD58 and HLA class II {2441}. *MSC* p.E116K mutations in cases with *DUSP22* rearrangement reverse the inhibitory effect of musculin over MYC {2442}. In about 5% of cases, rearrangement of *TP63* occurs as an inversion of 3q28, involving the partner gene *TBL1XR1* {3146,4189}. Copy-number abnormalities, including loss of 17p13 (*TP53*) {392,3541,4551}, are seen in a subset (30%) of cases {1323}. Gene expression profiling demonstrates that the molecular signature of ALK– ALCL shows some overlap with that of ALK+ ALCL {40,225,1736,3230,3263} but is distinct from that of peripheral T-cell lymphoma NOS {40, 1736}. Transcription factors such as IRF4 and MYC are essential for the survival of ALCL {4344}.

Macroscopic appearance

Not relevant

Histopathology

Involved tissues show complete or partial effacement by diffuse and cohesive infiltrates of tumour cells, which are large and pleomorphic with lobated vesicular nuclei and prominent nucleoli, similar to those observed in ALK+ ALCL, including the presence of hallmark cells. Multinucleated cells, including wreath-like cells, may also be present {1116,2886,3261, 3731}. A starry-sky pattern is occasionally observed, and mitotic figures are easily identified. In cases with partial lymph

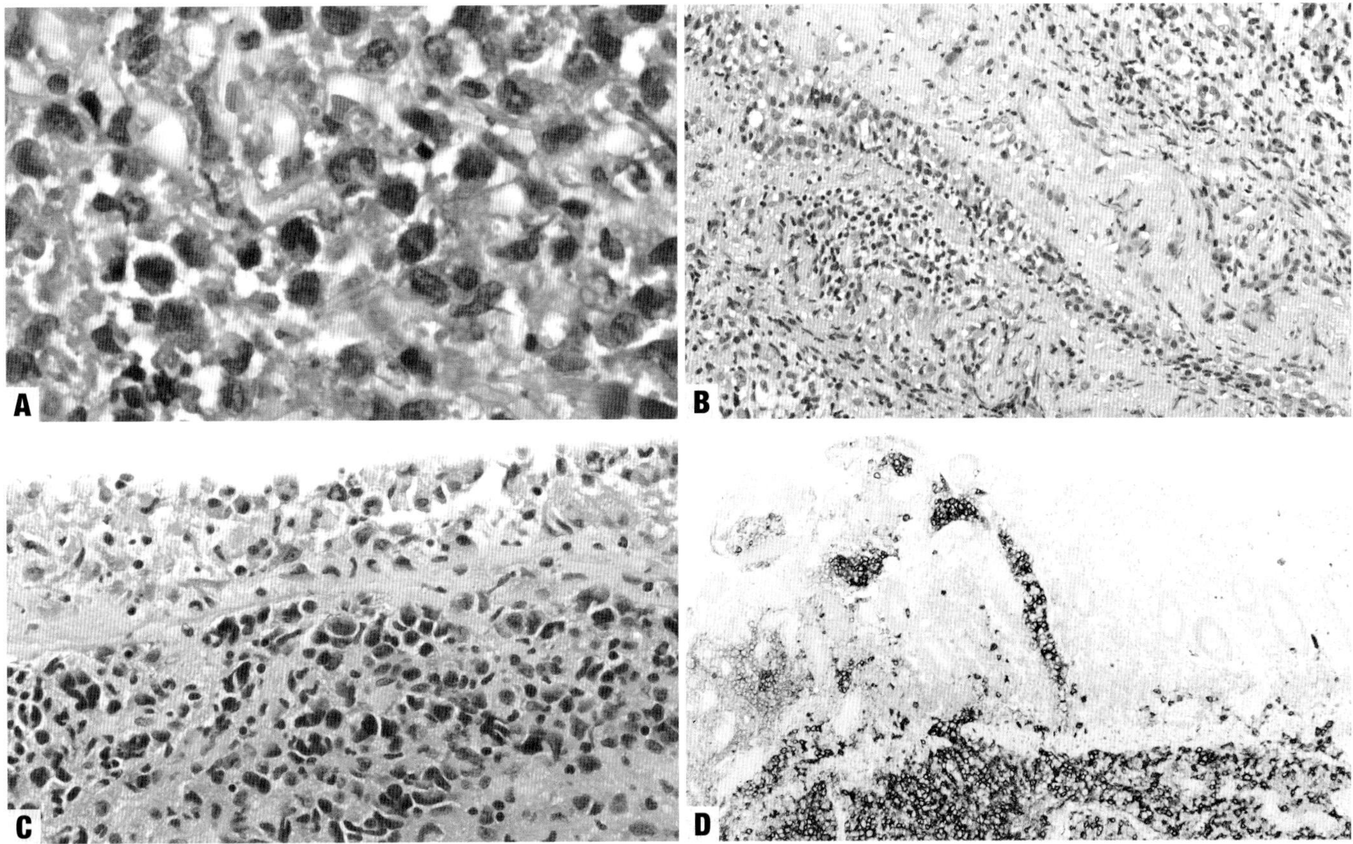

Fig. 5.121 ALK-negative anaplastic large cell lymphoma (ALCL). **A** Large anaplastic lymphoma cells, including hallmark cells, are seen in lung involved by ALK-negative ALCL. **B** ALCL infiltrating breast ducts in a patient with a remote history of chest burn. **C** Large pleomorphic lymphoma cells underlying the synovium. **D** CD30 highlights lymphoma cells within lymphovascular channels of the mucosa of a small bowel involved by ALK-negative ALCL.

node involvement, a sinusoidal or perifollicular pattern may be present {174}.

ALCLs with *DUSP22* rearrangement are characterized by neoplastic cells with a doughnut-cell appearance {2025} and a sheet-like growth pattern with reduced numbers of pleomorphic cells. A subset of cases with Hodgkin-like morphology may show aberrant expression of ERBB4 {3603}, whereas more anaplastic cells are seen in cases with *JAK2* rearrangement {1199}.

Immunohistochemistry

Neoplastic cells uniformly express CD30 with a membrane and Golgi pattern, although some cases treated with anti-CD30 brentuximab vedotin may lose CD30 expression {85}.

By definition, ALK is negative. CD2, CD3, CD5, and CD7 are expressed in < 50% of cases, whereas CD43, a marker not confined to T cells, may be the only positive marker. CD4 is less commonly expressed (70%), and CD8 expression is rare {3708}. Fewer than 20% of cases express T-cell receptors, mainly TCRαβ {96}, and occasional cases lack immunophenotypic evidence of T-cell lineage (null cell). Clusterin and IRF4 (MUM1) are expressed in most cases {2192,2906,3520}, whereas EMA is positive in < 50% of cases. One or several cytotoxic markers, including TIA1, granzyme B, or perforin, can be detected, except in cases with *DUSP22* rearrangement {3146}. LEF1 expression appears specific for *DUSP22*-rearranged cases {3375}. Nuclear phosphorylated STAT3 is expressed in approximately 50% of cases {837}, a feature in common with other T-cell lymphomas that reflects cytokine activation {2664}. Markers of immune evasion, PDL1, TGF-β, and IL-10, are also frequently expressed {168}. Notably, EBV is absent.

Differential diagnosis

ALK– ALCL needs to be distinguished from other malignancies expressing CD30, including classic Hodgkin lymphoma rich in Hodgkin cells, embryonal carcinoma, primary mediastinal large B-cell lymphoma {3249}, and myeloid sarcoma {3250}. ALK– ALCL should also be distinguished from primary cutaneous ALCL and breast implant–associated ALCL, which are localized forms of ALCL and clinically distinct. CD15 expression raises the possibility of classic Hodgkin lymphoma or peripheral T-cell lymphoma NOS {252}. Regional lymph nodes adjacent to primary cutaneous ALCL, lymphomatoid papulosis {1039}, mycosis fungoides / Sézary syndrome, and breast implant–associated ALCL {1183} may be difficult to distinguish from systemic ALK– ALCL.

Cytology

Neoplastic cells are large, usually 20–30 μm in air-dried smears, with abundant bluish and vacuolated cytoplasm with Wright–Giemsa staining. Nuclei are usually central and commonly lobated, with thin nuclear membranes and conspicuous single or multiple nucleoli {946}.

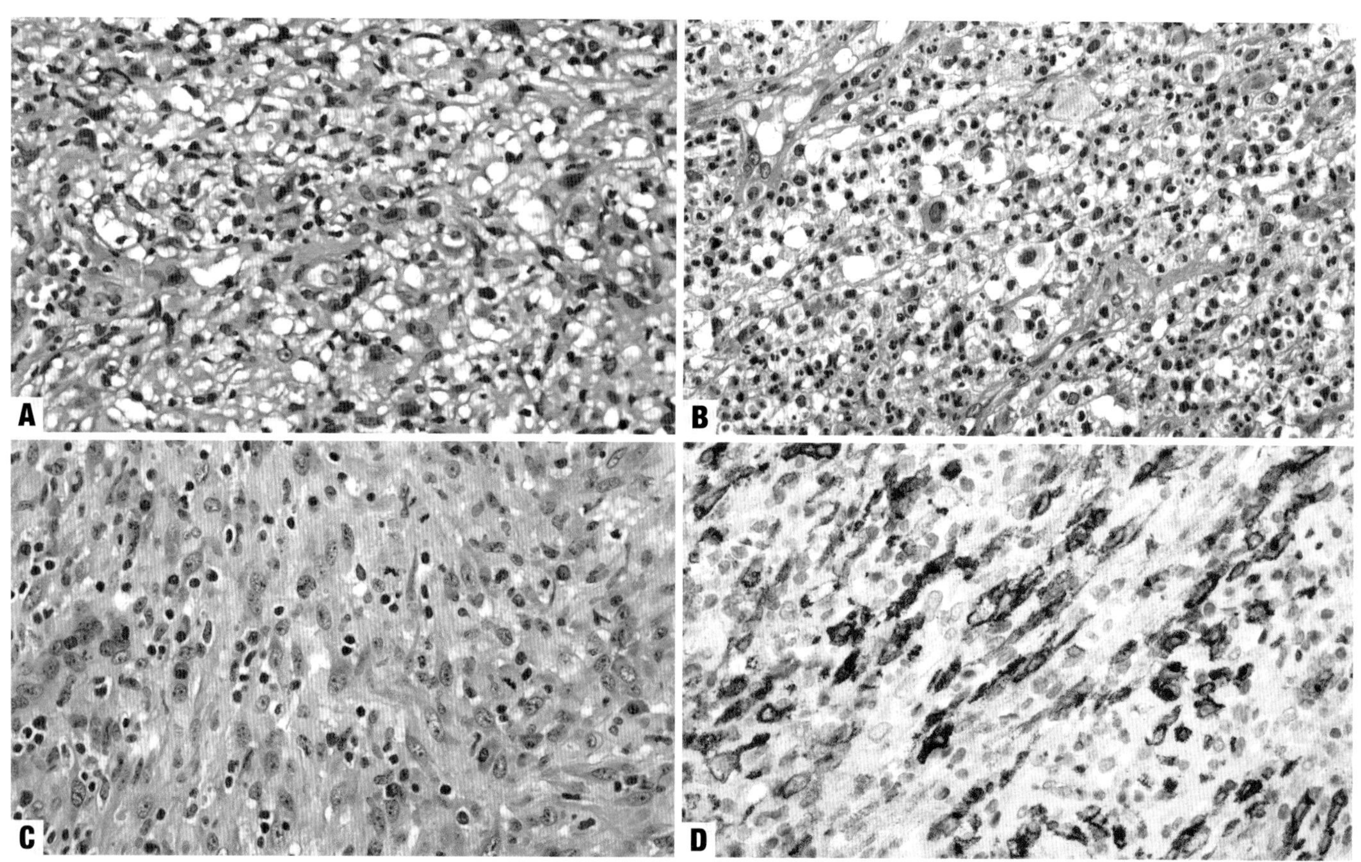

Fig. 5.122 ALK-negative anaplastic large cell lymphoma. **A** Scattered large lymphoma cells are admixed with small lymphocytes and numerous histiocytes. **B** The infiltrate is admixed with abundant neutrophils in the background. **C** Cases can have a sarcomatoid appearance, in which lymphoma cells are predominantly spindle-shaped. **D** CD30 highlights spindle-shaped lymphoma cells with a sarcomatoid appearance.

Diagnostic molecular pathology

TR gene rearrangement studies reveal a clonal T-cell population in about 80% of cases. Rearrangements of the *DUSP22* locus (20–30% of cases) and *TP63* (~5%) and *JAK1* and *STAT3* mutations (~30%) {913,948} can be detected by appropriate molecular methods {3027}.

Essential and desirable diagnostic criteria

Essential: complete or partial infiltration of lymph node or extranodal tissue by large pleomorphic cells with lobated nuclei and distinct nucleoli, including hallmark cells; uniform strong expression of CD30; absence of ALK protein expression or *ALK* rearrangement; negative for EBV.

Desirable: expression of T-cell markers and cytotoxic markers, albeit with frequent losses; clonal TR gene rearrangement.

Staging

The Cotswold modification {2369} of the Ann Arbor staging system is the standard anatomical staging system used.

Prognosis and prediction

The prognosis of systemic ALK– ALCL is worse than that of ALK+ ALCL, but better than that of peripheral T-cell lymphoma NOS using conventional chemotherapy {3593}, with a 5-year overall survival rate of approximately 50% {3736}. Outcomes are better when chemotherapy is combined with brentuximab vedotin {1130}. Initial reports suggested that *DUSP22* rearrangement was associated with survival comparable to that of ALK+ ALCL {3175}, but more recent studies have refuted a survival impact of *DUSP22* rearrangement {1493,3319}. Poor outcomes have been observed in patients with tumours bearing *TP63* rearrangements {3175,3146}, *TP53* deletion/mutation {392,2393,3404}, or overexpression of IL-2Rα {2332}.

Breast implant–associated anaplastic large cell lymphoma

Miranda RN
de Jong D
Di Napoli A
Oishi N
Ott G
Schmitt F

Definition

Breast implant–associated anaplastic large cell lymphoma (BIA-ALCL) is a mature CD30-positive T-cell lymphoma that arises in relation to a breast implant as an effusion confined by a fibrous capsule, and less commonly forming an invading mass.

ICD-O coding

9715/3 Breast implant–associated anaplastic large cell lymphoma

ICD-11 coding

2A90.B & XH05D8 Anaplastic large cell lymphoma, ALK-negative & Breast implant–associated anaplastic large cell lymphoma

Related terminology

Acceptable: seroma-associated anaplastic large cell lymphoma.

Subtype(s)

None

Localization

BIA-ALCL is most frequently restricted to the peri-implant space or as superficial deposits on the luminal side of the peri-implant fibrous capsule. BIA-ALCL can also present as a mass within or beyond the capsule, infiltrating the surrounding soft tissue or breast parenchyma. Regional lymph nodes may be involved {1183}. Rare cases of implant-associated anaplastic large cell lymphoma (ALCL) have been reported around implants in extramammary sites (e.g. gluteal implants) {3262,3707}.

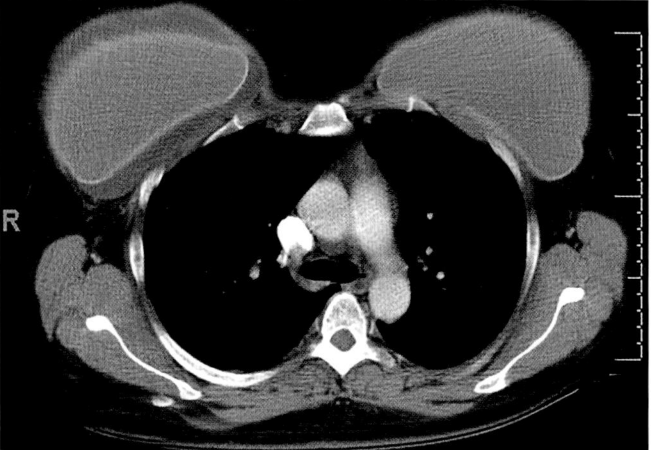

Fig. 5.123 Breast implant–associated anaplastic large cell lymphoma in peri-implant effusion. CT demonstrates fluid around a prosthetic implant on the right side. The left side is intact.

Clinical features

The median time from implant placement to presentation is approximately 10 years (range: 2–32 years) {2690A,890}. Most patients present with a unilateral effusion around the implant; the volume of effusion can be as high as 700 mL. B symptoms are typically absent {3325}. Approximately 5% of cases are bilateral {280A,2690A}. About 10–30% of patients present with a mass, and as many as 20% develop regional lymphadenopathy, most commonly in the axilla and supraclavicular fossa. Lymphadenopathy may be the first manifestation of disease where it can be misdiagnosed as Hodgkin lymphoma or systemic ALK-negative ALCL {1183}. Rarely, patients present with disseminated disease {2690A,1097}. Effusion is best detected with ultrasonography, whereas tumour mass assessment, lymphadenopathy assessment, and follow-up are better done by PET; mammography is suboptimal {27A}.

Epidemiology

The average age at diagnosis of BIA-ALCL is 50 years (range: 21 to > 80 years). It arises almost exclusively in women, including rare cases in transgender women {3165,889}. Although the vast majority of primary lymphomas of the breast are of B-cell lineage (mostly diffuse large B-cell lymphomas and extranodal marginal zone lymphomas {3951}), BIA-ALCL is a site-specific lymphoma and the most common lymphoma type associated with breast implants {2690A,890}. Reported incidence rates vary worldwide, with the highest rates in the USA, Europe, and Australia, and much lower rates in Latin America and Asia {1731}. Epidemiological risk studies show variable risk estimates, usually ranging from 1 in 3000 to 1 in 30 000 women with implants {890,4303,992,806,893}.

Etiology

BIA-ALCL is associated with macrotextured (as opposed to smooth-surface) implants {992,2477}. Evidence of an association with specific implant shell material is inconclusive; however, the surface roughness of textured implants is associated with the risk of developing BIA-ALCL {2477,3570}. Saline or silicone filling does not appear to have a pathogenetic role {2477,893}. Patients who receive implants after breast cancer surgery have a higher risk of developing BIA-ALCL than those who have implants for cosmetic purposes {806,2930}.

A genetic predisposition has been suggested, based on germline *TP53* mutations reported in 5 cases {2265,3155,27,378}. It has also been reported that women with *BRCA1* or *BRCA2* germline mutations may have a higher risk of BIA-ALCL (1 in 1200) {888}, although this finding needs independent validation {1731}.

Pathogenesis

The pathogenesis of BIA-ALCL involves immunological and molecular factors. The immunological events that contribute to

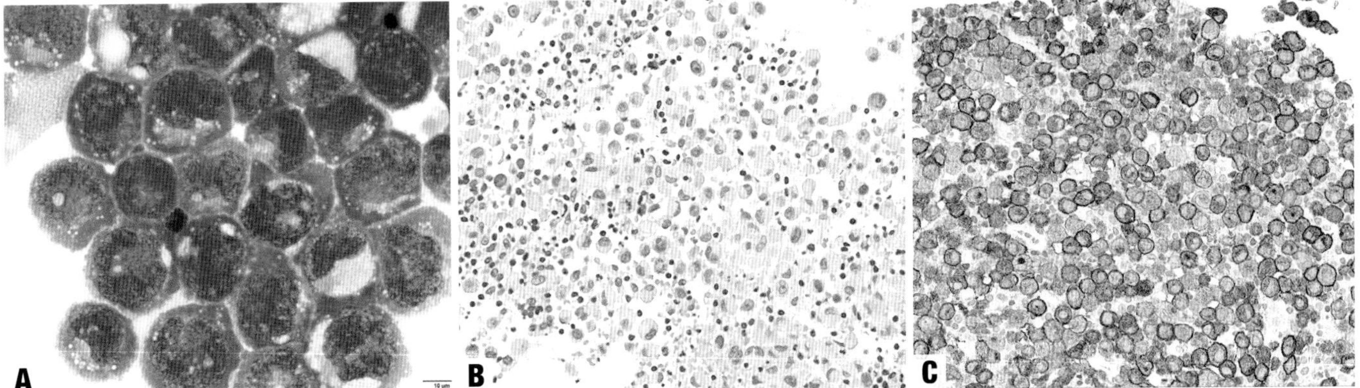

Fig. 5.124 Breast implant–associated anaplastic large cell lymphoma. **A** Cytological smear (Giemsa): large pleomorphic cells in a cytological smear of peri-implant fluid. Lymphoma cells have abundant vacuolated cytoplasm and large multilobated nuclei. **B** Cell block: numerous large neoplastic cells admixed with few inflammatory cells are noted. **C** CD30 immunohistochemistry demonstrates that most cells in the cell block are lymphoma cells. Only rare small lymphocytes are noted as negative.

BIA-ALCL are likely multifactorial and include direct and/or indirect stimulation driven by silicone shell material, shed silicone particles, and periprosthetic bacterial biofilm {1654,4281,3026}. Bacterial lipopolysaccharide antigens induce chemokines/cytokines, including IL-13, eotaxin, and IL-10, which induce a chronic T helper 17 (Th17) cell response more than a T helper 1 (Th1) cell response. A role for the T helper 2 (Th2) allergic inflammatory response {1654,1842,4400A,1844,944} has also been suggested.

Constitutive activation of the JAK/STAT3 pathway is pivotal, as supported by consistent expression of phosphorylated STAT3 and transcriptional activation of STAT3 target genes {3025, 2246A,2423,943}. Activating somatic mutations of *STAT3*, *STAT5B*, *JAK1*, and *JAK2*, as well as loss-of-function mutations of *SOCS1* and *SOCS3*, and/or genomic amplifications of JAK/STAT pathway genes, have been reported in more than half of the patients {3025,379,2237,2282,945,2423,3327}.

Other recurrent genetic alterations include point mutations in epigenetic modifiers (*KMT2C*, *KMT2D*, *CHD2*, *CREBBP*, *DNMT3A*) and *TP53* {945,2237}. Characteristic loss of chromosome 20 has also been detected in the majority of cases {2423}, with loss of 20q13.12-13.2 being highly specific for BIA-ALCL {2423} (see Table 5.18).

Focal amplification of *CD274* (*PDL1*) at 9p24.1 has been seen in about one third of the cases, with overexpression of PDL1 in over half of the cases {3916}. BIA-ALCL is consistently negative for gene rearrangements involving *ALK*, *DUSP22*, and *TP63* {2233,3025}. Like in other ALCLs, components of the T-cell receptor signalling pathway are downregulated {943}.

Macroscopic appearance

Macroscopic pathological assessment is best performed by en bloc resection of the intact capsule containing the implant and effusion. Fluid should be sent for flow cytometry and cytological examination, because in some cases the only evidence of lymphoma is in the effusion. Fixation of the capsule on a flat surface allows for optimal orientation and subsequent on-edge sectioning. Generous sampling is recommended when a grossly distinct lesion is not identified, and any floating material or fibrinous material attached to the implant or capsule should be submitted for histological evaluation {2451,1763}. Tumour masses are suggested by the presence of variable capsular thickening or readily apparent tumorous lesions. Assessment of the capsular resection margins is warranted for complete excision of infiltrating lesions. Fragmented capsules or incomplete capsulectomy may lead to recurrence or progression of disease {1097}.

Histopathology

Most cases of BIA-ALCL present as a seroma-confined disease. At capsulectomy, the tumour cells line the inner surface of the capsule as a distinct layer caught in a fibrinoid and highly necrotic meshwork. Infiltrating stages present as small clusters of tumour cells penetrating into the capsule and the tissues

Table 5.18 Molecular and cytogenetic aberrancies detected in breast implant–associated anaplastic large cell lymphoma

Recurrent molecular alterations	Frequency	References
JAK/STAT signalling		
STAT3	11–64%	{378,2237,3025,945,3327}
JAK1	7–44%	{3327,2237,3025}
SOCS1	3–20%	{945,3327,378,2237}
SOCS3	6%	{2237}
PTPN1	3–9%	{378,2237}
Epigenetic modifiers		
KMT2C	11–26%	{2237,3327}
CHD2	15%	{2237}
CREBBP	15%	{2237}
KMT2D	9%	{2237}
DNMT3A	6–20%	{945,2237}
HDAC2	6%	{2237}
TET2	3%	{2237}
Cell cycle / apoptosis		
TP53	11–20%	{945,378,2237,3327}
Chromosome		
Loss of 20q13.13	66%	{2423}

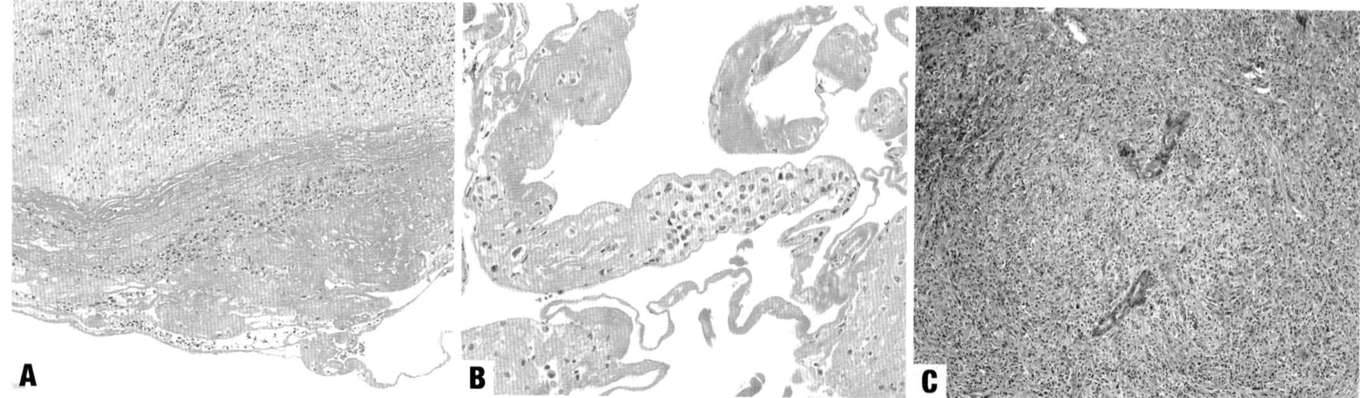

Fig. 5.125 Breast implant–associated anaplastic large cell lymphoma. **A** Tumour cells are found in a background of fibrinous material adjacent to the inner surface of a fibrous capsule. Although an inflammatory infiltrate with a large component of histiocytes is present in the capsular tissue, infiltration of tumour cells is absent. **B** Tumour cells in seroma fluid with strands of fibrin material. **C** Invasion into breast parenchyma. Remnants of breast ducts are extensively infiltrated by large lymphoma cells. This feature is associated with aggressive disease.

beyond (soft tissue, breast parenchyma, skin) or as a tumour-forming mass, both usually admixed with a reactive infiltrate of histiocytes and scattered eosinophils. Necrosis is usually prominent in early-stage as well as advanced-stage disease {3325, 946}. The neoplastic cells are large, with moderately abundant amphophilic, eosinophilic, or clear cytoplasm and oval to multilobated nuclei with small to prominent nucleoli with or without hallmark morphology. Silicone material can be identified focally throughout the capsule, usually with giant cell reaction.

Lymph node involvement, when present, is usually sinusoidal and less frequently diffuse, interfollicular, or perifollicular in an otherwise hyperplastic lymph node; some cases can mimic classic Hodgkin lymphoma or, out of context, systemic ALK-negative ALCL {1183}.

Immunophenotype

The immunophenotype is similar to ALK-negative ALCL with uniform strong expression of CD30. CD3, CD5, and CD7 are usually negative or only focally positive. The neoplastic cells commonly express CD4, CD43, CD25, IRF4 (MUM1), and GATA3, as well as cytotoxic markers (TIA1, granzyme B, and/or perforin). Approximately 20% of cases express surface T-cell receptor (either TCRαβ or TCRγδ) {3325}. Rare CD8+ or CD4/CD8 double-negative cases have been described {3325,946}. EBV-encoded small RNA (EBER), LMP1, and ALK are negative. The immunophenotype may be determined by flow cytometry but may be limited by the cell fragility and limited volume for testing {946}.

Differential diagnosis

Systemic ALCL involving the breast does not localize to the capsule {3325}. Diffuse large B-cell lymphoma, extranodal marginal zone lymphoma, and extranodal NK/T-cell lymphoma in women with breast implants have been described with a similar anatomical distribution to that of BIA-ALCL {3765A,1097}. Rare cases of EBV-positive fibrin-associated large B-cell lymphomas have been described around breast implants {2625,3443, 2666}. These may be misdiagnosed as BIA-ALCL, underpinning the importance of complete workup of suspected cases of BIA-ALCL, including the demonstration of T-cell features using immunohistochemistry and/or molecular TR gene rearrangement analysis. High-grade carcinomas such as those with medullary and pleomorphic patterns can be excluded through relevant immunohistochemical stains for epithelial markers.

Cytology

The primary diagnosis of BIA-ALCL is most often made on cytological aspirates of seroma fluid. The lymphoma cells show abundant, often vacuolated, basophilic cytoplasm and cytoplasmic blebs and large pleomorphic, oval, or lobated nuclei with

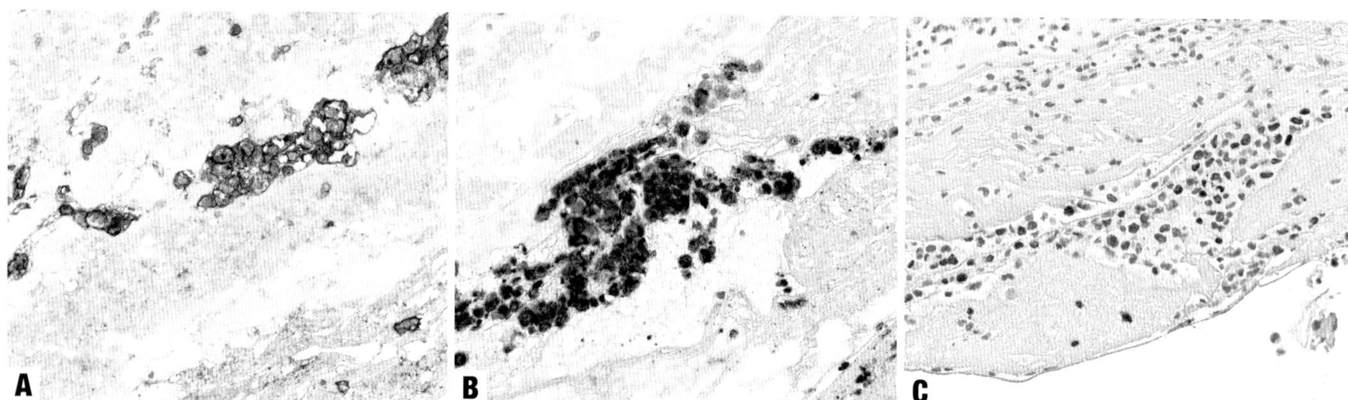

Fig. 5.126 Breast implant–associated anaplastic large cell lymphoma: immunohistochemistry. The tumour cells are positive for CD4 (**A**) and granzyme B (**B**). There is strong expression of phosphorylated STAT3 (**C**), consistent with constitutive activation of the JAK/STAT pathway.

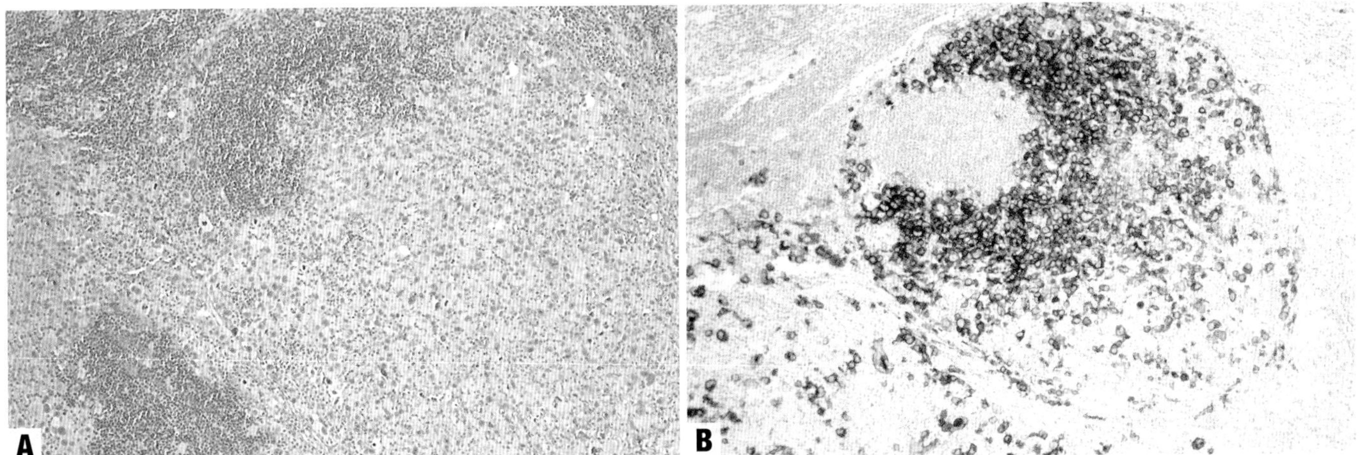

Fig. 5.127 Breast implant–associated anaplastic large cell lymphoma involving an axillary lymph node. **A** A remnant lymphoid follicle is partially surrounded by numerous large neoplastic cells in an axillary lymph node removed from a patient suspected of having breast implant–associated anaplastic large cell lymphoma. **B** Lymphoma cells positive for CD30 surround a lymphoid follicle, which is partially obliterated.

prominent nucleoli. Atypical mitotic figures can be observed. The background commonly shows necrosis and karyorrhexis. Cell block material can be used for both immunohistochemistry and molecular analyses {946,237}.

Diagnostic molecular pathology

Clonal TR gene rearrangement can be demonstrated in > 80% of cases. BIA-ALCL is consistently negative for gene rearrangements involving *ALK*, *DUSP22*, and *TP63* {2233,3025}.

Essential and desirable diagnostic criteria

Essential: a lymphoma restricted to the seroma surrounding a breast implant, or a tumour in association with a breast implant; large pleomorphic cells with lobated nuclei and distinct nucleoli; uniform strong expression of CD30; proven T-cell lineage, supported by the expression of one or more T-lineage markers and/or clonal TR (TCR) gene rearrangement.

Desirable: absence of ALK protein expression or *ALK* rearrangement; identification of lymphoma cells on the luminal side of the capsule on properly oriented sections.

Staging

The pathological T staging is as follows: T1 (tumour in fluid or confined to the inner surface of the capsule), T2 (superficial infiltration of the capsule), T3 (deep infiltration of the capsule by lymphoma cells admixed with inflammatory cells), and T4 (extension beyond the limits of the capsule into the soft tissue or into the breast parenchyma) {3325,760}. A disease-specific modification of the TNM system has been developed {760}. Clinical stage IIB, III, and IV disease includes regional lymph node involvement (N1) and distant lymph node involvement and disseminated disease (M1).

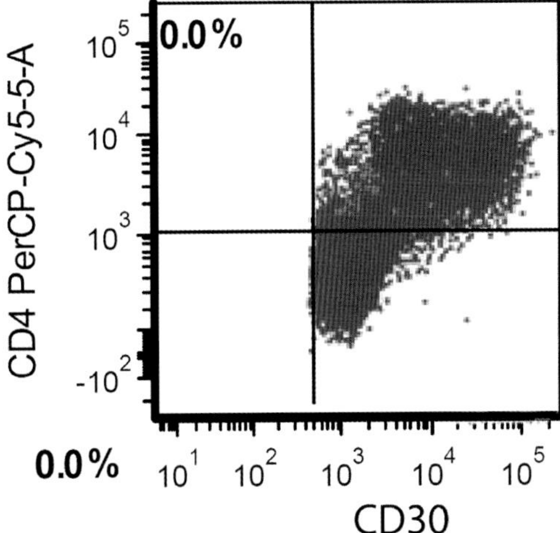

Fig. 5.128 Breast implant–associated anaplastic large cell lymphoma. Flow cytometry demonstrates that most cells coexpress CD4 and CD30 in a peri-implant effusion.

Prognosis and prediction

Most cases have an excellent outcome. Surgery is the cornerstone of therapy, with complete excision of the capsule and implant resulting in a 5-year overall survival rate of almost 100% in patients with effusion only {2690A,760}. The 5-year overall survival rate is 83.7% for patients with disease beyond the capsule and 75% for patients with lymph node involvement {1183}. The most important adverse prognostic factor is the presence of advanced disease with a non-resectable mass (T4) and disseminated disease (N1, M1); in these cases, systemic (immuno) chemotherapy as used for systemic nodal T-cell lymphomas is indicated.

Nodal T follicular helper cell lymphoma: Introduction

Attygalle AD
Alaggio R
Du MQ

Nodal T follicular helper (TFH) cell lymphomas (nTFHLs) represent a group of mature T-cell neoplasms with the phenotypic features and gene expression signature of TFH cells, a subset of effector T helper cells that reside predominantly in secondary lymphoid follicles and are essential for germinal centre formation, affinity maturation, and the development of high-affinity antibodies and memory B cells {451,1996}.

Although histopathological features define the individual entities within this group, there is considerable morphological overlap and interobserver variability. Characteristic histological features might not be sampled in core biopsies, and morphological plasticity at diagnosis and relapse is well recognized {1669}. The clinical and immunophenotypic overlap of the related entities {1669,972}, as well as similarities in their TFH gene signatures and mutation profiles, supported their unification into one group of related entities in the previous edition of the WHO classification of haematolymphoid tumours {972}. In the present edition, this concept has been propagated into the hierarchical design of the classification as a novel family/class of nTFHL and corresponding novel nomenclature, which is a step closer to their further unification as subtypes of a single entity.

nTFHL, angioimmunoblastic type, previously designated "angioimmunoblastic T-cell lymphoma", is the prototype, with a well-defined morphological, immunophenotypic, and mutation profile. In contrast, nTFHL, follicular type, and nTFHL-NOS, previously designated "follicular T-cell lymphoma" and "nodal peripheral T-cell lymphoma with TFH phenotype", respectively, represent less well studied nodal lymphomas that also express TFH molecules. The neoplastic T cells exhibit a spectrum of TFH-associated immunophenotypic markers, such as PD1, ICOS, CXCL13, CD10, BCL6, CXCR5, SAP, MAF, and CD200 {3534, 518, 2996, 899, 993, 2530, 1420, 173, 3456, 994, 2846, 3387}, with the first five being more commonly available in the diagnostic setting {261}. nTFHL-NOS – a diagnosis of exclusion, especially in relation to nTFHL, angioimmunoblastic type – often expresses only PD1 and ICOS, the less specific

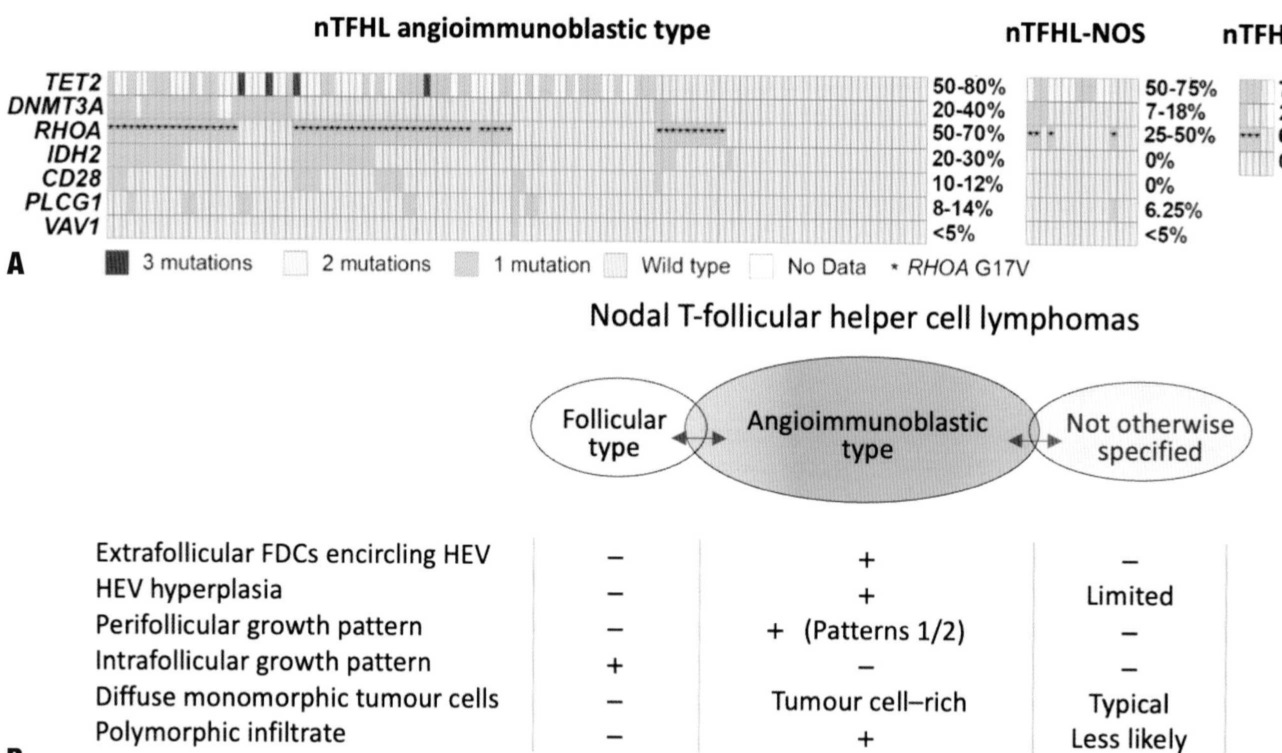

	Follicular type	Angioimmunoblastic type	Not otherwise specified
Extrafollicular FDCs encircling HEV	–	+	–
HEV hyperplasia	–	+	Limited
Perifollicular growth pattern	–	+ (Patterns 1/2)	–
Intrafollicular growth pattern	+	–	–
Diffuse monomorphic tumour cells	–	Tumour cell–rich	Typical
Polymorphic infiltrate	–	+	Less likely

Fig. 5.129 Comparison of mutation and morphology among nodal T follicular helper cell lymphoma entities. **A** Recurrent mutations in nodal T follicular helper cell lymphomas (nTFHLs). The heat-map data of nTFHL, angioimmunoblastic type, and nTFHL-NOS are from the Iqbal laboratory (nTFHL sequencing project), and the mutation frequencies are summarized from previous studies {518,4285,4141,3448,1543,4487}. The heat-map data and mutation frequencies of nTFHL, follicular type (nTFHL-F), are based on a previous study {972}. **B** The diagram represents the three entities within the umbrella group of nTFHLs and highlights the morphological overlap and plasticity between these lymphomas. Discriminatory histological features are tabulated. FDC, follicular dendritic cell; HEV, high endothelial venule.

TFH markers. Further studies may determine whether the current defining criterion of positivity for two TFH markers in addition to CD4 is sufficiently robust in excluding peripheral T-cell lymphoma NOS.

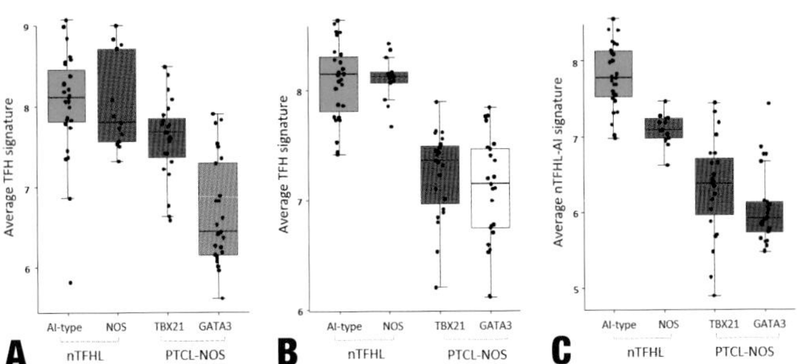

Fig. 5.130 Enriched expression of T follicular helper (TFH) cell–associated genes in nodal TFH cell lymphoma (nTFHL). Mean mRNA expression of pan-TFH genes (*CXCL13*, *MME* [*CD10*], *BCL6*, *CCR5*, *PDCD1*, *SH2D1A*) (**A**), median expression of TFH-associated genes {972} (**B**), and angioimmunoblastic-type (AI-type) diagnostic signature (**C**) in nTFHL entities and peripheral T-cell lymphoma (PTCL) molecular subtypes {1735,1736}.

An integrated approach to diagnosis is essential and requires the correlation of clinical, morphological, and immunophenotypic features, together with the integration of clonality and/or gene mutation profiles, especially when the morphology is not typical. Recommendations for reporting are listed in Box 5.06.

Box 5.06 Recommendations for reporting nodal T follicular helper cell lymphomas (nTFHLs)

- nTFHL-AI may be diagnosed on core or excision biopsies, provided the diagnostic criteria are fulfilled
- nTFHL-F often overlaps with nTFHL-AI, and its diagnosis is best based on excision biopsies
- nTFHL-NOS is a diagnosis of exclusion that should be based on excision biopsies only
- Use of the generic term "nTFHL", rather than nTFHL-NOS or nTFHL-F, is recommended when the diagnosis is based on core biopsies, to prevent misclassification due to insufficient sampling
- In the event of a change in morphology from one type to another across multiple biopsies or at relapse, the following comment is recommended: "This is consistent with a morphological variation of the patient's original nTFHL"

nTFHL-AI, nodal T follicular helper cell lymphoma, angioimmunoblastic type; nTFHL-F, nodal T follicular helper cell lymphoma, follicular type.

Nodal T follicular helper cell lymphoma, angioimmunoblastic type

Attygalle AD
Amador C
Du MQ
Iqbal J
Sakata-Yanagimoto M
Sewell WA
Tournilhac O

Definition

Nodal T follicular helper (TFH) cell lymphoma, angioimmunoblastic type (nTFHL-AI), is a neoplasm of mature T cells with a TFH phenotype, characterized by systemic disease and a polymorphous lymphoid infiltrate involving lymph nodes, accompanied by a prominent proliferation of high endothelial venules (HEVs) and follicular dendritic cells (FDCs).

ICD-O coding

9705/3 Nodal T follicular helper cell lymphoma, angioimmunoblastic type

ICD-11 coding

2A90.9 Angioimmunoblastic T-cell lymphoma

Related terminology

Acceptable: angioimmunoblastic T-cell lymphoma; follicular helper T-cell lymphoma, angioimmunoblastic type.

Not recommended: peripheral T-cell lymphoma; angioimmunoblastic lymphadenopathy with dysproteinaemia; immunoblastic lymphadenopathy; lymphogranulomatosis X.

Subtype(s)

None

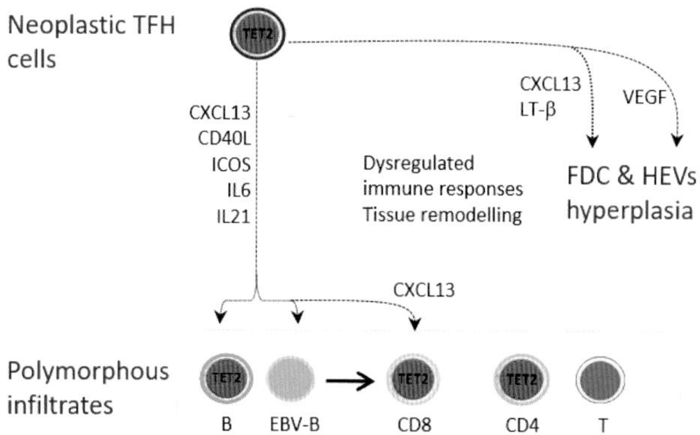

Fig. 5.131 Nodal T follicular helper (TFH) cell lymphoma (nTFHL), angioimmunoblastic type. Proposed pathogenesis. The neoplastic transformation of TFH cells and their clonal expansion are largely driven by oncogenic cooperation between mutations in DNA methylation regulators (*TET2*, *DNMT3A*, *IDH2*) and those involved in T-cell receptor signalling (*RHOA*, *VAV1*, *PLCG1*). The perturbed transcriptional programme in non-neoplastic B and T cells by *TET2* and *DNMT3A* mutations may dysregulate their immune responses. These are likely to be further exacerbated by exaggerated help from the neoplastic TFH cells and by EBV infection, together provoking prominent polymorphous infiltrates and remodelling the follicular dendritic cell (FDC) and high endothelial venule (HEV) meshworks seen in nTFHL, angioimmunoblastic type. *DNMT3A* mutation may frequently associate with *TET2* changes (not shown).

Localization

Most patients with nTFHL-AI present with generalized lymphadenopathy {2189,2816}. The spleen, liver, skin, and bone marrow are frequently involved. Leukaemic presentation is rare, but neoplastic T cells may be detected in the peripheral blood by flow cytometry.

Clinical features

Most patients present with constitutional B symptoms, advanced-stage disease, and variable but frequently generalized peripheral lymphadenopathy. Hepatosplenomegaly is frequent, and bone marrow involvement is observed in about 70% of cases {2816}. A pruritic maculopapular rash is common, whereas skin nodules with or without ulceration are infrequent. Other clinical findings include ascites, pleural effusions, and arthritis. Laboratory abnormalities that suggest immune dysregulation, including autoimmune haemolytic anaemia related to warm antibodies or cold agglutinins, thrombocytopenia, positive rheumatoid factor, cryoglobulinaemia, and anti–smooth muscle antibodies, are characteristic, albeit not universal. Although polyclonal hypergammaglobulinaemia is common, a monoclonal spike or hypogammaglobulinaemia may also occur. Leukocytosis is usually neutrophilic. The peripheral blood may show eosinophilia, lymphopenia, circulating atypical lymphoid cells, and circulating plasma cells {2189}.

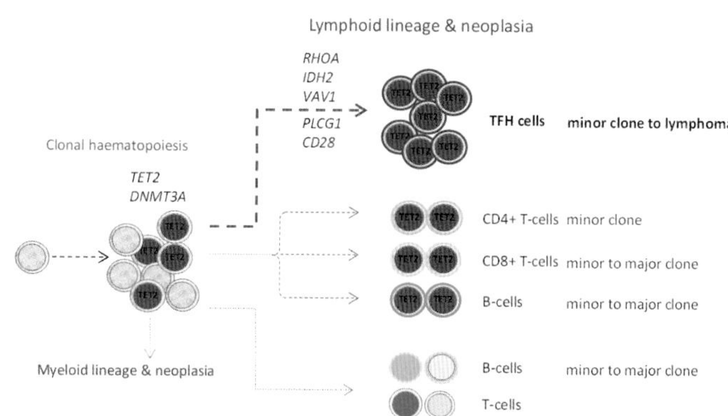

Fig. 5.132 Stepwise acquisition of genetic changes in the development of nodal T follicular helper (TFH) cell lymphoma (nTFHL), angioimmunoblastic type. *TET2* and *DNMT3A* mutations occur early in haematopoietic stem cells, and these mutations perturb transcription programmes and enhance stem cell renewal, resulting in clonal haematopoiesis. The mutated stem cells can differentiate into multiple lineage progenies, resulting in the presence of these early mutations in their progenies, including the neoplastic TFH-cell clone and a high proportion of non-neoplastic T and B cells. Further mutations in *RHOA* and others (as indicated) probably occur in committed CD4+ cells, driving TFH differentiation, malignant transformation, and clonal expansion, and are thus lymphoma-specific. In addition to the malignant TFH-cell clone, there are frequent variable minor, occasionally predominant, T-cell and B-cell clones in lymph nodes from patients with nTFHL, angioimmunoblastic type, which may harbour *TET2* mutations. *DNMT3A* mutation may frequently associate with *TET2* changes (not shown).

Epidemiology

nTFHL-AI is a disease of middle-aged and elderly individuals, and it has a slight male predilection. nTFHL-AI is the commonest type of node-based peripheral T-cell lymphoma, even considering the major variations in relative frequencies of mature T-cell and NK-cell lymphoma types in different geographical regions (e.g. Asia and Latin America versus the USA and Europe). nTFHL-AI generally accounts for 36% of the non-cutaneous T-cell lymphomas {4257,898,1067,3214}.

Etiology

Unknown

Pathogenesis

nTFHL-AI probably originates from TFH cells, because the lymphoma cells bear the characteristic TFH gene expression signature {899,1735}. The lymphomagenesis is largely driven by stepwise acquisition of somatic genetic changes, with *TET2* and *DNMT3A* mutations occurring early in haematopoietic stem cells. TET2, an α-ketoglutarate–dependent dioxygenase, oxidizes 5-methylcytosine successively to 5-carboxycytosine, promoting cytosine demethylation, while DNMT3A, a DNA methyltransferase, catalyses the production of 5-methylcytosine in CpG dinucleotides. *TET2* and *DNMT3A* mutations are loss-of-function changes, causing dysregulated DNA methylation, hence perturbing transcription programmes in the affected haematopoietic stem cells and their progenies, including B cells and CD4+ and CD8+ T cells {2066,3301}. The perturbed gene expression may promote stem cell renewal (clonal haematopoiesis), potentially favour TFH-cell differentiation, and dysregulate B- and T-cell interactions in peripheral lymphoid tissues, particularly in the presence of further genetic changes and immunological stimulations {3301}.

Other genetic changes identified in nTFHL-AI are confined to the lymphoma cells. *RHOA* mutation is seen in about 70% of nTFHL-AI cases {3534,3115,4504} and in about the same percentage of nTFHL-NOS {3534,4141,4327} and nTFHL, follicular type {2703,972}, but it is rarely present in PTCL-NOS {4327, 2996}. The p.G17V (NP_001655.1) is the most common mutated variant. *RHOA* encodes a small GTPase, and the mutation enables RhoA to interact with VAV1, an adaptor molecule downstream of T-cell receptor (TCR) signalling {1303}, and enhance

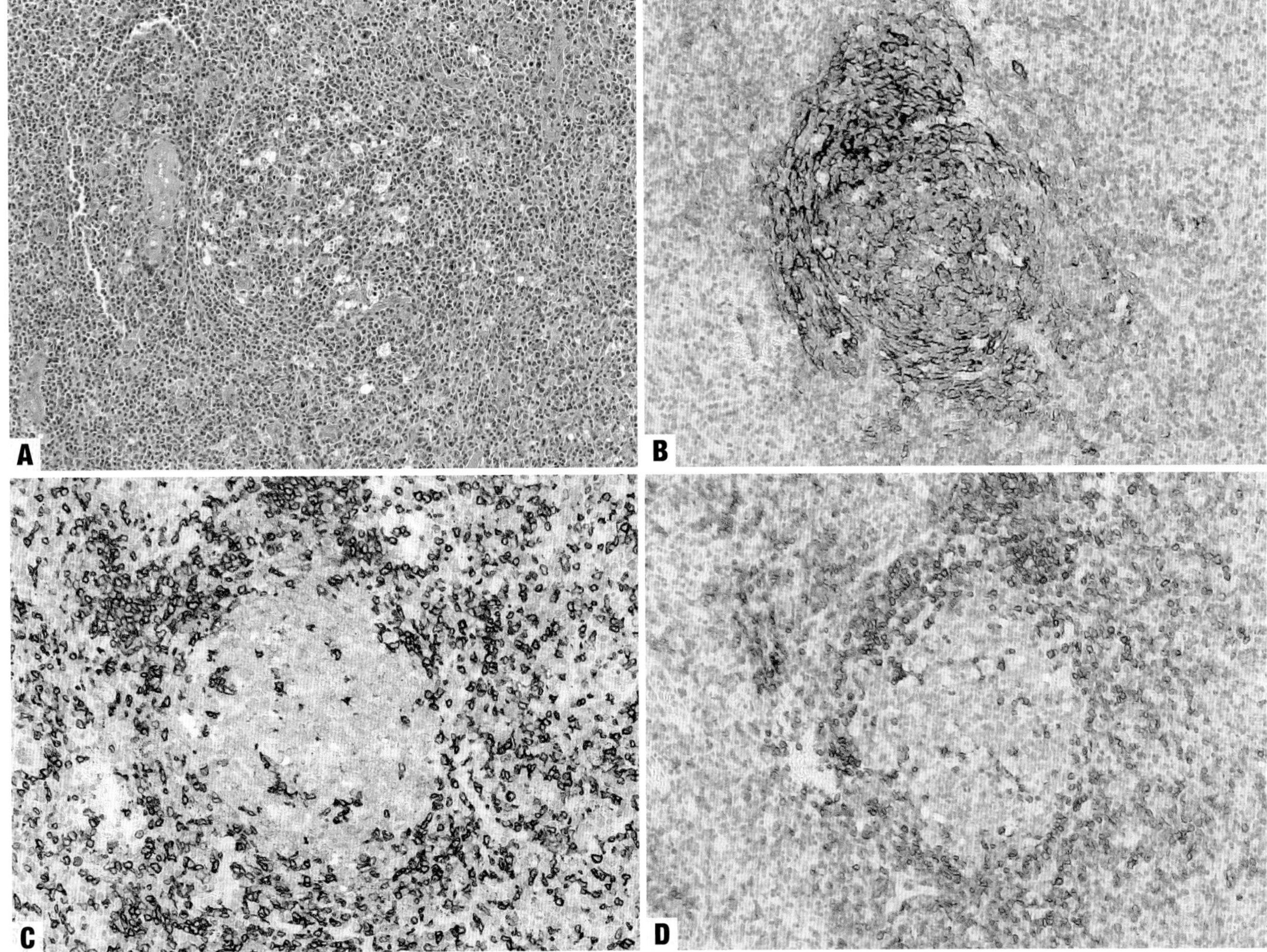

Fig. 5.133 Nodal T follicular helper cell lymphoma, angioimmunoblastic type, partial nodal involvement (pattern 1). **A** Large bare hyperplastic follicle. **B** CD21 immunostain highlights the lack of extrafollicular hyperplasia of follicular dendritic cells. **C** Strong CD10-positive neoplastic T cells spilling out from the outer rim of the hyperplastic follicle centre, in contrast to very weak CD10 in germinal-centre B cells. **D** PD1 immunostain highlights neoplastic T cells surrounding the hyperplastic follicle centre.

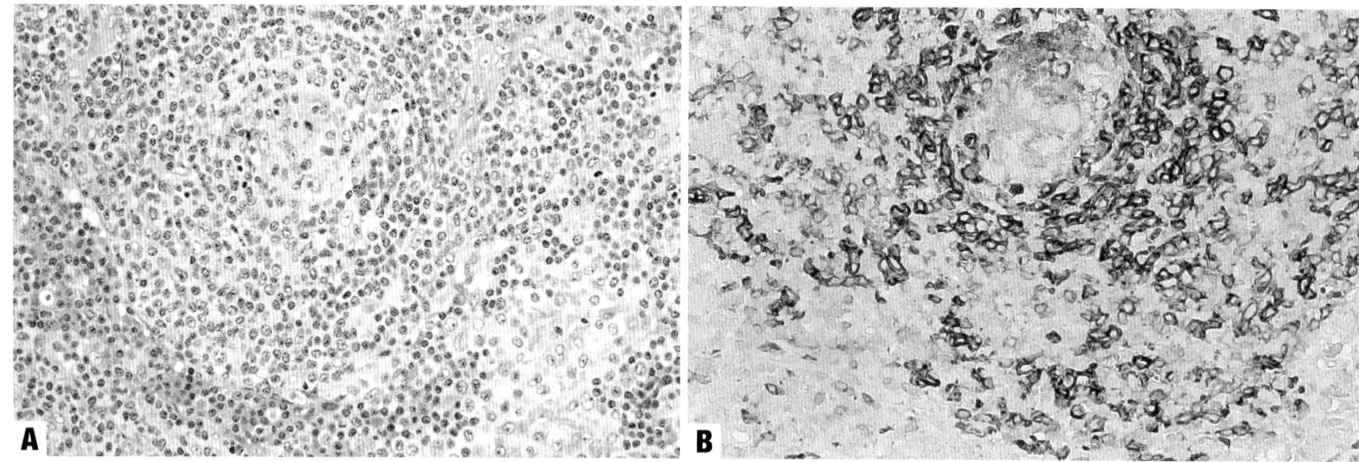

Fig. 5.134 Nodal T follicular helper cell lymphoma, angioimmunoblastic type (pattern 2). **A** An atretic follicle surrounded by clustered pale atypical lymphoid cells. **B** PD1 immunostain highlights perifollicular neoplastic T cells.

its function in signalling transduction {1258,2951,4}. Stronger TCR signalling conferred by the *RHOA* mutation in naïve CD4+ T cells may drive their preferential TFH differentiation and neoplastic transformation, together with perturbed gene expression (e.g. enhanced *BCL6* expression), by *TET2* and *DNMT3A* inactivation {2857,2970,813}.

IDH2 mutations are primarily seen in nTFHL-AI but rarely in nTFHL-NOS and nTFHL, follicular type, and they invariably affect p.R172, often concurrently with both *TET2* and *RHOA* mutations. *IDH2* encodes an isocitrate dehydrogenase, and the mutant IDH2 gains a neofunction, catalysing the production of 2-hydroxyglutarate, an oncometabolite that inhibits α-ketoglutarate–dependent dioxygenase {2272}. *IDH2* mutation defines a unique subset of nTFHL-AI cases, which are characterized molecularly by pronounced genome-wide promoter hypermethylation and enhanced expression of TFH genes, and histologically by medium-sized to large clear cells {4285,1543,3832}.

Furthermore, there are several other genetic changes that enhance TCR and costimulatory signalling. These include mutations in *VAV1*, *PLCG1*, and *FYN* downstream of TCR signalling {4141,1258,4,1543}, and gain-of-function alterations in *CD28* (mutation, *CTLA4*::*CD28*, *ICOS*::*CD28*) {4141,2262,4503,3448}, with *CD28* mutations conferring a poor prognosis {3448}. These genetic changes are infrequent and often concurrent with *RHOA*, *TET2*, and *DNMT3A* mutations, probably cooperating in their oncogenic activities. Nonetheless, these genetic changes can also be observed in PTCL-NOS and other T-cell lymphomas {4327,1543,705,383}.

Because the neoplastic cells bear TFH functionality, they may exert diverse immunological effects on non-neoplastic B and T cells, particularly in the presence of active immune responses {842}. The spatial expansion of neoplastic TFH cells may enable them to stimulate B cells and CD8+ T cells beyond the follicle centre, with dysregulated interactions due to their perturbed transcription programmes by *TET2* and *DNMT3A* mutations. Together, the exaggerated TFH function and dysregulated immune responses may provoke prominent polymorphous infiltrates, may remodel the FDC and HEV networks, and may even promote secondary clonal B- and T-cell proliferations {177,4487}.

Macroscopic appearance

Not relevant

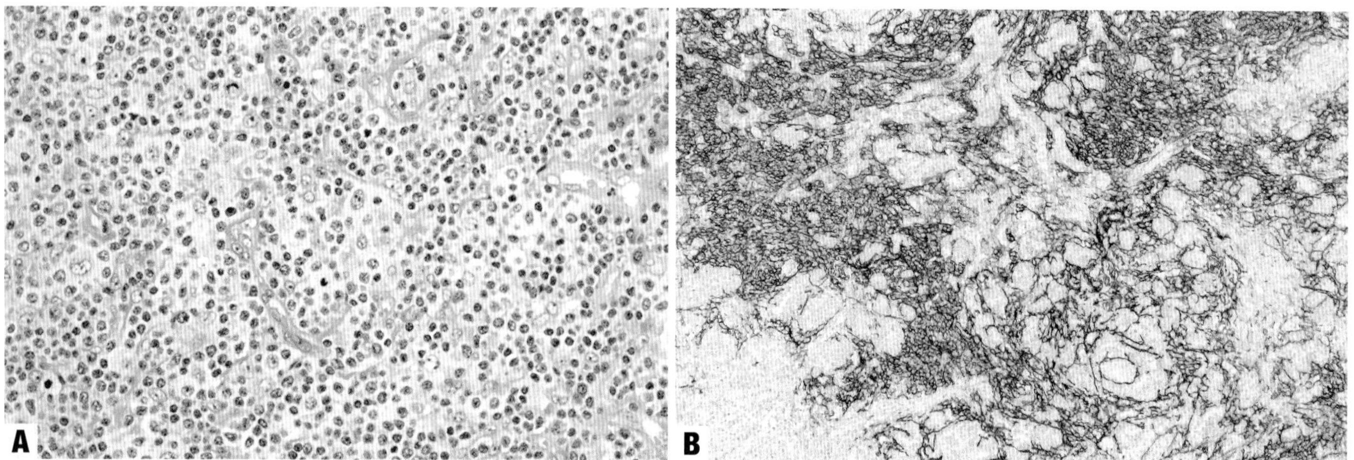

Fig. 5.135 Nodal T follicular helper cell lymphoma, angioimmunoblastic type, typical diffuse morphology (pattern 3). **A** The nodal architecture is effaced by a polymorphous infiltrate with clusters of medium-sized atypical pale to clear cells in the vicinity of hyperplastic marked high endothelial venules. **B** Florid CD21-positive hyperplastic follicular dendritic cell meshworks encircling high endothelial venules.

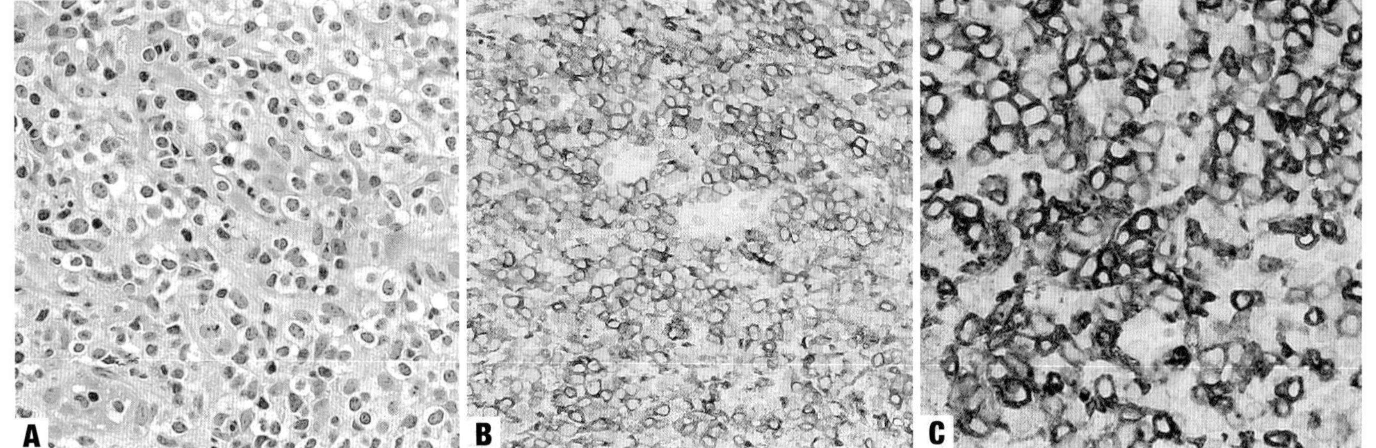

Fig. 5.136 Nodal T follicular helper cell lymphoma, angioimmunoblastic type, harbouring *IDH2* p.R172 mutation. **A** Clusters of characteristic atypical clear cells with distinct cell membranes amid hyperplastic high endothelial venules. **B** Neoplastic T cells are immunoreactive for PD1. **C** Characteristic strong CD10.

Histopathology

nTFHL-AI is characterized by partial or complete effacement of the lymph node architecture by a polymorphous infiltrate with frequent perinodal extension, with sparing of the peripheral cortical sinuses. The neoplastic T cells are often in the minority and frequently obscured by variable numbers of reactive small lymphocytes, immunoblasts, plasma cells, histiocytes, and eosinophils, and are better identified as clusters in the vicinity of hyperplastic and arborizing HEVs {173}. Neoplastic T cells are mostly small to medium-sized, with pale to clear cytoplasm and mild nuclear atypia. Conspicuous medium-sized to large clear cells with distinct cell membranes are a feature that appears to be specific to*IDH2* p.R172–mutant nTFHL-AI {3832}. Frequently, the presence of marked HEV proliferation with plump endothelial cells and hyalinized basement membranes, as well as expanded FDC meshworks, confers an eosinophilic appearance {978,3631}. Variable numbers of B immunoblasts, which may be positive or negative for EBV, are usually present in the paracortex. In some cases, prominent clusters of epithelioid histiocytes may mimic a reactive granulomatous process or the lymphoepithelioid variant of PTCL-NOS {1513}.

Three overlapping morphological patterns of nodal involvement have been described {173,174,3439}:

Pattern 1 mimics reactive follicular hyperplasia; it is characterized by partial lymph node involvement by hyperplastic follicles with large reactive follicle centres and often poorly defined mantle zones. Neoplastic T cells are inconspicuous. Immunohistochemistry is often needed to highlight the perifollicular distribution of the neoplastic T cells, which spill out from the rim of the follicle centre into the perifollicular area {174,3439}. The paracortex contains hyperplastic HEVs and a polymorphous infiltrate largely devoid of neoplastic cells.

Pattern 2 is characterized by a prominent perifollicular neoplastic T-cell infiltrate that effaces the normal nodal architecture except for a few residual atretic follicles.

Pattern 3 is characterized by the effacement of the nodal architecture with no identifiable follicular structures.

Overlapping patterns are often encountered in the same node and may vary in consecutive biopsies, not only at relapse but also in biopsies performed within weeks of one another {179,175}. Patterns 2 and 3 are encountered most frequently, but pattern 1 is usually observed in partially involved nodes of patients with otherwise disseminated disease that may be associated with typical immune manifestations {174}.

Tumour cell–rich nTFHL-AI is characterized by a monomorphic appearance, with abundant neoplastic T cells and a diminished inflammatory background. This morphology may be seen at relapse in cases where typical features of nTFHL-AI were present at diagnosis, suggesting histological progression {174}. FDC expansion, demonstrated by immunohistochemistry, is the only tenuous feature that discriminates tumour cell–rich nTFHL-AI from nTFHL-NOS {972,174}. A small number of nTFHLs harbouring *IDH2* p.R172, a mutation regarded as specific to nTFHL-AI, lack FDC proliferation despite showing HEV hyperplasia and diffuse infiltration of clear cells with strong TFH marker expression, further illustrating the biological continuum between these two entities {3832}.

nTFHL-AI often contains B-cell proliferations, commonly comprising variable numbers of immunoblasts and plasma cells. The immunoblastic proliferation may progress as secondary EBV-positive or (less frequently) EBV-negative diffuse large B-cell lymphoma {179,4550}. Rarely, clonal B-cell proliferations in the form of small lymphocytes and plasma cells may resemble nodal or extranodal marginal zone lymphoma {177,1848}. Plasma cells may also be abundant, in rare cases obscuring the neoplastic T cells. The plasma cells are mostly polyclonal, but they may be monoclonal {1689}. HRS-like cells may be encountered, mimicking classic Hodgkin lymphoma {174,2955}. These are not regarded as composite lymphomas, because there is no clear demarcation between the areas containing HRS-like cells and the more typical areas of nTFHL-AI.

The skin and bone marrow are the most frequently biopsied extranodal sites, but primary diagnosis is best made on an involved lymph node. Except when paratrabecular, marrow involvement may be difficult to differentiate from reactive lymphoid infiltrates, and interpretation is further hampered by secondary reactive marrow changes {176,1424,727}.

Immunophenotype

The neoplastic T cells are often positive for the pan–T-cell antigens CD2, CD3, and CD5, with variable loss of CD7 {2816}. Flow cytometry may reveal dim sCD3 expression {2399}.

The tumour cells are nearly always CD4-positive and CD8-negative {2816}. A characteristic feature is the expression of the TFH markers PD1 (CD279), ICOS, BCL6, CXCL13, and CD10, with varying levels of sensitivity (PD1 and ICOS being more sensitive than CD10 and CXCL13) and specificity (CD10 and CXCL13 being more specific than PD1 and ICOS). Strong PD1 staining is more specific. Only strong BCL6 expression is useful, because it is more specific, but sensitivity is low. Most cases express at least two TFH markers {261,2521,174}. In IDH2 p.R172–mutant cases, the neoplastic cells are often strongly positive for CD10 and CXCL13, and they can be highlighted by IDH2 immunohistochemistry when involving p.R172K {3832,1028}. The majority of nTFHL-AI cases harbouring *RHOA* p.G17V (NP_001655.1) express at least three TFH markers {3066}. Detection of an abnormal CD4/CD10+ or CD4 / bright PD1+ T-cell population by flow cytometry performed on tissue, bone marrow aspirate, or peripheral blood samples may help diagnosis {2399,4458}.

The TFH phenotype may be used to identify extranodal involvement. In the staging of bone marrow biopsies, strong PD1 expression is more specific for nTFHL-AI {1977}. For subtle infiltrates, immunohistochemistry is of limited value, but flow cytometry may help {2399}. The neoplastic TFH cells are EBV-negative, although very rare cases of EBV-positive nTFHL have been described {676,4575}.

Immunostains for CD21, CD23, or CD35 highlight the characteristic extrafollicular FDC proliferation that encircles HEVs. CD21 is usually the most reliable, but CD23 is more informative in occasional cases {174,4079}. Although a defining criterion, the FDC expansion may be subtle in pattern 1 (and occasionally in pattern 2) nTFHL-AI {173}.

B immunoblasts are highlighted by CD20, often with a range of staining intensities. EBV-positive B cells detected by in situ hybridization for EBV-encoded small RNA (EBER) are present in 66–81% of cases {898,175,4035}. Like the immunoblastic proliferations, the plasma cell expansions may be polytypic or monotypic, but unlike large B-cell proliferations, they are more often EBV-negative {174,4550,1689}.

The HRS-like cells often express CD30 and are variably positive for CD15 and EBV. Although the B-cell programme is often retained in these cells in most cases, some may have a phenotype more similar to that of classic Hodgkin lymphoma {174, 2955}. These HRS-like cells are usually rosetted by neoplastic TFH cells and are often accompanied by typical B immunoblasts. In addition to immunoblasts, CD30 may also be seen in a proportion of the neoplastic T cells {3062}. IgD-positive small B cells may reside as follicular aggregates {174}.

There are variable numbers of background reactive T cells, which at times can be very prominent. Although these are often a mixture of CD4-positive and CD8-positive subsets {3301}, occasionally cytotoxic T cells predominate. Clonal expansions of CD8-positive cytotoxic small to medium-sized T cells may obscure the underlying nTFHL-AI {177}.

Differential diagnosis

There are a wide range of differential diagnoses and potential misdiagnoses, including reactive follicular/paracortical

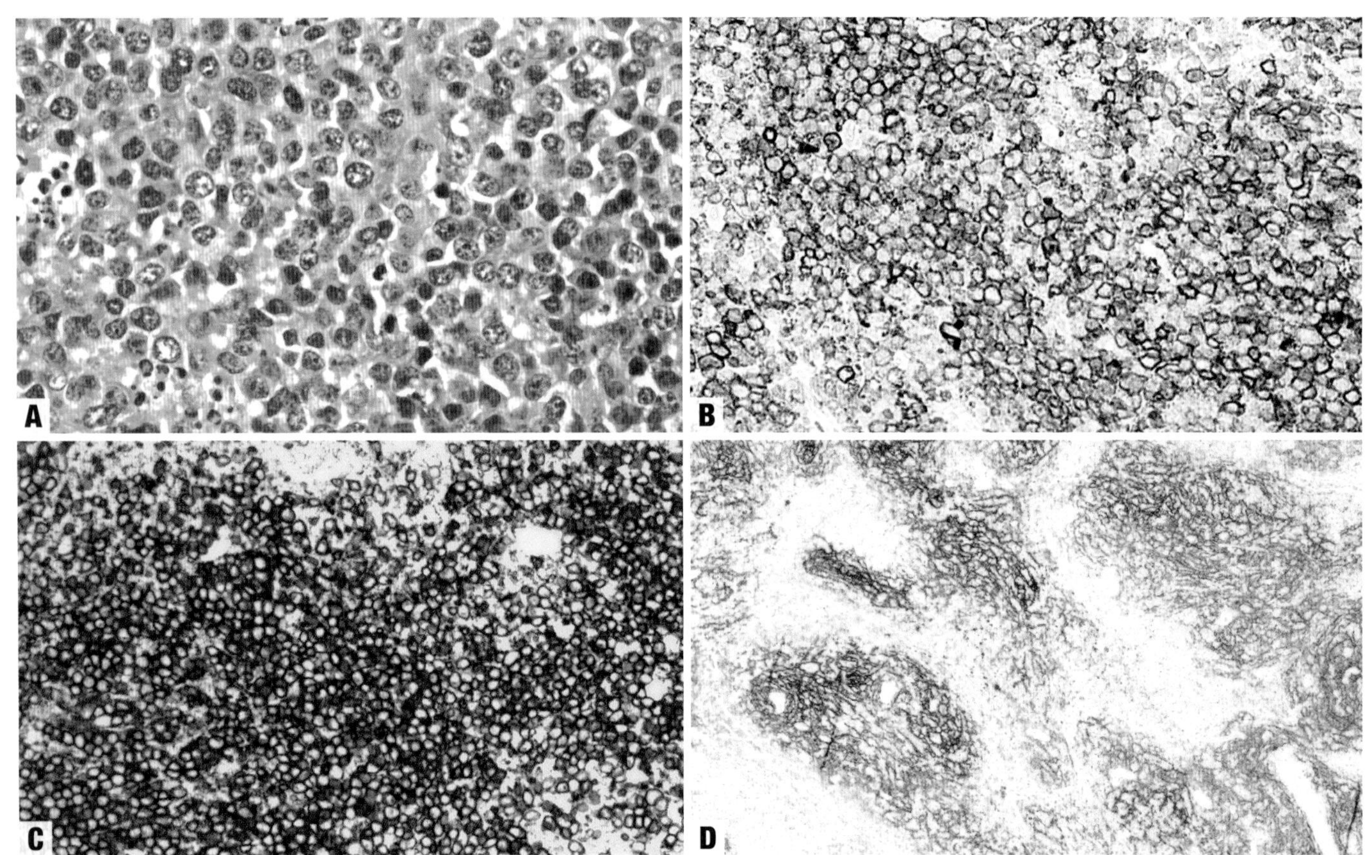

Fig. 5.137 Nodal T follicular helper cell lymphoma, angioimmunoblastic type, tumour cell–rich. **A** Monomorphic infiltrate of atypical lymphoid cells. **B,C** Neoplastic cells are strongly positive for PD1 (**B**) and for ICOS (**C**). **D** CD21-positive hyperplastic follicular dendritic meshworks.

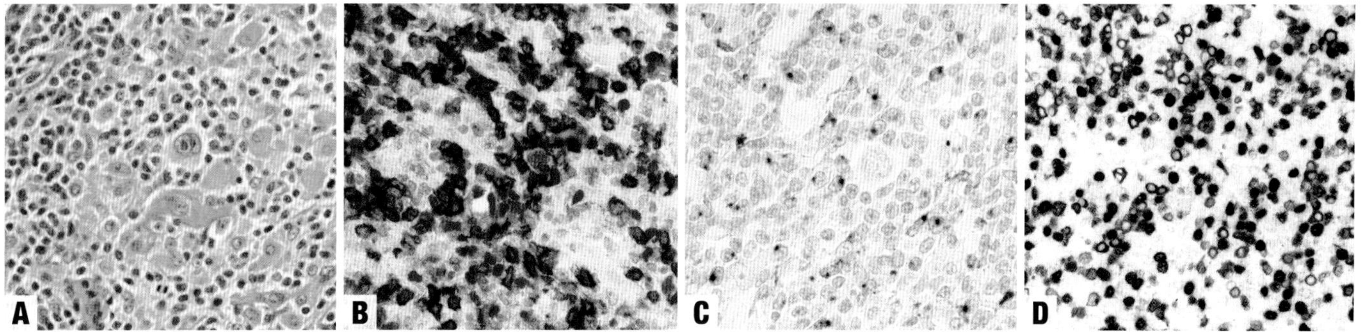

Fig. 5.138 Nodal T follicular helper cell lymphoma, angioimmunoblastic type. **A** An HRS-like cell ringed by medium-sized lymphoid cells. **B** CD10/PAX5 double immunostain highlights CD10-positive (brown, membranous) neoplastic T cells ringing a PAX5-positive (red, nuclear) HRS-like cell. **C** CXCL13 (cytoplasmic staining with paranuclear enhancement) is expressed by a proportion of neoplastic T cells including a few surrounding the HRS-like cell. **D** Double CD79a immunostain (brown, cytoplasmic) and in situ hybridization for EBV-encoded small RNA (EBER) (blue, nuclear) highlights EBV-positive and EBV-negative B immunoblasts.

hyperplasia, PTCL-NOS and its morphological variant lymphoepithelioid lymphoma, and (rarely) other mature T-cell neoplasms. In cases with secondary B-cell proliferations, differential diagnoses include polymorphic lymphoproliferative disorder (arising in immune deficiency and dysregulation), large B-cell lymphoma, plasmacytoma, marginal zone lymphoma, and classic Hodgkin lymphoma (see Table 5.19).

Cytology

FNA samples may be used for flow cytometry and diagnostic molecular investigations. Although FNA biopsies may yield cellular smears comprising a polymorphous infiltrate that reflects the cellular composition and architectural features of nTFHL-AI detected in lymph node tissue biopsies {2948}, an accurate diagnosis relies heavily on immunoarchitectural features with many potential pitfalls. Therefore, a diagnosis of nTFHL-AI based solely on FNA cytology is not recommended and should be confirmed by tissue biopsy.

Diagnostic molecular pathology

Demonstration of clonal TR gene rearrangement is useful when histopathological features are suspicious but not diagnostic. However, the clonally rearranged TR genes may not be detectable when the neoplastic cell content is low {974,1538}. Where

Table 5.19 Differential diagnoses for nodal T follicular helper (TFH) cell lymphoma, angioimmunoblastic type (nTFHL-AI) (continued on next page)

nTFHL-AI features	Mimics	Key features for differential diagnosis[a]
nTFHL-AI (pattern 1)	Reactive follicular hyperplasia Paracortical hyperplasia[b,c]	nTFHL-AI: • TFH cells (PD1+ [strong], CD10+/−) spill over the outer rim of follicle centres to the perifollicular area / paracortex Reactive follicular hyperplasia: • PD1+ TFH cells are within the follicle centres {2131} Paracortical hyperplasia: • Some weak PD1+ cells in paracortex and strong PD1+ TFH cells confined to follicle centres
nTFHL-AI with HRS-like cells	Classic Hodgkin lymphoma[b,c]	nTFHL-AI: • HRS-like cells usually (not always) have a relatively intact B-cell programme and are rosetted by neoplastic T cells with TFH phenotype • Favoured if B immunoblasts are present in addition to HRS cells Classic Hodgkin lymphoma: • Favoured if a mediastinal mass is present • Crippled B-cell programme in HRS cells; CD4+ T-cell rosettes may show weak to moderate (but not strong) PD1 expression and are CD10− {557}
	NLPHL, variant patterns[b,c]	nTFHL-AI: • TFH cells are atypical, medium-sized, often pale/clear, and often CD10+ • Extrafollicular FDCs encircle HEVs • Large B cells range from B immunoblasts to HRS-like cells, variably CD30+ and EBV+ and haphazardly distributed NLPHL: • PD1+ TFH cells may be numerous but normal-appearing and CD10− • May be T-cell/histiocyte–rich and small B cell–depleted, but eosinophils absent/rare • Large atypical neoplastic B cells are typically CD30−, rarely EBV+ • May be diffuse / focally nodular, but FDCs do not encircle HEVs

ATLL, adult T-cell leukaemia/lymphoma; FDC, follicular dendritic cell; HEV, high endothelial venule; IDD, immune deficiency/dysregulation; LPD, lymphoproliferative disorder; MF, mycosis fungoides; MZL, marginal zone lymphoma; NLPHL, nodular lymphocyte-predominant Hodgkin lymphoma; PTCL, peripheral T-cell lymphoma; SS, Sézary syndrome.
[a]An integrated approach is required {174}. [b]The characteristic clinical features, immune manifestations, flow cytometry, and mutation profile of nTFHL-AI are also useful in the differential diagnosis. [c]Detection of clonal TR (TCR) gene rearrangement supports a diagnosis of nTFHL-AI.

Table 5.19 Differential diagnoses for nodal T follicular helper (TFH) cell lymphoma, angioimmunoblastic type (nTFHL-AI) (continued)

nTFHL-AI features	Mimics	Key features for differential diagnosis[a]
nTFHL-AI with secondary clonal B-cell / plasma cell proliferations obscuring nTFHL-AI		
nTFHL-AI with secondary clonal large B-cell proliferations	Large B-cell lymphoma[b,c]	nTFHL-AI: • To be considered if large B cells are EBV+ • Favoured if atypical T cells with TFH phenotype are prominent in background and there is FDC expansion
nTFHL-AI with secondary EBV+ B-cell proliferations	Polymorphic LPD in IDD[b,c]	nTFHL-AI: • Detection of medium-sized, often pale to clear neoplastic T cells with TFH phenotype, which may be obscured by the (EBV+) B-cell proliferation Polymorphic LPD in IDD: • Highly suspicious of or confirmed IDD
nTFHL-AI with secondary clonal plasmacytic and small B-cell proliferations {177}	Prominent reactive TFH cells in nodal or extranodal (especially primary cutaneous) MZL[b,c] Plasmacytoma[b,c]	nTFHL-AI: • FDC hyperplasia encircling HEVs in lymph node Nodal/extranodal MZL • Favoured if disease is localized; disseminated disease does not help differentiate Plasmacytoma: • Aberrant plasma cell phenotype in plasmacytoma (CD19−, CD56+/−, and cyclin D1+/−), different from plasma cells in nTFHL-AI (CD19+, CD56−, and cyclin D1−)
nTFHL-AI with epithelioid granulomata +/− cytotoxic T-cell expansion {177}	PTCL-NOS, lymphoepithelioid morphological variant (Lennert lymphoma)[b]	nTFHL-AI: • Presence of neoplastic T cells with TFH phenotype • Granulomas may mask polymorphic infiltrates and HEV hyperplasia (pitfall) • May occasionally be obscured by clonal cytotoxic T-cell expansions (pitfall) PTCL-NOS, lymphoepithelioid variant: • Inactivated cytotoxic phenotype; lacks TFH phenotype and extrafollicular FDC hyperplasia {1513,2161}
Tumour cell–rich nTFHL-AI	nTFHL-NOS	nTFHL-AI: • TFH phenotype and FDC hyperplasia nTFHL-NOS: • TFH phenotype without FDC hyperplasia
	Lymphomatous ATLL (rare)[b] {1898}	nTFHL-AI: • Neoplastic cells may be CD25+ (focal) or negative • *RHOA* p.G17V mutation in 60–70%, usually associated with *TET2* mutations ATLL: • Mostly geographically restricted • No FDC expansion • Neoplastic cells are usually CD25+ (strong and diffuse), CD10−, and CXCL13− • HTLV-1+ serology • *RHOA* p.G17V mutations are rare, and co-occurrence with *TET2* mutations is very uncommon {1911}
	MF/SS secondarily involved lymph node[b]	MF/SS: • May express a variety of TFH markers (pitfall) {2674} • Cerebriform cytology • Dermatopathic change • *RHOA* mutations may occur, but p.G17V is rare {1911,3137} • Characteristics of the skin rash maybe helpful

ATLL, adult T-cell leukaemia/lymphoma; FDC, follicular dendritic cell; HEV, high endothelial venule; IDD, immune deficiency/dysregulation; LPD, lymphoproliferative disorder; MF, mycosis fungoides; MZL, marginal zone lymphoma; NLPHL, nodular lymphocyte-predominant Hodgkin lymphoma; PTCL, peripheral T-cell lymphoma; SS, Sézary syndrome.
[a]An integrated approach is required {174}. [b]The characteristic clinical features, immune manifestations, flow cytometry, and mutation profile of nTFHL-AI are also useful in the differential diagnosis. [c]Detection of clonal TR (TCR) gene rearrangement supports a diagnosis of nTFHL-AI.

consecutive specimens are available, comparative analyses are required to identify persistent – hence potentially lymphoma-related – TR gene rearrangements, discriminating those from oligoclonal/clonal populations of reactive T cells, which are often variable and minor, albeit occasionally predominant {974, 4487}. Clonal IG gene rearrangement is seen in about 30% of cases, largely due to EBV-infected B cells.

nTFHL-AI harbours a characteristic mutation profile with a subset of frequent changes confined to the lymphoma cells. *RHOA* mutation, mainly p.G17V (NP_001655.1), is seen in about 70% of nTFHL-AI cases. Its detection indicates the presence of the lymphoma clone, but it can be seen in specimens lacking apparent histological evidence of nTFHL-AI {974}. The clinical significance of its detection in premalignant lesions is unclear. *IDH2* mutation, often concurrent with *RHOA* p.G17V (NP_001655.1), is associated with a unique subset characterized histologically by clear cells {4285,3832,1028}. *TET2* and *DNMT3A* mutations occur early in haematopoietic stem cells, and their diagnostic value must be interpreted in conjunction with lymphoma-specific genetic changes. Therefore, in the assessment of an involved lymph node, the variant allele frequency is often much higher for *TET2* and *DNMT3A* than for *RHOA* and *IDH2*, because of the presence of *TET2* and *DNMT3A* mutations in non-neoplastic B and T cells.

Quantitative analysis of EBV viral load in peripheral blood is used to detect secondary EBV-positive B-cell proliferations at diagnosis/relapse and assess its response to therapy.

Essential and desirable diagnostic criteria

Typical (patterns 2 and 3) and tumour cell–rich nTFHL-AI

Essential: nodal disease; CD4-positive (occasionally CD4-negative), CD8-negative atypical lymphoid cells; extrafollicular FDC expansion and HEV hyperplasia (mild in tumour cell–rich cases).

Desirable: expression of at least two TFH markers, including strong PD1 (considered essential in cases of tumour cell–rich nTFHL-AI); clonal TR (TCR) gene rearrangement and/or *RHOA* p.G17V (NP_001655.1) or *IDH2* p.R172 mutation; EBV-positive B cells.

Partial nodal involvement (patterns 1 and 2)

Essential: nodal disease; perifollicular CD4+ (occasionally CD4−) and CD8− atypical T cells that express at least two TFH markers, including strong PD1; clonal TR (TCR) gene rearrangement and/or *RHOA* p.G17V or *IDH2* p.R172 mutation; if diagnostic criteria are not fulfilled because of insufficient sampling, rebiopsy is recommended.

Staging

Staging is performed according to the Lugano modification of the Ann Arbor staging system {688}.

Prognosis and prediction

The evolution is variable, but the prognosis is usually dismal, with a 3-year overall survival rate of about 50% {29,2273}. Nonetheless, there are occasional long-term survivors {179}. The male sex and concurrent *TET2*, *DNMT3A*, and *IDH2* mutations appear to be associated with an adverse prognosis {2816,2273,4427}. The Prognostic Index for Angioimmunoblastic T-cell Lymphoma (PIAI) is more discriminative than the International Prognostic Index (IPI) {1151}. A new nTFHL-AI score based on high B2M, high C-reactive protein, age ≥ 60 years, and an Eastern Cooperative Oncology Group (ECOG) performance status score of > 1 allows the separation of low-, intermediate-, and high-risk subgroups {29}.

Nodal T follicular helper cell lymphoma, follicular type

Attygalle AD
Amador C
Du MQ
Iqbal J
Sakata-Yanagimoto M
Tournilhac O

Definition

Nodal T follicular helper (TFH) cell lymphoma, follicular type (nTFHL-F), is a nodal peripheral T-cell lymphoma with a TFH phenotype that displays a follicular growth pattern and lacks the prominent high endothelial venules (HEVs) and extrafollicular follicular dendritic cell (FDC) meshworks characteristic of nodal TFH cell lymphoma, angioimmunoblastic type (nTFHL-AI).

ICD-O coding

9702/3 Nodal T follicular helper cell lymphoma, follicular type

ICD-11 coding

2A90.C & XH14S3 Peripheral T-cell lymphoma, NOS & Follicular T-cell lymphoma

Related terminology

Acceptable: follicular T-cell lymphoma (2017 WHO classification designation); follicular helper T-cell lymphoma, follicular type.

Not recommended: peripheral T-cell lymphoma NOS, follicular variant.

Subtype(s)

None

Localization

Disseminated nodal involvement is seen in 80–90% of cases; extranodal sites of involvement include the skin, liver, spleen, and bone marrow {972,1989,1657,1669,2703,2704}.

Clinical features

According to a small number of descriptive case reports, the clinical features of nTFHL-F resemble those of nTFHL-AI. Most patients present with advanced-stage disease and generalized lymphadenopathy, whereas a proportion develop skin rash and immune manifestations, such as polyclonal hypergammaglobulinaemia and a positive direct Coombs test {972,1989,1669,2703,2704}. Cases with localized stage I/II disease have also been reported {1669,2704}.

Epidemiology

nTFHL-F is rare, accounting for 1.8–2.6% of non-cutaneous peripheral T-cell lymphomas in one retrospective study and one prospective large study {4346,4427}. The median age of onset is 60–65 years, and there is a slight male predominance (M:F ratio: 1.05:1) {1989,1657,1669,2704}.

Etiology

Unknown

Pathogenesis

The genetic data for nTFHL-F are limited because of their rarity. Available data suggest a mutation profile similar to that of nTFHL-AI {972,2703}, with nTFHL-F further showing t(5;9)(q33;q22)/*ITK*::*SYK* in a proportion of cases {1669}, which is rarely seen in nTFHL-AI {178}.

Macroscopic appearance

Not relevant

Histopathology

The marked histological, clinical, immunophenotypic, transcriptomic, and genetic overlap with the other members of the nTFHL family suggests that nTFHL-F may represent a morphological pattern in the wider umbrella category of nTFHL rather than being a distinct entity {972}.

nTFHL-F is usually characterized by partial or complete effacement of the nodal architecture by a nodular/follicular proliferation of monotonous medium-sized lymphoid cells with moderate to abundant clear cytoplasm and round to slightly irregular nuclei {1669}. Two distinct growth patterns have been recognized.

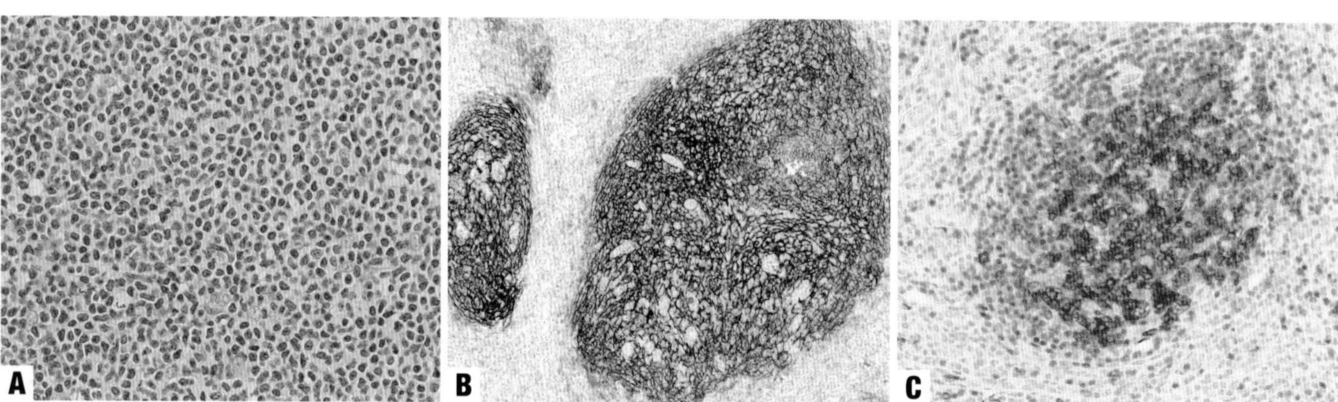

Fig. 5.139 Nodal T follicular helper cell lymphoma, follicular type, follicular lymphoma–like pattern. **A** Follicles composed of monotonous medium-sized lymphocytes with irregular nuclei; the large cell seen is a follicular dendritic cell. **B** CD21 immunostain highlights follicular dendritic cell meshworks confined to the follicles. **C** PAX5/CD10 double immunostain highlights PAX5-positive (brown, nuclear) mantle zone B cells rimming central CD10-positive (red, membranous), PAX5-negative neoplastic T cells.

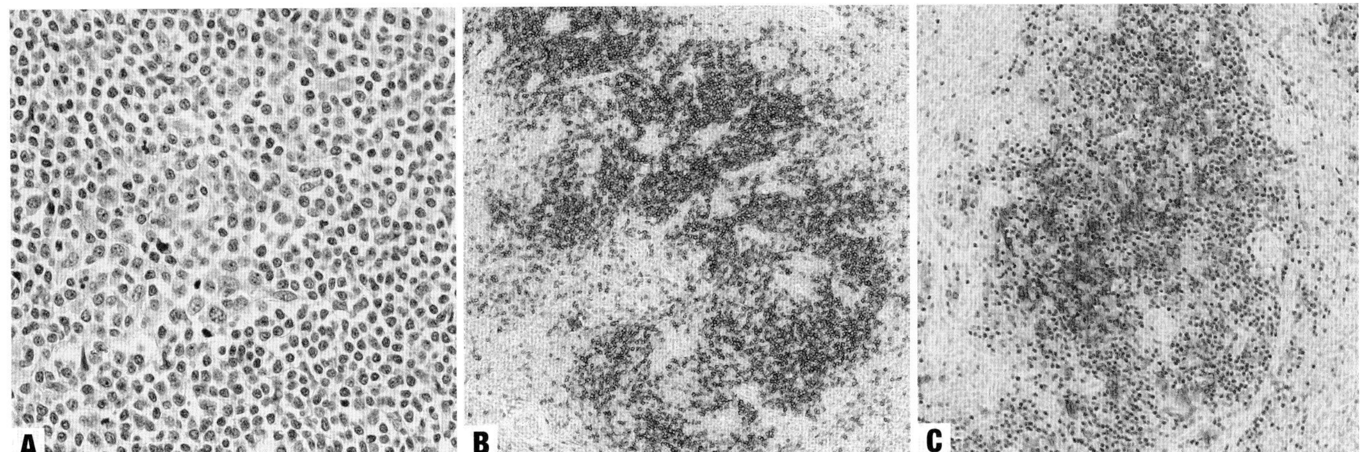

Fig. 5.140 Nodal T follicular helper cell lymphoma, follicular type, progressive transformation of germinal centres–like pattern. **A** Clusters of atypical lymphoid cells with pale cytoplasm amid small mantle zone–type lymphocytes. **B** IgD immunostain highlights the mantle zone B cells. **C** PAX5/CD10 double immunostain highlights PAX5-positive (brown, nuclear) mantle zone B cells surrounding clusters of CD10-positive (red, membranous), PAX5-negative neoplastic T cells.

One mimics follicular lymphoma, and the other mimics progressive transformation of germinal centres (PTGC). In the follicular lymphoma–like pattern, the neoplastic T cells form well-defined nodules surrounded by attenuated mantle zones {1669,900}. In the PTGC-like pattern, the nodules are reminiscent of PTGC, showing a moth-eaten appearance with clusters/aggregates of neoplastic T cells surrounded by small, mature, mantle zone–type lymphocytes {1669}. Both patterns are frequently observed in the same node. The interfollicular areas should lack HEV hyperplasia and the polymorphous infiltrate typical of nTFHL-AI. However, pure nTFHL-F is rare. Most cases classified as nTFHL-F show histological overlap with nTFHL-AI {1669, 2703,174}. Furthermore, nTFHL-F may relapse as typical nTFHL-AI, and vice versa {1669}. Scattered B immunoblasts may be seen. HRS-like cells may be distributed in the lymphocyte-rich PTGC-like nodules, as seen in a few cases {2795}.

Immunophenotype

The neoplastic T cells show an immunophenotype similar to that of nTFHL-AI. They are often positive for the pan–T-cell antigens CD2, CD3, and CD5, with variable loss of CD7. By flow cytometry, dim expression of sCD3 can be encountered {1669, 3853}. Most cases are positive for CD4 and negative for CD8 {1669}. The TFH markers PD1 (CD279), ICOS, BCL6, CXCL13, and CD10 are expressed, with varying levels of sensitivity. All cases express at least two of these TFH markers, with most cases expressing three or more. CD21, CD23, or CD35 immunostaining highlights FDC meshworks that may be expanded but confined to the nodules in both morphological patterns. The immunoblasts may be EBV-positive by EBV-encoded small RNA (EBER) in situ hybridization {1669}.

In the PTGC-like pattern, expression of CD10 and BCL6 by neoplastic T cells may be mistakenly attributed to B cells in the follicles, leading to misdiagnosis as follicular lymphoma. PAX5/CD10 double staining or direct comparison of single stains of consecutive sections may help in such cases. IgD-positive mantle zone–type small B cells surround clusters of neoplastic T cells within PTGC-like nodules {1669}. The HRS-like cells seen in the PTGC-like pattern are often CD30-positive, and they show variable expression of CD15, EBV, and B-cell antigens. The HRS-like cells are ringed by neoplastic T cells with a TFH phenotype {2795}.

Differential diagnosis

There is often morphological overlap with nTFHL-AI and considerable interobserver variation in the categorization of such cases. However, the more clinically significant differential diagnoses are follicular lymphoma and, in cases with HRS-like cells, classic Hodgkin lymphoma (lymphocyte-rich subtype) (see Table 5.20).

Table 5.20 Differential diagnoses for nodal T follicular helper (TFH) cell lymphoma, follicular type (nTFHL-F)

nTFHL-F growth pattern	Mimic	Key features for differential diagnosis (integrated approach required)[a]
Follicular lymphoma–like	Follicular lymphoma	nTFHL-F: • Comparison of CD10 and other TFH stains with CD20 shows that CD10+ cells are T cells; CD10/PAX5 double immunostaining may help
PTGC-like	Classic Hodgkin lymphoma	nTFHL-F: • HRS-like cells usually display a relatively intact B-cell programme (not always) • HRS-like cells rosetted by neoplastic T cells with TFH phenotype (CD10, if positive, is most helpful) Classic Hodgkin lymphoma: • Favoured if a mediastinal mass is present • Crippled B-cell programme in HRS cells • CD4+ T-cell rosettes may show weak to moderate (but not strong) PD1 expression and are CD10− {557}

PTGC, progressive transformation of germinal centres.
[a]Flow cytometry dim sCD3 and CD4+/CD10+ or CD4+/PD1+ T cells and detection of clonal TR (TCR) gene rearrangement and/or *RHOA* p.G17V point to nTFHL-F.

Cytology

Establishing a specific diagnosis by cytology is difficult, and not recommended. Samples may be used for flow cytometry and diagnostic molecular investigations.

Diagnostic molecular pathology

The molecular diagnostic strategies for nTFHL-AI also apply to nTFHL-F, with additional investigation of t(5;9)(q33;q22)/*ITK*::*SYK* where indicated {1669}.

Essential and desirable diagnostic criteria

Essential: nodal disease; follicular growth pattern (follicular lymphoma–like or PTGC-like); no extrafollicular expansion of FDCs; CD4+ (occasionally CD4−), CD8− atypical T cells that express at least two TFH markers, including strong PD1.

Desirable: lack of polymorphous infiltrate and HEV hyperplasia; clonal TR gene rearrangement.

Staging

Staging is performed according to the Lugano modification of the Ann Arbor staging system {688}.

Prognosis and prediction

The prognosis of nTFHL-F is uncertain. In two studies following up > 10 treated patients, the overall survival rate was 50–60% at 2 years {1669,2704}.

Nodal T follicular helper cell lymphoma NOS

Attygalle AD
Amador C
Du MQ
Iqbal J
Sakata-Yanagimoto M
Tournilhac O

Definition

Nodal T follicular helper (TFH) cell lymphoma (nTFHL) NOS is a nodal peripheral T-cell neoplasm with a TFH phenotype, demonstrated by the expression of CD4 and at least two TFH markers, that does not fulfil the required histopathological criteria for nTFHL, angioimmunoblastic type (nTFHL-AI) or nTFHL, follicular type.

ICD-O coding

9702/3 Nodal T follicular helper cell lymphoma, NOS

ICD-11 coding

2A90.C & XH6SR1 Mature T-cell lymphoma, specified types, nodal or systemic & Nodal peripheral T-cell lymphoma with T follicular helper phenotype

Related terminology

Acceptable: peripheral T-cell lymphoma with TFH phenotype; nodal peripheral T-cell lymphoma with TFH phenotype (2017 WHO classification designation); follicular helper T-cell lymphoma NOS.

Subtype(s)

None

Localization

nTFHL-NOS is characterized by disseminated disease with generalized lymphadenopathy and involvement of the spleen, liver, skin, and bone marrow, similar to nTFHL-AI.

Clinical features

In addition to lymphadenopathy, patients present with advanced-stage disease and may show autoimmune phenomena (Coombs positive haemolytic anaemia and polyclonal hypergammaglobulinaemia), as commonly seen in nTFHL-AI {972}.

Epidemiology

The true incidence of nTFHL-NOS is unknown.

Etiology

Unknown

Pathogenesis

Because the diagnostic criteria for nTFHL are evolving, there are limited genetic data from well-defined nTFHL-NOS cases available. Limited available data suggest that nTFHL-NOS and nTFHL-AI have a largely similar profile, except that *IDH2* mutations may be rare in the former {972}.

Macroscopic appearance

Not relevant

Histopathology

nTFHL-NOS is frequently characterized by effacement of the nodal architecture by a diffuse infiltrate of medium-sized to large lymphoid cells. Although it may show some morphological overlap with nTFHL-AI, it typically lacks a prominent polymorphous inflammatory background, high endothelial venule hyperplasia, and extrafollicular expansion of follicular dendritic cells. The lack of follicular dendritic cell expansion is the only tenuous distinguishing feature separating nTFHL-NOS from tumour cell–rich nTFHL-AI, suggesting they are part of a spectrum. In some cases, there is a T-zone pattern of involvement {43}. Secondary B-cell proliferations have not been well characterized.

Immunohistochemistry

By definition, cases are CD4-positive and show a minimum of two TFH markers (e.g. CD10, BCL6, PD1, ICOS, and CXCL13). Most cases of nTFHL-NOS express fewer TFH markers than nTFHL-AI, with the less specific PD1 and ICOS being positive most often {2521,261}. Although strong staining for PD1 provides a degree of specificity, the lack of specific markers may result in the inclusion of some cases better classified as peripheral T-cell lymphoma NOS {261}.

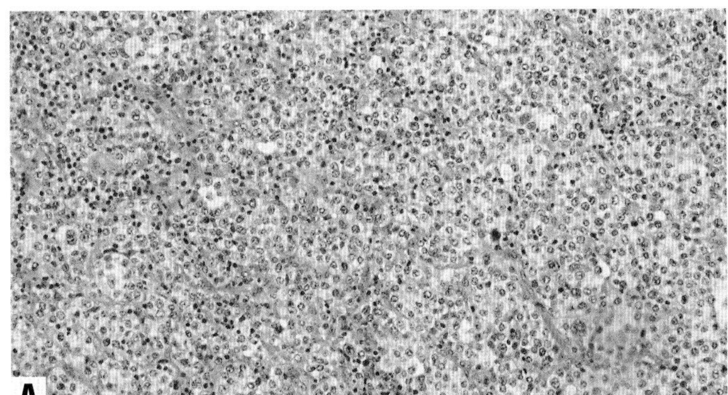

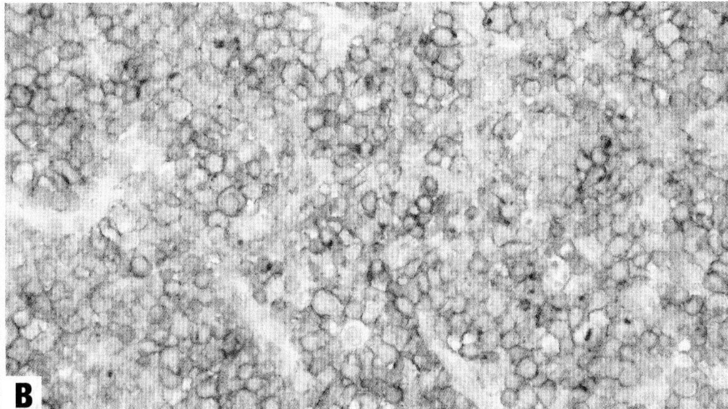

Fig. 5.141 Nodal T follicular helper cell lymphoma NOS. **A** Diffuse infiltrate of large atypical lymphoid cells. **B** The neoplastic T-cells express PD1.

Cytology

Samples may be used for immunophenotyping by flow cytometry and for diagnostic molecular investigations.

Diagnostic molecular pathology

The molecular diagnostic strategies for nTFHL-AI are also applicable to nTFHL-NOS. Detection of *RHOA* p.G17V (NP_001655.1) mutation, observed in as many as 60% of nTFHL-NOS cases, is a useful adjunct, because it supports the diagnosis of nTFHL over peripheral T-cell lymphoma NOS {972}.

Essential and desirable diagnostic criteria

Essential: nodal disease; effaced architecture or T-zone involvement by a morphologically atypical and/or immunophenotypically aberrant T-cell infiltrate (CD4+, CD8−) that expresses at least two TFH markers, including strong PD1; lack of extrafollicular hyperplasia of follicular dendritic cells, perifollicular distribution of neoplastic T cells, and follicular growth pattern.

Desirable: clonal TR gene rearrangement and/or *RHOA* p.G17V mutation.

Staging

Staging is performed according to the Lugano modification of the Ann Arbor staging system {688}.

Prognosis and prediction

Because of the rarity of nTFHL-NOS and its recent recognition in the WHO classification, clinical data on well-defined nTFHL-NOS, independent of the other nTFHLs, are limited. The survival of patients with nTFHL-NOS does not seem to differ from that of patients with nTFHL-AI {972,4507}.

Peripheral T-cell lymphoma NOS

Amador C
Iqbal J
Tan SY
Vega F
Weinstock DM

Definition

Peripheral T-cell lymphoma (PTCL) NOS is a heterogeneous category of nodal and extranodal mature T-cell lymphomas that cannot be assigned to a specific PTCL entity. Nodal T follicular helper (TFH) cell lymphomas and EBV-positive nodal T- and NK-cell lymphomas are excluded from this category.

ICD-O coding

9702/3 Peripheral T-cell lymphoma, NOS

ICD-11 coding

2A90.C Peripheral T-cell lymphoma, NOS

Related terminology

Not recommended: T-cell lymphoma NOS; peripheral T-cell lymphoma, pleomorphic small cell; peripheral T-cell lymphoma, pleomorphic medium and large cell; peripheral T-cell lymphoma, large cell.

Subtype(s)

None

Localization

Most patients present with advanced disease. Besides the lymph nodes, other sites can also be involved, including the bone marrow, liver, spleen, and extranodal tissues (most commonly the skin and gastrointestinal tract) {3416,4346,4257}. Leukaemic and CNS presentations are uncommon {2648}.

Clinical features

Patients most often present with lymphadenopathy and B symptoms. Paraneoplastic features such as eosinophilia, pruritus, or (rarely) haemophagocytic syndrome may be seen {3416}.

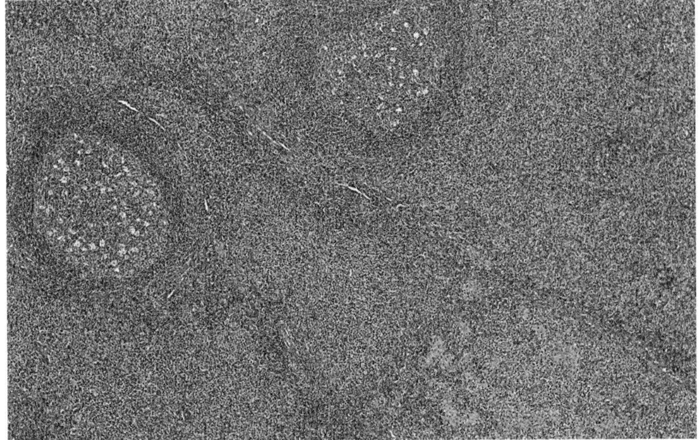

Fig. 5.142 Peripheral T-cell lymphoma NOS. Lymph node with a paracortical pattern of involvement. The lymphomatous infiltrate is located predominantly between residual reactive lymphoid follicles.

Epidemiology

PTCL-NOS is nearly always diagnosed in adults and shows a male predominance {4346}. These tumours account for as many as 35% of T-cell neoplasms {4257}, with some variation based on geography (20% in Asia, 28% in France, and 35% in North America) {4508,2232,4257}.

Etiology

Unknown

Pathogenesis

PTCL-NOS has complex karyotypes {2931}. Common abnormalities with a potential pathogenetic role include chromosomal gains of 7q and 7p, encompassing *CDK6* (7q21.2) and *CARD11* (7p22.2) {4008,2874,1260,1519}. Occasional cases show alterations involving the TR gene loci (mostly the TRA locus at 14q11.2), including t(14;19)(q11;q13) implicating *NECTIN2* (*PVRL2*) {81}, and t(6;14)(p25;q11.2) implicating *IRF4* in cytotoxic PTCL-NOS {1153,3780}. Next-generation sequencing studies have revealed frequent aberrations in tumour suppressor genes, including rearrangements of *TP63* {4189} and mutations and deletions of *CDKN2A*, *PTEN*, and *TP53* {1543, 4327,2607}, which are often associated with poor clinical outcomes. Codeletion of *CDKN2A*and *PTEN*, reported in 20% of cases, is a highly specific finding of PTCL-NOS that is rarely found in other mature T-cell neoplasms {2607}. Like other types of mature T-cell lymphomas, a subset of PTCL-NOS has alterations in *PLCG1*, *CD28*, and *VAV1* {4327,3448,4}.

Gene expression profiling studies have identified two molecular subtypes within PTCL-NOS: PTCL-TBX21 and PTCL-GATA3; these are characterized by overexpression of the transcription factors TBX21 (T-bet) and GATA3 (and corresponding target genes), respectively, and have different prognoses {1736,95}. Because these transcription factors regulate the T helper 1 (Th1) (TBX21) and T helper 2 (Th2) (GATA3) transcription programmes, it is postulated that these two molecular subtypes may represent neoplasms associated with aberrant Th1/2 differentiation. The PTCL-GATA3 molecular subtype is associated with high *MYC* expression, high proliferation, and aberrant PI3K activation, whereas in the PTCL-TBX21 subtype the NF-κB pathway is enriched. In addition, PTCL-GATA3 cases have a higher genomic complexity – in particular, genomic aberrations targeting tumour suppressor genes, including 17p deletion (*TP53*), 9p deletion (*CDKN2A*), and heterozygous 10p deletion (*PTEN*) – whereas PTCL-TBX21 is mainly characterized by mutations in epigenetic regulators (e.g. *TET2*, *DNMT3A*), suggesting distinct oncogenic pathways of tumorigenesis {1543}.

Within the PTCL-TBX21 molecular subtype, a subset of cases with a cytotoxic gene expression programme and more aggressive behaviour have been described {1736,1735}. This cytotoxic subset has not been entirely delineated yet, and additional studies are needed to distinguish it from non-cytotoxic PTCL-TBX21

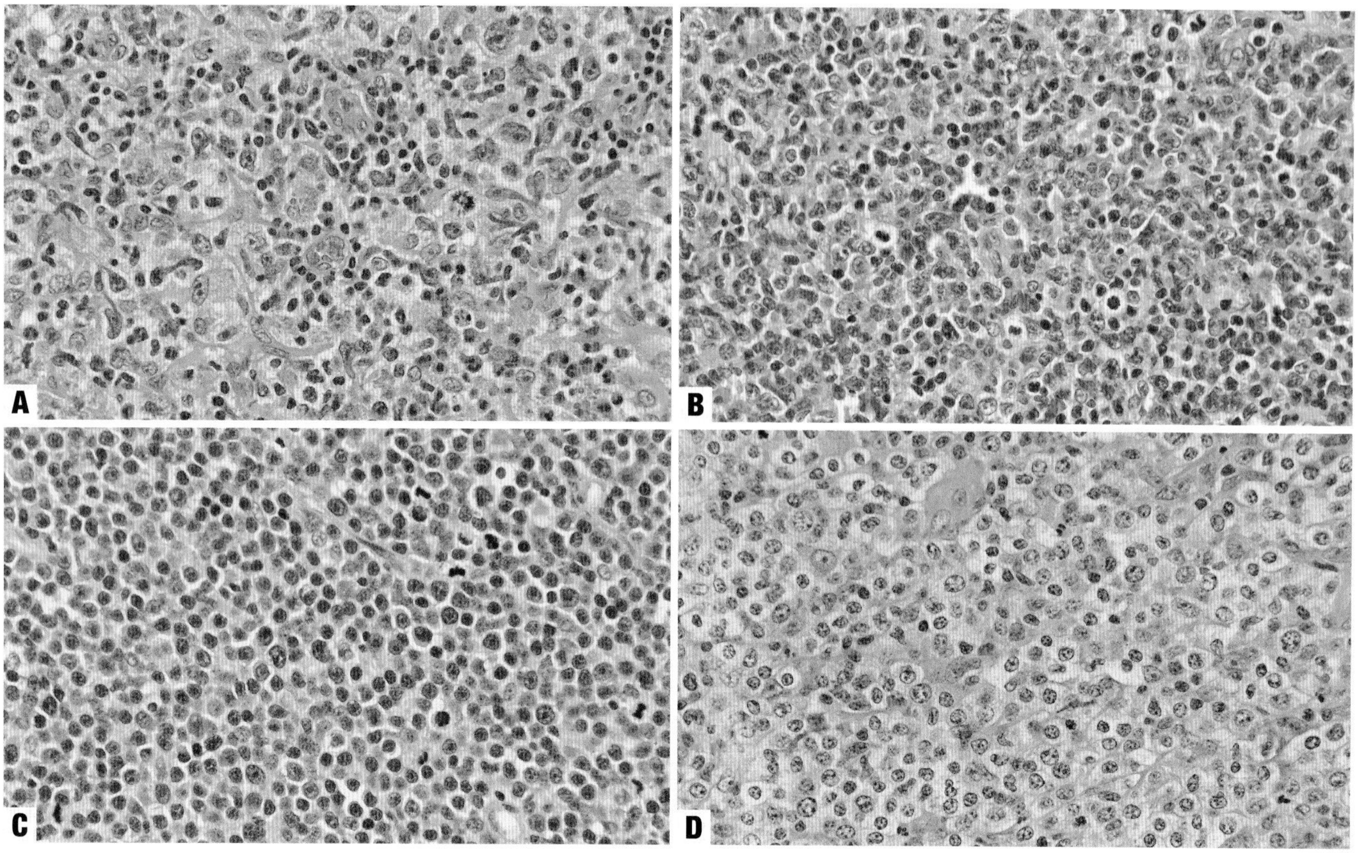

Fig. 5.143 Peripheral T-cell lymphoma NOS. The morphological spectrum of peripheral T-cell lymphoma NOS is broad, with highly variable tumour cell cytological characteristics and inflammatory background. **A** Large and anaplastic tumour cell morphology. **B** Pleomorphic tumour cell morphology. **C** Medium-sized monocytoid tumour cell morphology. **D** Clear tumour cell morphology.

cases and to establish its relationship with EBV-positive nodal T- and NK-cell lymphomas.

Macroscopic appearance

Not relevant

Histopathology

PTCL-NOS has highly variable cytological and morphological features. There is partial or complete effacement of the nodal architecture by paracortical or diffuse infiltrates. Most cases comprise medium-sized and/or large lymphoma cells with irregular, pleomorphic, hyperchromatic, or vesicular nuclei; prominent nucleoli; and many mitotic figures {1504,1762}. HRS-like cells can also be seen {1057}. Rare cases have a predominance of small to medium-sized lymphoid cells with clear cytoplasm. There is commonly an inflammatory background composed of variable proportions of small lymphocytes, eosinophils, plasma cells, large B cells (EBV-positive or -negative), and clusters of epithelioid histiocytes (see *Lymphoepithelioid lymphoma (Lennert lymphoma)*, below). An inflammatory background is much more frequent in the PTCL-TBX21 molecular subtype than in the PTCL-GATA3 molecular subtype {97}.

In the skin, the lymphomatous infiltrate in the dermis and subcutis often forms nodules, which may undergo central necrosis. Epidermotropism, angiocentricity, and adnexal involvement are sometimes seen {3167}. In the spleen, the pattern is variable, from solitary or multiple nodules to diffuse white pulp involvement with colonization of the periarteriolar sheaths or, in some cases, predominant infiltration of the red pulp.

Immunophenotype

PTCL-NOS is positive for pan–T-cell antigens, with frequent decreased expression of CD5 and CD7 {4346,4359}. It is more often CD4-positive than CD8-positive, and rare cases can be double-positive or double-negative. Most cases express TCR$\alpha\beta$,

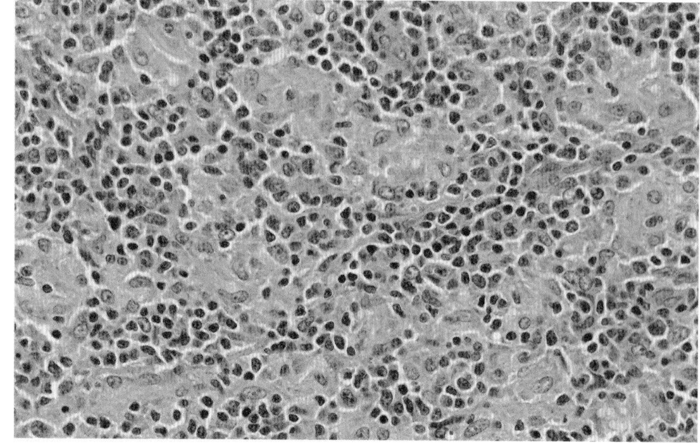

Fig. 5.144 Peripheral T-cell lymphoma NOS, lymphoepithelioid variant. Small, mildly atypical neoplastic cells are admixed with numerous epithelioid histiocytes, mimicking granulomatous inflammation.

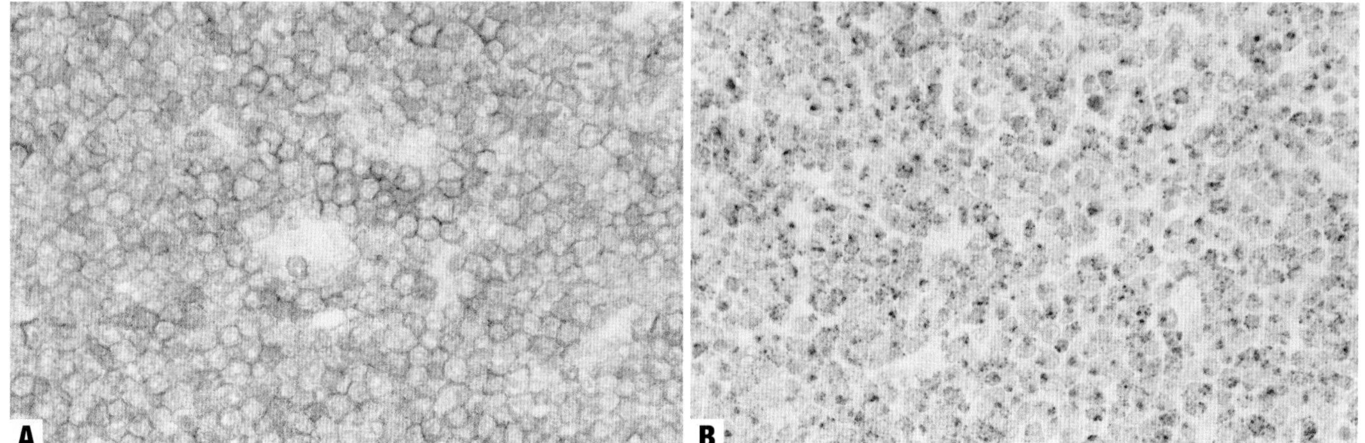

Fig. 5.145 Peripheral T-cell lymphoma NOS with cytotoxic phenotype. Neoplastic cells are positive for CD8 (**A**) and for TIA1 (**B**).

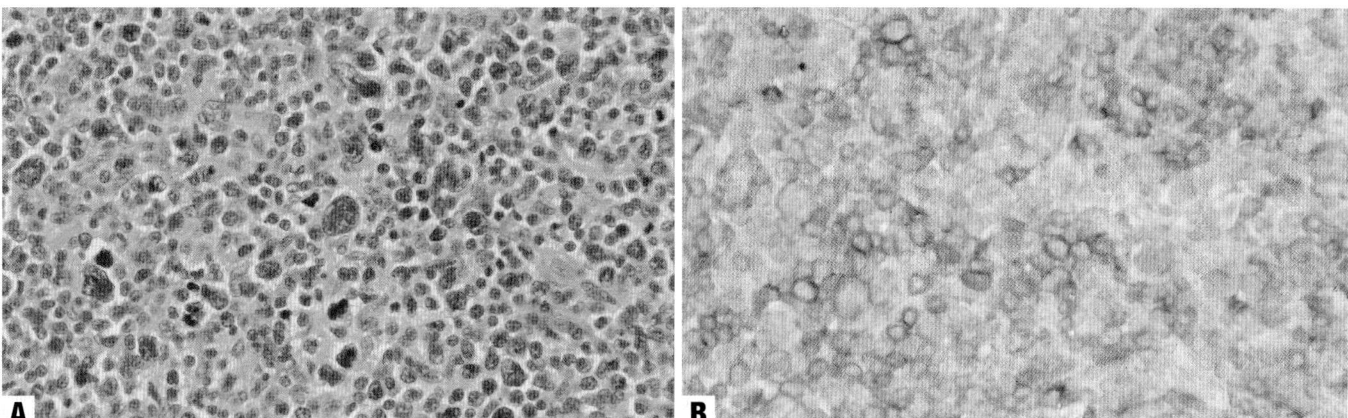

Fig. 5.146 Peripheral T-cell lymphoma NOS with CD30 positivity. **A** The neoplastic cells show significant variation in cell size, and nuclear pleomorphism. **B** CD30 immunohistochemistry shows variable and partial expression.

but rare cases are positive for TCRγδ or negative for both (T-cell receptor–silent). Expression of one or more cytotoxic markers is seen in 20–35% of cases, with TIA1 being more commonly expressed than granzyme B {4359,4477,160}. Concordant with the gene expression profiling findings, cases with cytotoxic marker expression are usually of the PTCL-TBX21 molecular

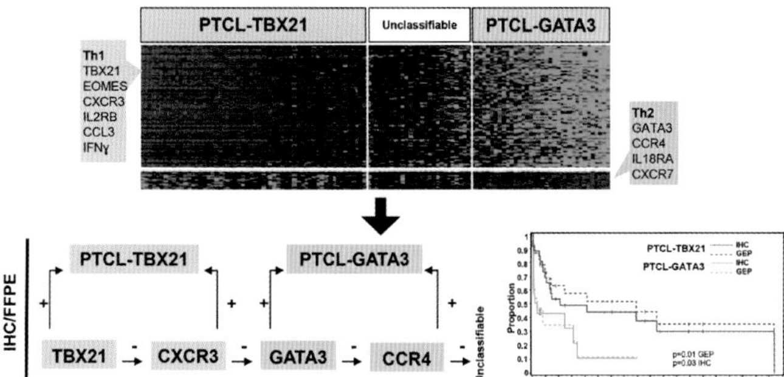

Fig. 5.147 Gene expression profiling (GEP) studies delineate two major molecular subtypes of peripheral T-cell lymphoma (PTCL) NOS, characterized by high expression of GATA3 and TBX21 and corresponding target genes, with distinct prognoses. An immunohistochemistry (IHC) algorithm using four immunostains (TBX21, CXCR3, GATA3, and CCR4) reproduces the molecular classification in an independent cohort and maintains the prognostic difference (dotted line, immunohistochemistry; solid line, GEP). FFPE, formalin-fixed, paraffin-embedded; Th1, T helper 1; Th2, T helper 2.

subtype, and it is rarely observed in the PTCL-GATA3 subtype {97}. CD56 is positive in a subset of cases, and cyclin D1 is expressed in rare cases {3784}. Aberrant B-cell marker (typically CD20) expression can be seen in rare cases {3346}. Scattered EBV-encoded small RNA (EBER)-positive B cells may be present.

The expression of a single TFH marker is still acceptable for the diagnosis of PTCL-NOS, but cases with diffuse positivity for two or more TFH markers should be diagnosed as nodal TFH cell lymphoma. CD30 expression is detected in > 25% of cases. When present, it is usually variable and is not uniformly and strongly positive, unlike the characteristic extensive strong staining in anaplastic large cell lymphomas {422,3514}. CD30 positivity (even weak expression) may have therapeutic utility where brentuximab vedotin is available {1636}. CD15 is present in about 5% of cases and may be coexpressed with CD30 {252}.

An immunohistochemical algorithm can be used to provide surrogate information on the molecular subtypes (PTCL-GATA3 and PTCL-TBX21) {97}. This algorithm begins with the determination of TBX21 expression and is followed, if needed, by the assessment of CXCR3, GATA3, and CCR4.

Lymphoepithelioid lymphoma (Lennert lymphoma)

This morphological variant is characterized by numerous epithelioid histiocytes that mimic granulomatous inflammation, often masking the neoplastic T cells. The tumour cells are usually small and mildly atypical, with irregular nuclei and mature coarse chromatin. Scattered larger immunoblasts or atypical HRS-like B cells (usually EBV-positive) can be encountered. The neoplastic cells typically have a non-activated cytotoxic phenotype (TIA1+ and granzyme B−), with expression of CD4 or CD8 {4346,1310,1513,2161}. Lymphomas with a lymphoepithelioid morphology and TFH immunophenotype should be classified as nodal TFH cell lymphoma {2161}. Lymphoepithelioid lymphoma has a better prognosis than other forms of PTCL-NOS {4346,1267}.

Differential diagnosis

The diagnosis of PTCL-NOS is essentially one of exclusion, and therefore all other types of PTCL should be considered (Table 5.21). In cases with HRS-like or scattered large B cells, the differential diagnosis includes classic Hodgkin lymphoma or T-cell/histiocyte–rich large B-cell lymphoma. Cases of PTCL-NOS that partially involve the lymph node, sparing lymphoid follicles, and are composed of clear cells can resemble nodal marginal zone lymphoma. PTCL-NOS also needs to be distinguished from several reactive conditions involving lymph nodes, including paracortical lymph node hyperplasia induced by viral infections (infectious mononucleosis) or drug reactions, autoimmune lymphoproliferative syndrome (ALPS), and Kikuchi–Fujimoto disease. The demonstration of a significant monoclonal T-cell population, often with an aberrant immunophenotype, is helpful to differentiate PTCL from these reactive entities.

Cytology

Not relevant

Diagnostic molecular pathology

Most cases show monoclonal rearrangement of the TR genes. *RHOA* p.G17V and *IDH2* p.R172 mutations, which are often present in nodal TFH cell lymphomas, are usually negative in PTCL-NOS.

Essential and desirable diagnostic criteria

Essential: presence of an abnormal T-cell infiltrate, which is morphologically or immunophenotypically aberrant and/or is monoclonal by ancillary studies; the tumour cells are negative or express only one TFH marker (to differentiate from nodal TFH cell lymphomas) and only show EBER in scattered B cells (to differentiate from EBV-positive nodal T- and NK-cell lymphoma); exclusion of other nodal or extranodal mature T- and NK-cell lymphomas (i.e. ALK+ anaplastic large cell

Table 5.21 Differential diagnosis of peripheral T-cell lymphoma NOS

Disease	Clinicopathological features	Molecular/genetic findings
Nodal TFH cell lymphoma, angioimmunoblastic type	Distinctive clinical syndrome[a] FDC hyperplasia (CD21/CD23), polymorphous inflammatory infiltrate, arborizing HEVs, EBV+/− B immunoblasts CD4+; expression of two or more TFH markers (CD10, BCL6, PD1, CXCL13, CXCR5, ICOS, SAP)	*RHOA* p.G17V and *IDH2* p.R172 mutations; lack of deletions of *CDKN2A* and *PTEN*; rare *TP53* deletions and/or mutations
Nodal TFH cell lymphoma NOS	CD4+; expression of two or more TFH markers (CD10, BCL6, PD1, CXCL13, CXCR5, ICOS, SAP) Lack of hyperplasia of FDCs and HEVs	*RHOA* p.G17V mutations in a subset; lack of deletions of *CDKN2A* and *PTEN*; rare *TP53* deletions and/or mutations
ALK− anaplastic large cell lymphoma	Large anaplastic (hallmark) cells, cohesive growth pattern, sinusoidal involvement CD30+ (strong and uniform); EMA+; cytotoxic granules+/−, CD4+/−; CD3−/+; CD43+; PAX5−; reduced T-cell surface antigen expression	*DUSP22* rearrangements (can also occur in PTCL-NOS); JAK-1 and STAT3 activation
Adult T-cell leukaemia/lymphoma	Mostly geographically restricted to areas in which HTLV-1 is endemic; hypercalcaemia; simultaneous opportunistic infections Presence of flower cells CD4+, CD25+, CD7−, CD30−/+, CCR4+, FOXP3−/+	Positive serological studies for HTLV-1; positive HTLV-1 integration studies; *CCR4* mutations and *IRF4* amplifications
EBV-positive nodal T- and NK-cell lymphoma	EBER positivity in most of the tumour cells Cytotoxic phenotype; CD56− (usually)	Positive TR gene rearrangements (cases with T-cell lineage); negative TR gene rearrangements (cases with NK-cell lineage)
Classic Hodgkin lymphoma	HRS cells in background of reactive T cells with normal phenotypic profile	Negative TR gene rearrangements / polyclonal T cells
T-cell/histiocyte–rich large B-cell lymphoma	Large CD20+ blasts in background of reactive T cells with normal phenotypic profile	Negative TR gene rearrangements / polyclonal T cells
Nodal marginal zone lymphoma	Neoplastic cells are B cells (CD20+); these small/medium-sized cells usually grow around follicles and into the interfollicular areas	Positive IG gene rearrangements
Paracortical hyperplasia	Expansion of T cells with normal phenotypic profile with mixed CD4 and CD8 populations; variable CD30 expression	Negative TR gene rearrangements / polyclonal T cells

EBER, EBV-encoded small RNA; FDC, follicular dendritic cell; HEV, high endothelial venule; nTFHL-AI, nodal TFH cell lymphoma, angioimmunoblastic type; PTCL, peripheral T-cell lymphoma; TFH, T follicular helper; +, nearly always positive; +/−, majority positive; −, negative; −/+, minority positive.
[a]Hepatosplenomegaly, skin rash, effusion, fever, polyclonal hypergammaglobulinaemia, and haemolytic anaemia.

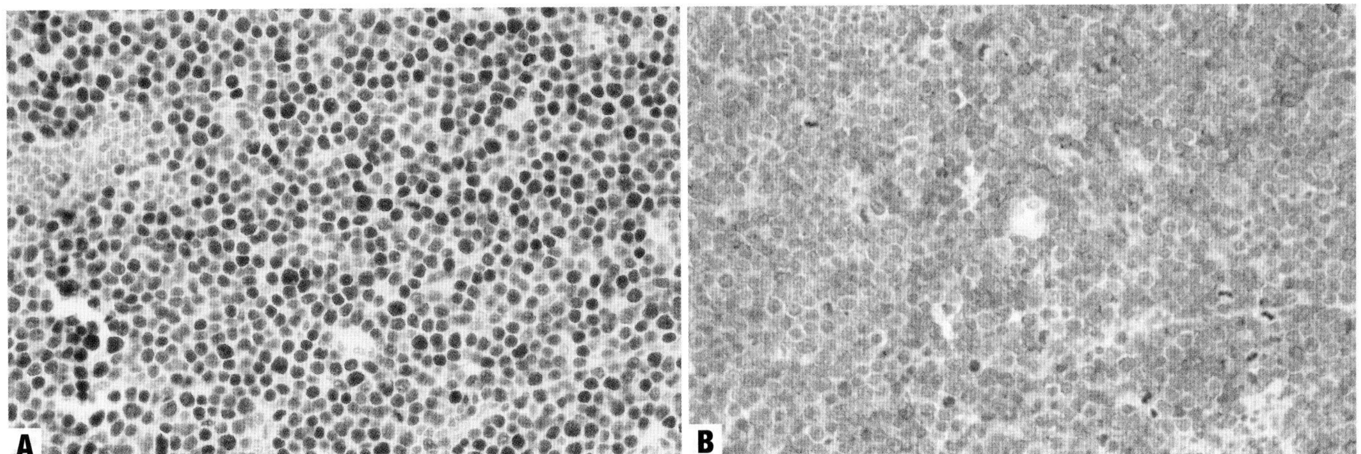

Fig. 5.148 Peripheral T-cell lymphoma NOS, GATA3 molecular subtype. The majority of the neoplastic cells are positive for GATA3 (**A**) and for CCR4 (**B**).

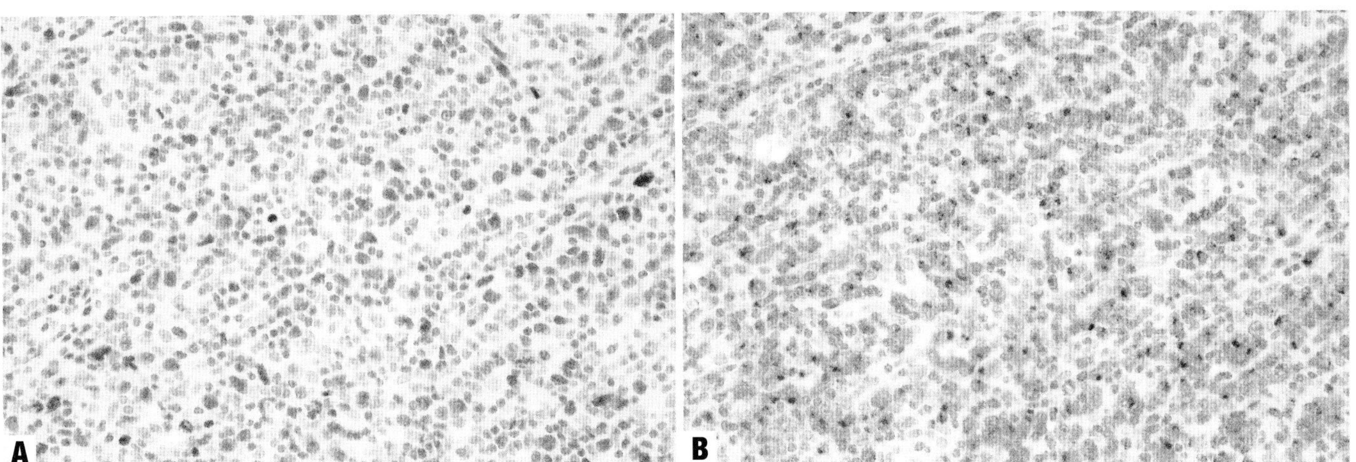

Fig. 5.149 Peripheral T-cell lymphoma NOS, TBX21 molecular subtype. The majority of the neoplastic cells are positive for TBX21 (**A**) and for CXCR3 (**B**).

lymphoma, ALK– anaplastic large cell lymphoma, adult T-cell leukaemia/lymphoma, extranodal NK/T-cell lymphoma).

Desirable: clonal TR gene rearrangements; establishment of the biological designation of PTCL-TBX21 or PTCL-GATA3.

Staging

Staging is performed according to the Lugano modification of the Ann Arbor staging system {688}.

Prognosis and prediction

These are aggressive lymphomas with a poor response to therapy, frequent relapses, and low survival rates {4346,4257, 1149}. The 5-year overall and failure-free survival rates for PTCL-NOS have been reported as 32% and 20% respectively {4346}. A high International Prognostic Index (IPI) score, PTCL-GATA3 molecular subtype, cytotoxic profile, increased numbers of transformed cells, CD30 expression in most or all cells, and abnormalities in tumour suppressor genes (e.g. deletion/mutations of *TP53* and *CDKN2A*) have been associated with poor prognosis {4189,1543,4327,2607,1736,97,4359,160,4305}.

EBV-positive nodal T- and NK-cell lymphoma

Ng S-B
Cheng CL
Kato S
Weinstock DM
Yamashita D

Definition

EBV-positive nodal T- and NK-cell lymphoma is an EBV-positive lymphoma of cytotoxic T- or NK-cell lineage, presenting primarily with nodal disease in adults.

ICD-O coding

9702/3 EBV-positive nodal T- and NK-cell lymphoma

ICD-11 coding

2B2Y Other specified mature T-cell or NK-cell neoplasms

Related terminology

Acceptable: nodal EBV+ cytotoxic T-cell lymphoma; nodal peripheral T-cell lymphoma, EBV-positive; primary nodal EBV-positive T/NK-cell lymphoma.

Not recommended: peripheral T-cell lymphoma NOS, EBV-positive.

Subtype(s)

None

Localization

The disease presents primarily in lymph nodes (most commonly cervical, inguinal, and axillary) but may also involve a limited number of extranodal sites. The liver and/or bone marrow are involved in 24–60% of cases; other extranodal sites, such as the skin and gastrointestinal tract, are less commonly involved {1797,1916,4477}. There is no reported nasal involvement.

Clinical features

Patients typically present with lymphadenopathy, advanced clinical stage (86–88% of cases), B symptoms (72–80%), high or high/intermediate International Prognostic Index (IPI) score (64–87%), and thrombocytopenia (53–62%) {1797,1916,2943, 4477}.

Fig. 5.150 EBV-positive nodal T- and NK-cell lymphoma. Low magnification shows a diffuse growth pattern with areas of necrosis.

Epidemiology

EBV-positive nodal T- and NK-cell lymphoma is a rare lymphoma type which occurs mostly in eastern Asia {3926,1917,1916,1459, 1797,1836,2943} and affects mainly older adults (median age: 61–64 years) although cases in younger adults have been reported. The M:F ratio is 1.5–3.8:1 {1797,1916,2943,4477}.

Etiology

EBV appears to play an important etiological role. The majority of cases show a type II EBV latency pattern, with expression of EBNA1, LMP1, and LMP2A and absence of EBNA2, although LMP1 protein expression is often undetectable {3926,4273}.

A minority of patients have concurrent autoimmune conditions, viral infections (e.g. HBV, HCV), or diabetes mellitus, which may impair immune responses and could contribute to the oncogenic transformation of EBV-infected cells {4477}.

Pathogenesis

According to a recent report of patients in Asia, the most commonly mutated gene in EBV-positive nodal T- and NK-cell lymphoma is *TET2* (64%), followed by *PIK3CD* (33%), *DDX3X* (20%), and *STAT3* (19%) {4273}. The lymphoma shows recurrent losses of 14q11.2 (including TR loci, and found in the majority of cases), 3q26.1, and 22q11.23, and recurrent gains of 6p22.1, 14q32.33, 3p14.1, and 22q11.23 {2943,4273}. Despite its aggressive behaviour, it demonstrates lower genomic instability than extranodal NK/T-cell lymphoma (ENKTL) and peripheral T-cell lymphoma NOS {4273}.

Gene expression profiling analysis has identified enriched expression of genes related to cytotoxic activation, IL-6/JAK/STAT3 signalling, cell cycle and genomic instability, immune-related pathways, and interferon-α/γ response {1459,2943, 4273}. NF-κB pathway–associated genes and proteins (*BIRC3*, *NFKB1*, and *CD27*) are overexpressed. CD274 (PDL1) is upregulated and correlates with IFN-γ, IL-6/JAK/STAT3, and NF-κB expression, although there is no gain of 9p24.1 {4273,2943}.

Macroscopic appearance

Not relevant

Histopathology

The lymph nodes show architectural effacement by a diffuse infiltrate of medium-sized to large lymphoid cells, often without prominent coagulative necrosis or angiocentric growth. The neoplastic cells are prototypically centroblastoid in appearance, resembling diffuse large B-cell lymphoma and distinct from the irregularly folded nuclei typical of ENKTL. Less frequently, the tumour has a pleomorphic or mixed-cell morphology {174,1797,1916,4477}.

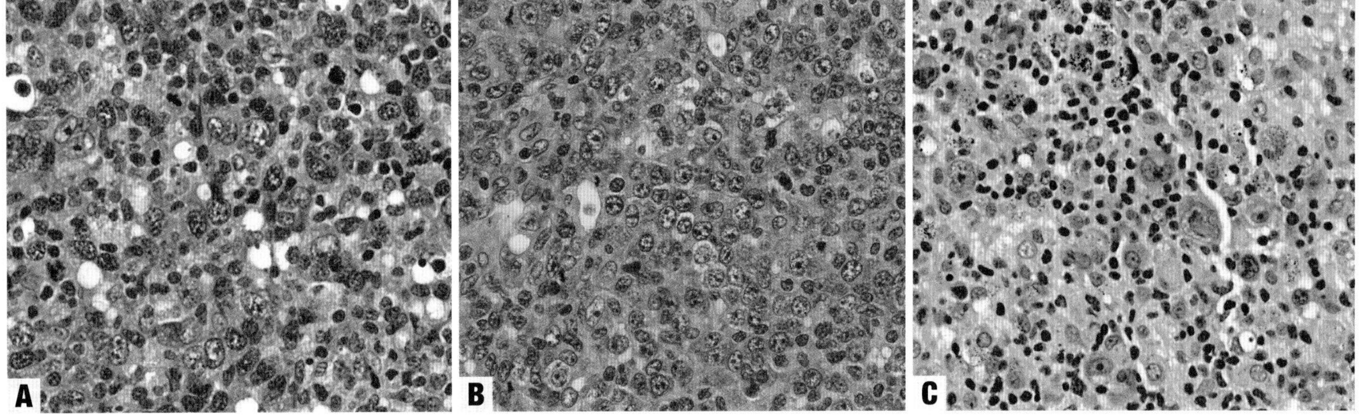

Fig. 5.151 EBV-positive nodal T- and NK-cell lymphoma. **A** High magnification shows a mixed population of small, medium, and large cells. **B** A diffuse infiltrate of relatively monotonous medium-sized to large cells with centroblastoid appearance. **C** In other cases, neoplastic cells appear large and pleomorphic, with abundant histiocytes and small lymphocytes in the background.

Immunohistochemistry and in situ hybridization

The tumour cells express pan–T-cell markers (such as CD3 and CD2) and cytotoxic molecules (TIA1, granzyme B, and perforin). CD8 and CD56 are positive in 63–72% and 7–22% of cases, respectively {1797,1916,2943,4477}. CD4 and CD5 are often negative {1797,1916,4477}.

This lymphoma is of T-cell lineage in > 80% of cases, based on T-cell receptor protein expression and/or clonal TR gene rearrangement {1797,1916,2943,4477}. TCRβ and TCRγ are expressed in 43–64% and 0–13% of cases, respectively. About 25% of T-cell tumours are negative for both TCRβ and TCRγ. A minority (< 20%) of tumours are of NK-cell lineage, lacking expression of TCRβ and TCRγ as well as clonal TR gene rearrangements. The majority of neoplastic cells are positive for EBV-encoded small RNA (EBER) by in situ hybridization.

Differential diagnosis

See Table 5.22.

Cytology

Not relevant

Diagnostic molecular pathology

Monoclonal TR gene rearrangement supports a T-cell lineage but is negative in tumours of NK-cell lineage.

Essential and desirable diagnostic criteria

Essential: a tumour primarily localized within lymph nodes but which may involve a limited number of extranodal sites (no nasal involvement); cytotoxic T-cell or NK-cell lymphoma; presence of EBER in the majority of neoplastic cells; exclusion of immune deficiency/dysregulation–associated T- and NK-cell lymphoproliferative diseases, ENKTL, systemic

Table 5.22 Differential diagnosis of EBV-positive T-cell and NK-cell lymphoproliferative diseases

Diagnostic criteria	EBV-positive nodal T- and NK-cell lymphoma	Extranodal NK/T-cell lymphoma	Systemic chronic active EBV disease	Systemic EBV-positive T-cell lymphoma of childhood	Aggressive NK-cell leukaemia	nTFHL-AI with large B cells
Age group	Adults	Adults	Children / young adults	Children / young adults	Young adults	Adults
Disease presentation	Nodal	Extranodal	Systemic proliferation involving bone marrow, liver, and/or spleen	Systemic proliferation involving bone marrow, liver, and/or spleen	Systemic proliferation involving bone marrow, liver, and spleen; lymph node involvement at presentation uncommon (20–26%) {2068,1742}	Commonly nodal
Nasal involvement	No	Very common	No	No	No	No
HLH at presentation	Uncommon (22%)	Uncommon (13%) {2306}	Common	Common	Common	No
Immunohisto-chemistry	CD8+ > CD4+, CD56−/+	CD4−, CD8−/+, CD56+/−	T-cell type (CD4+ > CD8+) NK-cell type (CD56+)	CD8+ > CD4+, CD56−	CD4−, CD8−, CD56+	CD4+, CD8−, CD56−, TFH markers+
Lineage of EBV+ tumour cells	T >> NK	NK > T	T or NK	T	NK	B

HLH, haemophagocytic lymphohistiocytosis; nTFHL-AI, nodal T follicular helper cell lymphoma, angioimmunoblastic type.

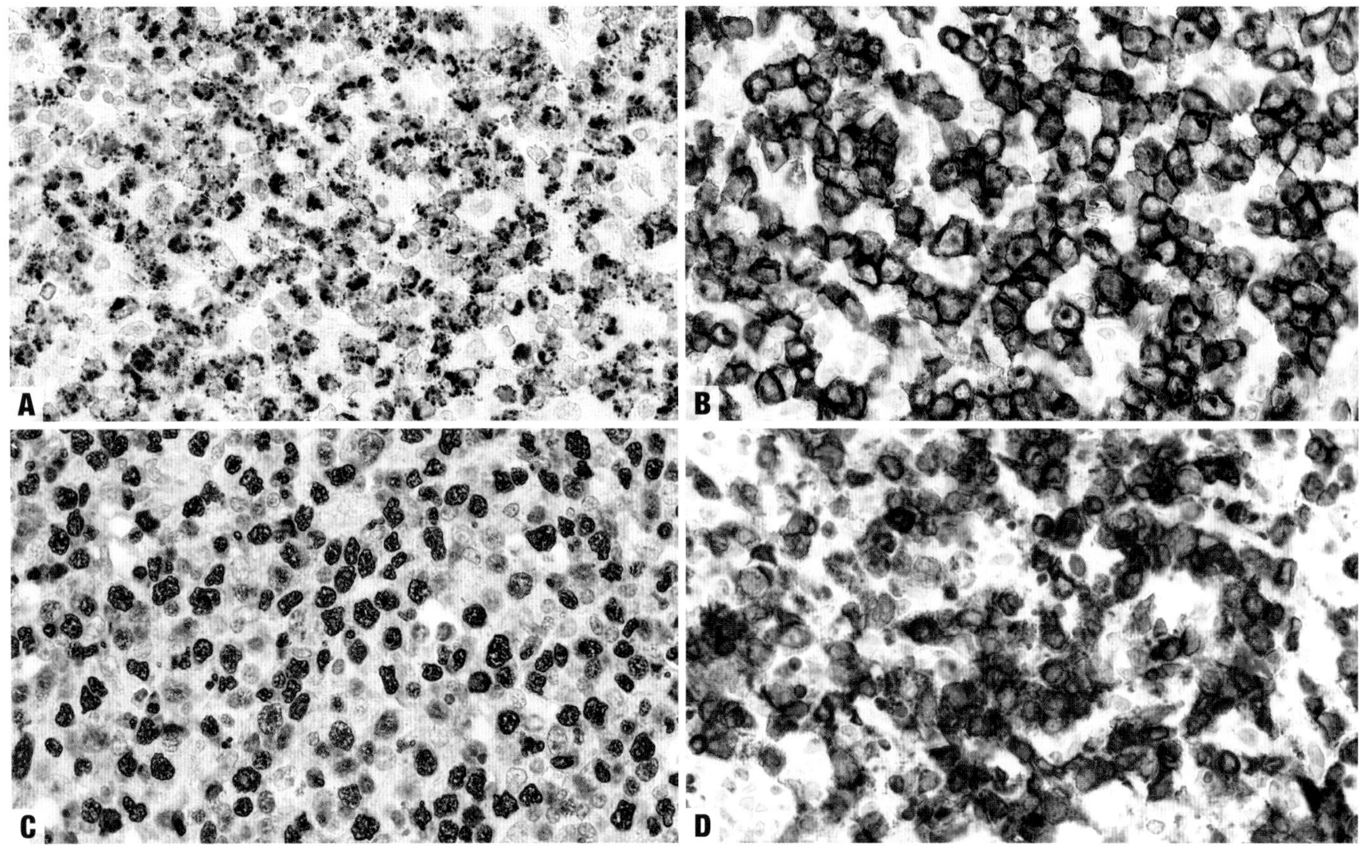

Fig. 5.152 EBV-positive nodal T- and NK-cell lymphoma. The neoplastic cells are positive for TIA1 (**A**) and positive for CD8 in approximately 80% of cases (**B**). **C** In situ hybridization identifies EBV-encoded small RNA (EBER) expression in the lymphoma cells. **D** In rare cases, TCRδ (clone H-41) is expressed.

EBV+ lymphoproliferative diseases of childhood, and aggressive NK-cell leukaemia with progression or secondary involvement of lymph nodes.

Staging

Staging is performed according to the Lugano classification, a modification of the Ann Arbor staging system {688}.

Prognosis and prediction

The median overall survival time (2.5–8.0 months) is worse than that of ENKTL (26–76 months) {1459,2308,1797,1916, 2009,2943,4477} and peripheral T-cell lymphoma NOS (16–20 months) {160,1916,1149,4477}.

Extranodal NK/T-cell lymphoma

Chuang S-S
Cheng CL
Huang YH
Kwong YL
Li GD
Ng S-B
Yamaguchi M
Zhao WL
Zhao S

Definition

Extranodal NK/T-cell lymphoma (ENKTL) is an extranodal lymphoma of NK- or T-cell lineage characterized by vascular damage and destruction, prominent necrosis, a cytotoxic phenotype, and an association with EBV.

ICD-O coding

9719/3 Extranodal NK/T-cell lymphoma

ICD-11 coding

2A90.6 Extranodal NK/T-cell lymphoma, nasal type

Related terminology

Acceptable: extranodal NK/T-cell lymphoma, nasal type; EBV-positive extranodal NK/T-cell lymphoma.

Not recommended: angiocentric lymphoma; lethal midline granuloma.

Subtype(s)

Clinical subtypes: nasal ENKTL; non-nasal (extranasal) ENKTL

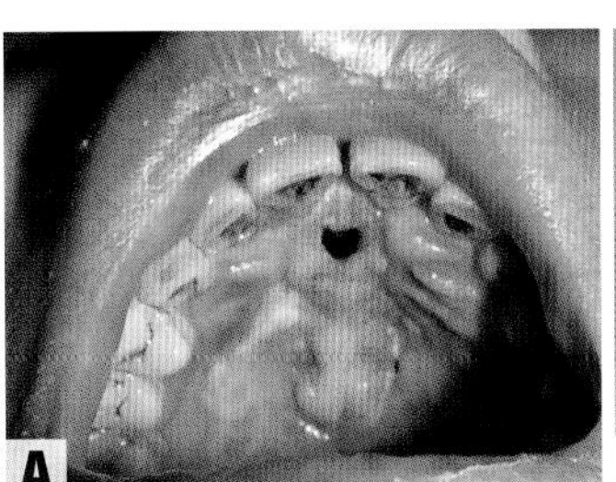

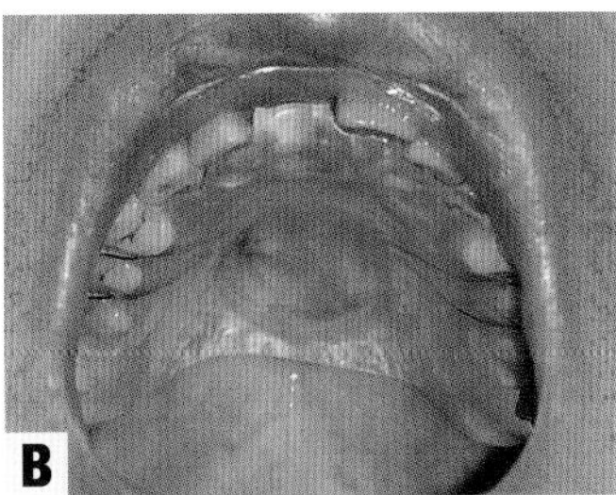

Fig. 5.153 Extranodal NK/T-cell lymphoma. **A** Perforation of the hard palate, with communication between the nasal and oral cavities. **B** The same patient after remission, with an oral obturator that restores normal ingestion and phonation.

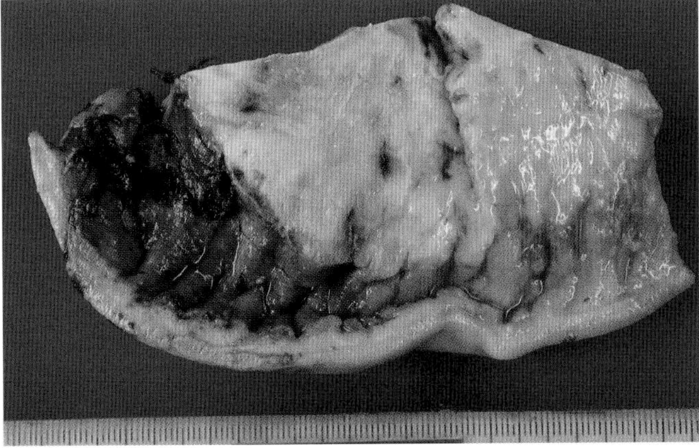

Fig. 5.154 Extranodal NK/T-cell lymphoma. Cut surface of a primary jejunal extranodal NK/T-cell lymphoma specimen showing full-thickness replacement by a fleshy tumour with extensive necrosis.

Localization

ENKTLs can be divided according to the site of primary tumour (not presentation) into two different clinical forms: nasal and non-nasal {620,2172,2170,3895,4095}. The nasal subtype accounts for about 80% of cases; the initially involved sites include the nasal cavity, nasopharynx, oropharynx, Waldeyer ring, epiglottis, and/or aryepiglottic fold. Lesions in the nasal cavity can invade externally into the face or erode the nasal floor, destroying and perforating the hard palate, resulting in the typical clinical appearance of so-called "lethal midline granuloma". Regional lymph nodes may be involved. In late stages, systemic spread can occur, with a predilection for the skin, gastrointestinal tract, testis, liver, spleen, and bone marrow.

The non-nasal subtype accounts for about 20% of cases {2009}. Presentation sites are those commonly involved in the advanced stages of nasal ENKTL, namely the skin, gastrointestinal tract, testis, and miscellaneous sites {2010,743,3895, 3275,3934,1802}. However, for apparently non-nasal cases, if overt or occult nasal involvement is found on clinical or radiological investigations (particularly by PET-CT), they should be reclassified as advanced nasal-subtype ENKTL instead of de novo non-nasal ENKTL {4093}.

Clinical features

Nasal ENKTLs present as nasal blockage, with discharge and bleeding. Involvement of paranasal sinuses leads to infections, and invasion into the orbit can result in visual problems. Perforation of the hard palate leads to communication between the nasal and oral cavities, severely impairing ingestion and phonation. In advanced stages, symptomatology is referable to the organs involved. B symptoms are common, and marrow infiltration may be accompanied by haemophagocytic syndrome with pancytopenia {2306}. Non-nasal ENKTLs are clinically similar to disseminated nasal ENKTLs {4096}. CNS involvement is rare, usually occurring in patients with advanced-stage disease {2007,1999}.

Epidemiology

ENKTL predominantly occurs in eastern Asia and among the Indigenous peoples of Central and South America {3333,181, 4509,4485,3880,2239,3993,744,541}. The incidence in other geographical areas, including Europe and the USA, as well as in other ethnicities, is low {847,1536}. The patients are most often adults (median age: 35–58 years), and there is a male predilection {620,183,4485,1802,4472}. The haplotypes *HLA-DPB1*, *HLA-DRB1*, and *IL18RAP* have been found to predispose eastern Asian populations (in China, including Hong Kong SAR, Macao SAR, and Taiwan; Singapore; Malaysia; and the Republic of Korea) to ENKTL, whereas the haplotype *HLA-A*02:01* appears to be protective in the Japanese population {1876, 2331,2354}.

Etiology

There is a very strong relationship between ENKTL and EBV infection {625,139,620,1064,3333}. The EBV predominantly occurs in a clonal episomal form in the tumour cells and exhibits a type II latency pattern (EBNA1+, LMP1+, LMP2A+, EBNA2−) {4157,3275,1871,625,1866,139,3333}. The EBV subtype in ENKTL is usually type A {1064,251,2748,4445} and commonly shows a deletion of 30 bp in the gene *LMP-1* {703,964,1064}.

ENKTL can occur in the setting of immunosuppression, including after transplantation {2176,1637,4091}. Other risk factors include lifestyle and environmental factors, with an increased risk reported among farmers, pesticide users, and those living near incinerators {4453}.

Pathogenesis

ENKTL demonstrates complex genomic alterations, and the most common chromosomal aberration is deletion of 6q21-25 {2888,1668,2943}, which harbours several candidate tumour suppressor genes, including *PRDM1*, *PTPRK*, *HACE1*, and *FOXO3* {1733,1894,678}. *PRDM1*, which is frequently inactivated by deletion, hypermethylation, and mutation, plays a role in NK-cell homeostasis {2140,989}.

Recurrent mutations identified in ENKTL include those in JAK/STAT pathway genes (*STAT3*, *JAK3*, *STAT5B*), epigenetic regulators (*BCOR*, *KMT2D*, *ARID1A*, *EP300*), tumour suppressor genes (*TP53*, *MGA*), and RNA helicase (*DDX3X*) {3335, 2102,2259,1803}. Constitutive activation of the JAK/STAT pathway through mutations and phosphorylation of JAK/STAT plays a crucial role in ENKTL pathogenesis and is a potential therapeutic target {802,1668,2102,423,2878}. Deregulation of other signalling pathways (e.g. NF-κB and PDGFR) and overexpression of genes (including *BIRC5*, *MYC*, *RUNX3*, *AURKA*, *EZH2*, and *CD274* [*PDL1*]) have also been identified {1668,1734, 2946,4481,3882,2872,3675,3788,4445}. Immune evasion has emerged as a critical pathway for the survival of ENKTL cells and may be a consequence of LMP1-driven or STAT3-driven upregulation of PDL1 {353,3788}.

ENKTL shows epigenetic alterations, including promoter hypermethylation of cell-cycle regulators (*CDKN2A*, *CDKN2B*, and *CDKN1A*) and tumour suppressor genes (*BCL2L11*, *DAPK1*, and *PTPN6*) {1933,2139}. EZH2, a histone methyltransferase, is phosphorylated by JAK-3 and functions as a transcriptional coactivator independently of its enzymatic activity to confer a proliferative advantage in ENKTL {4481,4479}. Deregulation of microRNAs, including miR-26, miR-101, miR-146a, miR-155, and mi-R21, may also play a pathogenetic role {4475,3103, 2947}.

A genomic and transcriptomic study has identified transcriptional defects at the *BART* microRNAs and the disruption of host *NHEJ1* by EBV integration into the host genome {3185}. Frequent intragenic deletions affecting *BART* microRNA clusters have been demonstrated in ENKTL and may reactivate the lytic cycle through the upregulation of BZLF1 and BRLF1, while averting viral production and subsequent cell lysis {3050}. Using a multiomics approach, three ENKTL molecular subtypes have been proposed: the tumour suppressor–immune modulator (TSIM) subtype, the MGA–BRDT (MB) subtype, and the HDAC9–EP300–ARID1A (HEA) subtype {4445}. The TSIM subtype is associated with JAK/STAT activation, *TP53* mutations, NK-cell origin, and PDL1 overexpression. It is characterized by the type II EBV latency programme and expression of the EBV lytic gene *BALF3*, which may increase genomic instability and result in malignant transformation. The MB subtype shows *MGA* mutations, MYC overexpression, type I EBV latency programme, and a poor outcome, whereas the HEA subtype is

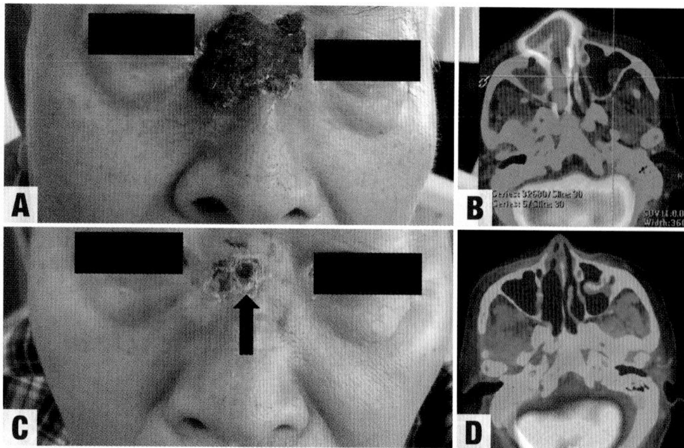

Fig. 5.155 Extranodal NK/T-cell lymphoma. **A** Involvement of the nasal cavity on presentation, with destruction of the nasal bridge and invasion of the overlying skin; PET-CT (**B**) shows a large hypermetabolic lesion. **C** Complete remission after chemotherapy, with a fistula (arrow) between the skin and nasal cavity; PET-CT (**D**) shows complete metabolic remission.

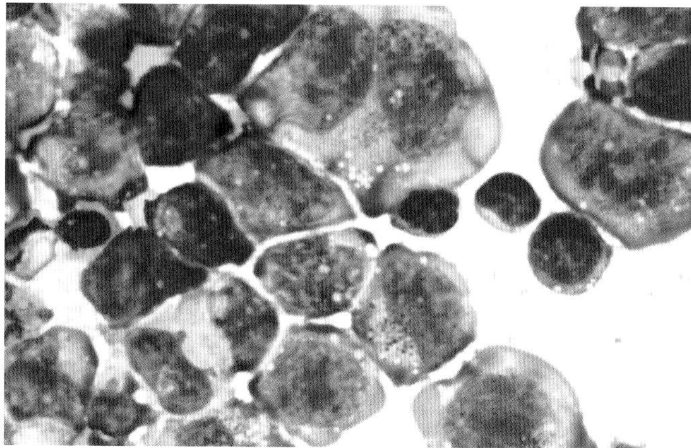

Fig. 5.156 Extranodal NK/T-cell lymphoma. Neoplastic cells in a pleural effusion with large and pleomorphic nuclei and azurophilic granules in the cytoplasm (Giemsa).

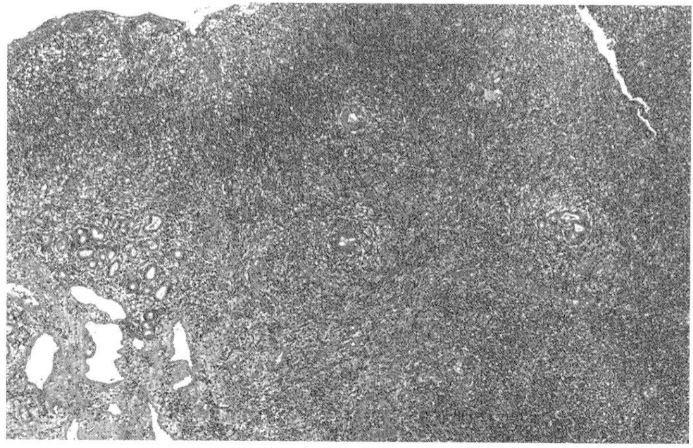

Fig. 5.157 Extranodal NK/T-cell lymphoma. Low magnification shows a diffuse lymphoid infiltrate in the nasal turbinate.

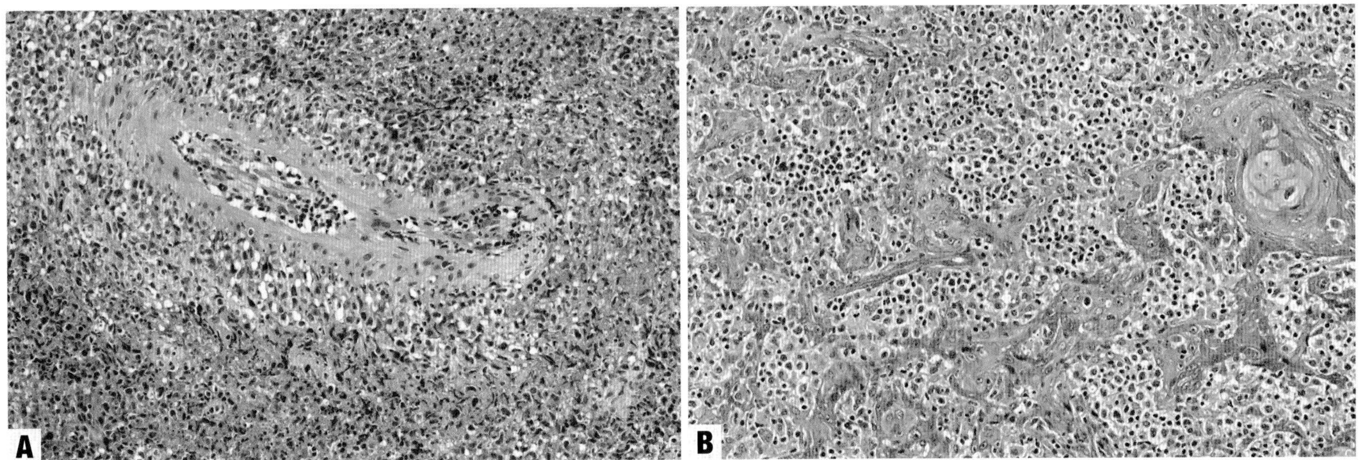

Fig. 5.158 Extranodal NK/T-cell lymphoma. **A** The neoplastic infiltrate has an angiocentric growth pattern. **B** Florid pseudoepitheliomatous hyperplasia mimicking squamous cell carcinoma.

characterized by histone acetylation, NF-κB activation, and a T-cell origin {4445}. In the HEA subtype, there is increased expression of the lytic gene *BNRF1*, encoding a partner of the histone chaperone complex, which may interact with *DAXX* to promote viral latency and cellular immortalization.

Macroscopic appearance

Involved extranodal tissues show a fleshy tumour often accompanied by necrosis and/or ulceration.

Histopathology

ENKTL shows a diffuse, dense, and permeative growth that is commonly but not invariably associated with coagulative necrosis and admixed apoptotic bodies. In mucosal and cutaneous sites, ulceration with superimposed inflammation is common. The overlying intact epithelium can show pseudoepitheliomatous hyperplasia, mimicking squamous cell carcinoma {2364, 4438}. Angiocentric-angiodestructive growth and fibrinoid changes in the blood vessels are common but not invariably present. There can be a heavy admixture of inflammatory cells (small lymphocytes, plasma cells, histiocytes, and eosinophils), mimicking an inflammatory process {1534}. Bone marrow involvement, which is uncommon, usually takes the form of interstitial infiltrate without discrete aggregates.

The cytological spectrum of the lymphoma cells is very broad, ranging from small cells to large and anaplastic cells. Medium-sized cells or mixed small and large cells are most common. The lymphoma cells often have irregularly folded nuclei and a moderate amount of pale to clear cytoplasm. The chromatin is granular, except in the very large cells, which often have vesicular nuclei. Nucleoli are generally inconspicuous or small. Mitotic figures are usually easily found. Histological progression with a predominance of large cells may occur at disease progression, relapse, or metastasis.

Immunohistochemistry and in situ hybridization

The cellular lineage of the tumour cells is either NK or T cell, as determined by the expression of sCD3, CD56, and T-cell receptor proteins, and by TR gene rearrangements {3275,2308, 3934,1802}. T-lineage tumours account for about 40% of cases {3275,3934,1802,1624}. The determination of NK- or T-cell lineage is not necessary for routine diagnosis because it is not of prognostic relevance.

In most cases, the tumour cells are positive for CD2, cCD3ε, and CD56, and negative for sCD3 (as demonstrated on fresh or frozen tissue) and CD5 {1765,621,1761}. However, a CD56-negative immunophenotype can be seen in about 20% of cases {3275,2308,1802}. CD43 and CD45RO are often positive, and

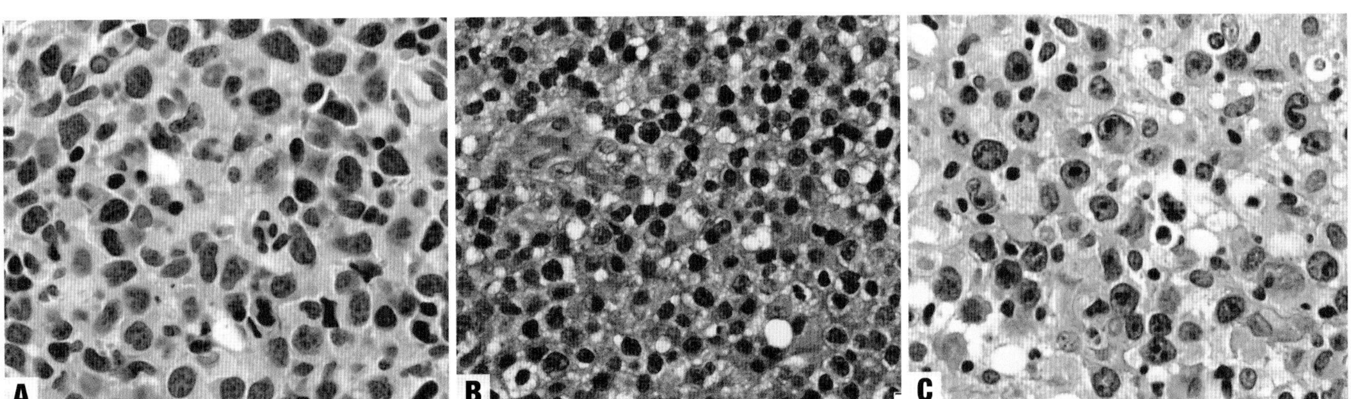

Fig. 5.159 Extranodal NK/T-cell lymphoma. The morphological spectrum is broad, showing pleomorphic medium to large neoplastic cells with irregular nuclear contours (**A**), small atypical lymphocytes with slightly irregular nuclear contours (**B**), and anaplastic large-cell morphology with prominent nucleoli (**C**).

CD7 is variably expressed. Other T and NK cell–associated antigens, including CD4, CD8, CD16, and CD57, are usually negative {3275}. Cases of T-cell lineage often express CD5, CD8, and T-cell receptor (TCRαβ or TCRγδ) and are often CD56-negative {3275,3934,1624}. Cytotoxic molecules (such as TIA1, granzyme B, and perforin) are positive {1064}. HLA-DR, CD25, FAS (CD95), FASL, CXCL13, IRF4 (MUM1), phosphorylated STAT3, and MATK are commonly expressed {2942, 3024,3957,3275}. Rare cases can exhibit aberrant expression of CD20 {1670,1667}. Approximately half of the cases variably express CD30, mainly in the larger cells {2308,2014,1802,1161, 1935}. PDL1 and CD38 are commonly expressed {4300,1810}.

In situ hybridization for EBV-encoded small RNA (EBER) demonstrates the presence of EBV in the majority of viable lymphoma cells.

Differential diagnosis

Table 5.23 lists the major distinguishing features of various lymphoproliferative lesions in the differential diagnosis of ENKTL {743,4526,1806,1677}.

Table 5.23 Differential diagnosis of extranodal NK/T-cell lymphoma (ENKTL)

Disease entity	Major distinguishing features vs ENKTL
EBV-positive nodal T- and NK-cell lymphoma	Predominant nodal localization of disease Coagulative necrosis and angioinvasion usually not prominent Neoplastic cells often large (resembling large B-cell lymphoma) Most cases exhibit T-cell rather than NK-cell phenotype
Aggressive NK-cell leukaemia	Predominately involves peripheral blood and bone marrow Prominent constitutional symptoms Always of NK-cell lineage by definition (whereas ENKTL comprises neoplasms of NK- or T-cell lineage)
Subcutaneous panniculitis-like T-cell lymphoma	In the skin, preferential infiltration of subcutaneous tissue with sparing of the dermis Often CD8+, CD56–, TCRαβ+ EBV–
Primary cutaneous gamma-delta T-cell lymphoma	Expression of TCRγδ by definition (contrasting with its extreme rarity in ENKTL) Usually EBV–
Systemic EBV-positive T-cell lymphoma of childhood	Paediatric and adolescent age group Presentation with systemic disease, including hepatosplenomegaly Lymphoid cells show T-cell phenotype
Monomorphic epitheliotropic intestinal T-cell lymphoma	Most commonly monomorphic infiltrate of medium-sized lymphoid cells (contrasting with the usually polymorphic infiltrate of ENKTL) Necrosis uncommon Often CD8+ (which is very uncommon in ENKTL) EBV–
Indolent NK-cell lymphoproliferative disorder of the gastrointestinal tract	Small lesion(s) in the gastrointestinal tract Usually superficial and non-destructive growth Medium-sized lymphoid cells with distinct eosinophilic cytoplasmic granules Always of NK-cell lineage by definition (whereas ENKTL comprises neoplasms of NK- or T-cell lineage) EBV–
Lymphomatoid granulomatosis	Predominant sites are lung, brain, kidney, and skin (all except skin uncommonly involved in ENKTL) Atypical cells are of B-cell lineage EBV+ in B cells
Granulomatosis with polyangiitis (Wegener granulomatosis)	Serum positive for cytoplasmic antineutrophilic cytoplasmic antibodies (c-ANCAs) or myeloperoxidase antibodies Poorly formed granulomas and microabscesses Necrotizing vasculitis involving arterioles, small arteries, and veins Lack of atypical lymphoid cell infiltrate Lack of lymphoid population with NK-cell or aberrant T-cell immunophenotype EBV–
Acute EBV-positive cytotoxic T-cell lymphoid hyperplasia of upper aerodigestive tract	Children and young adults Acute onset of symptoms, often including fever Atypical lymphoid infiltrate usually CD5+ and CD56– Complete remission within 1 month without cytotoxic therapy

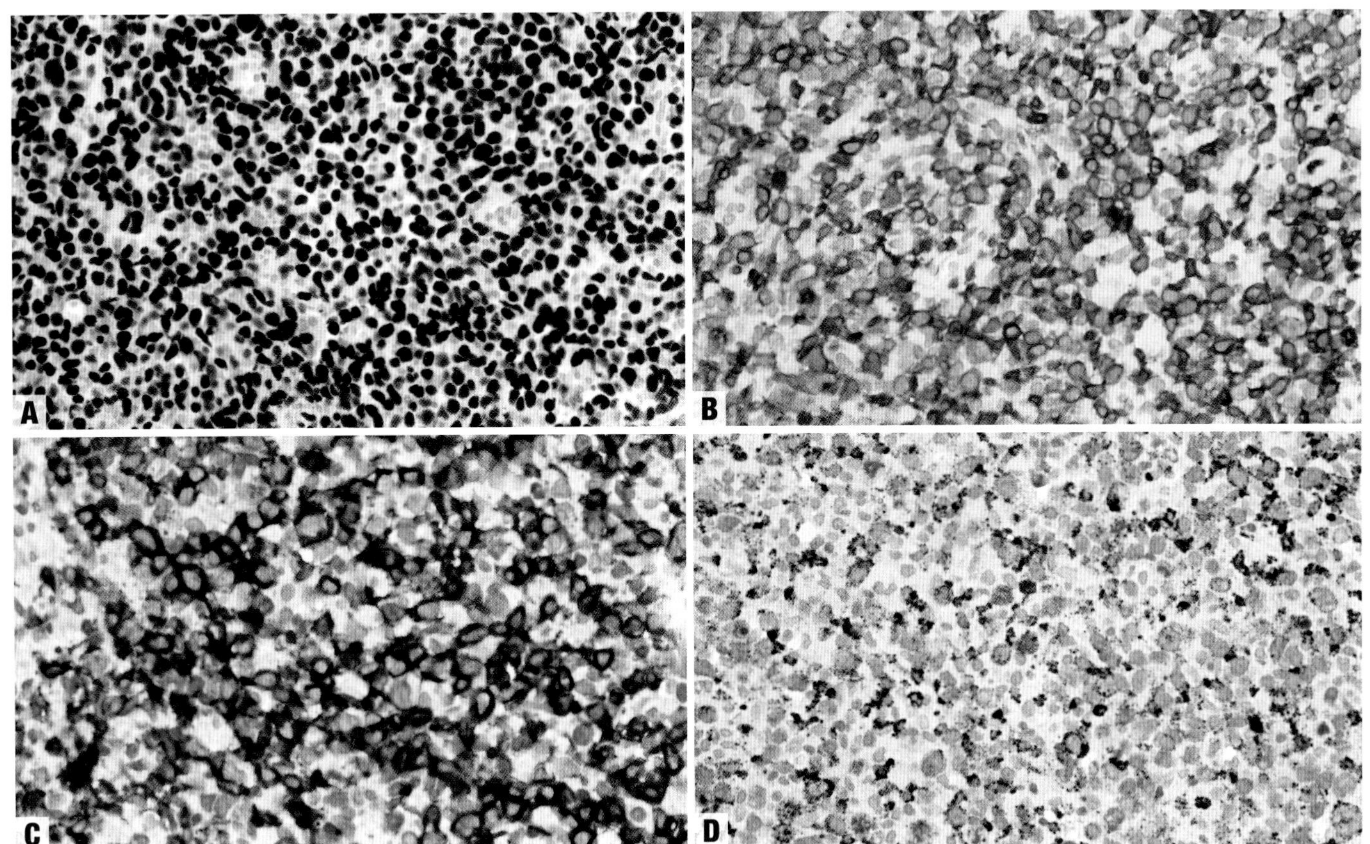

Fig. 5.160 Extranodal NK/T-cell lymphoma. **A** The majority of the neoplastic cells are positive for EBV-encoded small RNA (EBER). **B** Strong staining for cCD3ε is seen. **C** CD56 is expressed in the majority of cases. **D** TIA1 immunohistochemistry shows strong granular staining.

Cytology

Occasionally ENKTL may involve the pleural cavities, and the neoplastic cells seen in cytological preparations are usually large and anaplastic with fine to coarse azurophilic granules in the cytoplasm by Giemsa {2373}.

Diagnostic molecular pathology

In situ hybridization for EBER is positive in the majority of tumour cells. TR gene rearrangement studies may be performed for selected problematic cases {3934}.

Essential and desirable diagnostic criteria

Essential: infiltration of extranodal tissues by lymphoma cells with variable morphology; NK- or cytotoxic T-cell phenotype; majority of tumour cells positive for EBER.

Desirable: angiocentric growth and necrosis.

Staging

Staging is performed according to the Lugano classification {688}. FDG PET-CT is the standard and most accurate radiological staging investigation, because tumour cells of ENKTL are FDG-avid {1979,626,1978}.

Prognosis and prediction

With concurrent or sequential chemoradiotherapy with non–anthracycline-containing regimens, the 5-year overall survival rate is > 70% in patients with early-stage disease {2008,4473, 2175,3315,4472,2174}. L-asparaginase–containing regimens yield an overall response rate of about 80% in patients with advanced-stage disease {2175,4470,4295,4296}.

On presentation, age > 60 years, stage III/IV disease, distant nodal involvement, non-nasal clinical subtype disease, and quantifiable plasma EBV, incorporated into the prognostic index of natural killer lymphoma–EBV (PINK-E) index, predict an unfavourable outcome with non–anthracycline-containing regimens or radiotherapy with curative intent {2009}. Two parameters that reflect dynamic tumour load and chemosensitivity are plasma EBV DNA level {182,3896,1751,1864} and the metabolic phenotype of the tumour by PET-CT {626,1978}. If interim or end-of-treatment plasma EBV DNA and/or PET-CT findings are still positive, the outcome is inferior {1978,2177, 2004}.

Immune checkpoint inhibitors targeting the PD1/PDL1 axis have shown promise in the treatment of relapsed/refractory ENKTL {2173,2344,2006}. It has been proposed that PDL1 expression (in both the tumour cells and tumour-associated macrophages), immune microenvironment subtypes (classified according to FOXP3, PDL1, and CD68 immunohistochemistry), or somatic structural rearrangements in the 3′ untranslated region of *CD274* (*PDL1*) in tumour tissue may predict the response to immune checkpoint inhibitors {2344, 2006}.

EBV-positive T-cell and NK-cell lymphoid proliferations and lymphomas of childhood: Introduction

Chng WJ
Wood BL

Epstein–Barr virus (EBV)-associated lymphoproliferative diseases in the paediatric age group are a group of uncommon disorders characterized by EBV infection of T and NK cells. They are categorized into two major groups: systemic EBV-positive T-cell lymphoma of childhood and chronic active EBV (CAEBV) disease. Both occur with increased frequency in Asian people and in Native Americans from Central and South America and Mexico. Systemic EBV-positive T-cell lymphoma of childhood has a very fulminant clinical course, usually associated with haemophagocytic lymphohistiocytosis (see Box 5.07 for diagnostic criteria {1556}). CAEBV disease shows a broad range of clinical manifestations, from indolent, localized forms such as hydroa vacciniforme lymphoproliferative disorder and severe mosquito bite allergy to more systemic disease characterized by fever, hepatosplenomegaly, and lymphadenopathy, with or without cutaneous manifestations. Additionally, there is significant overlap in the morphological features of these conditions. Therefore, correlation with clinical features is critical for accurate diagnosis (see Table 5.24 for the differential diagnosis). EBV-positive haemophagocytic lymphohistiocytosis is a non-neoplastic and hyperinflammatory disorder triggered by EBV and shows significant overlap in the clinicopathological features with systemic EBV-positive T- and NK-cell lymphoproliferative diseases occurring in children and young adults. Therefore, the salient features of EBV-positive haemophagocytic lymphohistiocytosis have been included in the differential diagnosis table {1677,2013}.

Table 5.24 Clinical and pathological features of EBV-related T-cell and NK-cell lymphoproliferative diseases in childhood and related conditions

Diagnostic criteria	Severe mosquito bite allergy	Hydroa vacciniforme lymphoproliferative disorder (HV-LPD)	Systemic chronic active EBV (CAEBV) disease	Systemic EBV+ T-cell lymphoma (SEBVTCL) of childhood	EBV+ haemophagocytic lymphohistiocytosis (EBV+ HLH)
Localization	Cutaneous disease	Cutaneous (classic form) or systemic (multiorgan) disease	Systemic (multiorgan) disease	Systemic (multiorgan) disease	Systemic (multiorgan) disease
Age of onset	Children and young adults	Children / young adults, occasionally adults	Children / young adults, occasionally adults	Children / young adults, occasionally adults	Children and young adults
Clinical presentation	Fever and skin manifestations after mosquito bites	Recurring papulovesicular eruptions triggered by sun exposure, with or without systemic symptoms	Infectious mononucleosis–like symptoms (fever, lymphadenopathy, hepatosplenomegaly) for ≥ 3 months and/or HLH	Acute and fulminant (≤ 3 months) disease; systemic symptoms with fever, hepatosplenomegaly, and HLH Some arise in setting of CAEBV disease	Variable clinical manifestations, from nonspecific symptoms to acute disease with fever, systemic symptoms, and HLH
Morphology	Variable, small to large cells	Small to medium-sized cells	Variable, often small cells with minimal atypia	Variable, small to large cells, others small without atypia	Small cells without atypia
Lineage/phenotype of T cells	NK >> T	T > NK T cells (CD8 >> CD4)	T > NK T cells (CD4 > CD8)	T only T cells (CD8 >> CD4)	T >> NK (20%) T cells (CD8 >> CD4)
Clonality	Polyclonal (NK), monoclonal (T)	Monoclonal (T)	Monoclonal > oligoclonal or polyclonal	Monoclonal	Polyclonal >> monoclonal
Clinical behaviour	Protracted course Increased risk of HLH, CAEBV disease, ENKTL, or ANKL development	Relapsing and resolution by adolescence or adulthood (classic form) Some progress to systemic disease or lymphoma	Most have a progressive course, with organ complication, HLH, and/or acute transformation Some show an indolent clinical course	Aggressive disease with a fulminant clinical course resulting in multiorgan failure, sepsis, and death, usually within days to weeks of diagnosis	Varies from mild to severe or fatal disease
Treatment	Conservative treatment, HSCT	Conservative treatment Systemic HV-LPD may require HSCT	HLH-based protocols, HSCT	HLH-based protocols, HSCT	Conservative treatment, HLH-based protocol
Comments		Systemic HV-LPD needs to be distinguished from CAEBV disease without HV-LPD, because the latter has a poorer outcome	CAEBV with aggressive disease (≤ 3 months) should be diagnosed as SEBVTCL of childhood		Lack of karyotypic aberrations distinguish EBV+ HLH from SEBVTCL of childhood

ANKL, aggressive NK-cell leukaemia; ENKTL, extranodal NK/T-cell lymphoma; HLH, haemophagocytic lymphohistiocytosis; HSCT, haematopoietic stem cell transplantation.

Box 5.07 Clinical diagnostic criteria for haemophagocytic lymphohistiocytosis, which can be diagnosed if there is a mutation in a known causative gene or if at least five of the diagnostic criteria are met

1. Fever (peak temperature of > 38.5 °C for > 7 days)
2. Splenomegaly (spleen palpable > 30 mm below costal margin)
3. Cytopenia involving more than two cell lineages (haemoglobin < 9 g/dL [90 g/L], absolute neutrophil count < 100/µL [0.10 × 10^9/L], platelets < 100 000/µL [100 × 10^9/L])
4. Hypertriglyceridaemia (fasting triglycerides > 177 mg/dL [2.0 mmol/L] or > 3 standard deviations [SD] more than normal for age) or hypofibrinogenaemia (fibrinogen < 150 mg/dL [1.5 g/L] or > 3 SD less than normal for age)
5. Haemophagocytosis (in biopsy samples of bone marrow, spleen, or lymph nodes)
6. Low or absent NK-cell activity
7. Serum ferritin > 500 ng/mL (> 1123.5 pmol/L [ng/mL])
8. Elevated soluble CD25 (IL-2Ra) levels (> 2400 U/mL or very high for age)

Of note, although the diseases in this group most commonly affect the paediatric age groups, they can also occur in adults. This is especially true for CAEBV disease. There are some changes in the current edition of the WHO classification of haematolymphoid tumours, compared with the previous edition. Hydroa vacciniforme–like lymphoproliferative disorder is now known as hydroa vacciniforme lymphoproliferative disorder (HV-LPD), and two forms of HV-LPD are now recognized: the classic and systemic forms. Systemic HV-LPD is defined by the presence of persistent systemic symptoms of CAEBV disease or extracutaneous disease and should be distinguished from systemic CAEBV disease without HV-LPD. Severe mosquito bite allergy was previously understood to be derived from NK cells, but now it is recognized that a small subset is derived from T cells. Therefore, all of these entities, except for systemic EBV-positive T-cell lymphoma of childhood, can be derived from T or NK cells. The term "chronic active EBV infection" has been changed to "chronic active EBV disease" because it is a condition with an overall poor outcome and is not merely an infection. Lastly, the essential and desirable criteria for each disease are more clearly defined in this edition.

Severe mosquito bite allergy

Kimura H
Araujo I
Kato S
Ng S-B

Definition

Severe mosquito bite allergy is an EBV-positive NK-cell (or occasionally T-cell) lymphoproliferative disorder characterized by high fever and severe skin manifestations including bullae, ulcers, necrosis, and scarring after mosquito bites.

ICD-O coding

None

ICD-11 coding

2B0Y Other specified primary cutaneous mature T-cell or NK-cell lymphomas and lymphoproliferative disorders

Related terminology

Not recommended: hypersensitivity to mosquito bites.

Subtype(s)

None

Localization

Severe mosquito bite allergy is a skin-localized disease.

Clinical features

Severe mosquito bite allergy is characterized by high fever and severe skin manifestations after a mosquito (or, rarely, other insect)

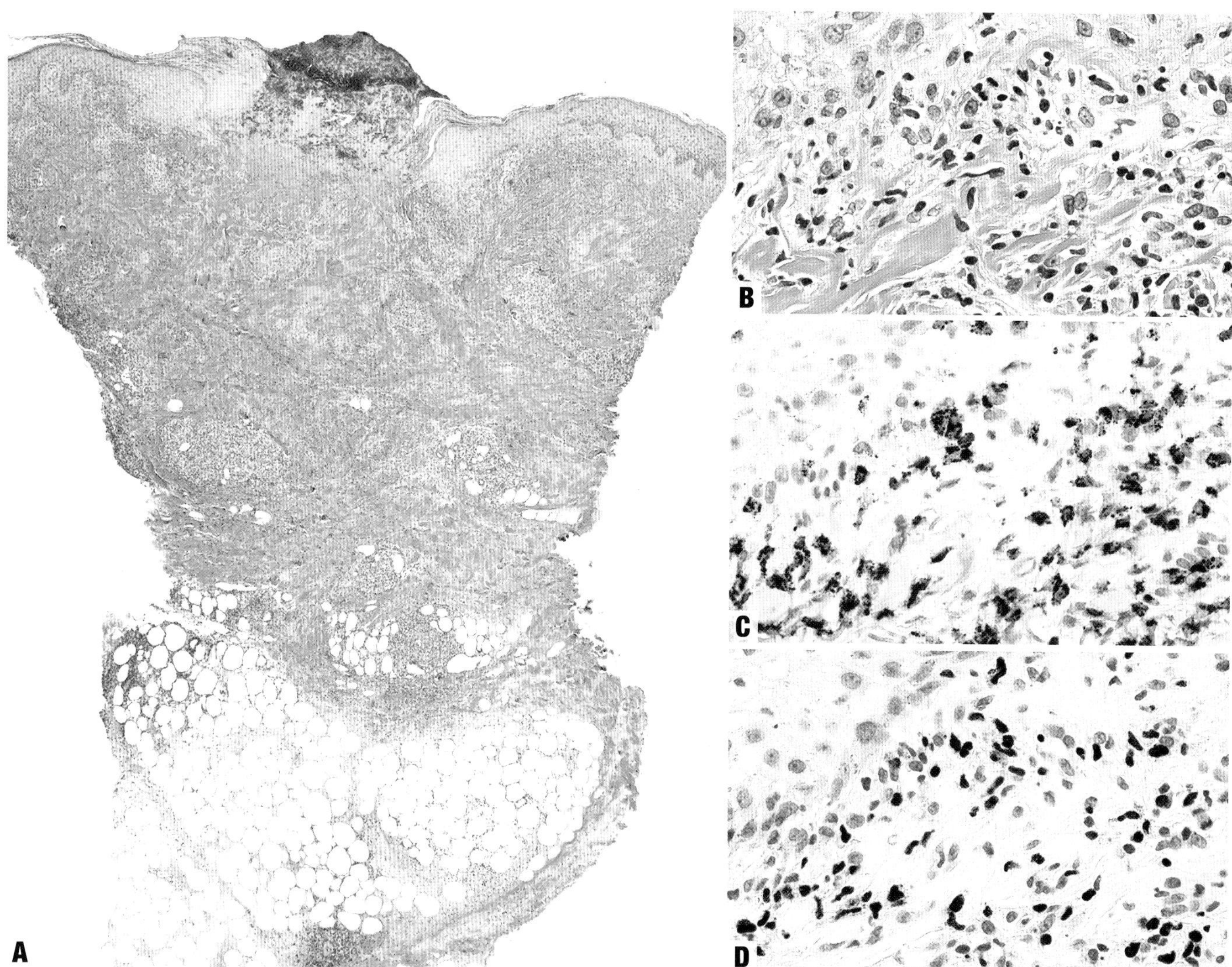

Fig. 5.161 Severe mosquito bite allergy. **A** Skin biopsy at the mosquito bite site showing epidermal necrosis and ulceration, with lymphocytic infiltrate in the dermis. **B** The dermal infiltrate consists of small to medium-sized atypical lymphoid cells. **C** The infiltrating lymphocytes are positive for TIA1. **D** In situ hybridization for EBV-encoded small RNA (EBER) highlights the atypical cells.

bite. The bite area develops blisters, bullae, induration, necrosis, and ulceration, leaving a scar that heals in 2–3 weeks. In addition to a strong local reaction, transient systemic symptoms such as fever, lymphadenopathy, and hepatic dysfunction may occur. Patients have high levels of IgE, EBV DNA, and EBV-infected large granular lymphocytes in the peripheral blood (NK-cell lymphocytosis) {1930,4037}. Some patients also exhibit hydroa vacciniforme–like eruptions in sun-exposed areas {2701,774}.

Epidemiology

Severe mosquito bite allergy is extremely rare. It is mostly reported from eastern Asia {1744,2021,2701,726,4574}, as well as from Mexico, Central America, and South America {3097,3526}. Most cases occur before the age of 20 years, predominantly in children aged < 10 years, and there is no sex predilection {4036}.

Etiology

Genetic background, environmental factors, and EBV strains may play an etiological role {2018}.

Pathogenesis

Severe mosquito bite allergy is a cutaneous form of chronic active EBV disease triggered by a mosquito bite. In the event of a mosquito bite, CD4+ T cells respond to mosquito salivary secretions and induce the reactivation of latently EBV-infected NK cells, which may induce inflammation {157,156}. Strong T helper 2 (Th2)-skewing immune dysregulation leads to high levels of serum IL-13 and IgE {2019,3977}. Basophil activation may also be involved in the development of intense skin reactions {3532}. Somatic mutations, including in *DDX3X*, are detected in EBV-positive cells, indicating that this may be a neoplastic disease {3050}.

Macroscopic appearance

The macroscopic appearance corresponds to the clinical features.

Histopathology

There is a variably dense infiltration of small, medium, and large atypical lymphoid cells, with a perivascular distribution in the dermis and subcutaneous tissue. An angiocentric and angiodestructive growth pattern is typically present in more advanced lesions, resulting in necrosis, ulceration, and bulla formation {4036}.

Immunohistochemistry and in situ hybridization

Most cases exhibit an NK-cell immunophenotype, and some exhibit a T-cell phenotype {2021}. NK cells are negative for sCD3 and T-cell receptor proteins, but are positive for CD3ε, CD16, CD56, and cytotoxic markers such as TIA1 and granzyme B. Lymphoid cells are positive for EBV-encoded small RNA (EBER) by in situ hybridization {2021}.

Differential diagnosis

Mosquito bites may occasionally cause severe erythema, swelling, and blistering in healthy people, but unlike in severe mosquito bite allergy, there is usually no fever or ulceration. Hydroa vacciniforme lymphoproliferative disorder is morphologically identical to severe mosquito bite allergy but is distinguished by the clinical manifestations. Patients with persistent systemic symptoms are classified as having systemic chronic active EBV disease {2019,2020,4468}.

Cytology

Not relevant

Diagnostic molecular pathology

Demonstration of clonality of the NK cells is not required for the diagnosis of severe mosquito bite allergy. However, identification of a clonal expansion is indicative of a malignant evolution {4468}.

Essential and desirable diagnostic criteria

Essential: high fever and severe skin manifestations after mosquito bites; bite site biopsy showing lymphoid infiltrate with an NK-cell or (less commonly) T-cell phenotype; EBER positivity.

Desirable: high circulating EBV DNA load; lack of T-cell receptor protein expression and/or clonal TR gene rearrangement in cases of NK-cell origin.

Staging

Not relevant

Prognosis and prediction

The disease is protracted and associated with an increased risk for haemophagocytic lymphohistiocytosis, chronic active EBV disease, aggressive NK-cell leukaemia, and extranodal NK/T-cell lymphoma {4036,2971,2021}. Late-onset disease (> 9 years of age) and expression of an EBV-encoded immediate early gene transcript, BZLF1, correlate with a poor prognosis {2701}.

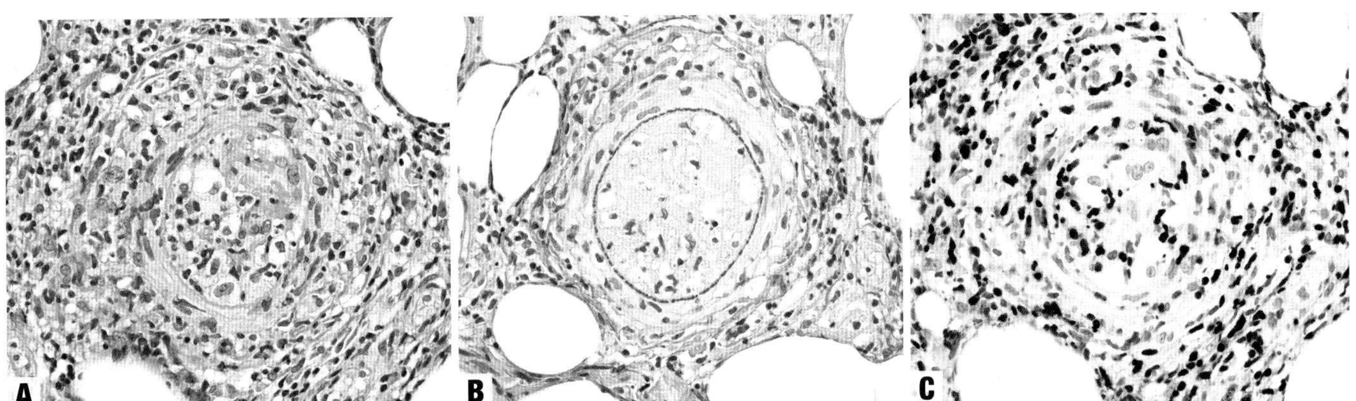

Fig. 5.162 Severe mosquito bite allergy. Small to medium-sized atypical cells show an angiocentric and angiodestructive growth pattern in H&E stain (**A**) and in a corresponding Victoria blue stain (**B**). The infiltrating lymphocytes are positive for EBV-encoded small RNA (EBER) by in situ hybridization (**C**).

Hydroa vacciniforme lymphoproliferative disorder

Kimura H
Araujo I
Chan JKC
Gru A
Plaza JA
Rao HL
Sangueza JM

Definition

Hydroa vacciniforme lymphoproliferative disorder (HV-LPD) is a cutaneous form of chronic active EBV disease that spans a range of behaviour, from the classic form with self-limited photodermatosis to the systemic form with extensive skin lesions and multiorgan involvement.

ICD-O coding

9725/1 Hydroa vacciniforme lymphoproliferative disorder

ICD-11 coding

2B0Y & XH0AK5 Other specified primary cutaneous mature T-cell or NK-cell lymphomas and lymphoproliferative disorders & Hydroa vacciniforme–like lymphoproliferative disorder

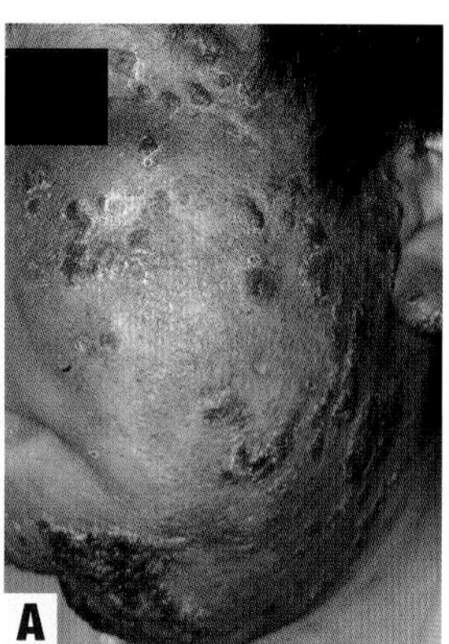

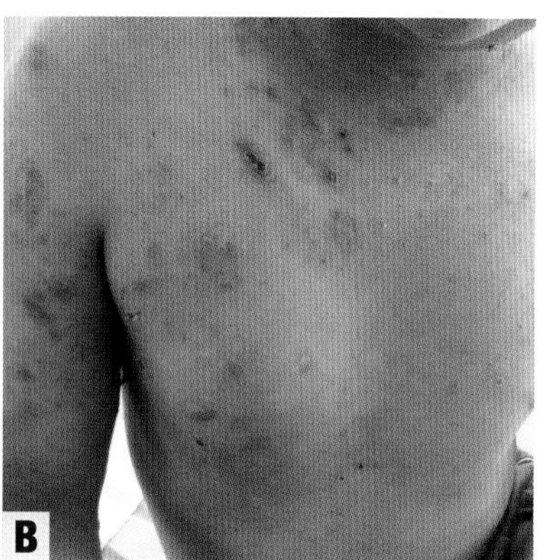

Fig. 5.163 Hydroa vacciniforme lymphoproliferative disorder. **A** In sun-exposed skin on the face, extensive papulovesicular eruptions with crusts, scars, and oedema are present. **B** In non–sun-exposed skin on arms and chest, lesions are limited.

Related terminology

Not recommended: severe hydroa vacciniforme; hydroa vacciniforme–like lymphoma; hydroa vacciniforme–like lymphoproliferative disorder.

Subtype(s)

Classic HV-LPD; systemic HV-LPD. (See Table 5.25.)

Localization

In the classic form, sun-exposed skin is involved. In the systemic form, there is often involvement of non–sun-exposed skin as well, in addition to multiorgan involvement (e.g. liver, spleen, lymph nodes, and very rarely, lung) {3337}.

Clinical features

Classic HV-LPD is characterized by recurring papulovesicular eruptions on sun-exposed skin that usually evolve to blisters and ulcers, leaving varioliform atrophic scars. The skin lesions often show seasonal variation, with recurrences in spring and summer. Although some cases resolve during adolescence, some have a more protracted course. In systemic HV-LPD, lesions are not clearly induced or exacerbated by sun exposure {2474}. As the disease progresses, there are severe and extensive skin lesions in sun-exposed and non–sun-exposed areas, accompanied by systemic manifestations, including fever, hepatosplenomegaly, hepatitis, lymphadenopathy, and haemophagocytic syndrome. Rare cases show an atypical clinical presentation including

Table 5.25 Major clinical and pathological features of hydroa vacciniforme lymphoproliferative disorder (HV-LPD)

Diagnostic criteria	Classic HV-LPD	Systemic HV-LPD
Skin lesions	Sun-exposed areas	Sun-exposed and non–sun-exposed areas
Extracutaneous disease	No	Yes
Persistent (≥ 3 months) systemic symptoms	No	Yes
EBV-infected cells	γδ T cells	αβ T cells
Features of systemic CAEBV: • Lymphadenopathy • Hepatosplenomegaly • Hepatitis • HLH	Absent	≥ 1 present
Ethnicity	More common in White populations	More common in non-White populations
EBV DNA levels in blood	Low	High
Cases with presence of T-cell clone	30%	83%
Prognosis and treatment	Good outcome, conservative treatment	High risk of disease progression, often requires haematopoietic stem cell transplantation

CAEBV, chronic active EBV; HLH, haemophagocytic lymphohistiocytosis (diagnosed when at least five of the following eight diagnostic criteria are met: fever, splenomegaly, cytopenia of at least two cell lines, hypertriglyceridaemia, hyperferritinaemia, haemophagocytosis, elevated soluble CD25 [IL-2Ra], and low/absent NK-cell activity).

prominent periorbital or lip oedema associated with systemic symptoms {2474,3267}. Clinical progression is heralded by a lack of improvement with photoprotection, severe facial and lip swelling, and systemic complications. Rare patients have concomitant severe mosquito bite allergy {1591}.

Epidemiology

HV-LPD is uncommon. It is seen mainly in children and adolescents from Asia (the Republic of Korea; Japan; Taiwan, China) and autochthonous populations of South and Central America (Guatemala, Peru) and Mexico, and it is rare in White populations. The median age is 16 years (range: 4–60 years). There is a slight male predilection (M:F ratio: 2:1) {2385,3337,3567,250,977}.

Etiology

EBV infection is a key factor, and genetic/ethnic predisposition may play a role {777}. An expansion of EBV-infected γδ T cells is well documented in the peripheral blood and blisters of patients with the classic form; αβ T cells are more common in the systemic form {4262,1591,4263}.

Pathogenesis

Most cases show clonal rearrangements of the TR genes, and EBV is usually present in a clonal form. Although LMP1 is often negative by immunohistochemistry, it can be detected in most cases by PCR in the peripheral blood, indicating type II EBV latency {2385,3337,3567,250,777,1426,4288,4455}.

Genetic and environmental factors appear to account for differences in the clinical behaviour of HV-LPD, which seems to be more indolent in White populations {777}. The mutation landscape of the disease is poorly characterized, and the presence of a T-cell clone does not predict the clinical behaviour of the disease {777}.

Macroscopic appearance

The macroscopic appearance corresponds to the clinical features.

Histopathology

The skin shows epidermal reticular degeneration evolving to intraepidermal vesiculation and sometimes ulceration. There is a perivascular and periadnexal infiltrate of atypical small to medium-sized lymphoid cells in the dermis, occasionally extending into the subcutis. Angiodestruction and necrosis are often present {2385,3337,3567,2475,2749}.

Immunohistochemistry and in situ hybridization

In most cases, the lymphoid cells have a CD8+ cytotoxic phenotype, expressing TIA1, granzyme B, or perforin. Variable expression of surface TCR is present. A higher prevalence of a CD4+ cytotoxic or double-positive CD4+/CD8+ phenotype has been reported in Chinese patients {2385,1452}. Less commonly, the lymphoid cells have an NK-cell phenotype (CD56+, CD5−, surface TCR−); such cases often show prominent subcutis involvement, morphologically mimicking subcutaneous panniculitis-like T-cell lymphoma {2385,3337,3567,1755}. Variable numbers of lymphoid cells show positive staining on in situ hybridization for EBV-encoded small RNA (EBER).

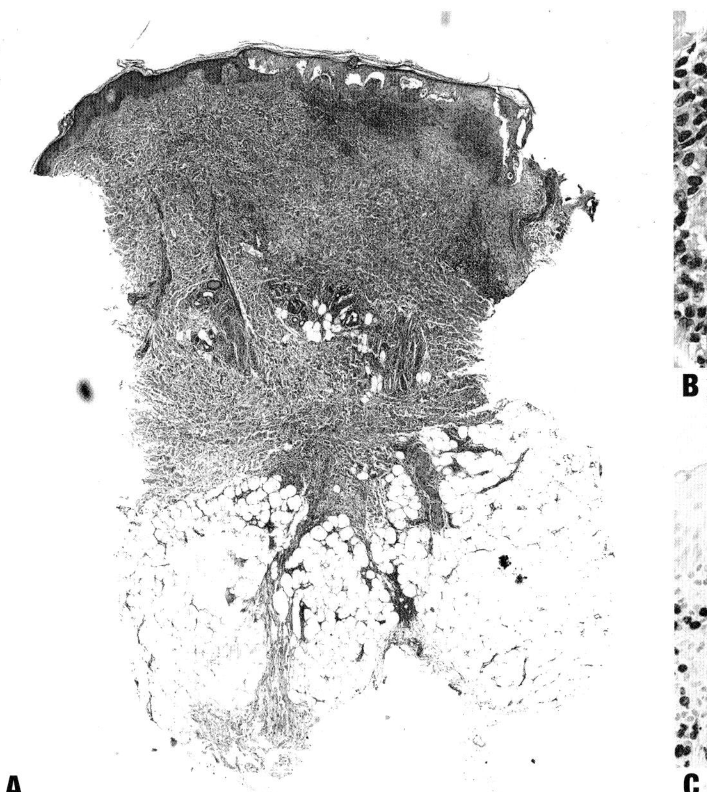

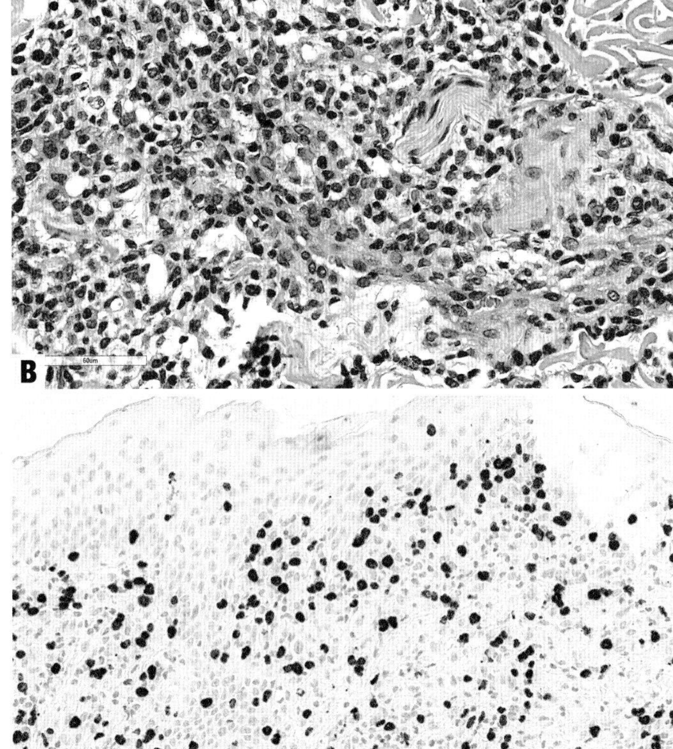

Fig. 5.164 Hydroa vacciniforme lymphoproliferative disorder. **A** At low magnification, the lymphoid infiltrate is centred in the dermis, showing a superficial and deep perivascular pattern involving the subcutaneous fat, with associated epidermal necrosis. **B** The lymphoid infiltrate is composed of a dense population of atypical lymphocytes of intermediate size. **C** The atypical cells are positive for EBV, as demonstrated by EBV-encoded small RNA (EBER) in situ hybridization.

Cytology
Not relevant

Diagnostic molecular pathology
In addition to in situ hybridization for EBER, demonstration of clonal TR gene rearrangements may help support the diagnosis.

Essential and desirable diagnostic criteria
Essential: papulovesicular skin eruption with or without photoexacerbation that heals with varioliform scarring; perivascular and periadnexal atypical lymphoid infiltrate of cytotoxic T or NK cells; EBER positivity; classic HV-LPD: no persistent systemic manifestations (i.e. fever, lymphadenopathy, hepatosplenomegaly, hepatitis, or haemophagocytic syndrome) or NK-cell lymphocytosis); systemic HV-LPD: at least one of the above-mentioned systemic manifestations, NK-cell lymphocytosis, or signs of extracutaneous disease.

Staging
None

Prognosis and prediction
The clinical course is variable. Classic HV-LPD often pursues a relapsing course, with complete resolution of the disease by adolescence or adulthood; this clinical outcome is apparently much more often seen in White populations {777}. Currently, there are no guidelines for the treatment of HV-LPD. For early-stage HV-LPD affecting children and young adults, conservative treatment with photoprotection and topical steroids may be used. Recent clinical studies suggest that systemic HV-LPD can be temporarily controlled with immunomodulators (thalidomide, antivirals, interferon), but only haematopoietic stem cell transplantation can lead to remission in patients with systemic disease or lymphoma {3497}. It is important to distinguish HV-LPD from systemic chronic active EBV disease without HV-LPD, because the latter is invariably fatal in the absence of haematopoietic stem cell transplantation {777}.

T-cell clonality, the number of EBV-positive cells, and the density of the lymphoid infiltrate do not correlate with the clinical course {3337,2701}. Late-onset disease (> 9 years of age) and expression of an EBV-encoded immediate early gene transcript, BZLF1, are correlated with a poor prognosis {2701}.

Systemic chronic active EBV disease

Araujo I
Kimura H
Liu WP
Sangüeza OP

Definition

Systemic chronic active EBV (CAEBV) disease is characterized by a systemic proliferation of polyclonal, oligoclonal, or (often) monoclonal EBV-positive T or NK cells, with symptoms persisting for > 3 months.

ICD-O coding

9725/1 Systemic chronic active EBV-positive disease

ICD-11 coding

2B0Y & XH6TZ4 Other specified primary cutaneous mature T-cell or NK-cell lymphomas and lymphoproliferative disorders & Systemic EBV-positive T-cell lymphoproliferative disease of childhood

Related terminology

Not recommended: chronic active EBV infection; severe chronic active EBV infection; chronic active EBV disease (T- and NK-cell phenotype); chronic active EBV infection of T- and NK-cell type, systemic form.

Subtype(s)

None

Localization

This systemic disease involves multiple sites, most commonly the spleen and the liver, followed by the bone marrow, lymph nodes, skin, and lungs {774,2020}.

Clinical features

Symptoms are caused by organ infiltration of EBV-infected T or NK cells and hypercytokinaemia from the reactive immune cells {2018,774}. Accompanying symptoms are fever, lymphadenopathy, hepatosplenomegaly, anaemia, thrombocytopenia, diarrhoea, uveitis, interstitial pneumonia, CNS involvement, myocarditis, and coronary aneurysm {3038,2020,2022}. Patients frequently present with haemophagocytic lymphohistiocytosis. Complications include multiorgan failure, hypersplenism, disseminated intravascular coagulation, and gastrointestinal ulcer/perforation. Some patients show skin manifestations such as severe mosquito bite allergy, hydroa vacciniforme lymphoproliferative disorder, and prominent lip or periorbital oedema {1934,4502}. The disease may evolve to malignant lymphoma or leukaemia {774,775}.

Epidemiology

Systemic CAEBV disease is uncommon and occurs mostly in children and young adults of eastern Asia {2020,2021,3021,1623,53}. It has also been reported in Central and South America {3650,3789A} but rarely in White populations. Systemic CAEBV disease is uncommon in adults. There is no sex predilection.

Etiology

The strong ethnic/geographical predisposition suggests that genetic polymorphisms in genes related to the immune response or EBV strains are responsible for the development of the disease {3038,2018}. Inherited immunodeficiency is unlikely in most cases, because germline mutations are rare {3050}.

Pathogenesis

EBV shows a type II latency programme with a lack of expression of the immunodominant antigens, thereby imparting an advantage in immune evasion {2017}. Somatic mutations in driver genes including *DDX3X* are detected in EBV-positive cells {3050}. These cells expand and may evolve to overt leukaemia or lymphoma. The EBV genome harbours frequent intragenic deletions (seen in 27 of 77 cases in a reported series), suggesting a unique role for these mutations in the development of the disease {3050}.

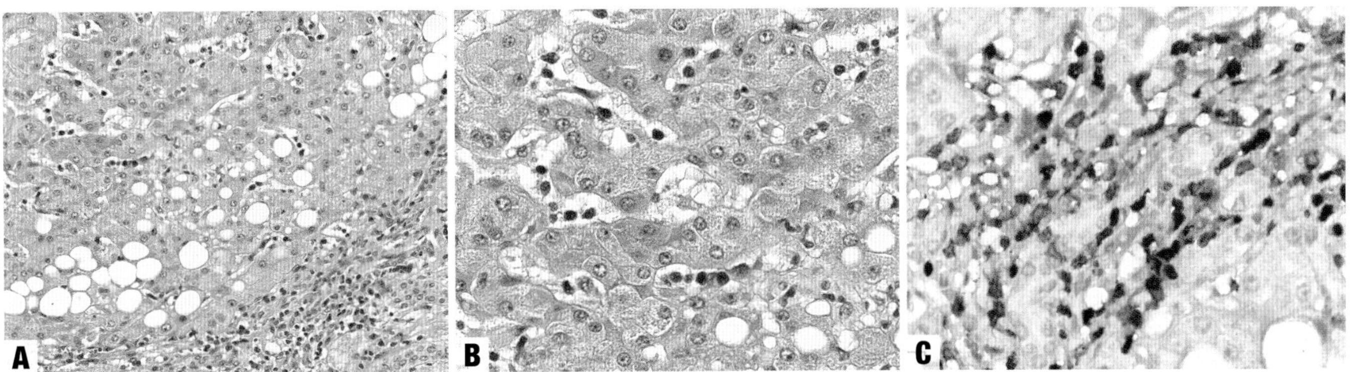

Fig. 5.165 Systemic chronic active EBV disease, liver involvement. **A** The neoplastic cells infiltrate the hepatic sinusoids and portal area. **B** The neoplastic cells infiltrating the hepatic sinusoids are small to medium-sized and lack cytological atypia. **C** Immunohistochemistry and EBV-encoded small RNA (EBER) in situ hybridization double staining: some of the EBER-positive cells (brown) are also positive for CD8 (red).

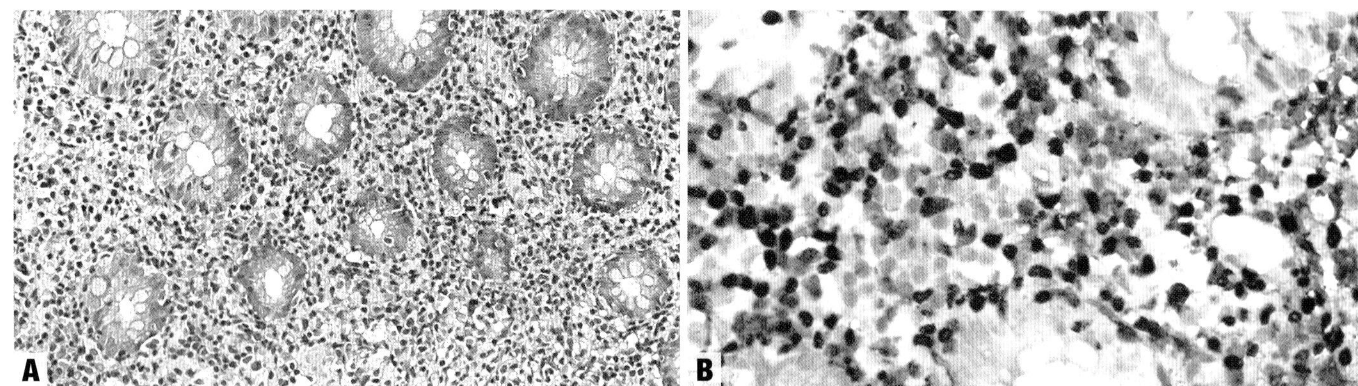

Fig. 5.166 Systemic chronic active EBV disease in intestine. **A** A dense lymphoid infiltrate is present in the mucosa. **B** Immunohistochemistry and EBV-encoded small RNA (EBER) in situ hybridization: some of the EBER-positive cells (brown) are also positive for CD3 (red).

Macroscopic appearance

Not relevant

Histopathology

The bone marrow, liver, and spleen are involved by a subtle or sinusoidal infiltrate of lymphoid cells, which are often small and without atypia. The lymph nodes frequently show paracortical hyperplasia and polymorphic proliferation of lymphoid cells admixed with other inflammatory cells. Haemophagocytosis is present in cases with haemophagocytic lymphohistiocytosis {1677,2013}.

Immunohistochemistry and in situ hybridization

The lymphoid cells are positive for CD3 and cytotoxic markers (TIA1, granzyme B) and are more commonly of T-cell than NK-cell lineage {2021}. T-lineage cells often express TCRαβ and CD4, and a minority are positive for CD8 and/or TCRγ {2019,2021}. CD56 may be expressed, particularly in NK-lineage cells. Some patients have EBV infection of both T cells and NK cells, as demonstrated by EBV-encoded small RNA (EBER) {3871,3007,3050}.

Cytology

Not relevant

Diagnostic molecular pathology

Systemic CAEBV disease is usually monoclonal, based on TR gene rearrangement or EBV clonality, but it can also be oligoclonal or polyclonal {2021}.

Essential and desirable diagnostic criteria

Essential: infectious mononucleosis–like symptoms persisting for > 3 months; increased EBV DNA in peripheral blood or EBER-positive cells in affected organs with evidence of EBV infection in T or NK cells; exclusion of known immunodeficiency, malignancy, or autoimmune disorders.

Staging

Not applicable

Prognosis and prediction

The prognosis is generally poor, although some patients have an indolent clinical course {2022,2021}. Cases with monomorphic and monoclonal proliferation have a poorer outcome than those with polymorphic and polyclonal proliferation {3021}. As the disease progresses, organ complications, haemophagocytic lymphohistiocytosis, and acute transformation (malignant lymphoma, leukaemia) can lead to death. Adult-onset cases are even more rapidly progressive {1747A,4502}. Onset age > 8 years and thrombocytopenia are risk factors for mortality {2022,1934}. Haematopoietic stem cell transplantation is currently the only curative treatment {2021,4502}, and non-myeloablative transplantation with reduced-intensity conditioning has shown good results {1379,1929}.

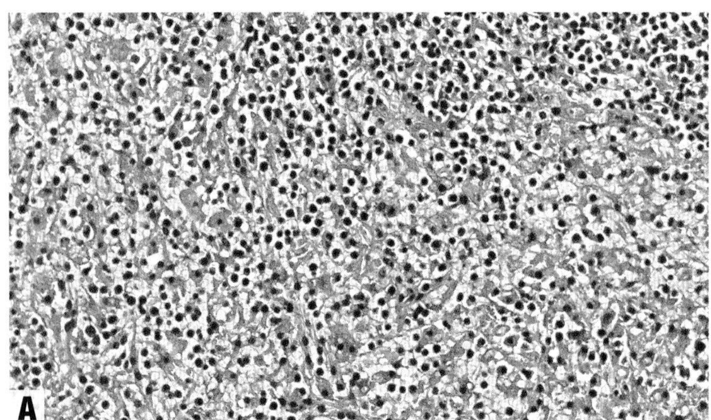

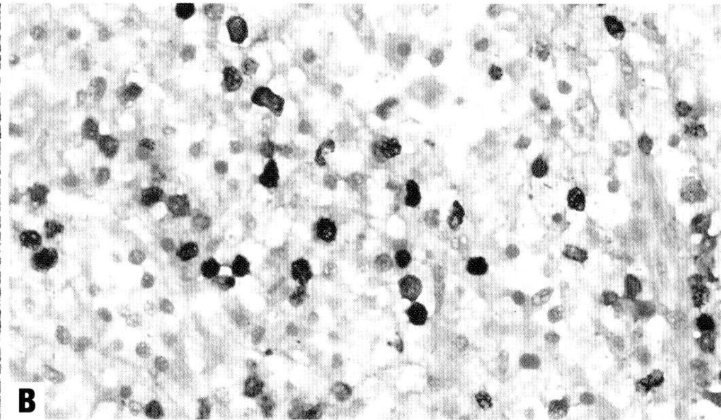

Fig. 5.167 Systemic chronic active EBV disease, spleen involvement. **A** The infiltrating lymphocytes of the red pulp are small to medium-sized, without atypia. **B** Immunohistochemistry and EBV-encoded small RNA (EBER) in situ hybridization double staining: some of the EBER-positive cells (brown) are also positive for CD3 (red).

Systemic EBV-positive T-cell lymphoma of childhood

Marcogliese AN
Araujo I
Liu WP
Ng S-B
Sangueza JM

Definition

Systemic EBV-positive T-cell lymphoma (SEBVTCL) of childhood is a clonal proliferation of EBV-infected cytotoxic T cells occurring in immunocompetent children and young adults, often associated with haemophagocytic lymphohistiocytosis (HLH), systemic symptoms, multiorgan involvement, and a rapidly fatal course.

ICD-O coding

9724/3 Systemic EBV-positive T-cell lymphoma of childhood

ICD-11 coding

2A90.4 Systemic Epstein–Barr virus–positive T-cell lymphoma of childhood

Related terminology

Not recommended: fulminant EBV-positive T-cell lymphoproliferative disorder of childhood; sporadic fatal infectious mononucleosis; severe chronic active EBV (CAEBV) infection; severe CAEBV with monoclonal EBV-positive T-cell proliferation; fatal EBV-associated haemophagocytic syndrome; fulminant haemophagocytic syndrome.

Subtype(s)

None

Localization

This disease is systemic and involves multiple sites, the most common being the spleen and the liver, followed by the bone marrow, lymph nodes, skin, and lungs {1992,2020,3336,3860, 3891}. CNS involvement is uncommon.

Clinical features

Previously healthy, immunocompetent individuals develop symptoms of infectious mononucleosis, with fever, general malaise, and/or upper respiratory symptoms after primary EBV infection. Within a period of weeks, the patients develop hepatosplenomegaly and liver failure, sometimes accompanied by lymphadenopathy and skin rash. Laboratory tests show pancytopenia, abnormal liver function tests, hyperferritinaemia, and high EBV viral loads, often with low or absent anti-VCA IgM antibodies. The disease is usually complicated by HLH, coagulopathy, multiorgan failure, and sepsis {3336,771,3442}. Some cases occur in the setting of well-documented systemic CAEBV disease {3336,1825,1868,771}.

Epidemiology

Most cases have been reported from Asia {1992,2020,3860, 3891,680}, but the disease has also been reported in autochthonous populations of Mexico, Central and South America, USA, and Europe {3336,774,771}. It occurs most often in children and young adults, although rare cases have been reported in older adults {4317}. There is no sex predilection {3891,4317}.

Etiology

The association with primary EBV infection and the geographical and ethnic predilection of the disease suggest an undefined genetic defect in the host immune response to EBV {776,2020, 3336,3891,771}. Some cases arise as a transformation and progression from systemic CAEBV disease.

Pathogenesis

EBV, present in a clonal episomal form {1825,1992,2020,3891}, belongs to type A EBV, either with wildtype *LMP1* or variant 30 bp deletion of *LMP1* {3891,1902}. Although some cases show cytogenetic abnormalities, no defining recurrent abnormalities have been described {771,667,2020,3766}. The molecular and phenotypic signature is similar to that of extranodal NK/T-cell lymphoma, with overexpression of p53, survivin, and EZH2. Gene expression profiling studies reveal distinctive enrichment of stem cell–related genes in SEBVTCL of childhood compared with extranodal NK/T-cell lymphoma {2944}.

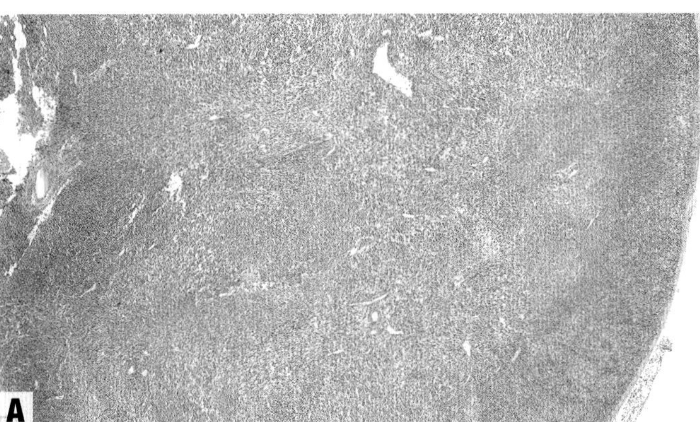

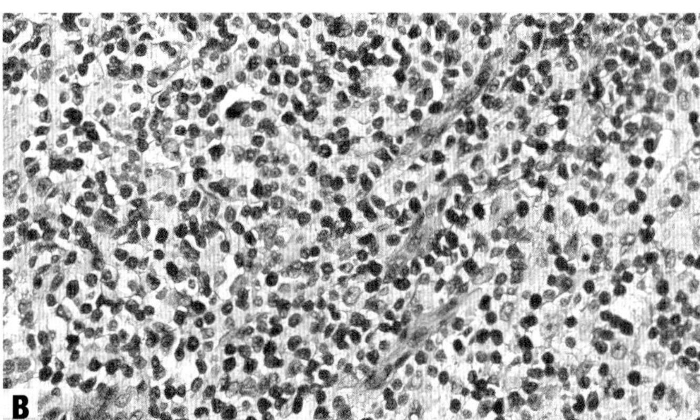

Fig. 5.168 Systemic EBV-positive T-cell lymphoma of childhood. **A** Low-magnification view of a lymph node showing partial preservation of the architecture and expanded interfollicular area. **B** At higher magnification, the infiltrating lymphocytes are pleomorphic and small to medium-sized, with darkly stained chromatin and irregular nuclei.

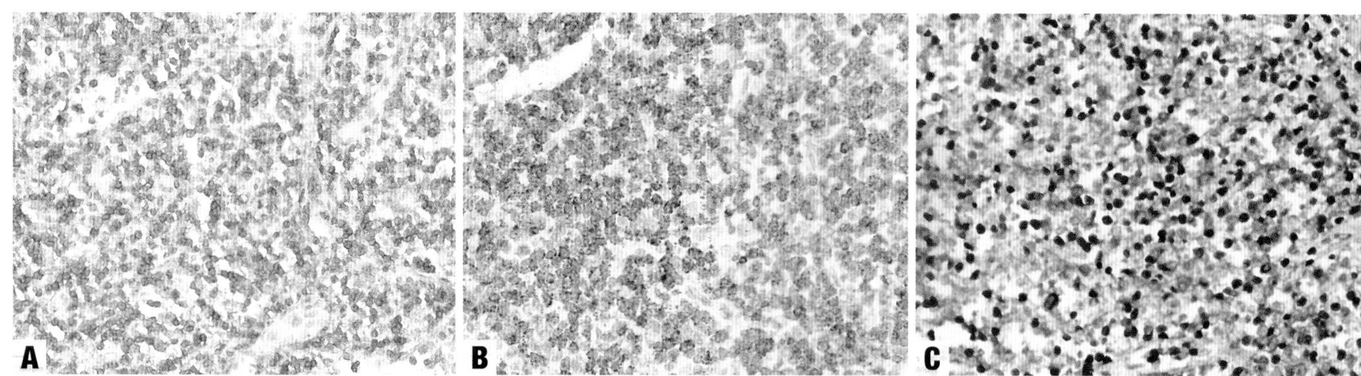

Fig. 5.169 Systemic EBV-positive T-cell lymphoma of childhood. The infiltrating lymphocytes are CD8-positive (**A**) and TIA1-positive (**B**). **C** Immunochemistry and EBV-encoded small RNA (EBER) in situ hybridization double staining shows EBER-positive cells (brown) that are also positive for CD8 (red).

Macroscopic appearance

Not relevant

Histopathology

The involved tissues show infiltration by lymphoid cells that can exhibit a broad cytological spectrum, ranging from small to large atypical lymphoid cells with hyperchromatic and irregular nuclei. However, small cells lacking significant cytological atypia are most common {3336,680,983}.

The liver shows mild to prominent portal and sinusoidal lymphoid infiltration, and cholestasis, steatosis, and necrosis can occur {4317,771,3336}. The spleen shows variable sinusoidal infiltration by abnormal lymphoid cells, accompanied by white pulp atrophy {3336,680}.

Lymph nodes, when involved, usually show distorted rather than effaced architecture, and open sinuses. The B-cell areas are depleted, and the paracortical areas are minimally to markedly expanded by a subtle to dense atypical lymphoid infiltrate. A variable degree of sinus histiocytosis with erythrophagocytosis may be present {771,3336}. Bone marrow biopsies usually show subtle lymphoid infiltrates with EBV-encoded small RNA (EBER) positivity and histiocytic proliferation with or without haemophagocytosis {771,4317}.

Immunohistochemistry and in situ hybridization

The neoplastic cells are typically CD2+ (bright), CD3+ (dim), CD56−, and TIA1+, with aberrant loss of CD5 and CD7. Most cases secondary to acute primary EBV infection are CD8+ {3336,983,771,680,774}, whereas cases arising in systemic CAEBV disease are usually CD4+ {1825,1868,3336,771}. Rare cases exhibit a CD4+, CD8+ phenotype {771,3336}. In situ hybridization for EBER shows that the majority of infiltrating lymphoid cells are positive.

Differential diagnosis

Differential diagnoses include other EBV-positive T- and NK-cell lymphoproliferative disorders such as systemic CAEBV disease {3021,4502}, EBV-positive nodal T- and NK-cell lymphoma, aggressive NK-cell leukaemia, and EBV-associated HLH {771,3766}. The distinction between EBV-positive HLH and SEBVTCL of childhood is often difficult, because aberrant T-cell immunophenotype and clonal TR gene rearrangements can be seen in both entities. The presence of a clonal cytogenetic abnormality would favour SEBVTCL of childhood {3766,1069}.

Cytology

Not relevant

Diagnostic molecular pathology

The diagnosis may be supported by clonal TR gene rearrangements. A few studies have demonstrated type A EBV {3336}.

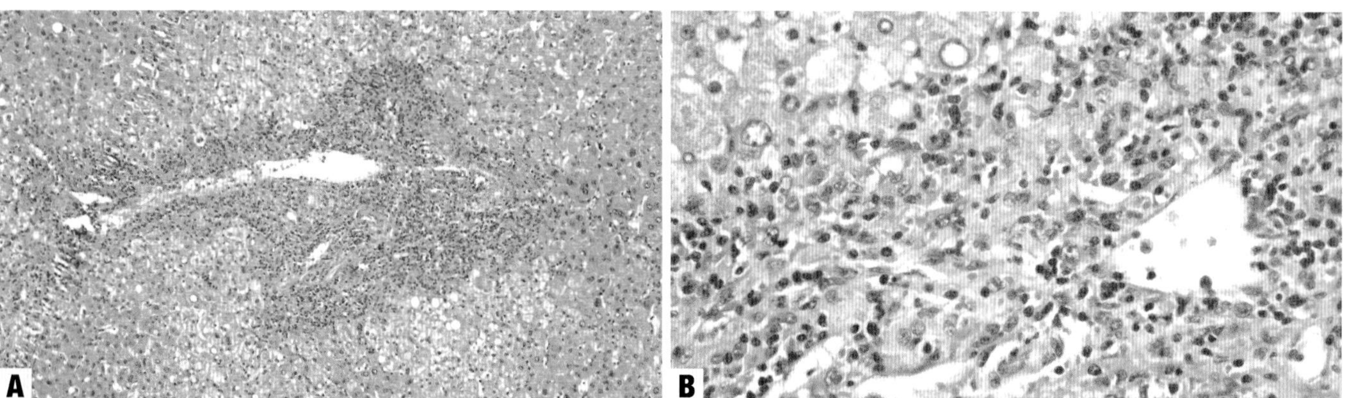

Fig. 5.170 Systemic EBV-positive T-cell lymphoma of childhood. **A** The neoplastic cells prominently infiltrate the portal area in the liver. **B** Higher magnification shows medium-sized neoplastic cells with irregular nuclei.

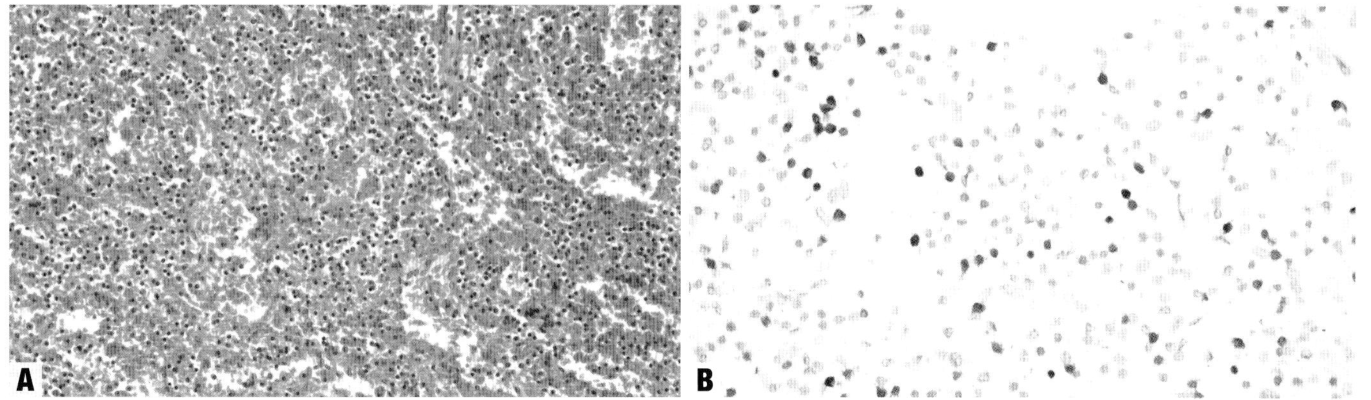

Fig. 5.171 Systemic EBV-positive T-cell lymphoma of childhood. **A** Splenic involvement shows splenic cords of red pulp infiltrated by small, bland-looking neoplastic lymphoid cells. **B** The neoplastic cells are positive for EBV-encoded small RNA (EBER).

Essential and desirable diagnostic criteria

Essential: acute presentation with fever and systemic symptoms; multiorgan infiltration by atypical T cells; EBV positivity; exclusion of known immunodeficiency.

Desirable: clonal TR gene rearrangements; HLH; hepatosplenomegaly.

Staging

Not relevant

Prognosis and prediction

This is an aggressive disease with a fulminant clinical course resulting in multiorgan failure, sepsis, and death, usually within days to weeks after diagnosis in most patients {771,774}. Some cases have been reported to respond to HLH-type protocols using etoposide and dexamethasone or multiagent chemotherapy followed by allogeneic haematopoietic stem cell transplantation {1556,1827,3766,4502,4510}. Monomorphic morphology and overexpression of cyclin E2 are associated with a poor prognosis {2945}.

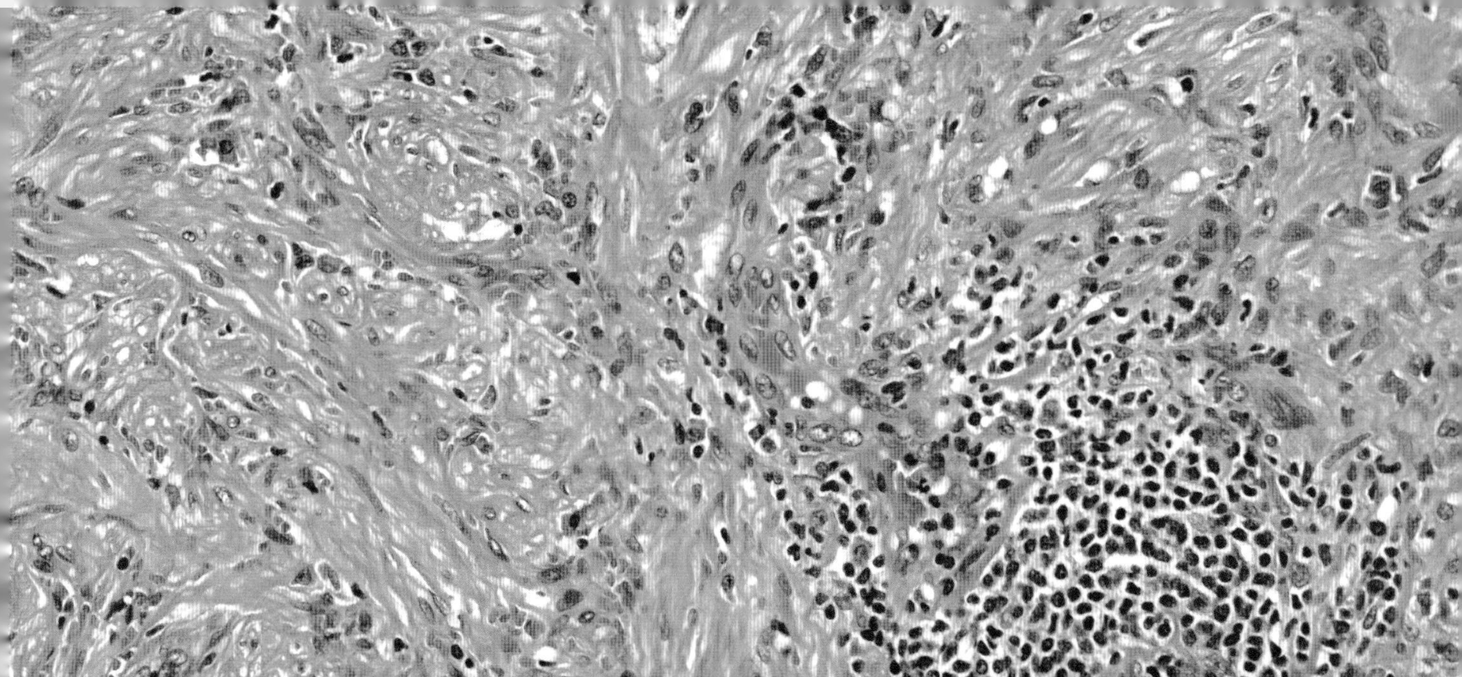

6

Stroma-derived neoplasms of lymphoid tissues

Edited by: Chan JKC, Naresh KN

Stroma-derived neoplasms of lymphoid tissues: Introduction

Chan JKC

The category of stroma-derived neoplasms of lymphoid tissues is introduced for the first time in this, the fifth edition of the WHO classification of haematolymphoid tumours. Mesenchymal tumours specific to lymph node (including intranodal palisaded myofibroblastoma) and spleen (including littoral cell angioma, splenic hamartoma, and sclerosing angiomatoid nodular transformation) are included. Various mesenchymal tumours and tumour-like lesions that can occur in lymph node or spleen but are not specific to these anatomical locations are only addressed briefly, in Table 6.01 and Table 6.02 (p. 786),

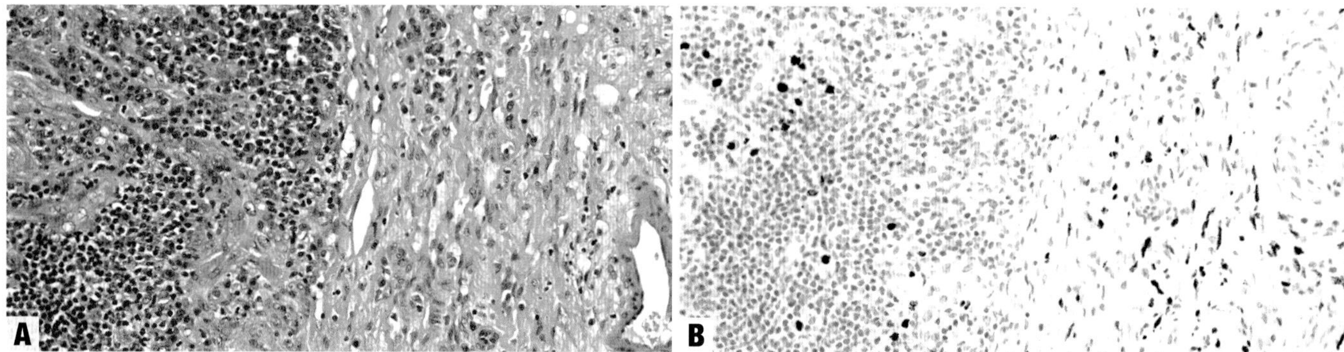

Fig. 6.01 Early Kaposi sarcoma in lymph node. **A** In the thickened capsule of the lymph node (right field), there are some thin-walled blood vessels, spindle cells, and plasma cells. Such features, in the appropriate setting, are highly suggestive of early Kaposi sarcoma. **B** Immunostaining for KSHV/HHV8 shows up positive cells in the nodal capsule, supporting a diagnosis of Kaposi sarcoma. Some KSHV/HHV8-positive lymphoid cells are also seen in the nodal parenchyma of this case (left field), attributable to KSHV/HHV8-associated multicentric Castleman disease.

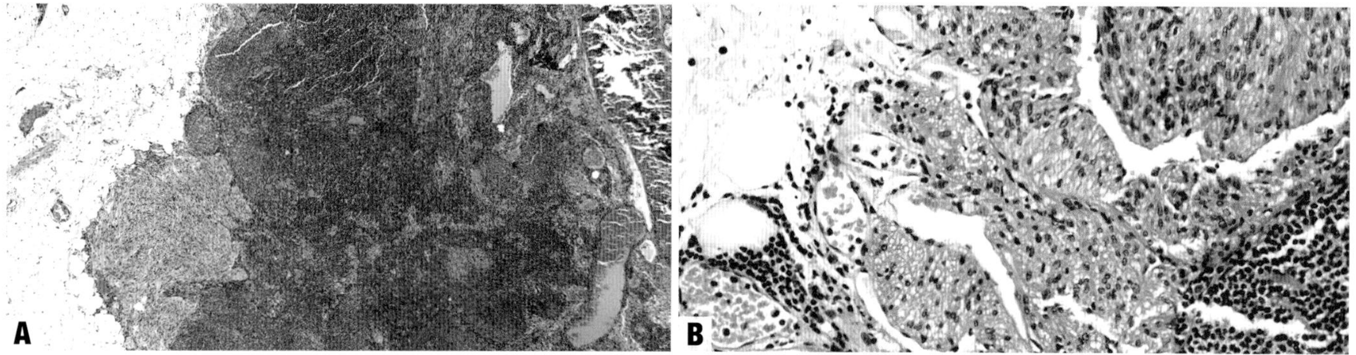

Fig. 6.02 Lymphangioleiomyomatosis of pelvic lymph node. **A** Lymphangioleiomyomatosis as an incidental finding in pelvic lymph node; nodular aggregates of spindle cells are present in the node. **B** The spindle cells show pale eosinophilic cytoplasm interspersed with occasional narrow, branching vascular (lymphatic) slits.

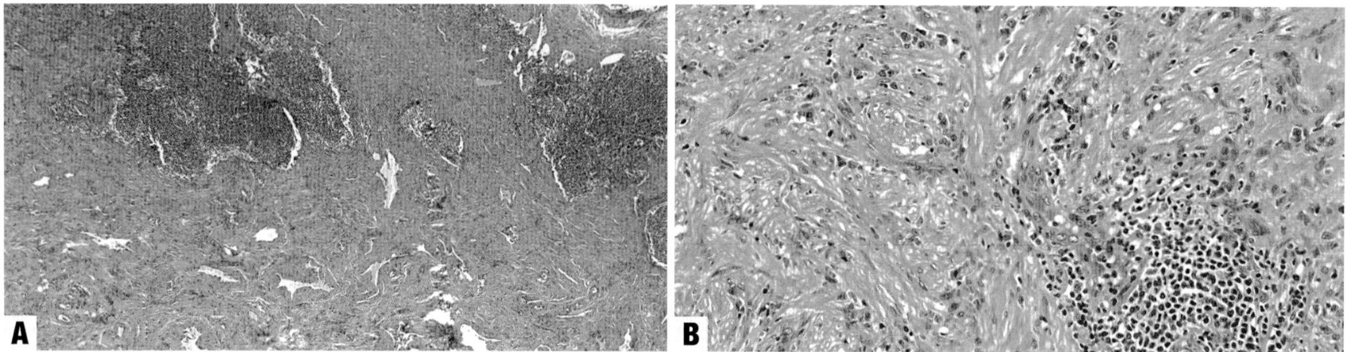

Fig. 6.03 Angiomyomatous hamartoma of lymph node. The nodal parenchyma shows variable replacement by fibrotic stroma (**A**), with scattered blood vessels and smooth muscle cells (**B**).

because these entities are covered in detail in the *Soft tissue and bone tumours* volume of this series.

In addition, follicular dendritic cell and fibroblastic reticular cell neoplasms have been moved from the "histiocytic and dendritic cell neoplasms" category to this new category, because follicular dendritic cells and fibroblastic reticular cells are not derived from haematopoietic stem cells but are of mesenchymal origin {389,4181,1789}. Given its distinctive clinicopathological features, EBV-positive inflammatory follicular dendritic cell sarcoma is now delineated as an entity separate from follicular dendritic cell sarcoma {1805}, and its name has been changed from "inflammatory pseudotumour-like follicular/fibroblastic dendritic cell sarcoma", a move first introduced in the fifth edition of the *Digestive system tumours* volume.

Table 6.01 Primary mesenchymal tumours and tumour-like lesions of lymph node

Entity	Salient features
Mesenchymal dendritic cell tumours	
Follicular dendritic cell sarcoma	See *Follicular dendritic cell sarcoma* (p. 787)
Fibroblastic reticular cell tumour	See *Fibroblastic reticular cell tumour* (p. 794)
Smooth muscle, myofibroblastic, and other stromal tumours and tumour-like lesions	
Intranodal palisaded myofibroblastoma	See *Intranodal palisaded myofibroblastoma* (p. 796)
Leiomyomatosis of lymph node	Partial or total replacement of nodal parenchyma by compact bundles of bland-looking smooth muscle cells; can occur as an isolated condition or as part of metastasizing uterine leiomyoma or leiomyomatosis peritonealis disseminata {3818,2188,2897,1627,3408,1653}
Angiomyolipoma	Retroperitoneal lymph nodes may rarely be involved by angiomyolipoma in association with renal angiomyolipoma {4089}
Lymphangioleiomyomatosis (lymphangiomyomatosis)	Nodal lymphangioleiomyomatosis is usually an incidental finding in pelvic/intra-abdominal lymph nodes of women undergoing gynaecological cancer surgery {4089}; it appears to be inconsequential and is not a harbinger of pulmonary lymphangioleiomyomatosis {3341,3636}
Inflammatory pseudotumour of lymph node	Inflammatory pseudotumour of lymph node is a rare lymphadenopathy occurring in young adults, who usually present with fever {3195}; it differs from inflammatory pseudotumour occurring in other sites {2165} Histologically, the pathological process predominantly involves the connective tissue framework of the node, with proliferation of spindle cells, blood vessels, and mononuclear cells, with or without phlebitis {3195,2165,883,2091}
Angiomyoid proliferation in association with Castleman disease	A benign proliferative process occurring in hyaline-vascular Castleman disease, featuring marked stromal overgrowth in the interfollicular zone, comprising venules and actin-positive spindle cells {2356,1756}
Lipomatosis	A non-neoplastic process of fatty replacement of most of the nodal parenchyma
Deciduosis	The abdominal lymph nodes show replacement by compact masses of decidual cells in pregnancy; a component of endometriosis can be present {500,162,828,2686}
Vascular tumours and tumour-like lesions	
Vascular transformation of sinuses	Reactive change in lymph node characterized by the conversion of nodal sinuses into complex, anastomosing, endothelium-lined vascular channels {4089,623,795}
Angiomyomatous hamartoma	Occurs almost exclusively in inguinal lymph nodes {618,4089,2711}; a proliferation of thick-walled blood vessels in nodal hilum blends into haphazardly disposed smooth muscle cells in a sclerotic stroma within the nodal parenchyma
Kaposi sarcoma	Nodal involvement by Kaposi sarcoma, a KSHV/HHV8-associated vascular tumour, occurs predominantly in the setting of immunodeficiency (particularly AIDS) and in the endemic form of Kaposi sarcoma {2994,4089} With overt involvement, nodules of spindly cells with interspersed vascular slits replace the nodal parenchyma Early lesions involve the nodal capsule with variable extension into fibrous trabeculae, featuring an increase in miniature vascular channels and spindle cells admixed with plasma cells {4089}
Haemangioma	Nodal haemangioma is either an incidental finding or presents as solitary lymphadenopathy; it comprises closely packed capillaries, veins, or cavernous blood vessels, or a combination of these {618,4089}
Haemangioendothelioma, including polymorphous haemangioendothelioma	Rarely, epithelioid haemangioendothelioma, spindle and epithelioid haemangioendothelioma, and polymorphous haemangioendothelioma can occur as primary lymph node lesions {618,3747,2907,2896}
Lymphangioma	Lymphangioma of lymph node is almost always accompanied by the involvement of surrounding soft tissues or other sites {4089}
Bacillary angiomatosis	A tumour-like vascular proliferation associated with *Bartonella henselae* infection, occurring in the setting of immunodeficiency {619,4089,618}
Angiolipomatous hamartoma in association with Castleman disease	A mass-forming lesion contiguous with hyaline-vascular Castleman disease, comprising fibroadipose tissue with scattered thick-walled blood vessels {4089,2470,74,2849}

Table 6.02 Primary mesenchymal tumours and tumour-like lesions of the spleen

Entity	Salient features
Mesenchymal dendritic cell tumours	
Follicular dendritic cell sarcoma	See *Follicular dendritic cell sarcoma* (p. 787)
EBV+ inflammatory follicular dendritic cell sarcoma	See *EBV-positive inflammatory follicular dendritic cell sarcoma* (p. 791)
Fibroblastic reticular cell tumour	See *Fibroblastic reticular cell tumour* (p. 794)
Smooth muscle, myofibroblastic, and other stromal tumours and tumour-like lesions	
Inflammatory pseudotumour	Inflammatory pseudotumour of the spleen is similar to that occurring in other sites {4003,2729} An important differential diagnosis is EBV+ inflammatory follicular dendritic cell sarcoma
EBV-associated smooth muscle tumour	EBV-associated smooth muscle tumour can rarely occur in the spleen, in the setting of immunodeficiency {113,3256,235}
Undifferentiated pleomorphic sarcoma	A highly aggressive sarcoma similar to its somatic soft tissue counterpart {4368,1531}
Vascular and vascular-stromal tumours and tumour-like lesions	
Littoral cell angioma	See *Littoral cell angioma* (p. 798)
Haemangioma and diffuse haemangiomatosis	Haemangioma is the commonest primary benign neoplasm of the spleen, and most cases are of the cavernous type {3566,3459} Diffuse haemangiomatosis is characterized by diffuse extensive splenic involvement {1015,868,3834}
Lymphangioma	Splenic lymphangioma is a solitary circumscribed tumour comprising lymphatic vascular channels {1730,3566}
Haemangioendothelioma	A low-grade malignant vascular neoplasm showing morphological features intermediate between those of haemangioma and angiosarcoma {4318,2319,2320}
Angiosarcoma	An aggressive malignant vascular neoplasm similar to its somatic soft tissue counterpart {1833,3566,1120,2933}
Splenic hamartoma	See *Splenic hamartoma* (p. 800)
Sclerosing angiomatoid nodular transformation	See *Sclerosing angiomatoid nodular transformation of spleen* (p. 802)
Bacillary angiomatosis	A tumour-like vascular proliferation associated with *Bartonella henselae* infection, occurring in the setting of immunodeficiency {4087,325}

Follicular dendritic cell sarcoma

Rech KL
Demicco EG
Gujral S
Hung YP
Macon WR
Picarsic J
Rossi ED
Schmitt F
Yin WH

Definition

Follicular dendritic cell sarcoma (FDCS) is a malignant neoplasm showing morphological and phenotypic characteristics of follicular dendritic cells (FDCs), which are stroma-derived cells normally found in germinal centres.

ICD-O coding

9758/3 Follicular dendritic cell sarcoma

ICD-11 coding

2B31.5 Follicular dendritic cell sarcoma

Related terminology

Acceptable: follicular dendritic cell tumour.

Subtype(s)

None

Localization

FDCS occurs in extranodal sites (in 58% of cases), lymph nodes (in 31%), or as concomitant nodal and extranodal disease (in 10%) {3601}. Extranodal disease occurs most commonly in the abdomen (particularly in the gastrointestinal tract and retroperitoneum) and upper aerodigestive tract, but it may occur at almost any extranodal site {4593,2304,1927}. Nodal disease is most common in cervical and abdominal lymph nodes {3601}.

Clinical features

Most patients present with a slow-growing, painless mass and/or isolated lymphadenopathy {3601,4418,2414}. Patients with abdominal disease may present with abdominal pain, and rare systemic symptoms can include fatigue, fever, and night sweats. FDCS can be associated with hyaline-vascular Castleman disease (HVCD) (see *Unicentric Castleman disease*, p. 319) or with autoimmune diseases (including paraneoplastic pemphigus / paraneoplastic autoimmune multiorgan syndrome and myasthenia gravis) {4284,4294,2254,2566}.

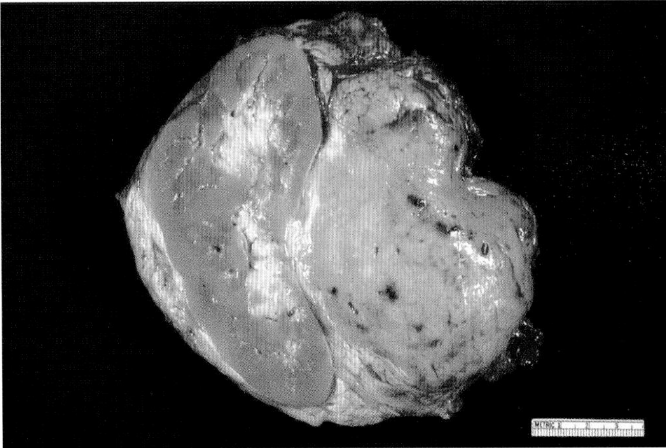

Fig. 6.04 Follicular dendritic cell sarcoma. A large, well-circumscribed tumour arising in the hilum of the kidney, showing a white bosselated cut surface.

Epidemiology

FDCS is rare {617,3237,121,2728,3190,4348} and can occur at any age (median: 50 years). There is no sex predilection. FDCS may be more frequent among certain ethnic groups or geographical locations, with the tumour being disproportionally frequently reported from eastern Asia {4418,3601}.

Etiology

A subset (< 20%) of cases are associated with HVCD {622, 2356,612,1105}, which can precede or co-occur with FDCS. The presence of dysplastic FDCs outside the follicles in HVCD is suggestive of transformation from this population, which may explain the association between HVCD and FDCS {4236, 1106}.

Pathogenesis

Non-neoplastic FDCs are derived from perivascular progenitors (vascular mural cells) rather than haematopoietic precursors {2120}. A hyperplasia–dysplasia–neoplasia model of FDC

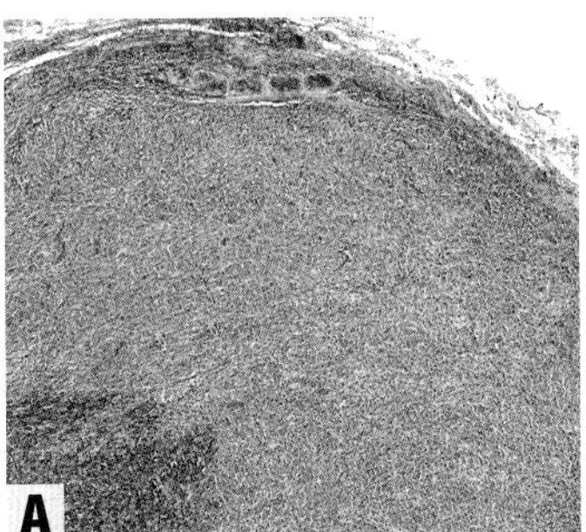

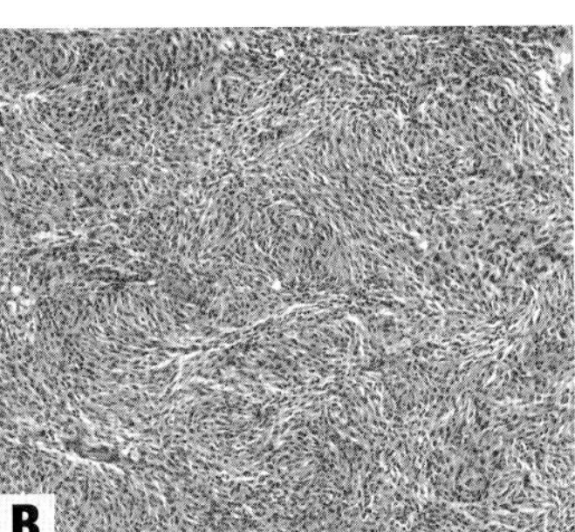

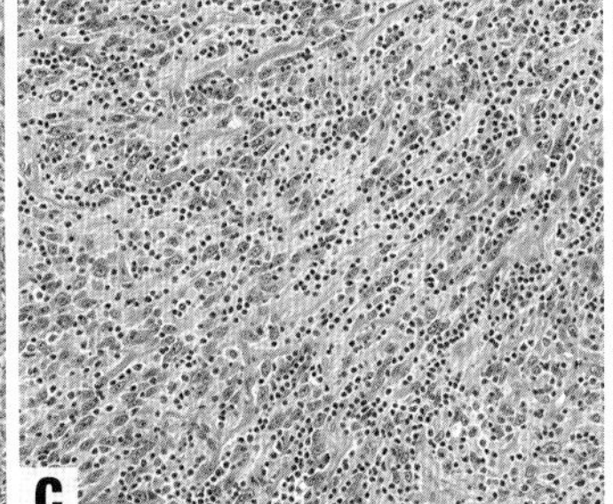

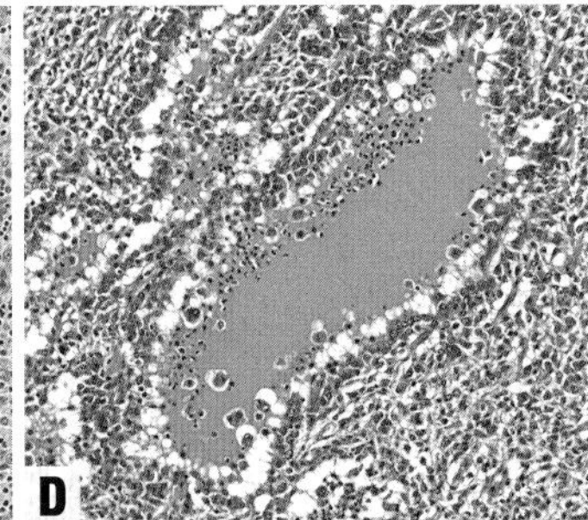

Fig. 6.05 Follicular dendritic cell sarcoma (FDCS). **A** FDCS in lymph node. Low-magnification view showing that the normal nodal architecture is completely effaced by a spindle cell neoplasm. **B** FDCS of tonsil. The tumour cells are arranged in a whorled or storiform pattern. **C** FDCS of soft tissue. Syncytial-appearing spindle cells are admixed with small lymphocytes. There is striking clustering of nuclei. **D** FDCS of the retroperitoneum. Pseudocystic spaces can be present.

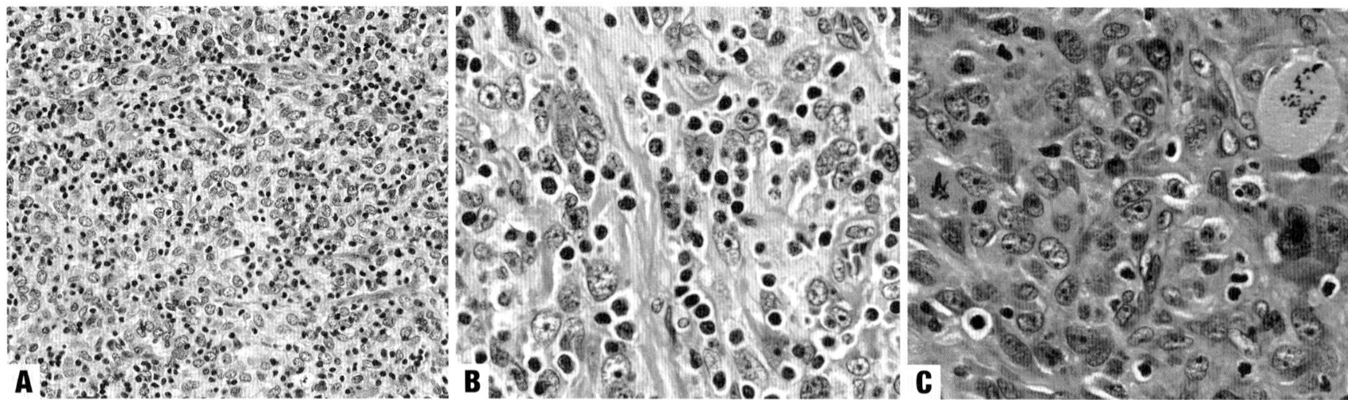

Fig. 6.06 Follicular dendritic cell sarcoma. **A** Tumour cells show an epithelioid morphology. **B** Follicular dendritic cell sarcoma of lymph node. Spindled to oval tumour cells have indistinct cell borders and distinct nucleoli. There are intermingled small lymphocytes. **C** Follicular dendritic cell sarcoma of the trachea. Some cases show significant nuclear pleomorphism and frequent mitoses.

proliferation has been proposed for the link between HVCD and FDCS, as supported by the shared clonality and EGFR (HER1) overexpression in dysplastic FDCs and FDCS {3883, 4226}.

Cytogenetic studies have shown a complex karyotype {3200}. Genomic studies show recurrent alterations in NF-κB pathway genes (*BIRC3*, *NFKBIA*, *TRAF3*, *SOCS3*, *CYLD*, and *TNFAIP3*) in 40–60% of cases, and in tumour suppressor genes (*CDKN2A*, *RB1*, and *TP53*) in 20–30% of cases {1416,114,2580}. A small subset of cases was reported to harbour IG rearrangement {671} or *BRAF* p.V600E mutation {1354}. Other uncommon genetic alterations include *HDGFRP3* (*HDGFL3*)::*SHC4* fusion {880}, focal deletion of *JAK2* and *BRAF* {2875}, and focal copy-number gain of *CD274* (*PDL1*) and *PDCD1LG2* (*PDL2*) {1416}. Transcriptomic analysis has shown highly specific expression of *FDCSP* and *SRGN*; a microenvironment enriched in T follicular helper (TFH) and T regulatory (Treg) cells; and upregulation of PD1, PDL1, and PDL2 {2193,2419}.

Macroscopic appearance

FDCS is usually well-circumscribed and sometimes encapsulated, with a bosselated or nodular appearance. Tumour size ranges from 10 to 150 mm depending upon the anatomical location, with the largest tumours reported in the abdomen and mediastinum {4418,3190,4593}. The cut surface is solid and tan to grey-white. Haemorrhage and necrosis can be seen in large tumours.

Histopathology

The neoplastic cells show a spindled, ovoid, or epithelioid cell morphology and are arranged in whorls, fascicles, syncytial sheets, and nodules, and in a storiform pattern. Several patterns can be seen in the same tumour. Tumour cells have moderate amounts of eosinophilic cytoplasm with indistinct cell borders, creating a syncytial appearance. The nuclei are elongated, with vesicular chromatin, delicate nuclear membranes, and small but distinct nucleoli. The nuclei tend to be unevenly spaced and clustered. Intranuclear pseudoinclusions are common. Binucleated forms reminiscent of benign FDCs may be present and represent a helpful diagnostic clue. Some cases may show prominent cytological atypia, with multinucleation and pleomorphic nuclei.

Typically, there is a light infiltrate of small lymphocytes among the tumour cells {1927}. Lymphoid aggregates can be seen at the periphery of the tumour or around blood vessels. Neutrophils or eosinophils may be seen, along with dilated and thick hyalinized blood vessels {4418,1927,359}.

Less common morphological features include epithelioid tumour cells with hyaline cytoplasm; clear cells; myxoid

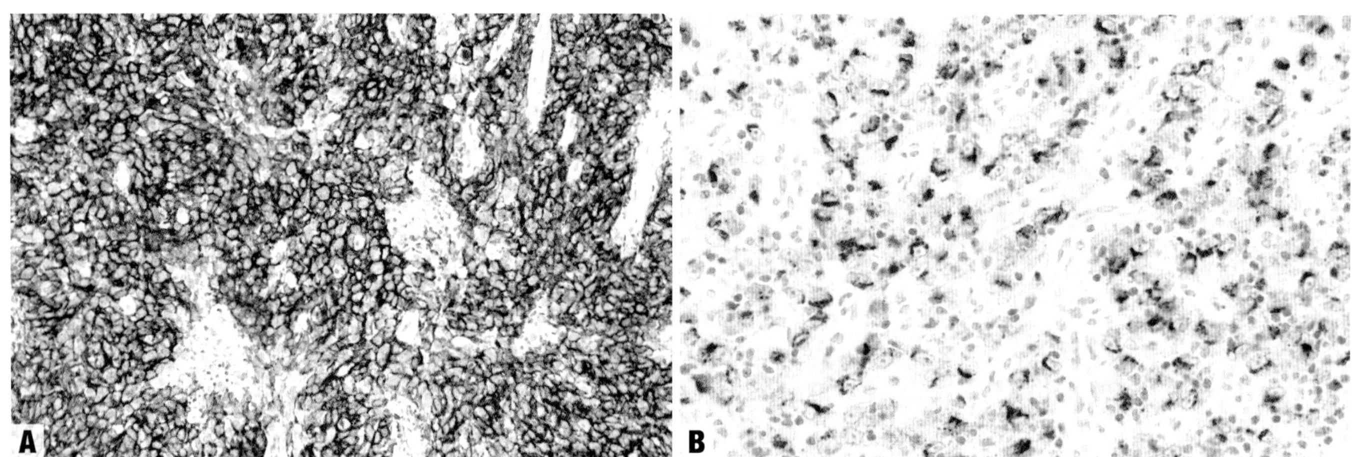

Fig. 6.07 Follicular dendritic cell sarcoma. **A** Tumour cells strongly and extensively express CD21. **B** CXCL13 is expressed with a paranuclear dot-like pattern.

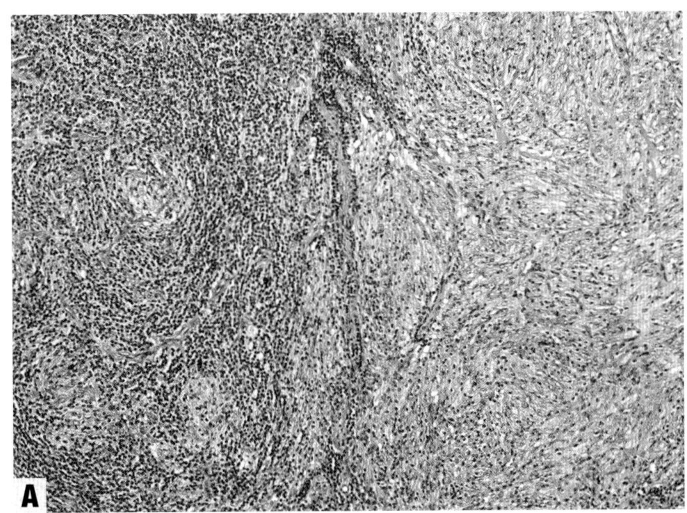
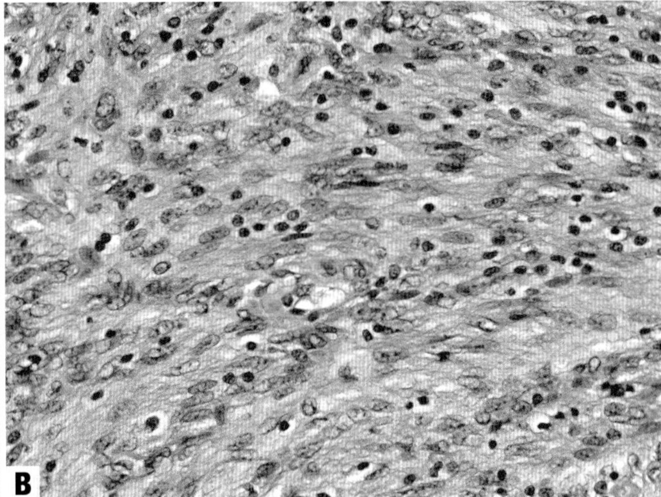

Fig. 6.08 Follicular dendritic cell sarcoma arising in association with hyaline-vascular Castleman disease. **A** The left field shows hyaline-vascular follicles in a background of small lymphocytes, consistent with hyaline-vascular Castleman disease. The right field shows sheets of spindly cells accompanied by a light infiltrate of small lymphocytes, consistent with follicular dendritic cell sarcoma. **B** The tumour comprises fascicles of spindly cells with elongated nuclei, vesicular chromatin, and small nucleoli. The spindly cells have indistinct cell borders, and the cytoplasm exhibits a fibrillary quality. There are admixed small lymphocytes.

stroma; fluid-filled cystic spaces; prominent fibrovascular septa; and admixed multinucleated, Reed–Sternberg–like or osteoclast-like giant cells {1422,617,3190,3191}. Cases showing jigsaw puzzle–like lobulation and perivascular spaces, mimicking thymoma or thymic carcinoma, have been reported {730}.

Immunohistochemistry

FDCS expresses antigens characteristic of normal FDCs, including CD21, CD23, CD35, clusterin, CXCL13, podoplanin (recognized by D2-40), and SSTR2 {3237,1422,3797,4520, 4227,858,1416,1106,3971}, and the newer markers FDCSP and SRGN {2419}. Among these markers, CXCL13, CD21, and clusterin are expressed most often (80–90% of cases) {1423,2419}. CXCL13 and the complement and Fc receptors (CD21, CD35, and CD23) show the highest specificity for FDCS {2419}. FDCS is also generally positive for fascin, PDL1, desmoplakin, EGFR, and vimentin {1422,1106}. There are occasional reports of positivity for CD4, CD30, CD31, CD45, CD68, CD163, claudin-4, EMA, lysozyme, S100, and vimentin {2376,1106}. Expression of CD20, cytokeratin, or thyroid transcription factor 1 (TTF1) is exceptional {1757,3237,2414}. The Ki-67 proliferation index is highly variable (5–70%) {1106}.

The admixed small lymphocytes can be predominantly T cells, predominantly B cells, or a mixture of T and B cells {617}. In almost half of all cases, an indolent T-lymphoblastic proliferation (see *Indolent T-lymphoblastic proliferation*, p. 649) is present {3012,2012}, with an infiltrate rich in TdT-positive cells that correlates with the occurrence of paraneoplastic manifestations {4284}.

Differential diagnosis

FDCS can mimic a wide variety of tumour types, such as unclassified pleomorphic sarcoma, meningioma, thymoma, thymic carcinoma, angiosarcoma, undifferentiated carcinoma, lymphoepithelial carcinoma, and gastrointestinal stromal tumour. The diagnostic problem can often be solved by applying a panel of immunohistochemical markers.

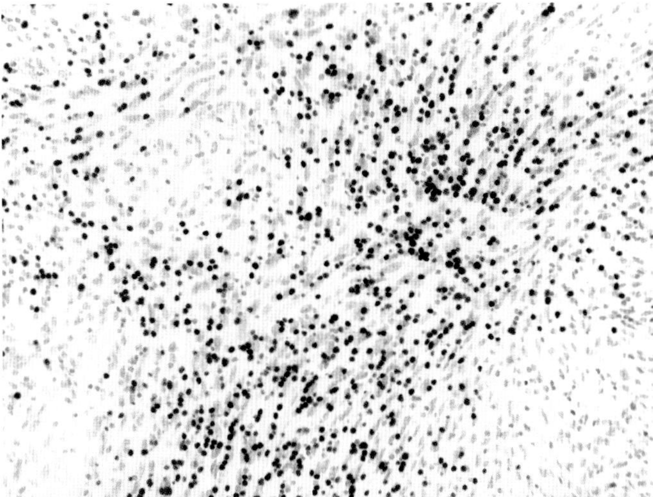

Fig. 6.09 Indolent T-lymphoblastic proliferation in follicular dendritic cell sarcoma. TdT staining highlights numerous immature T cells within the tumour lymphoid infiltrate of follicular dendritic cell sarcoma.

Cytology

Cytomorphological analysis coupled with ancillary techniques on fine-needle aspirate cell blocks is highly effective for diagnosis {3393,3030,3482}. Spindle to ovoid cells are arranged in clusters in a background of small lymphocytes. Single scattered tumour cells can also be seen. The cells show a moderate amount of cytoplasm and finely granular to vesicular nuclear chromatin with prominent nucleoli. Occasional intranuclear pseudoinclusions and nuclear grooves can be seen {3030}. Reed–Sternberg–like cells are sometimes observed {3393}. Small foci of necrosis and mitoses can be seen.

Diagnostic molecular pathology

Not clinically relevant

Essential and desirable diagnostic criteria

Essential: a tumour comprising spindled to ovoid cells with a storiform, fascicular, or whorled growth pattern; tumour cells with a syncytial appearance; small lymphocytes interspersed with tumour cells; positive immunostaining for two or more FDC markers; negative staining for lymphocyte-specific markers and generally negative staining for S100.

Staging

There is no established staging system for FDCS.

Prognosis and prediction

FDCS is a low- to intermediate-grade malignancy with a local recurrence rate of 28–40% and a distant metastasis rate of > 25% {617,3126,1891}. Metastasis may occur to other lymph nodes or by haematogenous spread to lung, liver, and bone {3601}. Surgery is potentially curative for early-stage disease, but recurrence and metastasis can occur many years after initial presentation {730}.

A simple stratification based on tumour size and histology was developed to predict the risk of recurrence: low risk, 16% (size < 50 mm, low- or high-grade histology); intermediate risk, 46% (size ≥ 50 mm, low-grade histology), and high risk, 73% (≥ 50 mm, high-grade histology). Mortality is low, except in the high-risk group (45%) {2304}. Other proposed poor prognostic factors include disseminated disease, extensive necrosis, a high mitotic rate (> 2 mitoses/mm^2), and significant nuclear pleomorphism {617,858,3193,3126,3601,2304}. Patients with complications of paraneoplastic autoimmune multiorgan syndrome experience high morbidity and mortality {4284}.

EBV-positive inflammatory follicular dendritic cell sarcoma

Li XQ
Cheuk W
Chuang S-S
Rech KL

Definition

EBV-positive inflammatory follicular dendritic cell sarcoma (FDCS) is an indolent malignant neoplasm characterized by neoplastic follicular dendritic cell (FDC) proliferation, a prominent lymphoplasmacytic infiltrate, and a consistent association with EBV.

ICD-O coding

9758/3 EBV-positive inflammatory follicular dendritic cell sarcoma

ICD-11 coding

2B31.Y Other specified histiocytic or dendritic cell neoplasms

Related terminology

Not recommended: inflammatory pseudotumour-like follicular/fibroblastic dendritic cell sarcoma; inflammatory pseudotumour-like follicular dendritic cell tumour; EBV-positive inflammatory pseudotumour.

Subtype(s)

None

Localization

EBV+ inflammatory FDCS occurs almost exclusively in the liver or spleen, sometimes with synchronous or metachronous involvement of both organs. It may uncommonly occur in the colon, tonsils, bronchus, pancreas, and mesentery {3118,1361, 2710,677,1939,1356,1805,1541}.

Clinical features

Patients with liver and/or splenic tumours are asymptomatic or present with abdominal distention or pain, sometimes accompanied by systemic symptoms such as malaise, weight loss, and low-grade fever. Laboratory investigations may reveal anaemia, elevated C-reactive protein, hypoalbuminaemia, hypergammaglobulinaemia, raised CA125, and (occasionally) peripheral eosinophilia {673,2321}. Patients with colonic tumours are asymptomatic or present with haematochezia or a positive faecal occult blood test. Tumours in the bronchus may cause obstructive symptoms. Rare patients present with paraneoplastic pemphigus {1805}.

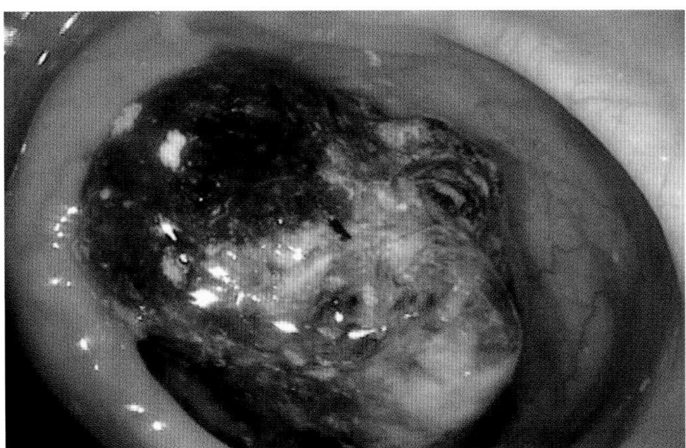

Fig. 6.10 Colonic EBV-positive inflammatory follicular dendritic cell sarcoma. Colonoscopy reveals a polypoid mass with superficial ulceration and haemorrhage.

Epidemiology

EBV+ inflammatory FDCS is rare, and most reported patients are Asian, raising the possibility of an ethnic predilection. It occurs predominantly in young to middle-aged adults (median age: 50–58 years), with marked female predominance, although a sex predilection is not evident for colonic tumours {1307,1805}.

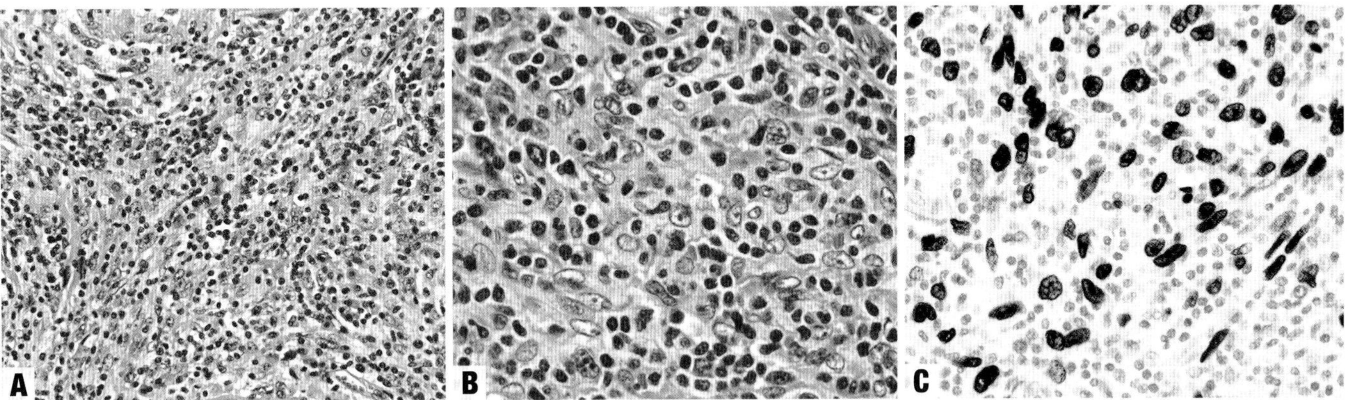

Fig. 6.11 EBV-positive inflammatory follicular dendritic cell sarcoma of spleen. **A** Spindle cells show a loose fascicular to storiform growth pattern and exhibit a range of nuclear atypia. The background is rich in lymphocytes and plasma cells. **B** The spindle cells show indistinct cell borders. The nuclei have thin nuclear membranes, vesicular chromatin, and distinct nucleoli. Binucleated cells are seen. Nuclear pleomorphism is relatively mild in this example. There are admixed lymphocytes and plasma cells. **C** On in situ hybridization for EBV-encoded small RNA (EBER), the neoplastic spindle cells are highlighted. Usually, the positive cells include bland-looking cells and overtly atypical cells.

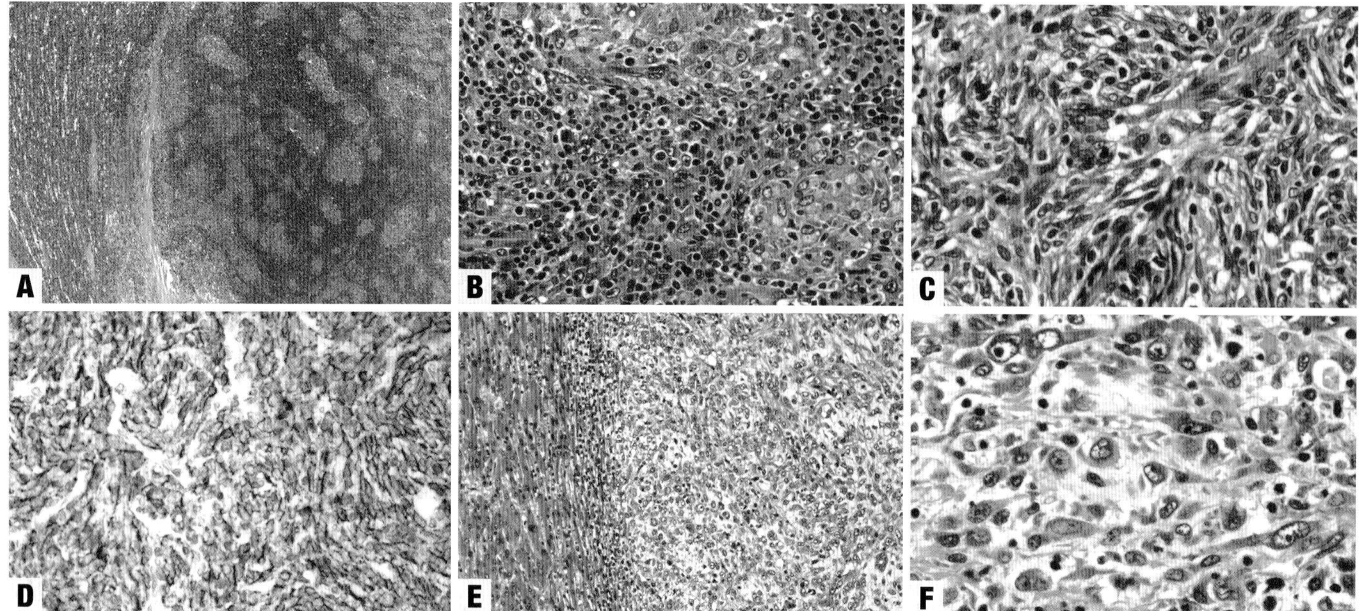

Fig. 6.12 EBV-positive inflammatory follicular dendritic cell sarcoma. A case of splenic involvement of follicular dendritic cell sarcoma in which the tumour is well demarcated from the surrounding splenic tissue by a fibrous pseudocapsule. **A** There are numerous coalescent non-caseating epithelioid granulomas within the lesion. **B** The scattered spindle to ovoid tumour cells are found within a prominent lymphoplasmacytic infiltrate between the granulomas. **C** High magnification of scattered spindle to ovoid tumour cells. **D** The tumour cells express CD21. **E,F** EBV-positive inflammatory follicular dendritic cell sarcoma involving the liver: synchronous involvement of the liver is present in the same case (**E**), and larger atypical cells with more pronounced pleomorphism are evident (**F**).

Etiology

EBV is a significant etiological factor. The neoplastic cells are consistently associated with clonal EBV genome, frequently with a 30 bp deletion or point mutations in exon 3 of *LMP-1* {3676,669,2293,1628}. Strain subtype A and the type f variant of the virus have been reported in a case series from southern China {2333}.

Pathogenesis

It has been postulated that the tumour may arise from a common EBV-infected mesenchymal cell that differentiates along the follicular or fibroblastic dendritic cell pathway {4177}. The genetic changes of the tumour have not been well characterized. Limited studies have reported copy-neutral loss of heterozygosity of 5q, gain of the X chromosome, and somatic mutations in some genes, mostly of uncertain clinical significance {2777,473}.

Macroscopic appearance

Tumours arising in the solid organs are often circumscribed, consisting of fleshy tan tissue often interspersed with foci of haemorrhage or necrosis. In tubular organs (colon and bronchus), the tumours form pedunculated or sessile polyps, with or without surface ulceration.

Histopathology

Neoplastic spindle to oval cells are singly dispersed or form loose whorled fascicles within a prominent lymphoplasmacytic infiltrate, sometimes accompanied by scattered reactive lymphoid follicles. However, tumour cell–rich areas, usually with a fascicular or storiform growth pattern, may be present or even dominant in rare cases. The tumour cells show indistinct cell borders, a scant to moderate amount of cytoplasm, and vesicular nuclei with stippled chromatin and small, centrally located distinct nucleoli. Nuclear atypia is highly variable, even within individual cases. Usually, there are bland-looking spindly cells admixed with overtly atypical cells with enlarged, irregularly folded or hyperchromatic nuclei. Some tumour cells may resemble Reed–Sternberg cells. Mitotic figures are rare. Necrosis and haemorrhage are often present and may be associated with a histiocytic reaction. The blood vessels frequently show fibrinoid deposits in the walls. Additional changes found in some cases include epithelioid granulomas, abundant eosinophils, xanthomatous cells, and monocytoid B-cell aggregates {2322,1805}.

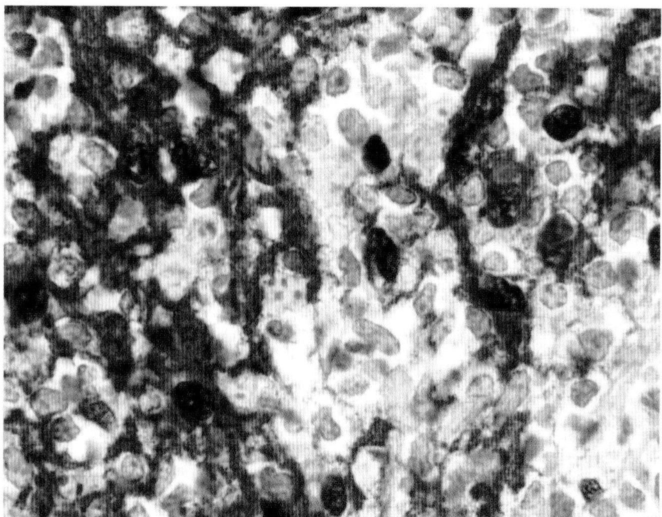

Fig. 6.13 EBV-positive inflammatory follicular dendritic cell sarcoma. Tumour cells are highlighted by dual labelling using EBV-encoded small RNA (EBER) in situ hybridization (brown) and CD21 immunostaining (red).

Table 6.03 Comparison of the epidemiological and clinical features of EBV-positive inflammatory follicular dendritic cell sarcoma and follicular dendritic cell sarcoma

Feature	EBV+ inflammatory follicular dendritic cell sarcoma	Follicular dendritic cell sarcoma
Epidemiology	Predominantly reported in Asian populations	No ethnic predilection
Sex	Female predilection	No sex predilection
Median age	55 years	50 years
Sites of disease	Predominantly spleen and liver; rarely colon (polyp), tonsils, bronchus, mesentery	Lymph node or practically any extranodal site, most commonly abdomen (including gastrointestinal tract, retroperitoneum) and upper aerodigestive tract (tonsil, nasopharynx, parapharynx)
Presentation	Most commonly presenting with splenomegaly or hepatomegaly; paraneoplastic pemphigus very rare	Lymphadenopathy or mass lesion attributable to extranodal disease; may be associated with autoimmune diseases, such as paraneoplastic pemphigus and myasthenia gravis
Constitutional symptoms	Present in a proportion of patients	Very rare
Predisposing conditions	Unknown	Hyaline-vascular Castleman disease in a proportion of cases
Histology	Dispersed tumour cells; many admixed lymphocytes and plasma cells	Compact spindly to oval tumour cells with indistinct cell borders; sprinkling of lymphocytes
Behaviour	Generally indolent; recurrence ~30%, distant metastasis uncommon	Variable; local recurrence 28–40%, distant metastasis > 25%
EBV association	Always present (by definition)	Extremely rare

Immunohistochemistry and in situ hybridization

The neoplastic cells often show variable staining for FDC markers, such as CD21, CD35, CD23, CXCL13, D2-40, and CNA.42, with the staining ranging from extensive to very focal. Rare cases may lack FDC markers but instead exhibit a fibroblastic/myoid immunophenotype (SMA+), suggesting fibroblastic reticular cell differentiation. LMP1 is frequently expressed. The background lymphocytes include a mixture of CD20+ B cells and CD3+ T cells. The plasma cells are polytypic, and they richly express IgG4 in some cases {728}.

In situ hybridization for EBV-encoded small RNA (EBER) is consistently positive, typically showing up slender, bland-looking nuclei as well as large pleomorphic nuclei.

Differential diagnosis

The major differential diagnoses include malignant lymphoma, inflammatory myofibroblastic tumour, and florid lymphoid hyperplasia or inflammatory polyp. A lack of cytological atypia in the lymphoid cells and the immunohistochemical demonstration of a mixture of T cells, B cells, and polytypic plasma cells do not support a diagnosis of malignant lymphoma. For inflammatory myofibroblastic tumour, the neoplastic spindle cells have well-defined amphophilic cytoplasm, express actin, often show translocation of receptor tyrosine kinase genes (most commonly *ALK*), and lack EBV. In fibroinflammatory lesions due to infection or reparative reaction (with inflammatory myofibroblastic tumour excluded), the spindle cells lack nuclear atypia, FDC markers, and EBV. Florid lymphoid hyperplasia or inflammatory polyp comprises predominantly lymphoid cells with no atypia, lacks a significant spindle cell component, and is usually EBV-negative. For the differential diagnosis with FDCS, see Table 6.03.

Cytology

Cytological preparations reveal hypercellular samples with dual populations of neoplastic spindle cells and chronic inflammatory cells. Tumour cells appear as syncytial groups, whorls, fascicles, or single cells, with variable nuclear atypia and prominent nucleoli. Multilobated and multinucleated forms can be seen {1387}.

Diagnostic molecular pathology

In situ hybridization for EBER is positive.

Essential and desirable diagnostic criteria

Essential: proliferation of atypical spindle to oval cells with indistinct cell borders, vesicular nuclei, and distinct nucleoli; accompanied by a rich lymphoplasmacytic infiltrate; expression of FDC or (rarely) fibroblastic/myoid markers; EBER-positive.

Staging

Not clinically relevant

Prognosis and prediction

Outcome data are limited, but tumours involving the liver or spleen are indolent, with a tendency to develop repeated intra-abdominal recurrences over many years. Rare distant metastases, including in lymph node, lung, and spine, can occur {694, 2321}. Tumours occurring in the liver have a worse prognosis than those occurring in the spleen. Based on several series on liver tumours, the recurrence rate is 29% and the tumour mortality rate is 10% {673,1307}. Tumours occurring in the colon, probably because of their polypoid nature and amenability to complete removal, have an excellent outcome {1805}.

Fibroblastic reticular cell tumour

Saygin C
Kaji S

Definition

Fibroblastic reticular cell tumour (FRCT) is a neoplasm of putative stromal fibroblastic reticular cell origin.

ICD-O coding

9759/3 Fibroblastic reticular cell tumour

ICD-11 coding

2B31.7 Fibroblastic reticular cell tumour

Related terminology

Acceptable: fibroblastic dendritic cell tumour; fibroblastic reticular cell sarcoma.

Not recommended: cytokeratin-positive interstitial reticulum cell tumour.

Subtype(s)

None

Localization

Isolated nodal disease is most common, but various extranodal sites can also be involved, such as the spleen, soft tissues, liver, lung, kidney, breast, adrenal gland, and bone {3601,857,613, 1890,2297,421}.

Clinical features

The most common presentation is lymphadenopathy or a newly developed mass. Rarely, FRCT is an incidental finding or occurs concurrently with another malignancy {3861,1851}.

Epidemiology

FRCT is rare, often presenting in the seventh decade of life (age range: 13–80 years, median: 61 years) {3601,2297}. There is no sex predilection.

Etiology

Unknown

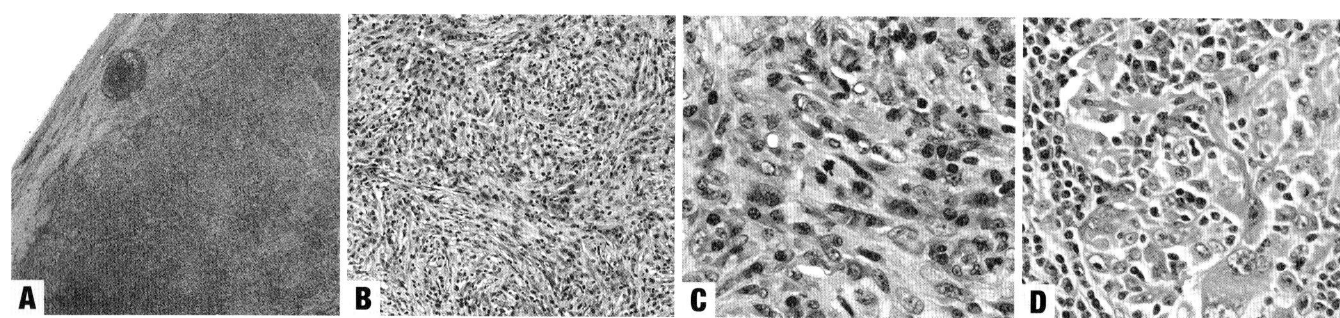

Fig. 6.14 Fibroblastic reticular cell tumour. **A** Lymph node showing total replacement by a spindle cell neoplasm. **B** Spindle cells are arranged in a storiform pattern, accompanied by a lymphoplasmacytic infiltrate. **C** The atypical spindle cells have indistinct cell borders and vesicular nuclei. A mitotic figure is also evident. **D** The tumour cells are round or polygonal and have vesicular nuclei and prominent nucleoli. The abundant cytoplasm is eosinophilic. Tumour cells are admixed with many small lymphocytes and plasma cells, and are closely associated with collagen fibres. The cytoplasm of some tumour cells is hyalinized and appears to merge into collagen fibres.

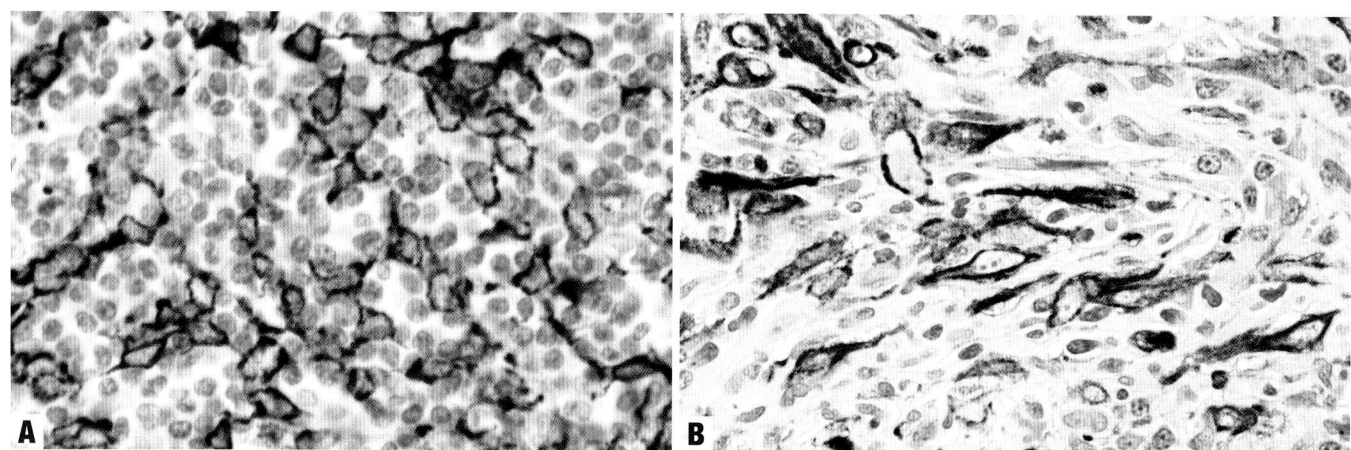

Fig. 6.15 Fibroblastic reticular cell tumour. **A** Positive immunostaining for cytokeratin, with a dendritic pattern. **B** Positive immunostaining for SMA; dendritic processes are evident.

Pathogenesis

Unknown

Macroscopic appearance

FRCT often forms a well-circumscribed tumour nodule. Tumour size is variable, ranging from 9 to 160 mm. Haemorrhage and necrosis can be present.

Histopathology

FRCTs are characterized by spindle to oval cells, often arranged in a whorled, fascicular, sheeting, or storiform pattern and accompanied by a lymphoplasmacytic infiltrate. The degree of nuclear pleomorphism is variable, and multinucleated or giant tumour cells may be admixed. Thus FRCT shows overlapping morphological features with follicular dendritic cell sarcoma and interdigitating dendritic cell sarcoma. A characteristic, but neither invariable nor pathognomonic, feature is the presence of intercellular collagen fibrils.

Ultrastructurally, the tumour cells show delicate cytoplasmic extensions and features reminiscent of myofibroblasts (elongated nuclei, filaments with occasional fusiform densities, moderate amounts of rough endoplasmic reticulum, well-developed desmosomal attachments in contiguous arrangements, and basal lamina–like material forming linear extracellular condensations) {121}.

Immunohistochemistry

The immunophenotype overlaps with that of myofibroblasts, with variable positivity for actin, desmin, and vimentin {725}. Two thirds of cases are cytokeratin-positive, with delicate cell processes being highlighted by the immunostain. L-caldesmon, fascin, vimentin, and EMA are often positive. The tumour should lack markers of follicular dendritic cell sarcoma (such as CD21 and CD35) and interdigitating dendritic cell sarcoma (S100), although there are rare reported cases with hybrid features of FRCT and follicular dendritic cell sarcoma {1823,1378}. In cytokeratin-positive FRCT cases, metastatic carcinoma should be considered in the differential diagnosis.

Cytology

Diagnosis requires histopathological examination.

Diagnostic molecular pathology

Not relevant

Essential and desirable diagnostic criteria

Essential: spindle to ovoid cells in whorls, fascicles, or sheets; interspersed small lymphocytes; positive immunostaining for one or more of the markers cytokeratin, actin, and desmin, with delicate cell processes being highlighted; negative staining for markers of follicular dendritic cells (CD21, CD23, CD35, CXCL13) and interdigitating dendritic cells (S100).

Staging

Not applicable

Prognosis and prediction

Most patients present with localized disease, which is associated with better survival than advanced disease {3601}. Among 21 reported patients with follow-up, 6 have died from disseminated disease {1851}.

Intranodal palisaded myofibroblastoma

Laskin WB
Miettinen M

Definition
Intranodal palisaded myofibroblastoma is a benign, lymph node–based smooth muscle / myofibroblastic stromal neoplasm.

ICD-O coding
8825/0 Intranodal palisaded myofibroblastoma

ICD-11 coding
2E84.Y Benign fibrogenic or myofibrogenic tumour of other specified sites

Related terminology
Acceptable: intranodal/nodal myofibroblastoma; nodal myofibroblastoma; palisaded myofibroblastoma.
Not recommended: intranodal haemorrhagic spindle cell tumour with amianthoid fibres.

Subtype(s)
None

Localization
Inguinal lymph nodes are principally involved {3889,4350,3477, 2678,2226}, with rare examples described in axillary, neck, submandibular, para-oesophageal, retroperitoneal, and mediastinal nodes {350,2226,1202,1655,3521,2950}.

Clinical features
Patients present with a solitary, rarely multicentric mass, which is slow-growing, painless or (less often) tender, and mobile {2950,351,2226}.

Epidemiology
The tumour occurs in patients aged 19–78 years {2950,351, 2226}, with peak incidence in the fifth and sixth decades of life

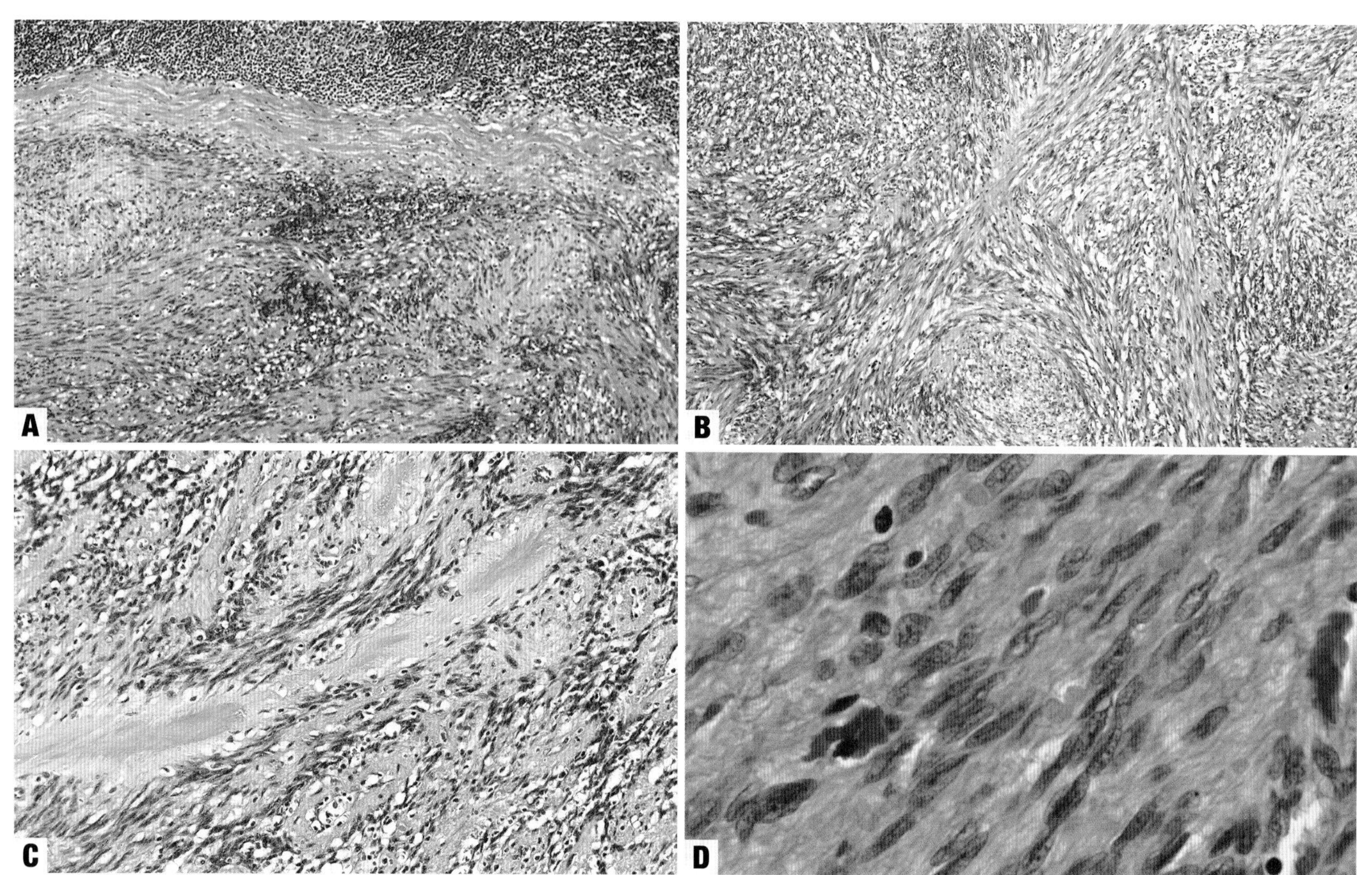

Fig. 6.16 Intranodal palisaded myofibroblastoma. **A** The tumour comprises densely packed spindly cells with vague nuclear palisading, accompanied by interstitial haemorrhage. Residual lymph node tissue is seen in the upper field. **B** Low-power view showing loose fascicular and whorled growth of spindled cells with extravasated erythrocytes. **C** Elongated collagenous body adjacent to vessels with thickened hyalinized walls. **D** Spindled cells with cytologically bland, focally wavy, elongated nuclei with an occasional longitudinal groove, and scattered rounded, pink intracytoplasmic inclusions.

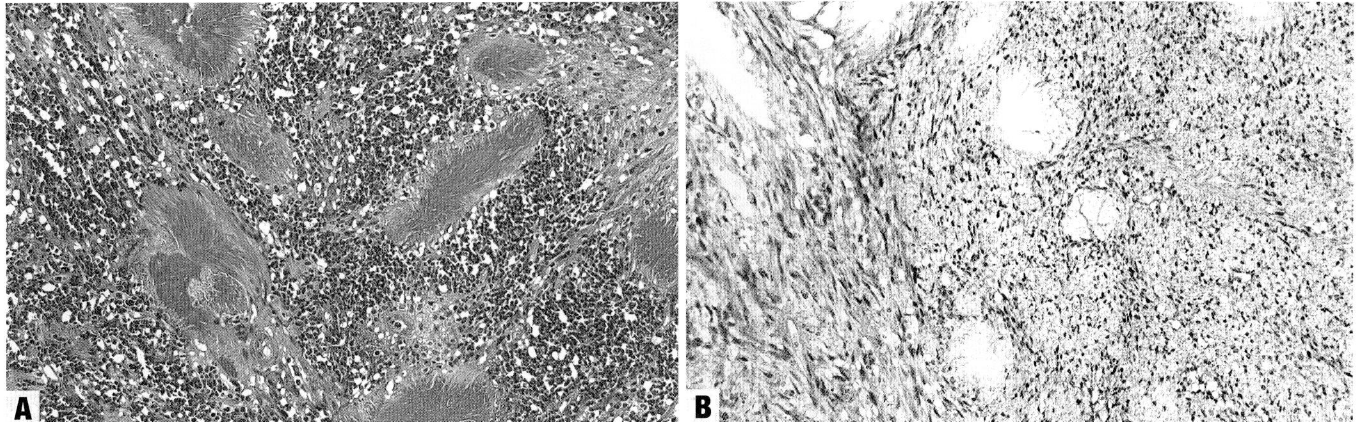

Fig. 6.17 Intranodal palisaded myofibroblastoma. **A** The spindle cell tumour is interspersed with brightly eosinophilic, starburst collagenous bodies. Prominent interstitial haemorrhage is present, mimicking a vascular tumour such as Kaposi sarcoma. **B** Immunostaining for β-catenin reveals abnormal nuclear localization of staining in the spindle cells.

{2950,2226}. The M:F ratio is 2:1 {2950,3477,2678,2226}, and there is no racial predilection {2950}.

Etiology

The etiology is unknown. It has been suggested that trauma, drainage of mutagenic factors, and/or inflammation potentially induce *CTNNB1* mutations in lymph node myoid stromal cells {4350,2226}.

Pathogenesis

Gain-of-function *CTNNB1* exon 3 missense mutations in codon 32, 33, 34, or 37 result in β-catenin–induced upregulation of cyclin D1 and cellular proliferation {2048,2226}.

Macroscopic appearance

Lymph nodes usually measure 6–50 mm {3889,4350,2678,2226}. The cut surface shows one or more tumour nodules separated from compressed lymphoid tissue by fibrous bands. Nodules are white-grey with dark-red haemorrhagic areas {2950,351}.

Histopathology

Tumour nodules are composed of moderately to highly cellular short fascicles, which are focally fibromatosis-like, and whorls of spindled cells. Variably shaped, dense collagenous bodies and vessels with hyalinized walls are present, on which the tumour cells may show vague nuclear palisading. The tumour cells have scant, lightly eosinophilic cytoplasm {3889,4350,2678, 815,3963,2226}. Perinuclear vacuoles and rounded, salmon-coloured intracytoplasmic inclusions are common {3889,4350, 2226}. The elongated, focally wavy nuclei are cytologically bland, and mitotic activity ranges from 0 to 8 mitoses/5 mm^2 {4350,2226}. The stromal matrix is finely collagenous to myxocollagenous, with extravasated erythrocytes and/or haemosiderin commonly encountered. A major differential diagnosis is Kaposi sarcoma.

Immunohistochemically, the tumour cells diffusely express vimentin, SMA, and MSA; variably express calponin, podoplanin (recognized by D2-40), factor XIIIa, nuclear β-catenin, and cyclin D1; and focally express desmin {3889,4350,3477,2678, 2226,750,2048,1595}. The Ki-67 proliferation index is < 5% {2048}. The tumour is negative for cytokeratins, S100, follicular dendritic cell markers (CD21, CD23, CD35), vascular markers (CD31, CD34, von Willebrand factor [factor VIII–related antigen]), and KSHV/HHV8 {2226,2950,3889,1886,1867,3521}.

Cytology

FNA reveals bland, tapered, spindled cells with nuclear grooves surrounding an acellular matrix, and haemosiderin deposits {4440,3793,2555}.

Diagnostic molecular pathology

Not clinically relevant

Essential and desirable diagnostic criteria

Essential: an intranodal benign spindle cell proliferation expressing actin(s); variably shaped dense collagenous bodies.
Desirable: nuclear β-catenin and/or cyclin D1 expression.

Staging

Not clinically relevant

Prognosis and prediction

Intranodal palisaded myofibroblastoma is a benign neoplasm with a postsurgical local recurrence rate of about 6% {2950}.

Littoral cell angioma

Michal M
Liu WP

Definition
Littoral cell angioma is a benign vascular tumour unique to the spleen, characterized by proliferation of vascular channels with a hybrid endothelial–histiocytic phenotype.

ICD-O coding
9120/0 Littoral cell angioma

ICD-11 coding
2E8Z Benign mesenchymal neoplasms, unspecified

Related terminology
None

Subtype(s)
None

Localization
This tumour is unique to the spleen.

Clinical features
Most patients are asymptomatic, with the tumour being discovered incidentally on imaging studies performed for another purpose. Symptomatic cases present with fever, abdominal pain, or signs of hypersplenism such as splenomegaly, thrombocytopenia, and anaemia {1122,3174,1005,808,1811,3451,3069, 3355}. The tumour is associated with concurrent epithelial or haematological malignancies in one third to two thirds of cases, as well as with systemic diseases often linked to immune dysregulation, such as inflammatory bowel disease and sarcoidosis {3174,368,808,1811,3451,3069,3355}. Incidental discovery of the splenic tumour during radiological evaluation or surgery for cancer may partly explain the former association.

Imaging
Imaging findings are nonspecific. Ultrasound usually shows multiple (rarely single) poorly defined, hypoechoic masses. The nodules are well circumscribed and low-attenuating on non-contrast CT, hypodense on arterial phase imaging, and isodense to spleen on delayed phase imaging. The lesions show low signal on T1-weighted MRI sequences, variable but often hyperintense signal on T2-weighted sequences, and heterogeneous peripheral arterial enhancement with delayed centripetal filling {1005, 3451,3069,3355,1266}.

Epidemiology
Littoral cell angioma of the spleen is very rare. It may occur at any age, but most typically arises in the fourth to seventh decade of life. There is no sex predilection {1122,3174,368,1005,3355}.

Etiology
Unknown

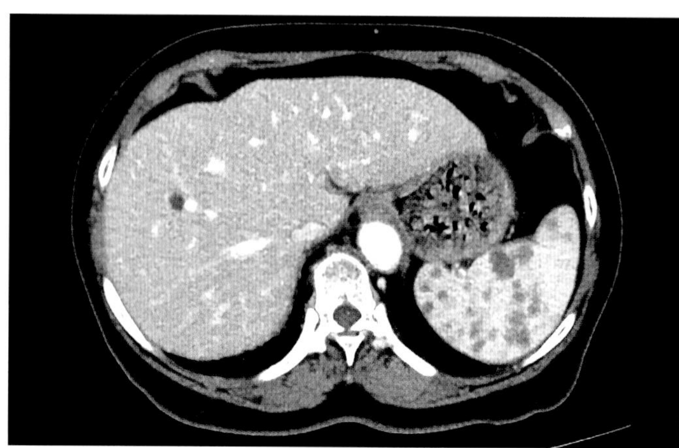

Fig. 6.18 Littoral cell angioma. Contrast-enhanced CT of the abdomen shows multiple well-demarcated and variably sized hypodense cystic masses throughout an enlarged spleen.

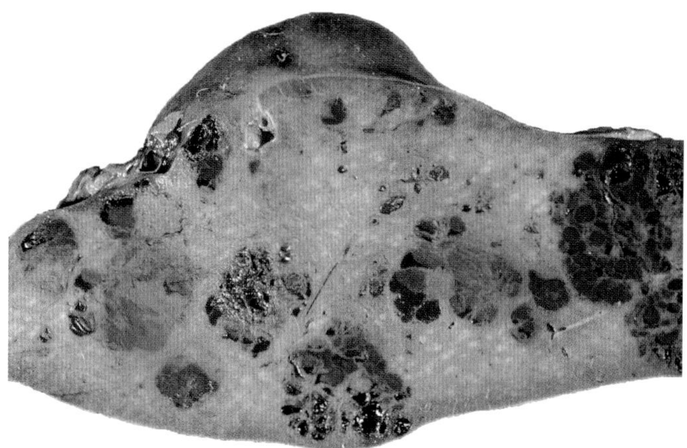

Fig. 6.19 Littoral cell angioma. Gross specimen with multiple well-demarcated and variably sized spongy nodules involving most of the splenic parenchyma.

Pathogenesis
The tumour is thought to originate from littoral cells lining the red pulp sinuses, but the exact mechanism is unclear.

Macroscopic appearance
Spleens are often enlarged, ranging from 145 to 3700 g in weight and from 95 to 220 mm in greatest dimension {1122, 3174}. Littoral cell angioma ranges from microscopic foci to extensive tumour involving the entire spleen. Solitary or (much more often) multiple variably sized, spongy and cystic nodules are seen on cut section of the spleen. They are well demarcated but unencapsulated, and expansile. The colour varies from dark red to brown and black {1122,3174,368,352,1005}.

Histopathology

Littoral cell angioma is a discrete lesion located within the red pulp, consisting of blood-filled, anastomosing vascular channels reminiscent of hypertrophied splenic sinuses. The vascular channels vary greatly in width and often are cystically dilated. They are lined by a single layer of protruding plump cuboidal or tall endothelial cells with ample eosinophilic cytoplasm. The cells often slough off into the lumina, and haemophagocytosis and intracytoplasmic haemosiderin granules may be seen, as well as eosinophilic hyaline globules {368,2679}. The cells sometimes form papillary fronds protruding into the vascular lumina. Mitotic figures are rare, and cellular atypia and tumour necrosis are absent {1122,3174,368,352,1005,2679}. Extramedullary haematopoiesis may be found.

Immunohistochemistry

Tumour cells express vascular markers, such as ERG, CD31, and von Willebrand factor (factor VIII–related antigen), as well as histiocytic markers, such as CD163, CD68, and lysozyme {1122,3174,368,352,1005}. Of note, WT1 and CD34 are often negative, as is the splenic littoral cell (sinus-lining cell) marker CD8 {3174,368,352,3060,3673}, whereas SIRPα, another marker of splenic littoral cells, is positive {3001}. CD207 (langerin), CD21, claudin-5, and VEGFR2 are expressed in most littoral cell angiomas but are negative in normal splenic sinuses {3174,3673,138}.

Cytology

Smears are composed of clusters of cuboidal to columnar-shaped cells with a low N:C ratio, eccentric nuclei, evenly distributed chromatin, and indistinct nucleoli. Intracytoplasmic haemosiderin pigment can be noted. However, FNAC is rarely performed, because of the high risk of complications {2871, 112}.

Diagnostic molecular pathology

Not relevant

Essential and desirable diagnostic criteria

Essential: circumscribed splenic tumour (often multiple) comprising variably sized vascular channels lined by plump endothelial cells with ample eosinophilic cytoplasm; immunohistochemical confirmation of dual endothelial and histiocytic phenotype.

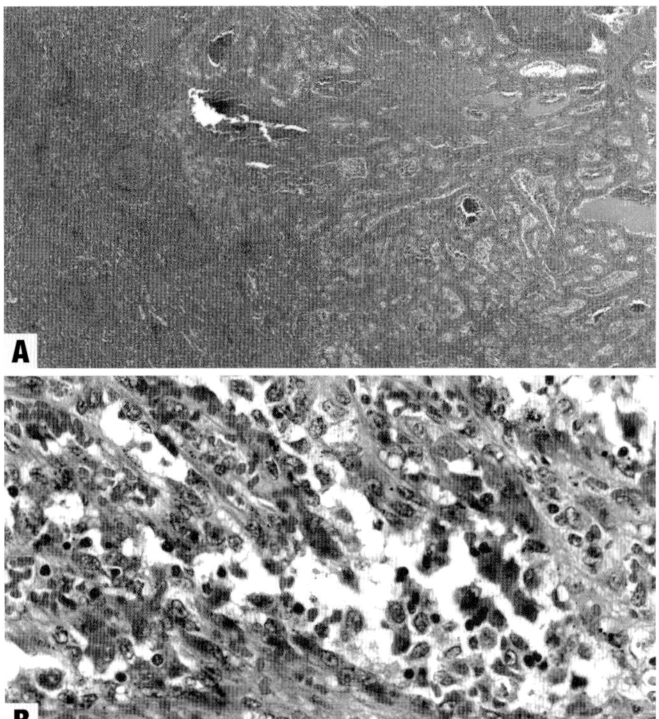

Fig. 6.20 Littoral cell angioma. **A** The tumour is located within the red splenic pulp and consists of blood-filled, anastomosing vascular spaces reminiscent of normal splenic sinuses. The vascular channels vary greatly in width and some are cystically dilated. **B** High-power view of the tumour cells, some of which show intracytoplasmic haemosiderin granules, whereas others exhibit small eosinophilic globules in their cytoplasm.

Staging

Not relevant

Prognosis and prediction

Littoral cell angioma is a benign tumour, but because of the risk of complications such as rupture or hypersplenism, splenectomy is usually performed {1122,3174,368,352,1005,3451, 3069}. Extremely rare cases capable of distant spread are more appropriately diagnosed as littoral cell haemangioendothelioma or angiosarcoma; these cases show either solid areas composed of bland neoplastic cells or vascular and solid structures containing atypical cells {1167,312,2224,3486}.

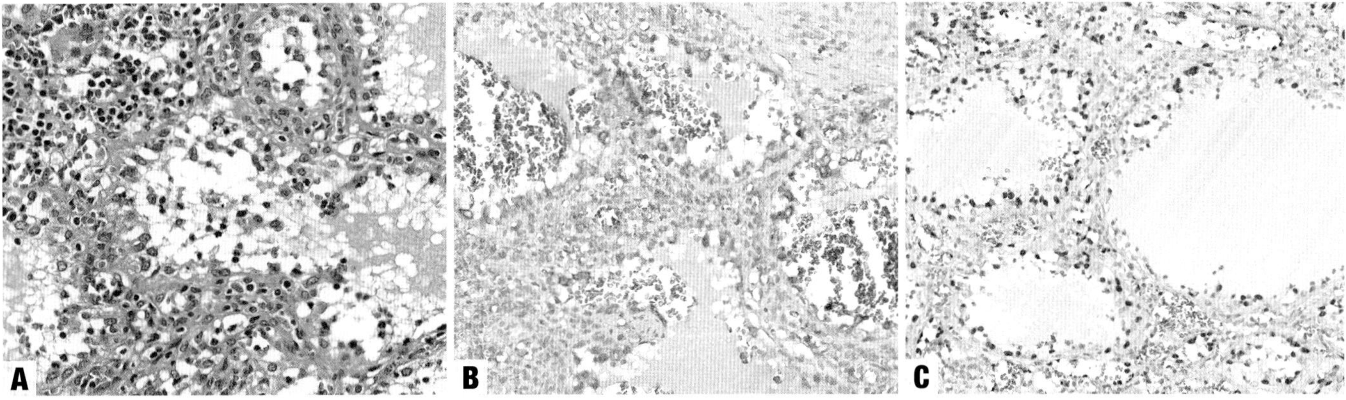

Fig. 6.21 Littoral cell angioma. **A** The vascular channels are lined by a single layer of protruding plump cuboidal or tall endothelial cells with ample eosinophilic cytoplasm. The cells often slough off into the lumina. **B** The histiocytic marker CD163 shows strong cytoplasmic staining. **C** The vascular marker ERG is strongly positive in tumour cell nuclei.

Splenic hamartoma

Cheuk W
Laskin WB

Definition
Splenic hamartoma is a benign circumscribed parenchymal lesion comprising disorganized red pulp elements without well-formed white pulp.

ICD-O coding
None

ICD-11 coding
3B81.0 Tumour-like conditions of spleen

Related terminology
Not recommended: splenoma.

Subtype(s)
None

Localization
Spleen

Clinical features
Most splenic hamartomas are incidental findings in splenectomy specimens or at autopsy {3750}. Approximately 20% of patients present with symptoms related to the mass lesion (such as abdominal discomfort and splenic rupture) or with haematological complications associated with hypersplenism (such as thrombocytopenia or anaemia) {1121,2249,3750}.

Epidemiology
Splenic hamartomas are uncommon, with reported incidence rates in autopsy series being 0.024–0.13% {3749,2199}. They occur in any age group (including in children), with a median age of 40 years {1121}, and exhibit no sex predilection {1539, 2249}.

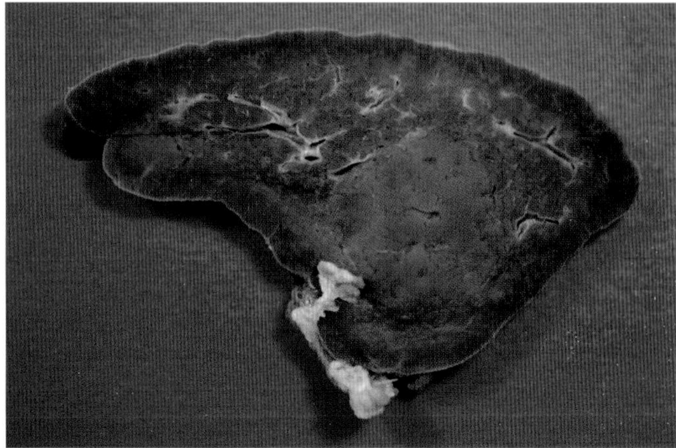

Fig. 6.22 Splenic hamartoma. The cut surfaces of the spleen reveal a well-circumscribed nodule that lacks the trabecular vessels seen in the surrounding normal spleen.

Etiology
The etiology is unknown. Rare cases occur in patients with tuberous sclerosis {871,4158,2520}. The reported association with solid or haematological malignancies may represent fortuitous discovery of the splenic hamartoma during radiological examinations or surgical explorations in these patients {3750, 1121}.

Pathogenesis
Splenic hamartoma has been postulated to represent a malformation, vascular neoplasm, or posttraumatic reactive lesion {3749,769,2249,3750}. Although the human androgen receptor (HUMARA) assay suggests a polyclonal lesion, clonal karyotypic abnormalities have been reported in 1 case {991,719}.

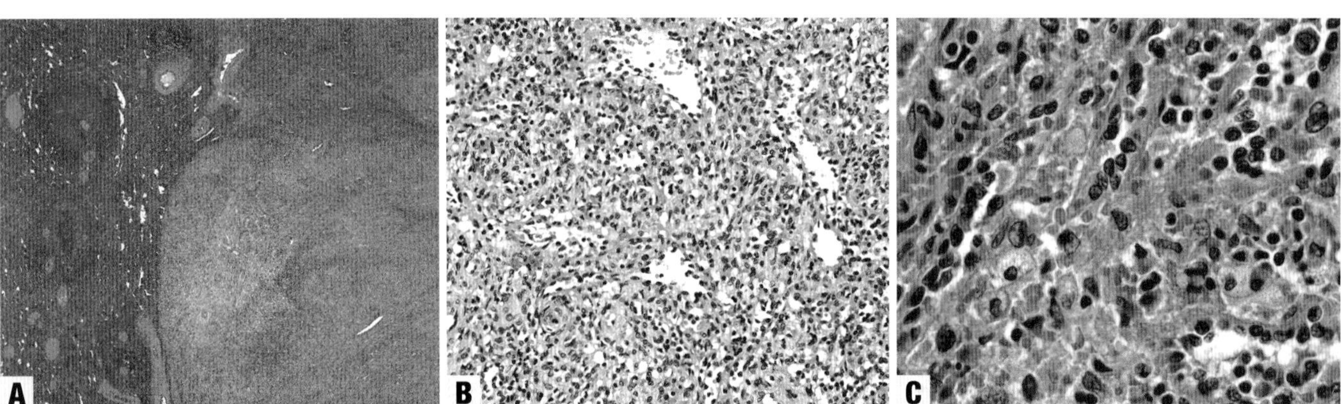

Fig. 6.23 Splenic hamartoma. **A** The lesion (right field) is well delineated from the normal splenic tissue (left field) and comprises irregularly scattered vascular channels lined by plump endothelium, reminiscent of splenic sinuses. **B** Histiocytes and stromal cells are found between the vascular channels. **C** At higher magnification, splenic sinus–type blood vessels are separated by many histiocytes (some foamy), architecturally reminiscent of disorganized red pulp tissue.

Macroscopic appearance

Splenic hamartomas are spherical and circumscribed but unencapsulated {1121}. Most are solitary, but some are multiple. They appear dark-red to greyish-white, with a median size of 50 mm (range: <10 mm to 200 mm) {2249,3750}.

Histopathology

Despite the sharp demarcation on gross examination, the border of splenic hamartoma is often not as well defined microscopically. The lesion is composed of irregularly dispersed sinusoidal vascular channels lined by plump endothelium and surrounded by loose aggregates of macrophages admixed with fibrovascular stroma, architecturally reminiscent of disorganized red pulp tissue. There is no well-formed white pulp, although lymphoid aggregates can be found {3565}. Additional features may include focal sclerosis, calcifications, haemorrhage, peliosis, plasmacytosis, extramedullary haematopoiesis, large aggregates of macrophages (histiocyte-rich variant), xanthomatous histiocytes, eosinophils, and mast cells {1121,2199}. Rarely, scattered bizarre cells featuring poorly defined cytoplasm and irregular nuclei with vesicular chromatin and variably prominent nucleoli are identified. Variable expression of cytokeratin, actin, or desmin in this population suggests accessory reticulum cell differentiation {695,2225,4498,683}.

Immunohistochemistry

Different types of blood vessels can be identified: splenic sinuses (CD8+, CD31+, CD34−), capillaries (CD34+, CD31+, CD8−), and small veins (CD34−, CD31+, CD8−) {4597,72}. Many admixed macrophages (CD68+, CD163+) are demonstrable.

Differential diagnosis

Major differential diagnoses include splenic haemangioma (proliferation of a single type of blood vessel; CD8−), sclerosing angiomatoid nodular transformation (multiple angiomatoid nodules surrounded by concentric collagen fibres, set in a sclerotic stroma), and EBV-positive inflammatory follicular dendritic cell sarcoma (proliferation of spindly cells with variable degrees of nuclear atypia in a lymphoplasmacytic background, lacking splenic sinus-type vasculature, positive for follicular dendritic cell markers and EBV).

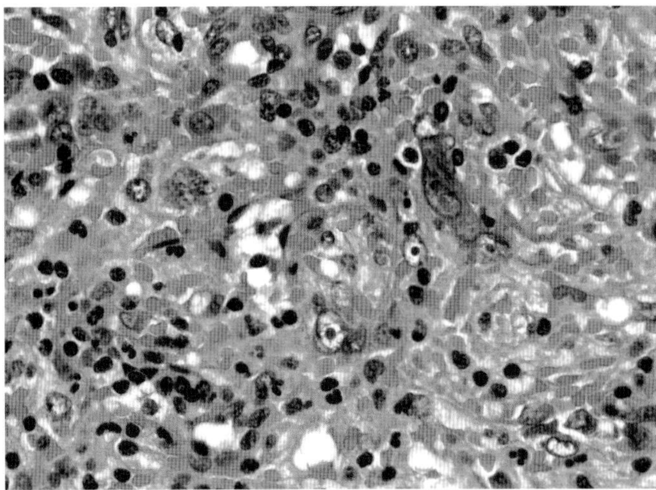

Fig. 6.24 Splenic hamartoma. An example with scattered bizarre stromal cells.

Cytology

Cytological features are nonspecific on FNAC {3359}.

Diagnostic molecular pathology

None

Essential and desirable diagnostic criteria

Essential: a circumscribed nodule in the spleen; composed of disorganized red pulp tissue, without a white pulp component.

Desirable: CD8 immunostain confirming the presence of disorganized splenic sinuses.

Staging

Not relevant

Prognosis and prediction

This benign lesion is curable by splenectomy.

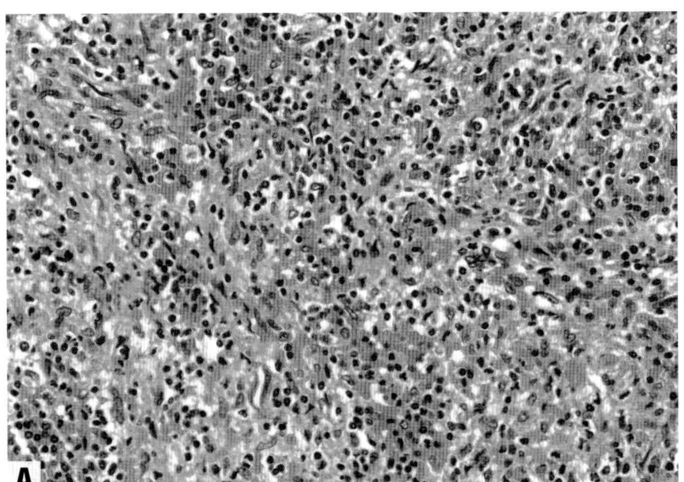

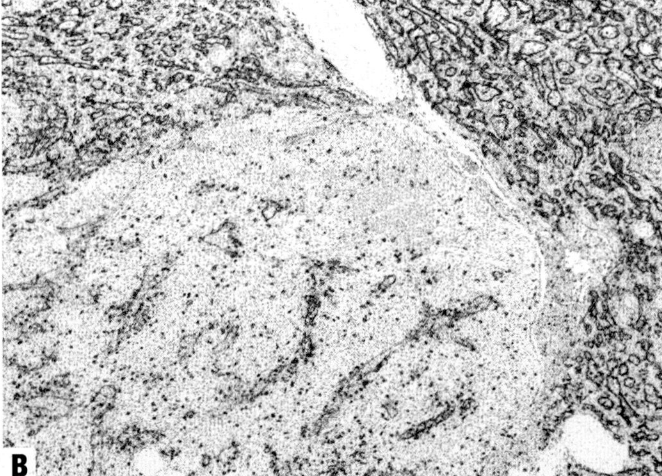

Fig. 6.25 Splenic hamartoma. **A** Vascular channels are admixed with stromal cells, histiocytes, and lymphocytes. Splenic sinus–type blood vessels are not evident on H&E staining. **B** Immunostaining for CD8, however, highlights the orderly splenic sinuses in the surrounding normal splenic tissue (upper field), and the more widely spaced, irregularly shaped sinuses in the hamartoma (lower field).

Sclerosing angiomatoid nodular transformation of spleen

Cheuk W
Medeiros LJ

Definition

Sclerosing angiomatoid nodular transformation (SANT) is a benign circumscribed lesion of the spleen composed of multiple angiomatoid nodules with intervening fibrosclerotic stroma.

ICD-O coding

9125/0 Sclerosing angiomatoid nodular transformation of spleen

ICD-11 coding

3B81.0 Tumour-like conditions of spleen

Related terminology

Not recommended: multinodular haemangioma.

Subtype(s)

None

Localization

Spleen

Clinical features

SANT is often asymptomatic, with 50–90% of cases detected incidentally by imaging studies. Some patients have symptoms, which are usually related to mass effects (abdominal discomfort, palpable mass) or hypersplenism (cytopenia, portal hypertension) {2542,951,1118,2975,1809,4493}. Growth retardation and splenic rupture have been rarely reported in children {2168, 3182}.

Epidemiology

SANT can occur in all age groups but most commonly affects middle-aged adults (median age: 46 years), and it has a female predilection (M:F ratio: 1:1.25–1.63) {1118,2975}. The incidence of SANT is unknown. SANT has been detected in as many as 15% of splenectomy specimens in some studies {4097}.

Etiology

The etiology is unknown. Roles for IgG4-related disease or EBV infection have been previously postulated, but these suggestions are not supported by current evidence {629,2975,3565}.

Pathogenesis

It has been hypothesized that fibrotic stromal proliferation from diverse causes may disrupt the local microcirculation, leading to transformation of red pulp into angiomatoid nodules {2542,951}. Assessment of clonality using the human androgen receptor (HUMARA) assay suggested that SANT is a polyclonal, reactive lesion {629}, but a recent study showed *CTNNB1* exon 3 deletions in SANT, suggesting that it is a benign neoplasm {4130}. Additional research is needed.

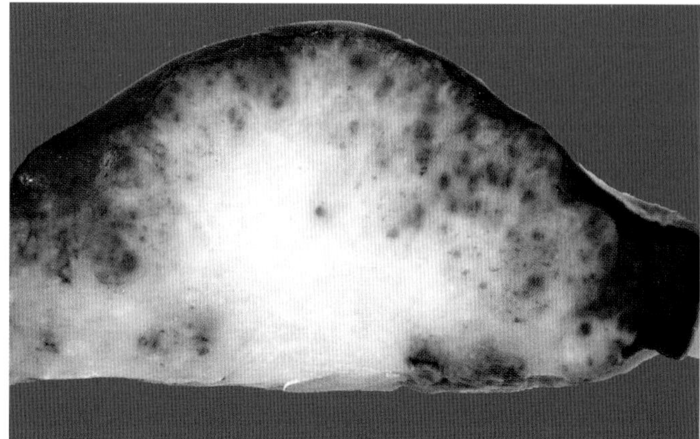

Fig. 6.26 Splenic sclerosing angiomatoid nodular transformation. The cut surface of the spleen shows a discrete bosselated lesion comprising red-brown nodules disposed in a firm, white, fibrotic background. The nodules are concentrated in the periphery.

Macroscopic appearance

SANT generally presents as a single, well-circumscribed, round to bosselated mass (mean diameter: 50 mm), or it may be composed of multiple such lesions (in 5–13% of cases) {544,2975}. There are multiple brown-red nodules, more numerous at the periphery of the lesion, delineated by intervening whitish fibrotic septa that converge to form a central stellate scar. These features manifest as a spoke-and-wheel pattern on enhanced CT or MRI {2336}.

Histopathology

Round or convoluted angiomatoid nodules, which can coalesce, are surrounded by concentric layers of collagen or fibrinoid material. The nodules are composed of slit-like, ectatic, or irregularly shaped vascular channels lined by attenuated or plump endothelial cells, with abundant red blood cells within or outside the vascular lumina. No cytological atypia or significant mitotic activity is found. The intervening stroma is densely fibrotic or composed of fibromyxoid tissue containing variable numbers of lymphocytes, plasma cells, eosinophils, and haemosiderin-laden macrophages. Immunohistochemical studies show a variable mixture of blood vessels as seen in splenic red pulp, including sinusoids (CD31+, CD8+, CD34–), capillaries (CD31+, CD8–, CD34+), and veins (CD31+, CD8–, CD34–).

Differential diagnosis

Splenic hamartoma lacks discrete angiomatoid nodules. Splenic haemangioma comprises a single type of vessels, namely capillaries (CD31+, CD8–, CD34+).

Cytology

Not relevant

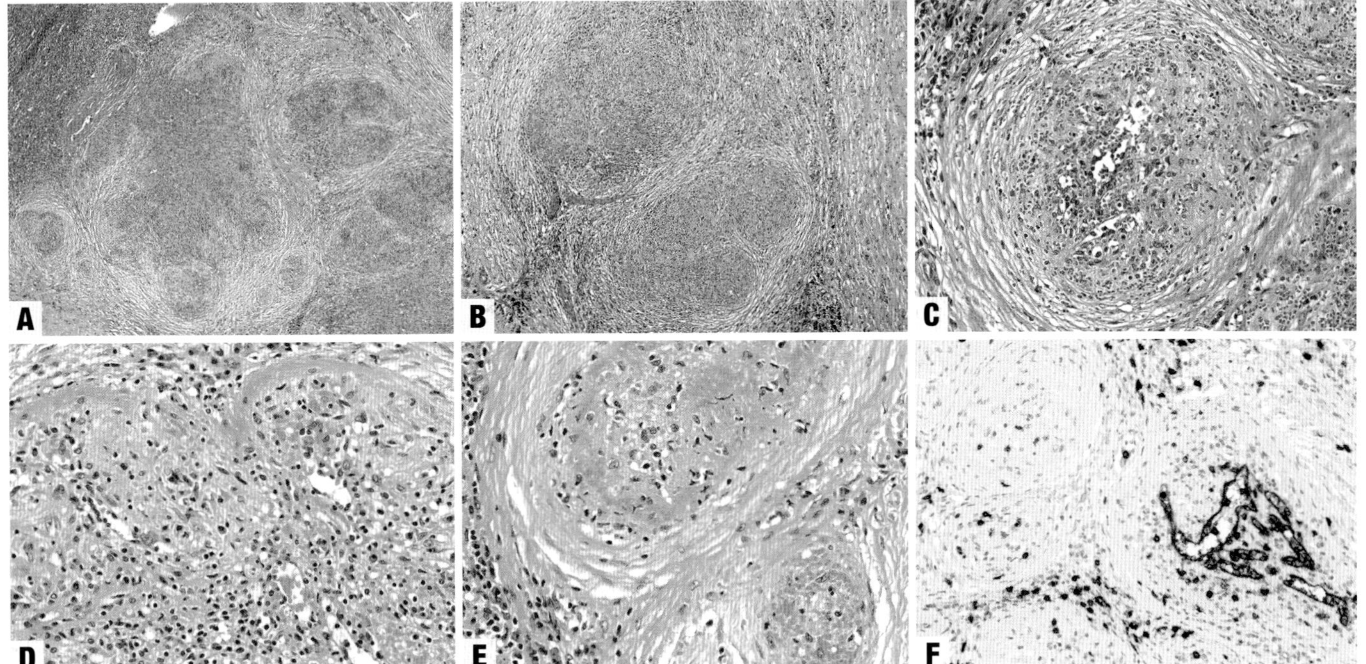

Fig. 6.27 Splenic sclerosing angiomatoid nodular transformation. **A** Multiple round or convoluted, sometimes coalescent, angiomatoid nodules occur in a sclerotic background. The individual nodules are surrounded by concentric rings of collagen fibres. Normal splenic tissue is seen in the upper-left corner. **B** Angiomatoid nodules occur in a sclerotic background with chronic inflammatory cell infiltration. **C** The angiomatoid nodule contains vascular channels reminiscent of splenic sinuses, accompanied by extravasation of red cells. It is surrounded by concentric rings of collagen fibres. **D** In the angiomatoid nodules, there are often some vascular channels reminiscent of splenic sinuses (sinusoids) mixed with other blood vessels, chronic inflammatory cells, and spindly cells in a fibrous stroma. **E** Some angiomatoid nodules show regressive changes, with few remaining blood vessels, haemorrhage, and fibrinoid deposits. **F** Immunostaining for CD8, a marker for splenic sinus lining cells, highlights the presence of splenic sinuses in at least some of the angiomatoid nodules.

Diagnostic molecular pathology

None

Essential and desirable diagnostic criteria

Essential: a circumscribed lesion in the spleen; multiple angiomatoid nodules comprising three types of blood vessels, with interspersed fibrosclerotic stroma.

Staging

Not relevant

Prognosis and prediction

Splenectomy or partial splenectomy is usually performed for diagnosis and/or symptomatic relief. No recurrence or metastasis has been reported {1118,2975}.

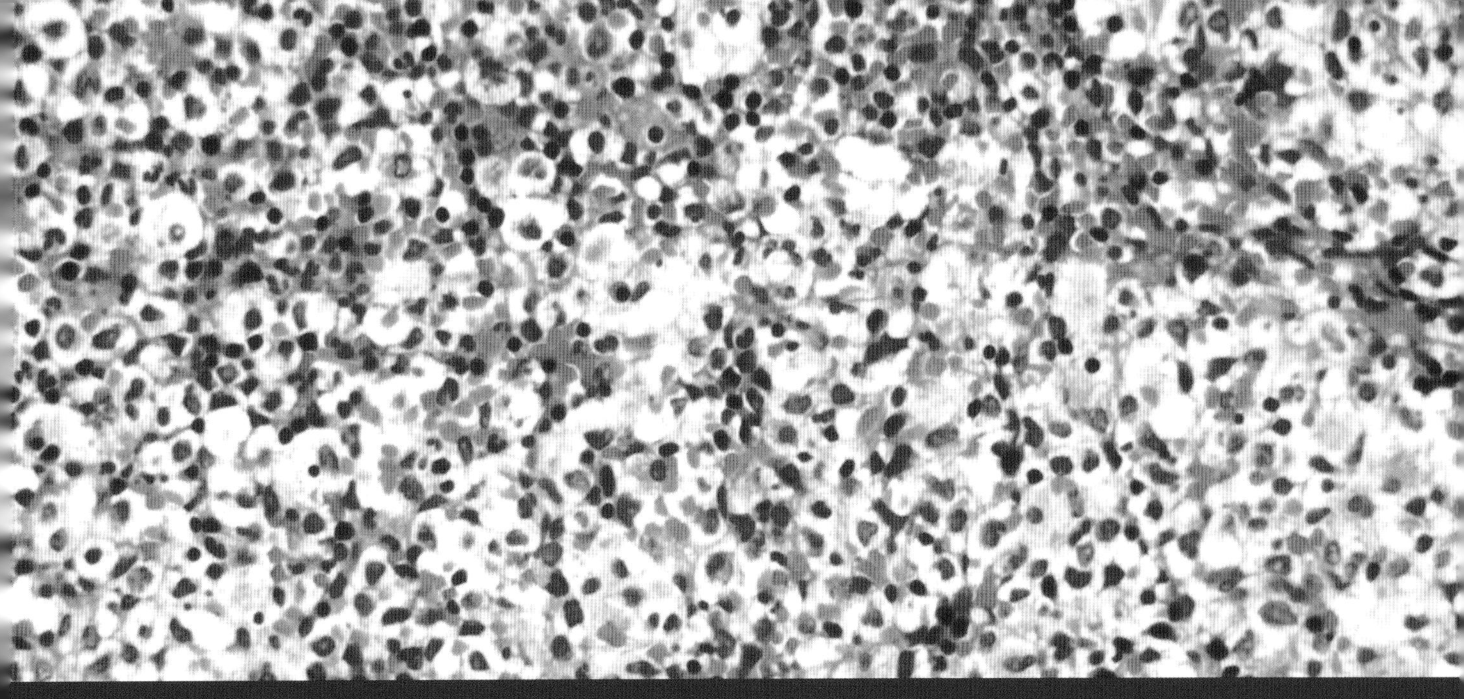

7

Genetic tumour syndromes associated with haematolymphoid tumours

Edited by: Akkari Y, Lax SF, Lazar AJ, Siebert R

Genetic tumour syndromes associated with haematolymphoid tumours: Introduction

Siebert R

Genetic predisposition is assumed for a variety of haematolymphoid neoplasms. Several epidemiological studies point to an increased incidence of haematolymphoid neoplasms in first- and second-degree relatives of patients with haematolymphoid malignancies. Notably, familial clustering does not necessarily imply a genetic predisposition; it can also indicate common exposures to pathogens, such as viruses associated with haematolymphoid neoplasms, chemical or physical hazards, or (particularly in lymphoid neoplasms) even antigens.

Associated familial risks vary depending on the entity. The conferred risk might be lineage- or even entity-specific or part of a broader cancer susceptibility. Entity-specific risks, such as in subsets of secondary myeloid neoplasms and proliferations, and also in lymphoid proliferations and lymphomas associated with immune deficiency and dysregulation, have been discussed in the sections describing these entities.

Generally, a genetic predisposition to haematolymphoid neoplasms, like to any cancer, can be distinguished in both syndromic and non-syndromic forms. Syndromic forms are characterized by recurrent and specific symptoms affecting organs other than the haematolymphoid system and can manifest as malformations, dysmorphisms, or developmental delay. Major syndromes associated with an increased risk of haematolymphoid neoplasms are presented in this chapter, namely Fanconi anaemia, ataxia–telangiectasia, Bloom syndrome, and RASopathies; other forms with syndromic features include *GATA2* deficiency, some forms of bone marrow failure syndrome, and disorders of telomere function. Common to all these named syndromes is their monogenic inheritance; however, constitutional chromosomal aberrations, as seen in Down syndrome and others, can be associated with an increased risk of haematolymphoid neoplasms.

The non-syndromic forms of genetic predisposition to haematolymphoid neoplasms can be divided into two overarching categories: monogenic and polygenic (i.e. mostly multifactorial). Among the monogenic forms, lymphomas and leukaemias form part of the spectrum of Li–Fraumeni and Li–Fraumeni–like syndromes associated with *TP53* and *CHEK2* variants, respectively. The majority of inborn errors of immunity predisposing to predominately lymphoid malignancies are also monogenic traits. Notwithstanding this, particularly in mature lymphoid neoplasms, monogenic predisposition seems to be rare, and a polygenic predisposition is assumed. Genes associated with such polygenic predisposition often include important factors of B- and T-cell regulation. Variants of these genes commonly also predispose to a spectrum of common immune disorders, which in turn increase the risk for mature lymphoid neoplasms, suggesting a multifactorial predisposition. Similarly, genomic variants linked to pathogen infection, like the sickle cell trait in asymptomatic malaria, have been associated with predisposition, in this example to Burkitt lymphoma.

Detection of a germline predisposition in haematolymphoid neoplasms is important not only for diagnostic categorization, as outlined in this volume, but also for treatment, surveillance, and family counselling. Some germline predispositions are associated with altered responses to therapy and increased toxicities. Moreover, a *TP53* germline variant confers an increased risk of radiation-induced secondary malignancies. In addition, first-degree relatives of germline variant carriers, depending on the underlying trait, can have an increased risk of the same disorders and could benefit from surveillance. It is therefore mandatory to consider genetic counselling and potentially initiate germline genetic testing in all patients for whom the clinical presentation, family history, or laboratory findings might point to a germline predisposition. Features that warrant germline genetic workup include the following:

- Diagnosis of a haematolymphoid neoplasm typically associated with germline predisposition as outlined in this volume
- A known germline predisposition to cancer in a family
- Fulfilment of the diagnostic criteria for any established cancer predisposition syndrome, like Li–Fraumeni syndrome, hereditary breast–ovarian cancer, familial colorectal cancer, etc.
- Occurrence of a haematolymphoid neoplasm in a patient with syndromic features (e.g. dysmorphisms, organ malformations, developmental disorder)
- Diagnosis of a haematolymphoid neoplasm in two first- or second-degree relatives within a family
- Diagnosis of two independent haematolymphoid neoplasms in the same person or a (non–therapy-induced) haematolymphoid neoplasm in a person with multiple or early-onset solid tumours
- Increased and unexplained treatment toxicity in a patient with haematolymphoid neoplasms
- Very early onset of a haematolymphoid neoplasm, as compared with the general epidemiology of the disease
- Detection of a pathogenic or likely pathogenic variant in the somatic workup of a neoplasm, if the variant affects a gene associated with germline cancer predisposition and sequencing findings are compatible with a germline origin

Germline genetic predisposition testing must take into account the fact that with many haematolymphoid neoplasms, samples usually assumed to be germline (including tissue samples, blood samples, and buccal swabs) can be contaminated by tumour cells, which can complicate molecular diagnostic characterization. In such cases, other sample sources (e.g. hair follicles or fingernail clippings) might be considered. Positive predictive values for genetic testing are currently based mostly on monogenic predisposition, although the application of polygenic risk scores might add to risk prediction in some diseases.

Fanconi anaemia

Kratz CP
Choi JK
Olson TS
Solomon DA

Definition

Fanconi anaemia (FA) is a clinically and genetically heterogeneous disorder caused by germline variants in the FA/BRCA DNA repair pathway, resulting in chromosomal breakage and hypersensitivity to crosslinking agents. Characteristic clinical features include developmental abnormalities in major organ systems, early-onset bone marrow failure, endocrine anomalies, and a high predisposition to cancer.

MIM numbering

227650 Fanconi anaemia, complementation group A; FANCA
300514 Fanconi anaemia, complementation group B; FANCB
227645 Fanconi anaemia, complementation group C; FANCC
605724 Fanconi anaemia, complementation group D1; FANCD1
227646 Fanconi anaemia, complementation group D2; FANCD2
600901 Fanconi anaemia, complementation group E; FANCE
603467 Fanconi anaemia, complementation group F; FANCF
614082 Fanconi anaemia, complementation group G; FANCG
609053 Fanconi anaemia, complementation group I; FANCI
609054 Fanconi anaemia, complementation group J; FANCJ
614083 Fanconi anaemia, complementation group L; FANCL
610832 Fanconi anaemia, complementation group N; FANCN
613390 Fanconi anaemia, complementation group O; FANCO
613951 Fanconi anaemia, complementation group P; FANCP
615272 Fanconi anaemia, complementation group Q; FANCQ
617244 Fanconi anaemia, complementation group R; FANCR
617883 Fanconi anaemia, complementation group S; FANCS
616435 Fanconi anaemia, complementation group T; FANCT
617247 Fanconi anaemia, complementation group U; FANCU
617243 Fanconi anaemia, complementation group V; FANCV
617784 Fanconi anaemia, complementation group W; FANCW

ICD-11 coding

3A70.0 Congenital aplastic anaemia

Related terminology

None

Subtype(s)

Complementation groups A, B, C, D1, D2, E, F, G, I, J, L, N, O, P, Q, R, S, T, U, V, and W

Localization

Manifestations of FA may develop in all organs and tissues.

Clinical features

FA is characterized by a range of physical abnormalities, progressive bone marrow failure, and an increased risk for cancer. Classic features include abnormal thumbs, absent radii, short stature, skin hyperpigmentation, abnormal facies (triangular face, microcephaly, microphthalmia), abnormal kidneys, and decreased fertility {911}, although the absence of these features

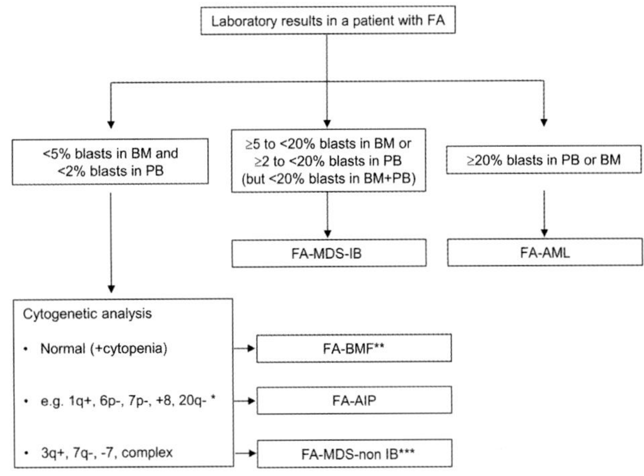

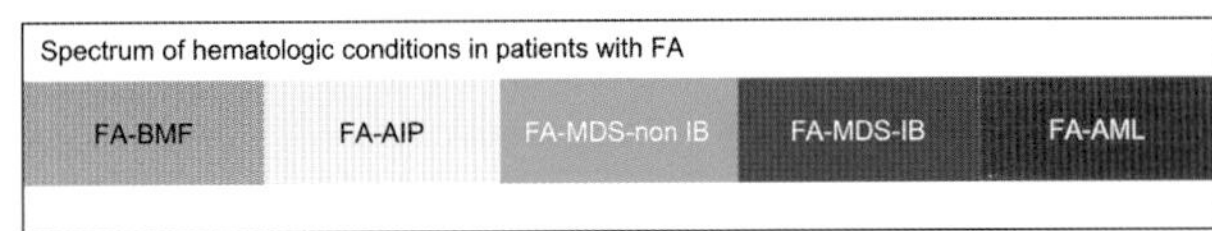

* all cytogenetic aberrations (exclusion: 3q+, 7q-, -7, complex)
**In cases with rapid rise in BM cellularity FA-MDS needs to be considered
*** In pediatric patients generally childhood myelodysplastic neoplasm with low blasts

Fig. 7.01 Fanconi anaemia (FA). Diagnostic algorithm for haematological conditions in patients with FA. BM, bone marrow; FA-AIP, aberration of indeterminate potential in a patient with FA; FA-AML, acute myeloid leukaemia in a patient with FA; FA-BMF, bone marrow failure in a patient with FA, a normal blast percentage, and normal cytogenetics; FA-MDS-IB, myelodysplastic neoplasm with increased blasts in a patient with FA; FA-MDS-non IB, myelodysplastic neoplasm without increased blasts in a patient with FA; PB, peripheral blood.

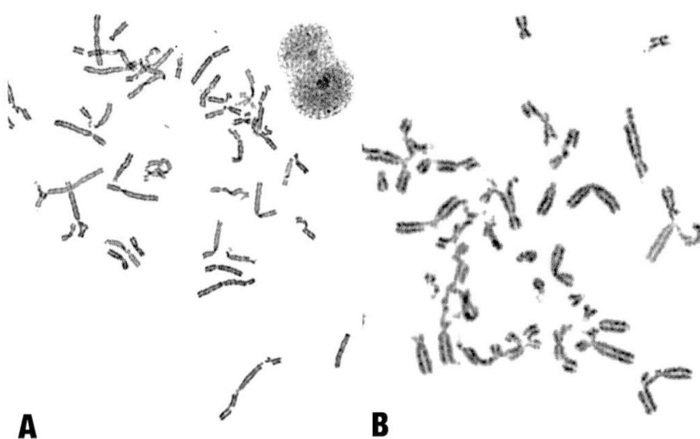

Fig. 7.02 Fanconi anaemia. **A,B** Lymphoblasts or skin fibroblasts from patients with Fanconi anaemia display chromosome breakage and radial formation when treated with DNA crosslinking agents such as mitomycin C or diepoxybutane (DEB).

does not exclude FA. The most common neoplasms associated with FA are myelodysplastic neoplasms, acute myeloid leukaemia, and squamous cell carcinoma of the head and neck. According to a recent study enrolling 421 patients, for all FA subgroups combined, the cancer-specific standardized incidence ratio for myeloid neoplasms was 445 (95% CI: 272–687) {1032}. By the age of 18 years, 10.6% of patients with FA developed any cancer {1032}.

Haematological conditions in patients with FA

A recently proposed classification {289} distinguishes between the following five categories:

1. FA-BMF (bone marrow failure in a patient with FA): normal blast percentage and normal cytogenetics in a patient with cytopenia; FA-BMF ranges from mild to severe (see Table 7.01).
2. FA-AIP (aberration of indeterminate potential in a patient with FA): normal blast percentage and one or more aberrations of indeterminate potential (these are clonal aberrations, such as duplication of 1q, that remain stable over a prolonged period of time without transformation).
3. FA-MDS (myelodysplastic neoplasm in a patient with FA) without increased blasts: normal blast percentage and clonal aberrations unambiguously associated with transformation (−7, 7q−, 3q+, complex).
4. FA-MDS with increased blasts: increased blast percentage in bone marrow (≥ 5% to < 20%) or in peripheral blood (≥ 2% to < 20%).
5. FA-AML (acute myeloid leukaemia in a patient with FA): defined by an increased blast percentage (≥ 20%) in bone marrow or peripheral blood.

Epidemiology

FA is most often an autosomal recessive disorder resulting from homozygous or compound heterozygous germline variants in the 21 different FANC genes. The two exceptions are complementation group B (*FANCB*), which is X-linked, and complementation group R (*RAD51*), which is autosomal dominant. The estimated carrier frequency for FA is 1 in 100–200 individuals, and the approximate syndrome incidence rate is 1 case per 130 000 live births {3466}.

Etiology

FA can be caused by germline pathogenic variants in at least 21 different genes, which result in mostly similar clinical phenotypes but with some differences, including varying cancer risks. Depending on the specific causative gene, FA is differentiated into complementation groups A–W (e.g. complementation group A is caused by a biallelic germline variant in *FANCA*).

Pathogenesis

The FANC genes encode proteins involved in the homologous recombination of DNA double-strand breaks and in the repair of DNA crosslinks. The deleterious variants in the FANC genes causative of FA result in impaired homologous recombination and crosslink repair, which drives chromosomal aberrations such as amplifications, deletions, and translocations that ultimately promote tumorigenesis {1229}.

Table 7.01 Severity of bone marrow failure

Test	Mild	Moderate	Severe
Absolute neutrophil count	< 1500/mm^3	< 1000/mm^3	< 500/mm^3
Platelets	50 000–150 000/mm^3	< 50 000/mm^3	< 20 000/mm^3
Haemoglobin	≥ 8 g/dL[a]	< 8 g/dL	< 8 g/dL

[a]Lower than normal for age but ≥ 8 g/dL.

Macroscopic appearance

Not relevant

Histopathology

FA-BMF mimics myelodysplastic neoplasms with low blasts (see *Childhood myelodysplastic neoplasm with low blasts*, p. 90) or severe aplastic anaemia. Dysgranulopoiesis and dysmegakaryopoiesis are histological indicators of progression to FA-MDS {751,1752}.

Cytology

Not relevant

Diagnostic molecular pathology

Diagnosis of FA has traditionally employed chromosomal breakage analysis performed on patient-derived cultures of either leukocytes from a peripheral blood sample or fibroblasts from a skin biopsy after treatment with an agent that induces DNA interstrand crosslinks, such as diepoxybutane (DEB) and/or mitomycin C (MMC). Mutation analysis of a constitutional DNA sample to assess for pathogenic variants or deletions in the FANC genes is a complementary diagnostic methodology that can identify the causative gene abnormality.

Essential and desirable diagnostic criteria

Essential: positive chromosomal breakage / radial formation (or cell-cycle) analysis after exposure of leukocyte or fibroblast cultures to crosslinking agents.

Desirable: pathogenic biallelic germline variants in a FANC gene, except *FANCB* and *RAD51* (*FANCR*), which require a monoallelic germline variant.

Staging

Not relevant

Prognosis and prediction

Haematopoietic stem cell transplantation using matched related and unrelated donors is highly efficacious for patients with FA-BMF; in particular, the use of haploidentical donors has resulted in markedly improved outcomes {3855}. Current preparative regimens for haematopoietic stem cell transplantation have eliminated the use of radiation and employ low doses of alkylating chemotherapy to lower the risks of secondary malignancies and organ toxicity. Treatment of patients with FA-MDS with increased blasts or FA-AML remains a challenge; outcomes are poor, and it often requires the initiation of transplant regimens during aplasia from induction chemotherapy {3179}.

Bloom syndrome

Elenitoba-Johnson KSJ
Attarbaschi A

Definition

Bloom syndrome is an autosomal recessive disorder characterized by perinatal growth deficiency, skin photosensitivity, typical facial features, insulin resistance, and immune deficiency leading to a marked increase in risk of early-onset cancer and the development of myeloid and lymphoid neoplasms. Loss-of-function variants of *BLM*, encoding RECQ, are the cause of Bloom syndrome.

MIM numbering

210900 Bloom syndrome; BLM

ICD-11 coding

4A01.31 DNA repair defects other than combined T-cell or B-cell immunodeficiencies

Related terminology

None

Subtype(s)

None

Localization

Not applicable

Clinical features

Affected individuals show abnormal growth, feeding difficulties, skin changes, immune deficiency, an increased risk of diabetes, and an increased risk of a variety of cancer types at a younger age, with a variety of haematological malignancies, including acute myeloid leukaemia (AML), lymphoblastic leukaemia/lymphoma (ALL/LBL), and lymphoma. Solid tumours and the development of multiple cancers of varying histology are common.

Leukaemia and lymphoma are the most commonly diagnosed malignancies {849}. For AML, the mean age at diagnosis is 18 years (range: 2–47 years), and for ALL/LBL it is 20 years (range: 5–40 years). The incidence of AML is higher than that of ALL/LBL, potentially because of preceding treatment-related myelodysplastic neoplasm. For lymphoma, the mean age at diagnosis is 22 years (range: 4–49 years), applying to B- and T-cell lymphomas, as well as (though rare) classic Hodgkin lymphoma. In approximately 75% of cases lymphoma is the first neoplasm, and in 25% it represents a second malignancy {849}.

Epidemiology

Bloom syndrome is extremely rare. In certain populations it has a high prevalence, and in the Ashkenazi Jewish population the estimated carrier frequency is 1 in 120 {3692}.

Etiology

Loss-of-function variants of *BLM* result in the absence of the functional BLM protein, which encodes a RECQ, leading to chromosome instability, excessive homologous recombination, and an increased number of sister chromatid exchanges {2617, 607}.

Pathogenesis

BLM is a component of a multisubunit complex of proteins, together with the Fanconi anaemia core complex and the mismatch repair protein MLH1. It functions as a 3′ to 5′ DNA helicase and is critical for the maintenance of genomic integrity {689}. BLM plays a critical role in T- and B-cell development {196} and immune integrity {197}. Although the numbers of B cells and T cells are normal in Bloom syndrome, there are significant impairments in T-cell function {3970}, as well as deficiencies of serum immunoglobulin class {947}, leading to the impairment of the adaptive immune system.

Macroscopic appearance

Not relevant

Histopathology

A variety of haematopoietic neoplasms, including AML, ALL/LBL, lymphoproliferative disorders, and lymphomas, are observed (see *Inborn error of immunity–associated lymphoid proliferations and lymphomas*, p. 573).

Cytology

Not relevant

Diagnostic molecular pathology

DNA sequencing analysis to demonstrate biallelic pathogenic variants in *BLM*

Essential and desirable diagnostic criteria

Essential: presence of a suggestive pattern of growth and medical problems; demonstration of biallelic pathogenic variants in *BLM*.

Staging

Not relevant

Prognosis and prediction

Affected individuals have many medical and health impairments, the most significant being skin abnormalities, problems associated with growth retardation, endocrine diseases, and an elevated risk of malignancies. Cancer surveillance is critical for individuals with Bloom syndrome. However, presymptomatic, early detection of leukaemia provides no proven additional value in terms of outcome, and monitoring by routine blood counts is therefore not recommended. Observation for signs and symptoms associated with lymphoma should be promptly followed by evaluation. The use of therapeutic radiation and some chemotherapeutic agents such as alkylating drugs may increase the risk of secondary malignancies and should be avoided if possible. Patients are especially prone to treatment-related toxicity and may need special vigilance when receiving standard or modified/reduced-intensity chemotherapy {849}. Nevertheless, as cure of leukaemias and lymphomas is possible in these patients, upfront de-escalation of chemotherapy with successive adaptations is currently recommended to reduce the risk of therapy-related fatalities.

Ataxia–telangiectasia

Elenitoba-Johnson KSJ
Attarbaschi A

Definition

Ataxia–telangiectasia (AT) is a rare autosomal recessive disease caused by germline variants in *ATM* leading to disease affecting multiple systems, which may manifest in infancy or early childhood. Characteristic disease manifestations include cerebellar degeneration with progressive ataxia, oculocutaneous telangiectasia, immunodeficiency, susceptibility to bronchopulmonary disease, and lymphoid tumours.

MIM numbering

208900 Ataxia–telangiectasia; AT

ICD-11 coding

4A01.31 DNA repair defects other than combined T-cell or B-cell immunodeficiencies

Related terminology

Not recommended: cerebello-oculocutaneous telangiectasia; immunodeficiency with ataxia–telangiectasia; Louis–Bar syndrome; Boder–Sedgwick syndrome.

Subtype(s)

None

Localization

Leukaemias affect bone marrow and peripheral blood. Occasionally, a mediastinal mass can be found in patients with T-lymphoblastic leukaemia. Lymphomas manifest with persistent lymphadenopathy. Extranodal lymphomatous involvement may also be observed. In patients with T-prolymphocytic leukaemia, peripheral blood lymphocytosis and splenomegaly are observed.

Clinical features

AT is a pleiotropic disorder with multiple manifestations, including immunodeficiency, neurological deficits, and an increased propensity for the development of cancer. As many as 10% of all people homozygous for pathogenic *ATM* variants develop a malignancy, with a 70- and 250-fold increased risk for leukaemias and lymphomas, respectively {2796}. The M:F ratio for lymphoid malignancies is approximately 1.4–2:1. The predisposition to leukaemia and lymphoma is observed from childhood, with a high propensity for the development of acute lymphoblastic leukaemia, which generally shows a higher frequency of unfavourable prognostic features than seen in non-AT cases, such as male sex, older age at presentation (median: 9 years), higher white blood cell count, and a mediastinal mass.

The prevalence of T-prolymphocytic leukaemia (T-PLL) is markedly higher in patients with AT, in whom it occurs in young adulthood, than in patients without AT, in whom it occurs at a median age of 69 years at diagnosis {3982}. The majority of the malignancies seen in younger patients with AT are of T-cell lineage, and a minor proportion are of B-cell lineage {3982}. The B-cell lymphomas are aggressive in nature and include diffuse large B-cell lymphoma and Burkitt lymphoma (see *Inborn error of immunity–associated lymphoid proliferations and lymphomas*, p. 573) {1061}. A rare case of Hodgkin lymphoma has been reported {3982}. Non-haematopoietic malignancies, including epithelial tumours, constitute 13–22% of all malignancies and can be seen in adolescents, with a median age of 17 years {3039,3982}. Myeloid malignancies are virtually absent {3982}.

Neurological deficits include cerebellar degeneration with progressive ataxia presenting in infancy, and oculocutaneous telangiectasia. The neurological symptoms include abnormal eye movements and dysarthria. Patients also exhibit growth retardation, hypogonadism, and elevated levels of AFP {3982}. Most patients develop sinopulmonary infections.

The differential diagnosis includes chronic ataxic syndromes {2571}, as well as disorders associated with deficiencies in DNA repair pathways, such as Cockayne syndrome, xeroderma pigmentosum, and Nijmegen breakage syndrome.

Epidemiology

AT is rare and is estimated to occur at a frequency of 1:40 000–100 000 live births {1277,4407,3911}. In some populations, the disease is reported to occur at even lower frequencies (1:300 000) {1341}. It tends to affect both sexes equally.

Etiology

AT is caused by germline pathogenic variants in *ATM* on 11q22.3 {3596}. Pathogenic nonsense variants, frameshift variants, missense indels, and structural variations have been described. Compound heterozygous variants have also been observed {2294}. The classic AT phenotype results from biallelic loss-of-function variants leading to loss of expression of the ATM protein or expression of a defective ATM protein {3564,2294}.

Pathogenesis

The protein encoded by *ATM* is a tumour suppressor. ATM is a high-molecular-weight (350 kDa) serine/threonine kinase member of the PI3K-related protein kinase (PIKK) family and is involved in the response to double-stranded DNA breaks {3596}. ATM phosphorylates critical protein substrates, including p53 and BRCA1 {230,539}, and plays a crucial functional role in controlling genome stability, cell-cycle checkpoint signalling, and apoptosis. A variant of *ATM* resulting in impaired protein function leads to defective DNA repair, chromosomal instability {3981}, and the deregulation of multiple pathways and biological processes (such as G1- to S-phase cell-cycle progression, cell growth, and apoptosis), which in turn results in an increased propensity for the development of cancer.

Macroscopic appearance

Tumours in AT resemble their sporadic counterparts.

Histopathology

The lymphoid malignancies that occur most frequently in AT include lymphoblastic leukaemia/lymphoma, T-PLL, diffuse large B-cell lymphoma, and (less frequently) Burkitt and Hodgkin lymphomas (see *Inborn error of immunity–associated lymphoid proliferations and lymphomas*, p. 573).

Immunophenotype

The phenotype of the lymphoid malignancies is identical to that of corresponding malignancies in patients without AT.

Cytology

The cytology mimics that observed in the corresponding lymphoid malignancies occurring in patients without AT.

Diagnostic molecular pathology

Cytogenetics

In routine metaphase preparations, individuals with AT show an increased frequency of chromosomal rearrangements that involve two different T-cell receptor (TR) loci (at 7p14, 7q34, or 14q11.2) and/or immunoglobulin (IG) loci (particularly IGH at 14q32). Clonal T-cell populations and T-PLL recurrently show t(14;14)(q11;q32) and inv(14)(q11q32) involving *TCL1A* and t(X;14)(q28;q11) involving *MTCP1* {3982}.

Molecular pathology

Monoclonal rearrangements of the TR genes (TRA/D, TRG, TRB) are detected in T-lineage lymphoblastic leukaemia/lymphoma, T-PLL, and other T-cell neoplasms. Monoclonal immunoglobulin gene (IGH, IGK, IGL) rearrangements are observed in B-cell neoplasms.

Essential and desirable diagnostic criteria

Essential: demonstration of homozygous or compound heterozygous pathogenic variants in *ATM*; the diagnostic criteria for lymphoid malignancies are the same as those used to establish the diagnosis of those entities in patients without AT.

Desirable: high AFP levels are not diagnostic but are observed in > 95% of patients.

Staging

Not relevant

Prognosis and prediction

AT has a poor prognosis. Many patients with AT succumb to progressive pulmonary disease or to cancer, with a median age at death of 25 years {834}. Patients with non-Hodgkin lymphomas and underlying AT have an inferior survival rate, with a larger proportion of therapy-related deaths and relapses than patients with non-Hodgkin lymphomas without AT. Nevertheless, because cure of lymphomas is possible in these patients, an upfront de-escalation of chemotherapy with successive adaptations is currently recommended to reduce the risk of therapy-related fatalities. Radiotherapy should be completely omitted.

RASopathies

Michaels PD
Petersen AK

Definition

The RASopathies are a diverse group of complex, multisystem disorders with etiologies arising from genes involved in the RAS/MAPK pathway.

MIM numbering

162200 Neurofibromatosis, type I; NF1
163950 Noonan syndrome 1; NS1
151100 LEOPARD syndrome 1; LPRD1
218040 Costello syndrome; CSTLO
115150 Cardiofaciocutaneous syndrome 1; CFC1
611431 Legius syndrome; LGSS

ICD-11 coding

LD2D.10 Neurofibromatosis type 1
LD2F.15 Noonan syndrome
LD2F.1Y Other specified syndromes with multiple structural anomalies, not of environmental origin
LD27.5 Genetic hamartoneoplastic syndromes affecting the skin

Related terminology

None

Subtype(s)

None

Localization

Not relevant

Clinical features

Each RASopathy has a distinct phenotype, although these phenotypes sometimes overlap. In descending order of incidence, RASopathies include neurofibromatosis type 1 (NF1), Noonan syndrome (NS), NS with multiple lentigines (formerly LEOPARD syndrome [multiple lentigines, electrocardiographic conduction abnormalities, ocular hypertelorism, pulmonic stenosis, abnormal genitalia, retardation of growth, and sensorineural deafness]), Costello syndrome, cardio-facial-cutaneous syndrome, and Legius syndrome.

NF1 is associated with café-au-lait spots, freckling, bone anomalies, and learning disabilities, as well as neurofibromas, which may be localized, diffuse, or plexiform. Plexiform neurofibromas carry a 10% lifetime risk of transformation to a malignant peripheral nerve sheath tumour. Of note, individuals with NF1 due to the NM_001042492.3(NF1):c.2970_2972del (p.M992del) variant do not have neurofibromas. Pilocytic astrocytomas / optic nerve gliomas occur in the first decade of life in ~20% of patients, but they often spontaneously regress. Individuals with NF1 also have an increased risk of other CNS tumours, sarcoma, gastrointestinal tumours, juvenile myelomonocytic leukaemia (JMML), and breast cancer. Approximately 15% of patients with NF1 have clinical features of NS.

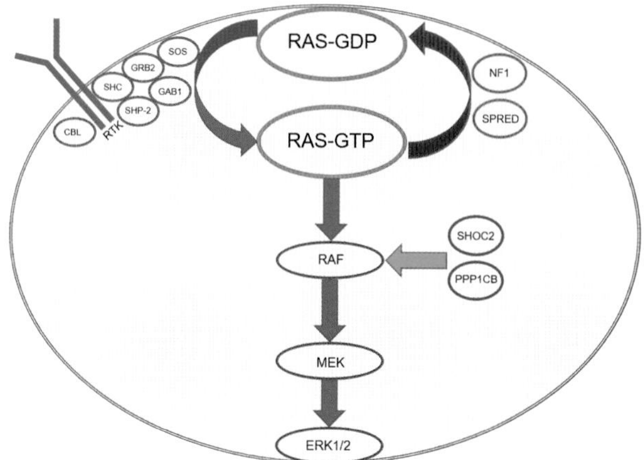

Fig. 7.03 The RAS/MAPK signalling pathway. Activation of the signalling pathway begins with a receptor tyrosine kinase (RTK) that autophosphorylates on tyrosine residues, creating docking sites for adapters such as SHC and GRB2 and relocalizing SOS to the membrane. SHP2 activates RAS by dephosphorylating several inhibitory phosphotyrosines, including the docking site for GAB1. RAS switches from a GDP-bound to a GTP-bound state, which begins the RAF/MEK/ERK phosphorylation cascade. RAS intrinsic GTPase activity hydrolyses GTP back to GDP. Neurofibromin (NF1) and SPRED negatively regulate RAS by accelerating conversion of RAS-GTP to RAS-GDP. SHOC2 and PPP1CB activate the signalling pathway by dephosphorylating an inhibitory residue on RAF. CBL drives RTK ubiquitination, thus turning off activating signals.

Legius syndrome is clinically indistinguishable from NF1 except there are no neurofibromas, and it often confers less oncological risk.

NS is associated with distinct facial features, congenital heart anomalies, short stature, coagulopathy, neurodevelopmental disability, and undescended testes, as well as ocular, lymphatic, and skeletal anomalies. Children with NS are thought to have an 8-fold increased risk of cancer relative to their peers, but the incidence is too low to justify routine surveillance. Embryonal rhabdomyosarcoma is rare but has been observed in patients with germline variants in *SOS1*. Myeloid neoplasms and JMML occur more commonly in *PTPN11*-associated and *CBL*-associated NS. Germline *PTPN11* variants at codons 61, 71, 72, and 76 appear to confer a particularly high risk. Lymphoblastic leukaemia/lymphoma and acute myeloid leukaemia (AML) are enriched in patients with *PTPN11*- and *RAF1*-related NS; these genes account for 93% of cases of NS with multiple lentigines. Hepatosplenomegaly is frequent and thought to be due to subclinical myeloid proliferations.

Costello syndrome and cardio-facial-cutaneous syndrome overlap clinically with NS, and their relative rarity makes incidence rates difficult to determine reliably. Costello syndrome confers the greatest malignancy risk, at three times that of NS.

Epidemiology

The cumulative incidence of RASopathies is estimated to be 1:1000 live births; however, it is likely to be higher than this given the high rate of missed diagnoses, particularly for mild forms of the diseases. NF1 and NS are estimated to occur in 1 in 2500 births, whereas Legius syndrome is exceedingly rare, with approximately 200 reported cases. The incidence of cardio-facial-cutaneous syndrome is estimated to be 1:200 000 live births. The incidence of Costello syndrome is approximately 1:300 000 live births.

Etiology

Genetic factors include germline variants in genes involved in the RAS/RAF/MEK/ERK (MAPK) pathway.

Pathogenesis

In vitro analysis has demonstrated increased circulating granulocyte–macrophage colony-forming unit (CFU-GM) progenitors, as well as MAPK hyperactivation, reflecting a constitutional predilection to myeloid cell proliferation {1272,349}. Abnormal apoptotic patterns of CD34-positive haematopoietic progenitors additionally give rise to increased cell survival in progenitors {4023}. In murine models, approximately 10% of *Nf1*+/– mice develop a JMML-like myeloproliferative neoplasm in their second year of life {1759}.

Macroscopic appearance

Not relevant

Histopathology

Bone marrow trephine biopsy reveals a hypercellular bone marrow, often with myeloid hyperplasia and rarely with erythroid hyperplasia. Dysgranulopoiesis is often minimal and, if identified, includes pseudo–Pelger–Huët cells or cells with cytoplasmic hypogranularity. Megakaryocytes are frequently decreased in number, with minimal dysplasia. Monocytes are often increased, but less so than in the peripheral blood. Blasts are increased but are below the threshold of 20%. Reticulin fibrosis may be present {1576,2958}. In the context of hypercellularity, a differential diagnosis would include myeloid neoplasms often seen in childhood, such as a myelodysplastic neoplasm, although dyspoiesis within RASopathy-associated myeloid neoplasms is minimal. AML is diagnosed if blasts are > 20%.

Cytology

Peripheral blood findings reveal leukocytosis (often < 100 × 10^9/L) with mildly left-shifted maturation, sustained monocytosis of ≥ 1 × 10^9/L, and blasts < 20%. Nucleated red blood cells are frequently identified within the peripheral blood {1576,2958}.

Diagnostic molecular pathology

Because somatic variants in the MAPK pathway are implicated in as many as 16% of all cancers and cluster in areas within genes that differ from those in RASopathies, assessment for germline variants should be undertaken in the context of appropriate genotype–phenotype correlation. Genetic analysis for the assessment of myeloid neoplasms in patients with a suspected RASopathy includes *NF1*, *NRAS*, *KRAS*, *PTPN11*, and *CBL*, which aid in the diagnosis of JMML in 85% of cases {3741,1205,3974,2401,2400}. However, multiple other genes may be involved, including *BRAF*, *CBL*, *HRAS*, *KRAS*, *MAP2K1* (*MEK1*), *MAP2K2* (*MEK2*), *MRAS*, *NRAS*, *PPP1CB*, *PTPN11*, *RAF1*, *RASA2*, *RIT1*, *RRAS*, *SHOC2*, *SOS1*, *SOS2*, and members of the SPRED and SPRY gene groups {3923}.

Essential and desirable diagnostic criteria

Essential: pathogenic variant in gene(s) associated with the RAS signalling pathway and/or a classic phenotype suggestive of a particular RASopathy (note that some phenotypes are associated with more than one RASopathy).

Desirable: correlation between expected oncological subtype and associated RASopathy.

Staging

Not relevant

Prognosis and prediction

RASopathy-associated JMML confers poor survival if untreated and carries a risk of transformation to an aggressive phenotype in ~33% of cases; however, patients with NS with *CBL* variants may demonstrate spontaneous remission of their myeloid neoplasm. Because of the evolution of RASopathy-associated myeloid neoplasms, haematopoietic stem cell transplantation remains the standard of care {3410}.

Contributors

ABLA, Oussama
Hospital for Sick Children
555 University Ave
Toronto ON M5G 1X8

ADES, Lionel*
Hôpital Saint-Louis
1 Av. Claude Vellefaux
75010 Paris

AHMED, Faiq
Basavatarakam Indo American Cancer
Hospital and Research Institute
Road No. 10, Banjara Hills
Hyderabad, Telangana 500034

AKINOLA, Norah Olubunmi
Obafemi Awolowo University
Department of Haematology and Immunology
Faculty of Basic Medical Sciences
02205 Ile-Ife

AKKARI, Yassmine
Nationwide Children's Hospital
575 Children's Crossroad
Columbus OH 43215

ALAGGIO, Rita
Sapienza Università di Roma
IRCCS Ospedale Pediatrico Bambino Gesù
Piazza di Sant'Onofrio, 4
00165 Rome RM

ALLENDE, Luis M.
Hospital Universitario 12 de Octubre
Av. de Córdoba
28041 Madrid

ALVAREZ-TWOSE, Iván
Virgen del Valle Hospital
Ctra. Cobisa, s/n
45071 Toledo

AMADOR, Catalina
University of Miami
1400 NW 12th Ave
Miami FL 33162

ANAGNOSTOPOULOS, Ioannis
Institute of Pathology
University of Würzburg
Josef-Schneider-Straße 2
97080 Würzburg

AOZASA, Katsuyuki
Osaka University
Graduate School of Medicine
2-2 Nakanoshima
Suita, Osaka 565-0871

APPERLEY, Jane F.
Imperial College London
Hammersmith Hospital, Du Cane Rd
London W12 0NN

ARAUJO, Iguaracyra
Federal University of Bahia
Av. Reitor Miguel Calmon, s/n
Vale do Canela
Salvador BA 40110-100

ARCAINI, Luca*
Division of Hematology, Fondazione IRCCS
Policlinico San Matteo; and
Department of Molecular Medicine,
University of Pavia
Viale Camillo Golgi 19
27100 Pavia PV

ARDESHNA, Kirit M.
University College London Hospitals
250 Euston Rd
London NW1 2PG

ASANO, Naoko
Nagano Prefectural Shinshu Medical Center
1332 Oaza Suzaka
Suzaka 382-8577

ATTARBASCHI, Andishe
St. Anna Children's Hospital
Kinderspitalgasse 6
1090 Vienna

ATTYGALLE, Ayoma D.
Royal Marsden Hospital
Fulham Rd
London SW3 6JJ

BACON, Chris M.
Newcastle University
Herschel Building, Brewery Ln
Newcastle upon Tyne NE1 7RU

BARRANS, Sharon Louise*
Leeds Cancer Centre
Level 3, Bexley Wing, St James's Hospital
Leeds LS9 7TF

BATCHELOR, Tracy*
Brigham and Women's Hospital
60 Fenwood Rd, Hale Building, 4th Floor
Boston MA 02115

BATTISTELLA, Maxime*
Hôpital Saint-Louis AP-HP
Université Paris Cité
1 Av. Claude Vellefaux
75010 Paris

BAUGHN, Linda B.*
Mayo Clinic
200 1st St SW
Rochester MN 55905

BEHDAD, Amir
Northwestern University
Northwestern Memorial Hospital
251 E Huron St, Galter 7-213F
Chicago IL 60611

BEJAR, Rafael*
University of California, San Diego
3855 Health Sciences Dr, MC 0820
La Jolla CA 92093

BERENTSEN, Sigbjørn
Helse Fonna Hospital Trust
Karmsundgata 120
5528 Haugesund

BERTI, Emilio
University of Milan, Fondazione Ca' Granda,
O.M.P., IRCCS &
Interdivisional Anatomic Pathology,
IRCCS MultiMedica
Via Francesco Sforza, 35
20122 Milan MI

BHAGAT, Govind
Columbia University Irving Medical Center
VC14-228, 630 W 168th St
New York NY 10032

BIANCHI, Giada*
Brigham and Women's Hospital
4 Blackfan Circle
Boston MA 02115

BLEDSOE, Jacob R.
Boston Children's Hospital
300 Longwood Ave
Boston MA 02115

* Indicates disclosure of interests (see p. 828).

BORCHMANN, Peter
University Hospital Cologne
Kerpener Str. 62
50937 Cologne

BORGES, Anita Maria
Centre for Oncopathology
Rectifier House, 570 Naigaum Cross Rd
Wadala
Mumbai 400028

BOWER, Mark*
Chelsea and Westminster Hospital
369 Fulham Rd
London SW10 9NH

BOYER, Daniel Frederick
University of Michigan
2800 Plymouth Rd, Building 36
Ann Arbor MI 48109

BULDINI, Barbara
University of Padua
Via Nicolò Giustiniani, 3
35128 Padua PD

BULLINGER, Lars*
Charité – Universitätsmedizin Berlin
Augustenburger Pl. 1
13353 Berlin

BURGER, Jan Andreas*
MD Anderson Cancer Center
1400 Holcombe Blvd
Houston TX 77030

BURKHARDT, Birgit
University Hospital Münster
Albert-Schweitzer-Campus 1
48149 Münster

BUSQUE, Lambert
OPTILAB-CHUM (HMR site)
5415 boul. de l'Assomption
Montréal QC H1T 2M4

BYCHKOV, Andrey
Kameda Medical Center
Department of Pathology
929 Higashi-cho
Kamogawa 296-8602

CALAMINICI, Mariarita
Barts Cancer Institute and
Barts Health NHS Trust
Pathology and Pharmacy Building
80 Newark St
London E1 2ES

CAMPBELL, Peter J.
Wellcome Sanger Institute
Wellcome Genome Campus
Hinxton CB10 1SA

CASSADAY, Ryan D.*
University of Washington School of Medicine
825 Eastlake Ave E
Seattle WA 98109

CAVÉ, Hélène
Hôpital universitaire Robert Debré AP-HP
Université Paris Cité
48 Bd Sérurier
75019 Paris

CAZZANIGA, Giovanni
University of Milano-Bicocca
Centro Ricerca Tettamanti
Via Elena Lucrezia Cornaro, 9
23891 Barzanò LC

CERF-BENSUSSAN, Nadine
Institut Imagine – Inserm U1183
Université Paris Cité
24 Bd du Montparnasse
75015 Paris

CESARMAN, Ethel
Weill Cornell Medicine
1300 York Ave, Room C410
New York NY 10065

CHADBURN, Amy*
Weill Cornell Medicine
525 E 68th St, St-709
New York NY 10021

CHAN, John K.C.
Queen Elizabeth Hospital
30 Gascoigne Rd
Kowloon, Hong Kong SAR

CHANDY, Mammen
Tata Medical Center
14 MAR(E-W), Newtown, Rajarhat
Kolkata 700160

CHANG, Kenneth Tou En*
KK Women's and Children's Hospital
100 Bukit Timah Rd
Singapore 229899

CHAPMAN, Jennifer R.
University of Miami
1120 NW 14th St #1403.26
Miami FL 33136

CHAPUY, Björn*
Charité – University Medical Center Berlin
Campus Benjamin Franklin
Hindenburgdamm 30
12203 Berlin

CHEN, Weina
UT Southwestern Medical Center
2330 Inwood Rd
Dallas TX 75390-9317

CHEN, Xueyan
University of Washington
1959 NE Pacific St
Seattle WA 98195

CHENG, Chee Leong
Singapore General Hospital
Department of Anatomical Pathology
Academia, Level 10, Diagnostics Tower
20 College Rd
Singapore 169856

CHEUK, Wah
Queen Elizabeth Hospital
Gascoigne Rd
Kowloon, Hong Kong SAR

CHIATTONE, Carlos*
Santa Casa Medical School
R. Pombal, 314
São Paulo SP 01253-010

CHIORAZZI, Nicholas
Feinstein Institutes for Medical Research
350 Community Dr
Manhasset NY 11030

CHNG, Wee Joo*
National University Cancer Institute
1E Kent Ridge Rd
Singapore 119228

CHOI, John Kim
University of Alabama at Birmingham
619 19th St S, WP P230N
Birmingham AL 35249

CHUANG, Shih-Sung*
Chi Mei Medical Center
901 Chang-Hwa Rd, Yung-Kang District
Tainan 71004

COLMENERO, Isabel
Hospital Infantil Universitario Niño Jesús
Av. de Menéndez Pelayo, 65
28009 Madrid

COOK, Lucy B.
Imperial College Healthcare NHS Trust
2nd Floor, Catherine Lewis Centre
Hammersmith Hospital, Du Cane Rd
London W12 0NN

COOPER, Wendy Anne
Royal Prince Alfred Hospital
NSW Health Pathology
Missenden Rd
Camperdown NSW 2050

CORBOY, Gregory Philip
Pathology Queensland
Block 7, Royal Brisbane and Women's Hospital
Herston QLD 4029

* Indicates disclosure of interests (see p. 828).

CORTES, Jorge*
Georgia Cancer Center at Augusta University
1410 Laney Walker Blvd, CN2222
Augusta GA 30912

COUPLAND, Sarah E.
Institute of Systems, Molecular and Integrative Biology, University of Liverpool
W Derby St, William Henry Duncan Building, 3rd Floor
Liverpool L7 8TX

COWAN, Andrew John*
University of Washington
617 Eastlake Ave E
Seattle WA 98109

COZZOLINO, Immacolata
University of Campania "Luigi Vanvitelli"
Via Luciano Armanni, 5
80138 Naples NA

CREE, Ian A.
International Agency for Research on Cancer
25 Av. Tony Garnier, CS 90627
69366 Lyon, CEDEX 07

CROSS, Nicholas C.P.*
University of Southampton
Salisbury NHS Foundation Trust
Salisbury SP2 8BJ

CZADER, Magdalena
Indiana University School of Medicine
350 E 11th St, Room 5034
Indianapolis IN 46202

D'AMORE, Emanuele S.G.
Ospedale San Bortolo di Vicenza
Viale Ferdinando Rodolfi
35123 Vicenza VI

DAVE, Sandeep S.
Duke Center for Genomic and Computational Biology
101 Science Dr
Durham NC 27708

DAVIES, Andrew John*
University of Southampton
Centre for Cancer Immunology, Southampton General Hospital
Southampton SO16 6YD

DAVIS, Kara L.*
Department of Pediatrics, Stanford University
Bass Center for Childhood Cancer and Blood Diseases
2078b Lokey Stem Cell Research Building
269 Campus Dr
Stanford CA 94305

DE JONG, Daphne*
Netherlands Cancer Institute /
Antoni van Leeuwenhoek Hospital
Plesmanlaan 121
1066 CX Amsterdam

DE VITO, Rita
Ospedale Pediatrico Bambino Gesù
Piazza di Sant'Onofrio, 4
00165 Rome RM

DECKERT, Martina
Faculty of Medicine and University Hospital Cologne
University of Cologne
Kerpener Str. 62
50924 Cologne

DEEG, H. Joachim*
Fred Hutchinson Cancer Center and University of Washington
1100 Fairview Ave N, D1-100
Seattle WA 98109

DELABIE, Jan
University Health Network and University of Toronto
200 Elizabeth St
Toronto ON M5G 2C4

DEMICCO, Elizabeth G.*
University of Toronto
Mount Sinai Hospital, 600 University Ave
Toronto ON M5G 1X5

DENTON, Erika R.E.
Norfolk and Norwich University Hospitals NHS Foundation Trust
Colney Ln
Norwich NR4 7UY

DESHPANDE, Vikram
Beth Israel Deaconess Medical Center
330 Brookline Ave
Boston MA 02215

DI NAPOLI, Arianna
Sapienza University of Rome
Sant'Andrea University Hospital
Via di Grottarossa, 1035
00189 Rome RM

DIEPSTRA, Arjan*
University Medical Center Groningen
Hanzeplein 1, PO Box 30.001
9700 RB Groningen

DIERICKX, Daan*
University Hospitals Leuven
Herestraat 49
3000 Leuven

DU, Ming-Qinq
University of Cambridge
Cellular and Molecular Pathology
Department of Pathology
PO Box 231, Level 3 Lab Block
Addenbrooke's Hospital, Hills Rd
Cambridge CB2 0QQ

DUNLEAVY, Kieron*
Lombardi Comprehensive Cancer Center
Georgetown University
3800 Reservoir Rd NW
Washington DC 20007

EDEN, Michael
Cambridge University Hospitals
NHS Foundation Trust
Hills Rd
Cambridge CB2 0QQ

EICHHORST, Barbara*
University of Cologne
Kerpener Str. 62
50937 Cologne

EISFELD, Ann-Kathrin*
Clara D. Bloomfield Center for Leukemia Outcomes Research
460 W 12th Ave, R806
Columbus OH 43210

ELENITOBA-JOHNSON, Kojo S.J.*
Memorial Sloan Kettering Cancer Center
1275 York Ave
New York NY 10021

ELGHETANY, M. Tarek
Texas Children's Hospital
Baylor College of Medicine
6621 Fannin St, WB1100
Houston TX 77030

EMILE, Jean-François
AP-HP and Versailles SQY University
9 Av. Charles de Gaulle
92104 Boulogne

ENNISHI, Daisuke*
Okayama University Hospital
2-5-1 Shikata-cho, Kita-ku
Okayama 700-8558

FAJGENBAUM, David C.*
University of Pennsylvania
3620 Hamilton Walk
Anatomy Chemistry Building, Suite 214
Philadelphia PA 19104

FARINHA, Pedro
BC Cancer
600 W 10th Ave
Vancouver BC V5Z 4E6

* Indicates disclosure of interests (see p. 828).

FERNÁNDEZ DE LARREA, Carlos*
Hospital Clínic de Barcelona, IDIBAPS
University of Barcelona
C. de Villarroel, 170
08036 Barcelona

FERRY, Judith A.
Massachusetts General Hospital
55 Fruit St
Boston MA 02114

FIELD, Andrew S.
University of NSW Sydney and
University of Notre Dame Medical Schools
Department of Anatomical Pathology
St Vincent's Hospital Sydney
Victoria St
Darlinghurst NSW 2010

FISHER, Kevin E.
Baylor College of Medicine
Texas Children's Hospital
6621 Fannin St
Houston TX 77030

FITZGIBBON, Jude*
Queen Mary University of London
3rd Floor, John Vane Science Centre
Barts Cancer Institute
Charterhouse Square
London EC1M 6BQ

FLANAGAN, Melina
West Virginia University School of Medicine
PO Box 9203
Morgantown WV 26506

FOGELSTRAND, Linda
Institute of Biomedicine, Sahlgrenska
Academy at University of Gothenburg
Sahlgrenska University Hospital
Bruna Stråket 16
413 45 Gothenburg

FONSECA, Anil Felix Angelo
Gandhi Medical College/TIMS
Hyderabad, Telangana

FONTENAY, Michaela*
Université Paris Cité, AP-HP, Hôpital Cochin
27 Rue du Faubourg Saint-Jacques
75014 Paris

FROMM, Jonathan R.*
University of Washington
825 Eastlake Ave E, G7800
Seattle WA 98109

GAMBACORTI-PASSERINI, Carlo
University of Milano-Bicocca
Via Cadore, 48
20900 Monza MB

GARCIA, Juan F.*
MD Anderson Cancer Center Madrid
C. de Arturo Soria, 270
28035 Madrid

GARNACHE OTTOU, Francine
EFS B/FC
8 Rue du Dr Jean-François Xavier Girod
25000 Besançon

GEDDIE, William Robert
University Health Network
48 Alexandra Blvd
Toronto ON M4R 1L7

GERMING, Ulrich
Heinrich Heine University Düsseldorf
Moorenstraße 5
40225 Düsseldorf

GERTZ, Morie
Mayo Clinic
200 1st St SW
Rochester MN 55905

GEYER, Julia
Weill Cornell Medicine
1300 York Ave
New York NY 10065

GILL, Anthony J.
Royal North Shore Hospital
Pacific Hwy
St Leonards NSW 2065

GIRAUDIER, Stephane
Hôpital Saint-Louis
Av. Claude Vellefaux
75010 Paris

GODLEY, Lucy A.
Northwestern University
303 E Superior St, Office 3-113
Chicago IL 60611

GOLDMAN-LÉVY, Gabrielle
International Agency for Research on Cancer
25 Av. Tony Garnier, CS 90627
69366 Lyon, CEDEX 07

GOPAL, Ajay K.*
University of Washington
825 Eastlake Ave E, CE3-300
Seattle WA 98109

GOPAL, Satish
National Cancer Institute
9609 Medical Center Dr
Rockville MD 20850

GRATZINGER, Dita
Stanford University School of Medicine
300 Pasteur Dr
Stanford CA 94305

GREENBERG, Peter L.*
Stanford Cancer Institute
875 Blake Wilbur Dr
Stanford CA 94305

GREIPP, Patricia T.*
Mayo Clinic
200 1st St SW
Rochester MN 55905

GRU, Alejandro
University of Virginia
415 Lane Rd
Charlottesville VA 22908

GUITART, Joan*
Feinberg School of Medicine
Northwestern University
NMH/Arkes Family Pavilion, Suite 1600
676 N Saint Clair St
Chicago IL 60611

GUJRAL, Sumeet
Tata Memorial Hospital, Mumbai
7, Charak, BPT Hospital Campus
Wadala East
Mumbai 400037

GUPTA, Ritu
All India Institute of Medical Sciences, Delhi
Room No. 239, Dr B.R.A. IRCH, AIIMS
Ansari Nagar
New Delhi 110029

HAASE, Detlef*
University Medical Center Göttingen
Robert-Koch-Straße 40
37075 Göttingen

HAFERLACH, Claudia*
MLL Munich Leukemia Laboratory
Max-Lebsche-Platz 31
81377 Munich

HAFERLACH, Torsten*
MLL Munich Leukemia Laboratory
Max-Lebsche-Platz 31
81377 Munich

HANSMANN, Martin-Leo
Institute of Pathology and Molecular Pathology
Heusnerstraße 40
42283 Wuppertal

HAROCHE, Julien
Hôpital Pitié Salpêtrière
47-83 Bd de l'Hôpital
75013 Paris

HARRIS, Marian H.
Boston Children's Hospital
300 Longwood Ave
Boston MA 02115

* Indicates disclosure of interests (see p. 828).

HARRISON, Christine J.
Translational and Clinical Research Institute
Newcastle University Centre for Cancer
Newcastle upon Tyne NE1 7RU

HARRISON, Claire Nicola*
Guy's and St Thomas' NHS Foundation Trust
Great Maze Pond
London SE1 9RT

HARTMANN, Sylvia
Goethe University
Theodor-Stern-Kai 7
60590 Frankfurt am Main

HEBEDA, Konnie M.
Radboudumc
PO Box 9101, r. 812
6500 HB Nijmegen

HERFARTH, Klaus*
University Hospital Heidelberg
Im Neuenheimer Feld 400
69120 Heidelberg

HERLING, Marco*
Leipzig University
Liebigstraße 22, Building 7
04103 Leipzig

HERMINE, Olivier
Necker Hospital AP-HP, Inserm U1163,
Imagine Institute, Université Paris Cité
24 Bd du Montparnasse
75015 Paris

HOANG-XUAN, Khe
Hôpital Universitaire Pitié Salpêtrière
Institut de Neurologie
47 Bd de l'Hôpital
75013 Paris

HOCHHAUS, Andreas*
Universitätsklinikum Jena
Am Klinikum 1
07740 Jena

HODGE, Jennelle C.
Indiana University School of Medicine
975 W Walnut St, IB-354
Indianapolis IN 46202

HU, Shimin
University of Texas
MD Anderson Cancer Center
1515 Holcombe Blvd
Houston TX 77030

HUANG, Xiao-Jun
Peking University
11 Xizhimen South St
Beijing 100044

HUANG, Yuhua
Sun Yat-sen University Cancer Center
Department of Pathology
No. 651 Dongfeng Road
Guangzhou 510060

HUNG, Yin Pun
Massachusetts General Hospital
55 Fruit St
Boston MA 02114

HUNGER, Stephen P.*
Children's Hospital of Philadelphia
3501 Civic Center Blvd, CTRB 3060
Philadelphia PA 19104

IDBAIH, Ahmed*
Sorbonne Université AP-HP, Institut du
Cerveau - Paris Brain Institute - ICM, Inserm,
CNRS, Hôpital de la Pitié Salpêtrière, DMU
Neurosciences, Service de Neuro-Oncologie
47-83 Bd de l'Hôpital
75013 Paris

INABA, Hiroto*
St. Jude Children's Research Hospital
262 Danny Thomas Pl, Mail Stop 260
Memphis TN 38105

INAGAKI, Hiroshi
Nagoya City University
1 Kawasumi, Mizuho-ku
Nagoya 467-8601

IQBAL, Javeed
University of Nebraska Medical Center
986842 Nebraska Medical Center
Omaha NE 68198-6842

ISHITSUKA, Kenji*
Kagoshima University
8-35-1 Sakuragaoka
Kagoshima 890-8544

ITO, Masafumi
Japanese Red Cross Nagoya Daiichi Hospital
Aichi Medical Center
3-35 Michishita-cho, Nakamura-ku
Nagoya 453-8511

ITZYKSON, Raphael
Hôpital Saint-Louis AP-HP
Université Paris Cité
1 Av. Claude Vellefaux
75010 Paris

IWAKI, Noriko
National Cancer Center Hospital
5-1-1 Tsukiji, Chuo-ku
Tokyo 104-0045

IWATSUKI, Keiji
Okayama University Graduate School of
Medicine, Dentistry and Pharmaceutical
Sciences
2-5-1 Shikata-cho, Kita-ku
Okayama 700-8558

JACQUES, Thomas S.*
UCL GOS Institute of Child Health
30 Guilford St
London WC1N 1EH

JAIN, Nitin*
University of Texas
MD Anderson Cancer Center
1515 Holcombe Blvd, Unit 428
Houston TX 77030

JAISWAL, Siddhartha*
Stanford University
240 Pasteur Dr
Stanford CA 94304

JANSEN, Joop H.
Radboud University Medical Center
Geert Grooteplein Zuid 8
6525 GA Nijmegen

JANSEN, Patty M.
Leiden University Medical Center
Albinusdreef 2
2333 ZA Leiden

JEON, Yoon Kyung
Seoul National University College of Medicine
Seoul National University Hospital
103 Daehak-ro, Jongno-gu
Seoul 03080

KADIN, Marshall E.
Warren Alpert Medical School of
Brown University
593 Eddy St
Providence RI 02903

KAJI, Sachiko
Japanese Red Cross Narita Hospital
90-1 Iida-cho, Narita
Chiba 286-8523

KAKKAR, Aanchal
All India Institute of Medical Sciences
Department of Pathology
New Delhi 110029

KANAGAL-SHAMANNA, Rashmi
MD Anderson Cancer Center
6565 MD Anderson Blvd, Suite Z3.5044
Houston TX 77030

* Indicates disclosure of interests (see p. 828).

KANTARJIAN, Hagop M.*
University of Texas
MD Anderson Cancer Center
1400 Holcombe Blvd, Unit 428
Leukemia Department
Houston TX 77030

KARADIMITRIS, Anastasios*
Centre for Haematology
Imperial College London and
Department of Haematology
Imperial College Healthcare NHS Trust
Hammersmith Hospital
Du Cane Rd
London W12 0NN

KARUBE, Kennosuke*
Nagoya University
Graduate School of Medicine
65 Tsurumai-cho, Showa-ku
Nagoya 466-8550

KATAOKA, Keisuke*
Keio University School of Medicine
35 Shinanomachi, Shinjuku-ku
Tokyo 160-8582

KATO, Seiichi
Aichi Cancer Center Hospital
1-1 Kanokoden, Chikusa-ku
Nagoya 464-8681

KEMPF, Werner
Kempf und Pfaltz Histologische Diagnostik
Affolternstrasse 56
8050 Zürich

KERSTEN, Marie José*
Amsterdam UMC
De Boelelaan 1117
1081 HV Amsterdam

KETTERLING, Rhett P.
Mayo Clinic
200 1st St SW
Rochester MN 55905

KHATTRY, Navin
Advanced Centre for Treatment Research
and Education in Cancer (ACTREC)
Tata Memorial Centre
Room No. 305, Paymaster Shodhika
Sector 22, Kharghar
Navi Mumbai 410210

KHOURY, Joseph David
University of Nebraska Medical Center
985900 Nebraska Medical Center
Omaha NE 68198

KIM, Ji Eun
Seoul National University
SNU-SMG Boramae Medical Center
Boramae-ro 5-gil
Seoul 07061

KIMURA, Hiroshi*
Nagoya University
Graduate School of Medicine
65 Tsurumai-cho, Showa-ku
Nagoya 466-8550

KLAPPER, Wolfram*
Department of Pathology
Hematopathology Section
University Hospital Schleswig-Holstein
Arnold-Heller-Straße 3, Haus U33
24105 Kiel

KOMROKJI, Rami*
H. Lee Moffitt Cancer Center
12902 Magnolia Dr
Tampa FL 33612

KOVACH, Alexandra Elizabeth
Children's Hospital Los Angeles
4650 Sunset Blvd, Mail Stop #32
Los Angeles CA 90027

KRATZ, Christian P.
Hannover Medical School
Carl-Neuberg-Straße 1
30625 Hannover

KRIDEL, Robert*
Princess Margaret Cancer Centre – UHN
610 University Ave
Toronto ON M5G 2M9

KRISTINSSON, Sigurdur Y.*
University of Iceland
Sturlugata 8
101 Reykjavik

KUMAR, Shaji*
Mayo Clinic
200 1st St SW
Rochester MN 55905

KÜPPERS, Ralf
University of Duisburg-Essen
Virchowstraße 173
45122 Essen

KUZU, Isinsu
Ankara University School of Medicine
Morphology Building, A.Adnan Saygun Cd.
No:35
06230 Ankara

KWONG, Yok-Lam*
Queen Mary Hospital
Pok Fu Lam Rd
Hong Kong SAR

LACASCE, Ann S.
Dana-Farber Cancer Institute
450 Brookline Ave, M227
Boston MA 02215

LAMANT-ROCHAIX, Laurence
Institut universitaire du cancer de
Toulouse Oncopole
1 Av. Irène Joliot-Curie
31059 Toulouse

LAMY, Thierry
Rennes University Hospital
Rue Henri le Guilloux
35033 Rennes

LANDGREN, Ola C.*
Sylvester Comprehensive Cancer Center
University of Miami
1120 NW 14th St, Clinical Research Building,
Room 650D
Miami FL 33136

LASKAR, Siddhartha
Tata Memorial Centre
Dr Ernest Borges Marg, Parel
Mumbai 400012

LASKIN, William Bradlyn
Yale School of Medicine
310 Cedar St
New Haven CT 06520-8023

LAX, Sigurd F.
General Hospital Graz II
Medical University of Graz
Göstinger Str. 22
8020 Graz

LAZAR, Alexander J.
University of Texas
MD Anderson Cancer Center
1515 Holcombe Blvd, Unit 85
Houston TX 77030

LAZZI, Stefano
Institute of Pathological Anatomy
University of Siena
6, Viale Bracci
53100 Siena SI

LENZ, Georg*
University Hospital Münster
Albert-Schweitzer-Campus 1
48149 Münster

LEONCINI, Lorenzo
University of Siena
Department of Medical Biotechnology
Pathological Anatomy Division
Via delle Scotte
53100 Siena SI

* Indicates disclosure of interests (see p. 828).

LEUNG, Nelson*
Mayo Clinic
200 1st St SW
Rochester MN 55905

LEVENTAKI, Vasiliki
University of Texas
MD Anderson Cancer Center
1515 Holcombe Blvd, Unit 0072
Houston TX 77030

LI, Gan Di
West China Hospital, Sichuan University
Guoxuexiang 37
Chengdu 610041

LI, Shaoying
University of Texas
MD Anderson Cancer Center
1515 Holcombe Blvd, Unit 0072
Houston TX 77030

LI, Xiao-Qiu
Fudan University Shanghai Cancer Center
270 Dong-An Rd
Shanghai 200032

LIM, Megan S.*
Memorial Sloan Kettering Cancer Center
1275 York Ave
New York NY 10065

LIN, Oscar*
Memorial Sloan Kettering Cancer Center
1275 York Ave
New York NY 10065

LIN, Pei
University of Texas
MD Anderson Cancer Center
1515 Holcombe Blvd, PO Box 72
Houston TX 77030

LIU, Wei-Ping
West China Hospital, Sichuan University
37 Guoxuexiang, Wuhou district
Chengdu, Sichuan 610041

LOCATELLI, Franco*
Bambino Gesù Children's Hospital
Piazza di Sant'Onofrio, 4
00165 Rome RM

LOEB, Keith R.
Fred Hutchinson Cancer Center
825 Eastlake Ave E (G7-910)
Seattle WA 98109

LOGHAVI, Sanam*
MD Anderson Cancer Center
6565 MD Anderson Blvd, Suite Z5.5036
Houston TX 77030

LOKUHETTY, Dilani
International Agency for Research on Cancer
25 Av. Tony Garnier, CS 90627
69366 Lyon, CEDEX 07

LORSBACH, Robert Brian
Cincinnati Children's Hospital Medical Center
University of Cincinnati College of Medicine
3333 Burnet Ave, ML 1035
Cincinnati OH 45229

LOSSOS, Izidore S.
University of Miami
1475 NW 12th Ave (D8-4)
Miami FL 33136

LOUGHRAN, Thomas P. Jr
University of Virginia
1300 Jefferson Park Ave
Charlottesville VA 22903

LOUISSAINT, Abner Jr
Massachusetts General Hospital
55 Fruit St, Warren 2
Boston MA 02114

MACON, William R.*
Mayo Clinic
200 1st St SW
Rochester MN 55905

MAKITA, Shinichi
National Cancer Center Hospital
5-1-1 Tsukiji, Chuo-ku
Tokyo 104-0045

MALESZEWSKI, Joseph J.
Mayo Clinic
200 1st St SW
Rochester MN 55905

MALHOTRA, Pankaj
Postgraduate Institute of Medical Education and Research
Sector 12
Chandigarh 160012

MARAFIOTI, Teresa
University College Hospital
60 Whitfield St
London WT1 4EU

MARCOGLIESE, Andrea Nicole
Baylor College of Medicine
1 Baylor Plaza
Houston TX 77030

MARUYAMA, Dai*
Cancer Institute Hospital of Japanese Foundation for Cancer Research
3-8-31 Ariake, Koto-ku
Tokyo 135-8550

MARX, Alexander
University Medical Centre Mannheim
Theodor-Kutzer-Ufer 1-3
68167 Mannheim

MATHEWS, Vikram
Christian Medical College
IDA Scudder Rd
Vellore 632004

MBULAITEYE, Sam M.
National Cancer Institute
9609 Medical Center Dr
Rockville MD 20850

MEDEIROS, L. Jeffrey
University of Texas
MD Anderson Cancer Center
1515 Holcombe Blvd
Houston TX 77030

MEIGNIN, Veronique*
Hôpital Saint-Louis
1 Av. Claude Vellefaux
75010 Paris

MEJSTRIKOVA, Ester*
2nd Faculty of Medicine
Motol University Hospital
V Úvalu 84
15006 Prague

MESA, Ruben*
Atrium Health Wake Forest Baptist Comprehensive Cancer Center
1 Medical Center Blvd, 11th Floor
Winston-Salem NC 27157-1082

MESHINCHI, Soheil
Fred Hutchinson Cancer Center
1100 Fairview Ave N
Seattle WA 98109

MICHAELS, Phillip Dane
Brigham and Women's Hospital
75 Francis St
Boston MA 02115

MICHAL, Michael
Charles University
Faculty of Medicine in Plzen
Alej Svobody 80
323 00 Plzen

MICHELOW, Pamela
University of the Witwatersrand and National Health Laboratory Service
PO Box 1038
Johannesburg 2000

* Indicates disclosure of interests (see p. 828).

MIETTINEN, Markku
National Cancer Institute / NIH
9000 Rockville Pike
Building 10, Room 2S235C
Bethesda MD 20892-0001

MILES, Rodney R.
University of Utah
15 Medical Dr N, E JMRB 2100
Salt Lake City UT 84112

MILOJKOVIC, Dragana
Imperial College London
Department of Haematology
Hammersmith Hospital, Du Cane Rd
London W12 0HS

MIRANDA, Roberto N.*
University of Texas
MD Anderson Cancer Center
1515 Holcombe Blvd
Houston TX 77030

MITTELDORF, Christina
University Medical Center Göttingen
Robert-Koch-Straße 40
37075 Göttingen

MIYAZAKI, Yasushi*
Atomic Bomb Disease Institute
Nagasaki University
1-12-4 Sakamoto
Nagasaki 852-8523

MIYOSHI, Hiroaki
Kurume University School of Medicine
67 Asahimachi
Kurume 830-0011

MOCH, Holger*
University of Zürich and
University Hospital Zürich
Schmelzbergstrasse 12
8091 Zürich

MOL, Jan A.
Stichting Hematon
Box 8152
3503 RD Utrecht

MOLINA, Thierry Jo
AP-HP, Hôpital Necker-Enfants Malades and
Robert Debré, Université Paris Cité
149 Rue de Sèvres
75015 Paris

MOLLEJO, Manuela
Hospital Universitario de Toledo
Av. del Río Guadiana, 1
45007 Toledo

MOMOSE, Shuji
Saitama Medical University
Saitama Medical Center
1981 Kamoda
Kawagoe 350-8550

MONTES-MORENO, Santiago*
Hospital Universitario Marqués de
Valdecilla / IDIVAL
Av. de Valdecilla, 25
39008 Santander

MORI, Tetsuya*
St. Marianna University School of Medicine
2-16-1 Sugao
Miyamae-ku, Kawasaki
Kanagawa 216-8511

MORICE, William G.
Mayo Clinic
200 1st St SW
Rochester MN 55905

NADEL, Bertrand*
Inserm CNRS AMU
Parc Scientifique de Luminy, Case 906
64 Av. de Luminy
13288 Marseille, CEDEX

NAGAI, Hirokazu*
National Hospital Organization
Nagoya Medical Center
4-1-1 Sannomaru, Naka-ku
Nagoya 460-0001

NAGANE, Motoo*
Kyorin University Faculty of Medicine
6-20-2 Shinkawa, Mitaka
Tokyo 181-8611

NAIR, Reena*
Tata Medical Center
14 MAR(E-W), Newtown
Kolkata 700160

NAKAMURA, Naoya*
Tokai University School of Medicine
143 Shimokasuya
Isehara 259-1193

NAKAZAWA, Atsuko
Saitama Children's Medical Center
1-2 Shintoshin, Chuo-ku
Saitama 330-8777

NARDI, Valentina
Massachusetts General Hospital
55 Fruit St, Warren 820 A
Boston MA 02114

NARESH, Kikkeri N.
Pathology, Clinical Research Division
Fred Hutchinson Cancer Center
1100 Fairview Ave N, Mail Stop G7-910
Seattle WA 98109

NARULA, Gaurav*
Tata Memorial Center
Homi Bhabha National Institute
Dr Ernest Borges Marg
Mumbai 400026

NASR, Samih H.
Mayo Clinic
200 1st St SW
Rochester MN 55905

NATKUNAM, Yasodha*
Stanford University
300 Pasteur Dr, L235
Stanford CA 94305

NEJATI, Reza
Fox Chase Cancer Center
333 Cottman Ave
Philadelphia PA 19111

NG, Siok-Bian
National University of Singapore
National University Hospital
5 Lower Kent Ridge Rd, Main Building, Level 3
Singapore 119074

NICHOLSON, Andrew Gordon*
Royal Brompton & Harefield
NHS Foundation Trust
Sydney St
London SW3 6NP

NICOLAE, Alina
Hautepierre Hospital
University Hospitals of Strasbourg
1 Av. Molière
67098 Strasbourg

OGAWA, Seishi*
Kyoto University
Yoshida Konoe-cho, Sakyo-ku
Kotyo 606-8315

OHGAMI, Robert Shigeo
University of Utah
500 Chipeta Way
Salt Lake City UT 84108

OISHI, Naoki
University of Yamanashi
1110 Shimokato
Chuo, Yamanashi 409-3898

OLAVARRIA, Eduardo
Imperial College London
Hammersmith Hospital, Du Cane Rd
London W12 0HS

* Indicates disclosure of interests (see p. 828).

OLSON, Timothy S.
Children's Hospital of Philadelphia
3615 Civic Center Blvd
Philadelphia PA 19104

ORGEL, Etan*
Cancer and Blood Disease Institute
Children's Hospital Los Angeles
4650 Sunset Blvd, Mail Stop #54
Los Angeles CA 90027

ORTONNE, Nicolas
AP-HP, Hopitaux Universitaires Henri Mondor
51 Av. du Maréchal de Lattre de Tassigny
94000 Créteil

OSCHLIES, Ilske
Department of Pathology
Hematopathology Section
University Hospital Schleswig-Holstein
Arnold-Heller-Straße 3, Haus U33
24105 Kiel

OTT, German
Department of Clinical Pathology
Robert-Bosch-Krankenhaus
Auerbachstraße 110
70376 Stuttgart

PADRON, Eric*
H. Lee Moffitt Cancer Center
12902 Magnolia Dr
Tampa FL 33612

PAIVA, Bruno*
Clinica Universidad de Navarra
Av. de Pio XII, 55
31008 Pamplona

PAN-HAMMARSTRÖM, Qiang
Karolinska Institutet
Division of Immunology, Department of Medical Biochemistry and Biophysics
171 77 Stockholm

PARIHAR, Mayur
Tata Medical Center
Cytogenetics Unit, North Lab
MAR(E-W), Newtown
Kolkata 700160

PARK, Sophie*
CHU Grenoble Alpes
Université Grenoble Alpes
CS 10217
38043 Grenoble, CEDEX 09

PARRENS, Marie
Bordeaux University Hospital
Av. Magellan
33604 Pessac (Bordeaux)

PATEL, Keyur*
MD Anderson Cancer Center
6565 MD Anderson Blvd, Unit 1062
Houston TX 77030

PATKAR, Nikhil V.*
Tata Memorial Center
Advanced Centre for Treatment, Research and Education in Cancer (ACTREC)
Room 4, CCE Building, Kharghar
Navi Mumbai 410210

PATNAIK, Mrinal*
Mayo Clinic
200 1st St SW
Rochester MN 55905

PAULLI, Marco
University of Pavia
Via Forlanini, 14
27100 Pavia PV

PEMMARAJU, Naveen*
University of Texas
MD Anderson Cancer Center
1515 Holcombe Blvd, Unit 0428
Houston TX 77030

PERCIVAL, Mary-Elizabeth*
University of Washington
825 Eastlake Ave E, LG-700
Seattle WA 98109

PETERSEN, Andrea K.
Legacy Health/Randall Children's Hospital and Washington State University
Elson S. Floyd College of Medicine
2801 N Gantenbein Ave
Portland OR 97227

PICARSIC, Jennifer
Cincinnati Children's Hospital Medical Center
Pathology and Lab Medicine
240 Albert Sabin Way, MLC 1035
Cincinnati OH 45229-3039

PILERI, Alessandro*
Dermatology Unit, IRCCS Azienda Ospedaliero-Universitaria di Bologna
Department of Medical and Surgical Sciences
University of Bologna
Via Giuseppe Massarenti, 1
40100 Bologna BO

PIMPINELLI, Nicola*
University of Florence Medical School
Hospital Palagi
Viale Michelangiolo, 41
50125 Florence FI

PLATZBECKER, Uwe*
University Hospital Leipzig
Liebigstraße 20
04103 Leipzig

PLAZA, Jose A.
Ohio State University Wexner Medical Center
930 Martha Morehouse Tower, 2050 Kenny Rd
Columbus OH 43221

PULITZER, Melissa
Memorial Sloan Kettering Cancer Center
1275 York Ave, C528
New York NY 10065

RABIN, Karen R.
Texas Children's Cancer Center
1102 Bates St, Suite 750.00
Houston TX 77030

RACA, Gordana
Children's Hospital Los Angeles
4650 Sunset Blvd, Mail Stop #173
Los Angeles CA 90027

RADERER, Markus*
Medical University of Vienna
Division of Oncology
Währinger Gürtel 18-20
1090 Vienna

RADICH, Jerald P.*
Fred Hutchinson Cancer Center
1100 Fairview Ave N
Seattle WA 98104

RAI, Kanti
Northwell Health Cancer Institute
410 Lakeville Rd, Suite 212
New Hyde Park NY 11042

RAJKUMAR, S. Vincent
Mayo Clinic
200 1st St SW
Rochester MN 55905

RANDEN, Ulla
Akershus University Hospital /
University of Oslo
Sykehusveien 25
1478 Lørenskog

RAO, Huilan
Sun Yat-sen University Cancer Center
No. 651 Dongfeng Road
Guangzhou 510060

RAWSTRON, Andy C.*
St James's Institute of Oncology
Bexley Wing, Beckett St
Leeds LS9 7TF

RECH, Karen L.
Mayo Clinic
200 1st St SW
Rochester MN 55902

* Indicates disclosure of interests (see p. 828).

ROBERTS, Irene A.G.
University of Oxford
MRC Weatherall Institute of Molecular Medicine
John Radcliffe Hospital
Oxford OX3 9DS

ROBSON, Alistair
IPOLFG - Serviço de Anatomia Patológica
R. Prof. Lima Basto
1099-023 Lisbon

ROCHFORD, Rosemary
University of Colorado
Anschutz Medical Campus
12800 E 19th Ave
Aurora CO 80045

ROSENQUIST, Richard
Karolinska Institutet
BioClinicum J10:20
171 76 Stockholm

ROSENWALD, Andreas
Institute of Pathology
University of Würzburg
Josef-Schneider-Straße 2
97080 Würzburg

ROSSI, Davide*
Oncology Institute of Southern Switzerland
Via Vincenzo Vela 6
6500 Bellinzona

ROSSI, Esther D.
Fondazione Policlinico Universitario Agostino Gemelli IRCCS
Largo Agostino Gemelli
00168 Rome RM

ROSSI, Sabrina
Bambino Gesù Children's Hospital
Piazza Sant'Onofrio, 4
00165 Rome RM

ROUS, Brian
NHS England
Victoria House, Capital Park
Fulbourn, Cambridge CB21 5XA

ROUSSELOT, Philippe*
Centre Hospitalier de Versailles
Université Paris-Saclay
177 Rue de Versailles
78150 Le Chesnay

RULE, Simon*
Plymouth University Medical School
John Bull Building
Plymouth PL6 8DH

RYMKIEWICZ, Grzegorz
Maria Sklodowska-Curie National Research Institute of Oncology
Roentgena 5
02-781 Warsaw

SABATTINI, Elena*
IRCCS Azienda Ospedaliero-Universitaria di Bologna
Via Giuseppe Massarenti, 9
40138 Bologna BO

SAHA, Vaskar
Tata Translational Cancer Research Centre
Tata Medical Center
Kolkata 700160

SAHM, Felix*
Heidelberg University and
German Cancer Research Center (DKFZ)
Im Neuenheimer Feld 224
69120 Heidelberg

SAID, Jonathan William
David Geffen School of Medicine
10833 Le Conte Ave
Los Angeles CA 90095

SAKATA-YANAGIMOTO, Mamiko*
University of Tsukuba
1-1-1 Tennodai, Tsukuba
Ibaraki 305-8575

SALLMAN, David A.*
H. Lee Moffitt Cancer Center
12902 Magnolia Dr
Tampa FL 33612

SANDER, Christian A.
Asklepios Klinik St. Georg
Lohmühlenstraße 5
20099 Hamburg

SANGIORGIO, Valentina Fabiola Ilenia
Royal London Hospital
Barts Health NHS Trust
Whitechapel Rd
London E1 1FR

SANGUEZA, J. Martin
Hospital Obrero No. 1 CNS, Hospital General
Av. 6 de Agosto 2700, Edificio Torre Cadeco
6541 La Paz

SANGÜEZA, Omar P.
Wake Forest University School of Medicine
Medical Center Blvd
Winston-Salem NC 27157-1072

SANTUCCI, Marco
University of Florence School of Human Health Sciences
Viale Gaetano Pieraccini, 6
50139 Florence FI

SARKOZY, Clementine
Institut Curie
35 Rue Dailly
92210 Saint-Cloud

SATO, Yasuharu
Okayama University
Graduate School of Health Sciences
2-5-1 Shikata-cho, Kita-ku
Okayama 700-8558

SATOU, Akira
Aichi Medical University Hospital
1-1 Yazakokarimata
Nagakute 480-1195

SAYED, Shahin
Aga Khan University
PO Box 30270
00100 Nairobi

SAYGIN, Caner
University of Chicago
5841 S Maryland Ave, MC 2115
Chicago IL 60637

SCHAFERNAK, Kristian Theo
Phoenix Children's Hospital
1919 E Thomas Rd
Phoenix AZ 85016

SCHMITT, Fernando
CINTESIS@RISE (Health Research Network);
Medical Faculty of the University of Porto;
Molecular Pathology Unit, Ipatimup
Rua Júlio Amaral de Carvalho 45
4200-135 Porto

SCHUH, Anna*
University of Oxford
Old Rd
Oxford OX3 7DJ

SEBERT, Marie
Hôpital Saint-Louis
1 Av. Claude Vellefaux
75010 Paris

SEMENZATO, Gianpietro C.*
University of Padua
Veneto Institute of Molecular Medicine
Via Giuseppe Orus, 2
35129 Padua PD

SENGAR, Manju
Tata Memorial Centre
Ernest Borges Rd, Parel
Mumbai 400012

SEWELL, William Arthur
Garvan Institute and
St Vincent's Hospital Sydney
Victoria St
Darlinghurst NSW 2010

* Indicates disclosure of interests (see p. 828).

SHANAFELT, Tait D.*
Stanford University
500 Pasteur Dr, Suite P354
Palo Alto CA 94305

SHIMADA, Kazuyuki*
Nagoya University
Graduate School of Medicine
65 Tsurumai-cho, Showa-ku
Nagoya 466-8550

SIEBERT, Reiner
Ulm University and
Ulm University Medical Center
Albert-Einstein-Allee 11
89081 Ulm

SLACK, Graham W.*
BC Cancer
600 W 10th Ave
Vancouver BC V5Z 4E6

SLAGER, Susan L.
Mayo Clinic
200 1st St SW
Rochester MN 55906

SOFFIETTI, Riccardo
University of Turin and
City of Health and Science Hospital, Turin
Via Cherasco, 15
10126 Turin TO

SOHANI, Aliyah R.*
Massachusetts General Hospital
55 Fruit St, WRN 219
Boston MA 02114

SOLARY, Eric*
Gustave Roussy
114 Rue Edouard Vaillant
94805 Villejuif

SOLOMON, David A.
University of California, San Francisco
513 Parnassus Ave, HSW 451
San Francisco CA 94143

SOROURI KHORASHAD, Jamshid
Imperial College London
Room 4N9, Centre for Haematology
4th Floor, Commonwealth Building
Hammersmith Hospital Campus
London W12 0NN

SOTLAR, Karl
University Institute of Pathology
Paracelsus Medical University of Salzburg
Müllner Hauptstraße 48
5020 Salzburg

SPIEKERMANN, Karsten*
Department of Medicine III
LMU University Hospital, LMU Munich
Marchioninistraße 15
81377 Munich

SRIGLEY, John R.
University of Toronto
Trillium Health Partners
2200 Eglinton Ave W
Mississauga ON L5M 2N1

STAMATOPOULOS, Kostas E.*
Institute of Applied Biosciences
6th km Charilaou-Thermis
57001 Thessaloniki

STEIDL, Christian*
University of British Columbia
675 W 10th Ave
Vancouver BC V5Z 1L3

STILGENBAUER, Stephan*
Ulm University
Albert-Einstein-Allee 23
89081 Ulm

SUBRAMANIAN, Papagudi Ganesan
Tata Memorial Centre
Advanced Centre for Treatment, Research
and Education in Cancer (ACTREC)
Plot No. 1 & 2, Sector 22, Kharghar
Navi Mumbai, Maharashtra 410210

SUKSWAI, Narittee
Chulalongkorn University
13 Rama IV Rd, Pathum Wan
Pathum Wan District
Bangkok 10330

SUZUKI, Ritsuro*
Shimane University
89-1 Enyacho
Izumo 693-8501

TAKAHASHI, Emiko
Aichi Medical University Hospital
1-1 Yazakokarimata
Nagakute 480-1195

TAKEUCHI, Kengo*
Japanese Foundation for Cancer Research
3-8-31 Ariake, Koto
Tokyo 135-8550

TALLINI, Giovanni
University of Bologna Medical Center
IRCCS Azienda Ospedaliero-Universitaria di
Bologna
Policlinico di Sant'Orsola
Via Giuseppe Massarenti, 9
40138 Bologna BO

TAMARU, Junichi*
Saitama Medical Center
Saitama Medical University
1981 Kamoda
Kawagoe, Saitama 350-8550

TAN, Puay Hoon
Luma Medical Centre
Royal Square Medical Centre
101 Irrawaddy Rd, #20-02 to 04
Singapore 329565

TAN, Soo Yong
National University of Singapore
Yong Loo Lin School of Medicine
NUH Main Building, Level 3
5 Lower Kent Ridge Rd
Singapore 119074

TEMBHARE, Prashant R.
Tata Memorial Centre
Advanced Centre for Treatment, Research
and Education in Cancer (ACTREC)
Sector 22, Utsav Chowk – CISF Rd, Owe
Camp, Kharghar
Navi Mumbai, Maharashtra 410210

THOMPSON, Lester D.R.
Head and Neck Pathology Consultations
22543 Ventura Blvd, Ste 22, PMB1034
Woodland Hills CA 91364

TIACCI, Enrico*
Institute of Hematology and
Center for Hemato-Oncology Research
University of Perugia, Department of Medicine
and Surgery, and Ospedale Santa Maria della
Misericordia (Blocco R, Piano 2)
Piazzale Giorgio Menghini, 8
06132 Perugia PG

TIRABOSCO, Roberto
Royal National Orthopaedic Hospital
Brockley Hill
Stanmore, Middlesex HA7 4LP

TOKURA, Yoshiki
Chutoen General Medical Center
1-1 Shobugaike
Kakegawa 436-8555

TOOZE, Reuben M.*
Leeds Institute of Molecular Medicine
St James's University Hospital
Leeds LS9 7TF

TORRELO, Antonio
Hospital Infantil Universitario Niño Jesús
Av. de Menéndez Pelayo, 65
28009 Madrid

* Indicates disclosure of interests (see p. 828).

TOURNILHAC, Olivier*
CHU de Clermont-Ferrand
1 Place Lucie et Raymond Aubrac
63000 Clermont-Ferrand

TRAVERSE-GLEHEN, Alexandra
Hospices Civils de Lyon/Université Lyon 1
Pierre-Bénite
69490 Lyon

TREON, Steven Peter*
Dana-Farber Cancer Institute
Harvard Medical School
450 Brookline Ave
Boston MA 02215

TRUEMPER, Lorenz H.
Universitätsmedizin Göttingen
Robert-Koch-Straße 40
37075 Göttingen

TSUKASAKI, Kunihiro*
International Medical Center
Saitama Medical University
1397-1 Yamane
Hidaka 350-1298

TSUZUKI, Toyonori
Aichi Medical University Hospital
1-1 Yazakokarimata
Nagakute 480-1195

TYNER, Jeffrey Wallace*
Oregon Health & Science University
3181 SW Sam Jackson Park Rd, KCRB 2122,
Mail code KR-HEM
Portland OR 97239

van RHEE, Frits
UAMS Winthrop P. Rockefeller Cancer Institute
4301 W Markham St #816
Little Rock AR 72205

VARGHESE, Abraham M.
Department of Haematology
St James's University Hospital
Level 3, Bexley Wing
Leeds LS9 7TF

VASSILIOU, George S.*
University of Cambridge
Wellcome-MRC Cambridge Stem Cell
Institute, Jeffrey Cheah Biomedical Centre
Puddicombe Way
Cambridge CB2 0AW

VEGA, Francisco*
University of Texas
MD Anderson Cancer Center
1515 Holcombe Blvd, Unit 1053
Houston TX 77030

VERGIER, Beatrice
CHU Bordeaux and Bordeaux University
Av. Magellan
33604 Pessac (Bordeaux)

VERMEER, Maarten H.*
Leiden University Medical Center
Albinusdreef 2, Room B1-Q93
2333 ZA Leiden

VERSTOVSEK, Srdan*
University of Texas
MD Anderson Cancer Center
1515 Holcombe Blvd
Houston TX 77030

VIELH, Philippe
Medipath and American Hospital of Paris
17 Rue Gazan
75014 Paris

WALKER, Brian A.*
Indiana University
975 W Walnut St
Indianapolis IN 46202

WANG, Huan-You*
University of California, San Diego
3855 Health Sciences Dr
La Jolla CA 92093

WANG, Michael*
University of Texas
MD Anderson Cancer Center
1515 Holcombe Blvd, Unit 429
Houston TX 77030

WANG, Wei
MD Anderson Cancer Center
1515 Holcombe Blvd, Unit 72
Houston TX 77030

WANG, Zhe
Fourth Military Medical University
169, Changle W Rd
Xi'an 710032

WASHINGTON, Mary K.
Vanderbilt University Medical Center
C-3321 MCN
Nashville TN 37232

WATANABE, Reiko
St. Marianna University School of Medicine
2-16-1 Sugao, Miyamae-ku, Kawasaki
Kanagawa 216-8511

WATANABE, Takashi
Mie University Graduate School of Medicine
2-174, Edobashi
Tsu 514-8507

WECHALEKAR, Ashutosh Dilip
University College London
Rowland Hill St
London NW3 2PF

WEIGERT, Oliver*
LMU Hospital
Marchioninistraße 15
81377 Munich

WEINSTOCK, David M.*
Dana-Farber Cancer Institute and
Harvard Medical School
450 Brookline Ave, Dana 510B
Boston MA 02215

WENIG, Bruce M.
Moffitt Cancer Center
12902 Magnolia Dr
Tampa FL 33612

WESTERMAN, David A.
Peter MacCallum Cancer Centre
305 Grattan St
Melbourne VIC 3000

WHITTAKER, Sean J.
St John's Institute of Dermatology
9th Floor, Tower Wing
Guy's Hospital, Great Maze Pond
London SE1 9RT

WILLEMZE, Rein
Leiden University Medical Center
Building 1, Albinusdreef 2
PO Box 9600
2333 ZA Leiden

WOESSMANN, Wilhelm
University Medical Center Hamburg-Eppendorf
Martinistraße 52, Building O45
20246 Hamburg

WOOD, Brent Lee*
Children's Hospital Los Angeles
4650 Sunset Blvd
Los Angeles CA 90027

WU, Catherine J.*
Dana-Farber Cancer Institute
Harvard Medical School
450 Brookline Ave, Dana 520C
Boston MA 02215

WU, David
University of Washington
825 Eastlake Ave E, SCCA G-7800
Seattle WA 98109

* Indicates disclosure of interests (see p. 828).

XERRI, Luc
Institut Paoli-Calmettes
232 Bd de Sainte-Marguerite
13273 Marseille

XIAO, Wenbin*
Memorial Sloan Kettering Cancer Center
1275 York Ave
New York NY 10065

YAMAGUCHI, Motoko*
Mie University Graduate School of Medicine
2-174, Edobashi
Tsu 514-8507

YAMAMOTO, Hidetaka
Kyushu University
3-1-1 Maidashi, Higashi-ku
Fukuoka 812-8582

YAMASHITA, Daisuke
Kobe City Medical Center General Hospital
2-1-1 Minatojima-Minamimachi, Chuo-ku
Kobe 650-0047

YANG, David T.
University of Wisconsin–Madison
600 Highland Ave, B4/251b
Madison WI 53705

YANG, Shenmiao
Peking University People's Hospital
Peking Institute of Hematology
11 Xizhimen Nan Street
Beijing 100044

YASUDA, Takahiko
Nagoya Medical Center
4-1-1 Sannomaru, Naka-ku
Nagoya 460-0001

YEUNG, Cecilia Chingsze
Fred Hutchinson Cancer Center
1100 Fairview Ave N
Seattle WA 98109

YIN, Wei-Hua
Peking University Shenzhen Hospital
1120 Lianhua Rd, Futian District
Shenzhen City, Guangdong Province
Shenzhen 518036

YOSHIDA, Akihiko
National Cancer Center Hospital
5-1-1 Tsukiji, Chuo-ku
Tokyo 104-0045

ZELGER, Bernhard
Praxis for Dermatology, specialized in Dermatopathology
Mariahilfpark 1 Top 006
6020 Innsbruck

ZEN, Yoh
King's College Hospital
Denmark Hill
London SE5 9RS

ZERBINI, Maria Claudia Nogueira
University of São Paulo Medical School
Av. Dr. Arnaldo, 455
São Paulo SP 01246-903

ZHAO, Sha
West China Hospital
37 Guoxuexiang
Chengdu 610041

ZHAO, Wei-Li
Institute of Hematology
197 Rui Jin Er Rd
Shanghai 200025

* Indicates disclosure of interests (see p. 828).

Declaration of interests

Dr Ades reports that his unit at Hôpital Saint-Louis benefits from research funding from Celgene.

Dr Arcaini reports receiving honoraria from EUSA Pharma and Novartis; receiving personal consultancy fees in his capacity as an advisory board member from Roche, Janssen-Cilag, Verastem, Incyte, EUSA Pharma, Celgene/BMS, Kite/Gilead, ADC Therapeutics, and Novartis; and receiving travel support from Roche.

Dr Barrans reports that her unit at Leeds Cancer Centre benefited from non-monetary support from HTG Molecular Diagnostics.

Dr Batchelor reports having received personal consultancy fees from GenomiCare and Champions Biotechnology, and that his institution received research support from Ono Pharmaceutical.

Dr Battistella reports receiving personal consultancy fees from Innate Pharma, and that his unit at Hôpital Saint-Louis benefited from research funding from Kyowa Kirin.

Dr Baughn reports that her unit at Mayo Clinic benefits from research funding from Genentech.

Dr Bejar reports holding stocks in Aptose Biosciences in his capacity as chief medical officer and senior vice president; receiving personal consultancy fees from Gilead Sciences and Epizyme; having received personal consultancy fees from Bristol Myers Squibb, Takeda, and Astex in his capacity as an advisory board member; and that his unit at the University of California, San Diego, benefits from research funding from Takeda and Celgene.

Dr Bianchi reports receiving personal consultancy fees from Prothena.

Dr Bower reports receiving personal consultancy fees from Gilead Sciences, ViiV Healthcare, and EUSA Pharma, and that his unit at Chelsea and Westminster Hospital benefits from research funding from GlaxoSmithKline and Sanofi.

Dr Bullinger reports that his unit at Charité – Universitätsmedizin Berlin benefits from research funding from Bayer and Jazz Pharmaceuticals; and receiving personal consultancy fees, honoraria, and support for travel from a number of pharmaceutical entities.

Dr Burger reports that his unit at MD Anderson Cancer Center benefited from clinical trial funding from Pharmacyclics, BeiGene, and AstraZeneca.

Dr Cassaday reports having received personal consultancy fees from Amgen, Kite Pharma / Gilead Sciences, and Pfizer in his capacity as an advisory board member, and that his unit at the University of Washington benefited from research funding from Merck and benefits from research funding from Amgen, Kite Pharma / Gilead Sciences, Pfizer, Servier, and Vanda Pharmaceuticals.

Dr Chadburn reports serving on the advisory board for Leica Biosystems and receiving personal consultancy fees from Boehringer Ingelheim.

Dr Chang reports that his unit at KK Women's and Children's Hospital benefits from research funding from Bayer (South East Asia).

Dr Chapuy reports that his unit at the University Medical Center Berlin benefits from research funding from Gilead Sciences, that he receives personal consultancy fees, honoraria, and support for travel from several pharmaceutical entities, and that he holds US patents #20170029904 and #20190292602.

Dr Chiattone reports having received personal consultancy fees from AbbVie, Janssen, and AstraZeneca.

Dr Chng reports receiving personal consultancy fees from MiRXES, and that his unit at the National University Cancer Institute benefited from research funding from Xian Janssen Pharmaceutical.

Dr Chuang reports that his unit at Chi Mei Medical Center benefited from research funding from Johnson & Johnson Taiwan Ltd.

Dr Cortes reports that his unit at Augusta University benefits from research funding from Novartis, Pfizer, Sun Pharma, AbbVie, and Bio-Path Holdings; receiving personal consultancy fees from a number of pharmaceutical entities; and holding stocks in Bio-Path Holdings.

Dr Cowan reports receiving personal consultancy fees from Janssen in his capacity as an advisory board member, and that his unit at the University of Washington benefits from research funding from Janssen, Bristol Myers Squibb, Sanofi-Aventis, Harpoon Therapeutics, Nektar, and AbbVie.

Dr Cross reports that his unit at the University of Southampton benefits from research funding from Novartis.

Dr Davis reports that her unit at the Bass Center for Childhood Cancer and Blood Diseases benefits from research funding from Jazz Pharmaceuticals.

Dr Davies reports having received honoraria for advisory work or speaker fees from Roche, Celgene/BMS, Kite/Gilead, AbbVie, Genmab, Janssen, AstraZeneca, Sobi, Prelude, and Incyte; his unit at Southampton General Hospital has received research funding from Roche, Celgene/BMS, MSD, Kite/Gilead, and AstraZeneca.

Dr de Jong reports that her unit at Amsterdam UMC / VUmc benefited from research funding from Celgene and Genmab.

Dr Deeg reports that his unit at Fred Hutchinson Cancer Center benefited from clinical trial support from Bristol Myers Squibb.

Dr Demicco reports that her unit at the University of Toronto benefited from research funding from Novartis.

Dr Diepstra reports that his unit at the University Medical Center Groningen benefits from research funding from Takeda.

Dr Dierickx reports that his unit at University Hospitals Leuven benefited from research funding from Roche.

Dr Dunleavy reports receiving consultancy fees from a number of pharmaceutical entities.

Dr Eichhorst reports serving on advisory boards for Janssen, AbbVie, Gilead, AstraZeneca, BeiGene, MSD, and Lilly; receiving personal speaker fees from Roche, AbbVie, BeiGene, AstraZeneca, and MSD; receiving honoraria from Roche, AbbVie, BeiGene, AstraZeneca, and MSD; receiving travel support from BeiGene; and receiving research support from Janssen, Gilead, Roche, AbbVie, BeiGene, and AstraZeneca.

Dr Eisfeld reports that her unit at the Clara D. Bloomfield Center benefits from research funding from the American Society of Hematology.

Dr Elenitoba-Johnson reports that his unit at the University of Pennsylvania benefits from research funding from Thermo Fisher Scientific, having a commercial interest in Genomenon in his capacity as a partner, and holding US patent #10590488 on novel methods to identify gene fusions in lymphoid neoplasms.

Dr Ennishi reports that his unit at Okayama University Hospital benefits from research funding from Chugai Pharmaceutical and Nippon Shinyaku, and holding patents WO2020/079591 and CA3115804.

Dr Fajgenbaum reports that his unit at the University of Pennsylvania benefits from research funding from EUSA Pharma and benefited from non-monetary support from Pfizer.

Dr Fernández de Larrea reports receiving personal consultancy fees and support for travel from Janssen, Amgen, Bristol Myers Squibb, Takeda, Sanofi, and The Binding Site; and that his unit at the Hospital Clínic de Barcelona benefits from research funding from Janssen, Amgen, Bristol Myers Squibb, and Takeda.

Dr Fitzgibbon reports that his unit at Queen Mary University of London benefited from research funding from Epizyme.

Dr Fontenay reports that her unit at Université Paris Cité benefited from research funding from Geron; and holding US patents #20200255912, #10662482, and #9675590.

Dr Fromm reports that his unit at the University of Washington benefits from research funding from Merck.

Dr Garcia reports that his unit at MD Anderson Cancer Center Madrid benefited from research funding from Roche Pharma.

Dr A.K. Gopal reports receiving personal consultancy fees from several pharmaceutical companies, and that his unit at the University of Washington benefits from research funding and non-monetary support from several pharmaceutical companies.

Dr Greenberg reports that his unit at the Stanford Cancer Institute benefits from research funding from Gilead Sciences, Celgene, H3 Biomedicine, and FibroGen.

Dr Greipp reports receiving consultancy fees from AbbVie in her capacity as a scientific advisory board member.

Dr Guitart reports that his unit at Feinberg School of Medicine benefited from research funding from Galderma, Elorac, and miRagen.

Dr Haase reports that his unit at University Medical Center Göttingen benefits from research funding from Celgene/BMS and Novartis.

Dr C. Haferlach reports being a salaried employee and part-owner of MLL Munich Leukemia Laboratory, and that her unit at MLL Munich Leukemia Laboratory benefits from funding from Illumina.

Dr T. Haferlach reports being a salaried employee and part-owner of MLL Munich Leukemia Laboratory, and that his unit at MLL Munich Leukemia Laboratory benefits from funding from Illumina.

Dr C.N. Harrison reports that her unit at Guy's and St Thomas' NHS Foundation Trust benefits from research funding from Novartis and from non-monetary support from Constellation Pharmaceuticals.

Dr Herfarth reports that his unit at University Hospital Heidelberg benefits from research funding from Roche Pharma.

Dr Herling reports that his unit at the University of Leipzig benefited from research funding from Janpix.

Dr Hochhaus reports that his unit at University Medical Center Jena benefits from clinical trial support from Bristol Myers Squibb, Novartis, Incyte, and Pfizer; and reports holding patent #20090306094 on BCR-ABL mutations.

Dr Hunger reports having received honoraria and support for travel from Amgen, and holding stocks in Amgen.

Dr Idbaih reports receiving personal consultancy fees from Novocure, LEO Pharma, Polytone Laser, Boehringer Ingelheim, and Novartis in his capacity as an advisory board member, and having received support for travel from Carthera. He reports that his unit at Sorbonne University benefits from research funding from Transgene, Sanofi, and Nutritheragene, and benefited from research funding from Carthera and Air Liquide.

Dr Inaba reports that his unit at St. Jude Children's Research Hospital benefits from research funding from Servier and from non-monetary support from Amgen and Incyte; and having received personal consultancy fees from Servier and Jazz Pharmaceuticals.

Dr Ishitsuka reports receiving personal consultancy fees from Daiichi Sankyo, and that his unit at Kagoshima University benefits from research funding from Ono Pharmaceutical and from honoraria from Kyowa Kirin.

Dr Jacques reports being a director and shareholder of Repath Ltd and a director, shareholder, and employee of Neuropath Ltd; and receiving fees for editorial work from Wiley.

Dr Jain reports receiving personal remuneration for an advisory role from Pharmacyclics, Janssen, AbbVie, Genentech, AstraZeneca, Bristol Myers Squibb, Adaptive Biotechnologies, Servier, Precision BioSciences, BeiGene, Cellectis, TG Therapeutics, and ADC Therapeutics.

Dr Jaiswal reports holding US patent #8562997.

Dr Kantarjian reports having received personal consultancy fees, and that his unit at MD Anderson Cancer Center benefits from research funding, from several pharmaceutical entities.

Dr Karadimitris reports receiving personal consultancy fees from SUDA Pharmaceuticals and that his unit at Imperial College London benefited from research funding from Celgene and GSK.

Dr Karube reports that his unit at Nagoya University benefits from research funding from Takeda Pharmaceuticals and Eisai. He also receives honoraria from a number of pharmaceutical entities.

Dr Kataoka reports that his unit at Keio University School of Medicine benefits from research funding from a number of pharmaceutical entities, receiving personal consultancy fees from a number of pharmaceutical entities, holding stocks in Asahi Genomics, and holding patents on a genetic test in T-cell lymphomas and a genetic test for PD-L1 genetic alterations.

Dr Kersten reports that her institution receives her consultancy fees from Kite Pharma / Gilead Sciences, Novartis, BMS/Celgene, Roche, Adicet Bio, and Miltenyi Biotec, and her travel support from BMS/Celgene and Roche; and that her department at Amsterdam UMC benefits from research funding from Kite Pharma / Gilead Sciences.

Dr Kimura reports that his unit at Nagoya University benefited from research funding from a number of pharmaceutical entities, and holding patent WO/2009/116266.

Dr Klapper reports that his unit at University Hospital Schleswig-Holstein benefits from research funding from Amgen, Regeneron, and Takeda.

Dr Komrokji reports that his unit at H. Lee Moffitt Cancer Center benefits from non-monetary support from Bristol Myers Squibb; receiving personal consultancy fees from Bristol Myers Squibb and Jazz Pharmaceuticals in his capacity as a speakers' bureau participant, as well as from AbbVie, Novartis, Accelleron, Geron, and Taiho; and holding stocks in AbbVie.

Dr Kridel reports that his unit at the Princess Margaret Cancer Centre benefits from research funding from Roche and AbbVie.

Dr Kristinsson reports that his unit at the University of Iceland benefited from research funding from Amgen and Bristol Myers Squibb.

Dr Kumar reports receiving personal consultancy fees from Oncopeptides, BeiGene, and Antengene; and that his unit at Mayo Clinic benefits from clinical trial funding from a number of pharmaceutical entities.

Dr Kwong reports receiving personal advisory fees from Amgen, Astellas, Bayer, BeiGene, Bristol Myers Squibb, Celgene, Gilead, Janssen, Merck Sharp & Dohme, Otsuka, Novartis, Roche, and Takeda, and that he has received research support from Merck Sharp & Dohme and Novartis.

Dr Landgren reports receiving personal consultancy fees from Amgen, Janssen, Sanofi, Celgene, and GSK in his capacity as a scientific advisory board member.

Dr Lenz reports receiving personal consultancy fees and non-monetary support from a number of pharmaceutical entities, and that his unit at University Hospital Münster benefits from research funding from a number of pharmaceutical entities.

Dr Leung reports owning NTC Consulting as a family business, and that his unit at Mayo Clinic benefits from research funding from Omeros.

Dr Lim reports that her former unit at the University of Pennsylvania benefits from research funding from Thermo Fisher Scientific; being a founding partner of Genomenon; holding patent US20150050274A1; and having provided expert testimony in relation to litigations on lymphoma diagnoses.

Dr O. Lin reports that his unit at Memorial Sloan Kettering Cancer Center benefited from research funding from Hologic.

Dr Locatelli reports having received speaking fees from Amgen, Novartis, Takeda, and Jazz Pharmaceuticals.

Dr Loghavi reports receiving personal consultancy fees from AbbVie, receiving research funding from Amgen, and owning stock in AbbVie

Dr Macon reports having attended an advisory board meeting organized by NanoString Technologies and having received partial salary support from Celgene for his role as central review pathologist for the ECOG/ACRIN E1412 clinical trial.

Dr Maruyama reports that his unit at the Japanese Foundation for Cancer Research benefited from research funding from Ono Pharma, Janssen, Eisai, Chugai, Kyowa Kirin, MSD, Zenyaku, Sanofi, SymBio, Takeda, AbbVie, AstraZeneca, Bristol Myers Squibb, Genmab, Novartis, Otsuka, Taiho, Pfizer, and Astellas, and receiving honoraria from Ono Pharma, Nippon Shinyaku, Janssen, Mundipharma, Eisai, Chugai, Kyowa Kirin, MSD, Zenyaku, Sanofi, SymBio, Takeda, AbbVie, AstraZeneca, Bristol Myers Squibb, Genmab, and Novartis.

Dr Meignin reports receiving personal consultancy fees from EUSA Pharma.

Dr Mejstrikova reports that her unit at Motol University Hospital benefits from research funding from Amgen.

Dr Mesa reports receiving personal consultancy fees from Novartis, Incyte, Blueprint Medicines, Geron, and Telios Pharma, as well as additional support for travel from Sierra, Bristol Myers Squibb, and CTI BioPharma; and that his unit at Mays Cancer Center benefited from research funding from Incyte, Bristol Myers Squibb, Celgene, CTI BioPharma, Sierra, and Blueprint Medicines.

Dr Miranda reports having received personal consultancy fees from Allergan in his capacity as a scientific advisory board member.

Dr Miyazaki reports that his unit at Nagasaki University benefits from research funding from Sumitomo Dainippon Pharma.

Dr Montes-Moreno reports that his unit at Hospital Universitario Marqués de Valdecilla benefits from research funding from Roche and Recordati Rare Diseases, and has benefited from research funding from Gilead Spain.

Dr Mori reports that his unit at St. Marianna University benefits from research funding and non-monetary support from Pfizer and benefited from Chugai Pharma and Takeda.

Dr Nadel reports that his unit at Inserm CNRS AMU benefited from research funding from Celgene/BMS.

Dr Nagai reports having received personal consultancy fees from AbbVie, AstraZeneca, Genmab, Janssen, Eli Lilly, Takeda, Kyowa Kirin, MSD, Eisai, Novartis, Ono Pharmaceutical, Sumitomo Dainippon, Chugai, Meiji Seika Pharma, Mundipharma, GSK, Bristol Myers Squibb, Nippon Shinyaku, and CSL Behring; and that his unit at Nagoya Medical Center benefits from research funding from AbbVie, AstraZeneca, BeiGene, Genmab, HUYA, Janssen, Eli Lilly, Takeda, Kyowa Kirin, MSD, Mitsubishi Tanabe, Chugai, Daiichi Sankyo, Celgene, Zenyaku Kogyo, Solasia Pharma, Ono Pharmaceutical, Nippon Shinyaku, Regeneron, and Haihe Biopharma.

Dr Nagane reports that his unit at Kyorin University benefited from research funding from Eisai, Chugai, MSD, Daiichi Sankyo, AbbVie, Pfizer, Astellas Pharma, Shionogi, Nippon Kayaku, Tsumura, Teijin Pharma, Bayer, Kyowa Kirin, Terumo, Mitsubishi Tanabe, Asahi Kasei Medical, Johnson & Johnson, and Otsuka; having received personal consultancy fees from Bristol Myers Squibb, Riemser, Ono Pharmaceutical, Novocure, Nippon Shinyaku, Ohara Pharmaceutical, AbbVie, and Daiichi Sankyo; and receiving honoraria from Chugai, Daiichi Sankyo, Ono Pharmaceutical, Nippon Kayaku, Sumitomo Dainippon, Eisai, Kyowa Kirin, Ohara Pharmaceutical, UCB Japan, and Novocure.

Dr Nair reports receiving personal consultancy fees from Dr Reddy's Laboratories in her capacity as an advisory board member.

Dr Nakamura reports that her unit at Tokai University School of Medicine benefits from research funding from Kyowa Kirin and Janssen, and receiving personal consultancy fees from Kyowa Kirin.

Dr Natkunam reports serving on the medical advisory boards of Leica Biosystems and Roche Tissue Diagnostics, for which she has received personal consultancy fees.

Dr Narula reports being on the scientific advisory board of ImmunoACT.

Dr Nicholson reports that his unit at Royal Brompton & Harefield NHS Foundation Trust benefited from research funding from Pfizer.

Dr Ogawa reports receiving personal consultancy fees from Kan Research Institute and Chordia Therapeutics; that his unit at Kyoto University benefited and benefits from research funding from Sumitomo Dainippon Pharma and Chordia Therapeutics, respectively; and holding stocks in RegCell, Asahi Genomics, and Chordia Therapeutics.

Dr Orgel reports having received personal consultancy fees from Jazz Pharmaceuticals.

Dr Padron reports that his unit at H. Lee Moffitt Cancer Center benefits from research funding from Kura Oncology, Bristol Myers Squibb, and Incyte.

Dr Paiva reports holding two patents, EP16196874.8/WO2018/083204 on "Bispecific antibody against BCMA and CD3 and an immunological drug for combined use in treating multiple myeloma" and EP18203878.6/WO2020/089437A1 on "Combination therapy", and that his unit at Clinica Universidad de Navarra benefits from research funding from BMS/Celgene, Roche, and Sanofi. He reports receiving personal consultancy fees from Bristol Myers Squibb, GSK, Janssen, Roche, Sanofi, and Takeda; research funding from AstraZeneca, BeiGene, Bristol Myers Squibb, GSK, Roche, and Sanofi; and honoraria from Adaptive Biotechnologies, Amgen, BD, Celgene/BMS, GSK, Janssen, Sanofi, and Roche.

Dr Park reports that her unit at CHU Grenoble Alpes benefits from research funding from Pfizer (past) and Takeda (current).

Dr Patel reports having received personal consultancy fees from Astellas Pharma and Novartis.

Dr Patkar reports that his unit at ACTREC, Tata Memorial Centre, receives research funding from Illumina.

Dr Patnaik reports that his unit at Mayo Clinic benefits from research funding from Stemline Therapeutics, Kura Oncology, Epigenetix, Polaris, and Solu Therapeutics.

Dr Pemmaraju reports that his unit at MD Anderson Cancer Center benefits from research funding from Affymetrix, and receiving personal consultancy fees and non-monetary support from a number of pharmaceutical entities.

Dr Percival reports that her unit at the University of Washington benefits from research funding from a number of pharmaceutical entities.

Dr Pileri reports receiving personal consultancy fees from Recordati Rare Diseases, Kyowa Kirin, and Stemline Menarini.

Dr Pimpinelli reports receiving consultancy fees for advisory boards and CME events from AbbVie, Bristol Myers Squibb, Kyowa Kirin, Novartis, Pierre Fabre, Recordati Rare Diseases, Sanofi, and Takeda.

Dr Platzbecker reports having received personal consultancy fees from Novartis, Takeda, Jazz Pharmaceuticals, Bristol Myers Squibb, Janssen, Curis, AbbVie, and Gilead Sciences in his capacity as an advisory board member, and that his unit at University Hospital Leipzig benefited from research funding from Jazz Pharmaceuticals, Curis, and Amgen.

Dr Raderer reports receiving honoraria from Celgene, Bristol Myers Squibb, Eli Lilly, Ipsen, Novartis, BeiGene, Janssen-Cilag, and Gilead Sciences.

Dr Radich reports having received personal consultancy fees from Cepheid and Bio-Rad, and, in his capacity as an advisory board member, from Novartis, Amgen, Genentech, Bristol Myers Squibb, and Takeda.

Dr Rawstron reports being a salaried technical advisor for Pharmacyclics, and that his unit at St James's Institute of Oncology benefits from research funding from AbbVie, Celgene, Janssen, Pharmacyclics, and Roche.

Dr D. Rossi reports having received personal consultancy fees and support for travel from, and that his unit at the Oncology Institute of Southern Switzerland benefits from unrestricted research funding from, AbbVie, Janssen, and AstraZeneca.

Dr Rousselot reports that his unit at Centre Hospitalier de Versailles benefited from research funding and drug supply (avelumab) from Pfizer.

Dr Rule reports having received personal consultancy fees from AstraZeneca, Acerta Pharma, Roche, Janssen, Pharmacyclics, Sunesis Pharmaceuticals, BeiGene, and Merck; that his unit at Plymouth University Medical School benefits from research funding from Janssen; and having provided expert testimony in a patent challenge with respect to the drug ibrutinib on behalf of the manufacturer Pharmacyclics.

Dr Sabattini reports having received speaker fees or personal consultancy fees for advisory board work from Recordati Rare Diseases, Kyowa Kirin, and Stemline Menarini.

Dr Sahm reports being a cofounder of Heidelberg Epignostix GmbH, a company specialized in methylation diagnostics.

Dr Sakata-Yanagimoto reports that her unit at the University of Tsukuba benefits from research funding from Bristol Myers Squibb, and receiving personal consultancy fees from Eisai.

Dr Sallman reports receiving personal consultancy fees from AbbVie, Agios, Magenta Therapeutics, Intellia Therapeutics, Novartis, Shattuck Labs, and Takeda in his capacity as an advisory board member, and from Bristol Myers Squibb and Incyte in his capacity as a speakers' bureau participant; that his unit at H. Lee Moffitt Cancer Center benefits from research funding from Jazz Pharmaceuticals and Aprea Therapeutics; and holding US patent #10071094.

Dr Schuh reports receiving personal consultancy fees from Roche, Janssen, AbbVie, BeiGene, and AstraZeneca; that her unit at the University of Oxford benefits from research funding from Janssen and AstraZeneca, and from non-monetary support from Illumina and Oxford Nanopore Technologies; and that her unit holds patent OUI 9742.

Dr Semenzato reports that his unit at the University of Padua and the Veneto Institute of Molecular Medicine benefited from research funding from Novartis, and having received non-monetary support from Roche.

Dr Shanafelt reports that his unit at Stanford University benefits from research funding from Pharmacyclics, Genentech, and AbbVie.

Dr Shimada reports that his unit at Nagoya University benefits from research funding from Otsuka Pharmaceutical Co.

Dr Slack reports having provided expert opinion in relation to litigation for plaintiffs in Roundup exposure cases.

Dr Sohani reports having provided expert opinion for various USA-based law firms in relation to litigation in lymphoma diagnosis and medical malpractice cases.

Dr Solary reports that his unit at Gustave Roussy benefited from research funding from Servier Laboratories.

Dr Spiekermann reports receiving speaker honoraria and/or travel grants and/or consultancy fees from AbbVie, Alexza, Bristol Myers Squibb, Gilead, Jazz Pharmaceuticals, LEO Pharma, MSD, Pfizer, Sanofi, Servier, Sobi, Stemline, and Takeda.

Dr Stamatopoulos reports that his unit at the Institute of Applied Biosciences benefits from research funding from Janssen, AbbVie, and AstraZeneca.

Dr Steidl reports having provided expert testimony for Bayer in relation to litigation for plaintiffs in pesticide exposure cases.

Dr Stilgenbauer reports that his unit at Ulm University benefits from research funding from a number of pharmaceutical entities, and receiving personal consultancy fees from AbbVie, Amgen, AstraZeneca, Bristol Myers Squibb, Celgene, Gilead Sciences, GSK, Hoffmann-La Roche, Janssen, Novartis, and Sunesis Pharmaceuticals.

Dr Suzuki reports that his unit at Shimane University benefits from research funding from Chugai, Kyowa Kirin, and Takeda.

Dr Takeuchi reports holding intellectual property rights on an ALK immunohistochemistry kit licensed to Nichirei Biosciences, and providing expert opinion on behalf of Nichirei Biosciences.

Dr Tamaru reports that his unit at Saitama Medical Center benefited from research support from Nichirei Biosciences.

Dr Tiacci reports holding a patent on the use of mutant BRAF as a biomarker of hairy cell leukaemia without any commercial revenues; receiving consultancy fees and non-monetary support from various pharmaceutical entities; and that his unit at the University of Perugia – Department of Medicine and Surgery and Ospedale Santa Maria della Misericordia benefits from funding from Roche and Kite/Gilead.

Dr Tooze reports that his unit at the Leeds Institute of Molecular Medicine benefits from non-monetary support from HTG Molecular Diagnostics.

Dr Tournilhac reports receiving personal consultancy fees from Takeda, and that his unit at CHU de Clermont-Ferrand benefited from support for travel from Takeda.

Dr Treon reports receiving personal consultancy fees from Janssen, AbbVie/ Pharmacyclics, and BeiGene; that his unit at Harvard Medical School benefits from research funding and non-monetary support from Janssen, AbbVie/ Pharmacyclics, BeiGene, Bristol Myers Squibb, and Eli Lilly; and holding patents on MYD88 and CXCR4 testing, and on HCK and IRAK inhibitors.

Dr Tsukasaki reports receiving personal consultancy fees from a number of pharmaceutical entities, and that his unit at Saitama Medical University benefits from research funding from Daiichi Sankyo, HUYABIO, Celgene, Chugai Pharma, Bayer, Eisai, and Kyowa Kirin.

Dr Tyner reports that his unit at Oregon Health & Science University benefits from research funding from a number of pharmaceutical entities, and having received personal consultancy fees from DAVA Oncology.

Dr Vassiliou reports receiving personal consultancy fees from STRM.BIO, and that his unit at the University of Cambridge benefited from research funding from Celgene.

Dr Vega reports having received research funding from CRISPR Therapeutics, Caribou Biosciences, Allogene, and Geron Corporation.

Dr Vermeer reports having received research funding from Kyowa, Takeda, and Helsinn.

Dr Verstovsek reports having received personal consultancy fees from Novartis and Blueprint Medicines.

Dr Walker reports that his unit at Indiana University benefits from research funding from Bristol Myers Squibb.

Dr H.-Y. Wang reports having received personal consultancy fees from Celgene.

Dr M. Wang reports receiving personal consultancy fees from a number of pharmaceutical entities, and that his unit at MD Anderson Cancer Center benefits from research funding from a number of pharmaceutical entities.

Dr Weigert reports receiving personal consultancy fees in his role as an advisory board member for BeiGene, Epizyme, Incyte, and Roche, and that his unit at LMU Hospital benefits from research funding from Incyte and Roche.

Dr Weinstock reports receiving personal consultancy fees from Bantam Pharmaceutical, ASELL, Secura Bio, AstraZeneca, and Daiichi Sankyo; that his unit at the Dana-Farber Cancer Institute benefits from research funding from Daiichi Sankyo, Verastem Oncology, and Abcuro; and owning stocks in Travera in his capacity as founder, and in Ajax Therapeutics.

Dr Wood reports receiving personal consultancy fees from Amgen and Beckman Coulter, and that his unit at Children's Hospital Los Angeles benefits from research funding from Novartis, Amgen, MacroGenics, BioSight, and Kite Pharma.

Dr C.J. Wu reports that her unit at Dana-Farber Cancer Institute benefited from research funding from Pharmacyclics, and holding equity shares in BioNTech.

Dr Xiao reports that his unit at Memorial Sloan Kettering Cancer Center benefited from research funding from Stemline Therapeutics.

Dr Yamaguchi reports that her unit at Mie University Graduate School of Medicine benefits from research funding from Chugai Pharmaceutical, Genmab, and Kyowa Kirin.

IARC/WHO Committee for the International Classification of Diseases for Oncology (ICD-O)

BRAY, Freddie
International Agency for Research on Cancer
25 Av. Tony Garnier, CS 90627
69366 Lyon, CEDEX 07

CREE, Ian A.
International Agency for Research on Cancer
25 Av. Tony Garnier, CS 90627
69366 Lyon, CEDEX 07

FERLAY, Jacques
International Agency for Research on Cancer
25 Av. Tony Garnier, CS 90627
69366 Lyon, CEDEX 07

GOLDMAN-LÉVY, Gabrielle
International Agency for Research on Cancer
25 Av. Tony Garnier, CS 90627
69366 Lyon, CEDEX 07

JAKOB, Robert
Classifications and Terminologies
World Health Organization (WHO)
Av. Appia 20
1211 Geneva

KRPELANOVA, Eva
Classifications and Terminologies
World Health Organization (WHO)
Av. Appia 20
1211 Geneva

LOKUHETTY, Dilani
International Agency for Research on Cancer
25 Av. Tony Garnier, CS 90627
69366 Lyon, CEDEX 07

ROUS, Brian
NHS England
Victoria House, Capital Park
Fulbourn, Cambridge CB21 5XA

WATANABE, Reiko
St. Marianna University School of Medicine
2-16-1 Sugao, Miyamae-ku, Kawasaki
Kanagawa 216-8511

ZNAOR, Ariana
International Agency for Research on Cancer
25 Av. Tony Garnier, CS 90627
69366 Lyon, CEDEX 07

Sources (Part B)

For the Part A source list, see p. 259 of the accompanying Part A book.

Note: For any figure, table, or box not listed below, the original source is this volume; the suggested source citation is

WHO Classification of Tumours Editorial Board. Haematolymphoid tumours. Lyon (France): International Agency for Research on Cancer; 2024. (WHO classification of tumours series, 5th ed.; vol. 11). https://publications.iarc.who.int/637.

Figures

4.01	Naresh KN
4.02	Naresh KN
4.03	Naresh KN
4.04	Naresh KN
4.05	Naresh KN
4.06	Naresh KN
4.07	Naresh KN
4.08	Chadburn A
4.09A–E	Ferry JA
4.10A–E	Louissaint A Jr
4.10F	Chan JKC
4.11A–C	Ferry JA
4.12A–E	Ferry JA
4.13A–E	Cheuk W
4.14A,B	Cheuk W
4.15A,B	Cheuk W
4.16A,B	Cheuk W
4.17A,C	Medeiros LJ
4.17B	Ferry JA
4.18A–C	Medeiros LJ
4.19	Adapted, with permission from Elsevier, from: Fajgenbaum DC, Uldrick TS, Bagg A, et al. International, evidence-based consensus diagnostic criteria for HHV-8-negative/idiopathic multicentric Castleman disease. Blood. 2017 Mar 23;129(12):1646–57. PMID:28087540.
4.20A,B	Chadburn A
4.20C	Ferry JA
4.21A,B	Chadburn A
4.22A–D	Chadburn A
4.23A,B	Wood BL
4.24A,B	Wood BL
4.25A,B	Kovach AE
4.26A–F	Gujral S
4.27A–C	Gujral S
4.28A–C	Harrison CJ
4.29	Lina Shao, Department of Pathology and Clinical Laboratories, University of Michigan, Ann Arbor MI
4.30	Lina Shao, Department of Pathology and Clinical Laboratories, University of Michigan, Ann Arbor MI
4.31A,B	Parihar M
4.31C	Lina Shao, Department of Pathology and Clinical Laboratories, University of Michigan, Ann Arbor MI
4.32	Rachel Dobson, University of Cambridge, Cambridge; and Du MQ
4.33A,B	Hodge JC
4.33C,D	Virginia Thurston, Atrium Health, Charlotte NC
4.34	Devon Chabot-Richards, University of New Mexico, Albuquerque NM
4.35A–C	Rachel Dobson, University of Cambridge, Cambridge; and Du MQ; and Adapted, with permission from Elsevier, from: Tasian SK, Loh ML, Hunger SP. Philadelphia chromosome-like acute lymphoblastic leukemia. Blood. 2017 Nov 9;130(19):2064–72. PMID:28972016; and Adapted, with permission from Elsevier, from: Iacobucci I, Li Y, Roberts KG, et al. Truncating erythropoietin receptor rearrangements in acute lymphoblastic leukemia. Cancer Cell. 2016 Feb 8;29(2):186–200. PMID:26859458; and Adapted, with permission from Elsevier, from: Roberts KG, Morin RD, Zhang J, et al. Genetic alterations activating kinase and cytokine receptor signaling in high-risk acute lymphoblastic leukemia. Cancer Cell. 2012 Aug 14;22(2):153–66. PMID:22897847; and Adapted, with permission from the Massachusetts Medical Society, from: Roberts KG, Li Y, Payne-Turner D, et al. Targetable kinase-activating lesions in Ph-like acute lymphoblastic leukemia. N Engl J Med. 2014 Sep 11;371(11):1005–15. PMID:25207766. Copyright © 2014 Massachusetts Medical Society.
4.36A,B	Tembhare PR
4.37A–C	Ketterling RP
4.38	Zi Chen, Department of Pathology, University of Cambridge, Cambridge; and Du MQ
4.39	Raca G
4.40	Francesco Cucco, Department of Pathology, University of Cambridge, Cambridge; and Du MQ
4.41	Maria Cardenas, Alexander Gout, Lu Wang, and David Wheeler, Molecular Pathology Department, St. Jude Children's Research Hospital, Memphis TN
4.42	Raca G
4.43	Maria-Myrsini Tzioni, Addenbrooke's Hospital, Cambridge; and Du MQ
4.44A–C	Tembhare PR
4.45	Leventaki V
4.46	Ketterling RP
4.47	Ketterling RP
4.48	Maria-Myrsini Tzioni, Addenbrooke's Hospital, Cambridge; and Du MQ
4.49	Tembhare PR
4.50	Rawstron AC
4.51	Rosenquist R
4.52	Burger JA
4.53	Sewell WA
4.54A,B	Ferry JA
4.55A–D	Ferry JA

4.56	Naresh KN
4.57A–D	Ott G
4.58A–D	Naresh KN
4.59A–D	Naresh KN
4.60A–C	Naresh KN
4.61	Stamatopoulos KE
4.62	Tiacci E
4.63	Lim MS
4.64	Lim MS
4.65A,B	Lim MS
4.65C	Molina TJ
4.65D	Tiacci E
4.66A–D	Tiacci E
4.67A	Lim MS
4.67B,C	Tiacci E
4.68	Rossi D
4.69	Ferry JA
4.70A,C	Lim MS
4.70B	Naresh KN
4.71	Lim MS
4.72A–C	Lim MS
4.72D	Traverse-Glehen A
4.73A–C	Traverse-Glehen A
4.74	Ferry JA
4.75A,B	Ferry JA
4.76A–C	Lim MS
4.77	Ferry JA
4.78A,B	Lin P
4.79A,B,E,F	Montes-Moreno S
4.79C,D	Lin P
4.80A–C	Montes-Moreno S
4.81A–D	Geddie WR
4.82	Montes-Moreno S
4.83	Raderer M
4.84	Du MQ
4.85	Du MQ
4.86A–D	Cheuk W
4.87A,B	Cheuk W
4.88A–D	Cheuk W
4.89A,B	Cheuk W
4.90A	Cheuk W
4.90B,C	Du MQ
4.91	Cheuk W
4.92A,C	Cynthia M. Magro, Department of Dermatology, Department of Pathology and Laboratory Medicine, Weill Cornell Medicine, New York NY
4.92B	Ferry JA
4.93A–G	Geyer J
4.94	Rossi D
4.95A–D	Natkunam Y
4.96A–C	Ferry JA
4.97A–F	Ferry JA
4.98	Natkunam Y
4.99	Natkunam Y
4.100	Natkunam Y
4.101A,B	Di Napoli A
4.102A–C	Oschlies I
4.103A–F	Di Napoli A
4.104A–C	Chan JKC
4.105	Xerri L
4.106	Nadel B
4.107A–C	Xerri L
4.108A,B	Ott G
4.109A–D	Chan JKC
4.110A–E	Marafioti T
4.111A–C	Xerri L
4.112A–E	Xerri L
4.113A–C	Xerri L
4.114A–D	Xerri L
4.115A	Xerri L
4.115B	Ott G
4.116A,B	Chan JKC
4.117	Chan JKC
4.118	Xerri L
4.119	Oschlies I
4.120A–C	Oschlies I
4.121A–E	Oschlies I
4.122	Karube K
4.123A–D	Chan JKC
4.124A	Karube K
4.124B–D	Chan JKC
4.125	Willemze R
4.126	Willemze R
4.127A–C	Oschlies I
4.128A–C	Oschlies I
4.129	Rosenquist R
4.130A–C	Lazzi S
4.131A	Lossos IS; and Daniel A. Sussman, Miller School of Medicine, University of Miami, Miami FL
4.131B	Lossos IS
4.132A–C	Ferry JA
4.133	Medeiros LJ
4.134	Ferry JA
4.135	Rosenquist R
4.136A–C	Klapper W
4.137A,D	Ferry JA
4.137B,C,E	Klapper W
4.138A,B	Medeiros LJ
4.139A,B	Klapper W
4.139C	Medeiros LJ
4.139D	Ferry JA
4.140A–C	Medeiros LJ
4.141A–D	Calaminici M
4.142A,B	Delabie J
4.142C,D	Ott G
4.143A–C	Delabie J
4.144A,B	Ott G
4.145A–D	Delabie J
4.146A–E	Ott G
4.147	Farinha P
4.148	Calaminici M
4.149A,C	Farinha P
4.149B,D	Sabattini E
4.150A,B	Farinha P
4.150C	Adapted, with permission, from: Li M, Liu Y, Wang Y, et al. Anaplastic variant of diffuse large B-cell lymphoma displays intricate genetic alterations and distinct biological features. Am J Surg Pathol. 2017 Oct;41(10):1322–32. PMID:28319526.
4.151A,B	Wang Z
4.152A,B	Sabattini E
4.153A–F	Farinha P
4.154A,D,F	Wang Z
4.154B,C,E	Farinha P
4.155A	Medeiros LJ
4.155B,C	Sabattini E
4.156A–D	Farinha P
4.157A,B	Sabattini E
4.157C	Farinha P
4.158A–D	Hartmann S
4.159A–D	Hartmann S
4.160	Du MQ; and Francesco Cucco, Department of Pathology, University of Cambridge, Cambridge
4.161A,F	Momose S
4.161B–E	Ott G
4.162A,B	Tooze RM
4.163A–E	Tooze RM
4.164	Ott G
4.165	Adapted, with permission, from: Medeiros LJ, editor. Ioachim's lymph node pathology. 5th ed. Philadelphia (PA): Wolters Kluwer; 2021.
4.166	Adapted, with permission, from: Medeiros LJ, editor. Ioachim's lymph node pathology. 5th ed. Philadelphia (PA): Wolters Kluwer; 2021.
4.167A,B	Molina TJ
4.168	Medeiros LJ
4.169	Medeiros LJ
4.170	Reprinted, with kind permission, from: Medeiros LJ, O'Malley DP, Caraway NP, et al. Tumors of the lymph nodes and spleen. Washington, DC: American Registry of Pathology; 2017. (AFIP atlas of tumor pathology, series 4; fascicle 25).
4.171A,B	Medeiros LJ
4.171C	Adapted, with permission, from: Medeiros LJ, editor. Ioachim's lymph node pathology. 5th ed. Philadelphia (PA): Wolters Kluwer; 2021.
4.172A–C	Schafernak KT
4.173A–E	Schafernak KT
4.174A,B	Siebert R
4.175A–D	Ott G
4.176A–C	Ott G
4.177	Klapper W
4.178	Klapper W
4.179A–D	Rymkiewicz G
4.180A–D	Anagnostopoulos I
4.181A,C,D	Anagnostopoulos I
4.181B	Deckert M
4.182A–C	Anagnostopoulos I
4.183A–C	Anagnostopoulos I
4.184A,C–E	Anagnostopoulos I
4.184B	Adapted, with permission, from: Medeiros LJ, editor. Ioachim's lymph node pathology. 5th ed. Philadelphia (PA): Wolters Kluwer; 2021.
4.185A,B	Medeiros LJ
4.186A,B	Anagnostopoulos I
4.187A,B	Anagnostopoulos I
4.188	Asano N
4.189	Chapman JR
4.190	Chan JKC
4.191	Chan JKC
4.192	Chan JKC
4.193A,B	Chan JKC
4.194	Chan JKC
4.195A,B	Boyer DF
4.195C,D	Cheuk W
4.196	Cheuk W
4.197A,B	Said JW
4.198	Ott G
4.199	Said JW
4.200A,B	Montes-Moreno S
4.201A–F	Montes-Moreno S

4.202	Chapuy B
4.203A,C–F	Deckert M
4.203B	Chan JKC
4.204A–D	Chan JKC
4.205A,B	Kuzu I
4.206A–C	Chan JKC
4.207A,D	Calaminici M
4.207B,C	Chan JKC
4.208A–D	Coupland SE
4.209A,B	Chan JKC
4.210A,B	Vermeer MH
4.211A,B	Oschlies I
4.212A–D	Oschlies I
4.213A,B	Ferry JA
4.213C	Ott G
4.214A,B	Takeuchi K
4.214C	Deckert M
4.215	Ferry JA
4.216	Takeuchi K
4.217	Shimada K
4.218A,B	Steidl C
4.219A–G	Traverse-Glehen A
4.219H–J	Nicolae A
4.220A	Traverse-Glehen A
4.220B–D	Nicolae A
4.221A–F	Nicolae A
4.222A–C	Traverse-Glehen A
4.223A	Ott G
4.223B	Leoncini L
4.224A–E	Lazzi S
4.224F	Leoncini L
4.225A,B	Reprinted from: Mbulaiteye SM, Devesa SS. Burkitt lymphoma incidence in five continents. Hemato. 2022;3(3):434–53. doi:10.3390/hemato3030030. https://creativecommons.org/licenses/by/4.0/.
4.226	Reprinted from: Mbulaiteye SM, Devesa SS. Burkitt lymphoma incidence in five continents. Hemato. 2022;3(3):434–53. doi:10.3390/hemato3030030. https://creativecommons.org/licenses/by/4.0/.
4.227	Adapted, with permission from Elsevier, from: Johnston WT, Erdmann F, Newton R, et al. Childhood cancer: estimating regional and global incidence. Cancer Epidemiol. 2021 Apr;71(Pt B):101662. PMID:31924557.
4.228	Reprinted from: Mbulaiteye SM, Devesa SS. Burkitt lymphoma incidence in five continents. Hemato. 2022;3(3):434–53. doi:10.3390/hemato3030030. https://creativecommons.org/licenses/by/4.0/.
4.229	Lazzi S
4.230A,C,D	Lazzi S
4.230B	Ott G
4.231A,B	Leoncini L
4.231C,D	Lazzi S
4.232	Ott G
4.233	Helena Barroca, Centro Hospitalar de São João, Alameda Prof. Hernâni Monteiro, Porto
4.234	Adapted, with permission from Springer Nature, from: Cesarman E, Damania B, Krown SE, et al. Kaposi sarcoma. Nat Rev Dis Primers. 2019 Jan 31;5(1):9. PMID:30705286.
4.235	Said JW
4.236	Said JW
4.237	Chadburn A
4.238A,B	Said JW
4.239	Chadburn A
4.240A,B,D	Said JW
4.240C	Vega F
4.241	Vega F
4.242A–D	Vega F
4.243A–C	Chan JKC
4.244A–C	Chan JKC
4.245A,B	Sato Y
4.245C	Natkunam Y
4.246A–D	Gratzinger D
4.247A–D	Natkunam Y
4.248A,B	Natkunam Y
4.249A–C	Sato Y
4.250A–D	Sato Y
4.251	Sato Y
4.252	Sato Y
4.253	Natkunam Y
4.254A–D	Sato Y
4.255A–G	Gratzinger D
4.256A,C–E	Chan JKC
4.256B	Gratzinger D
4.257A–C	Gratzinger D
4.258A,B	Gratzinger D
4.259A,B	Gratzinger D
4.260A–D	Chan JKC
4.261A–C	Chan JKC
4.262A,B	Adapted, by Küppers R, from: Weniger MA, Küppers R. Molecular biology of Hodgkin lymphoma. Leukemia. 2021 Apr;35(4):968–81. PMID:33686198. Creative Commons Attribution 4.0 International License, http://creativecommons.org/licenses/by/4.0/.
4.263	Reprinted, with kind permission, from: Tamaru J. Hodgkin lymphoma (HL). In: Kikuchi M, Mori S, editors. Atlas of malignant lymphomas. Tokyo (Japan): Bunkodo; 2004. pp. 281–92.
4.264A–D	Nicolae A
4.265A–F	Nicolae A
4.266A–C	Nicolae A
4.267	Fromm JR
4.268A,B	Nicolae A
4.268C	Reprinted, with kind permission, from: Tamaru J. Classic Hodgkin lymphoma. In: Nakamura S, Oshima K, Takeuchi K, et al., editors. Atlas of lymphoma V. Tokyo (Japan): Bunkodo; 2018. p. 274.
4.269A–C	Nicolae A
4.270A–F	Nicolae A
4.271A,B	Nicolae A
4.271C–G	Naresh KN
4.272A–D	Hebeda KM
4.273	Sohani AR
4.274	Natkunam Y
4.275A,B,D	Sohani AR
4.275C	Natkunam Y
4.276A,B	Sohani AR
4.276C,D	Natkunam Y
4.277A,B	Medeiros LJ
4.277C,D	Sohani AR
4.278	Tamaru J
4.279A	Sohani AR
4.279B–D	Natkunam Y
4.280	Adapted, with permission from Wiley, from: Tomkins O, Berentsen S, Arulogun S, et al. Daratumumab for disabling cold agglutinin disease refractory to B-cell directed therapy. Am J Hematol. 2020 Oct;95(10):E293–5. PMID:32652632. Republished with permission from patient and copyright owner. Copyright: John Wiley & Sons.
4.281	Ferry JA
4.282	Randen U
4.283A–C	Ferry JA
4.284A–D	Randen U
4.285A,B	Nasr SH
4.286A–D	Nasr SH
4.287A–C	Nasr SH
4.288	Adapted, with permission, from: Wechalekar AD, Gillmore JD, Hawkins PN. Systemic amyloidosis. Lancet. 2016 Jun 25;387(10038):2641–54. PMID:26719234.
4.289A,B	Gertz M
4.290	Adapted, with permission from S. Karger AG, Basel, from: Dittrich T, Kimmich C, Hegenbart U, et al. Prognosis and staging of AL amyloidosis. Acta Haematol. 2020;143(4):388–400. PMID:32570242; and Adapted, with permission, from: Dittrich T, Benner A, Kimmich C, et al. Performance analysis of AL amyloidosis cardiac biomarker staging systems with special focus on renal failure and atrial arrhythmia. Haematologica. 2019 Jul;104(7):1451–9. PMID:30655373.
4.291A–F	Nasr SH
4.292	Sewell WA
4.293A	Robert McKenna, Department of Laboratory Medicine and Pathology, University of Minnesota, Minneapolis MN
4.293B,C	Lucien Courtois, Laboratoire d'onco-hématologie, Institut Necker Enfants Malades, Paris; and Pierre Sujobert, Service d'hématologie biologique, Hôpital Lyon Sud, Pierre-Bénite, Équipe Lymphoma Immuno-biology, Faculté de Médecine Lyon Sud Charles Mérieux, Oullins

4.294A	Sewell WA
4.294B,C	Sohani AR
4.295A–F	Sohani AR
4.296A–C	Sohani AR
4.297A–C	Sohani AR
4.298A–D	Ferry JA
4.299A–D	Ferry JA
4.300	Kumar S
4.301A,B	Kumar S
4.302A,B	Kumar S
4.303A,B	Gujral S
4.304A,D	Baughn LB
4.305	Baughn LB
4.306	Baughn LB

5.01	Lim MS
5.02	Lim MS
5.03	Lim MS
5.04	Adapted, with permission from Elsevier, from: Elenitoba-Johnson KSJ, Wilcox R. A new molecular paradigm in mycosis fungoides and Sézary syndrome. Semin Diagn Pathol. 2017 Jan;34(1):15–21. PMID:28024703.
5.05	Chan JKC
5.06A–D	Chan JKC
5.07A–C	Chan JKC
5.08A	Chan JKC
5.08B	Gratzinger D
5.09	Gratzinger D
5.10A,D	Chan JKC
5.10B,C	Yang DT
5.11A	Chan JKC
5.11B	Gratzinger D
5.12A,B	Chan JKC
5.12C	Yang DT
5.13A–D	Ohgami RS
5.14A–E	Kovach AE
5.15A–C	Ott G
5.16	Kovach AE
5.17	Wood BL
5.18A–H	Tembhare PR
5.19	Chen X
5.20A–C	Ferry JA
5.21A–D	Chen X
5.22	Herling M
5.23A	Herling M
5.23B	Elenitoba-Johnson KSJ
5.24A–D	Morice WG
5.25	Morice WG
5.26	Gujral S
5.27	Reprinted from: Teramo A, Barilà G, Calabretto G, et al. Insights into genetic landscape of large granular lymphocyte leukemia. Front Oncol. 2020 Feb 18;10:152. PMID:32133291. Creative Commons Attribution License (CC BY).
5.28A–D	Morice WG
5.29	Morice WG
5.30	Morice WG
5.31	Reprinted, with permission, from: WHO. Human T-lymphotropic virus type 1: technical report, February 2020. Geneva (Switzerland): WHO; 2021. Available from: https://www.who.int/publications/i/item/9789240020221. Licence: CC BY-NC-SA 3.0 IGO.
5.32	Ferlay J, Ervik M, Lam F, et al. Global Cancer Observatory: Cancer Today [Internet]. Lyon (France): International Agency for Research on Cancer; 2020 [accessed 2024 Jan]. Available from: https://gco.iarc.who.int/today.
5.33	Karube K
5.34A,B	Karube K
5.35	Adapted, with permission, from: Imaizumi Y, Iwanaga M, Nosaka K, et al. Prognosis of patients with adult T-cell leukemia/lymphoma in Japan: a nationwide hospital-based study. Cancer Sci. 2020 Dec;111(12):4567–80. PMID:32976684.
5.36A,B	Karube K
5.37A–F	Karube K
5.38A	Chan JKC
5.38B–D	Karube K
5.39A,B	Karube K
5.40A,B	Karube K
5.41	Karube K
5.42	Elenitoba-Johnson KSJ
5.43A,B,D	Elenitoba-Johnson KSJ
5.43C	Geddie WR
5.44	Elenitoba-Johnson KSJ
5.45	Elenitoba-Johnson KSJ
5.46A,B	Chan JKC
5.47A–C	Suzuki R
5.48A,B	Suzuki R
5.48C	Chan JKC
5.49A	Marie Beylot-Barry, Hôpital Saint-André, CHU de Bordeaux, Translational Research In Oncodermatology and Orphan skin diseases (TRIO2), Bordeaux Institute of Oncology (BRIC) – Inserm U1312 / Université de Bordeaux, Bordeaux
5.49B	Vergier B
5.50A	Marie Beylot-Barry, Hôpital Saint-André, CHU de Bordeaux, Translational Research In Oncodermatology and Orphan skin diseases (TRIO2), Bordeaux Institute of Oncology (BRIC) – Inserm U1312 / Université de Bordeaux, Bordeaux
5.50B	Vergier B
5.51A–E	Vergier B
5.52A	Paul Craig, Gloucestershire Hospitals NHS Foundation Trust, Gloucestershire Cellular Pathology Laboratory, Cheltenham General Hospital, Cheltenham, Gloucestershire
5.52B	Kempf W
5.53A,B	Kempf W
5.54A–D	Kempf W
5.55A,B	Pimpinelli N
5.56A–C	Pimpinelli N
5.57A,B	Pulitzer M
5.58	Geddie WR
5.59	Geddie WR
5.60A,B	Pulitzer M
5.61A,B	Pulitzer M
5.62	Chan JKC
5.63	Kempf W
5.64	Kempf W
5.65	Kempf W
5.66	Kempf W
5.67A,B	Kempf W
5.68	Kempf W
5.69	Kempf W
5.70	Kempf W
5.71A,B	Kempf W
5.72A–C	Kempf W
5.73A,B	Willemze R
5.74A–C	Willemze R
5.75A–D	Willemze R
5.76A,B	Pulitzer M
5.77A,B	Pulitzer M
5.78	Pulitzer M
5.79	Pulitzer M
5.80	Pulitzer M
5.81	Berti E
5.82	Berti E
5.83A–C	Berti E
5.84	Berti E
5.85	Berti E
5.86	Berti E
5.87	Mitteldorf C
5.88A–E	Mitteldorf C
5.89	Mitteldorf C
5.90A	Reprinted, with permission from Elsevier, from: Perry AM, Warnke RA, Hu Q, et al. Indolent T-cell lymphoproliferative disease of the gastrointestinal tract. Blood. 2013 Nov 21;122(22):3599–606. PMID:24009234.
5.90B	Swerdlow SH, Campo E, Harris NL, et al., editors. WHO classification of tumours of haematopoietic and lymphoid tissues. Lyon (France): International Agency for Research on Cancer; 2017. (WHO classification of tumours series, 4th rev. ed.; vol. 2). https://publications.iarc.who.int/556.
5.91A–C	Bhagat G
5.92A–C	Bhagat G
5.93A,B	Chan JKC
5.94A–C	Chan JKC
5.95	Bhagat G
5.96	Bhagat G
5.97A,B	Bhagat G
5.98	Bhagat G
5.99A,B	Bhagat G
5.100A,B	Bhagat G
5.101A–C	Bhagat G
5.102A–C	Bhagat G
5.103	Bhagat G
5.104A–C	Bhagat G
5.105A,B	Chan JKC
5.106A,B	Chan JKC
5.107A,B	Chan JKC
5.108A–D	Chan JKC
5.109	Chan JKC
5.110A–C	Chan JKC
5.111A,B	Medeiros LJ
5.112A,B	Medeiros LJ
5.113A–D	Medeiros LJ
5.114	Elenitoba-Johnson KSJ

5.115	Elenitoba-Johnson KSJ
5.116	Elenitoba-Johnson KSJ
5.117A–D	Elenitoba-Johnson KSJ
5.118A,C,D	Elenitoba-Johnson KSJ
5.118B	Ott G
5.119	Cozzolino I
5.120A,C,D	Miranda RN
5.120B	Ott G
5.121A–D	Miranda RN
5.122A–D	Miranda RN
5.123	Miranda RN
5.124A	Miranda RN
5.124B,C	Ott G
5.125A,B	de Jong D
5.125C	Miranda RN
5.126A–C	de Jong D
5.127A,B	Miranda RN
5.128	Miranda RN
5.129A	Iqbal J
5.129B	Du MQ; Attygalle AD
5.130A–C	Iqbal J
5.131	Du MQ
5.132	Du MQ
5.133A–D	Attygalle AD
5.134A,B	Attygalle AD
5.135A,B	Attygalle AD
5.136A–C	Attygalle AD
5.137A–D	Attygalle AD
5.138A–D	Attygalle AD
5.139A–C	Attygalle AD
5.140A–C	Attygalle AD
5.141A,B	Amador C
5.142	Chan JKC
5.143A–D	Amador C
5.144	Amador C
5.145A,B	Amador C
5.146A,B	Amador C
5.147	Adapted, with permission from Elsevier, from: Amador C, Greiner TC, Heavican TB, et al. Reproducing the molecular subclassification of peripheral T-cell lymphoma-NOS by immunohistochemistry. Blood. 2019 Dec 12;134(24):2159–70. PMID:31562134.
5.148A,B	Amador C
5.149A,B	Amador C
5.150	Ng S-B
5.151A,C	Ng S-B
5.151B	Kato S
5.152A–D	Kato S
5.153A,B	Kwong YL
5.154	Chuang S-S
5.155A–D	Kwong YL
5.156	Chuang S-S
5.157	Chuang S-S
5.158A	Huang YH
5.158B	Ng S-B
5.159A	Chan JKC
5.159B	Chuang S-S
5.159C	Huang YH
5.160A	Chan JKC
5.160B–D	Huang YH
5.161A–D	Yuta Tsuyuki, Fujita Health University Hospital, Center for Clinical Pathology, Toyoake, Aichi
5.162A–C	Yuta Tsuyuki, Fujita Health University Hospital, Center for Clinical Pathology, Toyoake, Aichi
5.163A,B	Sangueza JM
5.164A–C	Sangueza JM
5.165A–C	Liu WP
5.166A,B	Liu WP
5.167A,B	Liu WP
5.168A,B	Liu WP
5.169A–C	Liu WP
5.170A,B	Liu WP
5.171A,B	Liu WP
6.01A,B	Chan JKC
6.02A,B	Chan JKC
6.03A,B	Chan JKC
6.04	Rech KL
6.05A–D	Yin WH
6.06A	Hung YP
6.06B,C	Yin WH
6.07A	Yin WH
6.07B	Rech KL
6.08A,B	Chan JKC
6.09	Rech KL
6.10	Jiang XN, Zhang Y, Xue T, et al. New clinicopathologic scenarios of EBV+ inflammatory follicular dendritic cell sarcoma: report of 9 extrahepatosplenic cases. Am J Surg Pathol. 2021 Jun 1;45(6):765–72. PMID:33264138.
6.11A–C	Cheuk W
6.12A–F	Li XQ
6.13	Chan JKC
6.14A–C	Chan JKC
6.14D	Kaji S
6.15A,B	Chan JKC
6.16A	Miettinen M
6.16B–D	Laskin WB
6.17A,B	Miettinen M
6.18	Liu WP
6.19	Chan JKC
6.20A	Michal M
6.20B	Chan JKC
6.21A–C	Michal M
6.22	Cheuk W
6.23A–C	Cheuk W
6.24	Cheuk W
6.25A,B	Cheuk W
6.26	Cheuk W
6.27A–F	Cheuk W
7.01	Reprinted, with kind permission, from: Behrens YL, Göhring G, Bawadi R, et al. A novel classification of hematologic conditions in patients with Fanconi anemia. Haematologica. 2021 Nov 1;106(11):3000–3. PMID:34196171.
7.02A,B	Stephen Moore and Susan Olson, School of Medicine, Oregon Health and Science University, Portland OR
7.03	Michaels PD

Tables

4.01	Naresh KN
4.02	Naresh KN
4.03	Naresh KN
4.04	Naresh KN
4.05	Naresh KN
4.06	Chadburn A
4.07	Louissaint A Jr
4.08	Cheuk W
4.09	Gujral S
4.10	Nardi V
4.11	Harris MH
4.12	Choi JK
4.13	Choi JK
4.14	Rosenquist R
4.16	Eichhorst B
4.17	Rai K
4.18	de Jong D
4.19	Tiacci E
4.20	Montes-Moreno S
4.21	Montes-Moreno S
4.22	Du MQ
4.23	Cheuk W
4.24	Adapted, with permission, from: Copie-Bergman C, Wotherspoon AC, Capella C, et al. Gela histological scoring system for post-treatment biopsies of patients with gastric MALT lymphoma is feasible and reliable in routine practice. Br J Haematol. 2013 Jan;160(1):47–52. PMID:23043300.
4.25	Natkunam Y
4.26	Xerri L
4.27	Klapper W
4.28	Klapper W
4.30	Rosenwald A
4.31	Medeiros LJ
4.32	Anagnostopoulos I
4.33	Anagnostopoulos I
4.34	Boyer DF
4.35	Montes-Moreno S
4.36	Coupland SE
4.37	Coupland SE
4.38	Oschlies I; Willemze R; Vergier B
4.39	Sarkozy C
4.40	Naresh KN
4.41	Said JW; Chadburn A; Vega F; Ferry JA
4.42	de Jong D
4.43	Natkunam Y; Dierickx D
4.44	de Jong D
4.45	Natkunam Y
4.46	Natkunam Y
4.47	Natkunam Y
4.48	Satou A
4.49	Natkunam Y
4.50	Natkunam Y
4.51	Gratzinger D
4.52	Gratzinger D
4.53	Nicolae A
4.54	Borges AM; Nicolae A; de Jong D
4.55	Natkunam Y
4.56	Naresh KN; Garcia JF
4.57	Natkunam Y
4.58	Natkunam Y
4.59	Natkunam Y

4.60 Randen U
4.61 Adapted, with permission from Elsevier, from: Rajkumar SV, Kyle RA, Therneau TM, et al. Serum free light chain ratio is an independent risk factor for progression in monoclonal gammopathy of undetermined significance. Blood. 2005 Aug 1;106(3):812–7. PMID:15855274.
4.62 Leung N
4.63 Sohani AR
4.64 de Jong D
4.65 Chng WJ
4.66 Naresh KN

5.01 Ng S-B
5.02 Allende LM
5.03 Adapted, with permission, from: Shimoyama M. Diagnostic criteria and classification of clinical subtypes of adult T-cell leukaemia-lymphoma. A report from the Lymphoma Study Group (1984-87). Br J Haematol. 1991 Nov;79(3):428–37. PMID:1751370.
5.04 Karube K
5.05 Kempf W
5.06 Vergier B
5.07 Kempf W
5.08 Adapted, with permission from Elsevier, from: Olsen E, Vonderheid E, Pimpinelli N, et al. Revisions to the staging and classification of mycosis fungoides and Sezary syndrome: a proposal of the International Society for Cutaneous Lymphomas (ISCL) and the cutaneous lymphoma task force of the European Organization of Research and Treatment of Cancer (EORTC). Blood. 2007 Sep 15;110(6):1713–22. PMID:17540844;
and
Elder DE, Massi D, Scolyer RA, et al., editors. WHO classification of skin tumours. Lyon (France): International Agency for Research on Cancer; 2018. (WHO classification of tumours series, 4th ed.; vol. 11). https://publications.iarc.who.int/560.
5.09 Kim JE
5.10 Kempf W
5.11 Willemze R
5.12 Berti E
5.13 Xiao W; Chan JKC
5.14 Medeiros LJ
5.15 Medeiros LJ
5.16 Medeiros LJ
5.17 Lim MS
5.18 de Jong D
5.19 Du MQ
5.20 Du MQ
5.21 Amador C
5.22 Ng S-B
5.23 Chan JKC
5.24 Ng S-B; Chng WJ
5.25 Ng S-B

6.01 Chan JKC
6.02 Chan JKC
6.03 Cheuk W

7.01 Reprinted, with kind permission from the Fanconi Anemia Research Fund, from: Fanconi Anemia Research Fund. Chapter 3: Clinical care of Fanconi anemia hematologic issues. In: Fanconi anemia clinical care guidelines. Eugene (OR): Fanconi Anemia Research Fund; [updated 2023 Jul]. Available from: https://www.fanconi.org/images/uploads/other/Chapter_3-_Hematologic_Issues_July2023.pdf

Boxes

4.01 Adapted from: Silkenstedt E, Dreyling M. Mantle cell lymphoma-advances in molecular biology, prognostication and treatment approaches. Hematol Oncol. 2021 Jun;39 Suppl 1:31–8. PMID:34105823.
4.02 Rosenwald A
4.03 Berentsen S
4.04 Adapted, with permission from the Lancet and Elsevier, from: Rajkumar SV, Dimopoulos MA, Palumbo A, et al. International Myeloma Working Group updated criteria for the diagnosis of multiple myeloma. Lancet Oncol. 2014 Nov;15(12):e538–48. PMID:25439696.
4.05 Adapted, with permission from the Lancet and Elsevier, from: Rajkumar SV, Dimopoulos MA, Palumbo A, et al. International Myeloma Working Group updated criteria for the diagnosis of multiple myeloma. Lancet Oncol. 2014 Nov;15(12):e538–48. PMID:25439696.
4.06 Sewell WA
4.07 Adapted, with permission from the Lancet and Elsevier, from: Rajkumar SV, Dimopoulos MA, Palumbo A, et al. International Myeloma Working Group updated criteria for the diagnosis of multiple myeloma. Lancet Oncol. 2014 Nov;15(12):e538–48. PMID:25439696.
4.08 Dispenzieri A. POEMS syndrome: 2019 update on diagnosis, risk-stratification, and management. Am J Hematol. 2019 Jul;94(7):812–27. PMID:31012139.
4.09 Adapted, with permission from Elsevier, from: Sykes DB, O'Connell C, Schroyens W. The TEMPI syndrome. Blood. 2020 Apr 9;135(15):1199–203. PMID:32108223.

5.01 Lim MS
5.02 Lim MS
5.03 Gratzinger D
5.05 Reprinted, with permission from Elsevier, from: Staber PB, Herling M, Bellido M, et al. Consensus criteria for diagnosis, staging, and treatment response assessment of T-cell prolymphocytic leukemia. Blood. 2019 Oct 3;134(14):1132–43. PMID:31292114.
5.06 Attygalle AD
5.07 Chng WJ

Images on the cover

Top left Fig. 6.18: Liu WP
Middle left Fig. 6.21A: Michal M
Bottom left Fig. 6.21B: Michal M
Top centre Fig. 4.69: Ferry JA
Middle centre Fig. 4.70A: Lim MS
Bottom centre Fig. 4.72A: Lim MS
Top right Fig. 5.22: Herling M
Middle right Fig. 5.19: Chen X
Bottom right Fig. 5.23B: Elenitoba-Johnson KSJ

Images on the chapter title pages

Chapter 4 Fig. 4.175C: Ott G
Chapter 5 Fig. 5.10D: Chan JKC
Chapter 6 Fig. 6.03B: Chan JKC
Chapter 7 Fig. 2.33A (in Part A): De Vito R

References (Part B)

For the Part A reference list, see p. 263 of the accompanying Part A book.

1. Aamot HV, Micci F, Holte H, et al. G-banding and molecular cytogenetic analyses of marginal zone lymphoma. Br J Haematol. 2005 Sep;130(6):890–901. PMID:16156859
2. Aarts WM, Willemze R, Bende RJ, et al. VH gene analysis of primary cutaneous B-cell lymphomas: evidence for ongoing somatic hypermutation and isotype switching. Blood. 1998 Nov 15;92(10):3857–64. PMID:9808579
3. Abate F, Ambrosio MR, Mundo L, et al. Distinct viral and mutational spectrum of endemic Burkitt lymphoma. PLoS Pathog. 2015 Oct 15;11(10):e1005158. PMID:26468873
4. Abate F, da Silva-Almeida AC, Zairis S, et al. Activating mutations and translocations in the guanine exchange factor VAV1 in peripheral T-cell lymphomas. Proc Natl Acad Sci U S A. 2017 Jan 24;114(4):764–9. PMID:28062691
5. Abboudi Z, Patel K, Naresh KN. Cyclin D1 expression in typical chronic lymphocytic leukaemia. Eur J Haematol. 2009 Sep;83(3):203–7. PMID:19467018
6. Abdallah N, Greipp P, Kapoor P, et al. Clinical characteristics and treatment outcomes of newly diagnosed multiple myeloma with chromosome 1q abnormalities. Blood Adv. 2020 Aug 11;4(15):3509–19. PMID:32750129
7. Abdel-Halim M, El-Nabarawy E, El Nemr R, et al. Frequency of hypopigmented mycosis fungoides in Egyptian patients presenting with hypopigmented lesions of the trunk. Am J Dermatopathol. 2015 Nov;37(11):834–40. PMID:26262921
8. AbdelRazek M, Stone JH. Neurologic features of immunoglobulin G4-related disease. Rheum Dis Clin North Am. 2017 Nov;43(4):621–31. PMID:29061247
9. Abdulla FR, Zhang W, Wu X, et al. Genomic analysis of cutaneous CD30-positive lymphoproliferative disorders. JID Innov. 2021 Nov 15;2(1):100068. PMID:34977845
10. Abdulla M, Hollander P, Pandzic T, et al. Cell-of-origin determined by both gene expression profiling and immunohistochemistry is the strongest predictor of survival in patients with diffuse large B-cell lymphoma. Am J Hematol. 2020 Jan;95(1):57–67. PMID:31659781
11. Abdul-Wahab A, Tang SY, Robson A, et al. Chromosomal anomalies in primary cutaneous follicle center cell lymphoma do not portend a poor prognosis. J Am Acad Dermatol. 2014 Jun;70(6):1010–20. PMID:24679486
12. Abe D, Nakaseko C, Takeuchi M, et al. Restrictive usage of monoclonal immunoglobulin lambda light chain germline in POEMS syndrome. Blood. 2008 Aug 1;112(3):836–9. PMID:18497319
13. Abolhassani H, Azizi G, Sharifi L, et al. Global systematic review of primary immunodeficiency registries. Expert Rev Clin Immunol. 2020 Jul;16(7):717–32. PMID:32720819
14. Abolhassani H, Hammarström L, Cunningham-Rundles C. Current genetic landscape in common variable immune deficiency. Blood. 2020 Feb 27;135(9):656–67. PMID:31942606
15. Abrey LE, Ben-Porat L, Panageas KS, et al. Primary central nervous system lymphoma: the Memorial Sloan-Kettering Cancer Center prognostic model. J Clin Oncol. 2006 Dec 20;24(36):5711–5. PMID:17116938
16. Abrey LE, DeAngelis LM, Yahalom J. Long-term survival in primary CNS lymphoma. J Clin Oncol. 1998 Mar;16(3):859–63. PMID:9508166
17. Abruzzo LV, Jaffe ES, Cotelingam JD, et al. T-cell lymphoblastic lymphoma with eosinophilia associated with subsequent myeloid malignancy. Am J Surg Pathol. 1992 Mar;16(3):236–45. PMID:1599015
18. AbuHilal M, Walsh S, Shear N. Associated hematolymphoid malignancies in patients with lymphomatoid papulosis: a Canadian retrospective study. J Cutan Med Surg. 2017 Nov/Dec;21(6):507–12. PMID:28614957
19. Achten R, Verhoef G, Vanuytsel L, et al. Histiocyte-rich, T-cell-rich B-cell lymphoma: a distinct diffuse large B-cell lymphoma subtype showing characteristic morphologic and immunophenotypic features. Histopathology. 2002 Jan;40(1):31–45. PMID:11903596
20. Achten R, Verhoef G, Vanuytsel L, et al. T-cell/histiocyte-rich large B-cell lymphoma: a distinct clinicopathologic entity. J Clin Oncol. 2002 Mar 1;20(5):1269–77. PMID:11870169
21. Adam M, Bekueretsion Y, Abubeker A, et al. Clinical characteristics and histopathological patterns of Hodgkin lymphoma and treatment outcomes at a tertiary cancer center in Ethiopia. JCO Glob Oncol. 2021 Feb;7:277–88. PMID:33591838
22. Adam P, Baumann R, Schmidt J, et al. The BCL2 E17 and SP66 antibodies discriminate 2 immunophenotypically and genetically distinct subgroups of conventionally BCL2-"negative" grade 1/2 follicular lymphomas. Hum Pathol. 2013 Sep;44(9):1817–26. PMID:23642737
23. Adam P, Czapiewski P, Colak S, et al. Prevalence of Achromobacter xylosoxidans in pulmonary mucosa-associated lymphoid tissue lymphoma in different regions of Europe. Br J Haematol. 2014 Mar;164(6):804–10. PMID:24372375
24. Adam P, Katzenberger T, Eifert M, et al. Presence of preserved reactive germinal centers in follicular lymphoma is a strong histopathologic indicator of limited disease stage. Am J Surg Pathol. 2005 Dec;29(12):1661–4. PMID:16327439
25. Adam P, Schiefer AI, Prill S, et al. Incidence of preclinical manifestations of mantle cell lymphoma and mantle cell lymphoma in situ in reactive lymphoid tissues. Mod Pathol. 2012 Dec;25(12):1629–36. PMID:22790016
26. Adams HJ, Nievelstein RA, Kwee TC. Systematic review on the additional value of 18F-fluoro-2-deoxy-D-glucose positron emission tomography in staging follicular lymphoma. J Comput Assist Tomogr. 2017 Jan;41(1):98–103. PMID:27560022
27. Adlard J, Burton C, Turton P. Increasing evidence for the association of breast implant-associated anaplastic large cell lymphoma and Li Fraumeni syndrome. Case Rep Genet. 2019 Jul 16;2019:5647940. PMID:31392066
27A. Adrada BE, Miranda RN, Rauch GM, et al. Breast implant-associated anaplastic large cell lymphoma: sensitivity, specificity, and findings of imaging studies in 44 patients. Breast Cancer Res Treat. 2014 Aug;147(1):1–14. PMID:25073777
28. Advani RH, Horning SJ, Hoppe RT, et al. Mature results of a phase II study of rituximab therapy for nodular lymphocyte-predominant Hodgkin lymphoma. J Clin Oncol. 2014 Mar 20;32(9):912–8. PMID:24516013
29. Advani RH, Skrypets T, Civallero M, et al. Outcomes and prognostic factors in angioimmunoblastic T-cell lymphoma: final report from the international T-cell Project. Blood. 2021 Jul 22;138(3):213–20. PMID:34292324
30. Afacan-Öztürk HB, Falay M, Albayrak M, et al. CD81 expression in the differential diagnosis of chronic lymphocytic leukemia. Clin Lab. 2019 Mar 1;65(3). PMID:30868852
31. Afshar-Sterle S, Zotos D, Bernard NJ, et al. Fas ligand-mediated immune surveillance by T cells is essential for the control of spontaneous B cell lymphomas. Nat Med. 2014 Mar;20(3):283–90. PMID:24487434
32. Agar NS, Wedgeworth E, Crichton S, et al. Survival outcomes and prognostic factors in mycosis fungoides/Sézary syndrome: validation of the revised International Society for Cutaneous Lymphomas/European Organisation for Research and Treatment of Cancer staging proposal. J Clin Oncol. 2010 Nov 1;28(31):4730–9. PMID:20855822
33. Agathangelidis A, Chatzidimitriou A, Gemenetzi K, et al. Higher-order connections between stereotyped subsets: implications for improved patient classification in CLL. Blood. 2021 Mar 11;137(10):1365–76. PMID:32992344
34. Agathangelidis A, Galigalidou C, Scarfò L, et al. Infrequent "chronic lymphocytic leukemia-specific" immunoglobulin stereotypes in aged individuals with or without low-count monoclonal B-cell lymphocytosis. Haematologica. 2021 Apr 1;106(4):1178–81. PMID:32586905
35. Agathangelidis A, Hadzidimitriou A, Rosenquist R, et al. Unlocking the secrets of immunoglobulin receptors in mantle cell lymphoma: implications for the origin and selection of the malignant cells. Semin Cancer Biol. 2011 Nov;21(5):299–307. PMID:21946621
36. Agathangelidis A, Ljungström V, Scarfò L, et al. Highly similar genomic landscapes in monoclonal B-cell lymphocytosis and ultra-stable chronic lymphocytic leukemia with low frequency of driver mutations. Haematologica. 2018 May;103(5):865–73. PMID:29449433
37. Agbay RL, Torres-Cabala CA, Patel KP, et al. Immunophenotypic shifts in primary cutaneous γδ T-cell lymphoma suggest antigenic modulation: a study of sequential biopsy specimens. Am J Surg Pathol. 2017 Apr;41(4):431–45. PMID:28248813
38. Agbuduwe C, Yang H, Gaglani J, et al. Clinical presentation and outcomes of solitary plasmacytoma in a tertiary hospital in the UK. Clin Med (Lond). 2020 Sep;20(5):e191–5. PMID:32934063
39. Aghamohammadi A, Parvaneh N, Tirgari F, et al. Lymphoma of mucosa-associated lymphoid tissue in common variable immunodeficiency. Leuk Lymphoma. 2006 Feb;47(2):343–6. PMID:16321869
40. Agnelli L, Mereu E, Pellegrino E, et al. Identification of a 3-gene model as a powerful diagnostic tool for the recognition of ALK-negative anaplastic large-cell lymphoma. Blood. 2012 Aug 9;120(6):1274–81. PMID:22740451
41. Agopian J, Navarro JM, Gac AC, et al. Agricultural pesticide exposure and the molecular connection to lymphomagenesis. J Exp Med. 2009 Jul 6;206(7):1473–83. PMID:19506050
42. Agostinelli C, Akarca AU, Ramsay A, et al. Novel markers in pediatric-type follicular lymphoma. Virchows Arch. 2019 Dec;475(6):771–9. PMID:31686194
43. Agostinelli C, Hartmann S, Klapper W, et al. Peripheral T cell lymphomas with follicular T helper phenotype: a new basket or a distinct entity? Revising Karl Lennert's personal archive. Histopathology. 2011 Oct;59(4):679–91. PMID:22014049
44. Agrawal R, Wang J. Pediatric follicular lymphoma: a rare clinicopathologic entity. Arch Pathol Lab Med. 2009 Jan;133(1):142–6. PMID:19123728
45. Aguilar C, Beltran B, Quiñones P, et al. Large B-cell lymphoma arising in cardiac myxoma or intracardiac fibrinous mass: a localized lymphoma usually associated with Epstein-Barr virus? Cardiovasc Pathol. 2015 Jan-Feb;24(1):60–4. PMID:25307939
46. Aguilar C, Laberiano C, Beltran B, et al. Clinicopathologic characteristics and survival of patients with primary effusion lymphoma. Leuk Lymphoma. 2020 Sep;61(9):2093–102. PMID:32449626
47. Aguilera NS, Tomaszewski MM, Moad JC, et al. Cutaneous follicle center lymphoma: a clinicopathologic study of 19 cases. Mod Pathol. 2001 Sep;14(9):828–35. PMID:11557777
48. Ahmadi SE, Rahimi S, Zarandi B, et al. MYC: a multipurpose oncogene with prognostic and therapeutic implications in blood malignancies. J Hematol Oncol. 2021 Aug 9;14(1):121. PMID:34372899
49. Ahn IE, Tian X, Ipe D, et al. Prediction of outcome in patients with chronic lymphocytic leukemia treated with ibrutinib: development and validation of a four-factor prognostic model. J Clin Oncol. 2021 Feb 20;39(6):576–85. PMID:33026937
50. Ahn IE, Underbayev C, Albitar A, et al. Clonal evolution leading to ibrutinib resistance in chronic lymphocytic leukemia. Blood. 2017 Mar 16;129(11):1469–79. PMID:28049639
51. Ahn JS, Yang DH, Duk Choi Y, et al. Clinical outcome of elderly patients with Epstein-Barr virus positive diffuse large B-cell lymphoma treated with a combination of rituximab and CHOP chemotherapy. Am J Hematol. 2013 Sep;88(9):774–9. PMID:23760676
52. Ahn SS, Song JJ, Park YB, et al. Malignancies in Korean patients with immunoglobulin G4-related disease. Int J Rheum Dis. 2017 Aug;20(8):1028–35. PMID:28544157
53. Ai J, Xie Z. Epstein-Barr virus-positive T/NK-cell lymphoproliferative diseases in Chinese mainland. Front Pediatr. 2018 Oct 9;6:289. PMID:30356785
54. Aiempanakit K, Amatawet C, Chiratikarnwong K, et al. Erythema multiforme-like cutaneous lesions in monomorphic epitheliotropic intestinal T-cell lymphoma: a rare case report. J Cutan Pathol. 2017 Feb;44(2):183–8. PMID:27862162
55. Akhtar S, Rauf MS, Khafaga Y, et al. Nodular lymphocyte-predominant Hodgkin lymphoma characteristics, management of primary and relapsed/refractory disease and outcome analysis: the first comprehensive report

from the Middle East. BMC Cancer. 2021 Apr 1;21(1):351. PMID:33794818
56. Akiyama M, Yasuoka H, Yamaoka K, et al. Enhanced IgG4 production by follicular helper 2 T cells and the involvement of follicular helper 1 T cells in the pathogenesis of IgG4-related disease. Arthritis Res Ther. 2016 Jul 13;18:167. PMID:27411315
57. Aktas Samur A, Minvielle S, Shammas M, et al. Deciphering the chronology of copy number alterations in multiple myeloma. Blood Cancer J. 2019 Mar 26;9(4):39. PMID:30914633
58. Al-Abbadi MA, Hattab EM, Tarawneh MS, et al. Primary testicular diffuse large B-cell lymphoma belongs to the nongerminal center B-cell-like subgroup: a study of 18 cases. Mod Pathol. 2006 Dec;19(12):1521–7. PMID:16998463
59. Aladily TN, Mansour A, Alsughayer A, et al. The utility of CD83, fascin and CD23 in the differential diagnosis of primary mediastinal large B-cell lymphoma versus classic Hodgkin lymphoma. Ann Diagn Pathol. 2019 Jun;40:72–6. PMID:31075666
60. Alame M, Cornillot E, Cacheux V, et al. The immune contexture of primary central nervous system diffuse large B cell lymphoma associates with patient survival and specific cell signaling. Theranostics. 2021 Jan 22;11(8):3565–79. PMID:33664848
61. Alberti-Violetti S, Fanoni D, Provasi M, et al. Primary cutaneous acral CD8 positive T-cell lymphoma with extra-cutaneous involvement: a long-standing case with an unexpected progression. J Cutan Pathol. 2017 Nov;44(11):964–8. PMID:28796362
62. Alberti-Violetti S, Torres-Cabala CA, Talpur R, et al. Clinicopathological and molecular study of primary cutaneous CD4+ small/medium-sized pleomorphic T-cell lymphoma. J Cutan Pathol. 2016 Dec;43(12):1121–30. PMID:27550169
63. Alderuccio JP, Olszewski AJ, Evens AM, et al. HIV-associated Burkitt lymphoma: outcomes from a US-UK collaborative analysis. Blood Adv. 2021 Jul 27;5(14):2852–62. PMID:34283175
64. Alderuccio JP, Zhao W, Desai A, et al. Risk factors for transformation to higher-grade lymphoma and its impact on survival in a large cohort of patients with marginal zone lymphoma from a single institution. J Clin Oncol. 2018 Oct 12; (Oct):JCO1800138. PMID:30312133
65. Alduaij W, Collinge B, Ben-Neriah S, et al. Molecular determinants of clinical outcomes in a real-world diffuse large B-cell lymphoma population. Blood. 2023 May 18;141(20):2493–507. PMID:36302166
66. Alegría-Landa V, Manzarbeitia F, Salvatierra Calderón MG, et al. Cutaneous intravascular natural killer/T cell lymphoma with peculiar immunophenotype. Histopathology. 2017 Dec;71(6):994–1002. PMID:28766736
67. Alexander TB, Gu Z, Iacobucci I, et al. The genetic basis and cell of origin of mixed phenotype acute leukaemia. Nature. 2018 Oct;562(7727):373–9. PMID:30209392
68. Alexanian S, Said J, Lones M, et al. KSHV/HHV8-negative effusion-based lymphoma, a distinct entity associated with fluid overload states. Am J Surg Pathol. 2013 Feb;37(2):241–9. PMID:23282971
69. Alexiou C, Kau RJ, Dietzfelbinger H, et al. Extramedullary plasmacytoma: tumor occurrence and therapeutic concepts. Cancer. 1999 Jun 1;85(11):2305–14. PMID:10357398
70. Alghisi A, Borghetti P, Maddalo M, et al. Radiotherapy for the treatment of solitary plasmacytoma: 7-year outcomes by a mono-institutional experience. J Cancer Res Clin Oncol. 2021 Jun;147(6):1773–9. PMID:33201300
71. Al Hamed R, Bazarbachi AH, Mohty M. Epstein-Barr virus-related post-transplant lymphoproliferative disease (EBV-PTLD) in the setting of allogeneic stem cell transplantation: a comprehensive review from pathogenesis to forthcoming treatment modalities. Bone Marrow Transplant. 2020 Jan;55(1):25–39. PMID:31089285
72. Ali TZ, Beyer G, Taylor M, et al. Splenic hamartoma: immunohistochemical and ultrastructural profile of two cases. Int J Surg Pathol. 2005 Jan;13(1):103–11. PMID:15735864
73. Alizadeh AA, Eisen MB, Davis RE, et al. Distinct types of diffuse large B-cell lymphoma identified by gene expression profiling. Nature. 2000 Feb 3;403(6769):503–11. PMID:10676951
74. Al-Jabi M, Tolnai G, McCaughey WT. Angiofollicular lymphoid hyperplasia in an angiolipomatous mass. Arch Pathol Lab Med. 1980 Jun;104(6):313–5. PMID:6892871
75. Aljurf M, Rawas F, Alnounou R, et al. Prevalence and relative proportions of CLL and non-CLL monoclonal B-cell lymphocytosis phenotypes in the Middle Eastern population. Hematol Oncol Stem Cell Ther. 2017 Mar;10(1):42–3. PMID:27842210
76. Allday MJ. How does Epstein-Barr virus (EBV) complement the activation of Myc in the pathogenesis of Burkitt's lymphoma? Semin Cancer Biol. 2009 Dec;19(6):366–76. PMID:19635566
77. Allen RC, Armitage RJ, Conley ME, et al. CD40 ligand gene defects responsible for X-linked hyper-IgM syndrome. Science. 1993 Feb 12;259(5097):990–3. PMID:7679801
78. Ally MS, Robson A. A review of the solitary cutaneous T-cell lymphomas. J Cutan Pathol. 2014 Sep;41(9):703–14. PMID:24666254
79. Al-Mansour M, Connors JM, Gascoyne RD, et al. Transformation to aggressive lymphoma in nodular lymphocyte-predominant Hodgkin's lymphoma. J Clin Oncol. 2010 Feb 10;28(5):793–9. PMID:20048177
80. Al-Mansour Z, Nelson BP, Evens AM. Post-transplant lymphoproliferative disease (PTLD): risk factors, diagnosis, and current treatment strategies. Curr Hematol Malig Rep. 2013 Sep;8(3):173–83. PMID:23737188
81. Almire C, Bertrand P, Ruminy P, et al. PVRL2 is translocated to the TRA@ locus in t(14;19)(q11;q13)-positive peripheral T-cell lymphomas. Genes Chromosomes Cancer. 2007 Nov;46(11):1011–8. PMID:17696193
82. Alon R, Shulman Z. Chemokine triggered integrin activation and actin remodeling events guiding lymphocyte migration across vascular barriers. Exp Cell Res. 2011 Mar 10;317(5):632–41. PMID:21376176
83. Alonso-Álvarez S, Magnano L, Alcoceba M, et al. Risk of, and survival following, histological transformation in follicular lymphoma in the rituximab era. A retrospective multicentre study by the Spanish GELTAMO group. Br J Haematol. 2017 Sep;178(5):699–708. PMID:28782811
84. Alonsozana EL, Stamberg J, Kumar D, et al. Isochromosome 7q: the primary cytogenetic abnormality in hepatosplenic gammadelta T cell lymphoma. Leukemia. 1997 Aug;11(8):1367–72. PMID:9264394
85. Al-Rohil RN, Torres-Cabala CA, Patel A, et al. Loss of CD30 expression after treatment with brentuximab vedotin in a patient with anaplastic large cell lymphoma: a novel finding. J Cutan Pathol. 2016 Dec;43(12):1161–6. PMID:27531242
86. Al-Saleem T, Al-Mondhiry H. Immunoproliferative small intestinal disease (IPSID): a model for mature B-cell neoplasms. Blood. 2005 Mar 15;105(6):2274–80. PMID:15542584
87. Al-Sawaf O, Zhang C, Lu T, et al. Minimal residual disease dynamics after venetoclax-obinutuzumab treatment: extended off-treatment follow-up from the randomized CLL14 study. J Clin Oncol. 2021 Dec 20;39(36):4049–60. PMID:34709929
88. Alsharif R, Dunleavy K. Burkitt lymphoma and other high-grade B-cell lymphomas with or without MYC, BCL2, and/or BCL6 rearrangements. Hematol Oncol Clin North Am. 2019 Aug;33(4):587–96. PMID:31229156
89. Altieri A, Bermejo JL, Hemminki K. Familial aggregation of lymphoplasmacytic lymphoma with non-Hodgkin lymphoma and other neoplasms. Leukemia. 2005 Dec;19(12):2342–3. PMID:16224483
90. Al-Toma A, Goerres MS, Meijer JW, et al. Human leukocyte antigen-DQ2 homozygosity and the development of refractory celiac disease and enteropathy-associated T-cell lymphoma. Clin Gastroenterol Hepatol. 2006 Mar;4(3):315–9. PMID:16527694
91. Al-Toma A, Verbeek WH, Hadithi M, et al. Survival in refractory coeliac disease and enteropathy-associated T-cell lymphoma: retrospective evaluation of single-centre experience. Gut. 2007 Oct;56(10):1373–8. PMID:17470479
92. Al-Tourah AJ, Gill KK, Chhanabhai M, et al. Population-based analysis of incidence and outcome of transformed non-Hodgkin's lymphoma. J Clin Oncol. 2008 Nov 10;26(32):5165–9. PMID:18838711
93. Alzouebi M, Goepel JR, Horsman JM, et al. Primary thyroid lymphoma: the 40 year experience of a UK lymphoma treatment centre. Int J Oncol. 2012 Jun;40(6):2075–80. PMID:22367111
94. Amaador K, Peeters H, Minnema MC, et al. Monoclonal gammopathy of renal significance (MGRS) histopathologic classification, diagnostic workup, and therapeutic options. Neth J Med. 2019 Sep;77(7):243–54. PMID:31582582
95. Amador C, Bouska A, Wright G, et al. Gene expression signatures for the accurate diagnosis of peripheral T-cell lymphoma entities in the routine clinical practice. J Clin Oncol. 2022 Dec 20;40(36):4261–75. PMID:35839444
96. Amador C, Feldman AL, How I. How I diagnose anaplastic large cell lymphoma. Am J Clin Pathol. 2021 Mar 15;155(4):479–97. PMID:33686426
97. Amador C, Greiner TC, Heavican TB, et al. Reproducing the molecular subclassification of peripheral T-cell lymphoma-NOS by immunohistochemistry. Blood. 2019 Dec 12;134(24):2159–70. PMID:31562134
98. Amato T, Abate F, Piccaluga P, et al. Clonality analysis of immunoglobulin gene rearrangement by next-generation sequencing in endemic Burkitt lymphoma suggests antigen drive activation of BCR as opposed to sporadic Burkitt lymphoma. Am J Clin Pathol. 2016 Jan;145(1):116–27. PMID:26712879
99. Ambrogio C, Martinengo C, Voena C, et al. NPM-ALK oncogenic tyrosine kinase controls T-cell identity by transcriptional regulation and epigenetic silencing in lymphoma cells. Cancer Res. 2009 Nov 15;69(22):8611–9. PMID:19887607
100. Ambrosio MR, De Falco G, Gozzetti A, et al. Plasmablastic transformation of a pre-existing plasmacytoma: a possible role for reactivation of Epstein Barr virus infection. Haematologica. 2014 Nov;99(11):e235–7. PMID:25193957
101. Ambrosio MR, Granai M, Lo Bello G, et al. How in-depth histological look may allow challenging diagnosis: the case of a primary in situ mantle cell neoplasm of the appendix. Hematol Oncol. 2018 Feb;36(1):376–8. PMID:28393378
102. Ambrosio MR, Lazzi S, Bello GL, et al. MYC protein expression scoring and its impact on the prognosis of aggressive B-cell lymphoma patients. Haematologica. 2019 Jan;104(1):e25–8. PMID:29954940
103. Ambrosio MR, Mundo L, Gazaneo S, et al. MicroRNAs sequencing unveils distinct molecular subgroups of plasmablastic lymphoma. Oncotarget. 2017 Oct 31;8(64):107356–73. PMID:29296171
104. Ambrosio MR, Piccaluga PP, Ponzoni M, et al. The alteration of lipid metabolism in Burkitt lymphoma identifies a novel marker: adipophilin. PLoS One. 2012;7(8):e44315. PMID:22952953
105. Amen F, Horncastle D, Elderfield K, et al. Absence of cyclin-D2 and Bcl-2 expression within the germinal centre type of diffuse large B-cell lymphoma identifies a very good prognostic subgroup of patients. Histopathology. 2007 Jul;51(1):70–9. PMID:17593082
106. Amé-Thomas P, Hoeller S, Artchounin C, et al. CD10 delineates a subset of human IL-4 producing follicular helper T cells involved in the survival of follicular lymphoma B cells. Blood. 2015 Apr 9;125(15):2381–5. PMID:25733581
107. Amin MB, Edge S, Greene F, et al., editors. AJCC cancer staging manual. 8th ed. New York (NY): Springer; 2017.
108. Amiot A, Allez M, Treton X, et al. High frequency of fatal haemophagocytic lymphohistiocytosis syndrome in enteropathy-associated T cell lymphoma. Dig Liver Dis. 2012 Apr;44(4):343–9. PMID:22100722
109. Anagnostopoulos I, Hansmann ML, Franssila K, et al. European Task Force on Lymphoma project on lymphocyte predominance Hodgkin disease: histologic and immunohistologic analysis of submitted cases reveals 2 types of Hodgkin disease with a nodular growth pattern and abundant lymphocytes. Blood. 2000 Sep 1;96(5):1889–99. PMID:10961891
110. Anand P, Guillaumet-Adkins A, Dimitrova V, et al. Single-cell RNA-seq reveals developmental plasticity with coexisting oncogenic states and immune evasion programs in ETP-ALL. Blood. 2021 May 6;137(18):2463–80. PMID:33227818
111. Anavi Y, Kaplinsky C, Calderon S, et al. Head, neck, and maxillofacial childhood Burkitt's lymphoma: a retrospective analysis of 31 patients. J Oral Maxillofac Surg. 1990 Jul;48(7):708–13. PMID:2358947
112. Anbardar MH, Kumar PV, Forootan HR. Littoral cell angioma of the spleen: cytological findings and review of the literature. J Cytol. 2017 Apr-Jun;34(2):121–4. PMID:28469325
113. Anbardar MH, Soleimani N, Safavi D, et al. Multifocal EBV-associated smooth muscle tumors in a patient with cytomegalovirus infection after liver transplantation: a case report from Shiraz, Iran. Diagn Pathol. 2022 Jan 7;17(1):3. PMID:34996501
114. Andersen EF, Paxton CN, O'Malley DP, et al. Genomic analysis of follicular dendritic cell sarcoma by molecular inversion probe array reveals tumor suppressor-driven biology. Mod Pathol. 2017 Sep;30(9):1321–34. PMID:28621320
115. Anderson JR, Armitage JO, Weisenburger DD. Epidemiology of the non-Hodgkin's lymphomas: distributions of the major subtypes differ by geographic locations. Non-Hodgkin's Lymphoma Classification Project. Ann Oncol. 1998 Jul;9(7):717–20. PMID:9739436
116. Anderson MA, Tam C, Lew TE, et al. Clinicopathological features and outcomes of progression of CLL on the BCL2 inhibitor venetoclax. Blood. 2017 Jun 22;129(25):3362–70. PMID:28473407
117. Andersson AK, Ma J, Wang J, et al. The landscape of somatic mutations in infant MLL-rearranged acute lymphoblastic leukemias. Nat Genet. 2015 Apr;47(4):330–7. PMID:25730765
118. Andersson EI, Tanahashi T, Sekiguchi N, et al. High incidence of activating STAT5B mutations in CD4-positive T-cell large granular lymphocyte leukemia. Blood. 2016 Nov

17;128(20):2465–8. PMID:27697773
119. Ando M, Sato Y, Takata K, et al. A20 (TNFAIP3) deletion in Epstein-Barr virus-associated lymphoproliferative disorders/ lymphomas. PLoS One. 2013;8(2):e56741. PMID:23418597
120. Andraos T, Ayoub Z, Nastoupil L, et al. Early stage extranodal follicular lymphoma: characteristics, management, and outcomes. Clin Lymphoma Myeloma Leuk. 2019 Jun;19(6):381–9. PMID:30935940
121. Andriko JW, Kaldjian EP, Tsokos M, et al. Reticulum cell neoplasms of lymph nodes: a clinicopathologic study of 11 cases with recognition of a new subtype derived from fibroblastic reticular cells. Am J Surg Pathol. 1998 Sep;22(9):1048–58. PMID:9737236
122. Andrulis M, Penzel R, Weichert W, et al. Application of a BRAF V600E mutation-specific antibody for the diagnosis of hairy cell leukemia. Am J Surg Pathol. 2012 Dec;36(12):1796–800. PMID:22531170
123. Angel-Korman A, Stern L, Angel Y, et al. The role of kidney transplantation in monoclonal Ig deposition disease. Kidney Int Rep. 2020 Mar 9;5(4):485–93. PMID:32274452
124. Angelopoulou MK, Siakantariz MP, Vassilakopoulos TP, et al. The splenic form of mantle cell lymphoma. Eur J Haematol. 2002 Jan;68(1):12–21. PMID:11952817
125. Angelova E, Audette C, Kovtun Y, et al. CD123 expression patterns and selective targeting with a CD123-targeted antibody-drug conjugate (IMGN632) in acute lymphoblastic leukemia. Haematologica. 2019 Apr;104(4):749–55. PMID:30361418
126. Angelova EA, Medeiros LJ, Wang W, et al. Clinicopathologic and molecular features in hairy cell leukemia-variant: single institutional experience. Mod Pathol. 2018 Nov;31(11):1717–32. PMID:29955146
127. Antoniadou F, Dimitrakopoulou A, Voutsinas PM, et al. Monomorphic epitheliotropic intestinal T-cell lymphoma in pleural effusion: a case report. Diagn Cytopathol. 2017 Nov;45(11):1050–4. PMID:28681573
128. Aoki T, Izutsu K, Suzuki R, et al. Prognostic significance of pleural or pericardial effusion and the implication of optimal treatment in primary mediastinal large B-cell lymphoma: a multicenter retrospective study in Japan. Haematologica. 2014 Dec;99(12):1817–25. PMID:25216682
129. Aoki Y, Jaffe ES, Chang Y, et al. Angiogenesis and hematopoiesis induced by Kaposi's sarcoma-associated herpesvirus-encoded interleukin-6. Blood. 1999 Jun 15;93(12):4034–43. PMID:10361100
130. Aozasa K, Takakuwa T, Nakatsuka S. Pyothorax-associated lymphoma: a lymphoma developing in chronic inflammation. Adv Anat Pathol. 2005 Nov;12(6):324–31. PMID:16330929
131. Aplan PD. Chromosomal translocations involving the MLL gene: molecular mechanisms. DNA Repair (Amst). 2006 Sep 8;5(9-10):1265–72. PMID:16797254
132. Appel BE, Chen L, Buxton AB, et al. Minimal treatment of low-risk, pediatric lymphocyte-predominant Hodgkin lymphoma: a report from the Children's Oncology Group. J Clin Oncol. 2016 Jul 10;34(20):2372–9. PMID:27185849
133. Aqel N, Barker F, Patel K, et al. In-situ mantle cell lymphoma–a report of two cases. Histopathology. 2008 Jan;52(2):256–60. PMID:18184277
134. Aqil B, Merritt BY, Elghetany MT, et al. Childhood nodal marginal zone lymphoma with unusual clinicopathologic and cytogenetic features for the pediatric variant: a case report. Pediatr Dev Pathol. 2015 Mar-Apr;18(2):167–71. PMID:25625642
135. Araf S, Wang J, Korfi K, et al. Genomic profiling reveals spatial intra-tumor heterogeneity in follicular lymphoma. Leukemia. 2018 May;32(5):1261–5. PMID:29568095
136. Araujo I, Coupland SE. Primary vitreoretinal lymphoma – a review. Asia Pac J Ophthalmol (Phila). 2017 May-Jun;6(3):283–9. PMID:28558176
137. Arber DA, Snyder DS, Fine M, et al. Myeloperoxidase immunoreactivity in adult acute lymphoblastic leukemia. Am J Clin Pathol. 2001 Jul;116(1):25–33. PMID:11447748
138. Arber DA, Strickler JG, Chen YY, et al. Splenic vascular tumors: a histologic, immunophenotypic, and virologic study. Am J Surg Pathol. 1997 Jul;21(7):827–35. PMID:9236839
139. Arber DA, Weiss LM, Albújar PF, et al. Nasal lymphomas in Peru. High incidence of T-cell immunophenotype and Epstein-Barr virus infection. Am J Surg Pathol. 1993 Apr;17(4):392–9. PMID:8388175
140. Arcaini L, Besson C, Frigeni M, et al. Interferon-free antiviral treatment in B-cell lymphoproliferative disorders associated with hepatitis C virus infection. Blood. 2016 Nov 24;128(21):2527–32. PMID:27605512
141. Arcaini L, Paulli M, Burcheri S, et al. Primary nodal marginal zone B-cell lymphoma: clinical features and prognostic assessment of a rare disease. Br J Haematol. 2007 Jan;136(2):301–4. PMID:17233821
142. Arcaini L, Rossi D, Paulli M. Splenic marginal zone lymphoma: from genetics to management. Blood. 2016 Apr 28;127(17):2072–81. PMID:26989207
143. Arcaini L, Zibellini S, Boveri E, et al. The BRAF V600E mutation in hairy cell leukemia and other mature B-cell neoplasms. Blood. 2012 Jan 5;119(1):188–91. PMID:22072557
144. Ardeshna KM, Qian W, Smith P, et al. Rituximab versus a watch-and-wait approach in patients with advanced-stage, asymptomatic, non-bulky follicular lymphoma: an open-label randomised phase 3 trial. Lancet Oncol. 2014 Apr;15(4):424–35. PMID:24602760
145. Ardeshna KM, Smith P, Norton A, et al. Long-term effect of a watch and wait policy versus immediate systemic treatment for asymptomatic advanced-stage non-Hodgkin lymphoma: a randomised controlled trial. Lancet. 2003 Aug 16;362(9383):516–22. PMID:12932382
146. Arenas DJ, Floess K, Kobrin D, et al. Increased mTOR activation in idiopathic multicentric Castleman disease. Blood. 2020 May 7;135(19):1673–84. PMID:32206779
147. Arisue N, Chagaluka G, Palacpac NMQ, et al. Assessment of mixed Plasmodium falciparum sera5 infection in endemic Burkitt lymphoma: a case-control study in Malawi. Cancers (Basel). 2021 Apr 2;13(7):1692. PMID:33918470
148. Armand M, Costopoulos M, Osman J, et al. Optimization of CSF biological investigations for CNS lymphoma diagnosis. Am J Hematol. 2019 Oct;94(10):1123–31. PMID:31328307
149. Arnulf B, Copie-Bergman C, Delfau-Larue MH, et al. Nonhepatosplenic gammadelta T-cell lymphoma: a subset of cytotoxic lymphomas with mucosal or skin localization. Blood. 1998 Mar 1;91(5):1723–31. PMID:9473239
150. Arons E, Adams S, Venzon DJ, et al. Class II human leucocyte antigen DRB1*11 in hairy cell leukaemia patients with and without haemolytic uraemic syndrome. Br J Haematol. 2014 Sep;166(5):729–38. PMID:24931452
151. Arons E, Kreitman RJ. Molecular variant of hairy cell leukemia with poor prognosis. Leuk Lymphoma. 2011 Jun;52 Suppl 2(Suppl 2):99–102. PMID:21599610
152. Arons E, Suntum T, Stetler-Stevenson M, et al. VH4-34+ hairy cell leukemia, a new variant with poor prognosis despite standard therapy. Blood. 2009 Nov 19;114(21):4687–95. PMID:19745070
153. Arthur SE, Jiang A, Grande BM, et al. Genome-wide discovery of somatic regulatory variants in diffuse large B-cell lymphoma. Nat Commun. 2018 Oct 1;9(1):4001. PMID:30275490
154. Aruffo A, Farrington M, Hollenbaugh D, et al. The CD40 ligand, gp39, is defective in activated T cells from patients with X-linked hyper-IgM syndrome. Cell. 1993 Jan 29;72(2):291–300. PMID:7678782
155. Arzoo KK, Bu X, Espina BM, et al. T-cell lymphoma in HIV-infected patients. J Acquir Immune Defic Syndr. 2004 Aug 15;36(5):1020–7. PMID:15247554
156. Asada H. Hypersensitivity to mosquito bites: a unique pathogenic mechanism linking Epstein-Barr virus infection, allergy and oncogenesis. J Dermatol Sci. 2007 Mar;45(3):153–60. PMID:17169531
157. Asada H, Saito-Katsuragi M, Niizeki H, et al. Mosquito salivary gland extracts induce EBV-infected NK cell oncogenesis via CD4 T cells in patients with hypersensitivity to mosquito bites. J Invest Dermatol. 2005 Nov;125(5):956–61. PMID:16297196
158. Asano J, Watanabe T, Oguchi T, et al. Association between immunoglobulin G4-related disease and malignancy within 12 years after diagnosis: an analysis after longterm followup. J Rheumatol. 2015 Nov;42(11):2135–42. PMID:26472416
159. Asano N, Oshiro A, Matsuo K, et al. Prognostic significance of T-cell or cytotoxic molecules phenotype in classical Hodgkin's lymphoma: a clinicopathologic study. J Clin Oncol. 2006 Oct 1;24(28):4626–33. PMID:16954517
160. Asano N, Suzuki R, Kagami Y, et al. Clinicopathologic and prognostic significance of cytotoxic molecule expression in nodal peripheral T-cell lymphoma, unspecified. Am J Surg Pathol. 2005 Oct;29(10):1284–93. PMID:16160469
161. Asano N, Yamamoto K, Tamaru J, et al. Age-related Epstein-Barr virus (EBV)-associated B-cell lymphoproliferative disorders: comparison with EBV-positive classic Hodgkin lymphoma in elderly patients. Blood. 2009 Mar 19;113(12):2629–36. PMID:19075188
162. Ashraf M, Boyd CB, Beresford WA. Ectopic decidual cell reaction in para-aortic and pelvic lymph nodes in the presence of cervical squamous cell carcinoma during pregnancy. J Surg Oncol. 1984 May;26(1):6–8. PMID:6727387
163. Ashrafi F, Shahidi S, Ebrahimi Z, et al. Outcome of rapamycin therapy for post-transplant-lymphoproliferative disorder after kidney transplantation: case series. Int J Hematol Oncol Stem Cell Res. 2015 Jan 1;9(1):26–32. PMID:25802698
164. Ashton-Key M, Diss TC, Pan L, et al. Molecular analysis of T-cell clonality in ulcerative jejunitis and enteropathy-associated T-cell lymphoma. Am J Pathol. 1997 Aug;151(2):493–8. PMID:9250161
165. Assaf C, Hummel M, Steinhoff M, et al. Early TCR-beta and TCR-gamma PCR detection of T-cell clonality indicates minimal tumor disease in lymph nodes of cutaneous T-cell lymphoma: diagnostic and prognostic implications. Blood. 2005 Jan 15;105(2):503–10. PMID:15459015
166. Atallah-Yunes SA, Murphy DJ, Noy A. HIV-associated Burkitt lymphoma. Lancet Haematol. 2020 Aug;7(8):e594–600. PMID:32735838
167. Atra A, Meller ST, Stevens RS, et al. Conservative management of follicular non-Hodgkin's lymphoma in childhood. Br J Haematol. 1998 Oct;103(1):220–3. PMID:9792312
168. Atsaves V, Tsesmetzis N, Chioureas D, et al. PD-L1 is commonly expressed and transcriptionally regulated by STAT3 and MYC in ALK-negative anaplastic large-cell lymphoma. Leukemia. 2017 Jul;31(7):1633–7. PMID:28344319
169. Attarbaschi A, Abla O, Arias Padilla L, et al. Rare non-Hodgkin lymphoma of childhood and adolescence: a consensus diagnostic and therapeutic approach to pediatric-type follicular lymphoma, marginal zone lymphoma, and nonanaplastic peripheral T-cell lymphoma. Pediatr Blood Cancer. 2020 Aug;67(8):e28416. PMID:32452165
170. Attarbaschi A, Beishuizen A, Mann G, et al. Children and adolescents with follicular lymphoma have an excellent prognosis with either limited chemotherapy or with a "Watch and wait" strategy after complete resection. Ann Hematol. 2013 Nov;92(11):1537–41. PMID:23665980
171. Attarbaschi A, Mann G, Strehl S, et al. Deletion of 11q23 is a highly specific nonrandom secondary genetic abnormality of ETV6/RUNX1-rearranged childhood acute lymphoblastic leukemia. Leukemia. 2007 Mar;21(3):584–6. PMID:17215856
172. Attard AA, Praveen P, Dunn PJ, et al. Epstein-Barr virus-positive mucocutaneous ulcer of the oral cavity: the importance of having a detailed clinical history to reach a correct diagnosis. Oral Surg Oral Med Oral Pathol Oral Radiol. 2012 Aug;114(2):e37–9. PMID:22769419
173. Attygalle A, Al-Jehani R, Diss TC, et al. Neoplastic T cells in angioimmunoblastic T-cell lymphoma express CD10. Blood. 2002 Jan 15;99(2):627–33. PMID:11781247
174. Attygalle AD, Cabeçadas J, Gaulard P, et al. Peripheral T-cell and NK-cell lymphomas and their mimics; taking a step forward - report on the lymphoma workshop of the XVIth meeting of the European Association for Haematopathology and the Society for Hematopathology. Histopathology. 2014 Jan;64(2):171–99. PMID:24128129
175. Attygalle AD, Chuang SS, Diss TC, et al. Distinguishing angioimmunoblastic T-cell lymphoma from peripheral T-cell lymphoma, unspecified, using morphology, immunophenotype and molecular genetics. Histopathology. 2007 Mar;50(4):498–508. PMID:17448026
176. Attygalle AD, Diss TC, Munson P, et al. CD10 expression in extranodal dissemination of angioimmunoblastic T-cell lymphoma. Am J Surg Pathol. 2004 Jan;28(1):54–61. PMID:14707864
177. Attygalle AD, Dobson R, Chak PK, et al. Parallel evolution of two distinct lymphoid proliferations in clonal haematopoiesis. Histopathology. 2022 Apr;80(5):847–58. PMID:35064935
178. Attygalle AD, Feldman AL, Dogan A. ITK/SYK translocation in angioimmunoblastic T-cell lymphoma. Am J Surg Pathol. 2013 Sep;37(9):1456–7. PMID:24076779
179. Attygalle AD, Kyriakou C, Dupuis J, et al. Histologic evolution of angioimmunoblastic T-cell lymphoma in consecutive biopsies: clinical correlation and insights into natural history and disease progression. Am J Surg Pathol. 2007 Jul;31(7):1077–88. PMID:17592275
180. Attygalle AD, Liu H, Shirali S, et al. Atypical marginal zone hyperplasia of mucosa-associated lymphoid tissue: a reactive condition of childhood showing immunoglobulin lambda light-chain restriction. Blood. 2004 Nov 15;104(10):3343–8. PMID:15256428
181. Au WY, Ma SY, Chim CS, et al. Clinicopathologic features and treatment outcome of mature T-cell and natural killer-cell lymphomas diagnosed according to the World Health Organization classification scheme: a single

center experience of 10 years. Ann Oncol. 2005 Feb;16(2):206–14. PMID:15668271
182. Au WY, Pang A, Choy C, et al. Quantification of circulating Epstein-Barr virus (EBV) DNA in the diagnosis and monitoring of natural killer cell and EBV-positive lymphomas in immunocompetent patients. Blood. 2004 Jul 1;104(1):243–9. PMID:15031209
183. Au WY, Weisenburger DD, Intragumtornchai T, et al. Clinical differences between nasal and extranasal natural killer/T-cell lymphoma: a study of 136 cases from the International Peripheral T-Cell Lymphoma Project. Blood. 2009 Apr 23;113(17):3931–7. PMID:19029440
184. Audouin J, Diebold J, Pallesen G. Frequent expression of Epstein-Barr virus latent membrane protein-1 in tumour cells of Hodgkin's disease in HIV-positive patients. J Pathol. 1992 Aug;167(4):381–4. PMID:1328576
185. Audouin J, Le Tourneau A, Molina T, et al. Patterns of bone marrow involvement in 58 patients presenting primary splenic marginal zone lymphoma with or without circulating villous lymphocytes. Br J Haematol. 2003 Aug;122(3):404–12. PMID:12877667
186. Auer F, Rüschendorf F, Gombert M, et al. Inherited susceptibility to pre B-ALL caused by germline transmission of PAX5 c.547G>A. Leukemia. 2014 May;28(5):1136–8. PMID:24287434
187. Aukema SM, Croci GA, Bens S, et al. Mantle cell lymphomas with concomitant MYC and CCND1 breakpoints are recurrently TdT positive and frequently show high-grade pathological and genetic features. Virchows Arch. 2021 Jul;479(1):133–45. PMID:33528622
188. Aukema SM, Hoster E, Rosenwald A, et al. Expression of TP53 is associated with the outcome of MCL independent of MIPI and Ki-67 in trials of the European MCL Network. Blood. 2018 Jan 25;131(4):417–20. PMID:29196411
189. Aukema SM, Kreuz M, Kohler CW, et al. Biological characterization of adult MYC-translocation-positive mature B-cell lymphomas other than molecular Burkitt lymphoma. Haematologica. 2014 Apr;99(4):726–35. PMID:24179151
190. Aukema SM, Siebert R, Schuuring E, et al. Double-hit B-cell lymphomas. Blood. 2011 Feb 24;117(8):2319–31. PMID:21119107
191. Aussedat G, Traverse-Glehen A, Stamatoullas A, et al. Composite and sequential lymphoma between classical Hodgkin lymphoma and primary mediastinal lymphoma/diffuse large B-cell lymphoma, a clinico-pathological series of 25 cases. Br J Haematol. 2020 Apr;189(2):244–56. PMID:32030731
192. Austin RM, Birdsong GG, Sidawy MK, et al. Fine needle aspiration is a feasible and accurate technique in the diagnosis of lymphoma. J Clin Oncol. 2005 Dec 10;23(35):9029–30. PMID:16339755
193. Au-Yeung RKH, Arias Padilla L, Zimmermann M, et al. Experience with provisional WHO-entities large B-cell lymphoma with IRF4-rearrangement and Burkitt-like lymphoma with 11q aberration in paediatric patients of the NHL-BFM group. Br J Haematol. 2020 Sep;190(5):753–63. PMID:32239695
194. Avet-Louseau H, Daviet A, Sauner S, et al. Chromosome 13 abnormalities in multiple myeloma are mostly monosomy 13. Br J Haematol. 2000 Dec;111(4):1116–7. PMID:11227093
195. Avitan-Hersh E, Stepensky P, Zaidman I, et al. Primary cutaneous clonal CD8+ T-cell lymphoproliferative disorder associated with immunodeficiency due to RAG1 mutation. Am J Dermatopathol. 2020 Jan;42(1):e11–5. PMID:31313695
196. Babbe H, Chester N, Leder P, et al. The Bloom's syndrome helicase is critical for development and function of the alpha-beta T-cell lineage. Mol Cell Biol. 2007 Mar;27(5):1947–59. PMID:17210642
197. Babbe H, McMenamin J, Hobeika E, et al. Genomic instability resulting from Blm deficiency compromises development, maintenance, and function of the B cell lineage. J Immunol. 2009 Jan 1;182(1):347–60. PMID:19109166
198. Baccarani M, Castagnetti F, Gugliotta G, et al. The proportion of different BCR-ABL1 transcript types in chronic myeloid leukemia. An international overview. Leukemia. 2019 May;33(5):1173–83. PMID:30675008
199. Baccarani M, Iacobucci I, Chiaretti S, et al. In Ph+BCR-ABL1P210+ acute lymphoblastic leukemia the e13a2 (B2A2) transcript is prevalent. Leukemia. 2020 Mar;34(3):929–31. PMID:31595038
200. Bacha D, Chelly B, Kilani H, et al. HHV8/EBV coinfection lymphoproliferative disorder: rare entity with a favorable outcome. Case Rep Hematol. 2017;2017:1578429. PMID:28280640
201. Bachy E, Maurer MJ, Habermann TM, et al. A simplified scoring system in de novo follicular lymphoma treated initially with immunochemotherapy. Blood. 2018 Jul 5;132(1):49–58. PMID:29666118
202. Bachy E, Seymour JF, Feugier P, et al. Sustained progression-free survival benefit of rituximab maintenance in patients with follicular lymphoma: long-term results of the PRIMA study. J Clin Oncol. 2019 Nov 1;37(31):2815–24. PMID:31339826
203. Bacon CM, Diss TC, Ye H, et al. Follicular lymphoma of the thyroid gland. Am J Surg Pathol. 2009 Jan;33(1):22–34. PMID:18830125
204. Bacon CM, Miller RF, Noursadeghi M, et al. Pathology of bone marrow in human herpes virus-8 (HHV8)-associated multicentric Castleman disease. Br J Haematol. 2004 Dec;127(5):585–91. PMID:15566362
205. Bacon CM, Ye H, Diss TC, et al. Primary follicular lymphoma of the testis and epididymis in adults. Am J Surg Pathol. 2007 Jul;31(7):1050–8. PMID:17592272
206. Baecklund E, Smedby KE, Sutton LA, et al. Lymphoma development in patients with autoimmune and inflammatory disorders–What are the driving forces? Semin Cancer Biol. 2014 Feb;24:61–70. PMID:24333759
207. Baens M, Finalet Ferreiro J, Tousseyn T, et al. t(X;14)(p11.4;q32.33) is recurrent in marginal zone lymphoma and up-regulates GPR34. Haematologica. 2012 Feb;97(2):184–8. PMID:22058210
208. Baer C, Kimura S, Rana MS, et al. CCL22 mutations drive natural killer cell lymphoproliferative disease by deregulating microenvironmental crosstalk. Nat Genet. 2022 May;54(5):637–48. PMID:35513723
209. Bagdi E, Diss TC, Munson P, et al. Mucosal intra-epithelial lymphocytes in enteropathy-associated T-cell lymphoma, ulcerative jejunitis, and refractory celiac disease constitute a neoplastic population. Blood. 1999 Jul 1;94(1):260–4. PMID:10381521
210. Bagherani N, Smoller BR. An overview of cutaneous T cell lymphomas. F1000Res. 2016 Jul 28;5:F1000 Faculty Rev-1882. PMID:27540476
211. Bagwan IN, Knee G, Abboudi Z, et al. Small intestinal presentation of nodular lymphocyte-predominant Hodgkin lymphoma with T cell/histiocyte-rich B cell lymphoma-like areas-with review of literature on extranodal presentation of this disease. J Hematop. 2010 Mar 24;3(1):29–34. PMID:21436871
212. Bai DY, Xie JL, Zheng YY, et al. [Paediatric nodal marginal zone lymphoma: a clinicopathological study of seven cases]. Zhonghua Bing Li Xue Za Zhi. 2019 May 8;48(5):369–72. Chinese. PMID:31104676
213. Bai RY, Dieter P, Peschel C, et al. Nucleophosmin-anaplastic lymphoma kinase of large-cell anaplastic lymphoma is a constitutively active tyrosine kinase that utilizes phospholipase C-gamma to mediate its mitogenicity. Mol Cell Biol. 1998 Dec;18(12):6951–61. PMID:9819383
214. Bai RY, Ouyang T, Miething C, et al. Nucleophosmin-anaplastic lymphoma kinase associated with anaplastic large-cell lymphoma activates the phosphatidylinositol 3-kinase/Akt antiapoptotic signaling pathway. Blood. 2000 Dec 15;96(13):4319–27. PMID:11110708
215. Bakhirev AG, Vasef MA, Zhang QY, et al. Fluorescence immunophenotyping and interphase cytogenetics (FICTION) detects BCL6 abnormalities, including gene amplification, in most cases of nodular lymphocyte-predominant Hodgkin lymphoma. Arch Pathol Lab Med. 2014 Apr;138(4):538–42. PMID:24678684
216. Bakr F, Wain EM, Barlow R, et al. Primary cutaneous CD4+ small/medium T-cell lymphoproliferative disorder or primary cutaneous marginal zone B-cell lymphoma? Two distinct entities with overlapping histopathological features. Am J Dermatopathol. 2021 Dec 1;43(12):e204–12. PMID:34231494
217. Bakr F, Wain EM, Wong S, et al. Prominent blasts in primary cutaneous CD4+ small/medium T-cell lymphoproliferative disorder. A reconsideration of diagnostic criteria. Am J Dermatopathol. 2021 Dec 1;43(12):e190–6. PMID:33989212
218. Balatzenko G, Guenova M, Kalinova I, et al. Simultaneous occurrence of ETV6-RUNX1 and BCR-ABL1 (e1a2) transcripts in a child with B-cell acute lymphoblastic leukemia. Cancer Genet. 2013 Mar;206(3):97–101. PMID:23491079
219. Baldassano MF, Bailey EM, Ferry JA, et al. Cutaneous lymphoid hyperplasia and cutaneous marginal zone lymphoma: comparison of morphologic and immunophenotypic features. Am J Surg Pathol. 1999 Jan;23(1):88–96. PMID:9888708
220. Baliakas P, Agathangelidis A, Hadzidimitriou A, et al. Not all IGHV3-21 chronic lymphocytic leukemias are equal: prognostic considerations. Blood. 2015 Jan 29;125(5):856–9. PMID:25634617
221. Baliakas P, Jeromin S, Iskas M, et al. Cytogenetic complexity in chronic lymphocytic leukemia: definitions, associations, and clinical impact. Blood. 2019 Mar 14;133(11):1205–16. PMID:30602617
222. Baliakas P, Kanellis G, Stavroyianni N, et al. The role of bone marrow biopsy examination at diagnosis of chronic lymphocytic leukemia: a reappraisal. Leuk Lymphoma. 2013 Nov;54(11):2377–84. PMID:23485170
223. Ball MK, Morris JM, Wood AJ, et al. Ventricle-predominant primary CNS lymphomas: clinical, radiological and pathological evaluation of five cases and review of the literature. Brain Tumor Pathol. 2020 Jan;37(1):22–30. PMID:31630277
224. Ballas LK, Metzger ML, Milgrom SA, et al. Nodular lymphocyte predominant Hodgkin lymphoma: executive summary of the American Radium Society appropriate use criteria. Leuk Lymphoma. 2021 May;62(5):1057–65. PMID:33274673
225. Ballester B, Ramuz O, Gisselbrecht C, et al. Gene expression profiling identifies molecular subgroups among nodal peripheral T-cell lymphomas. Oncogene. 2006 Mar 9;25(10):1560–70. PMID:16288225
226. Ballon G, Chen K, Perez R, et al. Kaposi sarcoma herpesvirus (KSHV) vFLIP oncoprotein induces B cell transdifferentiation and tumorigenesis in mice. J Clin Invest. 2011 Mar;121(3):1141–53. PMID:21339646
227. Baloda V, Wheeler SE, Murray DL, et al. Mu heavy chain disease with MYD88 L265P mutation: an unusual manifestation of lymphoplasmacytic lymphoma. Diagn Pathol. 2022 Aug 5;17(1):63. PMID:35932039
228. Bangham CR. CTL quality and the control of human retroviral infections. Eur J Immunol. 2009 Jul;39(7):1700–12. PMID:19582737
229. Bangham CRM, Matsuoka M. Human T-cell leukaemia virus type 1: parasitism and pathogenesis. Philos Trans R Soc Lond B Biol Sci. 2017 Oct 19;372(1732):372. PMID:28893939
230. Banin S, Moyal L, Shieh S, et al. Enhanced phosphorylation of p53 by ATM in response to DNA damage. Science. 1998 Sep 11;281(5383):1674–7. PMID:9733514
231. Banks PM, Chan J, Cleary ML, et al. Mantle cell lymphoma. A proposal for unification of morphologic, immunologic, and molecular data. Am J Surg Pathol. 1992 Jul;16(7):637–40. PMID:1530105
232. Bannard O, Horton RM, Allen CD, et al. Germinal center centroblasts transition to a centrocyte phenotype according to a timed program and depend on the dark zone for effective selection. Immunity. 2013 Nov 14;39(5):912–24. PMID:24184055
233. Banthia V, Jen A, Kacker A. Sporadic Burkitt's lymphoma of the head and neck in the pediatric population. Int J Pediatr Otorhinolaryngol. 2003 Jan;67(1):59–65. PMID:12560151
234. Barasch NJK, Liu YC, Ho J, et al. The molecular landscape and other distinctive features of primary cutaneous follicle center lymphoma. Hum Pathol. 2020 Dec;106:93–105. PMID:33045225
235. Barbashina V, Heller DS, Hameed M, et al. Splenic smooth-muscle tumors in children with acquired immunodeficiency syndrome: report of two cases of this unusual location with evidence of an association with Epstein-Barr virus. Virchows Arch. 2000 Feb;436(2):138–9. PMID:10755604
236. Barbat B, Jhaj R, Khurram D. Fatality in Kikuchi-Fujimoto disease: a rare phenomenon. World J Clin Cases. 2017 Feb 16;5(2):35–9. PMID:28255545
237. Barbé E, de Boer M, de Jong D. A practical cytological approach to the diagnosis of breast-implant associated anaplastic large cell lymphoma. Cytopathology. 2019 Jul;30(4):363–9. PMID:30628128
238. Barber KE, Harrison CJ, Broadfield ZJ, et al. Molecular cytogenetic characterization of TCF3 (E2A)/19p13.3 rearrangements in B-cell precursor acute lymphoblastic leukemia. Genes Chromosomes Cancer. 2007 May;46(5):478–86. PMID:17311319
239. Barber NA, Loberiza FR Jr, Perry AM, et al. Does functional imaging distinguish nodular lymphocyte-predominant Hodgkin lymphoma from T-cell/histiocyte-rich large B-cell lymphoma? Clin Lymphoma Myeloma Leuk. 2013 Aug;13(4):392–7. PMID:23773450
240. Bareau B, Rey J, Hamidou M, et al. Analysis of a French cohort of patients with large granular lymphocyte leukemia: a report on 229 cases. Haematologica. 2010 Sep;95(9):1534–41. PMID:20378561
241. Barete S, Mouawad R, Choquet S, et al. Skin manifestations and vascular endothelial growth factor levels in POEMS syndrome: impact of autologous hematopoietic stem cell transplantation. Arch Dermatol. 2010 Jun;146(6):615–23. PMID:20566924
242. Barilà G, Teramo A, Calabretto G, et al. STAT3 mutations impact on overall survival in large granular lymphocyte leukemia: a single-center experience of 205 patients. Leukemia. 2020 Apr;34(4):1116–24.

PMID:31740810
243. Barp A, Fedrigo M, Farina FM, et al. Carotid aneurism with acute dissection: an unusual case of IgG4-related diseases. Cardiovasc Pathol. 2016 Jan-Feb;25(1):59–62. PMID:26453089
244. Barraclough A, Bishton M, Cheah CY, et al. The diagnostic and therapeutic challenges of Grade 3B follicular lymphoma. Br J Haematol. 2021 Oct;195(1):15–24. PMID:33704790
245. Barrans S, Crouch S, Smith A, et al. Rearrangement of MYC is associated with poor prognosis in patients with diffuse large B-cell lymphoma treated in the era of rituximab. J Clin Oncol. 2010 Jul 10;28(20):3360–5. PMID:20498406
246. Barrans SL, Crouch S, Care MA, et al. Whole genome expression profiling based on paraffin embedded tissue can be used to classify diffuse large B-cell lymphoma and predict clinical outcome. Br J Haematol. 2012 Nov;159(4):441–53. PMID:22970711
247. Barrans SL, Fenton JA, Banham A, et al. Strong expression of FOXP1 identifies a distinct subset of diffuse large B-cell lymphoma (DLBCL) patients with poor outcome. Blood. 2004 Nov 1;104(9):2933–5. PMID:15238418
248. Barrena S, Almeida J, Del Carmen Garcia-Macias M, et al. Flow cytometry immunophenotyping of fine-needle aspiration specimens: utility in the diagnosis and classification of non-Hodgkin lymphomas. Histopathology. 2011 May;58(6):906–18. PMID:21438908
249. Barrio S, Shanafelt TD, Ojha J, et al. Genomic characterization of high-count MBL cases indicates that early detection of driver mutations and subclonal expansion are predictors of adverse clinical outcome. Leukemia. 2017 Jan;31(1):170–6. PMID:27469216
250. Barrionuevo C, Anderson VM, Zevallos-Giampietri E, et al. Hydroa-like cutaneous T-cell lymphoma: a clinicopathologic and molecular genetic study of 16 pediatric cases from Peru. Appl Immunohistochem Mol Morphol. 2002 Mar;10(1):7–14. PMID:11893040
251. Barrionuevo C, Zaharia M, Martinez MT, et al. Extranodal NK/T-cell lymphoma, nasal type: study of clinicopathologic and prognosis factors in a series of 78 cases from Peru. Appl Immunohistochem Mol Morphol. 2007 Mar;15(1):38–44. PMID:17536305
252. Barry TS, Jaffe ES, Sorbara L, et al. Peripheral T-cell lymphomas expressing CD30 and CD15. Am J Surg Pathol. 2003 Dec;27(12):1513–22. PMID:14657710
253. Barta SK, Samuel MS, Xue X, et al. Changes in the influence of lymphoma- and HIV-specific factors on outcomes in AIDS-related non-Hodgkin lymphoma. Ann Oncol. 2015 May;26(5):958–66. PMID:25632071
254. Barth TF, Müller S, Pawlita M, et al. Homogeneous immunophenotype and paucity of secondary genomic aberrations are distinctive features of endemic but not of sporadic Burkitt's lymphoma and diffuse large B-cell lymphoma with MYC rearrangement. J Pathol. 2004 Aug;203(4):940–5. PMID:15258997
255. Bartl R, Frisch B, Fateh-Moghadam A, et al. Histologic classification and staging of multiple myeloma. A retrospective and prospective study of 674 cases. Am J Clin Pathol. 1987 Mar;87(3):342–55. PMID:3825999
256. Bartlett NL, Wilson WH, Jung SH, et al. Dose-adjusted EPOCH-R compared with R-CHOP as frontline therapy for diffuse large B-cell lymphoma: clinical outcomes of the phase III intergroup trial Alliance/CALGB 50303. J Clin Oncol. 2019 Jul 20;37(21):1790–9. PMID:30939090
257. Baruchel A, Cayuela JM, Ballerini P, et al. The majority of myeloid-antigen-positive (My+) childhood B-cell precursor acute lymphoblastic leukaemias express TEL-AML1 fusion transcripts. Br J Haematol. 1997 Oct;99(1):101–6. PMID:9359509
258. Barwick BG, Neri P, Bahlis NJ, et al. Multiple myeloma immunoglobulin lambda translocations portend poor prognosis. Nat Commun. 2019 Apr 23;10(1):1911. PMID:31015454
259. Barzenje DA, Kolstad A, Ghanima W, et al. Long-term outcome of patients with solitary plasmacytoma treated with radiotherapy: a population-based, single-center study with median follow-up of 13.7 years. Hematol Oncol. 2018 Feb;36(1):217–23. PMID:28393375
260. Baseggio L, Traverse-Glehen A, Petinataud F, et al. CD5 expression identifies a subset of splenic marginal zone lymphomas with higher lymphocytosis: a clinico-pathological, cytogenetic and molecular study of 24 cases. Haematologica. 2010 Apr;95(4):604–12. PMID:20015887
261. Basha BM, Bryant SC, Rech KL, et al. Application of a 5 marker panel to the routine diagnosis of peripheral T-cell lymphoma with T-follicular helper phenotype. Am J Surg Pathol. 2019 Sep;43(9):1282–90. PMID:31283630
262. Bassarova A, Trøen G, Spetalen S, et al. Lymphoplasmacytic lymphoma and marginal zone lymphoma in the bone marrow: paratrabecular involvement as an important distinguishing feature. Am J Clin Pathol. 2015 Jun;143(6):797–806. PMID:25972321
263. Bassig BA, Au WY, Mang O, et al. Subtype-specific incidence rates of lymphoid malignancies in Hong Kong compared to the United States, 2001-2010. Cancer Epidemiol. 2016 Jun;42:15–23. PMID:26991956
264. Basso K. Biology of germinal center B cells relating to lymphomagenesis. Hemasphere. 2021 Jun 1;5(6):e582. PMID:34095765
265. Basso K, Dalla-Favera R. Germinal centres and B cell lymphomagenesis. Nat Rev Immunol. 2015 Mar;15(3):172–84. PMID:25712152
266. Basso K, Liso A, Tiacci E, et al. Gene expression profiling of hairy cell leukemia reveals a phenotype related to memory B cells with altered expression of chemokine and adhesion receptors. J Exp Med. 2004 Jan 5;199(1):59–68. PMID:14707115
267. Bastidas Torres AN, Cats D, Out-Luiting JJ, et al. Deregulation of JAK2 signaling underlies primary cutaneous CD8+ aggressive epidermotropic cytotoxic T-cell lymphoma. Haematologica. 2022 Mar 1;107(3):702–14. PMID:33792220
268. Bastidas Torres AN, Melchers RC, Van Grieken L, et al. Whole-genome profiling of primary cutaneous anaplastic large cell lymphoma. Haematologica. 2022 Jul 1;107(7):1619–32. PMID:34382383
269. Bata BM, Pulido JS, Patel SV, et al. Combined intraocular and systemic rituximab for ocular lymphoproliferative disorder with extranodal marginal zone lymphoma-type morphology after heart transplant. J AAPOS. 2018 Apr;22(2):159–61. PMID:29408337
270. Bataille R, Jégo G, Robillard N, et al. The phenotype of normal, reactive and malignant plasma cells. Identification of "many and multiple myelomas" and of new targets for myeloma therapy. Haematologica. 2006 Sep;91(9):1234–40. PMID:16956823
271. Bateman AC, Ashton-Key MR, Jogai S. Lymph node granulomas in immunoglobulin G4-related disease. Histopathology. 2015 Oct;67(4):557–61. PMID:25620085
272. Bates WD, Gray DW, Dada MA, et al. Lymphoproliferative disorders in Oxford renal transplant recipients. J Clin Pathol. 2003 Jun;56(6):439–46. PMID:12783971
273. Batista DA, Vonderheid EC, Hawkins A, et al. Multicolor fluorescence in situ hybridization (SKY) in mycosis fungoides and Sézary syndrome: search for recurrent chromosome abnormalities. Genes Chromosomes Cancer. 2006 Apr;45(4):383–91. PMID:16382449
274. Batlevi CL, Sha F, Alperovich A, et al. Follicular lymphoma in the modern era: survival, treatment outcomes, and identification of high-risk subgroups. Blood Cancer J. 2020 Jul 17;10(7):74. PMID:32678074
275. Battesti G, Ram-Wolff C, Dobos G, et al. Granulomatous slack skin: clinical retrospective study of 8 cases of the Cutaneous Lymphoma French Study Group. Eur J Cancer. 2021 Oct;156 Suppl 1:S35–6. PMID:34649654
276. Battistella M, Beylot-Barry M, Bachelez H, et al. Primary cutaneous follicular helper T-cell lymphoma: a new subtype of cutaneous T-cell lymphoma reported in a series of 5 cases. Arch Dermatol. 2012 Jul;148(7):832–9. PMID:22508770
277. Batton E, Alali M, Hageman JR, et al. Kikuchi-Fujimoto disease in children: an important diagnostic consideration for cervical lymphadenitis. Pediatr Ann. 2019 Oct 1;48(10):e406–11. PMID:31610000
278. Bauer M, Jasinski-Bergner S, Mandelboim O, et al. Epstein-Barr virus-associated malignancies and immune escape: the role of the tumor microenvironment and tumor cell evasion strategies. Cancers (Basel). 2021 Oct 16;13(20):5189. PMID:34680337
279. Baugh L, Brown N, Song JY, et al. Fibrin-associated, EBV-negative diffuse large B-cell lymphoma arising in atrial myxoma: expanding the spectrum of the entity. Int J Surg Pathol. 2022 Feb;30(1):39–45. PMID:33913371
280. Baum CL, Link BK, Neppalli VT, et al. Reappraisal of the provisional entity primary cutaneous CD4+ small/medium pleomorphic T-cell lymphoma: a series of 10 adult and pediatric patients and review of the literature. J Am Acad Dermatol. 2011 Oct;65(4):739–48. PMID:21641676
280A. Bautista-Quach MA, Nademanee A, Weisenburger DD, et al. Implant-associated primary anaplastic large-cell lymphoma with simultaneous involvement of bilateral breast capsules. Clin Breast Cancer. 2013 Dec;13(6):492–5. PMID:24267734
281. Beà S, Amador V. Role of SOX11 and genetic events cooperating with cyclin D1 in mantle cell lymphoma. Curr Oncol Rep. 2017 Jun;19(6):43. PMID:28466437
282. Beà S, Salaverria I, Armengol L, et al. Uniparental disomies, homozygous deletions, amplifications, and target genes in mantle cell lymphoma revealed by integrative high-resolution whole-genome profiling. Blood. 2009 Mar 26;113(13):3059–69. PMID:18984860
283. Beaty MW, Toro J, Sorbara L, et al. Cutaneous lymphomatoid granulomatosis: correlation of clinical and biologic features. Am J Surg Pathol. 2001 Sep;25(9):1111–20. PMID:11688570
284. Beaufils C, Fernandez I, Marchitto L, et al. Multicentric Castleman disease revealing complete signal transducer and activator of transcription 1 deficiency treated by JAK1/2 inhibition. J Allergy Clin Immunol Pract. 2021 Oct;9(10):3838–3840.e1. PMID:34217848
285. Beck JT, Hsu SM, Wijdenes J, et al. Brief report: alleviation of systemic manifestations of Castleman's disease by monoclonal anti-interleukin-6 antibody. N Engl J Med. 1994 Mar 3;330(9):602–5. PMID:8302342
286. Beckham TH, Yang JC, Chau KW, et al. Excellent outcomes with surgery or radiotherapy in the management of Castleman disease including a case of oligocentric disease. Clin Lymphoma Myeloma Leuk. 2020 Oct;20(10):685–9. PMID:32522439
287. Beekman R, Amador V, Campo E. SOX11, a key oncogenic factor in mantle cell lymphoma. Curr Opin Hematol. 2018 Jul;25(4):299–306. PMID:29738333
288. Behdad A, Griffin B, Chen YH, et al. PD-1 is highly expressed by neoplastic B-cells in Richter transformation. Br J Haematol. 2019 Apr;185(2):370–3. PMID:30028010
289. Behrens YL, Göhring G, Bawadi R, et al. A novel classification of hematologic conditions in patients with Fanconi anemia. Haematologica. 2021 Nov 1;106(11):3000–3. PMID:34196171
290. Behzadi F, Suh CH, Jo VY, et al. Imaging of IgG4-related disease in the head and neck: a systematic review, case series, and pathophysiology update. J Neuroradiol. 2021 Sep;48(5):369–78. PMID:33516733
291. Bein J, Thurner L, Hansmann ML, et al. Lymphocyte predominant cells of nodular lymphocyte predominant Hodgkin lymphoma interact with rosetting T cells in an immunological synapse. Am J Hematol. 2020 Dec;95(12):1495–502. PMID:32815561
292. Bekkenk MW, Geelen FA, van Voorst Vader PC, et al. Primary and secondary cutaneous CD30(+) lymphoproliferative disorders: a report from the Dutch Cutaneous Lymphoma Group on the long-term follow-up data of 219 patients and guidelines for diagnosis and treatment. Blood. 2000 Jun 15;95(12):3653–61. PMID:10845893
293. Bekkenk MW, Kluin PM, Jansen PM, et al. Lymphomatoid papulosis with a natural killer-cell phenotype. Br J Dermatol. 2001 Aug;145(2):318–22. PMID:11531801
294. Bekkenk MW, Vermeer MH, Jansen PM, et al. Peripheral T-cell lymphomas unspecified presenting in the skin: analysis of prognostic factors in a group of 82 patients. Blood. 2003 Sep 15;102(6):2213–9. PMID:12750155
295. Belhadj K, Reyes F, Farcet JP, et al. Hepatosplenic gammadelta T-cell lymphoma is a rare clinicopathologic entity with poor outcome: report on a series of 21 patients. Blood. 2003 Dec 15;102(13):4261–9. PMID:12907441
296. Belhouachi N, Xochelli A, Boudjoghra M, et al. Primary vitreoretinal lymphomas display a remarkably restricted immunoglobulin gene repertoire. Blood Adv. 2020 Apr 14;4(7):1357–66. PMID:32267931
297. Bell A, Rickinson AB. Epstein-Barr virus, the TCL-1 oncogene and Burkitt's lymphoma. Trends Microbiol. 2003 Nov;11(11):495–7. PMID:14607063
298. Bell JJ, Bhandoola A. The earliest thymic progenitors for T cells possess myeloid lineage potential. Nature. 2008 Apr 10;452(7188):764–7. PMID:18401411
299. Bellan C, Lazzi S, Hummel M, et al. Immunoglobulin gene analysis reveals 2 distinct cells of origin for EBV-positive and EBV-negative Burkitt lymphomas. Blood. 2005 Aug 1;106(3):1031–6. PMID:15840698
300. Bellanger D, Jacquemin V, Chopin M, et al. Recurrent JAK1 and JAK3 somatic mutations in T-cell prolymphocytic leukemia. Leukemia. 2014 Feb;28(2):417–9. PMID:24048415
301. Beltraminelli H, Leinweber B, Kerl H, et al. Primary cutaneous CD4+ small-/medium-sized pleomorphic T-cell lymphoma: a cutaneous nodular proliferation of pleomorphic T lymphocytes of undetermined significance? A study of 136 cases. Am J Dermatopathol. 2009 Jun;31(4):317–22. PMID:19461234
302. Beltraminelli H, Müllegger R, Cerroni L. Indolent CD8+ lymphoid proliferation of the ear: a phenotypic variant of the small-medium pleomorphic cutaneous T-cell lymphoma? J Cutan Pathol. 2010 Jan;37(1):81–4. PMID:19602068
303. Beltran BE, Castro D, Paredes S, et al. EBV-positive diffuse large B-cell lymphoma, not otherwise specified: 2020 update on diagnosis, risk-stratification and management.

Am J Hematol. 2020 Apr;95(4):435–45. PMID:32072672
304. Beltzung F, Ortonne N, Pelletier L, et al. Primary cutaneous CD4+ small/medium T-cell lymphoproliferative disorders: a clinical, pathologic, and molecular study of 60 cases presenting with a single lesion: a multicenter study of the French Cutaneous Lymphoma Study Group. Am J Surg Pathol. 2020 Jul;44(7):862–72. PMID:32271188
305. Belver L, Ferrando A. The genetics and mechanisms of T cell acute lymphoblastic leukaemia. Nat Rev Cancer. 2016 Jul 25;16(8):494–507. PMID:27451956
306. Bende RJ, Janssen J, Beentjes A, et al. Salivary gland mucosa-associated lymphoid tissue-type lymphoma from Sjögren's syndrome patients in the majority express rheumatoid factors affinity-selected for IgG. Arthritis Rheumatol. 2020 Aug;72(8):1330–40. PMID:32182401
307. Bende RJ, Slot LM, Hoogeboom R, et al. Stereotypic rheumatoid factors that are frequently expressed in mucosa-associated lymphoid tissue-type lymphomas are rare in the labial salivary glands of patients with Sjögren's syndrome. Arthritis Rheumatol. 2015 Apr;67(4):1074–83. PMID:25546553
308. Bender S, Javaugue V, Saintamand A, et al. Immunoglobulin variable domain high-throughput sequencing reveals specific novel mutational patterns in POEMS syndrome. Blood. 2020 May 14;135(20):1750–8. PMID:32243509
309. Bene MC, Castoldi G, Knapp W, et al. Proposals for the immunological classification of acute leukemias. Leukemia. 1995 Oct;9(10):1783–6. PMID:7564526
310. Benedetti D, Tissino E, Pozzo F, et al. NOTCH1 mutations are associated with high CD49d expression in chronic lymphocytic leukemia: link between the NOTCH1 and the NF-κB pathways. Leukemia. 2018 Mar;32(3):654–62. PMID:28935990
311. Benharroch D, Meguerian-Bedoyan Z, Lamant L, et al. ALK-positive lymphoma: a single disease with a broad spectrum of morphology. Blood. 1998 Mar 15;91(6):2076–84. PMID:9490693
312. Ben-Izhak O, Bejar J, Ben-Eliezer S, et al. Splenic littoral cell haemangioendothelioma: a new low-grade variant of malignant littoral cell tumour. Histopathology. 2001 Nov;39(5):469–75. PMID:11737304
313. Benner MF, Jansen PM, Meijer CJ, et al. Diagnostic and prognostic evaluation of phenotypic markers TRAF1, MUM1, BCL2 and CD15 in cutaneous CD30-positive lymphoproliferative disorders. Br J Dermatol. 2009 Jul;161(1):121–7. PMID:19416236
314. Benner MF, Willemze R. Applicability and prognostic value of the new TNM classification system in 135 patients with primary cutaneous anaplastic large cell lymphoma. Arch Dermatol. 2009 Dec;145(12):1399–404. PMID:20026848
315. Bennett JA, Oliva E, Nardi V, et al. Primary endometrial marginal zone lymphoma (MALT lymphoma): a unique clinicopathologic entity. Am J Surg Pathol. 2016 Sep;40(9):1217–23. PMID:27340748
316. Bennett JM, Catovsky D, Daniel MT, et al. Proposals for the classification of chronic (mature) B and T lymphoid leukaemias. J Clin Pathol. 1989 Jun;42(6):567–84. PMID:2738163
317. Benton EC, Crichton S, Talpur R, et al. A cutaneous lymphoma international prognostic index (CLIPi) for mycosis fungoides and Sezary syndrome. Eur J Cancer. 2013 Sep;49(13):2859–68. PMID:23735705
318. Beral V, Peterman T, Berkelman R, et al. AIDS-associated non-Hodgkin lymphoma. Lancet. 1991 Apr 6;337(8745):805–9. PMID:1672911
319. Berentsen S. Cold agglutinin disease. Hematology Am Soc Hematol Educ Program. 2016 Dec 2;2016(1):226–31. PMID:27913484
320. Berentsen S, Barcellini W, D'Sa S, et al. Cold agglutinin disease revisited: a multinational, observational study of 232 patients. Blood. 2020 Jul 23;136(4):480–8. PMID:32374875
321. Berentsen S, Ulvestad E, Langholm R, et al. Primary chronic cold agglutinin disease: a population based clinical study of 86 patients. Haematologica. 2006 Apr;91(4):460–6. PMID:16585012
322. Berg AN, Soma L, Clark BZ, et al. Evaluating breast lymphoplasmacytic infiltrates: a multiparameter immunohistochemical study, including assessment of IgG4. Hum Pathol. 2015 Aug;46(8):1162–70. PMID:26026200
323. Berger CL, Hanlon D, Kanada D, et al. The growth of cutaneous T-cell lymphoma is stimulated by immature dendritic cells. Blood. 2002 Apr 15;99(8):2929–39. PMID:11929784
324. Berger F, Felman P, Thieblemont C, et al. Non-MALT marginal zone B-cell lymphomas: a description of clinical presentation and outcome in 124 patients. Blood. 2000 Mar 15;95(6):1950–6. PMID:10706860
325. Berger TG, Koehler JE. Bacillary angiomatosis. AIDS Clin Rev. 1993:43–60. PMID:8217903
326. Berget E, Helgeland L, Molven A, et al. Detection of clonality in follicular lymphoma using formalin-fixed, paraffin-embedded tissue samples and BIOMED-2 immunoglobulin primers. J Clin Pathol. 2011 Jan;64(1):37–41. PMID:21030528
327. Berglund M, Thunberg U, Amini RM, et al. Evaluation of immunophenotype in diffuse large B-cell lymphoma and its impact on prognosis. Mod Pathol. 2005 Aug;18(8):1113–20. PMID:15920553
328. Bergsagel PL, Kuehl WM, Zhan F, et al. Cyclin D dysregulation: an early and unifying pathogenic event in multiple myeloma. Blood. 2005 Jul 1;106(1):296–303. PMID:15755896
329. Bermudez G, González de Villambrosía S, Martínez-López A, et al. Incidental and isolated follicular lymphoma in situ and mantle cell lymphoma in situ lack clinical significance. Am J Surg Pathol. 2016 Jul;40(7):943–9. PMID:26945339
330. Bernard A, Murphy SB, Melvin S, et al. Non-T, non-B lymphomas are rare in childhood and associated with cutaneous tumor. Blood. 1982 Mar;59(3):549–54. PMID:6977384
331. Bernd HW, Ziepert M, Thorns C, et al. Loss of HLA-DR expression and immunoblastic morphology predict adverse outcome in diffuse large B-cell lymphoma - analyses of cases from two prospective randomized clinical trials. Haematologica. 2009 Nov;94(11):1569–80. PMID:19880780
332. Berti E, Alessi E, Caputo R, et al. Reticulohistiocytoma of the dorsum. J Am Acad Dermatol. 1988 Aug;19(2 Pt 1):259–72. PMID:3049688
333. Berti E, Cerri A, Cavicchini S, et al. Primary cutaneous gamma/delta T-cell lymphoma presenting as disseminated pagetoid reticulosis. J Invest Dermatol. 1991 May;96(5):718–23. PMID:1827136
334. Berti E, Tomasini D, Vermeer MH, et al. Primary cutaneous CD8-positive epidermotropic cytotoxic T cell lymphomas. A distinct clinicopathological entity with an aggressive clinical behavior. Am J Pathol. 1999 Aug;155(2):483–92. PMID:10433941
335. Bertoni F, Conconi A, Capella C, et al. Molecular follow-up in gastric mucosa-associated lymphoid tissue lymphomas: early analysis of the LY03 cooperative trial. Blood. 2002 Apr 1;99(7):2541–4. PMID:11895791
336. Bertoni F, Rossi D, Raderer M, et al. Marginal zone lymphomas. Cancer J. 2020 Jul/Aug;26(4):336–47. PMID:32732678
337. Bertrand P, Bastard C, Maingonnat C, et al. Mapping of MYC breakpoints in 8q24 rearrangements involving non-immunoglobulin partners in B-cell lymphomas. Leukemia. 2007 Mar;21(3):515–23. PMID:17230227
338. Besch-Stokes JG, Costello CM, Severson KJ, et al. Primary cutaneous CD4+ small/medium T-cell lymphoproliferative disorder: diagnosis and management. J Am Acad Dermatol. 2022 May;86(5):1167–9. PMID:33915243
339. Besson C, Goubar A, Gabarre J, et al. Changes in AIDS-related lymphoma since the era of highly active antiretroviral therapy. Blood. 2001 Oct 15;98(8):2339–44. PMID:11588028
340. Besson C, Lancar R, Prevot S, et al. High risk features contrast with favorable outcomes in HIV-associated Hodgkin lymphoma in the modern cART era, ANRS CO16 LYMPHOVIR cohort. Clin Infect Dis. 2015 Nov 1;61(9):1469–75. PMID:26223997
341. Bethel KJ, Sharpe RW. Pathology of hairy-cell leukaemia. Best Pract Res Clin Haematol. 2003 Mar;16(1):15–31. PMID:12670462
342. Beylot-Barry M, Vergier B, Masquelier B, et al. The spectrum of cutaneous lymphomas in HIV infection: a study of 21 cases. Am J Surg Pathol. 1999 Oct;23(10):1208–16. PMID:10524521
343. Béziat V, Liu LL, Malmberg JA, et al. NK cell responses to cytomegalovirus infection lead to stable imprints in the human KIR repertoire and involve activating KIRs. Blood. 2013 Apr 4;121(14):2678–88. PMID:23325834
344. Bhargava P, Rushin JM, Rusnock EJ, et al. Pulmonary light chain deposition disease: report of five cases and review of the literature. Am J Surg Pathol. 2007 Feb;31(2):267–76. PMID:17255772
345. Bhavsar S, Liu YC, Gibson SE, et al. Mutational landscape of TdT+ large B-cell lymphomas supports their distinction from B-lymphoblastic neoplasms: a multiparameter study of a rare and aggressive entity. Am J Surg Pathol. 2022 Jan 1;46(1):71–82. PMID:34392269
346. Bhavsar T, Lee JC, Perner Y, et al. KSHV-associated and EBV-associated germinotropic lymphoproliferative disorder: new findings and review of the literature. Am J Surg Pathol. 2017 Jun;41(6):795–800. PMID:28248818
347. Bhavsar T, Vincent G, Durra H, et al. Primary amyloidosis involving mesenteric lymph nodes: diagnosis by fine-needle aspiration cytology. Acta Cytol. 2011;55(3):296–301. PMID:21525744
348. Bhoi S, Ljungström V, Baliakas P, et al. Prognostic impact of epigenetic classification in chronic lymphocytic leukemia: the case of subset #2. Epigenetics. 2016 Jun 2;11(6):449–55. PMID:27128508
349. Bhoj EJ, Yu Z, Guan Q, et al. Phenotypic predictors and final diagnoses in patients referred for RASopathy testing by targeted next-generation sequencing. Genet Med. 2017 Jun;19(6):715–8. PMID:27763634
350. Bhullar JS, Herschman BR, Dubay L. Intranodal palisaded myofibroblastoma: a new entity of axillary tumors. Am Surg. 2013 Jan;79(1):E19–21. PMID:23317593
351. Bhullar JS, Varshney N, Dubay L. Intranodal palisaded myofibroblastoma: a review of the literature. Int J Surg Pathol. 2013 Aug;21(4):337–41. PMID:23714684
352. Bi CF, Jiang LL, Li Z, et al. [Littoral cell angioma of spleen: a clinicopathologic study of 17 cases]. Zhonghua Bing Li Xue Za Zhi. 2007 Apr;36(4):239–43. Chinese. PMID:17706114
353. Bi XW, Wang H, Zhang WW, et al. PD-L1 is upregulated by EBV-driven LMP1 through NF-κB pathway and correlates with poor prognosis in natural killer/T-cell lymphoma. J Hematol Oncol. 2016 Oct 13;9(1):109. PMID:27737703
354. Bi Y, Huo Z, Liang Z, et al. Intravascular NK-cell lymphoma: a case report and review of the literature. Diagn Pathol. 2015 Jul 1;10:84. PMID:26126576
355. Bianchi G, Anderson KC, Harris NL, et al. The heavy chain diseases: clinical and pathologic features. Oncology (Williston Park). 2014 Jan;28(1):45–53. PMID:24683718
356. Bianchi G, Czarnecki PG, Ho M, et al. ROBO1 promotes homing, dissemination, and survival of multiple myeloma within the bone marrow microenvironment. Blood Cancer Discov. 2021 Jul;2(4):338–53. PMID:34268498
357. Bianchi G, Sohani AR. Heavy chain disease of the small bowel. Curr Gastroenterol Rep. 2018 Jan 25;20(1):3. PMID:29372346
358. Biasoli I, Stamatoullas A, Meignin V, et al. Nodular, lymphocyte-predominant Hodgkin lymphoma: a long-term study and analysis of transformation to diffuse large B-cell lymphoma in a cohort of 164 patients from the Adult Lymphoma Study Group. Cancer. 2010 Feb 1;116(3):631–9. PMID:20029973
359. Biddle DA, Ro JY, Yoon GS, et al. Extranodal follicular dendritic cell sarcoma of the head and neck region: three new cases, with a review of the literature. Mod Pathol. 2002 Jan;15(1):50–8. PMID:11796841
360. Bieliauskas S, Tubbs RR, Bacon CM, et al. Gamma heavy-chain disease: defining the spectrum of associated lymphoproliferative disorders through analysis of 13 cases. Am J Surg Pathol. 2012 Apr;36(4):534–43. PMID:22301495
361. Bienemann K, Borkhardt A, Klapper W, et al. High incidence of Epstein-Barr virus (EBV)-positive Hodgkin lymphoma and Hodgkin lymphoma-like B-cell lymphoproliferations with EBV latency profile 2 in children with interleukin-2-inducible T-cell kinase deficiency. Histopathology. 2015 Nov;67(5):607–16. PMID:25728094
362. Biggar RJ, Chaturvedi AK, Goedert JJ, et al. AIDS-related cancer and severity of immunosuppression in persons with AIDS. J Natl Cancer Inst. 2007 Jun 20;99(12):962–72. PMID:17565153
363. Biggar RJ, Henle W, Fleisher G, et al. Primary Epstein-Barr virus infections in African infants. I. Decline of maternal antibodies and time of infection. Int J Cancer. 1978 Sep 15;22(3):239–43. PMID:212369
364. Bikos V, Darzentas N, Hadzidimitriou A, et al. Over 30% of patients with splenic marginal zone lymphoma express the same immunoglobulin heavy variable gene: ontogenetic implications. Leukemia. 2012 Jul;26(7):1638–46. PMID:22222599
365. Binder M, Rajkumar SV, Ketterling RP, et al. Prognostic implications of abnormalities of chromosome 13 and the presence of multiple cytogenetic high-risk abnormalities in newly diagnosed multiple myeloma. Blood Cancer J. 2017 Sep 1;7(9):e600. PMID:28862698
366. Bink K, Haralambieva E, Kremer M, et al. Primary extramedullary plasmacytoma: similarities with and differences from multiple myeloma revealed by interphase cytogenetics. Haematologica. 2008 Apr;93(4):623–6. PMID:18326524
367. Birkeland SA, Hamilton-Dutoit S. Is posttransplant lymphoproliferative disorder (PTLD) caused by any specific immunosuppressive drug or by the transplantation per se? Transplantation. 2003 Sep 27;76(6):984–8. PMID:14508366
368. Bisceglia M, Sickel JZ, Giangaspero F, et al. Littoral cell angioma of the spleen: an additional report of four cases with emphasis

on the association with visceral organ cancers. Tumori. 1998 Sep-Oct;84(5):595–9. PMID:9862523
369. Bishnoi R, Bajwa R, Franke AJ, et al. Post-transplant lymphoproliferative disorder (PTLD): single institutional experience of 141 patients. Exp Hematol Oncol. 2017 Sep 29;6:26. PMID:29021921
370. Blackburn PR, Smadbeck JB, Znoyko I, et al. Cryptic and atypical KMT2A-USP2 and KMT2A-USP8 rearrangements identified by mate pair sequencing in infant and childhood leukemia. Genes Chromosomes Cancer. 2020 Jul;59(7):422–7. PMID:32196814
371. Blais ME, Louis I, Perreault C. T-cell development: an extrathymic perspective. Immunol Rev. 2006 Feb;209:103–14. PMID:16448537
372. Blaizot R, Ouattara E, Fauconneau A, et al. Infectious events and associated risk factors in mycosis fungoides/Sézary syndrome: a retrospective cohort study. Br J Dermatol. 2018 Dec;179(6):1322–8. PMID:30098016
373. Bledsoe JR, Ferry JA, Neyaz A, et al. IgG4-related lymphadenopathy: a comparative study of 41 cases reveals distinctive histopathologic features. Am J Surg Pathol. 2021 Feb 1;45(2):178–92. PMID:32889888
374. Bledsoe JR, Redd RA, Hasserjian RP, et al. The immunophenotypic spectrum of primary mediastinal large B-cell lymphoma reveals prognostic biomarkers associated with outcome. Am J Hematol. 2016 Oct;91(10):E436–41. PMID:27419920
375. Bledsoe JR, Wallace ZS, Deshpande V, et al. Atypical IgG4+ plasmacytic proliferations and lymphomas: characterization of 11 cases. Am J Clin Pathol. 2017 Sep 1;148(3):215–35. PMID:28821195
376. Bledsoe JR, Wallace ZS, Stone JH, et al. Lymphomas in IgG4-related disease: clinicopathologic features in a western population. Virchows Arch. 2018 May;472(5):839–52. PMID:29285637
377. Blombery P, Anderson MA, Gong JN, et al. Acquisition of the recurrent Gly101Val mutation in BCL2 confers resistance to venetoclax in patients with progressive chronic lymphocytic leukemia. Cancer Discov. 2019 Mar;9(3):342–53. PMID:30514704
378. Blombery P, Thompson E, Ryland GL, et al. Frequent activating STAT3 mutations and novel recurrent genomic abnormalities detected in breast implant-associated anaplastic large cell lymphoma. Oncotarget. 2018 Nov 16;9(90):36126–36. PMID:30546832
379. Blombery P, Thompson ER, Jones K, et al. Whole exome sequencing reveals activating JAK1 and STAT3 mutations in breast implant-associated anaplastic large cell lymphoma anaplastic large cell lymphoma. Haematologica. 2016 Sep;101(9):e387–90. PMID:27198716
380. Blombery P, Thompson ER, Nguyen T, et al. Multiple BCL2 mutations cooccurring with Gly101Val emerge in chronic lymphocytic leukemia progression on venetoclax. Blood. 2020 Mar 5;135(10):773–7. PMID:31951646
381. Blumenthal MJ, Cornejo Castro EM, Whitby D, et al. Evidence for altered host genetic factors in KSHV infection and KSHV-related disease development. Rev Med Virol. 2021 Mar;31(2):e2160. PMID:33043529
382. Bockorny B, Codreanu I, Dasanu CA. Hodgkin lymphoma as Richter transformation in chronic lymphocytic leukaemia: a retrospective analysis of world literature. Br J Haematol. 2012 Jan;156(1):50–66. PMID:22017478
383. Boddicker RL, Razidlo GL, Dasari S, et al. Integrated mate-pair and RNA sequencing identifies novel, targetable gene fusions in peripheral T-cell lymphoma. Blood. 2016 Sep 1;128(9):1234–45. PMID:27297792
384. Bodin K, Ellmerich S, Kahan MC, et al. Antibodies to human serum amyloid P component eliminate visceral amyloid deposits. Nature. 2010 Nov 4;468(7320):93–7. PMID:20962779
385. Bödör C, Alpár D, Marosvári D, et al. Molecular subtypes and genomic profile of primary central nervous system lymphoma. J Neuropathol Exp Neurol. 2020 Feb 1;79(2):176–83. PMID:31886867
386. Boer JM, Marchante JR, Evans WE, et al. BCR-ABL1-like cases in pediatric acute lymphoblastic leukemia: a comparison between DCOG/Erasmus MC and COG/St. Jude signatures. Haematologica. 2015 Sep;100(9):e354–7. PMID:26045294
387. Boer JM, Valsecchi MG, Hormann FM, et al. Favorable outcome of NUTM1-rearranged infant and pediatric B cell precursor acute lymphoblastic leukemia in a collaborative international study. Leukemia. 2021 Oct;35(10):2978–82. PMID:34211097
388. Boerma EG, Siebert R, Kluin PM, et al. Translocations involving 8q24 in Burkitt lymphoma and other malignant lymphomas: a historical review of cytogenetics in the light of todays knowledge. Leukemia. 2009 Feb;23(2):225–34. PMID:18923440
389. Bofill M, Akbar AN, Amlot PL. Follicular dendritic cells share a membrane-bound protein with fibroblasts. J Pathol. 2000 Jun;191(2):217–26. PMID:10861584
390. Bogusz AM, Bhargava P. Recurrent histiocytic necrotizing lymphadenitis with a long latency in a patient with autoimmunity: a case report and review of literature. Int J Surg Pathol. 2013 Jun;21(3):287–96. PMID:23204033
391. Bogusz AM, Seegmiller AC, Garcia R, et al. Plasmablastic lymphomas with MYC/IgH rearrangement: report of three cases and review of the literature. Am J Clin Pathol. 2009 Oct;132(4):597–605. PMID:19762538
392. Boi M, Rinaldi A, Kwee I, et al. PRDM1/BLIMP1 is commonly inactivated in anaplastic large T-cell lymphoma. Blood. 2013 Oct 10;122(15):2683–93. PMID:24004669
393. Bojanini L, Jiang L, Tun AJ, et al. Outcomes of hepatosplenic T-cell lymphoma: the Mayo Clinic experience. Clin Lymphoma Myeloma Leuk. 2021 Feb;21(2):106–112.e1. PMID:33160933
394. Bolen CR, Mattiello F, Herold M, et al. Treatment dependence of prognostic gene expression signatures in de novo follicular lymphoma. Blood. 2021 May 13;137(19):2704–7. PMID:33512481
395. Bolen CR, McCord R, Huet S, et al. Mutation load and an effector T-cell gene signature may distinguish immunologically distinct and clinically relevant lymphoma subsets. Blood Adv. 2017 Sep 27;1(22):1884–90. PMID:29296835
396. Bolli N, Maura F, Minvielle S, et al. Genomic patterns of progression in smoldering multiple myeloma. Nat Commun. 2018 Aug 22;9(1):3363. PMID:30135448
397. Bomken S, Haigh S, Bown N, et al. Cutaneous B-lymphoblastic lymphoma with IL3/IgH translocation presenting with hypereosinophilia and acute endocarditis. Pediatr Blood Cancer. 2015 Jun;62(6):1055–7. PMID:25382309
398. Bomze D, Sprecher E, Goldberg I, et al. Primary cutaneous B-cell lymphomas in children and adolescents: a SEER population-based study. Clin Lymphoma Myeloma Leuk. 2021 Dec;21(12):e1000–5. PMID:34417159
399. Bonato M, Pittaluga S, Tierens A, et al. Lymph node histology in typical and atypical chronic lymphocytic leukemia. Am J Surg Pathol. 1998 Jan;22(1):49–56. PMID:9422315
400. Bond J, Graux C, Lhermitte L, et al. Early response-based therapy stratification improves survival in adult early thymic precursor acute lymphoblastic leukemia: a Group for Research on Adult Acute Lymphoblastic Leukemia study. J Clin Oncol. 2017 Aug 10;35(23):2683–91. PMID:28605290
401. Bonfiglio F, Bruscaggin A, Guidetti F, et al. Genetic and phenotypic attributes of splenic marginal zone lymphoma. Blood. 2022 Feb 3;139(5):732–47. PMID:34653238
402. Bonnet A, Bossard C, Gabellier L, et al. Clinical presentation, outcome, and prognostic markers in patients with intravascular large B-cell lymphoma, a lymphoma study association (LYSA) retrospective study. Cancer Med. 2022 Oct;11(19):3602–11. PMID:35538643
403. Bonnichsen CR, Dearani JA, Maleszewski JJ, et al. Recurrent Ebstein-Barr virus-associated diffuse large B-cell lymphoma in an ascending aorta graft. Circulation. 2013 Sep 24;128(13):1481–3. PMID:24060945
404. Bonzheim I, Geissinger E, Roth S, et al. Anaplastic large cell lymphomas lack the expression of T-cell receptor molecules or molecules of proximal T-cell receptor signaling. Blood. 2004 Nov 15;104(10):3358–60. PMID:15297316
405. Bonzheim I, Giese S, Deuter C, et al. High frequency of MYD88 mutations in vitreoretinal B-cell lymphoma: a valuable tool to improve diagnostic yield of vitreous aspirates. Blood. 2015 Jul 2;126(1):76–9. PMID:25900979
406. Bonzheim I, Irmler M, Klier-Richter M, et al. Identification of C/EBPβ target genes in ALK+ anaplastic large cell lymphoma (ALCL) by gene expression profiling and chromatin immunoprecipitation. PLoS One. 2013 May 31;8(5):e64544. PMID:23741337
407. Bonzheim I, Salaverria I, Haake A, et al. A unique case of follicular lymphoma provides insights to the clonal evolution from follicular lymphoma in situ to manifest follicular lymphoma. Blood. 2011 Sep 22;118(12):3442–4. PMID:21940830
408. Bonzheim I, Sander P, Salmerón-Villalobos J, et al. The molecular hallmarks of primary and secondary vitreoretinal lymphoma. Blood Adv. 2022 Mar 8;6(5):1598–607. PMID:34448823
409. Booman M, Douwes J, Glas AM, et al. Mechanisms and effects of loss of human leukocyte antigen class II expression in immune-privileged site-associated B-cell lymphoma. Clin Cancer Res. 2006 May 1;12(9):2698–705. PMID:16675561
410. Booman M, Douwes J, Legdeur MC, et al. From brain to testis: immune escape and clonal selection in a B cell lymphoma with selective outgrowth in two immune sanctuaries [correction of sanctuariesy]. Haematologica. 2007 Jun;92(6):e69–71. PMID:17650453
411. Booman M, Szuhai K, Rosenwald A, et al. Genomic alterations and gene expression in primary diffuse large B-cell lymphomas of immune-privileged sites: the importance of apoptosis and immunomodulatory pathways. J Pathol. 2008 Oct;216(2):209–17. PMID:18729069
412. Boot MV, Schaapveld M, Van den Broek EC, et al. Pathology review identifies frequent misdiagnoses in recurrent classic Hodgkin lymphoma in a nationwide cohort: implications for clinical and epidemiological studies. Haematologica. 2023 May 1;108(5):1349–58. PMID:36263842
413. Booth CAG, Barkas N, Neo WH, et al. Ezh2 and Runx1 mutations collaborate to initiate lympho-myeloid leukemia in early thymic progenitors. Cancer Cell. 2018 Feb 12;33(2):274–291.e8. PMID:29438697
414. Borchmann S, Joffe E, Moskowitz CH, et al. Active surveillance for nodular lymphocyte-predominant Hodgkin lymphoma. Blood. 2019 May 16;133(20):2121–9. PMID:30770396
415. Borkhardt A, Wuchter C, Viehmann S, et al. Infant acute lymphoblastic leukemia - combined cytogenetic, immunophenotypical and molecular analysis of 77 cases. Leukemia. 2002 Sep;16(9):1685–90. PMID:12200682
416. Boroumand N, Ly TL, Sonstein J, et al. Microscopic diffuse large B-cell lymphoma (DLBCL) occurring in pseudocysts: Do these tumors belong to the category of DLBCL associated with chronic inflammation? Am J Surg Pathol. 2012 Jul;36(7):1074–80. PMID:22472958
417. Borowitz MJ, Croker BP, Metzgar RS. Lymphoblastic lymphoma with the phenotype of common acute lymphoblastic leukemia. Am J Clin Pathol. 1983 Mar;79(3):387–91. PMID:6338702
418. Borowitz MJ, Hunger SP, Carroll AJ, et al. Predictability of the t(1;19)(q23;p13) from surface antigen phenotype: implications for screening cases of childhood acute lymphoblastic leukemia for molecular analysis: a Pediatric Oncology Group study. Blood. 1993 Aug 15;82(4):1086–91. PMID:8353275
419. Borowitz MJ, Rubnitz J, Nash M, et al. Surface antigen phenotype can predict TEL-AML1 rearrangement in childhood B-precursor ALL: a Pediatric Oncology Group study. Leukemia. 1998 Nov;12(11):1764–70. PMID:9823952
420. Bosch X, Guilabert A, Miquel R, et al. Enigmatic Kikuchi-Fujimoto disease: a comprehensive review. Am J Clin Pathol. 2004 Jul;122(1):141–52. PMID:15272543
421. Bösmüller H, Klenske J, Bonzheim I, et al. Cytokeratin-positive interstitial reticulum cell tumor: recognition of a potential "in situ" pattern. Hum Pathol. 2016 Mar;49:15–21. PMID:26826404
422. Bossard C, Dobay MP, Parrens M, et al. Immunohistochemistry as a valuable tool to assess CD30 expression in peripheral T-cell lymphomas: high correlation with mRNA levels. Blood. 2014 Nov 6;124(19):2983–6. PMID:25224410
423. Bouchekioua A, Scourzic L, de Wever O, et al. JAK3 deregulation by activating mutations confers invasive growth advantage in extranodal nasal-type natural killer cell lymphoma. Leukemia. 2014 Feb;28(2):338–48. PMID:23689514
424. Boudová L, Torlakovic E, Delabie J, et al. Nodular lymphocyte-predominant Hodgkin lymphoma with nodules resembling T-cell/histiocyte-rich B-cell lymphoma: differential diagnosis between nodular lymphocyte-predominant Hodgkin lymphoma and T-cell/histiocyte-rich B-cell lymphoma. Blood. 2003 Nov 15;102(10):3753–8. PMID:12881319
425. Boué F, Gabarre J, Gisselbrecht C, et al. Phase II trial of CHOP plus rituximab in patients with HIV-associated non-Hodgkin's lymphoma. J Clin Oncol. 2006 Sep 1;24(25):4123–8. PMID:16896005
426. Boulanger E, Hermine O, Fermand JP, et al. Human herpesvirus 8 (HHV-8)-associated peritoneal primary effusion lymphoma (PEL) in two HIV-negative elderly patients. Am J Hematol. 2004 May;76(1):88–91. PMID:15114607
427. Boulland ML, Wechsler J, Bagot M, et al. Primary CD30-positive cutaneous T-cell lymphomas and lymphomatoid papulosis frequently express cytotoxic proteins. Histopathology. 2000 Feb;36(2):136–44. PMID:10672058
428. Bourbon E, Maucort-Boulch D, Fontaine J, et al. Clinicopathological features and survival in EBV-positive diffuse large B-cell lymphoma not otherwise specified. Blood Adv. 2021 Aug 24;5(16):3227–39. PMID:34427583
429. Bourgault-Rouxel AS, Loughran TP Jr, Zambello R, et al. Clinical spectrum of gammadelta+ T cell LGL leukemia: analysis of 20 cases. Leuk Res. 2008 Jan;32(1):45–8.

PMID:17544120
430. Bouroncle BA. Leukemic reticuloendotheliosis (hairy cell leukemia). Blood. 1979 Mar;53(3):412–36. PMID:367468
431. Bouska A, Bi C, Lone W, et al. Adult high-grade B-cell lymphoma with Burkitt lymphoma signature: genomic features and potential therapeutic targets. Blood. 2017 Oct 19;130(16):1819–31. PMID:28801451
432. Bouska A, Zhang W, Gong Q, et al. Combined copy number and mutation analysis identifies oncogenic pathways associated with transformation of follicular lymphoma. Leukemia. 2017 Jan;31(1):83–91. PMID:27389057
433. Boutboul D, Fadlallah J, Chawki S, et al. Treatment and outcome of unicentric Castleman disease: a retrospective analysis of 71 cases. Br J Haematol. 2019 Jul;186(2):269–73. PMID:31016730
434. Boveri E, Arcaini L, Merli M, et al. Bone marrow histology in marginal zone B-cell lymphomas: correlation with clinical parameters and flow cytometry in 120 patients. Ann Oncol. 2009 Jan;20(1):129–36. PMID:18718888
435. Bower K, Shah N. Primary CNS Burkitt lymphoma: a case report of a 55-year-old cerebral palsy patient. Case Rep Oncol Med. 2018 Jun 24;2018:5869135. PMID:30034894
436. Bower M, Newsom-Davis T, Naresh K, et al. Clinical features and outcome in HIV-associated multicentric Castleman's disease. J Clin Oncol. 2011 Jun 20;29(18):2481–6. PMID:21555697
437. Bowman RL, Busque L, Levine RL. Clonal hematopoiesis and evolution to hematopoietic malignancies. Cell Stem Cell. 2018 Feb 1;22(2):157–70. PMID:29395053
438. Boy SC, van Heerden MB, Raubenheimer EJ, et al. Plasmablastic lymphomas with light chain restriction - plasmablastic extramedullary plasmacytomas? J Oral Pathol Med. 2010 May;39(5):435–9. PMID:20537055
439. Boyer DF, Lindeman NI, Harris NL, et al. Peripheral T-cell lymphomas with cytotoxic phenotype in patients with chronic lymphocytic leukemia/small lymphocytic lymphoma. Am J Surg Pathol. 2014 Feb;38(2):279–88. PMID:24418862
440. Boyer DF, McKelvie PA, de Leval L, et al. Fibrin-associated EBV-positive large B-cell lymphoma: an indolent neoplasm with features distinct from diffuse large B-cell lymphoma associated with chronic inflammation. Am J Surg Pathol. 2017 Mar;41(3):299–312. PMID:28195879
441. Boyle EM, Deshpande S, Tytarenko R, et al. The molecular make up of smoldering myeloma highlights the evolutionary pathways leading to multiple myeloma. Nat Commun. 2021 Jan 12;12(1):293. PMID:33436579
442. Bracci PM, Benavente Y, Turner JJ, et al. Medical history, lifestyle, family history, and occupational risk factors for marginal zone lymphoma: the InterLymph Non-Hodgkin Lymphoma Subtypes Project. J Natl Cancer Inst Monogr. 2014 Aug;2014(48):52–65. PMID:25174026
443. Brady JL, Binkley MS, Hajj C, et al. Definitive radiotherapy for localized follicular lymphoma staged by 18F-FDG PET-CT: a collaborative study by ILROG. Blood. 2019 Jan 17;133(3):237–45. PMID:30446493
444. Braeuninger A, Küppers R, Strickler JG, et al. Hodgkin and Reed-Sternberg cells in lymphocyte predominant Hodgkin disease represent clonal populations of germinal center-derived tumor B cells. Proc Natl Acad Sci U S A. 1997 Aug 19;94(17):9337–42. PMID:9256483
445. Brar N, Butzmann A, Kumar J, et al. LIM domain only 2 (LMO2) expression distinguishes T-lymphoblastic leukemia/lymphoma from indolent T-lymphoblastic proliferations. Histopathology. 2020 Dec;77(6):984–8. PMID:32526041
446. Brar N, Spinner MA, Baker MC, et al. Increased double-negative αβ+ T-cells reveal adult-onset autoimmune lymphoproliferative syndrome in a patient with IgG4-related disease. Haematologica. 2022 Jan 1;107(1):347–50. PMID:34474549
447. Braun T, Glass M, Wahnschaffe L, et al. Micro-RNA networks in T-cell prolymphocytic leukemia reflect T-cell activation and shape DNA damage response and survival pathways. Haematologica. 2022 Jan 1;107(1):187–200. PMID:33543866
448. Braun T, Stachelscheid J, Bley N, et al. Noncanonical function of AGO2 augments T-cell receptor signaling in T-cell prolymphocytic leukemia. Cancer Res. 2022 May 3;82(9):1818–31. PMID:35259248
449. Bräuninger A, Küppers R, Spieker T, et al. Molecular analysis of single B cells from T-cell-rich B-cell lymphoma shows the derivation of the tumor cells from mutating germinal center B cells and exemplifies means by which immunoglobulin genes are modified in germinal center B cells. Blood. 1999 Apr 15;93(8):2679–87. PMID:10194448
450. Bräuninger A, Yang W, Wacker HH, et al. B-cell development in progressively transformed germinal centers: similarities and differences compared with classical germinal centers and lymphocyte-predominant Hodgkin disease. Blood. 2001 Feb 1;97(3):714–9. PMID:11157489
451. Breitfeld D, Ohl L, Kremmer E, et al. Follicular B helper T cells express CXC chemokine receptor 5, localize to B cell follicles, and support immunoglobulin production. J Exp Med. 2000 Dec 4;192(11):1545–52. PMID:11104797
452. Brenner I, Roth S, Puppe B, et al. Primary cutaneous marginal zone lymphomas with plasmacytic differentiation show frequent IgG4 expression. Mod Pathol. 2013 Dec;26(12):1568–76. PMID:23765244
453. Bretherick KL, Bu R, Gascoyne RD, et al. Elevated circulating t(14;18) translocation levels prior to diagnosis of follicular lymphoma. Blood. 2010 Dec 23;116(26):6146–7. PMID:21183699
454. Breza TS Jr, Zheng P, Porcu P, et al. Cutaneous marginal zone B-cell lymphoma in the setting of fluoxetine therapy: a hypothesis regarding pathogenesis based on in vitro suppression of T-cell-proliferative response. J Cutan Pathol. 2006 Jul;33(7):522–8. PMID:16872479
455. Brice SL, Jester JD, Friednash M, et al. Examination of cutaneous T-cell lymphoma for human herpesviruses by using the polymerase chain reaction. J Cutan Pathol. 1993 Aug;20(4):304–7. PMID:8227605
456. Bridoux F, Javaugue V, Bender S, et al. Unravelling the immunopathological mechanisms of heavy chain deposition disease with implications for clinical management. Kidney Int. 2017 Feb;91(2):423–34. PMID:27773425
457. Bridoux F, Leung N, Hutchison CA, et al. Diagnosis of monoclonal gammopathy of renal significance. Kidney Int. 2015 Apr;87(4):698–711. PMID:25607108
458. Brierley JD, Gospodarowicz MK, Wittekind C, editors. TNM classification of malignant tumours. 8th ed. Oxford (UK): Wiley-Blackwell; 2017.
459. Brimo F, Michel RP, Khetani K, et al. Primary effusion lymphoma: a series of 4 cases and review of the literature with emphasis on cytomorphologic and immunocytochemical differential diagnosis. Cancer. 2007 Aug 25;111(4):224–33. PMID:17554754
460. Bristeau-Leprince A, Mateo V, Lim A, et al. Human TCR alpha/beta+ CD4-CD8- double-negative T cells in patients with autoimmune lymphoproliferative syndrome express restricted Vbeta TCR diversity and are clonally related to CD8+ T cells. J Immunol. 2008 Jul 1;181(1):440–8. PMID:18566410
461. Brito-Babapulle V, Catovsky D. Inversions and tandem translocations involving chromosome 14q11 and 14q32 in T-prolymphocytic leukemia and T-cell leukemias in patients with ataxia telangiectasia. Cancer Genet Cytogenet. 1991 Aug;55(1):1–9. PMID:1913594
462. Brito-Babapulle V, Matutes E, Oscier D, et al. Chromosome abnormalities in hairy cell leukaemia variant. Genes Chromosomes Cancer. 1994 Jul;10(3):197–202. PMID:7522043
463. Brito-Zerón P, Ramos-Casals M, Bosch X, et al. The clinical spectrum of IgG4-related disease. Autoimmun Rev. 2014 Dec;13(12):1203–10. PMID:25151972
464. Britten O, Ragusa D, Tosi S, et al. MLL-rearranged acute leukemia with t(4;11)(q21;q23)-current treatment options. Is there a role for CAR-T cell therapy? Cells. 2019 Oct 29;8(11):1341. PMID:31671855
465. Broussard G, Damania B. KSHV: immune modulation and immunotherapy. Front Immunol. 2020 Feb 7;10:3084. PMID:32117196
466. Brown JR. Inherited susceptibility to chronic lymphocytic leukemia: evidence and prospects for the future. Ther Adv Hematol. 2013 Aug;4(4):298–308. PMID:23926461
467. Brown L, Cheng JT, Chen Q, et al. Site-specific recombination of the tal-1 gene is a common occurrence in human T cell leukemia. EMBO J. 1990 Oct;9(10):3343–51. PMID:2209547
468. Brown LM, Lonsdale A, Zhu A, et al. The application of RNA sequencing for the diagnosis and genomic classification of pediatric acute lymphoblastic leukemia. Blood Adv. 2020 Mar 10;4(5):930–42. PMID:32150610
469. Brown NA, Betz BL, Weigelin HC, et al. Evaluation of allele-specific PCR and immunohistochemistry for the detection of BRAF V600E mutations in hairy cell leukemia. Am J Clin Pathol. 2015 Jan;143(1):89–99. PMID:25511147
470. Browne P, Petrosyan K, Hernandez A, et al. The B-cell transcription factors BSAP, Oct-2, and BOB.1 and the pan-B-cell markers CD20, CD22, and CD79a are useful in the differential diagnosis of classic Hodgkin lymphoma. Am J Clin Pathol. 2003 Nov;120(5):767–77. PMID:14608905
471. Bruce-Brand C, Rigby J. Kaposi sarcoma with intravascular primary effusion lymphoma in the skin: a potential pitfall in HHV8 immunohistochemistry interpretation. Int J Surg Pathol. 2020 Dec;28(8):868–71. PMID:32460596
472. Brudno J, Tadmor T, Pittaluga S, et al. Discordant bone marrow involvement in non-Hodgkin lymphoma. Blood. 2016 Feb 25;127(8):965–70. PMID:26679865
473. Bruehl FK, Azzato E, Durkin L, et al. Inflammatory pseudotumor-like follicular/fibroblastic dendritic cell sarcomas of the spleen are EBV-associated and lack other commonly identifiable molecular alterations. Int J Surg Pathol. 2021 Jun;29(4):443–6. PMID:32787485
474. Bruford EA, Antonescu CR, Carroll AJ, et al. HUGO Gene Nomenclature Committee (HGNC) recommendations for the designation of gene fusions. Leukemia. 2021 Nov;35(11):3040–3. PMID:34615987
475. Brüggemann M, Kotrová M, Knecht H, et al. Standardized next-generation sequencing of immunoglobulin and T-cell receptor gene recombinations for MRD marker identification in acute lymphoblastic leukaemia; a EuroClonality-NGS validation study. Leukemia. 2019 Sep;33(9):2241–53. PMID:31243313
477. Brune V, Tiacci E, Pfeil I, et al. Origin and pathogenesis of nodular lymphocyte-predominant Hodgkin lymphoma as revealed by global gene expression analysis. J Exp Med. 2008 Sep 29;205(10):2251–68. PMID:18794340
478. Brunn A, Montesinos-Rongen M, Strack A, et al. Expression pattern and cellular sources of chemokines in primary central nervous system lymphoma. Acta Neuropathol. 2007 Sep;114(3):271–6. PMID:17641901
479. Brunn A, Nagel I, Montesinos-Rongen M, et al. Frequent triple-hit expression of MYC, BCL2, and BCL6 in primary lymphoma of the central nervous system and absence of a favorable MYC(low)BCL2 (low) subgroup may underlie the inferior prognosis as compared to systemic diffuse large B cell lymphomas. Acta Neuropathol. 2013 Oct;126(4):603–5. PMID:24061549
480. Bruzzi JF, Macapinlac H, Tsimberidou AM, et al. Detection of Richter's transformation of chronic lymphocytic leukemia by PET/CT. J Nucl Med. 2006 Aug;47(8):1267–73. PMID:16883004
481. Bryce AH, Ketterling RP, Gertz MA, et al. A novel report of cig-FISH and cytogenetics in POEMS syndrome. Am J Hematol. 2008 Nov;83(11):840–1. PMID:18839437
482. Brynes RK, Almaguer PD, Leathery KE, et al. Numerical cytogenetic abnormalities of chromosomes 3, 7, and 12 in marginal zone B-cell lymphomas. Mod Pathol. 1996 Oct;9(10):995–1000. PMID:8902837
483. Buchbinder R, Van Doornum S, Staples M, et al. Malignancy risk in Australian rheumatoid arthritis patients treated with anti-tumour necrosis factor therapy: analysis of the Australian Rheumatology Association Database (ARAD) prospective cohort study. BMC Musculoskelet Disord. 2015 Oct 20;16:309. PMID:26481039
484. Bueno C, Tejedor JR, Bashford-Rogers R, et al. Natural history and cell of origin of TC F3-ZN F384 and PTPN11 mutations in monozygotic twins with concordant BCP-ALL. Blood. 2019 Sep 12;134(11):900–5. PMID:31221673
485. Buettner M, Greiner A, Avramidou A, et al. Evidence of abortive plasma cell differentiation in Hodgkin and Reed-Sternberg cells of classical Hodgkin lymphoma. Hematol Oncol. 2005 Sep-Dec;23(3-4):127–32. PMID:16342298
486. Bug S, Dürig J, Oyen F, et al. Recurrent loss, but lack of mutations, of the SMARCB1 tumor suppressor gene in T-cell prolymphocytic leukemia with TCL1A-TCRAD juxtaposition. Cancer Genet Cytogenet. 2009 Jul;192(1):44–7. PMID:19480937
487. Bugarin C, Sarno J, Palmi C, et al. Fine tuning of surface CRLF2 expression and its associated signaling profile in childhood B-cell precursor acute lymphoblastic leukemia. Haematologica. 2015 Jun;100(6):e229–32. PMID:25862705
488. Bunn PA Jr, Schechter GP, Jaffe E, et al. Clinical course of retrovirus-associated adult T-cell lymphoma in the United States. N Engl J Med. 1983 Aug 4;309(5):257–64. PMID:6602943
489. Burg G, Kempf W, Cozzio A, et al. WHO/EORTC classification of cutaneous lymphomas 2005: histological and molecular aspects. J Cutan Pathol. 2005 Nov;32(10):647–74. PMID:16293178
490. Burg G, Kempf W, Kazakov DV, et al. Pyogenic lymphoma of the skin: a peculiar variant of primary cutaneous neutrophil-rich CD30+ anaplastic large-cell lymphoma. Clinicopathological study of four cases and review of the literature. Br J Dermatol. 2003 Mar;148(3):580–6. PMID:12653754
491. Burger JA. Treatment of chronic lymphocytic leukemia. N Engl J Med. 2020 Jul 30;383(5):460–73. PMID:32726532
492. Burger JA, Barr PM, Robak T, et al.

Long-term efficacy and safety of first-line ibrutinib treatment for patients with CLL/SLL: 5 years of follow-up from the phase 3 RESONATE-2 study. Leukemia. 2020 Mar;34(3):787–98. PMID:31628428
493. Burger JA, Li KW, Keating MJ, et al. Leukemia cell proliferation and death in chronic lymphocytic leukemia patients on therapy with the BTK inhibitor ibrutinib. JCI Insight. 2017 Jan 26;2(2):e89904. PMID:28138560
494. Burger JA, Quiroga MP, Hartmann E, et al. High-level expression of the T-cell chemokines CCL3 and CCL4 by chronic lymphocytic leukemia B cells in nurselike cell cocultures and after BCR stimulation. Blood. 2009 Mar 26;113(13):3050–8. PMID:19074730
495. Burke AP, Andriko JA, Virmani R. Anaplastic large cell lymphoma (CD 30+), T-phenotype, in the heart of an HIV-positive man. Cardiovasc Pathol. 2000 Jan-Feb;9(1):49–52. PMID:10739907
496. Burmeister T, Gökbuget N, Schwartz S, et al. Clinical features and prognostic implications of TCF3-PBX1 and ETV6-RUNX1 in adult acute lymphoblastic leukemia. Haematologica. 2010 Feb;95(2):241–6. PMID:19713226
497. Burmeister T, Schwartz S, Bartram CR, et al. Patients' age and BCR-ABL frequency in adult B-precursor ALL: a retrospective analysis from the GMALL study group. Blood. 2008 Aug 1;112(3):918–9. PMID:18650471
498. Burmeister T, Schwartz S, Taubald A, et al. Atypical BCR-ABL mRNA transcripts in adult acute lymphoblastic leukemia. Haematologica. 2007 Dec;92(12):1699–702. PMID:18055996
499. Burmester GR, Panaccione R, Gordon KB, et al. Adalimumab: long-term safety in 23 458 patients from global clinical trials in rheumatoid arthritis, juvenile idiopathic arthritis, ankylosing spondylitis, psoriatic arthritis, psoriasis and Crohn's disease. Ann Rheum Dis. 2013 Apr;72(4):517–24. PMID:22562972
500. Burnett RA, Millan D. Decidual change in pelvic lymph nodes: a source of possible diagnostic error. Histopathology. 1986 Oct;10(10):1089–92. PMID:3536713
501. Burns A, Alsolami R, Becq J, et al. Whole-genome sequencing of chronic lymphocytic leukaemia reveals distinct differences in the mutational landscape between IgHVmut and IgHVunmut subgroups. Leukemia. 2018 Feb;32(2):332–42. PMID:28584254
502. Burns MA, Place AE, Stevenson KE, et al. Identification of prognostic factors in childhood T-cell acute lymphoblastic leukemia: results from DFCI ALL Consortium Protocols 05-001 and 11-001. Pediatr Blood Cancer. 2021 Jan;68(1):e28719. PMID:33026184
503. Buske C, Hoster E, Dreyling M, et al. The Follicular Lymphoma International Prognostic Index (FLIPI) separates high-risk from intermediate- or low-risk patients with advanced-stage follicular lymphoma treated front-line with rituximab and the combination of cyclophosphamide, doxorubicin, vincristine, and prednisone (R-CHOP) with respect to treatment outcome. Blood. 2006 Sep 1;108(5):1504–8. PMID:16690968
504. Bussot L, Chevalier S, Cristante J, et al. Adverse outcome in follicular lymphoma is associated with MYC rearrangements but not MYC extra copies. Br J Haematol. 2021 Jul;194(2):382–92. PMID:34155628
505. Bustoros M, Sklavenitis-Pistofidis R, Park J, et al. Genomic profiling of smoldering multiple myeloma identifies patients at a high risk of disease progression. J Clin Oncol. 2020 Jul 20;38(21):2380–9. PMID:32442065
506. Butsch F, Kind P, Bräuninger W. Bilateral indolent epidermotropic CD8-positive lymphoid proliferations of the ear. J Dtsch Dermatol Ges. 2012 Mar;10(3):195–6. PMID:22142195
507. Butzmann A, Kumar J, Sridhar K, et al. A review of genetic abnormalities in unicentric and multicentric Castleman disease. Biology (Basel). 2021 Mar 24;10(4):251. PMID:33804823
508. Buxbaum JN, Genega EM, Lazowski P, et al. Infiltrative nonamyloidotic monoclonal immunoglobulin light chain cardiomyopathy: an underappreciated manifestation of plasma cell dyscrasias. Cardiology. 2000;93(4):220–8. PMID:11025347
509. Buxton J, Leen C, Goodlad JR. Polymorphic lymphoid proliferations occurring in HIV-positive patients: report of a case responding to HAART. Virchows Arch. 2012 Jul;461(1):93–8. PMID:22706705
510. Bylsma LC, Gulbech Ording A, Rosenthal A, et al. Occurrence, thromboembolic risk, and mortality in Danish patients with cold agglutinin disease. Blood Adv. 2019 Oct 22;3(20):2980–5. PMID:31648316
511. Byun JH, Park SE, Nam SO, et al. Three children of meningoencephalitis with Kikuchi necrotizing lymphadenitis. Brain Dev. 2018 Mar;40(3):251–5. PMID:29050838
512. Cady FM, Morice WG. Flow cytometric assessment of T-cell chronic lymphoproliferative disorders. Clin Lab Med. 2007 Sep;27(3):513–32, vi. PMID:17658405
513. Cady FM, O'Neill BP, Law ME, et al. Del(6)(q22) and BCL6 rearrangements in primary CNS lymphoma are indicators of an aggressive clinical course. J Clin Oncol. 2008 Oct 10;26(29):4814–9. PMID:18645192
514. Cahill N, Bergh AC, Kanduri M, et al. 450K-array analysis of chronic lymphocytic leukemia cells reveals global DNA methylation to be relatively stable over time and similar in resting and proliferative compartments. Leukemia. 2013 Jan;27(1):150–8. PMID:22922567
515. Cai ZR, Chen ML, Weinstock MA, et al. Incidence trends of primary cutaneous T-cell lymphoma in the US from 2000 to 2018: a SEER population data analysis. JAMA Oncol. 2022 Nov 1;8(11):1690–2. PMID:36048455
516. Caillard S, Lelong C, Pessione F, et al. Post-transplant lymphoproliferative disorders occurring after renal transplantation in adults: report of 230 cases from the French Registry. Am J Transplant. 2006 Nov;6(11):2735–42. PMID:17049061
517. Caillard S, Porcher R, Provot F, et al. Post-transplantation lymphoproliferative disorder after kidney transplantation: report of a nationwide French registry and the development of a new prognostic score. J Clin Oncol. 2013 Apr 1;31(10):1302–9. PMID:23423742
518. Cairns RA, Iqbal J, Lemonnier F, et al. IDH2 mutations are frequent in angioimmunoblastic T-cell lymphoma. Blood. 2012 Feb 23;119(8):1901–3. PMID:22215888
519. Calado DP, Sasaki Y, Godinho SA, et al. The cell-cycle regulator c-Myc is essential for the formation and maintenance of germinal centers. Nat Immunol. 2012 Nov;13(11):1092–100. PMID:23001146
520. Calaminici M, Piper K, Lee AM, et al. CD23 expression in mediastinal large B-cell lymphomas. Histopathology. 2004 Dec;45(6):619–24. PMID:15569053
521. Calgüneri M, Oztürk MA, Ozbalkan Z, et al. Frequency of lymphadenopathy in rheumatoid arthritis and systemic lupus erythematosus. J Int Med Res. 2003 Jul-Aug;31(4):345–9. PMID:12964513
522. Call TG, Norman AD, Hanson CA, et al. Incidence of chronic lymphocytic leukemia and high-count monoclonal B-cell lymphocytosis using the 2008 guidelines. Cancer. 2014 Jul 1;120(13):2000–5. PMID:24711224
523. Callet-Bauchu E, Baseggio L, Felman P, et al. Cytogenetic analysis delineates a spectrum of chromosomal changes that can distinguish non-MALT marginal zone B-cell lymphomas among mature B-cell entities: a description of 103 cases. Leukemia. 2005 Oct;19(10):1818–23. PMID:16094418
524. Caltharp SA, Qayed M, Park SI. Atypical marginal zone hyperplasia is a mimic for lymphoma in pediatric transplant recipients: report of two patients. Pediatr Dev Pathol. 2015 Sep-Oct;18(5):416–21. PMID:25955878
525. Calvo KR, Price S, Braylan RC, et al. JMML and RALD (Ras-associated autoimmune leukoproliferative disorder): common genetic etiology yet clinically distinct entities. Blood. 2015 Apr 30;125(18):2753–8. PMID:25691160
526. Camacho FI, Algara P, Mollejo M, et al. Nodal marginal zone lymphoma: a heterogeneous tumor: a comprehensive analysis of a series of 27 cases. Am J Surg Pathol. 2003 Jun;27(6):762–71. PMID:12766579
527. Camacho FI, García JF, Cigudosa JC, et al. Aberrant Bcl6 protein expression in mantle cell lymphoma. Am J Surg Pathol. 2004 Aug;28(8):1051–6. PMID:15252312
528. Camacho FI, Mollejo M, Mateo MS, et al. Progression to large B-cell lymphoma in splenic marginal zone lymphoma: a description of a series of 12 cases. Am J Surg Pathol. 2001 Oct;25(10):1268–76. PMID:11688461
529. Camilleri-Broët S, Davi F, Feuillard J, et al. AIDS-related primary brain lymphomas: histopathologic and immunohistochemical study of 51 cases. Hum Pathol. 1997 Mar;28(3):367–74. PMID:9042803
530. Campana D, Coustan-Smith E. Minimal residual disease studies by flow cytometry in acute leukemia. Acta Haematol. 2004;112(1-2):8–15. PMID:15178999
531. Campbell J, Seymour JF, Matthews J, et al. The prognostic impact of bone marrow involvement in patients with diffuse large cell lymphoma varies according to the degree of infiltration and presence of discordant marrow involvement. Eur J Haematol. 2006 Jun;76(6):473–80. PMID:16529599
532. Campbell JJ, Clark RA, Watanabe R, et al. Sezary syndrome and mycosis fungoides arise from distinct T-cell subsets: a biologic rationale for their distinct clinical behaviors. Blood. 2010 Aug 5;116(5):767–71. PMID:20484084
533. Campo E, Cymbalista F, Ghia P, et al. TP53 aberrations in chronic lymphocytic leukemia: an overview of the clinical implications of improved diagnostics. Haematologica. 2018 Dec;103(12):1956–68. PMID:30442727
534. Campo E, Miquel R, Krenacs L, et al. Primary nodal marginal zone lymphomas of splenic and MALT type. Am J Surg Pathol. 1999 Jan;23(1):59–68. PMID:9888704
535. Campo E, Rule S. Mantle cell lymphoma: evolving management strategies. Blood. 2015 Jan 1;125(1):48–55. PMID:25499451
536. Campos KR, Santos FLN, da Silva Brito V, et al. Line immunoassay for confirmation and discrimination of human T-cell lymphotropic virus infections in inconclusive western blot serum samples from Brazil. J Clin Microbiol. 2019 Dec 23;58(1):e01384-19. PMID:31597749
537. Camus V, Rossi C, Sesques P, et al. Outcomes after first-line immunochemotherapy for primary mediastinal B-cell lymphoma: a LYSA study. Blood Adv. 2021 Oct 12;5(19):3862–72. PMID:34461634
538. Canioni D, Arnulf B, Asso-Bonnet M, et al. Nasal natural killer lymphoma associated with Epstein-Barr virus in a patient infected with human immunodeficiency virus. Arch Pathol Lab Med. 2001 May;125(5):660–2. PMID:11300939
539. Canman CE, Lim DS, Cimprich KA, et al. Activation of the ATM kinase by ionizing radiation and phosphorylation of p53. Science. 1998 Sep 11;281(5383):1677–9. PMID:9733515
540. Cannon T, Mobarek D, Wegge J, et al. Hairy cell leukemia: current concepts. Cancer Invest. 2008 Oct;26(8):860–5. PMID:18798068
541. Cao C, Feng J, Gu H, et al. Distribution of lymphoid neoplasms in Northwest China: analysis of 3244 cases according to WHO classification in a single institution. Ann Diagn Pathol. 2018 Jun;34:60–5. PMID:29661730
542. Cao F, Zhao H, Li Y, et al. Clinicopathological and phenotypic features of chronic NK cell lymphocytosis identified among patients with asymptomatic lymphocytosis. Int J Lab Hematol. 2015 Dec;37(6):783–90. PMID:26234181
543. Cao X, Medeiros LJ, Xia Y, et al. Clinicopathologic features and outcomes of lymphoplasmacytic lymphoma patients with monoclonal IgG or IgA paraprotein expression. Leuk Lymphoma. 2016 May;57(5):1104–13. PMID:26421453
544. Cao Z, Wang Q, Li J, et al. Multifocal sclerosing angiomatoid nodular transformation of the spleen: a case report and review of literature. Diagn Pathol. 2015 Jul 11;10:95. PMID:26159169
545. Capello D, Rossi D, Gaidano G. Post-transplant lymphoproliferative disorders: molecular basis of disease histogenesis and pathogenesis. Hematol Oncol. 2005 Jun;23(2):61–7. PMID:16216037
546. Caprini E, Cristofoletti C, Arcelli D, et al. Identification of key regions and genes important in the pathogenesis of Sezary syndrome by combining genomic and expression microarrays. Cancer Res. 2009 Nov 1;69(21):8438–46. PMID:19843862
547. Carbone A. The spectrum of AIDS-related lymphoproliferative disorders. Adv Clin Path. 1997 Jan;1(1):13–9. PMID:10352465
548. Carbone A, Gloghini A. "Intrafollicular neoplasia" of nodular lymphocyte predominant Hodgkin lymphoma: description of a hypothetic early step of the disease. Hum Pathol. 2012 May;43(5):619–28. PMID:22209342
549. Carbone A, Santoro A. How I treat: diagnosing and managing "in situ" lymphoma. Blood. 2011 Apr 14;117(15):3954–60. PMID:21224472
550. Carbone A, Spina M, Gloghini A, et al. Nodular lymphocyte predominant Hodgkin lymphoma with non-invasive or early invasive growth pattern suggests an early step of the disease with a highly favorable outcome. Am J Hematol. 2013 Feb;88(2):161–2. PMID:23349009
551. Carbone A, Vaccher E, Gloghini A. Hematologic cancers in individuals infected by HIV. Blood. 2022 Feb 17;139(7):995–1012. PMID:34469512
552. Carbone PP, Berard CW, Bennett JM, et al. NIH clinical staff conference. Burkitt's tumor. Ann Intern Med. 1969 Apr;70(4):817–32. PMID:4306129
553. Carbonnel F, d'Almagne H, Lavergne A, et al. The clinicopathological features of extensive small intestinal CD4 T cell infiltration. Gut. 1999 Nov;45(5):662–7. PMID:10517900
554. Cardenas-de la Garza JA, Esquivel-Valerio JA, Arvizu-Rivera RI, et al. Flushing out a plasmacytoma in a patient with POEMS and AESOP syndromes. Lancet. 2020 Aug 29;396(10251):e21. PMID:32861309
555. Cardenas-Garcia J, Talwar A, Shah R, et al. Update in primary pulmonary lymphomas. Curr Opin Pulm Med. 2015 Jul;21(4):333–7. PMID:25978630
556. Cardoso CC, Auat M, Santos-Pirath IM, et al. The importance of CD39, CD43, CD81, and CD95 expression for differentiating B cell lymphoma by flow cytometry.

Cytometry B Clin Cytom. 2018 May;94(3):451–8. PMID:28509416
557. Carey CD, Gusenleitner D, Lipschitz M, et al. Topological analysis reveals a PD-L1-associated microenvironmental niche for Reed-Sternberg cells in Hodgkin lymphoma. Blood. 2017 Nov 30;130(22):2420–30. PMID:28893733
558. Cario G, Leoni V, Conter V, et al. BCR-ABL1-like acute lymphoblastic leukemia in childhood and targeted therapy. Haematologica. 2020 Sep 1;105(9):2200–4. PMID:33054045
559. Carlotti E, Wrench D, Matthews J, et al. Transformation of follicular lymphoma to diffuse large B-cell lymphoma may occur by divergent evolution from a common progenitor cell or by direct evolution from the follicular lymphoma clone. Blood. 2009 Apr 9;113(15):3553–7. PMID:19202129
560. Carlsen ED, Bhavsar S, Cook JR, et al. IRTA1 positivity helps identify a MALT-lymphoma-like subset of primary cutaneous marginal zone lymphomas, largely but not exclusively defined by IgM expression. J Cutan Pathol. 2022 Jan;49(1):55–60. PMID:34309899
561. Carlsen ED, Swerdlow SH, Cook JR, et al. Class-switched primary cutaneous marginal zone lymphomas are frequently IgG4-positive and have features distinct from IgM-positive cases. Am J Surg Pathol. 2019 Oct;43(10):1403–12. PMID:31464711
562. Carrasquillo JA, Chen CC, Price S, et al. 18F-FDG PET imaging features of patients with autoimmune lymphoproliferative syndrome. Clin Nucl Med. 2019 Dec;44(12):949–55. PMID:31689275
563. Carroll AJ, Shago M, Mikhail FM, et al. Masked hypodiploidy: hypodiploid acute lymphoblastic leukemia (ALL) mimicking hyperdiploid ALL in children: a report from the Children's Oncology Group. Cancer Genet. 2019 Oct;238:62–8. PMID:31425927
564. Carvajal-Cuenca A, Sua LF, Silva NM, et al. In situ mantle cell lymphoma: clinical implications of an incidental finding with indolent clinical behavior. Haematologica. 2012 Feb;97(2):270–8. PMID:22058203
565. Casadei B, Argnani L, Morigi A, et al. Treatment and outcomes of primary mediastinal B cell lymphoma: a three-decade monocentric experience with 151 patients. Ann Hematol. 2021 Sep;100(9):2261–8. PMID:33305333
566. Casamayor-Polo L, López-Nevado M, Paz-Artal E, et al. Immunologic evaluation and genetic defects of apoptosis in patients with autoimmune lymphoproliferative syndrome (ALPS). Crit Rev Clin Lab Sci. 2021 Jun;58(4):253–74. PMID:33356695
567. Cassidy DP, Vega F, Chapman JR. Epstein-Barr virus-positive extranodal marginal zone lymphoma of bronchial-associated lymphoid tissue in the posttransplant setting: an immunodeficiency-related (posttransplant) lymphoproliferative disorder? Am J Clin Pathol. 2017 Dec 20;149(1):42–9. PMID:29228090
568. Cassim S, Antel K, Chetty DR, et al. Diffuse large B-cell lymphoma in a South African cohort with a high HIV prevalence: an analysis by cell-of-origin, Epstein-Barr virus infection and survival. Pathology. 2020 Jun;52(4):453–9. PMID:32305135
569. Castelli R, Schiavon R, Preti C, et al. HIV-related lymphoproliferative diseases in the era of combination antiretroviral therapy. Cardiovasc Hematol Disord Drug Targets. 2020;20(3):175–80. PMID:32294049
570. Castelli R, Wu MA, Arquati M, et al. High prevalence of splenic marginal zone lymphoma among patients with acquired C1 inhibitor deficiency. Br J Haematol. 2016 Mar;172(6):902–8. PMID:26728240
571. Castillo JJ, Beltran BE, Malpica L, et al. Anaplastic lymphoma kinase-positive large B-cell lymphoma (ALK+ LBCL): a systematic review of clinicopathological features and management. Leuk Lymphoma. 2021 Dec;62(12):2845–53. PMID:34151703
572. Castillo JJ, Bibas M, Miranda RN. The biology and treatment of plasmablastic lymphoma. Blood. 2015 Apr 9;125(15):2323–30. PMID:25636338
573. Castillo JJ, Itchaki G, Gustine JN, et al. A matched case-control study comparing features, treatment and outcomes between patients with non-IgM lymphoplasmacytic lymphoma and Waldenström macroglobulinemia. Leuk Lymphoma. 2020 Jun;61(6):1388–94. PMID:31992103
574. Castor A, Nilsson L, Astrand-Grundström I, et al. Distinct patterns of hematopoietic stem cell involvement in acute lymphoblastic leukemia. Nat Med. 2005 Jun;11(6):630–7. PMID:15908956
575. Casulo C, Byrtek M, Dawson KL, et al. Early relapse of follicular lymphoma after rituximab plus cyclophosphamide, doxorubicin, vincristine, and prednisone defines patients at high risk for death: an analysis from the National LymphoCare Study. J Clin Oncol. 2015 Aug 10;33(23):2516–22. PMID:26124482
576. Catassi C, Bearzi I, Holmes GK. Association of celiac disease and intestinal lymphomas and other cancers. Gastroenterology. 2005 Apr;128(4 Suppl 1):S79–86. PMID:15825131
577. Cavalli F, Ceriani L, Zucca E. Functional imaging using 18-fluorodeoxyglucose PET in the management of primary mediastinal large B-cell lymphoma: the contributions of the International Extranodal Lymphoma Study Group. Am Soc Clin Oncol Educ Book. 2016;35:e368–75. PMID:27249743
578. Cavé H, Cacheux V, Raynaud S, et al. ETV6 is the target of chromosome 12p deletions in t(12;21) childhood acute lymphocytic leukemia. Leukemia. 1997 Sep;11(9):1459–64. PMID:9305598
579. Caviglia GP, Sciacca C, Abate ML, et al. Chronic hepatitis C virus infection and lymphoproliferative disorders: mixed cryoglobulinemia syndrome, monoclonal gammopathy of undetermined significance, and B-cell non-Hodgkin lymphoma. J Gastroenterol Hepatol. 2015 Apr;30(4):742–7. PMID:25351042
580. Cavo M, San-Miguel J, Usmani SZ, et al. Prognostic value of minimal residual disease negativity in myeloma: combined analysis of POLLUX, CASTOR, ALCYONE, and MAIA. Blood. 2022 Feb 10;139(6):835–44. PMID:34289038
581. Cawley JC, Burns GF, Hayhoe FG. A chronic lymphoproliferative disorder with distinctive features: a distinct variant of hairy-cell leukaemia. Leuk Res. 1980;4(6):547–59. PMID:7206776
582. Cazals-Hatem D, Lepage E, Brice P, et al. Primary mediastinal large B-cell lymphoma. A clinicopathologic study of 141 cases compared with 916 nonmediastinal large B-cell lymphomas, a GELA ("Groupe d'Etude des Lymphomes de l'Adulte") study. Am J Surg Pathol. 1996 Jul;20(7):877–88. PMID:8669537
583. Cazzaniga G, De Lorenzo P, Alten J, et al. Predictive value of minimal residual disease in Philadelphia-chromosome-positive acute lymphoblastic leukemia treated with imatinib in the European intergroup study of post-induction treatment of Philadelphia-chromosome-positive acute lymphoblastic leukemia, based on immunoglobulin/T-cell receptor and BCR/ABL1 methodologies. Haematologica. 2018 Jan;103(1):107–15. PMID:29079599
584. Cellier C, Patey N, Mauvieux L, et al. Abnormal intestinal intraepithelial lymphocytes in refractory sprue. Gastroenterology. 1998 Mar;114(3):471–81. PMID:9496937
585. Cerhan JR. Epidemiology of follicular lymphoma. Hematol Oncol Clin North Am. 2020 Aug;34(4):631–46. PMID:32586570
586. Cerhan JR, Berndt SI, Vijai J, et al. Genome-wide association study identifies multiple susceptibility loci for diffuse large B cell lymphoma. Nat Genet. 2014 Nov;46(11):1233–8. PMID:25261932
587. Cerhan JR, Habermann TM. Epidemiology of marginal zone lymphoma. Ann Lymphoma. 2021 Mar;5(Mar):5. PMID:33829216
588. Cerhan JR, Kricker A, Paltiel O, et al. Medical history, lifestyle, family history, and occupational risk factors for diffuse large B-cell lymphoma: the InterLymph Non-Hodgkin Lymphoma Subtypes Project. J Natl Cancer Inst Monogr. 2014 Aug;2014(48):15–25. PMID:25174023
589. Ceriani L, Milan L, Martelli M, et al. Metabolic heterogeneity on baseline 18FDG-PET/CT scan is a predictor of outcome in primary mediastinal B-cell lymphoma. Blood. 2018 Jul 12;132(2):179–86. PMID:29720487
590. Cerroni L, Arzberger E, Pütz B, et al. Primary cutaneous follicle center cell lymphoma with follicular growth pattern. Blood. 2000 Jun 15;95(12):3922–8. PMID:10845929
591. Cerroni L, El-Shabrawi-Caelen L, Fink-Puches R, et al. Cutaneous spindle-cell B-cell lymphoma: a morphologic variant of cutaneous large B-cell lymphoma. Am J Dermatopathol. 2000 Aug;22(4):299–304. PMID:10949453
592. Cerroni L, Massone C, Kutzner H, et al. Intravascular large T-cell or NK-cell lymphoma: a rare variant of intravascular large cell lymphoma with frequent cytotoxic phenotype and association with Epstein-Barr virus infection. Am J Surg Pathol. 2008 Jun;32(6):891–8. PMID:18425045
593. Cerroni L, Zöchling N, Pütz B, et al. Infection by Borrelia burgdorferi and cutaneous B-cell lymphoma. J Cutan Pathol. 1997 Sep;24(8):457–61. PMID:9331890
594. Cesarman E, Chadburn A, Rubinstein PG. KSHV/HHV8-mediated hematologic diseases. Blood. 2022 Feb 17;139(7):1013–25. PMID:34479367
595. Cesarman E, Chang Y, Moore PS, et al. Kaposi's sarcoma-associated herpesvirus-like DNA sequences in AIDS-related body-cavity-based lymphomas. N Engl J Med. 1995 May 4;332(18):1186–91. PMID:7700311
596. Cesarman E, Damania B, Krown SE, et al. Kaposi sarcoma. Nat Rev Dis Primers. 2019 Jan 31;5(1):9. PMID:30705286
597. Cessna MH, Hartung L, Tripp S, et al. Hairy cell leukemia variant: fact or fiction. Am J Clin Pathol. 2005 Jan;123(1):132–8. PMID:15762289
598. Cetinözman F, Jansen PM, Vermeer MH, et al. Differential expression of programmed death-1 (PD-1) in Sézary syndrome and mycosis fungoides. Arch Dermatol. 2012 Dec;148(12):1379–85. PMID:23247480
599. Cetinözman F, Jansen PM, Willemze R. Expression of programmed death-1 in primary cutaneous CD4-positive small/medium-sized pleomorphic T-cell lymphoma, cutaneous pseudo-T-cell lymphoma, and other types of cutaneous T-cell lymphoma. Am J Surg Pathol. 2012 Jan;36(1):109–16. PMID:21989349
600. Chadburn A, Abdul-Nabi AM, Teruya BS, et al. Lymphoid proliferations associated with human immunodeficiency virus infection. Arch Pathol Lab Med. 2013 Mar;137(3):360–70. PMID:23451747
601. Chadburn A, Cesarman E, Liu YF, et al. Molecular genetic analysis demonstrates that multiple posttransplantation lymphoproliferative disorders occurring in one anatomic site in a single patient represent distinct primary lymphoid neoplasms. Cancer. 1995 Jun 1;75(11):2747–56. PMID:7743481
602. Chadburn A, Chen JM, Hsu DT, et al. The morphologic and molecular genetic categories of posttransplantation lymphoproliferative disorders are clinically relevant. Cancer. 1998 May 15;82(10):1978–87. PMID:9587133
603. Chadburn A, Hyjek E, Mathew S, et al. KSHV-positive solid lymphomas represent an extra-cavitary variant of primary effusion lymphoma. Am J Surg Pathol. 2004 Nov;28(11):1401–16. PMID:15489644
604. Chadburn A, Hyjek EM, Tam W, et al. Immunophenotypic analysis of the Kaposi sarcoma herpesvirus (KSHV; HHV-8)-infected B cells in HIV+ multicentric Castleman disease (MCD). Histopathology. 2008 Nov;53(5):513–24. PMID:18983461
605. Chadburn A, Metroka C, Mouradian J. Progressive lymph node histology and its prognostic value in patients with acquired immunodeficiency syndrome and AIDS-related complex. Hum Pathol. 1989 Jun;20(6):579–87. PMID:2722179
606. Chadburn A, Said J, Gratzinger D, et al. HHV8/KSHV-positive lymphoproliferative disorders and the spectrum of plasmablastic and plasma cell neoplasms: 2015 SH/EAHP Workshop Report-Part 3. Am J Clin Pathol. 2017 Feb 1;147(2):171–87. PMID:28395104
607. Chaganti RS, Schonberg S, German J. A manyfold increase in sister chromatid exchanges in Bloom's syndrome lymphocytes. Proc Natl Acad Sci U S A. 1974 Nov;71(11):4508–12. PMID:4140506
608. Chaganti S, Illidge T, Barrington S, et al. Guidelines for the management of diffuse large B-cell lymphoma. Br J Haematol. 2016 Jul;174(1):43–56. PMID:27196701
609. Challagundla P, Medeiros LJ, Kanagal-Shamanna R, et al. Differential expression of CD200 in B-cell neoplasms by flow cytometry can assist in diagnosis, subclassification, and bone marrow staging. Am J Clin Pathol. 2014 Dec;142(6):837–44. PMID:25389338
610. Chamuleau MED, Burggraaff CN, Nijland M, et al. Treatment of patients with MYC rearrangement positive large B-cell lymphoma with R-CHOP plus lenalidomide: results of a multicenter HOVON phase II trial. Haematologica. 2020 Dec 1;105(12):2805–12. PMID:33256379
611. Chan A, Scarpa Carniello JV, Gao Q, et al. Role of flow cytometric immunophenotyping for classic Hodgkin lymphoma in small biopsy and cytology specimens. Arch Pathol Lab Med. 2022 Apr 1;146(4):462–8. PMID:34293084
612. Chan AC, Chan KW, Chan JK, et al. Development of follicular dendritic cell sarcoma in hyaline-vascular Castleman's disease of the nasopharynx: tracing its evolution by sequential biopsies. Histopathology. 2001 Jun;38(6):510–8. PMID:11422494
613. Chan AC, Serrano-Olmo J, Erlandson RA, et al. Cytokeratin-positive malignant tumors with reticulum cell morphology: a subtype of fibroblastic reticulum cell neoplasm? Am J Surg Pathol. 2000 Jan;24(1):107–16. PMID:10632494
614. Chan FC, Mottok A, Gerrie AS, et al. Prognostic model to predict post-autologous stem-cell transplantation outcomes in classical Hodgkin lymphoma. J Clin Oncol. 2017 Nov 10;35(32):3722–33. PMID:28898161
615. Chan JK. Natural killer cell neoplasms. Anat Pathol. 1998;3:77–145. PMID:10389582
616. Chan JK, Chan AC, Cheuk W, et al. Type II enteropathy-associated T-cell lymphoma: a distinct aggressive lymphoma with frequent γδ T-cell receptor expression. Am J Surg Pathol. 2011 Oct;35(10):1557–69. PMID:21921780
617. Chan JK, Fletcher CD, Nayler SJ, et al. Follicular dendritic cell sarcoma.

Clinicopathologic analysis of 17 cases suggesting a malignant potential higher than currently recognized. Cancer. 1997 Jan 15;79(2):294–313. PMID:9010103

618. Chan JK, Frizzera G, Fletcher CD, et al. Primary vascular tumors of lymph nodes other than Kaposi's sarcoma. Analysis of 39 cases and delineation of two new entities. Am J Surg Pathol. 1992 Apr;16(4):335–50. PMID:1373579

619. Chan JK, Lewin KJ, Lombard CM, et al. Histopathology of bacillary angiomatosis of lymph node. Am J Surg Pathol. 1991 May;15(5):430–7. PMID:2035737

620. Chan JK, Sin VC, Wong KF, et al. Nonnasal lymphoma expressing the natural killer cell marker CD56: a clinicopathologic study of 49 cases of an uncommon aggressive neoplasm. Blood. 1997 Jun 15;89(12):4501–13. PMID:9192774

621. Chan JK, Tsang WY, Ng CS. Clarification of CD3 immunoreactivity in nasal T/natural killer cell lymphomas: the neoplastic cells are often CD3 epsilon+. Blood. 1996 Jan 15;87(2):839–41. PMID:8555511

622. Chan JK, Tsang WY, Ng CS. Follicular dendritic cell tumor and vascular neoplasm complicating hyaline-vascular Castleman's disease. Am J Surg Pathol. 1994 May;18(5):517–25. PMID:8172326

623. Chan JK, Warnke RA, Dorfman R. Vascular transformation of sinuses in lymph nodes. A study of its morphological spectrum and distinction from Kaposi's sarcoma. Am J Surg Pathol. 1991 Aug;15(8):732–43. PMID:2069211

624. Chan JK, Wong KC, Ng CS. A fatal case of multicentric Kikuchi's histiocytic necrotizing lymphadenitis. Cancer. 1989 May 1;63(9):1856–62. PMID:2784712

625. Chan JK, Yip TT, Tsang WY, et al. Detection of Epstein-Barr viral RNA in malignant lymphomas of the upper aerodigestive tract. Am J Surg Pathol. 1994 Sep;18(9):938–46. PMID:8067515

626. Chan WK, Au WY, Wong CY, et al. Metabolic activity measured by F-18 FDG PET in natural killer-cell lymphoma compared to aggressive B- and T-cell lymphomas. Clin Nucl Med. 2010 Aug;35(8):571–5. PMID:20631501

627. Chandran R, Gardiner SK, Fenske TS, et al. Survival trends in T cell prolymphocytic leukemia: a SEER database analysis. Leuk Lymphoma. 2016;57(4):942–4. PMID:26292711

628. Chandran R, Gardiner SK, Smith SD, et al. Improved survival in hairy cell leukaemia over three decades: a SEER database analysis of prognostic factors. Br J Haematol. 2013 Nov;163(3):407–9. PMID:23889044

629. Chang KC, Lee JC, Wang YC, et al. Polyclonality in sclerosing angiomatoid nodular transformation of the spleen. Am J Surg Pathol. 2016 Oct;40(10):1343–51. PMID:27526296

630. Chang KC, Wang YC, Hung LY, et al. Monoclonality and cytogenetic abnormalities in hyaline vascular Castleman disease. Mod Pathol. 2014 Jun;27(6):823–31. PMID:24201121

631. Chang KL, Kamel OW, Arber DA, et al. Pathologic features of nodular lymphocyte predominance Hodgkin's disease in extranodal sites. Am J Surg Pathol. 1995 Nov;19(11):1313–24. PMID:7573694

632. Chang LW, Patrone CC, Yang W, et al. An integrated data resource for genomic analysis of cutaneous T-cell lymphoma. J Invest Dermatol. 2018 Dec;138(12):2681–3. PMID:29981755

633. Chang SH, Luo S, Thomas TS, et al. Obesity and the transformation of monoclonal gammopathy of undetermined significance to multiple myeloma: a population-based cohort study. J Natl Cancer Inst. 2016 Dec 31;109(5):djw264. PMID:28040690

634. Chanudet E, Ye H, Ferry J, et al. A20 deletion is associated with copy number gain at the TNFA/B/C locus and occurs preferentially in translocation-negative MALT lymphoma of the ocular adnexa and salivary glands. J Pathol. 2009 Feb;217(3):420–30. PMID:19006194

635. Chanudet E, Zhou Y, Bacon CM, et al. Chlamydia psittaci is variably associated with ocular adnexal MALT lymphoma in different geographical regions. J Pathol. 2006 Jul;209(3):344–51. PMID:16583361

636. Chao C, Silverberg MJ, Xu L, et al. A comparative study of molecular characteristics of diffuse large B-cell lymphoma from patients with and without human immunodeficiency virus infection. Clin Cancer Res. 2015 Mar 15;21(6):1429–37. PMID:25589617

637. Chao C, Xu L, Silverberg MJ, et al. Stromal immune infiltration in HIV-related diffuse large B-cell lymphoma is associated with HIV disease history and patient survival. AIDS. 2015 Sep 24;29(15):1943–51. PMID:26355571

638. Chapman J, Gentles AJ, Sujoy V, et al. Gene expression analysis of plasmablastic lymphoma identifies downregulation of B-cell receptor signaling and additional unique transcriptional programs. Leukemia. 2015 Nov;29(11):2270–3. PMID:25921246

639. Chapman JR, Alvarez JP, White K, et al. Unusual variants of follicular lymphoma: case-based review. Am J Surg Pathol. 2020 Mar;44(3):329–39. PMID:31688142

640. Chapman JR, Bouska AC, Zhang W, et al. EBV-positive HIV-associated diffuse large B cell lymphomas are characterized by JAK/STAT (STAT3) pathway mutations and unique clinicopathologic features. Br J Haematol. 2021 Sep;194(5):870–8. PMID:34272731

641. Chapuy B, Roemer MG, Stewart C, et al. Targetable genetic features of primary testicular and primary central nervous system lymphomas. Blood. 2016 Feb 18;127(7):869–81. PMID:26702065

642. Chapuy B, Stewart C, Dunford AJ, et al. Author correction: Molecular subtypes of diffuse large B cell lymphoma are associated with distinct pathogenic mechanisms and outcomes. Nat Med. 2018 Aug;24(8):1290–1. PMID:29955182

643. Chapuy B, Stewart C, Dunford AJ, et al. Genomic analyses of PMBL reveal new drivers and mechanisms of sensitivity to PD-1 blockade. Blood. 2019 Dec 26;134(26):2369–82. PMID:31697821

644. Chapuy B, Stewart C, Dunford AJ, et al. Molecular subtypes of diffuse large B cell lymphoma are associated with distinct pathogenic mechanisms and outcomes. Nat Med. 2018 May;24(5):679–90. PMID:29713087

645. Charalabopoulos K, Charalabopoulos A, Binolis J, et al. Is implant pacemaker a physicochemical cause triggering Kikuchi-Fujimoto disease? In Vivo. 2002 Jan-Feb;16(1):73–6. PMID:11980366

646. Charli-Joseph Y, Kashani-Sabet M, McCalmont TH, et al. Association of a proposed new staging system for folliculotropic mycosis fungoides with prognostic variables in a US cohort. JAMA Dermatol. 2021 Feb 1;157(2):157–65. PMID:33295938

647. Chatterjee G, Dudakia V, Ghogale S, et al. Expression of CD304/neuropilin-1 in adult B-cell lymphoblastic leukemia/lymphoma and its utility for the measurable residual disease assessment. Int J Lab Hematol. 2021 Oct;43(5):990–9. PMID:33432783

648. Chatterjee G, Gujral S, Subramanian PG, et al. Clinical relevance of multicolour flow cytometry in plasma cell disorders. Indian J Hematol Blood Transfus. 2017 Sep;33(3):303–15. PMID:28824230

649. Chatterjee M, Osborne J, Bestetti G, et al. Viral IL-6-induced cell proliferation and immune evasion of interferon activity. Science. 2002 Nov 15;298(5597):1432–5. PMID:12434062

650. Chaudhary S, Brown N, Song JY, et al. Relative frequency and clinicopathologic characteristics of MYC-rearranged follicular lymphoma. Hum Pathol. 2021 Aug;114:19–27. PMID:33964277

651. Chauveau B, Le Loarer F, Bacci J, et al. [Indolent T-lymphoblastic proliferation in association with localized Castleman disease: a case report]. Ann Pathol. 2019 Feb;39(1):29–35. French. PMID:30554835

652. Chavez JC, Sandoval-Sus J, Horna P, et al. Lymphomatoid granulomatosis: a single institution experience and review of the literature. Clin Lymphoma Myeloma Leuk. 2016 Aug;16 Suppl:S170–4. PMID:27521314

653. Cheah CY, Wirth A, Seymour JF. Primary testicular lymphoma. Blood. 2014 Jan 23;123(4):486–93. PMID:24282217

654. Cheminant M, Bruneau J, Malamut G, et al. NKp46 is a diagnostic biomarker and may be a therapeutic target in gastrointestinal T-cell lymphoproliferative diseases: a CELAC study. Gut. 2019 Aug;68(8):1396–405. PMID:30448772

655. Chen BJ, Chapuy B, Ouyang J, et al. PD-L1 expression is characteristic of a subset of aggressive B-cell lymphomas and virus-associated malignancies. Clin Cancer Res. 2013 Jul 1;19(13):3462–73. PMID:23674495

656. Chen BJ, Wang RC, Ho CH, et al. Primary effusion lymphoma in Taiwan shows two distinctive clinicopathological subtypes with rare human immunodeficiency virus association. Histopathology. 2018 May;72(6):930–44. PMID:29206290

657. Chen C, Gong Y, Yang Y, et al. Clinicopathological and molecular genomic features of monomorphic epitheliotropic intestinal T-cell lymphoma in the Chinese population: a study of 20 cases. Diagn Pathol. 2021 Dec 12;16(1):114. PMID:34895266

658. Chen CN, Wang Z, Jiang Y, et al. [Monomorphic epitheliotropic intestinal T-cell lymphoma: a clinicopathological analysis of twelve cases]. Zhonghua Bing Li Xue Za Zhi. 2020 Jan 8;49(1):17–21. Chinese. PMID:31914529

659. Chen D, Camponeschi A, Nordlund J, et al. RAG1 co-expression signature identifies ETV6-RUNX1-like B-cell precursor acute lymphoblastic leukemia in children. Cancer Med. 2021 Jun;10(12):3997–4003. PMID:33987955

660. Chen D, Sandford G, Nicholas J. Intracellular signaling mechanisms and activities of human herpesvirus 8 interleukin-6. J Virol. 2009 Jan;83(2):722–33. PMID:18987143

661. Chen DB, Liu XY, Kong FZ, et al. Risk factors evaluation of post-transplant lymphoproliferative disorders after allogeneic haematopoietic stem cell transplantation with comparison between paediatric and adult. J Clin Pathol. 2021 Nov;74(11):697–703. PMID:34011618

662. Chen DB, Song QJ, Chen YX, et al. Clinicopathologic spectrum and EBV status of post-transplant lymphoproliferative disorders after allogeneic hematopoietic stem cell transplantation. Int J Hematol. 2013 Jan;97(1):117–24. PMID:23255160

663. Chen GL, Xia ZG, Jin J, et al. Characterization of artificial pneumothorax-unrelated pyothorax-associated lymphoma. J Oncol. 2021 Jan 25;2021:3869438. PMID:33564306

664. Chen J, Feng J, Xiao H, et al. Indolent T-lymphoblastic proliferation associated with Castleman disease and low grade follicular dendric cell sarcoma: report of a case and review of literature. Int J Clin Exp Pathol. 2019 Apr 1;12(4):1497–505. PMID:31933967

665. Chen J, Petrus M, Bamford R, et al. Increased serum soluble IL-15Rα levels in T-cell large granular lymphocyte leukemia. Blood. 2012 Jan 5;119(1):137–43. PMID:22049515

666. Chen JS, Coustan-Smith E, Suzuki T, et al. Identification of novel markers for monitoring minimal residual disease in acute lymphoblastic leukemia. Blood. 2001 Apr 1;97(7):2115–20. PMID:11264179

667. Chen JS, Tzeng CC, Tsao CJ, et al. Clonal karyotype abnormalities in EBV-associated hemophagocytic syndrome. Haematologica. 1997 Sep-Oct;82(5):572–6. PMID:9407723

668. Chen L, Al-Kzayer LF, Liu T, et al. IFR4/MUM1-positive lymphoma in Waldeyer ring with co-expression of CD5 and CD10. Pediatr Blood Cancer. 2017 Feb;64(2):311–4. PMID:27616053

669. Chen TC, Kuo TT, Ng KF. Follicular dendritic cell tumor of the liver: a clinicopathologic and Epstein-Barr virus study of two cases. Mod Pathol. 2001 Apr;14(4):354–60. PMID:11301353

670. Chen W, Gong QX, Li X, et al. [Clinicopathological study of large B-cell lymphoma with IRF4 rearrangement]. Zhonghua Bing Li Xue Za Zhi. 2020 Oct 8;49(10):1003–8. Chinese. PMID:32992413

671. Chen W, Lau SK, Fong D, et al. High frequency of clonal immunoglobulin receptor gene rearrangements in sporadic histiocytic/dendritic cell sarcomas. Am J Surg Pathol. 2009 Jun;33(6):863–73. PMID:19145200

672. Chen X, Cherian S. Immunophenotypic characterization of T-cell prolymphocytic leukemia. Am J Clin Pathol. 2013 Nov;140(5):727–35. PMID:24124154

673. Chen Y, Shi H, Li H, et al. Clinicopathological features of inflammatory pseudotumour-like follicular dendritic cell tumour of the abdomen. Histopathology. 2016 May;68(6):858–65. PMID:26332157

674. Chen YH, Gao J, Fan G, et al. Nuclear expression of sox11 is highly associated with mantle cell lymphoma but is independent of t(11;14)(q13;q32) in non-mantle cell B-cell neoplasms. Mod Pathol. 2010 Jan;23(1):105–12. PMID:19801969

675. Chen YH, Tallman MS, Goolsby C, et al. Immunophenotypic variations in hairy cell leukemia. Am J Clin Pathol. 2006 Feb;125(2):251–9. PMID:16393677

676. Chen YP, Jones D, Chen TY, et al. Epstein-Barr virus present in T cells or B cells shows differential effects on hemophagocytic symptoms associated with outcome in T-cell lymphomas. Leuk Lymphoma. 2014 Sep;55(9):2038–47. PMID:24180328

677. Chen YR, Lee CL, Lee YC, et al. Inflammatory pseudotumour-like follicular dendritic cell tumour of the colon with plasmacytosis mimicking EBV-positive lymphoproliferative disorder. Pathology. 2020 Jun;52(4):484–8. PMID:32327214

678. Chen YW, Guo T, Shen L, et al. Receptor-type tyrosine-protein phosphatase κ directly targets STAT3 activation for tumor suppression in nasal NK/T-cell lymphoma. Blood. 2015 Mar 5;125(10):1589–600. PMID:25612622

679. Chen Z, Hu S, Wang SA, et al. Chronic myeloid leukemia presenting in lymphoblastic crisis, a differential diagnosis with Philadelphia-positive B-lymphoblastic leukemia. Leuk Lymphoma. 2020 Dec;61(12):2831–8. PMID:32700989

680. Chen Z, Wang M, Guan P, et al. Comparison of systemic EBV-positive T-cell and NK-cell lymphoproliferative diseases of childhood based on classification evolution: new classification, old problems. Am J Surg Pathol. 2020 Aug;44(8):1061–72. PMID:32317607

681. Cheng CY, Sheng WH, Lo YC, et al. Clinical presentations, laboratory results and outcomes of patients with Kikuchi's disease: emphasis on the association between recurrent Kikuchi's disease and autoimmune diseases. J

Microbiol Immunol Infect. 2010 Oct;43(5):366–71. PMID:21075702
682. Cheng J, Klairmont MM, Choi JK. Peripheral blood flow cytometry for the diagnosis of pediatric acute leukemia: highly reliable with rare exceptions. Pediatr Blood Cancer. 2019 Jan;66(1):e27453. PMID:30255571
683. Cheng N, Chen J, Pan Y, et al. Splenic hamartoma with bizarre stromal cells: a case report and literature review. Diagn Pathol. 2018 Jan 22;13(1):8. PMID:29378604
684. Cheng S, Guo A, Lu P, et al. Functional characterization of BTK(C481S) mutation that confers ibrutinib resistance: exploration of alternative kinase inhibitors. Leukemia. 2015 Apr;29(4):895–900. PMID:25189416
685. Cheon H, Xing JC, Moosic KB, et al. Genomic landscape of TCRαβ and TCRγδ T-large granular lymphocyte leukemia. Blood. 2022 May 19;139(20):3058–72. PMID:35015834
686. Chesi M, Kuehl WM, Bergsagel PL. Recurrent immunoglobulin gene translocations identify distinct molecular subtypes of myeloma. Ann Oncol. 2000;11 Suppl 1:131–5. PMID:10707795
687. Cheson BD, Ansell S, Schwartz L, et al. Refinement of the Lugano classification lymphoma response criteria in the era of immunomodulatory therapy. Blood. 2016 Nov 24;128(21):2489–96. PMID:27574190
688. Cheson BD, Fisher RI, Barrington SF, et al. Recommendations for initial evaluation, staging, and response assessment of Hodgkin and non-Hodgkin lymphoma: the Lugano classification. J Clin Oncol. 2014 Sep 20;32(27):3059–68. PMID:25113753
689. Chester N, Babbe H, Pinkas J, et al. Mutation of the murine Bloom's syndrome gene produces global genome destabilization. Mol Cell Biol. 2006 Sep;26(17):6713–26. PMID:16914751
690. Chetaille B, Bertucci F, Finetti P, et al. Molecular profiling of classical Hodgkin lymphoma tissues uncovers variations in the tumor microenvironment and correlations with EBV infection and outcome. Blood. 2009 Mar 19;113(12):2765–3775. PMID:19096012
691. Chetty R, Pulford K, Jones M, et al. SCL/Tal-1 expression in T-acute lymphoblastic leukemia: an immunohistochemical and genotypic study. Hum Pathol. 1995 Sep;26(9):994–8. PMID:7672800
692. Cheuk W, Chan AC, Chan JK, et al. Metallic implant-associated lymphoma: a distinct subgroup of large B-cell lymphoma related to pyothorax-associated lymphoma? Am J Surg Pathol. 2005 Jun;29(6):832–6. PMID:15897752
693. Cheuk W, Chan JK. Kuttner tumor of the submandibular gland: fine-needle aspiration cytologic findings of seven cases. Am J Clin Pathol. 2002 Jan;117(1):103–8. PMID:11791589
694. Cheuk W, Chan JK, Shek TW, et al. Inflammatory pseudotumor-like follicular dendritic cell tumor: a distinctive low-grade malignant intra-abdominal neoplasm with consistent Epstein-Barr virus association. Am J Surg Pathol. 2001 Jun;25(6):721–31. PMID:11395549
695. Cheuk W, Lee AK, Arora N, et al. Splenic hamartoma with bizarre stromal cells. Am J Surg Pathol. 2005 Jan;29(1):109–14. PMID:15613862
696. Cheuk W, Tam FK, Chan AN, et al. Idiopathic cervical fibrosis–a new member of IgG4-related sclerosing diseases: report of 4 cases, 1 complicated by composite lymphoma. Am J Surg Pathol. 2010 Nov;34(11):1678–85. PMID:20871392
697. Cheuk W, Wong KO, Wong CS, et al. Consistent immunostaining for cyclin D1 can be achieved on a routine basis using a newly available rabbit monoclonal antibody. Am J Surg Pathol. 2004 Jun;28(6):801–7. PMID:15166673
698. Cheuk W, Yuen HK, Chan JK. Chronic sclerosing dacryoadenitis: part of the spectrum of IgG4-related Sclerosing disease? Am J Surg Pathol. 2007 Apr;31(4):643–5. PMID:17414116
699. Cheuk W, Yuen HK, Chu SY, et al. Lymphadenopathy of IgG4-related sclerosing disease. Am J Surg Pathol. 2008 May;32(5):671–81. PMID:18344866
700. Cheung KJ, Horsman DE, Gascoyne RD. The significance of TP53 in lymphoid malignancies: mutation prevalence, regulation, prognostic impact and potential as a therapeutic target. Br J Haematol. 2009 Aug;146(3):257–69. PMID:19500100
701. Cheung KJ, Johnson NA, Affleck JG, et al. Acquired TNFRSF14 mutations in follicular lymphoma are associated with worse prognosis. Cancer Res. 2010 Nov 15;70(22):9166–74. PMID:20884631
702. Cheung MC, Bailey D, Pennell N, et al. In situ localization of follicular lymphoma: evidence for subclinical systemic disease with detection of an identical BCL-2/IGH fusion gene in blood and lymph node. Leukemia. 2009 Jun;23(6):1176–9. PMID:19212334
703. Chiang AK, Wong KY, Liang AC, et al. Comparative analysis of Epstein-Barr virus gene polymorphisms in nasal T/NK-cell lymphomas and normal nasal tissues: implications on virus strain selection in malignancy. Int J Cancer. 1999 Jan 29;80(3):356–64. PMID:9935174
704. Chiattone CS, Gabus R, Pavlovsky MA, et al. Management of chronic lymphocytic leukemia in less-resourced countries. Cancer J. 2021 Jul-Aug;27(4):314–9. PMID:34398558
705. Chiba S, Sakata-Yanagimoto M. Advances in understanding of angioimmunoblastic T-cell lymphoma. Leukemia. 2020 Oct;34(10):2592–606. PMID:32704161
706. Chigrinova E, Rinaldi A, Kwee I, et al. Two main genetic pathways lead to the transformation of chronic lymphocytic leukemia to Richter syndrome. Blood. 2013 Oct 10;122(15):2673–82. PMID:24004666
707. Chihara D, Arons E, Stetler-Stevenson M, et al. Randomized phase II study of first-line cladribine with concurrent or delayed rituximab in patients with hairy cell leukemia. J Clin Oncol. 2020 May 10;38(14):1527–38. PMID:32109194
708. Chihara D, Ito H, Matsuda T, et al. Differences in incidence and trends of haematological malignancies in Japan and the United States. Br J Haematol. 2014 Feb;164(4):536–45. PMID:24245986
709. Chihara D, Westin JR, Miranda RN, et al. Dose adjusted-EPOCH-R and mediastinal disease may improve outcomes for patients with gray-zone lymphoma. Br J Haematol. 2017 Nov;179(3):503–6. PMID:27378601
710. Chihara T, Wada N, Ikeda J, et al. Frequency of intravascular large B-cell lymphoma in Japan: study of the Osaka Lymphoma Study Group. J Hematol Oncol. 2011 Apr 11;4:14. PMID:21481222
711. Child FJ, Russell-Jones R, Woolford AJ, et al. Absence of the t(14;18) chromosomal translocation in primary cutaneous B-cell lymphoma. Br J Dermatol. 2001 Apr;144(4):735–44. PMID:11298531
712. Chilton L, Buck G, Harrison CJ, et al. High hyperdiploidy among adolescents and adults with acute lymphoblastic leukaemia (ALL): cytogenetic features, clinical characteristics and outcome. Leukemia. 2014 Jul;28(7):1511–8. PMID:24352198
713. Chiorazzi N, Ferrarini M. B cell chronic lymphocytic leukemia: lessons learned from studies of the B cell antigen receptor. Annu Rev Immunol. 2003;21:841–94. PMID:12615894
714. Chiorazzi N, Rai KR, Ferrarini M. Chronic lymphocytic leukemia. N Engl J Med. 2005 Feb 24;352(8):804–15. PMID:15728813
715. Chiron D, Di Liberto M, Martin P, et al. Cell-cycle reprogramming for PI3K inhibition overrides a relapse-specific C481S BTK mutation revealed by longitudinal functional genomics in mantle cell lymphoma. Cancer Discov. 2014 Sep;4(9):1022–35. PMID:25082755
716. Chisholm KM, Bangs CD, Bacchi CE, et al. Expression profiles of MYC protein and MYC gene rearrangement in lymphomas. Am J Surg Pathol. 2015 Mar;39(3):294–303. PMID:25581730
717. Chisholm KM, Mohlman J, Liew M, et al. IRF4 translocation status in pediatric follicular and diffuse large B-cell lymphoma patients enrolled in Children's Oncology Group trials. Pediatr Blood Cancer. 2019 Aug;66(8):e27770. PMID:31012208
718. Chittal SM, Caveriviere P, Schwarting R, et al. Monoclonal antibodies in the diagnosis of Hodgkin's disease. The search for a rational panel. Am J Surg Pathol. 1988 Jan;12(1):9–21. PMID:2827535
719. Chiu A, Czader M, Cheng L, et al. Clonal X-chromosome inactivation suggests that splenic cord capillary hemangioma is a true neoplasm and not a subtype of splenic hamartoma. Mod Pathol. 2011 Jan;24(1):108–16. PMID:20852592
720. Chiu BC, Dave BJ, Blair A, et al. Agricultural pesticide use and risk of t(14;18)-defined subtypes of non-Hodgkin lymphoma. Blood. 2006 Aug 15;108(4):1363–9. PMID:16621961
721. Chiu BC, Soni L, Gapstur SM, et al. Obesity and risk of non-Hodgkin lymphoma (United States). Cancer Causes Control. 2007 Aug;18(6):677–85. PMID:17484069
722. Chng WJ, Dispenzieri A, Chim CS, et al. IMWG consensus on risk stratification in multiple myeloma. Leukemia. 2014 Feb;28(2):269–77. PMID:23974982
723. Chng WJ, Huang GF, Chung TH, et al. Clinical and biological implications of MYC activation: a common difference between MGUS and newly diagnosed multiple myeloma. Leukemia. 2011 Jun;25(6):1026–35. PMID:21468039
724. Cho I, Yoon N, Hyeon J, et al. Comparison of the Lymph2Cx assay and Hans algorithm in determining the cell-of-origin of diffuse large B-cell lymphomas, not otherwise specified. Appl Immunohistochem Mol Morphol. 2020 Nov/Dec;28(10):731–40. PMID:32287077
725. Cho J, Gong G, Choe G, et al. Extrafollicular reticulum cells in pathologic lymph nodes. J Korean Med Sci. 1994 Feb;9(1):9–15. PMID:7520705
726. Cho JH, Kim HS, Ko YH, et al. Epstein-Barr virus infected natural killer cell lymphoma in a patient with hypersensitivity to mosquito bite. J Infect. 2006 Jun;52(6):e173–6. PMID:16246422
727. Cho YU, Chi HS, Park CJ, et al. Distinct features of angioimmunoblastic T-cell lymphoma with bone marrow involvement. Am J Clin Pathol. 2009 May;131(5):640–6. PMID:19369622
728. Choe JY, Go H, Jeon YK, et al. Inflammatory pseudotumor-like follicular dendritic cell sarcoma of the spleen: a report of six cases with increased IgG4-positive plasma cells. Pathol Int. 2013 May;63(5):245–51. PMID:23714251
729. Choi J, Goh G, Walradt T, et al. Genomic landscape of cutaneous T cell lymphoma. Nat Genet. 2015 Sep;47(9):1011–9. PMID:26192916
730. Choi PC, To KF, Lai FM, et al. Follicular dendritic cell sarcoma of the neck: report of two cases complicated by pulmonary metastases. Cancer. 2000 Aug 1;89(3):664–72. PMID:10931467
731. Choi YK, Yang JH, Ahn SY, et al. Retroperitoneal fibrosis in the era of immunoglobulin G4-related disease. Kidney Res Clin Pract. 2019 Mar 31;38(1):42–8. PMID:30754935
732. Chong LC, Ben-Neriah S, Slack GW, et al. High-resolution architecture and partner genes of MYC rearrangements in lymphoma with DLBCL morphology. Blood Adv. 2018 Oct 23;2(20):2755–65. PMID:30348671
733. Chong Y, Kang CS. Causative agents of Kikuchi-Fujimoto disease (histiocytic necrotizing lymphadenitis): a meta-analysis. Int J Pediatr Otorhinolaryngol. 2014 Nov;78(11):1890–7. PMID:25200851
734. Chonghaile TN, Roderick JE, Glenfield C, et al. Maturation stage of T-cell acute lymphoblastic leukemia determines BCL-2 versus BCL-XL dependence and sensitivity to ABT-199. Cancer Discov. 2014 Sep;4(9):1074–87. PMID:24994123
735. Choquet S, Leblond V, Herbrecht R, et al. Efficacy and safety of rituximab in B-cell post-transplantation lymphoproliferative disorders: results of a prospective multicenter phase 2 study. Blood. 2006 Apr 15;107(8):3053–7. PMID:16254143
736. Choquet S, Trappe R, Leblond V, et al. CHOP-21 for the treatment of post-transplant lymphoproliferative disorders (PTLD) following solid organ transplantation. Haematologica. 2007 Feb;92(2):273–4. PMID:17296588
737. Chott A, Haedicke W, Mosberger I, et al. Most CD56+ intestinal lymphomas are CD8+CD5-T-cell lymphomas of monomorphic small to medium size histology. Am J Pathol. 1998 Nov;153(5):1483–90. PMID:9811340
738. Chott A, Vonderheid EC, Olbricht S, et al. The dominant T cell clone is present in multiple regressing skin lesions and associated T cell lymphomas of patients with lymphomatoid papulosis. J Invest Dermatol. 1996 Apr;106(4):696–700. PMID:8618007
739. Choudhari R, Minero VG, Menotti M, et al. Redundant and nonredundant roles for Cdc42 and Rac1 in lymphomas developed in NPM-ALK transgenic mice. Blood. 2016 Mar 10;127(10):1297–306. PMID:26747246
740. Christe L, Veloza L, Gros L, et al. HHV8-negative primary effusion-based large B-cell lymphoma in a patient with chronic myeloid leukemia, BCR:ABL1-positive under dasatinib treatment: report of a new case and literature review. Diagn Cytopathol. 2022 Dec;50(12):E351–6. PMID:35916333
741. Chu CC, Catera R, Hatzi K, et al. Chronic lymphocytic leukemia antibodies with a common stereotypic rearrangement recognize nonmuscle myosin heavy chain IIA. Blood. 2008 Dec 15;112(13):5122–9. PMID:18812466
742. Chu PG, Huang Q, Weiss LM. Incidental and concurrent malignant lymphomas discovered at the time of prostatectomy and prostate biopsy: a study of 29 cases. Am J Surg Pathol. 2005 May;29(5):693–9. PMID:15832096
743. Chuang SS, Chang ST, Chuang WY, et al. NK-cell lineage predicts poor survival in primary intestinal NK-cell and T-cell lymphomas. Am J Surg Pathol. 2009 Aug;33(8):1230–40. PMID:19561449
744. Chuang SS, Chen SW, Chang ST, et al. Lymphoma in Taiwan: review of 1347 neoplasms from a single institution according to the 2016 revision of the World Health Organization classification. J Formos Med Assoc. 2017 Aug;116(8):620–5. PMID:28003113
745. Chung SS, Kim E, Park JH, et al. Hematopoietic stem cell origin of BRAFV600E mutations in hairy cell leukemia. Sci Transl Med. 2014 May 28;6(238):238ra71. PMID:24871132
746. Churchill HR, Roncador G, Warnke RA, et al. Programmed death 1 expression in variant

immunoarchitectural patterns of nodular lymphocyte predominant Hodgkin lymphoma: comparison with CD57 and lymphomas in the differential diagnosis. Hum Pathol. 2010 Dec;41(12):1726–34. PMID:20825974
747. Ciccocioppo R, Croci GA, Biagi F, et al. Intestinal T-cell lymphoma with enteropathy-associated T-cell lymphoma-like features arising in the setting of adult autoimmune enteropathy. Hematol Oncol. 2018 Apr;36(2):481–8. PMID:29446107
748. Ciccone M, Agostinelli C, Rigolin GM, et al. Proliferation centers in chronic lymphocytic leukemia: correlation with cytogenetic and clinicobiological features in consecutive patients analyzed on tissue microarrays. Leukemia. 2012 Mar;26(3):499–508. PMID:21941366
749. Cimmino A, Calin GA, Fabbri M, et al. miR-15 and miR-16 induce apoptosis by targeting BCL2. Proc Natl Acad Sci U S A. 2005 Sep 27;102(39):13944–9. PMID:16166262
750. Cimpean AM, Raica M. Intranodal hemorrhagic spindle cell tumor with amianthoid fibers - report of a case with emphasis to mast cell reaction and d2-40 expression. In Vivo. 2013 May-Jun;27(3):395–9. PMID:23606697
751. Cioc AM, Wagner JE, MacMillan ML, et al. Diagnosis of myelodysplastic syndrome among a cohort of 119 patients with Fanconi anemia: morphologic and cytogenetic characteristics. Am J Clin Pathol. 2010 Jan;133(1):92–100. PMID:20023263
752. Cirillo E, Prencipe MR, Giardino G, et al. Clinical phenotype, immunological abnormalities, and genomic findings in patients with DiGeorge spectrum phenotype without 22q11.2 deletion. J Allergy Clin Immunol Pract. 2020 Oct;8(9):3112–20. PMID:32668295
753. Cirillo M, Borchmann S. An update on disease biomarkers for Hodgkin lymphoma. Expert Rev Hematol. 2020 May;13(5):481–8. PMID:32193957
754. Clark Schneider KM, Banks PM, Collie AM, et al. Dual expression of MYC and BCL2 proteins predicts worse outcomes in diffuse large B-cell lymphoma. Leuk Lymphoma. 2016 Jul;57(7):1640–8. PMID:26421520
755. Clarke CA, Glaser SL, Keegan TH, et al. Neighborhood socioeconomic status and Hodgkin's lymphoma incidence in California. Cancer Epidemiol Biomarkers Prev. 2005 Jun;14(6):1441–7. PMID:15941953
756. Clavel J, Hémon D, Mandereau L, et al. Farming, pesticide use and hairy-cell leukemia. Scand J Work Environ Health. 1996 Aug;22(4):285–93. PMID:8881017
757. Clavel J, Mandereau L, Cordier S, et al. Hairy cell leukaemia, occupation, and smoking. Br J Haematol. 1995 Sep;91(1):154–61. PMID:7577624
758. Claviez A, Meyer U, Dominick C, et al. MALT lymphoma in children: a report from the NHL-BFM Study Group. Pediatr Blood Cancer. 2006 Aug;47(2):210–4. PMID:16123999
759. Claviez A, Tiemann M, Lüders H, et al. Impact of latent Epstein-Barr virus infection on outcome in children and adolescents with Hodgkin's lymphoma. J Clin Oncol. 2005 Jun 20;23(18):4048–56. PMID:15961758
760. Clemens MW, Medeiros LJ, Butler CE, et al. Complete surgical excision is essential for the management of patients with breast implant-associated anaplastic large-cell lymphoma. J Clin Oncol. 2016 Jan 10;34(2):160–8. PMID:26628470
762. Clemente MJ, Wlodarski MW, Makishima H, et al. Clonal drift demonstrates unexpected dynamics of the T-cell repertoire in T-large granular lymphocyte leukemia. Blood. 2011 Oct 20;118(16):4384–93. PMID:21865345
763. Clemmensen SB, Harris JR, Mengel-From J, et al. Familial risk and heritability of hematologic malignancies in the Nordic Twin Study of Cancer. Cancers (Basel). 2021 Jun 16;13(12):3023. PMID:34208754
764. Clipson A, Barrans S, Zeng N, et al. The prognosis of MYC translocation positive diffuse large B-cell lymphoma depends on the second hit. J Pathol Clin Res. 2015 Mar 30;1(3):125–33. PMID:27347428
765. Clipson A, Wang M, de Leval L, et al. KLF2 mutation is the most frequent somatic change in splenic marginal zone lymphoma and identifies a subset with distinct genotype. Leukemia. 2015 May;29(5):1177–85. PMID:25428260
766. Clot G, Jares P, Giné E, et al. A gene signature that distinguishes conventional and leukemic nonnodal mantle cell lymphoma helps predict outcome. Blood. 2018 Jul 26;132(4):413–22. PMID:29769262
767. Cobbers JM, Wolter M, Reifenberger J, et al. Frequent inactivation of CDKN2A and rare mutation of TP53 in PCNSL. Brain Pathol. 1998 Apr;8(2):263–76. PMID:9546285
768. Cocks M, Porcu P, Wick MR, et al. Recent advances in cutaneous T-cell lymphoma: diagnostic and prognostic considerations. Surg Pathol Clin. 2019 Sep;12(3):783–803. PMID:31352988
769. Coe JI, von Drashek SC. Hamartoma of the spleen: a report of four cases. Am J Pathol. 1952 Jul-Aug;28(4):663–71. PMID:14943802
770. Coffey AJ, Brooksbank RA, Brandau O, et al. Host response to EBV infection in X-linked lymphoproliferative disease results from mutations in an SH2-domain encoding gene. Nat Genet. 1998 Oct;20(2):129–35. PMID:9771704
771. Coffey AM, Lewis A, Marcogliese AN, et al. A clinicopathologic study of the spectrum of systemic forms of EBV-associated T-cell lymphoproliferative disorders of childhood: a single tertiary care pediatric institution experience in North America. Pediatr Blood Cancer. 2019 Aug;66(8):e27798. PMID:31099136
772. Cohen C, El-Karoui K, Alyanakian MA, et al. Light and heavy chain deposition disease associated with CH1 deletion. Clin Kidney J. 2015 Apr;8(2):237–9. PMID:25815184
773. Cohen C, Royer B, Javaugue V, et al. Bortezomib produces high hematological response rates with prolonged renal survival in monoclonal immunoglobulin deposition disease. Kidney Int. 2015 Nov;88(5):1135–43. PMID:26176826
774. Cohen JI, Iwatsuki K, Ko YH, et al. Epstein-Barr virus NK and T cell lymphoproliferative disease: report of a 2018 international meeting. Leuk Lymphoma. 2020 Apr;61(4):808–19. PMID:31833428
775. Cohen JI, Jaffe ES, Dale JK, et al. Characterization and treatment of chronic active Epstein-Barr virus disease: a 28-year experience in the United States. Blood. 2011 Jun 2;117(22):5835–49. PMID:21454450
776. Cohen JI, Kimura H, Nakamura S, et al. Epstein-Barr virus-associated lymphoproliferative disease in non-immunocompromised hosts: a status report and summary of an international meeting, 8-9 September 2008. Ann Oncol. 2009 Sep;20(9):1472–82. PMID:19515747
777. Cohen JI, Manoli I, Dowdell K, et al. Hydroa vacciniforme-like lymphoproliferative disorder: an EBV disease with a low risk of systemic illness in whites. Blood. 2019 Jun 27;133(26):2753–64. PMID:31064750
778. Cohen OC, Ismael A, Pawarova B, et al. Longitudinal strain is an independent predictor of survival and response to therapy in patients with systemic AL amyloidosis. Eur Heart J. 2022 Jan 31;43(4):333–41. PMID:34472567
779. Colleoni GW, Bridge JA, Garicochea B, et al. ATIC-ALK: a novel variant ALK gene fusion in anaplastic large cell lymphoma resulting from the recurrent cryptic chromosomal inversion, inv(2)(p23q35). Am J Pathol. 2000 Mar;156(3):781–9. PMID:10702393
780. Collinge B, Ben-Neriah S, Chong L, et al. The impact of MYC and BCL2 structural variants in tumors of DLBCL morphology and mechanisms of false-negative MYC IHC. Blood. 2021 Apr 22;137(16):2196–208. PMID:33120427
781. Colombat M, Stern M, Groussard O, et al. Pulmonary cystic disorder related to light chain deposition disease. Am J Respir Crit Care Med. 2006 Apr 1;173(7):777–80. PMID:16399989
782. Colomo L, Loong F, Rives S, et al. Diffuse large B-cell lymphomas with plasmablastic differentiation represent a heterogeneous group of disease entities. Am J Surg Pathol. 2004 Jun;28(6):736–47. PMID:15166665
783. Colomo L, López-Guillermo A, Perales M, et al. Clinical impact of the differentiation profile assessed by immunophenotyping in patients with diffuse large B-cell lymphoma. Blood. 2003 Jan 1;101(1):78–84. PMID:12393466
784. Colović N, Perunicić M, Jurisić V, et al. Specific skin lesions in hairy cell leukemia at presentation: case report and review of literature. Med Oncol. 2010 Jun;27(2):559–61. PMID:19533422
785. Colt JS, Davis S, Severson RK, et al. Residential insecticide use and risk of non-Hodgkin's lymphoma. Cancer Epidemiol Biomarkers Prev. 2006 Feb;15(2):251–7. PMID:16492912
786. Comeaux EQ, Mullighan CG. TP53 mutations in hypodiploid acute lymphoblastic leukemia. Cold Spring Harb Perspect Med. 2017 Mar 1;7(3):a026286. PMID:28003275
787. Comenzo RL, Zhou P, Fleisher M, et al. Seeking confidence in the diagnosis of systemic AL (Ig light-chain) amyloidosis: patients can have both monoclonal gammopathies and hereditary amyloid proteins. Blood. 2006 May 1;107(9):3489–91. PMID:16439680
788. Comfere NI, Gonzalez Santiago TM, Peters MS, et al. Cutaneous extramedullary plasmacytoma: clinical, prognostic, and interphase cytogenetic analysis. Am J Dermatopathol. 2013 May;35(3):357–63. PMID:23000906
789. Conconi A, Bertoni F, Pedrinis E, et al. Nodal marginal zone B-cell lymphomas may arise from different subsets of marginal zone B lymphocytes. Blood. 2001 Aug 1;98(3):781–6. PMID:11468179
790. Conconi A, Franceschetti S, Aprile von Hohenstaufen K, et al. Histologic transformation in marginal zone lymphomas. Ann Oncol. 2015 Nov;26(11):2329–35. PMID:26400898
790A. Condoluci A, Rossi D. Biology and treatment of Richter transformation. Front Oncol. 2022 Mar 22;12:829983. PMID:35392219
791. Condoluci A, Rossi D, Zucca E, et al. Toward a risk-tailored therapeutic policy in mantle cell lymphoma. Curr Oncol Rep. 2018 Aug 22;20(10):79. PMID:30132080
792. Condoluci A, Terzi di Bergamo L, Langerbeins P, et al. International prognostic score for asymptomatic early-stage chronic lymphocytic leukemia. Blood. 2020 May 21;135(21):1859–69. PMID:32267500
793. Cong P, Raffeld M, Teruya-Feldstein J, et al. In situ localization of follicular lymphoma: description and analysis by laser capture microdissection. Blood. 2002 May 1;99(9):3376–82. PMID:11964306
794. Conter V, Valsecchi MG, Buldini B, et al. Early T-cell precursor acute lymphoblastic leukaemia in children treated in AIEOP centres with AIEOP-BFM protocols: a retrospective analysis. Lancet Haematol. 2016 Feb;3(2):e80–6. PMID:26853647
795. Cook PD, Czerniak B, Chan JK, et al. Nodular spindle-cell vascular transformation of lymph nodes. A benign process occurring predominantly in retroperitoneal lymph nodes draining carcinomas that can simulate Kaposi's sarcoma or metastatic tumor. Am J Surg Pathol. 1995 Sep;19(9):1010–20. PMID:7661274
796. Cools J, Wlodarska I, Somers R, et al. Identification of novel fusion partners of ALK, the anaplastic lymphoma kinase, in anaplastic large-cell lymphoma and inflammatory myofibroblastic tumor. Genes Chromosomes Cancer. 2002 Aug;34(4):354–62. PMID:12112524
797. Copie-Bergman C, Cuillière-Dartigues P, Baia M, et al. MYC-IG rearrangements are negative predictors of survival in DLBCL patients treated with immunochemotherapy: a GELA/LYSA study. Blood. 2015 Nov 26;126(22):2466–74. PMID:26373676
798. Copie-Bergman C, Gaulard P, Lavergne-Slove A, et al. Proposal for a new histological grading system for post-treatment evaluation of gastric MALT lymphoma. Gut. 2003 Nov;52(11):1656. PMID:14570741
799. Copie-Bergman C, Gaulard P, Maouche-Chrétien L, et al. The MAL gene is expressed in primary mediastinal large B-cell lymphoma. Blood. 1999 Nov 15;94(10):3567–75. PMID:10552968
800. Copie-Bergman C, Niedobitek G, Mangham DC, et al. Epstein-Barr virus in B-cell lymphomas associated with chronic suppurative inflammation. J Pathol. 1997 Nov;183(3):287–92. PMID:9422983
801. Copie-Bergman C, Wotherspoon AC, Capella C, et al. Gela histological scoring system for post-treatment biopsies of patients with gastric MALT lymphoma is feasible and reliable in routine practice. Br J Haematol. 2013 Jan;160(1):47–52. PMID:23043300
802. Coppo P, Gouilleux-Gruart V, Huang Y, et al. STAT3 transcription factor is constitutively activated and is oncogenic in nasal-type NK/T-cell lymphoma. Leukemia. 2009 Sep;23(9):1667–78. PMID:19421230
803. Corbingi A, Innocenti I, Tomasso A, et al. Monoclonal gammopathy and serum immunoglobulin levels as prognostic factors in chronic lymphocytic leukaemia. Br J Haematol. 2020 Sep;190(6):901–8. PMID:32712965
804. Corcoran MM, Mould SJ, Orchard JA, et al. Dysregulation of cyclin dependent kinase 6 expression in splenic marginal zone lymphoma through chromosome 7q translocations. Oncogene. 1999 Nov 4;18(46):6271–7. PMID:10597225
805. Corcos D. Oncogenic potential of the B-cell antigen receptor and its relevance to heavy chain diseases and other B-cell neoplasias: a new model. Res Immunol. 1990 Jul-Aug;141(6):543–53. PMID:2284498
806. Cordeiro PG, Ghione P, Ni A, et al. Risk of breast implant associated anaplastic large cell lymphoma (BIA-ALCL) in a cohort of 3546 women prospectively followed long term after reconstruction with textured breast implants. J Plast Reconstr Aesthet Surg. 2020 May;73(5):841–6. PMID:32008941
807. Cordel N, Tressières B, D'Incan M, et al. Frequency and risk factors for associated lymphomas in patients with lymphomatoid papulosis. Oncologist. 2016 Jan;21(1):76–83. PMID:26668250
808. Cordesmeyer S, Pützler M, Titze U, et al. Littoral cell angioma of the spleen in a patient with previous pulmonary sarcoidosis: a TNF-α related pathogenesis? World J Surg Oncol. 2011 Sep 19;9:106. PMID:21929754
809. Cording S, Lhermitte L, Malamut G, et al. Oncogenic landscape of lymphomagenesis in coeliac disease. Gut. 2022 Mar;71(3):497–508. PMID:33579790
810. Cordo' V, van der Zwet JCG, Canté-Barrett K, et al. T-cell acute lymphoblastic leukemia: a roadmap to targeted therapies. Blood Cancer Discov. 2020 Nov 24;2(1):19–31.

PMID:34661151
811. Correia S, Bridges R, Wegner F, et al. Sequence variation of Epstein-Barr virus: viral types, geography, codon usage, and diseases. J Virol. 2018 Oct 29;92(22):e01132-18. PMID:30111570
812. Corrente F, Bellesi S, Metafuni E, et al. Role of flow-cytometric immunophenotyping in prediction of BCR/ABL1 gene rearrangement in adult B-cell acute lymphoblastic leukemia. Cytometry B Clin Cytom. 2018 May;94(3):468–76. PMID:29220871
813. Cortes JR, Ambesi-Impiombato A, Couronné L, et al. RHOA G17V induces T follicular helper cell specification and promotes lymphomagenesis. Cancer Cell. 2018 Feb 12;33(2):259–273.e7. PMID:29398449
814. Corti M, Villafañe M, Minue G, et al. Clinical features of AIDS patients with Hodgkin's lymphoma with isolated bone marrow involvement: report of 12 cases at a single institution. Cancer Biol Med. 2015 Mar;12(1):41–5. PMID:25859410
815. Cosenza UM, Galati G, Zofrea P, et al. Clinical and biological features of an intranodal palisaded myofibroblastoma. Anticancer Res. 2006 May-Jun;26 3B:2349–52. PMID:16821615
816. Costa D, Granada I, Espinet B, et al. Balanced and unbalanced translocations in a multicentric series of 2843 patients with chronic lymphocytic leukemia. Genes Chromosomes Cancer. 2022 Jan;61(1):37–43. PMID:34414624
817. Costa D, Queralt R, Aymerich M, et al. High levels of chromosomal imbalances in typical and small-cell variants of T-cell prolymphocytic leukemia. Cancer Genet Cytogenet. 2003 Nov;147(1):36–43. PMID:14580769
818. Coulter TI, Chandra A, Bacon CM, et al. Clinical spectrum and features of activated phosphoinositide 3-kinase δ syndrome: a large patient cohort study. J Allergy Clin Immunol. 2017 Feb;139(2):597–606.e4. PMID:27555459
819. Coupland SE, Damato B. Understanding intraocular lymphomas. Clin Exp Ophthalmol. 2008 Aug;36(6):564–78. PMID:18954321
820. Coupland SE, Hummel M, Müller HH, et al. Molecular analysis of immunoglobulin genes in primary intraocular lymphoma. Invest Ophthalmol Vis Sci. 2005 Oct;46(10):3507–14. PMID:16186327
821. Coupland SE, Krause L, Delecluse HJ, et al. Lymphoproliferative lesions of the ocular adnexa. Analysis of 112 cases. Ophthalmology. 1998 Aug;105(8):1430–41. PMID:9709754
822. Courtois L, Sujobert P. Morphologic features of μ-heavy-chain disease. Blood. 2017 Jul 27;130(4):558. PMID:28751360
823. Courts C, Montesinos-Rongen M, Brunn A, et al. Recurrent inactivation of the PRDM1 gene in primary central nervous system lymphoma. J Neuropathol Exp Neurol. 2008 Jul;67(7):720–7. PMID:18596541
824. Courville EL, Sohani AR, Hasserjian RP, et al. Diverse clinicopathologic features in human herpesvirus 8-associated lymphomas lead to diagnostic problems. Am J Clin Pathol. 2014 Dec;142(6):816–29. PMID:25389336
825. Courville EL, Yohe S, Chou D, et al. EBV-negative monomorphic B-cell post-transplant lymphoproliferative disorders are pathologically distinct from EBV-positive cases and frequently contain TP53 mutations. Mod Pathol. 2016 Oct;29(10):1200–11. PMID:27443517
826. Coustan-Smith E, Mullighan CG, Onciu M, et al. Early T-cell precursor leukaemia: a subtype of very high-risk acute lymphoblastic leukaemia. Lancet Oncol. 2009 Feb;10(2):147–56. PMID:19147408
827. Coustan-Smith E, Sancho J, Hancock ML, et al. Clinical importance of minimal residual disease in childhood acute lymphoblastic leukemia. Blood. 2000 Oct 15;96(8):2691–6. PMID:11023499
828. Covell LM, Disciullo AJ, Knapp RC. Decidual change in pelvic lymph nodes in the presence of cervical squamous cell carcinoma during pregnancy. Am J Obstet Gynecol. 1977 Mar 15;127(6):674–6. PMID:842598
829. Cowan AJ, Allen C, Barac A, et al. Global burden of multiple myeloma: a systematic analysis for the Global Burden of Disease Study 2016. JAMA Oncol. 2018 Sep 1;4(9):1221–7. PMID:29800065
830. Cozzolino I, Varone V, Picardi M, et al. CD10, BCL6, and MUM1 expression in diffuse large B-cell lymphoma on FNA samples. Cancer Cytopathol. 2016 Feb;124(2):135–43. PMID:26414904
831. Craig VJ, Cogliatti SB, Arnold I, et al. B-cell receptor signaling and CD40 ligand-independent T cell help cooperate in Helicobacter-induced MALT lymphomagenesis. Leukemia. 2010 Jun;24(6):1186–96. PMID:20428202
832. Crane GM, Powell H, Kostadinov R, et al. Primary CNS lymphoproliferative disease, mycophenolate and calcineurin inhibitor usage. Oncotarget. 2015 Oct 20;6(32):33849–66. PMID:26460822
833. Crapanzano JP, Lin O. Cytologic findings of marginal zone lymphoma. Cancer. 2003 Oct 25;99(5):301–9. PMID:14579297
834. Crawford TO, Skolasky RL, Fernandez R, et al. Survival probability in ataxia telangiectasia. Arch Dis Child. 2006 Jul;91(7):610–1. PMID:16790721
835. Creasey T, Enshaei A, Nebral K, et al. Single nucleotide polymorphism array-based signature of low hypodiploidy in acute lymphoblastic leukemia. Genes Chromosomes Cancer. 2021 Sep;60(9):604–15. PMID:33938069
836. Cree IA, Tan PH, Travis WD, et al. Counting mitoses: SI(ze) matters! Mod Pathol. 2021 Sep;34(9):1651–7. PMID:34079071
837. Crescenzo R, Abate F, Lasorsa E, et al. Convergent mutations and kinase fusions lead to oncogenic STAT3 activation in anaplastic large cell lymphoma. Cancer Cell. 2015 Apr 13;27(4):516–32. PMID:25873174
838. Criado I, Rodríguez-Caballero A, Gutiérrez ML, et al. Low-count monoclonal B-cell lymphocytosis persists after seven years of follow up and is associated with a poorer outcome. Haematologica. 2018 Jul;103(7):1198–208. PMID:29567775
839. Criel A, Michaux L, De Wolf-Peeters C. The concept of typical and atypical chronic lymphocytic leukaemia. Leuk Lymphoma. 1999 Mar;33(1-2):33–45. PMID:10194119
840. Croci GA, Hoster E, Beà S, et al. Reproducibility of histologic prognostic parameters for mantle cell lymphoma: cytology, Ki67, p53 and SOX11. Virchows Arch. 2020 Aug;477(2):259–67. PMID:31975037
841. Crotty R, Hu K, Stevenson K, et al. Simultaneous identification of cell of origin, translocations, and hotspot mutations in diffuse large B-cell lymphoma using a single RNA-sequencing assay. Am J Clin Pathol. 2021 Apr 26;155(5):748–54. PMID:33258912
842. Crotty S. T follicular helper cell biology: a decade of discovery and diseases. Immunity. 2019 May 21;50(5):1132–48. PMID:31117010
843. Crowson AN, Baschinsky DY, Kovatich A, et al. Granulomatous eccrinotropic lymphomatoid papulosis. Am J Clin Pathol. 2003 May;119(5):731–9. PMID:12760293
844. Crowther-Swanepoel D, Broderick P, Di Bernardo MC, et al. Common variants at 2q37.3, 8q24.21, 15q21.3 and 16q24.1 influence chronic lymphocytic leukemia risk. Nat Genet. 2010 Feb;42(2):132–6. PMID:20062064
845. Crowther-Swanepoel D, Corre T, Lloyd A, et al. Inherited genetic susceptibility to monoclonal B-cell lymphocytosis. Blood. 2010 Dec 23;116(26):5957–60. PMID:20855867
846. Csernus B, Timár B, Fülöp Z, et al. Mutational analysis of IgVH and BCL-6 genes suggests thymic B-cells origin of mediastinal (thymic) B-cell lymphoma. Leuk Lymphoma. 2004 Oct;45(10):2105–10. PMID:15370257
847. Cuadra-Garcia I, Proulx GM, Wu CL, et al. Sinonasal lymphoma: a clinicopathologic analysis of 58 cases from the Massachusetts General Hospital. Am J Surg Pathol. 1999 Nov;23(11):1356–69. PMID:10555004
848. Cucco F, Barrans S, Sha C, et al. Distinct genetic changes reveal evolutionary history and heterogeneous molecular grade of DLBCL with MYC/BCL2 double-hit. Leukemia. 2020 May;34(5):1329–41. PMID:31844144
849. Cunniff C, Bassetti JA, Ellis NA. Bloom's syndrome: clinical spectrum, molecular pathogenesis, and cancer predisposition. Mol Syndromol. 2017 Jan;8(1):4–23. PMID:28232778
850. Curiel-Olmo S, Mondéjar R, Almaraz C, et al. Splenic diffuse red pulp small B-cell lymphoma displays increased expression of cyclin D3 and recurrent CCND3 mutations. Blood. 2017 Feb 23;129(8):1042–5. PMID:28069605
851. Curry J, O'steen L, Morris CG, et al. Long-term outcomes after definitive radiation therapy for solitary plasmacytoma. Am J Clin Oncol. 2020 Oct;43(10):709–13. PMID:32739971
852. Curry JL, Prieto VG, Jones DM, et al. Transient iatrogenic immunodeficiency-related B-cell lymphoproliferative disorder of the skin in a patient with mycosis fungoides/Sézary syndrome. J Cutan Pathol. 2011 Mar;38(3):295–7. PMID:19889052
853. da Cunha CB, Oliveira C, Wen X, et al. De novo expression of CD44 variants in sporadic and hereditary gastric cancer. Lab Invest. 2010 Nov;90(11):1604–14. PMID:20856229
854. da Silva Almeida AC, Abate F, Khiabanian H, et al. The mutational landscape of cutaneous T cell lymphoma and Sézary syndrome. Nat Genet. 2015 Dec;47(12):1465–70. PMID:26551667
855. Dagklis A, Ponzoni M, Govi S, et al. Immunoglobulin gene repertoire in ocular adnexal lymphomas: hints on the nature of the antigenic stimulation. Leukemia. 2012 Apr;26(4):814–21. PMID:22024723
856. Dalal NH, Dores GM, Curtis RE, et al. Cause-specific mortality in individuals with lymphoplasmacytic lymphoma/Waldenström macroglobulinaemia, 2000-2016. Br J Haematol. 2020 Jun;189(6):1107–18. PMID:32090327
857. Dalia S, Jaglal M, Chervenick P, et al. Clinicopathologic characteristics and outcomes of histiocytic and dendritic cell neoplasms: the Moffitt Cancer Center experience over the last twenty five years. Cancers (Basel). 2014 Nov 14;6(4):2275–95. PMID:25405526
858. Dalia S, Shao H, Sagatys E, et al. Dendritic cell and histiocytic neoplasms: biology, diagnosis, and treatment. Cancer Control. 2014 Oct;21(4):290–300. PMID:25310210
859. Dallenbach FE, Stein H. Expression of T-cell-receptor beta chain in Reed-Sternberg cells. Lancet. 1989 Oct 7;2(8667):828–30. PMID:2477655
860. Dal Maso L, Franceschi S. Hepatitis C virus and risk of lymphoma and other lymphoid neoplasms: a meta-analysis of epidemiologic studies. Cancer Epidemiol Biomarkers Prev. 2006 Nov;15(11):2078–85. PMID:17119031
861. Damle RN, Wasil T, Fais F, et al. Ig V gene mutation status and CD38 expression as novel prognostic indicators in chronic lymphocytic leukemia. Blood. 1999 Sep 15;94(6):1840–7. PMID:10477712
862. Damm-Welk C, Kutscher N, Zimmermann M, et al. Quantification of minimal disseminated disease by quantitative polymerase chain reaction and digital polymerase chain reaction for NPM-ALK as a prognostic factor in children with anaplastic large cell lymphoma. Haematologica. 2020 Aug;105(8):2141–9. PMID:31649129
863. d'Amore ES, Menin A, Bonoldi E, et al. Anaplastic large cell lymphomas: a study of 75 pediatric patients. Pediatr Dev Pathol. 2007 May-Jun;10(3):181–91. PMID:17535098
864. Daniels J, Doukas PG, Escala MEM, et al. Cellular origins and genetic landscape of cutaneous gamma delta T cell lymphomas. Nat Commun. 2020 Apr 14;11(1):1806. PMID:32286303
865. Daniels JA, Lederman HM, Maitra A, et al. Gastrointestinal tract pathology in patients with common variable immunodeficiency (CVID): a clinicopathologic study and review. Am J Surg Pathol. 2007 Dec;31(12):1800–12. PMID:18043034
866. Danon AD, Krishnan J, Frizzera G. Morpho-immunophenotypic diversity of Castleman's disease, hyaline-vascular type: with emphasis on a stroma-rich variant and a new pathogenetic hypothesis. Virchows Arch A Pathol Anat Histopathol. 1993;423(5):369–82. PMID:8116226
867. D'Antonio A, Boscaino A, Addesso M, et al. KSHV- and EBV-associated germinotropic lymphoproliferative disorder: a rare lymphoproliferative disease of HIV patient with plasmablastic morphology, indolent course and favourable response to therapy. Leuk Lymphoma. 2007 Jul;48(7):1444–7. PMID:17613780
868. D'Antonio A, Boscaino A, De Dominicis G, et al. Splenic hemangiomatosis. A report of two cases and review of literature. Adv Clin Path. 2002 Jul-Oct;6(3-4):119–24. PMID:19757634
869. Dao LN, Hanson CA, Dispenzieri A, et al. Bone marrow histopathology in POEMS syndrome: a distinctive combination of plasma cell, lymphoid, and myeloid findings in 87 patients. Blood. 2011 Jun 16;117(24):6438–44. PMID:21385854
870. D'Arcy ME, Beachler DC, Pfeiffer RM, et al. Tumor necrosis factor inhibitors and the risk of cancer among older Americans with rheumatoid arthritis. Cancer Epidemiol Biomarkers Prev. 2021 Nov;30(11):2059–67. PMID:34426413
871. Darden JW, Teeslink R, Parrish A. Hamartoma of the spleen: a manfestation of tuberous sclerosis. Am Surg. 1975 Sep;41(9):564–6. PMID:1166974
872. Dargent JL, Tinton N, Trimech M, et al. Lymph node involvement by enteropathy-like indolent NK-cell proliferation. Virchows Arch. 2021 Jun;478(6):1197–202. PMID:32696224
873. Daroontum T, Kohno K, Eladl AE, et al. Comparison of Epstein-Barr virus-positive mucocutaneous ulcer associated with treated lymphoma or methotrexate in Japan. Histopathology. 2018 Jun;72(7):1115–27. PMID:29314151
874. Das DK. Serous effusions in malignant lymphomas: a review. Diagn Cytopathol. 2006 May;34(5):335–47. PMID:16604559
875. Dasgupta Y, Golovine K, Nieborowska-Skorska M, et al. Drugging DNA repair to target T-ALL cells. Leuk Lymphoma. 2018 Jul;59(7):1746–9. PMID:29115896
876. Daum S, Weiss D, Hummel M, et al. Frequency of clonal intraepithelial T lymphocyte proliferations in enteropathy-type intestinal T cell lymphoma, coeliac disease, and refractory sprue. Gut. 2001 Dec;49(6):804–12. PMID:11709515
877. Dave SS, Fu K, Wright GW, et al. Molecular diagnosis of Burkitt's lymphoma. N Engl J Med. 2006 Jun 8;354(23):2431–42. PMID:16760443
878. Dave SS, Wright G, Tan B, et al. Prediction of survival in follicular lymphoma based

on molecular features of tumor-infiltrating immune cells. N Engl J Med. 2004 Nov 18;351(21):2159–69. PMID:15548776

879. Davies A, Cummin TE, Barrans S, et al. Gene-expression profiling of bortezomib added to standard chemoimmunotherapy for diffuse large B-cell lymphoma (REMoDL-B): an open-label, randomised, phase 3 trial. Lancet Oncol. 2019 May;20(5):649–62. PMID:30948276

880. Davila JI, Starr JS, Attia S, et al. Comprehensive genomic profiling of a rare thyroid follicular dendritic cell sarcoma. Rare Tumors. 2017 Sep 15;9(2):6834. PMID:28975018

881. Davis AR, Stone SL, Oran AR, et al. Targeted massively parallel sequencing of mature lymphoid neoplasms: assessment of empirical application and diagnostic utility in routine clinical practice. Mod Pathol. 2021 May;34(5):904–21. PMID:33311649

882. Davis JL, Viciana AL, Ruiz P. Diagnosis of intraocular lymphoma by flow cytometry. Am J Ophthalmol. 1997 Sep;124(3):362–72. PMID:9439362

883. Davis RE, Warnke RA, Dorfman RF. Inflammatory pseudotumor of lymph nodes. Additional observations and evidence for an inflammatory etiology. Am J Surg Pathol. 1991 Aug;15(8):744–56. PMID:2069212

884. Davis TH, Morton CC, Miller-Cassman R, et al. Hodgkin's disease, lymphomatoid papulosis, and cutaneous T-cell lymphoma derived from a common T-cell clone. N Engl J Med. 1992 Apr 23;326(17):1115–22. PMID:1532439

885. de Baaij LR, Berkhof J, van de Water JM, et al. A new and validated clinical prognostic model (EPI) for enteropathy-associated T-cell lymphoma. Clin Cancer Res. 2015 Jul 1;21(13):3013–9. PMID:25779949

886. de Boer CJ, Schuuring E, Dreef E, et al. Cyclin D1 protein analysis in the diagnosis of mantle cell lymphoma. Blood. 1995 Oct 1;86(7):2715–23. PMID:7670110

887. de Boer CJ, van Krieken JH, Kluin-Nelemans HC, et al. Cyclin D1 messenger RNA overexpression as a marker for mantle cell lymphoma. Oncogene. 1995 May 4;10(9):1833–40. PMID:7753558

888. de Boer M, Hauptmann M, Hijmering NJ, et al. Increased prevalence of BRCA1/2 mutations in women with macrotextured breast implants and anaplastic large cell lymphoma of the breast. Blood. 2020 Sep 10;136(11):1368–72. PMID:32452517

889. de Boer M, van der Sluis WB, de Boer JP, et al. Breast implant-associated anaplastic large-cell lymphoma in a transgender woman. Aesthet Surg J. 2017 Sep 1;37(8):NP83–7. PMID:29036941

890. de Boer M, van Leeuwen FE, Hauptmann M, et al. Breast implants and the risk of anaplastic large-cell lymphoma in the breast. JAMA Oncol. 2018 Mar 1;4(3):335–41. PMID:29302687

891. de Jong D, Roemer MG, Chan JK, et al. B-cell and classical Hodgkin lymphomas associated with immunodeficiency: 2015 SH/EAHP Workshop Report-Part 2. Am J Clin Pathol. 2017 Feb 1;147(2):153–70. PMID:28395108

892. de Jong MME, Kellermayer Z, Papazian N, et al. The multiple myeloma microenvironment is defined by an inflammatory stromal cell landscape. Nat Immunol. 2021 Jun;22(6):769–80. PMID:34017122

893. De Jong WH, Panagiotakos D, Proykova A, et al. Final opinion on the safety of breast implants in relation to anaplastic large cell lymphoma: report of the Scientific Committee on Health, Emerging and Environmental Risks (SCHEER). Regul Toxicol Pharmacol. 2021 Oct;125:104982. PMID:34214611

894. de la Garza Bravo MM, Patel KP, Loghavi S, et al. Shared clonality in distinctive lesions of lymphomatoid papulosis and mycosis fungoides occurring in the same patients suggests a common origin. Hum Pathol. 2015 Apr;46(4):558–69. PMID:25666664

895. de Leval L, Bonnet C, Copie-Bergman C, et al. Diffuse large B-cell lymphoma of Waldeyer's ring has distinct clinicopathologic features: a GELA study. Ann Oncol. 2012 Dec;23(12):3143–51. PMID:22700993

896. de Leval L, Ferry JA, Falini B, et al. Expression of bcl-6 and CD10 in primary mediastinal large B-cell lymphoma: evidence for derivation from germinal center B cells? Am J Surg Pathol. 2001 Oct;25(10):1277–82. PMID:11688462

897. de Leval L, Harris NL, Longtine J, et al. Cutaneous B-cell lymphomas of follicular and marginal zone types: use of Bcl-6, CD10, Bcl-2, and CD21 in differential diagnosis and classification. Am J Surg Pathol. 2001 Jun;25(6):732–41. PMID:11395550

898. de Leval L, Parrens M, Le Bras F, et al. Angioimmunoblastic T-cell lymphoma is the most common T-cell lymphoma in two distinct French information data sets. Haematologica. 2015 Sep;100(9):e361–4. PMID:26045291

899. de Leval L, Rickman DS, Thielen C, et al. The gene expression profile of nodal peripheral T-cell lymphoma demonstrates a molecular link between angioimmunoblastic T-cell lymphoma (AITL) and follicular helper T (TFH) cells. Blood. 2007 Jun 1;109(11):4952–63. PMID:17284527

900. de Leval L, Savilo E, Longtine J, et al. Peripheral T-cell lymphoma with follicular involvement and a CD4+/bcl-6+ phenotype. Am J Surg Pathol. 2001 Mar;25(3):395–400. PMID:11224611

901. de Mascarel A, Belleannée G, Stanislas S, et al. Mucosal intraepithelial T-lymphocytes in refractory celiac disease: a neoplastic population with a variable CD8 phenotype. Am J Surg Pathol. 2008 May;32(5):744–51. PMID:18360280

902. de Mel S, Li JB, Abid MB, et al. The utility of flow cytometry in differentiating NK/T cell lymphoma from indolent and reactive NK cell proliferations. Cytometry B Clin Cytom. 2018 Jan;94(1):159–68. PMID:28431200

903. De Roos AJ, Davis S, Colt JS, et al. Residential proximity to industrial facilities and risk of non-Hodgkin lymphoma. Environ Res. 2010 Jan;110(1):70–8. PMID:19840879

904. de Sanjose S, Benavente Y, Vajdic CM, et al. Hepatitis C and non-Hodgkin lymphoma among 4784 cases and 6269 controls from the International Lymphoma Epidemiology Consortium. Clin Gastroenterol Hepatol. 2008 Apr;6(4):451–8. PMID:18387498

905. de Souza A, Camilleri MJ, Wada DA, et al. Clinical, histopathologic, and immunophenotypic features of lymphomatoid papulosis with CD8 predominance in 14 pediatric patients. J Am Acad Dermatol. 2009 Dec;61(6):993–1000. PMID:19577330

906. de Souza A, el-Azhary RA, Camilleri MJ, et al. In search of prognostic indicators for lymphomatoid papulosis: a retrospective study of 123 patients. J Am Acad Dermatol. 2012 Jun;66(6):928–37. PMID:21982062

907. De Souza A, Ferry JA, Burghart DR, et al. IgG4 expression in primary cutaneous marginal zone lymphoma: a multicenter study. Appl Immunohistochem Mol Morphol. 2018 Aug;26(7):462–7. PMID:28151793

908. de Waal EG, Leene M, Veeger N, et al. Progression of a solitary plasmacytoma to multiple myeloma. A population-based registry of the northern Netherlands. Br J Haematol. 2016 Nov;175(4):661–7. PMID:27605358

909. De Zen L, Orfao A, Cazzaniga G, et al. Quantitative multiparametric immunophenotyping in acute lymphoblastic leukemia: correlation with specific genotype. I. ETV6/AML1 ALLs identification. Leukemia. 2000 Jul;14(7):1225–31. PMID:10914546

910. Dearden CE, Matutes E, Cazin B, et al. High remission rate in T-cell prolymphocytic leukemia with CAMPATH-1H. Blood. 2001 Sep 15;98(6):1721–6. PMID:11535503

911. de Chadarévian JP, Vekemans M, Bernstein M. Fanconi's anemia, medulloblastoma, Wilms' tumor, horseshoe kidney, and gonadal dysgenesis. Arch Pathol Lab Med. 1985 Apr;109(4):367–9. PMID:2985019

912. Deckert M, Brunn A, Montesinos-Rongen M, et al. Primary lymphoma of the central nervous system–a diagnostic challenge. Hematol Oncol. 2014 Jun;32(2):57–67. PMID:23949943

913. DeCoster RC, Clemens MW, Di Napoli A, et al. Cellular and molecular mechanisms of breast implant-associated anaplastic large cell lymphoma. Plast Reconstr Surg. 2021 Jan 1;147(1):30e–41e. PMID:33370049

914. DeCoteau JF, Butmarc JR, Kinney MC, et al. The t(2;5) chromosomal translocation is not a common feature of primary cutaneous CD30+ lymphoproliferative disorders: comparison with anaplastic large-cell lymphoma of nodal origin. Blood. 1996 Apr 15;87(8):3437–41. PMID:8605362

915. Deenen NJ, Koens L, Jaspars EH, et al. Pitfalls in diagnosing primary cutaneous aggressive epidermotropic CD8+ T-cell lymphoma. Br J Dermatol. 2019 Feb;180(2):411–2. PMID:30259963

916. de Fijter JW. Cancer and mTOR inhibitors in transplant recipients. Transplantation. 2017 Jan;101(1):45–55. PMID:27547865

917. De Keersmaecker K, Marynen P, Cools J. Genetic insights in the pathogenesis of T-cell acute lymphoblastic leukemia. Haematologica. 2005 Aug;90(8):1116–27. PMID:16079112

918. Del Giudice I, Matutes E, Morilla R, et al. The diagnostic value of CD123 in B-cell disorders with hairy or villous lymphocytes. Haematologica. 2004 Mar;89(3):303–8. PMID:15020268

919. Del Giudice I, Osuji N, Dexter T, et al. B-cell prolymphocytic leukemia and chronic lymphocytic leukemia have distinctive gene expression signatures. Leukemia. 2009 Nov;23(11):2160–7. PMID:19641528

920. Del Poeta G, Maurillo L, Venditti A, et al. Clinical significance of CD38 expression in chronic lymphocytic leukemia. Blood. 2001 Nov 1;98(9):2633–9. PMID:11675331

921. Delabesse E, Bernard M, Meyer V, et al. TAL1 expression does not occur in the majority of T-ALL blasts. Br J Haematol. 1998 Jul;102(2):449–57. PMID:9695959

922. Delabie J, Holte H, Vose JM, et al. Enteropathy-associated T-cell lymphoma: clinical and histological findings from the international peripheral T-cell lymphoma project. Blood. 2011 Jul 7;118(1):148–55. PMID:21566094

923. Delecluse HJ, Anagnostopoulos I, Dallenbach F, et al. Plasmablastic lymphomas of the oral cavity: a new entity associated with the human immunodeficiency virus infection. Blood. 1997 Feb 15;89(4):1413–20. PMID:9028965

924. Deleeuw RJ, Zettl A, Klinker E, et al. Whole-genome analysis and HLA genotyping of enteropathy-type T-cell lymphoma reveals 2 distinct lymphoma subtypes. Gastroenterology. 2007 May;132(5):1902–11. PMID:17484883

925. D'Elios MM, Amedei A, Del Prete G. Helicobacter pylori antigen-specific T-cell responses at gastric level in chronic gastritis, peptic ulcer, gastric cancer and low-grade mucosa-associated lymphoid tissue (MALT) lymphoma. Microbes Infect. 2003 Jul;5(8):723–30. PMID:12814773

926. Delsol G, Lamant L, Mariamé B, et al. A new subtype of large B-cell lymphoma expressing the ALK kinase and lacking the 2; 5 translocation. Blood. 1997 Mar 1;89(5):1483–90. PMID:9057627

927. Demehri S, Paschka P, Schultheis B, et al. e8a2 BCR-ABL: more frequent than other atypical BCR-ABL variants? Leukemia. 2005 Apr;19(4):681–4. PMID:15703785

928. Demirkesen C, Tüzüner N, Esen T, et al. The expression of IgM is helpful in the differentiation of primary cutaneous diffuse large B cell lymphoma and follicle center lymphoma. Leuk Res. 2011 Sep;35(9):1269–72. PMID:21700336

929. Den Boer ML, van Slegtenhorst M, De Menezes RX, et al. A subtype of childhood acute lymphoblastic leukaemia with poor treatment outcome: a genome-wide classification study. Lancet Oncol. 2009 Feb;10(2):125–34. PMID:19138562

930. Derringer GA, Thompson LD, Frommelt RA, et al. Malignant lymphoma of the thyroid gland: a clinicopathologic study of 108 cases. Am J Surg Pathol. 2000 May;24(5):623–39. PMID:10800981

931. Desai M, Liu S, Parker S. Clinical characteristics, prognostic factors, and survival of 393 patients with mycosis fungoides and Sézary syndrome in the southeastern United States: a single-institution cohort. J Am Acad Dermatol. 2015 Feb;72(2):276–85. PMID:25458019

932. Deschênes M, Michel RP, Tabah R, et al. Fine-needle aspiration cytology of Castleman disease: case report with review of the literature. Diagn Cytopathol. 2008 Dec;36(12):904–8. PMID:18855889

933. Deshmukh M, Elderfield K, Rahemtulla A, et al. Immunophenotype of neoplastic plasma cells in AL amyloidosis. J Clin Pathol. 2009 Aug;62(8):724–30. PMID:19638544

934. Deshpande PA, Srivastava VM, Mani S, et al. Atypical BCR-ABL1 fusion transcripts in adult B-acute lymphoblastic leukemia, including a novel fusion transcript-e8a1. Leuk Lymphoma. 2016 Oct;57(10):2481–4. PMID:26942999

935. Deshpande V, Zen Y, Chan JK, et al. Consensus statement on the pathology of IgG4-related disease. Mod Pathol. 2012 Sep;25(9):1181–92. PMID:22596100

936. De Silva NS, Klein U. Dynamics of B cells in germinal centres. Nat Rev Immunol. 2015 Mar;15(3):137–48. PMID:25656706

937. de-Thé G. Epstein-Barr virus behavior in different populations and implications for control of Epstein-Barr virus-associated tumors. Cancer Res. 1976 Feb;36(2 pt 2):692–5. PMID:1253156

938. Devilard E, Bertucci F, Trempat P, et al. Gene expression profiling defines molecular subtypes of classical Hodgkin's disease. Oncogene. 2002 May 2;21(19):3095–102. PMID:12082542

939. Dheilly E, Battistello E, Katanayeva N, et al. Cathepsin S regulates antigen processing and T cell activity in non-Hodgkin lymphoma. Cancer Cell. 2020 May 11;37(5):674–689.e12. PMID:32330455

940. Dhodapkar MV, Li CY, Lust JA, et al. Clinical spectrum of clonal proliferations of T-large granular lymphocytes: a T-cell clonopathy of undetermined significance? Blood. 1994 Sep 1;84(5):1620–7. PMID:8068951

941. Di Bernardo MC, Crowther-Swanepoel D, Broderick P, et al. A genome-wide association study identifies six susceptibility loci for chronic lymphocytic leukemia. Nat Genet. 2008 Oct;40(10):1204–10. PMID:18758461

942. Di Giacomo D, La Starza R, Gorello P, et al. 14q32 rearrangements deregulating BCL11B mark a distinct subgroup of T-lymphoid and myeloid immature acute leukemia. Blood. 2021 Sep 2;138(9):773–84. PMID:33876209

943. Di Napoli A, De Cecco L, Piccaluga PP,

et al. Transcriptional analysis distinguishes breast implant-associated anaplastic large cell lymphoma from other peripheral T-cell lymphomas. Mod Pathol. 2019 Feb;32(2):216–30. PMID:30206415
944. Di Napoli A, Greco D, Scafetta G, et al. IL-10, IL-13, Eotaxin and IL-10/IL-6 ratio distinguish breast implant-associated anaplastic large-cell lymphoma from all types of benign late seromas. Cancer Immunol Immunother. 2021 May;70(5):1379–92. PMID:33146828
945. Di Napoli A, Jain P, Duranti E, et al. Targeted next generation sequencing of breast implant-associated anaplastic large cell lymphoma reveals mutations in JAK/STAT signalling pathway genes, TP53 and DNMT3A. Br J Haematol. 2018 Mar;180(5):741–4. PMID:27859003
946. Di Napoli A, Pepe G, Giarnieri E, et al. Cytological diagnostic features of late breast implant seromas: from reactive to anaplastic large cell lymphoma. PLoS One. 2017 Jul 17;12(7):e0181097. PMID:28715445
947. Diaz A, Vogiatzi MG, Sanz MM, et al. Evaluation of short stature, carbohydrate metabolism and other endocrinopathies in Bloom's syndrome. Horm Res. 2006;66(3):111–7. PMID:16763388
948. Díaz de la Pinta FJ, Rodríguez Moreno M, Salgado RN, et al. Anaplastic large cell lymphomas with the 6p25.3 rearrangement are a heterogeneous group of tumours with a diverse molecular background. Hum Pathol. 2023 Jul;137:71–8. PMID:37127078
949. Dictor M, Ek S, Sundberg M, et al. Strong lymphoid nuclear expression of SOX11 transcription factor defines lymphoblastic neoplasms, mantle cell lymphoma and Burkitt's lymphoma. Haematologica. 2009 Nov;94(11):1563–8. PMID:19880779
950. Diebold J, Anderson JR, Armitage JO, et al. Diffuse large B-cell lymphoma: a clinicopathologic analysis of 444 cases classified according to the updated Kiel classification. Leuk Lymphoma. 2002 Jan;43(1):97–104. PMID:11908742
951. Diebold J, Le Tourneau A, Marmey B, et al. Is sclerosing angiomatoid nodular transformation (SANT) of the splenic red pulp identical to inflammatory pseudotumour? Report of 16 cases. Histopathology. 2008 Sep;53(3):299–310. PMID:18643852
952. Diefenbach CS, Li H, Hong F, et al. Evaluation of the International Prognostic Score (IPS-7) and a Simpler Prognostic Score (IPS-3) for advanced Hodgkin lymphoma in the modern era. Br J Haematol. 2015 Nov;171(4):530–8. PMID:26343802
953. Diepstra A, Niens M, Vellenga E, et al. Association with HLA class I in Epstein-Barr-virus-positive and with HLA class III in Epstein-Barr-virus-negative Hodgkin's lymphoma. Lancet. 2005 Jun 25;365(9478):2216–24. PMID:15978930
954. Dierickx D, Habermann TM. Post-transplantation lymphoproliferative disorders in adults. N Engl J Med. 2018 Feb 8;378(6):549–62. PMID:29414277
955. Dierickx D, Tousseyn T, Morscio J, et al. Validation of prognostic scores in post-transplantation lymphoproliferative disorders. J Clin Oncol. 2013 Sep 20;31(27):3443–4. PMID:23960181
956. Dierickx D, Tousseyn T, Sagaert X, et al. Single-center analysis of biopsy-confirmed posttransplant lymphoproliferative disorder: incidence, clinicopathological characteristics and prognostic factors. Leuk Lymphoma. 2013 Nov;54(11):2433–40. PMID:23442063
957. Dierlamm J, Rosenberg C, Stul M, et al. Characteristic pattern of chromosomal gains and losses in marginal zone B cell lymphoma detected by comparative genomic hybridization. Leukemia. 1997 May;11(5):747–58. PMID:9180302
958. Dietrich S, Pircher A, Endris V, et al. BRAF inhibition in hairy cell leukemia with low-dose vemurafenib. Blood. 2016 Jun 9;127(23):2847–55. PMID:26941398
959. Dijkman R, Tensen CP, Jordanova ES, et al. Array-based comparative genomic hybridization analysis reveals recurrent chromosomal alterations and prognostic parameters in primary cutaneous large B-cell lymphoma. J Clin Oncol. 2006 Jan 10;24(2):296–305. PMID:16330669
960. Dimitriades VR, Devlin V, Pittaluga S, et al. DOCK 8 deficiency, EBV+ lymphomatoid granulomatosis, and intrafamilial variation in presentation. Front Pediatr. 2017 Feb 28;5:38. PMID:28293550
961. Dimopoulos MA, Hamilos G. Solitary bone plasmacytoma and extramedullary plasmacytoma. Curr Treat Options Oncol. 2002 Jun;3(3):255–9. PMID:12057071
962. Dimopoulos MA, Moreau P, Terpos E, et al. Multiple myeloma: EHA-ESMO Clinical Practice Guidelines for diagnosis, treatment and follow-up. Ann Oncol. 2021 Mar;32(3):309–22. PMID:33549387
963. Dinmohamed AG, Visser O, Doorduijn JK, et al. Treatment and survival of patients with primary effusion lymphoma in the Netherlands: a population-based analysis, 2002-2015. Hemasphere. 2018 Oct;2(5):e143. PMID:30887007
964. Dirnhofer S, Angeles-Angeles A, Ortiz-Hidalgo C, et al. High prevalence of a 30-base pair deletion in the Epstein-Barr virus (EBV) latent membrane protein 1 gene and of strain type B EBV in Mexican classical Hodgkin's disease and reactive lymphoid tissue. Hum Pathol. 1999 Jul;30(7):781–7. PMID:10414496
965. Disanto MG, Ambrosio MR, Rocca BJ, et al. Optimal minimal panels of immunohistochemistry for diagnosis of B-cell lymphoma for application in countries with limited resources and for triaging cases before referral to specialist centers. Am J Clin Pathol. 2016 May;145(5):687–95. PMID:27247372
966. Dispenzieri A. POEMS syndrome: 2019 update on diagnosis, risk-stratification, and management. Am J Hematol. 2019 Jul;94(7):812–27. PMID:31012139
967. Dispenzieri A. POEMS syndrome: 2021 update on diagnosis, risk-stratification, and management. Am J Hematol. 2021 Jul 1;96(7):872–88. PMID:34000085
968. Dispenzieri A, Fajgenbaum DC. Overview of Castleman disease. Blood. 2020 Apr 16;135(16):1353–64. PMID:32106302
968A. Dispenzieri A, Gertz MA, Kyle RA, et al. Serum cardiac troponins and N-terminal pro-brain natriuretic peptide: a staging system for primary systemic amyloidosis. J Clin Oncol. 2004 Sep 15;22(18):3751–7. PMID:15365071
969. Dispenzieri A, Kyle RA, Lacy MQ, et al. POEMS syndrome: definitions and long-term outcome. Blood. 2003 Apr 1;101(7):2496–506. PMID:12456500
970. Diss TC, Wotherspoon AC, Speight P, et al. B-cell monoclonality, Epstein Barr virus, and t(14;18) in myoepithelial sialadenitis and low-grade B-cell MALT lymphoma of the parotid gland. Am J Surg Pathol. 1995 May;19(5):531–6. PMID:7726362
970A. Dittrich T, Benner A, Kimmich C, et al. Performance analysis of AL amyloidosis cardiac biomarker staging systems with special focus on renal failure and atrial arrhythmia. Haematologica. 2019 Jul;104(7):1451–9. PMID:30655373
970B. Dittrich T, Kimmich C, Hegenbart U, et al. Prognosis and staging of AL amyloidosis. Acta Haematol. 2020;143(4):388–400. PMID:32570242
971. Djokic M, Le Beau MM, Swinnen LJ, et al. Post-transplant lymphoproliferative disorder subtypes correlate with different recurring chromosomal abnormalities. Genes Chromosomes Cancer. 2006 Mar;45(3):313–8. PMID:16283619
972. Dobay MP, Lemonnier F, Missiaglia E, et al. Integrative clinicopathological and molecular analyses of angioimmunoblastic T-cell lymphoma and other nodal lymphomas of follicular helper T-cell origin. Haematologica. 2017 Apr;102(4):e148–51. PMID:28082343
973. Dobos G, de Masson A, Ram-Wolff C, et al. Epidemiological changes in cutaneous lymphomas: an analysis of 8593 patients from the French Cutaneous Lymphoma Registry. Br J Dermatol. 2021 Jun;184(6):1059–67. PMID:33131055
974. Dobson R, Du PY, Rásó-Barnett L, et al. Early detection of T-cell lymphoma with T follicular helper phenotype by RHOA mutation analysis. Haematologica. 2022 Feb 1;107(2):489–99. PMID:33567811
975. Dobson R, Venkatraman L, Cucco F, et al. In situ follicular neoplasia in a young post-liver transplant patient. Pathol Int. 2023 Jan;73(1):58–60. PMID:36504425
976. Dobson R, Wotherspoon A, Liu SA, et al. Widespread in situ follicular neoplasia in patients who subsequently developed follicular lymphoma. J Pathol. 2022 Apr;256(4):369–77. PMID:34957565
977. Doeden K, Molina-Kirsch H, Perez E, et al. Hydroa-like lymphoma with CD56 expression. J Cutan Pathol. 2008 May;35(5):488–94. PMID:17976208
978. Dogan A, Attygalle AD, Kyriakou C. Angioimmunoblastic T-cell lymphoma. Br J Haematol. 2003 Jun;121(5):681–91. PMID:12780782
979. Dogan A, Burke JS, Goteri G, et al. Micronodular T-cell/histiocyte-rich large B-cell lymphoma of the spleen: histology, immunophenotype, and differential diagnosis. Am J Surg Pathol. 2003 Jul;27(7):903–11. PMID:12826882
980. Dogan A, Du M, Koulis A, et al. Expression of lymphocyte homing receptors and vascular addressins in low-grade gastric B-cell lymphomas of mucosa-associated lymphoid tissue. Am J Pathol. 1997 Nov;151(5):1361–9. PMID:9358762
981. Doglioni C, Ponzoni M, Ferreri AJ, et al. Gastric lymphoma: the histology report. Dig Liver Dis. 2011 Mar;43 Suppl 4:S310–8. PMID:21459337
982. Döhner H, Stilgenbauer S, Benner A, et al. Genomic aberrations and survival in chronic lymphocytic leukemia. N Engl J Med. 2000 Dec 28;343(26):1910–6. PMID:11136261
983. Dojcinov SD, Fend F, Quintanilla-Martinez L. EBV-Positive lymphoproliferations of B- T- and NK-cell derivation in non-immunocompromised hosts. Pathogens. 2018 Mar 7;7(1):28. PMID:29518976
984. Dojcinov SD, Venkataraman G, Pittaluga S, et al. Age-related EBV-associated lymphoproliferative disorders in the western population: a spectrum of reactive lymphoid hyperplasia and lymphoma. Blood. 2011 May 5;117(18):4726–35. PMID:21385849
985. Dojcinov SD, Venkataraman G, Raffeld M, et al. EBV positive mucocutaneous ulcer–a study of 26 cases associated with various sources of immunosuppression. Am J Surg Pathol. 2010 Mar;34(3):405–17. PMID:20154586
986. Dölken G, Dölken L, Hirt C, et al. Age-dependent prevalence and frequency of circulating t(14;18)-positive cells in the peripheral blood of healthy individuals. J Natl Cancer Inst Monogr. 2008; (39):44–7. PMID:18648002
987. Domchek SM, Hecht JL, Fleming MD, et al. Lymphomas of the breast: primary and secondary involvement. Cancer. 2002 Jan 1;94(1):6–13. PMID:11815954
988. Dominguez-Sola D, Kung J, Holmes AB, et al. The FOXO1 transcription factor instructs the germinal center dark zone program. Immunity. 2015 Dec 15;43(6):1064–74. PMID:26620759
989. Dong G, Li Y, Lee L, et al. Genetic manipulation of primary human natural killer cells to investigate the functional and oncogenic roles of PRDM1. Haematologica. 2021 Sep 1;106(9):2427–38. PMID:32732362
990. Dong N, Castillo Tokumori F, Isenalumhe L, et al. Large granular lymphocytic leukemia - a retrospective study of 319 cases. Am J Hematol. 2021 Jul 1;96(7):772–80. PMID:33819354
991. Donner LR, Marcussen S, Dobin SM. A clonal dic(16;21)(p13.1;p11.2)del(16)(q11.1), with gains of several chromosomes and monosomy 21, in a case of splenic hamartoma: evidence for its neoplastic, not hamartomatous, origin. Cancer Genet Cytogenet. 2005 Mar;157(2):160–3. PMID:15721639
992. Doren EL, Miranda RN, Selber JC, et al. U.S. epidemiology of breast implant-associated anaplastic large cell lymphoma. Plast Reconstr Surg. 2017 May;139(5):1042–50. PMID:28157769
993. Dorfman DM, Brown JA, Shahsafaei A, et al. Programmed death-1 (PD-1) is a marker of germinal center-associated T cells and angioimmunoblastic T-cell lymphoma. Am J Surg Pathol. 2006 Jul;30(7):802–10. PMID:16819321
994. Dorfman DM, Shahsafaei A. CD200 (OX-2 membrane glycoprotein) is expressed by follicular T helper cells and in angioimmunoblastic T-cell lymphoma. Am J Surg Pathol. 2011 Jan;35(1):76–83. PMID:21164290
995. Dorfman DM, Shahsafaei A, Alonso MA. Utility of CD200 immunostaining in the diagnosis of primary mediastinal large B cell lymphoma: comparison with MAL, CD23, and other markers. Mod Pathol. 2012 Dec;25(12):1637–43. PMID:22899296
996. Dorfman RF, Berry GJ. Kikuchi's histiocytic necrotizing lymphadenitis: an analysis of 108 cases with emphasis on differential diagnosis. Semin Diagn Pathol. 1988 Nov;5(4):329–45. PMID:3217625
997. Dowdell KC, Niemela JE, Price S, et al. Somatic FAS mutations are common in patients with genetically undefined autoimmune lymphoproliferative syndrome. Blood. 2010 Jun 24;115(25):5164–9. PMID:20360470
998. Dreyling M, Ghielmini M, Rule S, et al. Newly diagnosed and relapsed follicular lymphoma: ESMO Clinical Practice Guidelines for diagnosis, treatment and follow-up. Ann Oncol. 2021 Mar;32(3):298–308. PMID:33249059
999. Driessen GJ, van Zelm MC, van Hagen PM, et al. B-cell replication history and somatic hypermutation status identify distinct pathophysiologic backgrounds in common variable immunodeficiency. Blood. 2011 Dec 22;118(26):6814–23. PMID:22042693
1000. D'Sa S, Kersten MJ, Castillo JJ, et al. Investigation and management of IgM and Waldenström-associated peripheral neuropathies: recommendations from the IWWM-8 consensus panel. Br J Haematol. 2017 Mar;176(5):728–42. PMID:28198999
1001. D'Souza A, Hayman SR, Buadi F, et al. The utility of plasma vascular endothelial growth factor levels in the diagnosis and follow-up of patients with POEMS syndrome. Blood. 2011 Oct 27;118(17):4663–5. PMID:21881050
1002. D'Souza A, Lacy M, Gertz M, et al. Long-term outcomes after autologous stem cell transplantation for patients with POEMS syndrome (osteosclerotic myeloma): a single-center

experience. Blood. 2012 Jul 5;120(1):56–62. PMID:22611150

1003. Du H, Shi L, Chen P, et al. Prohibitin is involved in patients with IgG4 related disease. PLoS One. 2015 May 1;10(5):e0125331. PMID:25932630

1004. Du J, Chisholm KM, Tsuchiya K, et al. Lineage switch in an infant B-lymphoblastic leukemia with t(1;11)(p32;q23); KMT2A/EPS15, following blinatumomab therapy. Pediatr Dev Pathol. 2021 Jul-Aug;24(4):378–82. PMID:33749383

1005. Du J, Shen Q, Yin H, et al. Littoral cell angioma of the spleen: report of three cases and literature review. Int J Clin Exp Pathol. 2015 Jul 1;8(7):8516–20. PMID:26339427

1006. Du MQ. MALT lymphoma : recent advances in aetiology and molecular genetics. J Clin Exp Hematop. 2007 Nov;47(2):31–42. PMID:18040143

1007. Du MQ. MALT lymphoma: a paradigm of NF-κB dysregulation. Semin Cancer Biol. 2016 Aug;39:49–60. PMID:27452667

1008. Du MQ. MALT lymphoma: genetic abnormalities, immunological stimulation and molecular mechanism. Best Pract Res Clin Haematol. 2017 Mar-Jun;30(1-2):13–23. PMID:28288707

1009. Du MQ, Atherton JC. Molecular subtyping of gastric MALT lymphomas: implications for prognosis and management. Gut. 2006 Jun;55(6):886–93. PMID:16698756

1010. Du MQ, Diss TC, Liu H, et al. KSHV- and EBV-associated germinotropic lymphoproliferative disorder. Blood. 2002 Nov 1;100(9):3415–8. PMID:12384445

1011. Du MQ, Liu H, Diss TC, et al. Kaposi sarcoma-associated herpesvirus infects monotypic (IgM lambda) but polyclonal naive B cells in Castleman disease and associated lymphoproliferative disorders. Blood. 2001 Apr 1;97(7):2130–6. PMID:11264181

1012. Du MQ, Xu CF, Diss TC, et al. Intestinal dissemination of gastric mucosa-associated lymphoid tissue lymphoma. Blood. 1996 Dec 15;88(12):4445–51. PMID:8977236

1013. Dubois S, Viailly PJ, Mareschal S, et al. Next-generation sequencing in diffuse large B-cell lymphoma highlights molecular divergence and therapeutic opportunities: a LYSA study. Clin Cancer Res. 2016 Jun 15;22(12):2919–28. PMID:26819451

1014. Ducharme O, Beylot-Barry M, Pham-Ledard A, et al. Mutations of the B-cell receptor pathway confer chemoresistance in primary cutaneous diffuse large B-cell lymphoma leg type. J Invest Dermatol. 2019 Nov;139(11):2334–2342.e8. PMID:31150604

1015. Dufau JP, le Tourneau A, Audouin J, et al. Isolated diffuse hemangiomatosis of the spleen with Kasabach-Merritt-like syndrome. Histopathology. 1999 Oct;35(4):337–44. PMID:10564388

1016. Dufva O, Kankainen M, Kelkka T, et al. Aggressive natural killer-cell leukemia mutational landscape and drug profiling highlight JAK-STAT signaling as therapeutic target. Nat Commun. 2018 Apr 19;9(1):1567. PMID:29674644

1017. Dühren-von Minden M, Übelhart R, Schneider D, et al. Chronic lymphocytic leukaemia is driven by antigen-independent cell-autonomous signalling. Nature. 2012 Sep 13;489(7415):309–12. PMID:22885698

1018. Dumas G, Prendki V, Haroche J, et al. Kikuchi-Fujimoto disease: retrospective study of 91 cases and review of the literature. Medicine (Baltimore). 2014 Nov;93(24):372–82. PMID:25500707

1019. Dun KA, Vanhaeften R, Batt TJ, et al. BCR-ABL1 gene rearrangement as a subclonal change in ETV6-RUNX1-positive B-cell acute lymphoblastic leukemia. Blood Adv. 2016 Nov 30;1(2):132–8. PMID:29296806

1020. Dunleavy K, Fanale MA, Abramson JS, et al. Dose-adjusted EPOCH-R (etoposide, prednisone, vincristine, cyclophosphamide, doxorubicin, and rituximab) in untreated aggressive diffuse large B-cell lymphoma with MYC rearrangement: a prospective, multicentre, single-arm phase 2 study. Lancet Haematol. 2018 Dec;5(12):e609–17. PMID:30501868

1021. Dunleavy K, Pittaluga S, Maeda LS, et al. Dose-adjusted EPOCH-rituximab therapy in primary mediastinal B-cell lymphoma. N Engl J Med. 2013 Apr 11;368(15):1408–16. PMID:23574119

1022. Duns G, Viganò E, Ennishi D, et al. Characterization of DLBCL with a PMBL gene expression signature. Blood. 2021 Jul 15;138(2):136–48. PMID:33684939

1023. Dunsmore KP, Winter SS, Devidas M, et al. Children's Oncology Group AALL0434: a phase III randomized clinical trial testing nelarabine in newly diagnosed T-cell acute lymphoblastic leukemia. J Clin Oncol. 2020 Oct 1;38(28):3282–93. PMID:32813610

1024. Dupin N, Diss TL, Kellam P, et al. HHV-8 is associated with a plasmablastic variant of Castleman disease that is linked to HHV-8-positive plasmablastic lymphoma. Blood. 2000 Feb 15;95(4):1406–12. PMID:10666218

1025. Duployez N, Boudry-Labis E, Decool G, et al. Diagnosis of intrachromosomal amplification of chromosome 21 (iAMP21) by molecular cytogenetics in pediatric acute lymphoblastic leukemia. Clin Case Rep. 2015 Oct;3(10):814–6. PMID:26509013

1026. Duployez N, Jamrog LA, Fregona V, et al. Germline PAX5 mutation predisposes to familial B-cell precursor acute lymphoblastic leukemia. Blood. 2021 Mar 11;137(10):1424–8. PMID:33036026

1027. Dupré L, Aiuti A, Trifari S, et al. Wiskott-Aldrich syndrome protein regulates lipid raft dynamics during immunological synapse formation. Immunity. 2002 Aug;17(2):157–66. PMID:12196287

1028. Dupuy A, Lemonnier F, Fataccioli V, et al. Multiple ways to detect IDH2 mutations in angioimmunoblastic T-cell lymphoma from immunohistochemistry to next-generation sequencing. J Mol Diagn. 2018 Sep;20(5):677–85. PMID:29981867

1029. Durandy A, Kracker S. Increased activation of PI3 kinase-δ predisposes to B-cell lymphoma. Blood. 2020 Feb 27;135(9):638–43. PMID:31942637

1030. Durham BH, Getta B, Dietrich S, et al. Genomic analysis of hairy cell leukemia identifies novel recurrent genetic alterations. Blood. 2017 Oct 5;130(14):1644–8. PMID:28801450

1031. Durot E, Tomowiak C, Michallet AS, et al. Transformed Waldenström macroglobulinaemia: clinical presentation and outcome. A multi-institutional retrospective study of 77 cases from the French Innovative Leukemia Organization (FILO). Br J Haematol. 2017 Nov;179(3):439–48. PMID:28770576

1032. Dutzmann CM, Spix C, Popp I, et al. Cancer in children with Fanconi anemia and ataxia-telangiectasia-a nationwide register-based cohort study in Germany. J Clin Oncol. 2022 Jan 1;40(1):32–9. PMID:34597127

1033. Dworzak MN, Buldini B, Gaipa G, et al. AIEOP-BFM consensus guidelines 2016 for flow cytometric immunophenotyping of pediatric acute lymphoblastic leukemia. Cytometry B Clin Cytom. 2018 Jan;94(1):82–93. PMID:28187514

1034. Dyer MJ, Akasaka T, Capasso M, et al. Immunoglobulin heavy chain locus chromosomal translocations in B-cell precursor acute lymphoblastic leukemia: rare clinical curios or potent genetic drivers? Blood. 2010 Feb 25;115(8):1490–9. PMID:20042721

1035. Dyhdalo KS, Lanigan C, Tubbs RR, et al. Immunoarchitectural patterns of germinal center antigens including LMO2 assist in the differential diagnosis of marginal zone lymphoma vs follicular lymphoma. Am J Clin Pathol. 2013 Aug;140(2):149–54. PMID:23897248

1036. Eberle FC, Mani H, Jaffe ES. Histopathology of Hodgkin's lymphoma. Cancer J. 2009 Mar-Apr;15(2):129–37. PMID:19390308

1037. Eberle FC, Rodriguez-Canales J, Wei L, et al. Methylation profiling of mediastinal gray zone lymphoma reveals a distinctive signature with elements shared by classical Hodgkin's lymphoma and primary mediastinal large B-cell lymphoma. Haematologica. 2011 Apr;96(4):558–66. PMID:21454882

1038. Eberle FC, Salaverria I, Steidl C, et al. Gray zone lymphoma: chromosomal aberrations with immunophenotypic and clinical correlations. Mod Pathol. 2011 Dec;24(12):1586–97. PMID:21822207

1039. Eberle FC, Song JY, Xi L, et al. Nodal involvement by cutaneous CD30-positive T-cell lymphoma mimicking classical Hodgkin lymphoma. Am J Surg Pathol. 2012 May;36(5):716–25. PMID:22367293

1040. Ebied A, Thanh Huan V, Makram OM, et al. The role of primary lymph node sites in survival and mortality prediction in Hodgkin lymphoma: a SEER population-based retrospective study. Cancer Med. 2018 Apr;7(4):953–65. PMID:29520977

1041. Eckert C, Parker C, Moorman AV, et al. Risk factors and outcomes in children with high-risk B-cell precursor and T-cell relapsed acute lymphoblastic leukaemia: combined analysis of ALLR3 and ALL-REZ BFM 2002 clinical trials. Eur J Cancer. 2021 Jul;151:175–89. PMID:34010787

1042. Edelmann J, Holzmann K, Tausch E, et al. Genomic alterations in high-risk chronic lymphocytic leukemia frequently affect cell cycle key regulators and NOTCH1-regulated transcription. Haematologica. 2020 May;105(5):1379–90. PMID:31467127

1043. Edinger JT, Kant JA, Swerdlow SH. Cutaneous marginal zone lymphomas have distinctive features and include 2 subsets. Am J Surg Pathol. 2010 Dec;34(12):1830–41. PMID:21107089

1044. Edlefsen KL, Greisman HA, Yi HS, et al. Early lymph node involvement by mantle cell lymphoma limited to the germinal center: report of a case with a novel "follicular in situ" growth pattern. Am J Clin Pathol. 2011 Aug;136(2):276–81. PMID:21757601

1045. Egan LJ, Walsh SV, Stevens FM, et al. Celiac-associated lymphoma. A single institution experience of 30 cases in the combination chemotherapy era. J Clin Gastroenterol. 1995 Sep;21(2):123–9. PMID:8583077

1046. Egawa N, Fukayama M, Kawaguchi K, et al. Relapsing oral and colonic ulcers with monoclonal T-cell infiltration. A low grade mucosal T-lymphoproliferative disease of the digestive tract. Cancer. 1995 Apr 1;75(7):1728–33. PMID:8826934

1047. Egg D, Schwab C, Gabrysch A, et al. Increased risk for malignancies in 131 affected CTLA4 mutation carriers. Front Immunol. 2018 Sep 10;9:2012. PMID:30250467

1048. Eibel H, Kraus H, Sic H, et al. B cell biology: an overview. Curr Allergy Asthma Rep. 2014 May;14(5):434. PMID:24633618

1049. Eichenauer DA, Fuchs M, Pluetschow A, et al. Phase 2 study of rituximab in newly diagnosed stage IA nodular lymphocyte-predominant Hodgkin lymphoma: a report from the German Hodgkin Study Group. Blood. 2011 Oct 20;118(16):4363–5. PMID:21828141

1050. Eichenauer DA, Kreissl S, Bühnen I, et al. PET-2-guided escalated BEACOPP for advanced nodular lymphocyte-predominant Hodgkin lymphoma: a subgroup analysis of the randomized German Hodgkin Study Group HD18 study. Ann Oncol. 2021 Jun;32(6):807–10. PMID:33667668

1051. Eichenauer DA, Plütschow A, Fuchs M, et al. Long-term follow-up of patients with nodular lymphocyte-predominant Hodgkin lymphoma treated in the HD7 to HD15 trials: a report from the German Hodgkin Study Group. J Clin Oncol. 2020 Mar 1;38(7):698–705. PMID:31626571

1052. Eichenauer DA, Plütschow A, Schröder L, et al. Relapsed and refractory nodular lymphocyte-predominant Hodgkin lymphoma: an analysis from the German Hodgkin Study Group. Blood. 2018 Oct 4;132(14):1519–25. PMID:30064977

1053. Ek S, Dictor M, Jerkeman M, et al. Nuclear expression of the non B-cell lineage Sox11 transcription factor identifies mantle cell lymphoma. Blood. 2008 Jan 15;111(2):800–5. PMID:17934069

1054. Ekström Smedby K, Vajdic CM, Falster M, et al. Autoimmune disorders and risk of non-Hodgkin lymphoma subtypes: a pooled analysis within the InterLymph Consortium. Blood. 2008 Apr 15;111(8):4029–38. PMID:18263783

1055. El Behery R, Laurini JA, Weisenburger DD, et al. Follicular large cleaved cell (centrocytic) lymphoma: an unrecognized variant of follicular lymphoma. Hum Pathol. 2018 Feb;72:180–90. PMID:29170017

1056. El Hussein S, Patel KP, Fang H, et al. Genomic and immunophenotypic landscape of aggressive NK-cell leukemia. Am J Surg Pathol. 2020 Sep;44(9):1235–43. PMID:32590457

1057. Eladl AE, Satou A, Elsayed AA, et al. Clinicopathological study of 30 cases of peripheral T-cell lymphoma with Hodgkin and Reed-Sternberg-like B-cells from Japan. Am J Surg Pathol. 2017 Apr;41(4):506–16. PMID:28125450

1058. el-Azhary RA, Gibson LE, Kurtin PJ, et al. Lymphomatoid papulosis: a clinical and histopathologic review of 53 cases with leukocyte immunophenotyping, DNA flow cytometry, and T-cell receptor gene rearrangement studies. J Am Acad Dermatol. 1994 Feb;30(2 Pt 1):210–8. PMID:8288780

1059. Eldfors S, Kuusanmäki H, Kontro M, et al. Idelalisib sensitivity and mechanisms of disease progression in relapsed TCF3-PBX1 acute lymphoblastic leukemia. Leukemia. 2017 Jan;31(1):51–7. PMID:27461063

1060. Elenitoba-Johnson KS, Gascoyne RD, Lim MS, et al. Homozygous deletions at chromosome 9p21 involving p16 and p15 are associated with histologic progression in follicle center lymphoma. Blood. 1998 Jun 15;91(12):4677–85. PMID:9616165

1061. Elenitoba-Johnson KS, Jaffe ES. Lymphoproliferative disorders associated with congenital immunodeficiencies. Semin Diagn Pathol. 1997 Feb;14(1):35–47. PMID:9044508

1062. Elenitoba-Johnson KS, Kumar S, Lim MS, et al. Marginal zone B-cell lymphoma with monocytoid B-cell lymphocytes in pediatric patients without immunodeficiency. A report of two cases. Am J Clin Pathol. 1997 Jan;107(1):92–8. PMID:8980374

1063. Elenitoba-Johnson KS, Wilcox R. A new molecular paradigm in mycosis fungoides and Sézary syndrome. Semin Diagn Pathol. 2017 Jan;34(1):15–21. PMID:28024703

1064. Elenitoba-Johnson KS, Zarate-Osorno A, Meneses A, et al. Cytotoxic granular protein expression, Epstein-Barr virus strain type, and latent membrane protein-1 oncogene deletions in nasal T-lymphocyte/natural killer cell lymphomas from Mexico. Mod Pathol. 1998 Aug;11(8):754–61. PMID:9720504

1065. El Hussein S, Khoury JD, Medeiros LJ. B-prolymphocytic leukemia: Is it time to retire this entity? Ann Diagn Pathol. 2021 Oct;54:151790. PMID:34293709

1066. Elkaim E, Neven B, Bruneau J, et al. Clinical and immunologic phenotype associated with activated phosphoinositide 3-kinase δ syndrome 2: a cohort study. J Allergy Clin Immunol. 2016 Jul;138(1):210–218.e9. PMID:27221134

1067. Ellin F, Landström J, Jerkeman M, et al. Real-world data on prognostic factors and treatment in peripheral T-cell lymphomas: a study from the Swedish Lymphoma Registry. Blood. 2014 Sep 4;124(10):1570–7. PMID:25006130

1068. Ellington TD, Henley SJ, Wilson RJ, et al. Trends in solitary plasmacytoma, extramedullary plasmacytoma, and plasma cell myeloma incidence and myeloma mortality by racial-ethnic group, United States 2003-2016. Cancer Med. 2021 Jan;10(1):386–95. PMID:33270992

1069. El-Mallawany NK, Curry CV, Allen CE. Haemophagocytic lymphohistiocytosis and Epstein-Barr virus: a complex relationship with diverse origins, expression and outcomes. Br J Haematol. 2022 Jan;196(1):31–44. PMID:34169507

1070. El Shabrawi-Caelen L, Kerl H, Cerroni L. Lymphomatoid papulosis: reappraisal of clinicopathologic presentation and classification into subtypes A, B, and C. Arch Dermatol. 2004 Apr;140(4):441–7. PMID:15096372

1071. Elshiekh M, Naresh KN. Lymphoproliferative disorders and lymphoreticular malignancies in the setting of immunodeficiency. Diagn Histopathol (Oxf). 2018;24(7):246–56. doi:10.1016/j.mpdhp.2018.05.008.

1072. Elsner RA, Shlomchik MJ. Germinal center and extrafollicular B cell responses in vaccination, immunity, and autoimmunity. Immunity. 2020 Dec 15;53(6):1136–50. PMID:33326765

1073. Elstrom RL, Andreadis C, Aqui NA, et al. Treatment of PTLD with rituximab or chemotherapy. Am J Transplant. 2006 Mar;6(3):569–76. PMID:16468968

1074. Emmanuel B, Kawira E, Ogwang MD, et al. African Burkitt lymphoma: age-specific risk and correlations with malaria biomarkers. Am J Trop Med Hyg. 2011 Mar;84(3):397–401. PMID:21363976

1075. Enciso-Mora V, Broderick P, Ma Y, et al. A genome-wide association study of Hodgkin's lymphoma identifies new susceptibility loci at 2p16.1 (REL), 8q24.21 and 10p14 (GATA3). Nat Genet. 2010 Dec;42(12):1126–30. PMID:21037568

1076. Engelhard M, Brittinger G, Huhn D, et al. Subclassification of diffuse large B-cell lymphomas according to the Kiel classification: distinction of centroblastic and immunoblastic lymphomas is a significant prognostic risk factor. Blood. 1997 Apr 1;89(7):2291–7. PMID:9116271

1077. Engels EA, Pfeiffer RM, Goedert JJ, et al. Trends in cancer risk among people with AIDS in the United States 1980-2002. AIDS. 2006 Aug 1;20(12):1645–54. PMID:16868446

1078. Engels EA, Pittaluga S, Whitby D, et al. Immunoblastic lymphoma in persons with AIDS-associated Kaposi's sarcoma: a role for Kaposi's sarcoma-associated herpesvirus. Mod Pathol. 2003 May;16(5):424–9. PMID:12748248

1079. Engels K, Jungnickel B, Tobollik S, et al. Expression of activation-induced cytidine deaminase in malignant lymphomas infiltrating the bone marrow. Appl Immunohistochem Mol Morphol. 2008 Dec;16(6):521–9. PMID:18776814

1080. Ennishi D, Jiang A, Boyle M, et al. Double-hit gene expression signature defines a distinct subgroup of germinal center B-cell-like diffuse large B-cell lymphoma. J Clin Oncol. 2019 Jan 20;37(3):190–201. PMID:30523716

1081. Ennishi D, Mottok A, Ben-Neriah S, et al. Genetic profiling of MYC and BCL2 in diffuse large B-cell lymphoma determines cell-of-origin-specific clinical impact. Blood. 2017 May 18;129(20):2760–70. PMID:28351934

1082. Ennishi D, Takeuchi K, Yokoyama M, et al. CD5 expression is potentially predictive of poor outcome among biomarkers in patients with diffuse large B-cell lymphoma receiving rituximab plus CHOP therapy. Ann Oncol. 2008 Nov;19(11):1921–6. PMID:18573805

1083. Enno A, Catovsky D, O'Brien M, et al. 'Prolymphocytoid' transformation of chronic lymphocytic leukaemia. Br J Haematol. 1979 Jan;41(1):9–18. PMID:420739

1084. Enok Bonong PR, Zahreddine M, Buteau C, et al. Factors associated with post-transplant active Epstein-Barr virus infection and lymphoproliferative disease in hematopoietic stem cell transplant recipients: a systematic review and meta-analysis. Vaccines (Basel). 2021 Mar 19;9(3):288. PMID:33808928

1085. Enshaei A, Vora A, Harrison CJ, et al. Defining low-risk high hyperdiploidy in patients with paediatric acute lymphoblastic leukaemia: a retrospective analysis of data from the UKALL97/99 and UKALL2003 clinical trials. Lancet Haematol. 2021 Nov;8(11):e828–39. PMID:34715050

1086. Ensor HM, Schwab C, Russell LJ, et al. Demographic, clinical, and outcome features of children with acute lymphoblastic leukemia and CRLF2 deregulation: results from the MRC ALL97 clinical trial. Blood. 2011 Feb 17;117(7):2129–36. PMID:21106984

1087. Enzan N, Kitadate A, Tanaka A, et al. Incisional random skin biopsy, not punch biopsy, is an appropriate method for diagnosis of intravascular large B-cell lymphoma: a clinicopathological study of 25 patients. Br J Dermatol. 2019 Jul;181(1):200–1. PMID:30609011

1088. Epling-Burnette PK, Bai F, Wei S, et al. ERK couples chronic survival of NK cells to constitutively activated Ras in lymphoproliferative disease of granular lymphocytes (LDGL). Oncogene. 2004 Dec 9;23(57):9220–9. PMID:15516985

1089. Epling-Burnette PK, Liu JH, Catlett-Falcone R, et al. Inhibition of STAT3 signaling leads to apoptosis of leukemic large granular lymphocytes and decreased Mcl-1 expression. J Clin Invest. 2001 Feb;107(3):351–62. PMID:11160159

1090. Epling-Burnette PK, Painter JS, Chaurasia P, et al. Dysregulated NK receptor expression in patients with lymphoproliferative disease of granular lymphocytes. Blood. 2004 May 1;103(9):3431–9. PMID:14726391

1091. Epstein EH Jr, Levin DL, Croft JD Jr, et al. Mycosis fungoides. Survival, prognostic features, response to therapy, and autopsy findings. Medicine (Baltimore). 1972 Jan;51(1):61–72. PMID:5009530

1092. Espinet B, Ferrer A, Bellosillo B, et al. Distinction between asymptomatic monoclonal B-cell lymphocytosis with cyclin D1 overexpression and mantle cell lymphoma: from molecular profiling to flow cytometry. Clin Cancer Res. 2014 Feb 15;20(4):1007–19. PMID:24352646

1093. Ettersperger J, Montcuquet N, Malamut G, et al. Interleukin-15-dependent T-cell-like innate intraepithelial lymphocytes develop in the intestine and transform into lymphomas in celiac disease. Immunity. 2016 Sep 20;45(3):610–25. PMID:27612641

1094. Eun S, Jeon YK, Jang JJ. Hepatocellular carcinoma with immature T-cell (T-lymphoblastic) proliferation. J Korean Med Sci. 2010 Feb;25(2):309–12. PMID:20119589

1095. Evangelista-Leite D, Affonso Madaloso B, Shouta Yamashita B, et al. Treating chronic diarrhea: a systematic review on immunoproliferative small intestinal disease (IPSID). PLoS One. 2021 Jul 16;16(7):e0253695. PMID:34270561

1096. Evans AG, Rothberg PG, Burack WR, et al. Evolution to plasmablastic lymphoma evades CD19-directed chimeric antigen receptor T cells. Br J Haematol. 2015 Oct;171(2):205–9. PMID:26084925

1097. Evans MG, Medeiros LJ, Marques-Piubelli ML, et al. Breast implant-associated anaplastic large cell lymphoma: clinical follow-up and analysis of sequential pathologic specimens of untreated patients shows persistent or progressive disease. Mod Pathol. 2021 Dec;34(12):2148–53. PMID:34155351

1098. Evans PA, Pott Ch, Groenen PJ, et al. Significantly improved PCR-based clonality testing in B-cell malignancies by use of multiple immunoglobulin gene targets. Report of the BIOMED-2 Concerted Action BHM4-CT98-3936. Leukemia. 2007 Feb;21(2):207–14. PMID:17170731

1099. Evens AM, Antillón M, Aschebrook-Kilfoy B, et al. Racial disparities in Hodgkin's lymphoma: a comprehensive population-based analysis. Ann Oncol. 2012 Aug;23(8):2128–37. PMID:22241896

1100. Evens AM, Choquet S, Kroll-Desrosiers AR, et al. Primary CNS posttransplant lymphoproliferative disease (PTLD): an international report of 84 cases in the modern era. Am J Transplant. 2013 Jun;13(6):1512–22. PMID:23721553

1101. Eyre TA, Khan D, Hall GW, et al. Anaplastic lymphoma kinase-positive anaplastic large cell lymphoma: current and future perspectives in adult and paediatric disease. Eur J Haematol. 2014 Dec;93(6):455–68. PMID:24766435

1102. Eyre TA, Schuh A. An update for Richter syndrome - new directions and developments. Br J Haematol. 2017 Aug;178(4):508–20. PMID:28439883

1103. Fabbri G, Khiabanian H, Holmes AB, et al. Genetic lesions associated with chronic lymphocytic leukemia transformation to Richter syndrome. J Exp Med. 2013 Oct 21;210(11):2273–88. PMID:24127483

1104. Facchetti F, de Wolf-Peeters C, van den Oord JJ, et al. Plasmacytoid monocytes (so-called plasmacytoid T-cells) in Kikuchi's lymphadenitis. An immunohistologic study. Am J Clin Pathol. 1989 Jul;92(1):42–50. PMID:2787597

1105. Facchetti F, Lorenzi L. Follicular dendritic cells and related sarcoma. Semin Diagn Pathol. 2016 Sep;33(5):262–76. PMID:27318412

1106. Facchetti F, Pileri SA, Lorenzi L, et al. Histiocytic and dendritic cell neoplasms: what have we learnt by studying 67 cases. Virchows Arch. 2017 Oct;471(4):467–89. PMID:28695297

1107. Fais F, Ghiotto F, Hashimoto S, et al. Chronic lymphocytic leukemia B cells express restricted sets of mutated and unmutated antigen receptors. J Clin Invest. 1998 Oct 15;102(8):1515–25. PMID:9788964

1108. Fajgenbaum DC. Novel insights and therapeutic approaches in idiopathic multicentric Castleman disease. Blood. 2018 Nov 29;132(22):2323–30. PMID:30487129

1109. Fajgenbaum DC, Langan RA, Japp AS, et al. Identifying and targeting pathogenic PI3K/AKT/mTOR signaling in IL-6-blockade-refractory idiopathic multicentric Castleman disease. J Clin Invest. 2019 Aug 13;129(10):4451–63. PMID:31408438

1110. Fajgenbaum DC, Uldrick TS, Bagg A, et al. International, evidence-based consensus diagnostic criteria for HHV-8-negative/idiopathic multicentric Castleman disease. Blood. 2017 Mar 23;129(12):1646–57. PMID:28087540

1111. Fajgenbaum DC, van Rhee F, Nabel CS. HHV-8-negative, idiopathic multicentric Castleman disease: novel insights into biology, pathogenesis, and therapy. Blood. 2014 May 8;123(19):2924–33. PMID:24622327

1112. Falchook GS, Vega F, Dang NH, et al. Hepatosplenic gamma-delta T-cell lymphoma: clinicopathological features and treatment. Ann Oncol. 2009 Jun;20(6):1080–5. PMID:19237479

1113. Falini B. Anaplastic large cell lymphoma: pathological, molecular and clinical features. Br J Haematol. 2001 Sep;114(4):741–60. PMID:11564061

1114. Falini B, Agostinelli C, Bigerna B, et al. IRTA1 is selectively expressed in nodal and extranodal marginal zone lymphomas. Histopathology. 2012 Nov;61(5):930–41. PMID:22716304

1115. Falini B, Flenghi L, Pileri S, et al. PG-M1: a new monoclonal antibody directed against a fixative-resistant epitope on the macrophage-restricted form of the CD68 molecule. Am J Pathol. 1993 May;142(5):1359–72. PMID:7684194

1116. Falini B, Pileri S, Zinzani PL, et al. ALK+ lymphoma: clinico-pathological findings and outcome. Blood. 1999 Apr 15;93(8):2697–706. PMID:10194450

1117. Falini B, Tiacci E, Liso A, et al. Simple diagnostic assay for hairy cell leukaemia by immunocytochemical detection of annexin A1 (ANXA1). Lancet. 2004 Jun 5;363(9424):1869–70. PMID:15183626

1118. Falk GA, Nooli NP, Morris-Stiff G, et al. Sclerosing angiomatoid nodular transformation (SANT) of the spleen: case report and review of the literature. Int J Surg Case Rep. 2012;3(10):492–500. PMID:22858789

1119. Falk RH, Alexander KM, Liao R, et al. AL (light-chain) cardiac amyloidosis: a review of diagnosis and therapy. J Am Coll Cardiol. 2016 Sep 20;68(12):1323–41. PMID:27634125

1120. Falk S, Krishnan J, Meis JM. Primary angiosarcoma of the spleen. A clinicopathologic study of 40 cases. Am J Surg Pathol. 1993 Oct;17(10):959–70. PMID:8372948

1121. Falk S, Stutte HJ. Hamartomas of the spleen: a study of 20 biopsy cases. Histopathology. 1989 Jun;14(6):603–12. PMID:2759557

1122. Falk S, Stutte HJ, Frizzera G. Littoral cell angioma. A novel splenic vascular lesion demonstrating histiocytic differentiation. Am J Surg Pathol. 1991 Nov;15(11):1023–33. PMID:1928554

1123. Fallah M, Kharazmi E, Pukkala E, et al. Familial risk of non-Hodgkin lymphoma by sex, relationship, age at diagnosis and histology: a joint study from five Nordic countries. Leukemia. 2016 Feb;30(2):373–8. PMID:26442613

1124. Fallah M, Liu X, Ji J, et al. Autoimmune diseases associated with non-Hodgkin lymphoma: a nationwide cohort study. Ann Oncol. 2014 Oct;25(10):2025–30. PMID:25081899

1125. Fallah M, Liu X, Ji J, et al. Hodgkin lymphoma after autoimmune diseases by age at diagnosis and histological subtype. Ann Oncol. 2014 Jul;25(7):1397–404. PMID:24718892

1126. Famà R, Bomben R, Rasi S, et al. Ibrutinib-naïve chronic lymphocytic leukemia lacks Bruton tyrosine kinase mutations associated with treatment resistance. Blood. 2014 Dec 11;124(25):3831–3. PMID:25498455

1127. Familiades J, Bousquet M, Lafage-Pochitaloff M, et al. PAX5 mutations occur frequently in adult B-cell progenitor acute lymphoblastic leukemia and PAX5 haploinsufficiency is associated with BCR-ABL1 and TCF3-PBX1 fusion genes: a GRAALL study. Leukemia. 2009 Nov;23(11):1989–98. PMID:19587702

1128. Fan L, Miao Y, Wu YJ, et al. Expression patterns of CD200 and CD148 in leukemic

B-cell chronic lymphoproliferative disorders and their potential value in differential diagnosis. Leuk Lymphoma. 2015;56(12):3329–35. PMID:25791119
1129. Fan Z, Natkunam Y, Bair E, et al. Characterization of variant patterns of nodular lymphocyte predominant Hodgkin lymphoma with immunohistologic and clinical correlation. Am J Surg Pathol. 2003 Oct;27(10):1346–56. PMID:14508396
1130. Fanale MA, Horwitz SM, Forero-Torres A, et al. Brentuximab vedotin in the front-line treatment of patients with CD30+ peripheral T-cell lymphomas: results of a phase I study. J Clin Oncol. 2014 Oct 1;32(28):3137–43. PMID:25135998
1131. Fang H, Beird HC, Wang SA, et al. T-prolymphocytic leukemia: TCL1 or MTCP1 rearrangement is not mandatory to establish diagnosis. Leukemia. 2023 Sep;37(9):1919–21. PMID:37443196
1132. Fang H, Kapoor P, Gonsalves WI, et al. Defining lymphoplasmacytic lymphoma: Does MYD88L265P define a pathologically distinct entity among patients with an IgM paraprotein and bone marrow-based low-grade B-cell lymphomas with plasmacytic differentiation? Am J Clin Pathol. 2018 Jul 3;150(2):168–76. PMID:29868855
1133. Fang H, Wang W, El Hussein S, et al. B-cell lymphoma/leukaemia 11B (BCL11B) expression status helps distinguish early T-cell precursor acute lymphoblastic leukaemia/ lymphoma (ETP-ALL/LBL) from other subtypes of T-cell ALL/LBL. Br J Haematol. 2021 Sep;194(6):1034–8. PMID:34402058
1134. Fang W, Zhang J, Hong S, et al. EBV-driven LMP1 and IFN-γ up-regulate PD-L1 in nasopharyngeal carcinoma: implications for oncotargeted therapy. Oncotarget. 2014 Dec 15;5(23):12189–202. PMID:25361008
1135. Fanoni D, Corti L, Alberti-Violetti S, et al. Array-based CGH of primary cutaneous CD8+ aggressive EPIDERMO-tropic cytotoxic T-cell lymphoma. Genes Chromosomes Cancer. 2018 Dec;57(12):622–9. PMID:30307677
1136. Farah N, Kirkwood AA, Rahman S, et al. Prognostic impact of the absence of biallelic deletion at the TRG locus for pediatric patients with T-cell acute lymphoblastic leukemia treated on the Medical Research Council UK Acute Lymphoblastic Leukemia 2003 trial. Haematologica. 2018 Jul;103(7):e288–92. PMID:29519867
1137. Farcet JP, Gaulard P, Marolleau JP, et al. Hepatosplenic T-cell lymphoma: sinusal/sinusoidal localization of malignant cells expressing the T-cell receptor gamma delta. Blood. 1990 Jun 1;75(11):2213–9. PMID:2140703
1138. Farooq U, Choudhary S, McLeod MP, et al. Adenopathy and extensive skin patch overlying a plasmacytoma (AESOP) syndrome. J Clin Aesthet Dermatol. 2012 Nov;5(11):25–7. PMID:23198009
1139. Farren TW, Sadanand KS, Agrawal SG. Highly sensitive and accurate assessment of minimal residual disease in chronic lymphocytic leukemia using the novel CD160-ROR1 assay. Front Oncol. 2020 Dec 3;10:597730. PMID:33344247
1140. Farstad IN, Johansen FE, Vlatkovic L, et al. Heterogeneity of intraepithelial lymphocytes in refractory sprue: potential implications of CD30 expression. Gut. 2002 Sep;51(3):372–8. PMID:12171959
1141. Fasching K, Panzer S, Haas OA, et al. Presence of clone-specific antigen receptor gene rearrangements at birth indicates an in utero origin of diverse types of early childhood acute lymphoblastic leukemia. Blood. 2000 Apr 15;95(8):2722–4. PMID:10753857
1142. Fasulo SM, Narvaneni S, Kumar V, et al. Lytic bone lesion: an unusual presentation of hairy cell leukemia. Cureus. 2021 Jan 28;13(1):e12959. PMID:33659114
1143. Fattizzo B, Rosa J, Giannotta JA, et al. The physiopathology of T- cell acute lymphoblastic leukemia: focus on molecular aspects. Front Oncol. 2020 Feb 28;10:273. PMID:32185137
1144. Favre R, Manzoni D, Traverse-Glehen A, et al. Usefulness of CD200 in the differential diagnosis of SDRPL, SMZL, and HCL. Int J Lab Hematol. 2018 Aug;40(4):e59–62. PMID:29659173
1145. Fawzy MM, Abd El-hafez A, El-Ashwah S, et al. Isolated myeloperoxidase immunohistochemical expression in bone marrow biopsy depicts clinical outcomes in adults with typical B-acute lymphoblastic leukemia. Asian Pac J Cancer Prev. 2021 Jul 1;22(7):2143–52. PMID:34319037
1146. Fayand A, Boutboul D, Galicier L, et al. Epidemiology of Castleman disease associated with AA amyloidosis: description of 2 new cases and literature review. Amyloid. 2019 Dec;26(4):197–202. PMID:31364863
1147. Fazi C, Scarfò L, Pecciarini L, et al. General population low-count CLL-like MBL persists over time without clinical progression, although carrying the same cytogenetic abnormalities of CLL. Blood. 2011 Dec 15;118(25):6618–25. PMID:21876118
1148. Fazio G, Bardini M, De Lorenzo P, et al. Recurrent genetic fusions redefine MLL germ line acute lymphoblastic leukemia in infants. Blood. 2021 Apr 8;137(14):1980–4. PMID:33512459
1149. Federico M, Bellei M, Marcheselli L, et al. Peripheral T cell lymphoma, not otherwise specified (PTCL-NOS). A new prognostic model developed by the International T cell Project Network. Br J Haematol. 2018 Jun;181(6):760–9. PMID:29672827
1150. Federico M, Caballero Barrigón MD, Marcheselli L, et al. Rituximab and the risk of transformation of follicular lymphoma: a retrospective pooled analysis. Lancet Haematol. 2018 Aug;5(8):e359–67. PMID:30078408
1151. Federico M, Rudiger T, Bellei M, et al. Clinicopathologic characteristics of angioimmunoblastic T-cell lymphoma: analysis of the international peripheral T-cell lymphoma project. J Clin Oncol. 2013 Jan 10;31(2):240–6. PMID:22869878
1152. Feely MM, Gonzalo DH, Corbera M, et al. IgG4-related cholecystitis presenting as biliary malignancy: report of three cases. J Gastrointest Surg. 2014 Sep;18(9):1710–5. PMID:24944152
1153. Feldman AL, Law M, Remstein ED, et al. Recurrent translocations involving the IRF4 oncogene locus in peripheral T-cell lymphomas. Leukemia. 2009 Mar;23(3):574–80. PMID:18987657
1154. Feldman AL, Law ME, Inwards DJ, et al. PAX5-positive T-cell anaplastic large cell lymphomas associated with extra copies of the PAX5 gene locus. Mod Pathol. 2010 Apr;23(4):593–602. PMID:20118907
1155. Feldman AL, Vasmatzis G, Asmann YW, et al. Novel TRAF1-ALK fusion identified by deep RNA sequencing of anaplastic large cell lymphoma. Genes Chromosomes Cancer. 2013 Nov;52(11):1097–102. PMID:23999969
1156. Felgar RE, Furth EE, Wasik MA, et al. Histiocytic necrotizing lymphadenitis (Kikuchi's disease): in situ end-labeling, immunohistochemical, and serologic evidence supporting cytotoxic lymphocyte-mediated apoptotic cell death. Mod Pathol. 1997 Mar;10(3):231–41. PMID:9071731
1157. Felgar RE, Steward KR, Cousar JB, et al. T-cell-rich large-B-cell lymphomas contain non-activated CD8+ cytolytic T cells, show increased tumor cell apoptosis, and have lower Bcl-2 expression than diffuse large-B-cell lymphomas. Am J Pathol. 1998 Dec;153(6):1707–15. PMID:9846961
1158. Felice MS, Gallego MS, Alonso CN, et al. Prognostic impact of t(1;19)/ TCF3-PBX1 in childhood acute lymphoblastic leukemia in the context of Berlin-Frankfurt-Münster-based protocols. Leuk Lymphoma. 2011 Jul;52(7):1215–21. PMID:21534874
1159. Fend F, Cabecadas J, Gaulard P, et al. Early lesions in lymphoid neoplasia: conclusions based on the Workshop of the XV. Meeting of the European Association of Hematopathology and the Society of Hematopathology, in Uppsala, Sweden. J Hematop. 2012 Sep;5(3). PMID:24307917
1160. Fend F, Ferreri AJ, Coupland SE. How we diagnose and treat vitreoretinal lymphoma. Br J Haematol. 2016 Jun;173(5):680–92. PMID:27133587
1161. Feng Y, Rao H, Lei Y, et al. CD30 expression in extranodal natural killer/T-cell lymphoma, nasal type among 622 cases of mature T-cell and natural killer-cell lymphoma at a single institution in South China. Chin J Cancer. 2017 May 10;36(1):43. PMID:28486951
1162. Ferlay J, Colombet M, Soerjomataram I, et al. Estimating the global cancer incidence and mortality in 2018: GLOBOCAN sources and methods. Int J Cancer. 2019 Apr 15;144(8):1941–53. PMID:30350310
1163. Ferlay J, Ervik M, Lam F, et al. Global Cancer Observatory: Cancer Today [Internet]. Lyon (France): International Agency for Research on Cancer; 2020. Available from: https://gco.iarc.who.int/today.
1164. Fermand JP, Bridoux F, Kyle RA, et al. How I treat monoclonal gammopathy of renal significance (MGRS). Blood. 2013 Nov 21;122(22):3583–90. PMID:24108460
1165. Fermand JP, Brouet JC, Danon F, et al. Gamma heavy chain "disease": heterogeneity of the clinicopathologic features. Report of 16 cases and review of the literature. Medicine (Baltimore). 1989 Nov;68(6):321–35. PMID:2509855
1166. Fernández de Larrea C, Kyle R, Rosiñol L, et al. Primary plasma cell leukemia: consensus definition by the International Myeloma Working Group according to peripheral blood plasma cell percentage. Blood Cancer J. 2021 Dec 2;11(12):192. PMID:34857730
1167. Fernandez S, Cook GW, Arber DA. Metastasizing splenic littoral cell hemangioendothelioma. Am J Surg Pathol. 2006 Aug;30(8):1036–40. PMID:16861977
1168. Fernàndez V, Salamero O, Espinet B, et al. Genomic and gene expression profiling defines indolent forms of mantle cell lymphoma. Cancer Res. 2010 Feb 15;70(4):1408–18. PMID:20124476
1169. Fernandez-Pol S, Costa HA, Steiner DF, et al. High-throughput sequencing of subcutaneous panniculitis-like T-cell lymphoma reveals candidate pathogenic mutations. Appl Immunohistochem Mol Morphol. 2019 Nov/ Dec;27(10):740–8. PMID:31702703
1170. Ferrando AA, Neuberg DS, Staunton J, et al. Gene expression signatures define novel oncogenic pathways in T cell acute lymphoblastic leukemia. Cancer Cell. 2002 Feb;1(1):75–87. PMID:12086890
1171. Ferrara G, Cusano F, Robson A, et al. Primary cutaneous marginal zone B-cell lymphoma with anetoderma: spontaneous involution plus de novo clonal expansion. J Cutan Pathol. 2011 Apr;38(4):342–5. PMID:21219395
1172. Ferrara G, Di Blasi A, Zalaudek I, et al. Regarding the algorithm for the diagnosis of early mycosis fungoides proposed by the International Society for Cutaneous Lymphomas: suggestions from routine histopathology practice. J Cutan Pathol. 2008 Jun;35(6):549–53. PMID:18201238
1173. Ferreiro JF, Morscio J, Dierickx D, et al. EBV-positive and EBV-negative posttransplant diffuse large B cell lymphomas have distinct genomic and transcriptomic features. Am J Transplant. 2016 Feb;16(2):414–25. PMID:26780579
1174. Ferreiro JF, Morscio J, Dierickx D, et al. Post-transplant molecularly defined Burkitt lymphomas are frequently MYC-negative and characterized by the 11q-gain/loss pattern. Haematologica. 2015 Jul;100(7):e275–9. PMID:25795716
1175. Ferreri AJ, Blay JY, Reni M, et al. Prognostic scoring system for primary CNS lymphomas: the International Extranodal Lymphoma Study Group experience. J Clin Oncol. 2003 Jan 15;21(2):266–72. PMID:12525518
1176. Ferreri AJ, Campo E, Seymour JF, et al. Intravascular lymphoma: clinical presentation, natural history, management and prognostic factors in a series of 38 cases, with special emphasis on the 'cutaneous variant'. Br J Haematol. 2004 Oct;127(2):173–83. PMID:15461623
1177. Ferreri AJ, Ciceri F, Brandes AA, et al. MATILDE chemotherapy regimen for primary CNS lymphoma: results at a median follow-up of 12 years. Neurology. 2014 Apr 15;82(15):1370–3. PMID:24634458
1178. Ferreri AJ, Dognini GP, Bairey O, et al. The addition of rituximab to anthracycline-based chemotherapy significantly improves outcome in 'western' patients with intravascular large B-cell lymphoma. Br J Haematol. 2008 Oct;143(2):253–7. PMID:18699850
1179. Ferreri AJ, Dognini GP, Campo E, et al. Variations in clinical presentation, frequency of hemophagocytosis and clinical behavior of intravascular lymphoma diagnosed in different geographical regions. Haematologica. 2007 Apr;92(4):486–92. PMID:17488659
1180. Ferreri AJ, Dognini GP, Govi S, et al. Can rituximab change the usually dismal prognosis of patients with intravascular large B-cell lymphoma? J Clin Oncol. 2008 Nov 1;26(31):5134–6. PMID:18838697
1181. Ferreri AJ, Guidoboni M, Ponzoni M, et al. Evidence for an association between Chlamydia psittaci and ocular adnexal lymphomas. J Natl Cancer Inst. 2004 Apr 21;96(8):586–94. PMID:15100336
1182. Ferreri AJ, Ponzoni M, Guidoboni M, et al. Regression of ocular adnexal lymphoma after Chlamydia psittaci-eradicating antibiotic therapy. J Clin Oncol. 2005 Aug 1;23(22):5067–73. PMID:15968003
1183. Ferrufino-Schmidt MC, Medeiros LJ, Liu H, et al. Clinicopathologic features and prognostic impact of lymph node involvement in patients with breast implant-associated anaplastic large cell lymphoma. Am J Surg Pathol. 2018 Mar;42(3):293–305. PMID:29194092
1184. Ferry JA, Deshpande V. IgG4-related disease in the head and neck. Semin Diagn Pathol. 2012 Nov;29(4):235–44. PMID:23068303
1185. Ferry JA, Fung CY, Zukerberg L, et al. Lymphoma of the ocular adnexa: a study of 353 cases. Am J Surg Pathol. 2007 Feb;31(2):170–84. PMID:17255761
1186. Ferry JA, Harris NL, Young RH, et al. Malignant lymphoma of the testis, epididymis, and spermatic cord. A clinicopathologic study of 69 cases with immunophenotypic analysis. Am J Surg Pathol. 1994 Apr;18(4):376–90. PMID:8141430
1187. Ferry JA, Sohani AR, Longtine JA, et al. HHV8-positive, EBV-positive Hodgkin lymphoma-like large B-cell lymphoma and

HHV8-positive intravascular large B-cell lymphoma. Mod Pathol. 2009 May;22(5):618–26. PMID:19287457
1188. Ferry JA, Zukerberg LR, Harris NL. Florid progressive transformation of germinal centers. A syndrome affecting young men, without early progression to nodular lymphocyte predominance Hodgkin's disease. Am J Surg Pathol. 1992 Mar;16(3):252–8. PMID:1599017
1189. Feuerhake F, Kutok JL, Monti S, et al. NFkappaB activity, function, and target-gene signatures in primary mediastinal large B-cell lymphoma and diffuse large B-cell lymphoma subtypes. Blood. 2005 Aug 15;106(4):1392–9. PMID:15870177
1190. Fierro MT, Comessatti A, Quaglino P, et al. Expression pattern of chemokine receptors and chemokine release in inflammatory erythroderma and Sézary syndrome. Dermatology. 2006;213(4):284–92. PMID:17135733
1191. Finalet Ferreiro J, Rouhigharabaei L, Urbankova H, et al. Integrative genomic and transcriptomic analysis identified candidate genes implicated in the pathogenesis of hepatosplenic T-cell lymphoma. PLoS One. 2014 Jul 24;9(7):e102977. PMID:25057852
1192. Finkin S, Hartweger H, Oliveira TY, et al. Protein amounts of the MYC transcription factor determine germinal center B cell division capacity. Immunity. 2019 Aug 20;51(2):324–336.e5. PMID:31350178
1193. Fiori S, Todisco E, Ramadan S, et al. HHV8-negative effusion-based large B cell lymphoma arising in chronic myeloid leukemia patients under dasatinib treatment: a report of two cases. Biology (Basel). 2021 Feb 14;10(2):152. PMID:33672947
1194. Fischer K, Al-Sawaf O, Bahlo J, et al. Venetoclax and obinutuzumab in patients with CLL and coexisting conditions. N Engl J Med. 2019 Jun 6;380(23):2225–36. PMID:31166681
1195. Fischer K, Bahlo J, Fink AM, et al. Long-term remissions after FCR chemoimmunotherapy in previously untreated patients with CLL: updated results of the CLL8 trial. Blood. 2016 Jan 14;127(2):208–15. PMID:26486789
1196. Fischer U, Forster M, Rinaldi A, et al. Genomics and drug profiling of fatal TCF3-HLF-positive acute lymphoblastic leukemia identifies recurrent mutation patterns and therapeutic options. Nat Genet. 2015 Sep;47(9):1020–9. PMID:26214592
1197. Fischer U, Yang JJ, Ikawa T, et al. Cell fate decisions: the role of transcription factors in early B-cell development and leukemia. Blood Cancer Discov. 2020 Nov;1(3):224–33. PMID:33392513
1198. Fisher GH, Rosenberg FJ, Straus SE, et al. Dominant interfering Fas gene mutations impair apoptosis in a human autoimmune lymphoproliferative syndrome. Cell. 1995 Jun 16;81(6):935–46. PMID:7540117
1199. Fitzpatrick MJ, Massoth LR, Marcus C, et al. JAK2 rearrangements are a recurrent alteration in CD30+ systemic T-cell lymphomas with anaplastic morphology. Am J Surg Pathol. 2021 Jul 1;45(7):895–904. PMID:34105517
1200. Fitzsimmons L, Boyce AJ, Wei W, et al. Coordinated repression of BIM and PUMA by Epstein-Barr virus latent genes maintains the survival of Burkitt lymphoma cells. Cell Death Differ. 2018 Feb;25(2):241–54. PMID:28960205
1201. Flann S, Orchard GE, Wain EM, et al. Three cases of lymphomatoid papulosis with a CD56+ immunophenotype. J Am Acad Dermatol. 2006 Nov;55(5):903–6. PMID:17052504
1202. Fletcher CD, Stirling RW. Intranodal myofibroblastoma presenting in the submandibular region: evidence of a broader clinical and histological spectrum. Histopathology. 1990 Mar;16(3):287–93. PMID:2332214
1203. Flores-Montero J, de Tute R, Paiva B, et al. Immunophenotype of normal vs. myeloma plasma cells: toward antibody panel specifications for MRD detection in multiple myeloma. Cytometry B Clin Cytom. 2016 Jan;90(1):61–72. PMID:26100534
1204. Florindez JA, Alderuccio JP, Reis IM, et al. Splenic marginal zone lymphoma: a US population-based survival analysis (1999-2016). Cancer. 2020 Nov 1;126(21):4706–16. PMID:32767702
1205. Flotho C, Valcamonica S, Mach-Pascual S, et al. RAS mutations and clonality analysis in children with juvenile myelomonocytic leukemia (JMML). Leukemia. 1999 Jan;13(1):32–7. PMID:10049057
1206. Foà R, Bassan R, Vitale A, et al. Dasatinib-blinatumomab for Ph-positive acute lymphoblastic leukemia in adults. N Engl J Med. 2020 Oct 22;383(17):1613–23. PMID:33085860
1207. Fonseca FP, Robinson L, van Heerden MB, et al. Oral plasmablastic lymphoma: a clinicopathological study of 113 cases. J Oral Pathol Med. 2021 Jul;50(6):594–602. PMID:34091967
1208. Fonseca R, Barlogie B, Bataille R, et al. Genetics and cytogenetics of multiple myeloma: a workshop report. Cancer Res. 2004 Feb 15;64(4):1546–58. PMID:14989251
1209. Fonseca R, Bergsagel PL, Drach J, et al. International Myeloma Working Group molecular classification of multiple myeloma: spotlight review. Leukemia. 2009 Dec;23(12):2210–21. PMID:19798094
1210. Fonseca R, Debes-Marun CS, Picken EB, et al. The recurrent IgH translocations are highly associated with nonhyperdiploid variant multiple myeloma. Blood. 2003 Oct 1;102(7):2562–7. PMID:12805059
1211. Fonseca R, Oken MM, Harrington D, et al. Deletions of chromosome 13 in multiple myeloma identified by interphase FISH usually denote large deletions of the q arm or monosomy. Leukemia. 2001 Jun;15(6):981–6. PMID:11417487
1212. Fonseca R, Van Wier SA, Chng WJ, et al. Prognostic value of chromosome 1q21 gain by fluorescent in situ hybridization and increase CKS1B expression in myeloma. Leukemia. 2006 Nov;20(11):2034–40. PMID:17024118
1213. Fontanilles M, Marguet F, Bohers É, et al. Non-invasive detection of somatic mutations using next-generation sequencing in primary central nervous system lymphoma. Oncotarget. 2017 Jul 18;8(29):48157–68. PMID:28636991
1214. Forconi F, Raspadori D, Lenoci M, et al. Absence of surface CD27 distinguishes hairy cell leukemia from other leukemic B-cell malignancies. Haematologica. 2005 Feb;90(2):266–8. PMID:15710587
1215. Forconi F, Sahota SS, Raspadori D, et al. Hairy cell leukemia: at the crossroad of somatic mutation and isotype switch. Blood. 2004 Nov 15;104(10):3312–7. PMID:15284115
1216. Forconi F, Sahota SS, Raspadori D, et al. Tumor cells of hairy cell leukemia express multiple clonally related immunoglobulin isotypes via RNA splicing. Blood. 2001 Aug 15;98(4):1174–81. PMID:11493467
1217. Forconi F, Sozzi E, Rossi D, et al. Selective influences in the expressed immunoglobulin heavy and light chain gene repertoire in hairy cell leukemia. Haematologica. 2008 May;93(5):697–705. PMID:18387977
1218. Ford AM, Fasching K, Panzer-Grümayer ER, et al. Origins of "late" relapse in childhood acute lymphoblastic leukemia with TEL-AML1 fusion genes. Blood. 2001 Aug 1;98(3):558–64. PMID:11468150
1219. Ford AM, Pombo-de-Oliveira MS, McCarthy KP, et al. Monoclonal origin of concordant T-cell malignancy in identical twins. Blood. 1997 Jan 1;89(1):281–5. PMID:8978302
1220. Forero A, Moore PS, Sarkar SN. Role of IRF4 in IFN-stimulated gene induction and maintenance of Kaposi sarcoma-associated herpesvirus latency in primary effusion lymphoma cells. J Immunol. 2013 Aug 1;191(3):1476–85. PMID:23804715
1221. Foshat M, Stewart J, Khoury JD, et al. Accuracy of diagnosing mantle cell lymphoma and identifying its variants on fine-needle aspiration biopsy. Cancer Cytopathol. 2019 Feb;127(1):44–51. PMID:30452126
1222. Foss FM, Horwitz SM, Civallero M, et al. Incidence and outcomes of rare T cell lymphomas from the T Cell Project: hepatosplenic, enteropathy associated and peripheral gamma delta T cell lymphomas. Am J Hematol. 2020 Feb;95(2):151–5. PMID:31709579
1223. Foss HD, Anagnostopoulos I, Araujo I, et al. Anaplastic large-cell lymphomas of T-cell and null-cell phenotype express cytotoxic molecules. Blood. 1996 Nov 15;88(10):4005–11. PMID:8916967
1224. Fournier B, Balducci E, Duployez N, et al. B-ALL with t(5;14)(q31;q32); IGH-IL3 rearrangement and eosinophilia: a comprehensive analysis of a peculiar IGH-rearranged B-ALL. Front Oncol. 2019 Dec 10;9:1374. PMID:31921638
1225. Fraga M, Brousset P, Schlaifer D, et al. Bone marrow involvement in anaplastic large cell lymphoma. Immunohistochemical detection of minimal disease and its prognostic significance. Am J Clin Pathol. 1995 Jan;103(1):82–9. PMID:7817951
1226. Fraga M, Sánchez-Verde L, Forteza J, et al. T-cell/histiocyte-rich large B-cell lymphoma is a disseminated aggressive neoplasm: differential diagnosis from Hodgkin's lymphoma. Histopathology. 2002 Sep;41(3):216–29. PMID:12207783
1227. Frampton M, da Silva Filho MI, Broderick P, et al. Variation at 3p24.1 and 6q23.3 influences the risk of Hodgkin's lymphoma. Nat Commun. 2013;4:2549. PMID:24149102
1228. Franco V, Florena AM, Campesi G. Intrasinusoidal bone marrow infiltration: a possible hallmark of splenic lymphoma. Histopathology. 1996 Dec;29(6):571–5. PMID:8971565
1229. Frappart PO, Lee Y, Lamont J, et al. BRCA2 is required for neurogenesis and suppression of medulloblastoma. EMBO J. 2007 Jun 6;26(11):2732–42. PMID:17476307
1230. Frauenfeld L, Bonzheim I, Wirths S, et al. Clonal evolution of chronic lymphocytic leukemia to Langerhans cell histiocytosis: a case report. Virchows Arch. 2019 Dec;475(6):795–8. PMID:31317311
1231. Frauenfeld L, Castrejon-de-Anta N, Ramis-Zaldivar JE, et al. Diffuse large B-cell lymphomas in adults with aberrant coexpression of CD10, BCL6, and MUM1 are enriched in IRF4 rearrangements. Blood Adv. 2022 Apr 12;6(7):2361–72. PMID:34654055
1232. Freedman A, Jacobsen E. Follicular lymphoma: 2020 update on diagnosis and management. Am J Hematol. 2020 Mar;95(3):316–27. PMID:31814159
1233. Freeman CL, Kridel R, Moccia AA, et al. Early progression after bendamustine-rituximab is associated with high risk of transformation in advanced stage follicular lymphoma. Blood. 2019 Aug 29;134(9):761–4. PMID:31300404
1234. Fresquet V, Robles EF, Parker A, et al. High-throughput sequencing analysis of the chromosome 7q32 deletion reveals IRF5 as a potential tumour suppressor in splenic marginal-zone lymphoma. Br J Haematol. 2012 Sep;158(6):712–26. PMID:22816737
1235. Friedman J, Schattner A, Shvidel L, et al. Characterization of T-cell large granular lymphocyte leukemia associated with Sjogren's syndrome-an important but under-recognized association. Semin Arthritis Rheum. 2006 Apr;35(5):306–11. PMID:16616153
1236. Frismantas V, Dobay MP, Rinaldi A, et al. Ex vivo drug response profiling detects recurrent sensitivity patterns in drug-resistant acute lymphoblastic leukemia. Blood. 2017 Mar 16;129(11):e26–37. PMID:28122742
1237. Fritz A, Percy C, Jack A, et al., editors. International classification of diseases for oncology (ICD-O). 3rd ed. 1st rev. Geneva (Switzerland): World Health Organization; 2013.
1238. Frizzera G, Banks PM, Massarelli G, et al. A systemic lymphoproliferative disorder with morphologic features of Castleman's disease. Pathological findings in 15 patients. Am J Surg Pathol. 1983 Apr;7(3):211–31. PMID:6837832
1239. Fromm JR, Edlefsen KL, Cherian S, et al. Flow cytometric features of incidental indolent T lymphoblastic proliferations. Cytometry B Clin Cytom. 2020 May;98(3):282–7. PMID:31571375
1240. Fromm JR, Kussick SJ, Wood BL. Identification and purification of classical Hodgkin cells from lymph nodes by flow cytometry and flow cytometric cell sorting. Am J Clin Pathol. 2006 Nov;126(5):764–80. PMID:17050074
1241. Fromm JR, Thomas A, Wood BL. Characterization and purification of neoplastic cells of nodular lymphocyte predominant Hodgkin lymphoma from lymph nodes by flow cytometry and flow cytometric cell sorting. Am J Pathol. 2017 Feb;187(2):304–17. PMID:27998726
1242. Fromm JR, Thomas A, Wood BL. Flow cytometry can diagnose classical Hodgkin lymphoma in lymph nodes with high sensitivity and specificity. Am J Clin Pathol. 2009 Mar;131(3):322–32. PMID:19228638
1243. Frontzek F, Staiger AM, Zapukhlyak M, et al. Molecular and functional profiling identifies therapeutically targetable vulnerabilities in plasmablastic lymphoma. Nat Commun. 2021 Aug 31;12(1):5183. PMID:34465776
1244. Frost BM, Forestier E, Gustafsson G, et al. Translocation t(12;21) is related to in vitro cellular drug sensitivity to doxorubicin and etoposide in childhood acute lymphoblastic leukemia. Blood. 2004 Oct 15;104(8):2452–7. PMID:15217836
1245. Fu K, Weisenburger DD, Greiner TC, et al. Cyclin D1-negative mantle cell lymphoma: a clinicopathologic study based on gene expression profiling. Blood. 2005 Dec 15;106(13):4315–21. PMID:16123218
1246. Fu S, Wang M, Lairson DR, et al. Trends and variations in mantle cell lymphoma incidence from 1995 to 2013: a comparative study between Texas and National SEER areas. Oncotarget. 2017 Nov 3;8(68):112516–29. PMID:29348844
1247. Fuhrmann S, Schabath R, Möricke A, et al. Expression of CD56 defines a distinct subgroup in childhood T-ALL with inferior outcome. Results of the ALL-BFM 2000 trial. Br J Haematol. 2018 Oct;183(1):96–103. PMID:30028023
1248. Fuji S, Yamaguchi T, Inoue Y, et al. Development of a modified prognostic index for patients with aggressive adult T-cell leukemia-lymphoma aged 70 years or younger: possible risk-adapted management strategies including allogeneic transplantation. Haematologica. 2017 Jul;102(7):1258–65. PMID:28341734
1249. Fujikura K, Yamashita D, Sakamoto R, et al. Intravascular NK/T-cell lymphoma: clinicopathological and integrated molecular analysis of two cases provides a clue to disease pathogenesis. J Clin Pathol. 2019 Sep;72(9):642–6. PMID:31123138
1250. Fujikura K, Yamashita D, Yoshida M, et al. Cytogenetic complexity and heterogeneity in intravascular lymphoma. J Clin Pathol. 2021

Apr;74(4):244–50. PMID:32763919
1251. Fujimoto A, Hiramoto N, Yamasaki S, et al. Risk factors and predictive scoring system for post-transplant lymphoproliferative disorder after hematopoietic stem cell transplantation. Biol Blood Marrow Transplant. 2019 Jul;25(7):1441–9. PMID:30794929
1252. Fujimoto A, Ishida F, Izutsu K, et al. Allogeneic stem cell transplantation for patients with aggressive NK-cell leukemia. Bone Marrow Transplant. 2021 Feb;56(2):347–56. PMID:32778688
1253. Fujimoto M, Haga H, Okamoto M, et al. EBV-associated diffuse large B-cell lymphoma arising in the chest wall with surgical mesh implant. Pathol Int. 2008 Oct;58(10):668–71. PMID:18801089
1254. Fujimoto M, Kaku Y, Hirata M, et al. EBV-positive mucocutaneous ulcer with small lymphocytic infiltration mimicking nonspecific ulceration. Am J Surg Pathol. 2021 May 1;45(5):694–700. PMID:33739792
1255. Fujimoto S, Koga T, Kawakami A, et al. Tentative diagnostic criteria and disease severity classification for Castleman disease: a report of the research group on Castleman disease in Japan. Mod Rheumatol. 2018 Jan;28(1):161–7. PMID:28880697
1256. Fujimoto S, Sakai T, Kawabata H, et al. Is TAFRO syndrome a subtype of idiopathic multicentric Castleman disease? Am J Hematol. 2019 Sep;94(9):975–83. PMID:31222819
1257. Fujimoto Y, Kojima Y, Yamaguchi K. Cervical subacute necrotizing lymphadenitis. A new clinicopathological entity. Naika. 1972;20:920–7.
1258. Fujisawa M, Sakata-Yanagimoto M, Nishizawa S, et al. Activation of RHOA-VAV1 signaling in angioimmunoblastic T-cell lymphoma. Leukemia. 2018 Mar;32(3):694–702. PMID:28832024
1259. Fujiwara M, Morales AV, Seo K, et al. Clonal identity and differences in primary cutaneous B-cell lymphoma occurring at different sites or time points in the same patient. Am J Dermatopathol. 2013 Feb;35(1):11–8. PMID:22588547
1260. Fujiwara SI, Yamashita Y, Nakamura N, et al. High-resolution analysis of chromosome copy number alterations in angioimmunoblastic T-cell lymphoma and peripheral T-cell lymphoma, unspecified, with single nucleotide polymorphism-typing microarrays. Leukemia. 2008 Oct;22(10):1891–8. PMID:18633432
1261. Fukushima T, Nomura S, Shimoyama M, et al. Japan Clinical Oncology Group (JCOG) prognostic index and characterization of long-term survivors of aggressive adult T-cell leukaemia-lymphoma (JCOG0902A). Br J Haematol. 2014 Sep;166(5):739–48. PMID:24931507
1262. Funkhouser AW, Katzman PJ, Sickel JZ, et al. CD30-positive anaplastic large cell lymphoma (ALCL) of T-cell lineage in a 14-month-old infant with perinatally acquired HIV-1 infection. J Pediatr Hematol Oncol. 1998 Nov-Dec;20(6):556–9. PMID:9856678
1263. Furudoï A, Gros A, Stanislas S, et al. Spleen histologic appearance in common variable immunodeficiency: analysis of 17 cases. Am J Surg Pathol. 2016 Jul;40(7):958–67. PMID:27158760
1264. Fuster C, Martín-Garcia D, Balagué O, et al. Cryptic insertions of the immunoglobulin light chain enhancer region near CCND1 in t(11;14)-negative mantle cell lymphoma. Haematologica. 2020 Aug;105(8):e408–11. PMID:31753927
1265. Gadoury-Levesque V, Dong L, Su R, et al. Frequency and spectrum of disease-causing variants in 1892 patients with suspected genetic HLH disorders. Blood Adv. 2020 Jun 23;4(12):2578–94. PMID:32542393
1266. Gaetke-Udager K, Wasnik AP, Kaza RK, et al. Multimodality imaging of splenic lesions and the role of non-vascular, image-guided intervention. Abdom Imaging. 2014 Jun;39(3):570–87. PMID:24525666
1267. Gafencu GA, Selicean SE, Petrushev B, et al. Clinicopathological analysis of a case series of peripheral T-cell lymphomas, not otherwise specified, of lymphoepithelioid variant (Lennert's lymphoma). A Central European single-center study. Hum Pathol. 2016 Jul;53:192–4. PMID:27016488
1268. Gaidano G, Carbone A, Pastore C, et al. Frequent mutation of the 5' noncoding region of the BCL-6 gene in acquired immunodeficiency syndrome-related non-Hodgkin's lymphomas. Blood. 1997 May 15;89(10):3755–62. PMID:9160681
1269. Gaikwad AS, Donohue RE, Elghetany MT, et al. Expression of CD25 is a specific and relatively sensitive marker for the Philadelphia chromosome (BCR-ABL1) translocation in pediatric B acute lymphoblastic leukemia. Int J Clin Exp Pathol. 2014 Aug 15;7(9):6225–30. PMID:25337274
1270. Gailllard B, Cornillet-Lefebvre P, Le QH, et al. Clinical and biological features of B-cell neoplasms with CDK6 translocations: an association with a subgroup of splenic marginal zone lymphomas displaying frequent CD5 expression, prolymphocytic cells, and TP53 abnormalities. Br J Haematol. 2021 Apr;193(1):72–82. PMID:33314017
1271. Gaine ME, Sharpe DJ, Smith JS, et al. GATA2 regulates the erythropoietin receptor in t(12;21) ALL. Oncotarget. 2017 Aug 2;8(39):66061–74. PMID:29029492
1272. Gaipa G, Bugarin C, Cianci P, et al. Peripheral blood cells from children with RASopathies show enhanced spontaneous colonies growth in vitro and hyperactive RAS signaling. Blood Cancer J. 2015 Jul 17;5(7):e324. PMID:26186557
1273. Galán J, Martin I, Carmona I, et al. The utility of multiparametric flow cytometry in the detection of primary effusion lymphoma (PEL). Cytometry B Clin Cytom. 2019 Sep;96(5):375–8. PMID:29669178
1274. Gale J, Simmonds PD, Mead GM, et al. Enteropathy-type intestinal T-cell lymphoma: clinical features and treatment of 31 patients in a single center. J Clin Oncol. 2000 Feb;18(4):795–803. PMID:10673521
1275. Gale KB, Ford AM, Repp R, et al. Backtracking leukemia to birth: identification of clonotypic gene fusion sequences in neonatal blood spots. Proc Natl Acad Sci U S A. 1997 Dec 9;94(25):13950–4. PMID:9391133
1276. Galindo LM, Garcia FU, Hanau CA, et al. Fine-needle aspiration biopsy in the evaluation of lymphadenopathy associated with cutaneous T-cell lymphoma (mycosis fungoides/Sézary syndrome). Am J Clin Pathol. 2000 Jun;113(6):865–71. PMID:10874888
1277. Gall DG, Chapman D, Kelly M, et al. Na+ transport in jejunal crypt cells. Gastroenterology. 1977 Mar;72(3):452–6. PMID:137828
1278. Gallo V, Cirillo E, Prencipe R, et al. Clinical, immunological, and functional characterization of six patients with very high IgM levels. J Clin Med. 2020 Mar 17;9(3):818. PMID:32192142
1279. Gambineri E, Ciullini Mannurita S, Hagin D, et al. Clinical, immunological, and molecular heterogeneity of 173 patients with the phenotype of immune dysregulation, polyendocrinopathy, enteropathy, X-linked (IPEX) syndrome. Front Immunol. 2018 Nov 1;9:2411. PMID:30443250
1280. Gammon B, Robson A, Deonizio J, et al. CD8(+) granulomatous cutaneous T-cell lymphoma: a potential association with immunodeficiency. J Am Acad Dermatol. 2014 Sep;71(3):555–60. PMID:24813299
1281. Ganapathi KA, Jobanputra V, Iwamoto F, et al. The genetic landscape of dural marginal zone lymphomas. Oncotarget. 2016 Jul 12;7(28):43052–61. PMID:27248180
1282. Gandemer V, Chevret S, Petit A, et al. Excellent prognosis of late relapses of ETV6/RUNX1-positive childhood acute lymphoblastic leukemia: lessons from the FRALLE 93 protocol. Haematologica. 2012 Nov;97(11):1743–50. PMID:22580999
1283. Gao J, Behdad A, Ji P, et al. EBV-negative aggressive NK-cell leukemia/lymphoma: a clinical and pathological study from a single institution. Mod Pathol. 2017 Aug;30(8):1100–15. PMID:28548121
1284. Gao J, Gauerke SJ, Martinez-Escala ME, et al. Bone marrow involvement by subcutaneous panniculitis-like T-cell lymphoma: a report of three cases. Mod Pathol. 2014 Jun;27(6):800–7. PMID:24201122
1285. Gao J, Peterson L, Nelson B, et al. Immunophenotypic variations in mantle cell lymphoma. Am J Clin Pathol. 2009 Nov;132(5):699–706. PMID:19846810
1286. Gao Q, Ryan SL, Iacobucci I, et al. The genomic landscape of acute lymphoblastic leukemia with intrachromosomal amplification of chromosome 21. Blood. 2023 Aug 24;142(8):711–23. PMID:37216686
1287. Gao Y, Moonis G, Cunnane ME, et al. Lacrimal gland masses. AJR Am J Roentgenol. 2013 Sep;201(3):W371-81. PMID:23971467
1288. Garand R, Goasguen J, Brizard A, et al. Indolent course as a relatively frequent presentation in T-prolymphocytic leukaemia. Groupe Français d'Hématologie Cellulaire. Br J Haematol. 1998 Nov;103(2):488–94. PMID:9827924
1289. Garbe C, Stein H, Dienemann D, et al. Borrelia burgdorferi-associated cutaneous B cell lymphoma: clinical and immunohistologic characterization of four cases. J Am Acad Dermatol. 1991 Apr;24(4):584–90. PMID:2033136
1290. Garcés JJ, Simicek M, Vicari M, et al. Transcriptional profiling of circulating tumor cells in multiple myeloma: a new model to understand disease dissemination. Leukemia. 2020 Feb;34(2):589–603. PMID:31595039
1291. Garces S, Khoury JD, Kanagal-Shamanna R, et al. Chronic lymphocytic leukemia with proliferation centers in bone marrow is associated with younger age at initial presentation, complex karyotype, and TP53 disruption. Hum Pathol. 2018 Dec;82:215–31. PMID:30086334
1292. García JF, Mollejo M, Fraga M, et al. Large B-cell lymphoma with Hodgkin's features. Histopathology. 2005 Jul;47(1):101–10. PMID:15982329
1293. Garcia M, Konoplev S, Morosan C, et al. MALT lymphoma involving the kidney: a report of 10 cases and review of the literature. Am J Clin Pathol. 2007 Sep;128(3):464–73. PMID:17709321
1294. García-Barchino MJ, Sarasquete ME, Panizo C, et al. Richter transformation driven by Epstein-Barr virus reactivation during therapy-related immunosuppression in chronic lymphocytic leukaemia. J Pathol. 2018 May;245(1):61–73. PMID:29464716
1295. Garcia-Herrera A, Song JY, Chuang SS, et al. Nonhepatosplenic γδ T-cell lymphomas represent a spectrum of aggressive cytotoxic T-cell lymphomas with a mainly extranodal presentation. Am J Surg Pathol. 2011 Aug;35(8):1214–25. PMID:21753698
1296. Garcia-Reyero J, Martinez Magunacelaya N, Gonzalez de Villambrosia S, et al. Diagnostic value of bone marrow core biopsy patterns in lymphoplasmacytic lymphoma/Waldenström macroglobulinaemia and description of its mutational profiles by targeted NGS. J Clin Pathol. 2020 Sep;73(9):571–7. PMID:31980558
1297. Garcia-Reyero J, Martinez Magunacelaya N, Gonzalez de Villambrosia S, et al. Genetic lesions in MYC and STAT3 drive oncogenic transcription factor overexpression in plasmablastic lymphoma. Haematologica. 2021 Apr 1;106(4):1120–8. PMID:32273478
1298. Garcia-Sanz R, Montoto S, Torrequebrada A, et al. Waldenström macroglobulinaemia: presenting features and outcome in a series with 217 cases. Br J Haematol. 2001 Dec;115(3):575–82. PMID:11736938
1299. Garnache Ottou F, Chandesris MO, Lhermitte L, et al. Peripheral blood 8 colour flow cytometry monitoring of hairy cell leukaemia allows detection of high-risk patients. Br J Haematol. 2014 Jul;166(1):50–9. PMID:24661013
1300. Gasparini VR, Binatti A, Coppe A, et al. A high definition picture of somatic mutations in chronic lymphoproliferative disorder of natural killer cells. Blood Cancer J. 2020 Apr 22;10(4):42. PMID:32321919
1301. Gassmann W, Löffler H, Thiel E, et al. Morphological and cytochemical findings in 150 cases of T-lineage acute lymphoblastic leukaemia in adults. Br J Haematol. 1997 May;97(2):372–82. PMID:9163604
1302. Gatta G, Capocaccia R, Botta L, et al. Burden and centralised treatment in Europe of rare tumours: results of RARECAREnet-a population-based study. Lancet Oncol. 2017 Aug;18(8):1022–39. PMID:28687376
1303. Gaud G, Lesourne R, Love PE. Regulatory mechanisms in T cell receptor signalling. Nat Rev Immunol. 2018 Aug;18(8):485–97. PMID:29789755
1304. Gaulard P, Zafrani ES, Mavier P, et al. Peripheral T-cell lymphoma presenting as predominant liver disease: a report of three cases. Hepatology. 1986 Sep-Oct;6(5):864–8. PMID:3530944
1305. Gayden T, Sepulveda FE, Khuong-Quang DA, et al. Germline HAVCR2 mutations altering TIM-3 characterize subcutaneous panniculitis-like T cell lymphomas with hemophagocytic lymphohistiocytic syndrome. Nat Genet. 2018 Dec;50(12):1650–7. PMID:30374066
1306. GBD 2017 Childhood Cancer Collaborators. The global burden of childhood and adolescent cancer in 2017: an analysis of the Global Burden of Disease Study 2017. Lancet Oncol. 2019 Sep;20(9):1211–25. PMID:31371206
1307. Ge R, Liu C, Yin X, et al. Clinicopathologic characteristics of inflammatory pseudotumor-like follicular dendritic cell sarcoma. Int J Clin Exp Pathol. 2014 Apr 15;7(5):2421–9. PMID:24966952
1308. Gebauer N, Künstner A, Ketzer J, et al. Genomic insights into the pathogenesis of Epstein-Barr virus-associated diffuse large B-cell lymphoma by whole-genome and targeted amplicon sequencing. Blood Cancer J. 2021 May 26;11(5):102. PMID:34039950
1309. Geer M, Roberts E, Shango M, et al. Multicentre retrospective study of intravascular large B-cell lymphoma treated at academic institutions within the United States. Br J Haematol. 2019 Jul;186(2):255–62. PMID:31044423
1310. Geissinger E, Odenwald T, Lee SS, et al. Nodal peripheral T-cell lymphomas and, in particular, their lymphoepithelioid (Lennert's) variant are often derived from CD8(+) cytotoxic T-cells. Virchows Arch. 2004 Oct;445(4):334–43. PMID:15480768
1311. Gelebart P, Hegazy SA, Wang P, et al. Aberrant expression and biological significance of Sox2, an embryonic stem cell transcriptional factor, in ALK-positive anaplastic large cell lymphoma. Blood Cancer J. 2012 Aug 10;2(8):e82.

PMID:22885405
1312. Geller S, Hollmann TJ, Horwitz SM, et al. C-C chemokine receptor 4 expression in CD8+ cutaneous T-cell lymphomas and lymphoproliferative disorders, and its implications for diagnosis and treatment. Histopathology. 2020 Jan;76(2):222–32. PMID:31355940
1313. Geller S, Lebowitz E, Pulitzer MP, et al. Outcomes and prognostic factors in African American and black patients with mycosis fungoides/Sézary syndrome: retrospective analysis of 157 patients from a referral cancer center. J Am Acad Dermatol. 2020 Aug;83(2):430–9. PMID:31499157
1314. Gellrich S, Rutz S, Golembowski S, et al. Primary cutaneous follicle center cell lymphomas and large B cell lymphomas of the leg descend from germinal center cells. A single cell polymerase chain reaction analysis. J Invest Dermatol. 2001 Dec;117(6):1512–20. PMID:11886516
1315. Genescà E, Morgades M, Montesinos P, et al. Unique clinico-biological, genetic and prognostic features of adult early T-cell precursor acute lymphoblastic leukemia. Haematologica. 2020 Jun;105(6):e294–7. PMID:31537688
1316. Gentry M, Bodo J, Durkin L, et al. Performance of a commercially available MAL antibody in the diagnosis of primary mediastinal large B-cell lymphoma. Am J Surg Pathol. 2017 Feb;41(2):189–94. PMID:27879516
1317. Georgesen C, Magro C. Lymphomatoid papulosis in children and adolescents: a clinical and histopathologic retrospective cohort. Ann Diagn Pathol. 2020 Jun;46:151486. PMID:32172217
1318. Gerami P, Rosen S, Kuzel T, et al. Folliculotropic mycosis fungoides: an aggressive variant of cutaneous T-cell lymphoma. Arch Dermatol. 2008 Jun;144(6):738–46. PMID:18559762
1319. Gerami P, Wickless SC, Querfeld C, et al. Cutaneous involvement with marginal zone lymphoma. J Am Acad Dermatol. 2010 Jul;63(1):142–5. PMID:20462658
1320. Gerami P, Wickless SC, Rosen S, et al. Applying the new TNM classification system for primary cutaneous lymphomas other than mycosis fungoides and Sézary syndrome in primary cutaneous marginal zone lymphoma. J Am Acad Dermatol. 2008 Aug;59(2):245–54. PMID:18486274
1321. Gérard L, Bérezné A, Galicier L, et al. Prospective study of rituximab in chemotherapy-dependent human immunodeficiency virus associated multicentric Castleman's disease: ANRS 117 CastlemaB Trial. J Clin Oncol. 2007 Aug 1;25(22):3350–6. PMID:17664482
1322. Gérard L, Michot JM, Burcheri S, et al. Rituximab decreases the risk of lymphoma in patients with HIV-associated multicentric Castleman disease. Blood. 2012 Mar 8;119(10):2228–33. PMID:22223822
1323. Gerbe A, Alame M, Dereure O, et al. Systemic, primary cutaneous, and breast implant-associated ALK-negative anaplastic large-cell lymphomas present similar biologic features despite distinct clinical behavior. Virchows Arch. 2019 Aug;475(2):163–74. PMID:30953147
1324. Gerdes J, Van Baarlen J, Pileri S, et al. Tumor cell growth fraction in Hodgkin's disease. Am J Pathol. 1987 Sep;128(3):390–3. PMID:3307442
1325. Gerstner ER, Carson KA, Grossman SA, et al. Long-term outcome in PCNSL patients treated with high-dose methotrexate and deferred radiation. Neurology. 2008 Jan 29;70(5):401–2. PMID:18227422
1326. Gesk S, Klapper W, Martín-Subero JI, et al. A chromosomal translocation in cyclin D1-negative/cyclin D2-positive mantle cell lymphoma fuses the CCND2 gene to the IGK locus. Blood. 2006 Aug 1;108(3):1109–10. PMID:16861358
1327. Geyer JT, Ferry JA, Harris NL, et al. Florid reactive lymphoid hyperplasia of the lower female genital tract (lymphoma-like lesion): a benign condition that frequently harbors clonal immunoglobulin heavy chain gene rearrangements. Am J Surg Pathol. 2010 Feb;34(2):161–8. PMID:20087162
1328. Geyer JT, Ferry JA, Longtine JA, et al. Characteristics of cutaneous marginal zone lymphomas with marked plasmacytic differentiation and a T cell-rich background. Am J Clin Pathol. 2010 Jan;133(1):59–69. PMID:20023259
1329. Geyer JT, Niesvizky R, Jayabalan DS, et al. IgG4 plasma cell myeloma: new insights into the pathogenesis of IgG4-related disease. Mod Pathol. 2014 Mar;27(3):375–81. PMID:24030741
1330. Gherardi RK, Bélec L, Soubrier M, et al. Overproduction of proinflammatory cytokines imbalanced by their antagonists in POEMS syndrome. Blood. 1996 Feb 15;87(4):1458–65. PMID:8608236
1331. Ghia P, Prato G, Scielzo C, et al. Monoclonal CD5+ and CD5- B-lymphocyte expansions are frequent in the peripheral blood of the elderly. Blood. 2004 Mar 15;103(6):2337–42. PMID:14630808
1332. Ghodke K, Shet T, Epari S, et al. A retrospective study of correlation of morphologic patterns, MIB1 proliferation index, and survival analysis in 134 cases of plasmacytoma. Ann Diagn Pathol. 2015 Jun;19(3):117–23. PMID:25842207
1333. Ghoneima A, Cooke J, Shaw E, et al. Human herpes virus 8-positive germinotropic lymphoproliferative disorder: first case diagnosed in the UK, literature review and discussion of treatment options. BMJ Case Rep. 2020 Sep 2;13(9):e231640. PMID:32878845
1334. Ghosh A, Pradhan SV, Talwar OP. Castleman's disease - hyaline vascular type - clinical, cytological and histological features with review of literature. Indian J Pathol Microbiol. 2010 Apr-Jun;53(2):244–7. PMID:20551525
1335. Ghosh S, Köstel Bal S, Edwards ESJ, et al. Extended clinical and immunological phenotype and transplant outcome in CD27 and CD70 deficiency. Blood. 2020 Dec 3;136(23):2638–55. PMID:32603431
1336. Giachino C, Padovan E, Lanzavecchia A. Kappa+lambda+ dual receptor B cells are present in the human peripheral repertoire. J Exp Med. 1995 Mar 1;181(3):1245–50. PMID:7869042
1337. Giannini C, Dogan A, Salomão DR. CNS lymphoma: a practical diagnostic approach. J Neuropathol Exp Neurol. 2014 Jun;73(6):478–94. PMID:24806301
1338. Gibson JF, Alpdogan O, Subtil A, et al. Hematopoietic stem cell transplantation for primary cutaneous γδ T-cell lymphoma and refractory subcutaneous panniculitis-like T-cell lymphoma. J Am Acad Dermatol. 2015 Jun;72(6):1010–5.e5. PMID:25981001
1339. Gibson SE, Swerdlow SH, Craig FE, et al. EBV-positive extranodal marginal zone lymphoma of mucosa-associated lymphoid tissue in the posttransplant setting: a distinct type of posttransplant lymphoproliferative disorder? Am J Surg Pathol. 2011 Jun;35(6):807–15. PMID:21552113
1340. Gibson SE, Swerdlow SH, Ferry JA, et al. Reassessment of small lymphocytic lymphoma in the era of monoclonal B-cell lymphocytosis. Haematologica. 2011 Aug;96(8):1144–52. PMID:21546505
1341. Gilad S, Bar-Shira A, Harnik R, et al. Ataxia-telangiectasia: founder effect among north African Jews. Hum Mol Genet. 1996 Dec;5(12):2033–7. PMID:8968760
1342. Giles FJ, O'Brien SM, Keating MJ. Chronic lymphocytic leukemia in (Richter's) transformation. Semin Oncol. 1998 Feb;25(1):117–25. PMID:9482533
1343. Gill KZ, Iwamoto F, Allen A, et al. MYC protein expression in primary diffuse large B-cell lymphoma of the central nervous system. PLoS One. 2014 Dec 5;9(12):e114398. PMID:25479599
1344. Giménez N, Martínez-Trillos A, Montraveta A, et al. Mutations in the RAS-BRAF-MAPK-ERK pathway define a specific subgroup of patients with adverse clinical features and provide new therapeutic options in chronic lymphocytic leukemia. Haematologica. 2019 Mar;104(3):576–86. PMID:30262568
1345. Giné E, Martinez A, Villamor N, et al. Expanded and highly active proliferation centers identify a histological subtype of chronic lymphocytic leukemia ("accelerated" chronic lymphocytic leukemia) with aggressive clinical behavior. Haematologica. 2010 Sep;95(9):1526–33. PMID:20421272
1346. Gion Y, Doi M, Nishimura Y, et al. PD-L1 expression is associated with the spontaneous regression of patients with methotrexate-associated lymphoproliferative disorders. Cancer Med. 2022 Jan;11(2):417–32. PMID:34842351
1347. Gion Y, Iwaki N, Takata K, et al. Clinicopathological analysis of methotrexate-associated lymphoproliferative disorders: comparison of diffuse large B-cell lymphoma and classical Hodgkin lymphoma types. Cancer Sci. 2017 Jun;108(6):1271–80. PMID:28380678
1348. Girodon F, Bergoin E, Favre B, et al. Hypereosinophilia in acute B-lineage lymphoblastic leukaemia. Br J Haematol. 2005 Jun;129(5):568. PMID:15916678
1349. Gitelson E, Al-Saleem T, Robu V, et al. Pediatric nodal marginal zone lymphoma may develop in the adult population. Leuk Lymphoma. 2010 Jan;51(1):89–94. PMID:19863176
1350. Giuffrè C, Cicinelli MV, Marchese A, et al. Clinical experience in a large cohort of patients with vitreoretinal lymphoma in a single center. Ocul Immunol Inflamm. 2021 Apr 3;29(3):472–8. PMID:32845738
1351. Giza A, Gałązka K, Jońca M, et al. Subcutaneous panniculitis-like T-cell lymphoma (SPTCL) with probable mesentery involvement with associated hemophagocytic syndrome (HPS) - how to treat it? J Dermatolog Treat. 2022 Aug;33(5):2674–6. PMID:32924664
1352. Gladden AB, Woolery R, Aggarwal P, et al. Expression of constitutively nuclear cyclin D1 in murine lymphocytes induces B-cell lymphoma. Oncogene. 2006 Feb 16;25(7):998–1007. PMID:16247460
1353. Gloghini A, Dolcetti R, Carbone A. Lymphomas occurring specifically in HIV-infected patients: from pathogenesis to pathology. Semin Cancer Biol. 2013 Dec;23(6):457–67. PMID:23999127
1354. Go H, Jeon YK, Huh J, et al. Frequent detection of BRAF(V600E) mutations in histiocytic and dendritic cell neoplasms. Histopathology. 2014 Aug;65(2):261–72. PMID:24720374
1355. Goatly A, Bacon CM, Nakamura S, et al. FOXP1 abnormalities in lymphoma: translocation breakpoint mapping reveals insights into deregulated transcriptional control. Mod Pathol. 2008 Jul;21(7):902–11. PMID:18487996
1356. Goh L, Teo NZ, Wang LM. Beware the inflammatory cell-rich colonic polyp: a rare case of EBV-positive inflammatory pseudotumour-like follicular dendritic cell sarcoma with increased IgG4-positive plasma cells. Pathology. 2020 Oct;52(6):713–7. PMID:32814623
1357. Goicoechea I, Puig N, Cedena MT, et al. Deep MRD profiling defines outcome and unveils different modes of treatment resistance in standard- and high-risk myeloma. Blood. 2021 Jan 7;137(1):49–60. PMID:32693406
1358. Goldin LR, Björkholm M, Kristinsson SY, et al. Highly increased familial risks for specific lymphoma subtypes. Br J Haematol. 2009 Jun;146(1):91–4. PMID:19438470
1359. Goldstone AH, Richards SM, Lazarus HM, et al. In adults with standard-risk acute lymphoblastic leukemia, the greatest benefit is achieved from a matched sibling allogeneic transplantation in first complete remission, and an autologous transplantation is less effective than conventional consolidation/maintenance chemotherapy in all patients: final results of the International ALL Trial (MRC UKALL XII/ECOG E2993). Blood. 2008 Feb 15;111(4):1827–33. PMID:18048644
1360. Golling P, Cozzio A, Dummer R, et al. Primary cutaneous B-cell lymphomas - clinicopathological, prognostic and therapeutic characterisation of 54 cases according to the WHO-EORTC classification and the ISCL/EORTC TNM classification system for primary cutaneous lymphomas other than mycosis fungoides and Sezary syndrome. Leuk Lymphoma. 2008 Jun;49(6):1094–103. PMID:18569636
1361. Gong S, Auer I, Duggal R, et al. Epstein-Barr virus-associated inflammatory pseudotumor presenting as a colonic mass. Hum Pathol. 2015 Dec;46(12):1956–61. PMID:26477709
1362. Gong S, Crane GM, McCall CM, et al. Expanding the spectrum of EBV-positive marginal zone lymphomas: a lesion associated with diverse immunodeficiency settings. Am J Surg Pathol. 2018 Oct;42(10):1306–16. PMID:29957733
1363. Gong Z, Xie W, Wang W, et al. T-lymphoid or T/myeloid blast phase of chronic myeloid leukemia in the era of tyrosine kinase inhibitor therapy: a report of 14 cases. Int J Lab Hematol. 2017 Apr;39(2):e45–50. PMID:27863007
1364. Gong Z, Zhou T, Liu H, et al. Genotype-phenotype correlation of unusual BCR-ABL1 transcripts in Philadelphia chromosome-positive leukaemia. Br J Haematol. 2020 Jun;189(5):e207–11. PMID:32237084
1365. Gonsalves WI, Jevremovic D, Nandakumar B, et al. Enhancing the R-ISS classification of newly diagnosed multiple myeloma by quantifying circulating clonal plasma cells. Am J Hematol. 2020 Mar;95(3):310–5. PMID:31867775
1366. Gonzalez de Villambrosia S, Bastos M, Palanca JM, et al. BCL2 translocation in high grade B cell lymphoma (NOS, DH/TH) is associated with reduced progression free survival. Leuk Lymphoma. 2022 Jan;63(1):101–8. PMID:34510996
1367. Gonzalez-Aguilar A, Idbaih A, Boisselier B, et al. Recurrent mutations of MYD88 and TBL1XR1 in primary central nervous system lymphomas. Clin Cancer Res. 2012 Oct 1;18(19):5203–11. PMID:22837180
1368. González-Barca E, Domingo-Domenech E, Capote FJ, et al. Prospective phase II trial of extended treatment with rituximab in patients with B-cell post-transplant lymphoproliferative disease. Haematologica. 2007 Nov;92(11):1489–94. PMID:18024397
1369. Gonzalez-Farre B, Martinez D, Lopez-Guerra M, et al. HHV8-related lymphoid proliferations: a broad spectrum of lesions from reactive lymphoid hyperplasia to overt lymphoma. Mod Pathol. 2017 May;30(5):745–60. PMID:28084335
1370. Gonzalez-Farre B, Ramis-Zaldivar JE, Castrejón de Anta N, et al. Intravascular large B-cell lymphoma genomic profile is characterized by alterations in genes regulating NF-κB and immune checkpoints. Am J Surg Pathol.

2023 Feb 1;47(2):202–11. PMID:36221796
1371. Gonzalez-Farre B, Ramis-Zaldivar JE, Salmeron-Villalobos J, et al. Burkitt-like lymphoma with 11q aberration: a germinal center-derived lymphoma genetically unrelated to Burkitt lymphoma. Haematologica. 2019 Sep;104(9):1822–9. PMID:30733272
1372. Goodlad JR. Spindle-cell B-cell lymphoma presenting in the skin. Br J Dermatol. 2001 Aug;145(2):313–7. PMID:11531800
1373. Goodlad JR, Davidson MM, Hollowood K, et al. Primary cutaneous B-cell lymphoma and Borrelia burgdorferi infection in patients from the Highlands of Scotland. Am J Surg Pathol. 2000 Sep;24(9):1279–85. PMID:10976703
1374. Goodlad JR, Krajewski AS, Batstone PJ, et al. Primary cutaneous diffuse large B-cell lymphoma: prognostic significance of clinicopathological subtypes. Am J Surg Pathol. 2003 Dec;27(12):1538–45. PMID:14657713
1375. Goodlad JR, Krajewski AS, Batstone PJ, et al. Primary cutaneous follicular lymphoma: a clinicopathologic and molecular study of 16 cases in support of a distinct entity. Am J Surg Pathol. 2002 Jun;26(6):733–41. PMID:12023577
1376. Goodman AM, Jeong AR, Phillips A, et al. Novel somatic alterations in unicentric and idiopathic multicentric Castleman disease. Eur J Haematol. 2021 Dec;107(6):642–9. PMID:34431136
1377. Gopal S, Gross TG. How I treat Burkitt lymphoma in children, adolescents, and young adults in sub-Saharan Africa. Blood. 2018 Jul 19;132(3):254–63. PMID:29769263
1378. Goto N, Tsurumi H, Takami T, et al. Cytokeratin-positive fibroblastic reticular cell tumor with follicular dendritic cell features: a case report and review of the literature. Am J Surg Pathol. 2015 Apr;39(4):573–80. PMID:25768257
1379. Gotoh K, Ito Y, Shibata-Watanabe Y, et al. Clinical and virological characteristics of 15 patients with chronic active Epstein-Barr virus infection treated with hematopoietic stem cell transplantation. Clin Infect Dis. 2008 May 15;46(10):1525–34. PMID:18419486
1380. Gotti D, Danesi M, Calabresi A, et al. Clinical characteristics, incidence, and risk factors of HIV-related Hodgkin lymphoma in the era of combination antiretroviral therapy. AIDS Patient Care STDS. 2013 May;27(5):259–65. PMID:23600703
1381. Gouveia MH, Otim I, Ogwang MD, et al. Endemic Burkitt Lymphoma in second-degree relatives in Northern Uganda: in-depth genome-wide analysis suggests clues about genetic susceptibility. Leukemia. 2021 Apr;35(4):1209–13. PMID:33051549
1382. Goyal A, Goyal K, Bohjanen K, et al. Epidemiology of primary cutaneous γδ T-cell lymphoma and subcutaneous panniculitis-like T-cell lymphoma in the U.S.A. from 2006 to 2015: a Surveillance, Epidemiology, and End Results-18 analysis. Br J Dermatol. 2019 Oct;181(4):848–50. PMID:30951189
1383. Goyal T, Ondrejka SL, Bodo J, et al. Lack of activation-induced cytidine deaminase expression in in situ follicular neoplasia. Haematologica. 2021 Apr 1;106(4):1212–5. PMID:32817287
1384. Goyal T, Thakral B, Wang SA, et al. T-cell large granular lymphocytic leukemia and coexisting B-cell lymphomas: a study from the Bone Marrow Pathology Group. Am J Clin Pathol. 2018 Jan 29;149(2):164–71. PMID:29365010
1385. Gradowski JF, Jaffe ES, Warnke RA, et al. Follicular lymphomas with plasmacytic differentiation include two subtypes. Mod Pathol. 2010 Jan;23(1):71–9. PMID:19838161
1386. Gradowski JF, Sargent RL, Craig FE, et al. Chronic lymphocytic leukemia/small lymphocytic lymphoma with cyclin D1 positive proliferation centers do not have CCND1 translocations or gains and lack SOX11 expression. Am J Clin Pathol. 2012 Jul;138(1):132–9. PMID:22706868
1387. Granados R, Aramburu JA, Rodríguez JM, et al. Cytopathology of a primary follicular dendritic cell sarcoma of the liver of the inflammatory pseudotumor-like type. Diagn Cytopathol. 2008 Jan;36(1):42–6. PMID:18064686
1388. Granai M, Amato T, Di Napoli A, et al. IGHV mutational status of nodal marginal zone lymphoma by NGS reveals distinct pathogenic pathways with different prognostic implications. Virchows Arch. 2020 Jul;477(1):143–50. PMID:31802229
1389. Granai M, Lazzi S. Early pattern of large B-cell lymphoma with IRF4 rearrangement. Blood. 2020 Aug 6;136(6):769. PMID:32761226
1390. Granai M, Lazzi S, Mancini V, et al. Burkitt lymphoma with a granulomatous reaction: an M1/Th1-polarised microenvironment is associated with controlled growth and spontaneous regression. Histopathology. 2022 Jan;80(2):430–42. PMID:33948980
1391. Grande BM, Gerhard DS, Jiang A, et al. Genome-wide discovery of somatic coding and noncoding mutations in pediatric endemic and sporadic Burkitt lymphoma. Blood. 2019 Mar 21;133(12):1313–24. PMID:30617194
1392. Grange F, Bekkenk MW, Wechsler J, et al. Prognostic factors in primary cutaneous large B-cell lymphomas: a European multicenter study. J Clin Oncol. 2001 Aug 15;19(16):3602–10. PMID:11504742
1393. Grange F, Beylot-Barry M, Courville P, et al. Primary cutaneous diffuse large B-cell lymphoma, leg type: clinicopathologic features and prognostic analysis in 60 cases. Arch Dermatol. 2007 Sep;143(9):1144–50. PMID:17875875
1394. Grange F, Joly P, Barbe C, et al. Improvement of survival in patients with primary cutaneous diffuse large B-cell lymphoma, leg type, in France. JAMA Dermatol. 2014 May;150(5):535–41. PMID:24647650
1395. Grange F, Petrella T, Beylot-Barry M, et al. Bcl-2 protein expression is the strongest independent prognostic factor of survival in primary cutaneous large B-cell lymphomas. Blood. 2004 May 15;103(10):3662–8. PMID:14726400
1396. Gratzinger D, de Jong D, Jaffe ES, et al. T- and NK-cell lymphomas and systemic lymphoproliferative disorders and the immunodeficiency setting: 2015 SH/EAHP Workshop Report-Part 4. Am J Clin Pathol. 2017 Feb 1;147(2):188–203. PMID:28395105
1397. Gratzinger D, Jaffe ES, Chadburn A, et al. Primary/congenital immunodeficiency: 2015 SH/EAHP Workshop Report-Part 5. Am J Clin Pathol. 2017 Feb 1;147(2):204–16. PMID:28395106
1398. Graux C, Cools J, Michaux L, et al. Cytogenetics and molecular genetics of T-cell acute lymphoblastic leukemia: from thymocyte to lymphoblast. Leukemia. 2006 Sep;20(9):1496–510. PMID:16826225
1399. Greaves M. A causal mechanism for childhood acute lymphoblastic leukaemia. Nat Rev Cancer. 2018 Aug;18(8):471–84. PMID:29784935
1400. Greaves MF. Biological models for leukaemia and lymphoma. IARC Sci Publ. 2004;(157):351–72. PMID:15055306
1401. Green MR, Alizadeh AA. Common progenitor cells in mature B-cell malignancies: implications for therapy. Curr Opin Hematol. 2014 Jul;21(4):333–40. PMID:24811163
1402. Green MR, Gentles AJ, Nair RV, et al. Hierarchy in somatic mutations arising during genomic evolution and progression of follicular lymphoma. Blood. 2013 Feb 28;121(9):1604–11. PMID:23297126
1403. Green MR, Kihira S, Liu CL, et al. Mutations in early follicular lymphoma progenitors are associated with suppressed antigen presentation. Proc Natl Acad Sci U S A. 2015 Mar 10;112(10):E1116–25. PMID:25713363
1404. Green MR, Monti S, Rodig SJ, et al. Integrative analysis reveals selective 9p24.1 amplification, increased PD-1 ligand expression, and further induction via JAK2 in nodular sclerosing Hodgkin lymphoma and primary mediastinal large B-cell lymphoma. Blood. 2010 Oct 28;116(17):3268–77. PMID:20628145
1405. Green MR, Rodig S, Juszczynski P, et al. Constitutive AP-1 activity and EBV infection induce PD-L1 in Hodgkin lymphomas and post-transplant lymphoproliferative disorders: implications for targeted therapy. Clin Cancer Res. 2012 Mar 15;18(6):1611–8. PMID:22271878
1406. Green TM, Young KH, Visco C, et al. Immunohistochemical double-hit score is a strong predictor of outcome in patients with diffuse large B-cell lymphoma treated with rituximab plus cyclophosphamide, doxorubicin, vincristine, and prednisone. J Clin Oncol. 2012 Oct 1;30(28):3460–7. PMID:22665537
1407. Greenblatt D, Ally M, Child F, et al. Indolent CD8(+) lymphoid proliferation of acral sites: a clinicopathologic study of six patients with some atypical features. J Cutan Pathol. 2013 Feb;40(2):248–58. PMID:23189944
1408. Greenough A, Dave SS. New clues to the molecular pathogenesis of Burkitt lymphoma revealed through next-generation sequencing. Curr Opin Hematol. 2014 Jul;21(4):326–32. PMID:24867287
1409. Greiner A, Knörr C, Qin Y, et al. Low-grade B cell lymphomas of mucosa-associated lymphoid tissue (MALT-type) require CD40-mediated signaling and Th2-type cytokines for in vitro growth and differentiation. Am J Pathol. 1997 May;150(5):1583–93. PMID:9137085
1410. Greipp PR, Leong T, Bennett JM, et al. Plasmablastic morphology–an independent prognostic factor with clinical and laboratory correlates: Eastern Cooperative Oncology Group (ECOG) myeloma trial E9486 report by the ECOG Myeloma Laboratory Group. Blood. 1998 Apr 1;91(7):2501–7. PMID:9516151
1411. Greipp PR, San Miguel J, Durie BG, et al. International staging system for multiple myeloma. J Clin Oncol. 2005 May 20;23(15):3412–20. PMID:15809451
1412. Greisser J, Palmedo G, Sander C, et al. Detection of clonal rearrangement of T-cell receptor genes in the diagnosis of primary cutaneous CD30 lymphoproliferative disorders. J Cutan Pathol. 2006 Nov;33(11):711–5. PMID:17083688
1413. Grever MR. How I treat hairy cell leukemia. Blood. 2010 Jan 7;115(1):21–8. PMID:19843881
1414. Grever MR, Abdel-Wahab O, Andritsos LA, et al. Consensus guidelines for the diagnosis and management of patients with classic hairy cell leukemia. Blood. 2017 Feb 2;129(5):553–60. PMID:27903528
1415. Grewal JS, Smith LB, Winegarden JD 3rd, et al. Highly aggressive ALK-positive anaplastic large cell lymphoma with a leukemic phase and multi-organ involvement: a report of three cases and a review of the literature. Ann Hematol. 2007 Jul;86(7):499–508. PMID:17396261
1416. Griffin GK, Sholl LM, Lindeman NI, et al. Targeted genomic sequencing of follicular dendritic cell sarcoma reveals recurrent alterations in NF-κB regulatory genes. Mod Pathol. 2016 Jan;29(1):67–74. PMID:26564005
1417. Griffin GK, Weirather JL, Roemer MGM, et al. Spatial signatures identify immune escape via PD-1 as a defining feature of T-cell/histiocyte-rich large B-cell lymphoma. Blood. 2021 Mar 11;137(10):1353–64. PMID:32871584
1418. Grimaldi JC, Meeker TC. The t(5;14) chromosomal translocation in a case of acute lymphocytic leukemia joins the interleukin-3 gene to the immunoglobulin heavy chain gene. Blood. 1989 Jun;73(8):2081–5. PMID:2499362
1419. Gritti C, Dastot H, Soulier J, et al. Transgenic mice for MTCP1 develop T-cell prolymphocytic leukemia. Blood. 1998 Jul 15;92(2):368–73. PMID:9657733
1420. Grogg KL, Attygalle AD, Macon WR, et al. Angioimmunoblastic T-cell lymphoma: a neoplasm of germinal-center T-helper cells? Blood. 2005 Aug 15;106(4):1501–2. PMID:16079436
1421. Grogg KL, Jung S, Erickson LA, et al. Primary cutaneous CD4-positive small/medium-sized pleomorphic T-cell lymphoma: a clonal T-cell lymphoproliferative disorder with indolent behavior. Mod Pathol. 2008 Jun;21(6):708–15. PMID:18311111
1422. Grogg KL, Lae ME, Kurtin PJ, et al. Clusterin expression distinguishes follicular dendritic cell tumors from other dendritic cell neoplasms: report of a novel follicular dendritic cell marker and clinicopathologic data on 12 additional follicular dendritic cell tumors and 6 additional interdigitating dendritic cell tumors. Am J Surg Pathol. 2004 Aug;28(8):988–98. PMID:15252304
1423. Grogg KL, Macon WR, Kurtin PJ, et al. A survey of clusterin and fascin expression in sarcomas and spindle cell neoplasms: strong clusterin immunostaining is highly specific for follicular dendritic cell tumor. Mod Pathol. 2005 Feb;18(2):260–6. PMID:15467709
1424. Grogg KL, Morice WG, Macon WR. Spectrum of bone marrow findings in patients with angioimmunoblastic T-cell lymphoma. Br J Haematol. 2007 Jun;137(5):416–22. PMID:17488486
1425. Gross TG, Bucuvalas JC, Park JR, et al. Low-dose chemotherapy for Epstein-Barr virus-positive post-transplantation lymphoproliferative disease in children after solid organ transplantation. J Clin Oncol. 2005 Sep 20;23(27):6481–8. PMID:16170157
1426. Gru AA, Jaffe ES. Cutaneous EBV-related lymphoproliferative disorders. Semin Diagn Pathol. 2017 Jan;34(1):60–75. PMID:27988064
1427. Gru AA, Kim J, Pulitzer M, et al. The use of central pathology review with digital slide scanning in advanced-stage mycosis fungoides and Sézary syndrome: a multi-institutional and international pathology study. Am J Surg Pathol. 2018 Jun;42(6):726–34. PMID:29543675
1428. Gruber M, Bozic I, Leshchiner I, et al. Growth dynamics in naturally progressing chronic lymphocytic leukaemia. Nature. 2019 Jun;570(7762):474–9. PMID:31142838
1429. Grygalewicz B, Woroniecka R, Rymkiewicz G, et al. The 11q-gain/loss aberration occurs recurrently in MYC-negative Burkitt-like lymphoma with 11q aberration, as well as MYC-positive Burkitt lymphoma and MYC-positive high-grade B-cell lymphoma, NOS. Am J Clin Pathol. 2017 Dec 20;149(1):17–28. PMID:29272887
1430. Gu J, Reynolds A, Fang L, et al. Coexistence of iAMP21 and ETV6-RUNX1 fusion in an adolescent with B cell acute lymphoblastic leukemia: literature review of six additional cases. Mol Cytogenet. 2016 Nov 21;9:84. PMID:27895713
1431. Gu SX, Pan Z, Xu ML. Thinking outside the cavity: effusion lymphoma primary to bone marrow. Clin Case Rep. 2021 May 20;9(5):e04100. PMID:34026143
1432. Gu Z, Churchman M, Roberts K, et al. Genomic analyses identify recurrent MEF2D fusions in acute lymphoblastic leukaemia. Nat Commun. 2016 Nov 8;7:13331. PMID:27824051

1433. Gu Z, Churchman ML, Roberts KG, et al. PAX5-driven subtypes of B-progenitor acute lymphoblastic leukemia. Nat Genet. 2019 Feb;51(2):296–307. PMID:30643249

1434. Gualco G, Natkunam Y, Bacchi CE. The spectrum of B-cell lymphoma, unclassifiable, with features intermediate between diffuse large B-cell lymphoma and classical Hodgkin lymphoma: a description of 10 cases. Mod Pathol. 2012 May;25(5):661–74. PMID:22222636

1435. Guenzel AJ, Smadbeck JB, Golden CL, et al. Clinical utility of next generation sequencing to detect IGH/IL3 rearrangements [t(5;14)(q31.1;q32.1)] in B-lymphoblastic leukemia/lymphoma. Ann Diagn Pathol. 2021 Aug;53:151761. PMID:33991782

1436. Guerrini F, Paolicchi M, Ghio F, et al. The droplet digital PCR: a new valid molecular approach for the assessment of B-RAF V600E mutation in hairy cell leukemia. Front Pharmacol. 2016 Oct 13;7:363. PMID:27790140

1437. Guièze R, Liu VM, Rosebrock D, et al. Mitochondrial reprogramming underlies resistance to BCL-2 inhibition in lymphoid malignancies. Cancer Cell. 2019 Oct 14;36(4):369–384.e13. PMID:31543463

1438. Guièze R, Robbe P, Clifford R, et al. Presence of multiple recurrent mutations confers poor trial outcome of relapsed/refractory CLL. Blood. 2015 Oct 29;126(18):2110–7. PMID:26316624

1439. Guillet S, Gérard L, Meignin V, et al. Classic and extracavitary primary effusion lymphoma in 51 HIV-infected patients from a single institution. Am J Hematol. 2016 Feb;91(2):233–7. PMID:26799611

1440. Guilloton F, Caron G, Ménard C, et al. Mesenchymal stromal cells orchestrate follicular lymphoma cell niche through the CCL2-dependent recruitment and polarization of monocytes. Blood. 2012 Mar 15;119(11):2556–67. PMID:22289889

1441. Guisado-Vasco P, Arranz-Saez R, Canales M, et al. Stage IV and age over 45 years are the only prognostic factors of the International Prognostic Score for the outcome of advanced Hodgkin lymphoma in the Spanish Hodgkin Lymphoma Study Group series. Leuk Lymphoma. 2012 May;53(5):812–9. PMID:22185637

1442. Guitart J. HIV-1 and an HTLV-II-associated cutaneous T-cell lymphoma. N Engl J Med. 2000 Jul 27;343(4):303–4. PMID:10928885

1443. Guitart J, Deonizio J, Bloom T, et al. High incidence of gastrointestinal tract disorders and autoimmunity in primary cutaneous marginal zone B-cell lymphomas. JAMA Dermatol. 2014 Apr;150(4):412–8. PMID:24500411

1444. Guitart J, Magro C. Cutaneous T-cell lymphoid dyscrasia: a unifying term for idiopathic chronic dermatoses with persistent T-cell clones. Arch Dermatol. 2007 Jul;143(7):921–32. PMID:17638739

1445. Guitart J, Martinez-Escala ME, Subtil A, et al. Primary cutaneous aggressive epidermotropic cytotoxic T-cell lymphomas: reappraisal of a provisional entity in the 2016 WHO classification of cutaneous lymphomas. Mod Pathol. 2017 May;30(5):761–72. PMID:28128277

1446. Guitart J, Querfeld C. Cutaneous CD30 lymphoproliferative disorders and similar conditions: a clinical and pathologic prospective on a complex issue. Semin Diagn Pathol. 2009 Aug;26(3):131–40. PMID:20043512

1447. Guitart J, Weisenburger DD, Subtil A, et al. Cutaneous γδ T-cell lymphomas: a spectrum of presentations with overlap with other cytotoxic lymphomas. Am J Surg Pathol. 2012 Nov;36(11):1656–65. PMID:23073324

1448. Guiter C, Dusanter-Fourt I, Copie-Bergman C, et al. Constitutive STAT6 activation in primary mediastinal large B-cell lymphoma. Blood. 2004 Jul 15;104(2):543–9. PMID:15044251

1449. Gujral S, Badrinath Y, Kumar A, et al. Immunophenotypic profile of acute leukemia: critical analysis and insights gained at a tertiary care center in India. Cytometry B Clin Cytom. 2009 May;76(3):199–205. PMID:18803279

1450. Gulia A, Saggini A, Wiesner T, et al. Clinicopathologic features of early lesions of primary cutaneous follicle center lymphoma, diffuse type: implications for early diagnosis and treatment. J Am Acad Dermatol. 2011 Nov;65(5):991–1000. PMID:21704419

1451. Gunawardana J, Chan FC, Telenius A, et al. Recurrent somatic mutations of PTPN1 in primary mediastinal B cell lymphoma and Hodgkin lymphoma. Nat Genet. 2014 Apr;46(4):329–35. PMID:24531327

1452. Guo N, Chen Y, Wang Y, et al. Clinicopathological categorization of hydroa vacciniforme-like lymphoproliferative disorder: an analysis of prognostic implications and treatment based on 19 cases. Diagn Pathol. 2019 Jul 17;14(1):82. PMID:31315684

1453. Guo RJ, Bahmanyar M, Minden MD, et al. CD33, not early precursor T-cell phenotype, is associated with adverse outcome in adult T-cell acute lymphoblastic leukaemia. Br J Haematol. 2016 Mar;172(5):823–5. PMID:26123477

1454. Gupta GK, Jaffe ES, Pittaluga S. A study of PD-L1 expression in intravascular large B cell lymphoma: correlation with clinical and pathological features. Histopathology. 2019 Aug;75(2):282–6. PMID:30938862

1455. Guru Murthy GS, Pondaiah SK, Abedin S, et al. Incidence and survival of T-cell acute lymphoblastic leukemia in the United States. Leuk Lymphoma. 2019 May;60(5):1171–8. PMID:30407885

1456. Gustine JN, Meid K, Dubeau T, et al. Serum IgM level as predictor of symptomatic hyperviscosity in patients with Waldenström macroglobulinaemia. Br J Haematol. 2017 Jun;177(5):717–25. PMID:28485115

1457. Gutierrez A, Dahlberg SE, Neuberg DS, et al. Absence of biallelic TCRgamma deletion predicts early treatment failure in pediatric T-cell acute lymphoblastic leukemia. J Clin Oncol. 2010 Aug 20;28(24):3816–23. PMID:20644084

1458. Gutierrez M, Bladek P, Goksu B, et al. T-cell prolymphocytic leukemia: diagnosis, pathogenesis, and treatment. Int J Mol Sci. 2023 Jul 28;24(15):12106. PMID:37569479

1459. Ha SY, Sung J, Ju H, et al. Epstein-Barr virus-positive nodal peripheral T cell lymphomas: clinicopathologic and gene expression profiling study. Pathol Res Pract. 2013 Jul;209(7):448–54. PMID:23735590

1460. Haas OA, Borkhardt A. Hyperdiploidy: the longest known, most prevalent, and most enigmatic form of acute lymphoblastic leukemia in children. Leukemia. 2022 Dec;36(12):2769–83. PMID:36266323

1461. Habermehl GK, Durkin L, Hsi ED. A tissue counterpart to monoclonal B-cell lymphocytosis. Arch Pathol Lab Med. 2021 Dec 1;145(12):1544–51. PMID:33720326

1462. Hachisuga T, Ookuma Y, Fukuda K, et al. Detection of Epstein-Barr virus DNA from a lymphoma-like lesion of the uterine cervix. Gynecol Oncol. 1992 Jul;46(1):69–73. PMID:1321783

1463. Hadzidimitriou A, Agathangelidis A, Darzentas N, et al. Is there a role for antigen selection in mantle cell lymphoma? Immunogenetic support from a series of 807 cases. Blood. 2011 Sep 15;118(11):3088–95. PMID:21791422

1464. Hafezi N, Zaki-Dizaji M, Nirouei M, et al. Clinical, immunological, and genetic features in 780 patients with autoimmune lymphoproliferative syndrome (ALPS) and ALPS-like diseases: a systematic review. Pediatr Allergy Immunol. 2021 Oct;32(7):1519–32. PMID:33963613

1465. Hagemeijer A, Graux C. ABL1 rearrangements in T-cell acute lymphoblastic leukemia. Genes Chromosomes Cancer. 2010 Apr;49(4):299–308. PMID:20073070

1466. Hagen JW, Magro CM. Indolent CD8+ lymphoid proliferation of the face with eyelid involvement. Am J Dermatopathol. 2014 Feb;36(2):137–41. PMID:24556898

1467. Haghighi B, Smoller BR, LeBoit PE, et al. Pagetoid reticulosis (Woringer-Kolopp disease): an immunophenotypic, molecular, and clinicopathologic study. Mod Pathol. 2000 May;13(5):502–10. PMID:10824921

1468. Hagiwara M, Takata K, Shimoyama Y, et al. Primary cutaneous T-cell lymphoma of unspecified type with cytotoxic phenotype: clinicopathological analysis of 27 patients. Cancer Sci. 2009 Jan;100(1):33–41. PMID:19018763

1469. Hales EC, Taub JW, Matherly LH. New insights into Notch1 regulation of the PI3K-AKT-mTOR1 signaling axis: targeted therapy of γ-secretase inhibitor resistant T-cell acute lymphoblastic leukemia. Cell Signal. 2014 Jan;26(1):149–61. PMID:24140475

1470. Halldórsdóttir AM, Sander B, Göransson H, et al. High-resolution genomic screening in mantle cell lymphoma–specific changes correlate with genomic complexity, the proliferation signature and survival. Genes Chromosomes Cancer. 2011 Feb;50(2):113–21. PMID:21117067

1471. Hallek M, Cheson BD, Catovsky D, et al. Guidelines for the diagnosis and treatment of chronic lymphocytic leukemia: a report from the International Workshop on Chronic Lymphocytic Leukemia updating the National Cancer Institute-Working Group 1996 guidelines. Blood. 2008 Jun 15;111(12):5446–56. PMID:18216293

1472. Hallek M, Cheson BD, Catovsky D, et al. iwCLL guidelines for diagnosis, indications for treatment, response assessment, and supportive management of CLL. Blood. 2018 Jun 21;131(25):2745–60. PMID:29540348

1473. Hallermann C, Kaune KM, Gesk S, et al. Molecular cytogenetic analysis of chromosomal breakpoints in the IGH, MYC, BCL6, and MALT1 gene loci in primary cutaneous B-cell lymphomas. J Invest Dermatol. 2004 Jul;123(1):213–9. PMID:15191563

1474. Hamada T, Iwatsuki K. Cutaneous lymphoma in Japan: a nationwide study of 1733 patients. J Dermatol. 2014 Jan;41(1):3–10. PMID:24438138

1475. Hamadani M, Kanate AS, DiGilio A, et al. Allogeneic hematopoietic cell transplantation for aggressive NK cell leukemia. A Center for International Blood and Marrow Transplant Research analysis. Biol Blood Marrow Transplant. 2017 May;23(5):853–6. PMID:28161608

1476. Hamadeh F, MacNamara S, Bacon CM, et al. Gamma heavy chain disease lacks the MYD88 L265p mutation associated with lymphoplasmacytic lymphoma. Haematologica. 2014 Sep;99(9):e154–5. PMID:24859878

1477. Hamadeh F, MacNamara SP, Aguilera NS, et al. MYD88 L265P mutation analysis helps define nodal lymphoplasmacytic lymphoma. Mod Pathol. 2015 Apr;28(4):564–74. PMID:25216226

1478. Hamblin TJ, Davis Z, Gardiner A, et al. Unmutated Ig V(H) genes are associated with a more aggressive form of chronic lymphocytic leukemia. Blood. 1999 Sep 15;94(6):1848–54. PMID:10477713

1479. Hamilton SN, Wai ES, Tan K, et al. Treatment and outcomes in patients with primary cutaneous B-cell lymphoma: the BC Cancer Agency experience. Int J Radiat Oncol Biol Phys. 2013 Nov 15;87(4):719–25. PMID:24001373

1480. Hamilton-Dutoit SJ, Raphael M, Audouin J, et al. In situ demonstration of Epstein-Barr virus small RNAs (EBER 1) in acquired immunodeficiency syndrome-related lymphomas: correlation with tumor morphology and primary site. Blood. 1993 Jul 15;82(2):619–24. PMID:8392401

1481. Hammer RD, Glick AD, Greer JP, et al. Splenic marginal zone lymphoma. A distinct B-cell neoplasm. Am J Surg Pathol. 1996 May;20(5):613–26. PMID:8619426

1482. Hämmerl L, Colombet M, Rochford R, et al. The burden of Burkitt lymphoma in Africa. Infect Agent Cancer. 2019 Aug 1;14:17. PMID:31388351

1483. Hamoudi R, Diss TC, Oksenhendler E, et al. Distinct cellular origins of primary effusion lymphoma with and without EBV infection. Leuk Res. 2004 Apr;28(4):333–8. PMID:15109530

1484. Han X, Bueso-Ramos CE. Precursor T-cell acute lymphoblastic leukemia/lymphoblastic lymphoma and acute biphenotypic leukemias. Am J Clin Pathol. 2007 Apr;127(4):528–44. PMID:17369128

1485. Hanahan D, Weinberg RA. Hallmarks of cancer: the next generation. Cell. 2011 Mar 4;144(5):646–74. PMID:21376230

1486. Hanamura I, Stewart JP, Huang Y, et al. Frequent gain of chromosome band 1q21 in plasma-cell dyscrasias detected by fluorescence in situ hybridization: incidence increases from MGUS to relapsed myeloma and is related to prognosis and disease progression following tandem stem-cell transplantation. Blood. 2006 Sep 1;108(5):1724–32. PMID:16705089

1487. Hanchard B. Adult T-cell leukemia/lymphoma in Jamaica: 1986-1995. J Acquir Immune Defic Syndr Hum Retrovirol. 1996;13 Suppl 1:S20–5. PMID:8797699

1488. Handgretinger R, Geiselhart A, Moris A, et al. Pure red-cell aplasia associated with clonal expansion of granular lymphocytes expressing killer-cell inhibitory receptors. N Engl J Med. 1999 Jan 28;340(4):278–84. PMID:9920952

1489. Hang JF, Yuan CT, Chang KC, et al. Targeted next-generation sequencing reveals a wide morphologic and immunophenotypic spectrum of monomorphic epitheliotropic intestinal T-cell lymphoma. Am J Surg Pathol. 2022 Sep 1;46(9):1207–18. PMID:35551151

1490. Hans CP, Weisenburger DD, Greiner TC, et al. Confirmation of the molecular classification of diffuse large B-cell lymphoma by immunohistochemistry using a tissue microarray. Blood. 2004 Jan 1;103(1):275–82. PMID:14504078

1491. Hansmann ML, Fellbaum C, Hui PK, et al. Progressive transformation of germinal centers with and without association to Hodgkin's disease. Am J Clin Pathol. 1990 Feb;93(2):219–26. PMID:2405631

1492. Hansmann ML, Stein H, Fellbaum C, et al. Nodular paragranuloma can transform into high-grade malignant lymphoma of B type. Hum Pathol. 1989 Dec;20(12):1169–75. PMID:2591946

1493. Hapgood G, Ben-Neriah S, Mottok A, et al. Identification of high-risk DUSP22-rearranged ALK-negative anaplastic large cell lymphoma. Br J Haematol. 2019 Aug;186(3):e28–31. PMID:30873584

1494. Haque AK, Myers JL, Hudnall SD, et al. Pulmonary lymphomatoid granulomatosis in acquired immunodeficiency syndrome: lesions with Epstein-Barr virus infection. Mod Pathol. 1998 Apr;11(4):347–56. PMID:9578085

1495. Harada A, Oguchi M, Terui Y, et al. Radiation therapy for localized duodenal low-grade follicular lymphoma. J Radiat Res. 2016 Jul;57(4):412–7. PMID:27009323

1496. Haralambieva E, Pulford KA, Lamant L,

et al. Anaplastic large-cell lymphomas of B-cell phenotype are anaplastic lymphoma kinase (ALK) negative and belong to the spectrum of diffuse large B-cell lymphomas. Br J Haematol. 2000 Jun;109(3):584–91. PMID:10886208

1497. Haralambieva E, Rosati S, van Noesel C, et al. Florid granulomatous reaction in Epstein-Barr virus-positive nonendemic Burkitt lymphomas: report of four cases. Am J Surg Pathol. 2004 Mar;28(3):379–83. PMID:15104301

1498. Hardell L, Eriksson M, Nordstrom M. Exposure to pesticides as risk factor for non-Hodgkin's lymphoma and hairy cell leukemia: pooled analysis of two Swedish case-control studies. Leuk Lymphoma. 2002 May;43(5):1043–9. PMID:12148884

1499. Harigai M. Lymphoproliferative disorders in patients with rheumatoid arthritis in the era of widespread use of methotrexate: a review of the literature and current perspective. Mod Rheumatol. 2018 Jan;28(1):1–8. PMID:28758827

1500. Harris J, Cherry D, Lazarchick J. Follicular lymphoma with PAS-positive amorphous material: report of two cases. Ann Clin Lab Sci. 2002 Summer;32(3):299–304. PMID:12175094

1501. Harris MH, Czuchlewski DR, Arber DA, et al. Genetic testing in the diagnosis and biology of acute leukemia. Am J Clin Pathol. 2019 Aug 1;152(3):322–46. PMID:31367767

1502. Harris NL. Lymphoid proliferations of the salivary glands. Am J Clin Pathol. 1999 Jan;111(1 Suppl 1):S94–103. PMID:9894474

1503. Harris NL, Jaffe ES, Diebold J, et al. World Health Organization classification of neoplastic diseases of the hematopoietic and lymphoid tissues: report of the Clinical Advisory Committee meeting-Airlie House, Virginia, November 1997. J Clin Oncol. 1999 Dec;17(12):3835–49. PMID:10577857

1504. Harris NL, Jaffe ES, Stein H, et al. A revised European-American classification of lymphoid neoplasms: a proposal from the International Lymphoma Study Group. Blood. 1994 Sep 1;84(5):1361–92. PMID:8068936

1505. Harrison CJ. Blood Spotlight on iAMP21 acute lymphoblastic leukemia (ALL), a high-risk pediatric disease. Blood. 2015 Feb 26;125(9):1383–6. PMID:25608562

1506. Harrison CJ, Haas O, Harbott J, et al. Detection of prognostically relevant genetic abnormalities in childhood B-cell precursor acute lymphoblastic leukaemia: recommendations from the Biology and Diagnosis Committee of the International Berlin-Frankfürt-Münster study group. Br J Haematol. 2010 Oct;151(2):132–42. PMID:20701601

1507. Harrison CJ, Moorman AV, Barber KE, et al. Interphase molecular cytogenetic screening for chromosomal abnormalities of prognostic significance in childhood acute lymphoblastic leukaemia: a UK Cancer Cytogenetics Group Study. Br J Haematol. 2005 May;129(4):520–30. PMID:15877734

1508. Harrison CJ, Moorman AV, Schwab C, et al. An international study of intrachromosomal amplification of chromosome 21 (iAMP21): cytogenetic characterization and outcome. Leukemia. 2014 May;28(5):1015–21. PMID:24166298

1509. Harrison CJ, Schwab C. Constitutional abnormalities of chromosome 21 predispose to iAMP21-acute lymphoblastic leukaemia. Eur J Med Genet. 2016 Mar;59(3):162–5. PMID:26836400

1510. Hart DN, Baker BW, Inglis MJ, et al. Epstein-Barr viral DNA in acute large granular lymphocyte (natural killer) leukemic cells. Blood. 1992 Apr 15;79(8):2116–23. PMID:1314113

1511. Hart M, Thakral B, Yohe S, et al. EBV-positive mucocutaneous ulcer in organ transplant recipients: a localized indolent posttransplant lymphoproliferative disorder. Am J Surg Pathol. 2014 Nov;38(11):1522–9. PMID:25007145

1512. Hartge P, Colt JS, Severson RK, et al. Residential herbicide use and risk of non-Hodgkin lymphoma. Cancer Epidemiol Biomarkers Prev. 2005 Apr;14(4):934–7. PMID:15824166

1513. Hartmann S, Agostinelli C, Klapper W, et al. Revising the historical collection of epithelioid cell-rich lymphomas of the Kiel Lymph Node Registry: What is Lennert's lymphoma nowadays? Histopathology. 2011 Dec;59(6):1173–82. PMID:22175897

1514. Hartmann S, Döring C, Jakobus C, et al. Nodular lymphocyte predominant Hodgkin lymphoma and T cell/histiocyte rich large B cell lymphoma–endpoints of a spectrum of one disease? PLoS One. 2013 Nov 11;8(11):e78812. PMID:24244368

1515. Hartmann S, Döring C, Vucic E, et al. Array comparative genomic hybridization reveals similarities between nodular lymphocyte predominant Hodgkin lymphoma and T cell/histiocyte rich large B cell lymphoma. Br J Haematol. 2015 May;169(3):415–22. PMID:25644177

1516. Hartmann S, Eichenauer DA, Plütschow A, et al. Histopathological features and their prognostic impact in nodular lymphocyte-predominant Hodgkin lymphoma–a matched pair analysis from the German Hodgkin Study Group (GHSG). Br J Haematol. 2014 Oct;167(2):238–42. PMID:24965443

1517. Hartmann S, Eichenauer DA, Plütschow A, et al. The prognostic impact of variant histology in nodular lymphocyte-predominant Hodgkin lymphoma: a report from the German Hodgkin Study Group (GHSG). Blood. 2013 Dec 19;122(26):4246–52. PMID:24100447

1518. Hartmann S, Eray M, Döring C, et al. Diffuse large B cell lymphoma derived from nodular lymphocyte predominant Hodgkin lymphoma presents with variable histopathology. BMC Cancer. 2014 May 13;14:332. PMID:24885870

1519. Hartmann S, Gesk S, Scholtysik R, et al. High resolution SNP array genomic profiling of peripheral T cell lymphomas, not otherwise specified, identifies a subgroup with chromosomal aberrations affecting the REL locus. Br J Haematol. 2010 Feb;148(3):402–12. PMID:19863542

1520. Hartmann S, Goncharova O, Portyanko A, et al. CD30 expression in neoplastic T cells of follicular T cell lymphoma is a helpful diagnostic tool in the differential diagnosis of Hodgkin lymphoma. Mod Pathol. 2019 Jan;32(1):37–47. PMID:30140037

1521. Hartmann S, Jakobus C, Rengstl B, et al. Spindle-shaped CD163+ rosetting macrophages replace CD4+ T-cells in HIV-related classical Hodgkin lymphoma. Mod Pathol. 2013 May;26(5):648–57. PMID:23307058

1522. Hartmann S, Plütschow A, Mottok A, et al. The time to relapse correlates with the histopathological growth pattern in nodular lymphocyte predominant Hodgkin lymphoma. Am J Hematol. 2019 Nov;94(11):1208–13. PMID:31396979

1523. Hartmann S, Scharf S, Steiner Y, et al. Landscape of 4D cell interaction in Hodgkin and non-Hodgkin lymphomas. Cancers (Basel). 2021 Oct 17;13(20):5208. PMID:34680356

1524. Hartmann S, Schuhmacher B, Rausch T, et al. Highly recurrent mutations of SGK1, DUSP2 and JUNB in nodular lymphocyte predominant Hodgkin lymphoma. Leukemia. 2016 Apr;30(4):844–53. PMID:26658840

1525. Hartmann S, Tousseyn T, Döring C, et al. Macrophages in T cell/histiocyte rich large B cell lymphoma strongly express metal-binding proteins and show a bi-activated phenotype. Int J Cancer. 2013 Dec 1;133(11):2609–18. PMID:23686423

1526. Hartmann S, Winkelmann R, Metcalf RA, et al. Immunoarchitectural patterns of progressive transformation of germinal centers with and without nodular lymphocyte-predominant Hodgkin lymphoma. Hum Pathol. 2015 Nov;46(11):1655–61. PMID:26410017

1527. Harvey RC, Tasian SK. Clinical diagnostics and treatment strategies for Philadelphia chromosome-like acute lymphoblastic leukemia. Blood Adv. 2020 Jan 14;4(1):218–28. PMID:31935290

1528. Hasenclever D, Diehl V. A prognostic score for advanced Hodgkin's disease. International Prognostic Factors Project on Advanced Hodgkin's Disease. N Engl J Med. 1998 Nov 19;339(21):1506–14. PMID:9819449

1529. Hashimoto A, Chiba N, Tsuno H, et al. Incidence of malignancy and the risk of lymphoma in Japanese patients with rheumatoid arthritis compared to the general population. J Rheumatol. 2015 Apr;42(4):564–71. PMID:25593236

1530. Hashimoto M, Yamashita Y, Mori N. Immunohistochemical detection of CD79a expression in precursor T cell lymphoblastic lymphoma/leukaemias. J Pathol. 2002 Jul;197(3):341–7. PMID:12115880

1531. Hashmi A, Podgaetz E, Richards ML. Laparoscopic resection of an undifferentiated pleomorphic splenic sarcoma. JSLS. 2010 Jul-Sep;14(3):426–30. PMID:21333202

1532. Hassab-El-Naby HM, El-Khalawany MA. Hypopigmented mycosis fungoides in Egyptian patients. J Cutan Pathol. 2013 Apr;40(4):397–404. PMID:23379648

1533. Hasselblom S, Ridell B, Sigurdardottir M, et al. Low rather than high Ki-67 protein expression is an adverse prognostic factor in diffuse large B-cell lymphoma. Leuk Lymphoma. 2008 Aug;49(8):1501–9. PMID:18766962

1534. Hasserjian RP, Harris NL. NK-cell lymphomas and leukemias: a spectrum of tumors with variable manifestations and immunophenotype. Am J Clin Pathol. 2007 Jun;127(6):860–8. PMID:17509983

1535. Havelange V, Ameye G, Théate I, et al. The peculiar 11q-gain/loss aberration reported in a subset of MYC-negative high-grade B-cell lymphomas can also occur in a MYC-rearranged lymphoma. Cancer Genet. 2016 Mar;209(3):117–8. PMID:26776268

1536. Haverkos BM, Pan Z, Gru AA, et al. Extranodal NK/T cell lymphoma, nasal type (ENKTL-NT): an update on epidemiology, clinical presentation, and natural history in North American and European cases. Curr Hematol Malig Rep. 2016 Dec;11(6):514–27. PMID:27778143

1537. Haws BT, Cui W, Persons DL, et al. Clinical and pathologic correlation of increased MYC gene copy number in diffuse large B-cell lymphoma. Clin Lymphoma Myeloma Leuk. 2016 Dec;16(12):679–83. PMID:27633159

1538. Hayashida M, Maekawa F, Chagi Y, et al. Combination of multicolor flow cytometry for circulating lymphoma cells and tests for the RHOAG17V and IDH2R172 hot-spot mutations in plasma cell-free DNA as liquid biopsy for the diagnosis of angioimmunoblastic T-cell lymphoma. Leuk Lymphoma. 2020 Oct;61(10):2389–98. PMID:32476550

1539. Hayes TC, Britton HA, Mewborne EB, et al. Symptomatic splenic hamartoma: case report and literature review. Pediatrics. 1998 May;101(5):E10. PMID:9565443

1540. He H, Cheng L, Weiss LM, et al. Clinical outcome of incidental pelvic node malignant B-cell lymphomas discovered at the time of radical prostatectomy. Leuk Lymphoma. 2007 Oct;48(10):1976–80. PMID:17917966

1541. He H, Xue Q, Tan F, et al. A rare case of primary pulmonary inflammatory pseudotumor-like follicular dendritic cell sarcoma successfully treated by lobectomy. Ann Transl Med. 2021 Jan;9(1):77. PMID:33553370

1542. He R, Ding W, Viswanatha DS, et al. PD-1 expression in chronic lymphocytic leukemia/small lymphocytic lymphoma (CLL/SLL) and large B-cell Richter transformation (DLBCL-RT): a characteristic feature of DLBCL-RT and potential surrogate marker for clonal relatedness. Am J Surg Pathol. 2018 Jul;42(7):843–54. PMID:29762141

1543. Heavican TB, Bouska A, Yu J, et al. Genetic drivers of oncogenic pathways in molecular subgroups of peripheral T-cell lymphoma. Blood. 2019 Apr 11;133(15):1664–76. PMID:30782609

1544. Hebert J, Cayuela JM, Berkeley J, et al. Candidate tumor-suppressor genes MTS1 (p16INK4A) and MTS2 (p15INK4B) display frequent homozygous deletions in primary cells from T- but not from B-cell lineage acute lymphoblastic leukemias. Blood. 1994 Dec 15;84(12):4038–44. PMID:7994022

1545. Hebraud B, Leleu X, Lauwers-Cances V, et al. Deletion of the 1p32 region is a major independent prognostic factor in young patients with myeloma: the IFM experience on 1195 patients. Leukemia. 2014 Mar;28(3):675–9. PMID:23892719

1546. Heerema NA, Carroll AJ, Devidas M, et al. Intrachromosomal amplification of chromosome 21 is associated with inferior outcomes in children with acute lymphoblastic leukemia treated in contemporary standard-risk children's oncology group studies: a report from the children's oncology group. J Clin Oncol. 2013 Sep 20;31(27):3397–402. PMID:23940221

1547. Heilgeist A, McClanahan F, Ho AD, et al. Prognostic value of the Follicular Lymphoma International Prognostic Index score in marginal zone lymphoma: an analysis of clinical presentation and outcome in 144 patients. Cancer. 2013 Jan 1;119(1):99–106. PMID:22736411

1548. Hein D, Dreisig K, Metzler M, et al. The preleukemic TCF3-PBX1 gene fusion can be generated in utero and is present in ≈0.6% of healthy newborns. Blood. 2019 Oct 17;134(16):1355–8. PMID:31434706

1549. Heise N, De Silva NS, Silva K, et al. Germinal center B cell maintenance and differentiation are controlled by distinct NF-κB transcription factor subunits. J Exp Med. 2014 Sep 22;211(10):2103–18. PMID:25180063

1550. Hellmuth JC, Louissaint A Jr, Szczepanowski M, et al. Duodenal-type and nodal follicular lymphomas differ by their immune microenvironment rather than their mutation profiles. Blood. 2018 Oct 18;132(16):1695–702. PMID:30126979

1551. Hendershot L, Bole D, Köhler G, et al. Assembly and secretion of heavy chains that do not associate posttranslationally with immunoglobulin heavy chain-binding protein. J Cell Biol. 1987 Mar;104(3):761–7. PMID:3102505

1552. Hendrickson PG, Doráis JA, Grow EJ, et al. Conserved roles of mouse DUX and human DUX4 in activating cleavage-stage genes and MERVL/HERVL retrotransposons. Nat Genet. 2017 Jun;49(6):925–34. PMID:28459457

1553. Heng TS, Painter MW, Immunological Genome Project Consortium. The Immunological Genome Project: networks of gene expression in immune cells. Nat Immunol. 2008 Oct;9(10):1091–4. PMID:18800157

1554. Henn A, Michel L, Fite C, et al. Sézary syndrome without erythroderma. J Am Acad Dermatol. 2015 Jun;72(6):1003–9.e1. PMID:25981000

1555. Henopp T, Quintanilla-Martínez L, Fend F, et al. Prevalence of follicular lymphoma in situ in consecutively analysed reactive lymph nodes. Histopathology. 2011 Jul;59(1):139–42. PMID:21771030

1556. Henter JI, Horne A, Aricó M, et al. HLH-2004: Diagnostic and therapeutic guidelines for hemophagocytic lymphohistiocytosis. Pediatr Blood Cancer. 2007 Feb;48(2):124–31. PMID:16937360

1557. Hentrich M, Müller M, Wyen C, et al. Characteristics and outcome of human immunodeficiency virus (HIV)-associated primary effusion lymphoma as observed in the German HIV-related lymphoma cohort study. Br J Haematol. 2021 Aug;194(3):642–6. PMID:33959944

1558. Herber M, Mertz P, Dieudonné Y, et al. Primary immunodeficiencies and lymphoma: a systematic review of literature. Leuk Lymphoma. 2020 Feb;61(2):274–84. PMID:31580160

1559. Herbst H, Dallenbach F, Hummel M, et al. Epstein-Barr virus latent membrane protein expression in Hodgkin and Reed-Sternberg cells. Proc Natl Acad Sci U S A. 1991 Jun 1;88(11):4766–70. PMID:1647016

1560. Herbst H, Niedobitek G, Kneba M, et al. High incidence of Epstein-Barr virus genomes in Hodgkin's disease. Am J Pathol. 1990 Jul;137(1):13–8. PMID:2164775

1561. Herglotz J, Unrau L, Hauschildt F, et al. Essential control of early B-cell development by Mef2 transcription factors. Blood. 2016 Feb 4;127(5):572–81. PMID:26660426

1562. Herishanu Y, Pérez-Galán P, Liu D, et al. The lymph node microenvironment promotes B-cell receptor signaling, NF-kappaB activation, and tumor proliferation in chronic lymphocytic leukemia. Blood. 2011 Jan 13;117(2):563–74. PMID:20940416

1563. Herling CD, Abedpour N, Weiss J, et al. Clonal dynamics towards the development of venetoclax resistance in chronic lymphocytic leukemia. Nat Commun. 2018 Feb 20;9(1):727. PMID:29463802

1564. Herling M, Khoury JD, Washington LT, et al. A systematic approach to diagnosis of mature T-cell leukemias reveals heterogeneity among WHO categories. Blood. 2004 Jul 15;104(2):328–35. PMID:15044256

1565. Herling M, Patel KA, Teitell MA, et al. High TCL1 expression and intact T-cell receptor signaling define a hyperproliferative subset of T-cell prolymphocytic leukemia. Blood. 2008 Jan 1;111(1):328–37. PMID:17890451

1566. Hernandez L, Fest T, Cazorla M, et al. p53 gene mutations and protein overexpression are associated with aggressive variants of mantle cell lymphomas. Blood. 1996 Apr 15;87(8):3351–9. PMID:8605352

1567. Hernández L, Pinyol M, Hernández S, et al. TRK-fused gene (TFG) is a new partner of ALK in anaplastic large cell lymphoma producing two structurally different TFG-ALK translocations. Blood. 1999 Nov 1;94(9):3265–8. PMID:10556217

1568. Hernandez-Trujillo VP, Scalchunes C, Cunningham-Rundles C, et al. Autoimmunity and inflammation in X-linked agammaglobulinemia. J Clin Immunol. 2014 Aug;34(6):627–32. PMID:24909997

1569. Herndier BG, Sanchez HC, Chang KL, et al. High prevalence of Epstein-Barr virus in the Reed-Sternberg cells of HIV-associated Hodgkin's disease. Am J Pathol. 1993 Apr;142(4):1073–9. PMID:8386441

1570. Herndon TM, Chen SS, Saba NS, et al. Direct in vivo evidence for increased proliferation of CLL cells in lymph nodes compared to bone marrow and peripheral blood. Leukemia. 2017 Jun;31(6):1340–7. PMID:28074063

1571. Herold T, Schneider S, Metzeler KH, et al. Adults with Philadelphia chromosome-like acute lymphoblastic leukemia frequently have IGH-CRLF2 and JAK2 mutations, persistence of minimal residual disease and poor prognosis. Haematologica. 2017 Jan;102(1):130–8. PMID:27561722

1572. Herreman A, Dierickx D, Morscio J, et al. Clinicopathological characteristics of post-transplant lymphoproliferative disorders of T-cell origin: single-center series of nine cases and meta-analysis of 147 reported cases. Leuk Lymphoma. 2013 Oct;54(10):2190–9. PMID:23402267

1573. Herrera GA, Teng J, Turbat-Herrera EA, et al. Understanding mesangial pathobiology in AL-amyloidosis and monoclonal Ig light chain deposition disease. Kidney Int Rep. 2020 Jul 21;5(11):1870–93. PMID:33163710

1574. Hertzberg L, Vendramini E, Ganmore I, et al. Down syndrome acute lymphoblastic leukemia, a highly heterogeneous disease in which aberrant expression of CRLF2 is associated with mutated JAK2: a report from the International BFM Study Group. Blood. 2010 Feb 4;115(5):1006–17. PMID:19965641

1575. Hervé M, Xu K, Ng YS, et al. Unmutated and mutated chronic lymphocytic leukemias derive from self-reactive B cell precursors despite expressing different antibody reactivity. J Clin Invest. 2005 Jun;115(6):1636–43. PMID:15902303

1576. Hess JL, Zutter MM, Castleberry RP, et al. Juvenile chronic myelogenous leukemia. Am J Clin Pathol. 1996 Feb;105(2):238–48. PMID:8607451

1577. Hetet G, Dastot H, Baens M, et al. Recurrent molecular deletion of the 12p13 region, centromeric to ETV6/TEL, in T-cell prolymphocytic leukemia. Hematol J. 2000;1(1):42–7. PMID:11920168

1578. Hiddemann W, Barbui AM, Canales MA, et al. Immunochemotherapy with obinutuzumab or rituximab for previously untreated follicular lymphoma in the GALLIUM study: influence of chemotherapy on efficacy and safety. J Clin Oncol. 2018 Aug 10;36(23):2395–404. PMID:29856692

1579. Hiemcke-Jiwa LS, Ten Dam-van Loon NH, Leguit RJ, et al. Potential diagnosis of vitreoretinal lymphoma by detection of MYD88 mutation in aqueous humor with ultrasensitive droplet digital polymerase chain reaction. JAMA Ophthalmol. 2018 Oct 1;136(10):1098–104. PMID:30027272

1580. Higgins JP, Warnke RA. CD30 expression is common in mediastinal large B-cell lymphoma. Am J Clin Pathol. 1999 Aug;112(2):241–7. PMID:10439805

1581. Higgins L, Nasr SH, Said SM, et al. Kidney involvement of patients with Waldenström macroglobulinemia and other IgM-producing B cell lymphoproliferative disorders. Clin J Am Soc Nephrol. 2018 Jul 6;13(7):1037–46. PMID:29848505

1582. Higuchi T, Matsuo K, Hashida Y, et al. Epstein-Barr virus-positive pyothorax-associated lymphoma expresses CCL17 and CCL22 chemokines that attract CCR4-expressing regulatory T cells. Cancer Lett. 2019 Jul 1;453:184–92. PMID:30953706

1583. Hill BT, Tubbs RR, Smith MR. Complete remission of CD30-positive diffuse large B-cell lymphoma in a patient with post-transplant lymphoproliferative disorder and end-stage renal disease treated with single-agent brentuximab vedotin. Leuk Lymphoma. 2015 May;56(5):1552–3. PMID:24717110

1584. Hill HA, Qi X, Jain P, et al. Genetic mutations and features of mantle cell lymphoma: a systematic review and meta-analysis. Blood Adv. 2020 Jul 14;4(13):2927–38. PMID:32598477

1585. Hill QA, Hill A, Berentsen S. Defining autoimmune hemolytic anemia: a systematic review of the terminology used for diagnosis and treatment. Blood Adv. 2019 Jun 25;3(12):1897–906. PMID:31235526

1586. Hill QA, Rawstron AC, de Tute RM, et al. Outcome prediction in plasmacytoma of bone: a risk model utilizing bone marrow flow cytometry and light-chain analysis. Blood. 2014 Aug 21;124(8):1296–9. PMID:24939658

1587. Hilton LK, Tang J, Ben-Neriah S, et al. The double-hit signature identifies double-hit diffuse large B-cell lymphoma with genetic events cryptic to FISH. Blood. 2019 Oct 31;134(18):1528–32. PMID:31527075

1588. Hindsø TG, Esmaeli B, Holm F, et al. International multicentre retrospective cohort study of ocular adnexal marginal zone B-cell lymphoma. Br J Ophthalmol. 2020 Mar;104(3):357–62. PMID:31177189

1589. Hirabayashi S, Butler ER, Ohki K, et al. Clinical characteristics and outcomes of B-ALL with ZNF384 rearrangements: a retrospective analysis by the Ponte di Legno Childhood ALL Working Group. Leukemia. 2021 Nov;35(11):3272–7. PMID:33692463

1590. Hirabayashi S, Ohki K, Nakabayashi K, et al. ZNF384-related fusion genes define a subgroup of childhood B-cell precursor acute lymphoblastic leukemia with a characteristic immunotype. Haematologica. 2017 Jan;102(1):118–29. PMID:27634205

1591. Hirai Y, Yamamoto T, Kimura H, et al. Hydroa vacciniforme is associated with increased numbers of Epstein-Barr virus-infected γδT cells. J Invest Dermatol. 2012 May;132(5):1401–8. PMID:22297643

1592. Hirakawa K, Fuchigami T, Nakamura S, et al. Primary gastrointestinal T-cell lymphoma resembling multiple lymphomatous polyposis. Gastroenterology. 1996 Sep;111(3):778–82. PMID:8780585

1593. Hirano K, Tada M, Sasahira N, et al. Incidence of malignancies in patients with IgG4-related disease. Intern Med. 2014;53(3):171–6. PMID:24492683

1594. Hirt C, Camargo MC, Yu KJ, et al. Risk of follicular lymphoma associated with BCL2 translocations in peripheral blood. Leuk Lymphoma. 2015;56(9):2625–9. PMID:25549806

1595. Hisaoka M, Hashiomoto H, Daimaru Y. Intranodal palisaded myofibroblastoma with so-called amianthoid fibers: a report of two cases with a review of the literature. Pathol Int. 1998 Apr;48(4):307–12. PMID:9648161

1596. Hjalgrim H, Askling J, Rostgaard K, et al. Characteristics of Hodgkin's lymphoma after infectious mononucleosis. N Engl J Med. 2003 Oct 2;349(14):1324–32. PMID:14523140

1597. Hjalgrim H, Askling J, Sørensen P, et al. Risk of Hodgkin's disease and other cancers after infectious mononucleosis. J Natl Cancer Inst. 2000 Sep 20;92(18):1522–8. PMID:10995808

1598. Hjalgrim H, Rostgaard K, Johnson PC, et al. HLA-A alleles and infectious mononucleosis suggest a critical role for cytotoxic T-cell response in EBV-related Hodgkin lymphoma. Proc Natl Acad Sci U S A. 2010 Apr 6;107(14):6400–5. PMID:20308568

1599. Ho HE, Cunningham-Rundles C. Non-infectious complications of common variable immunodeficiency: updated clinical spectrum, sequelae, and insights to pathogenesis. Front Immunol. 2020 Feb 7;11:149. PMID:32117289

1600. Ho YH, Wang JL, DeLelys ME, et al. Gamma heavy chain disease: cytological diagnosis of a rare lymphoid malignancy facilitated by correlation with key laboratory findings. Cytopathology. 2014 Aug;25(4):270–3. PMID:25180407

1601. Hockley SL, Else M, Morilla A, et al. The prognostic impact of clinical and molecular features in hairy cell leukaemia variant and splenic marginal zone lymphoma. Br J Haematol. 2012 Aug;158(3):347–54. PMID:22594855

1602. Hockley SL, Giannouli S, Morilla A, et al. Insight into the molecular pathogenesis of hairy cell leukaemia, hairy cell leukaemia variant and splenic marginal zone lymphoma, provided by the analysis of their IGH rearrangements and somatic hypermutation patterns. Br J Haematol. 2010 Feb;148(4):666–9. PMID:19863540

1603. Hockley SL, Morilla A, Else M, et al. Higher expression levels of activation-induced cytidine deaminase distinguish hairy cell leukemia from hairy cell leukemia-variant and splenic marginal zone lymphoma. Leukemia. 2010 May;24(5):1084–6. PMID:20237507

1604. Hodak E, Amitay-Laish I, Atzmony L, et al. New insights into folliculotropic mycosis fungoides (FMF): a single-center experience. J Am Acad Dermatol. 2016 Aug;75(2):347–55. PMID:27245278

1605. Hodgson K, Ferrer G, Montserrat E, et al. Chronic lymphocytic leukemia and autoimmunity: a systematic review. Haematologica. 2011 May;96(5):752–61. PMID:21242190

1606. Hoefnagel JJ, Dijkman R, Basso K, et al. Distinct types of primary cutaneous large B-cell lymphoma identified by gene expression profiling. Blood. 2005 May 1;105(9):3671–8. PMID:15308563

1607. Hoefnagel JJ, Vermeer MH, Jansen PM, et al. Bcl-2, Bcl-6 and CD10 expression in cutaneous B-cell lymphoma: further support for a follicle centre cell origin and differential diagnostic significance. Br J Dermatol. 2003 Dec;149(6):1183–91. PMID:14674895

1608. Hoefnagel JJ, Vermeer MH, Jansen PM, et al. Primary cutaneous marginal zone B-cell lymphoma: clinical and therapeutic features in 50 cases. Arch Dermatol. 2005 Sep;141(9):1139–45. PMID:16172311

1609. Hoeller S, Tzankov A, Pileri SA, et al. Epstein-Barr virus-positive diffuse large B-cell lymphoma in elderly patients is rare in western populations. Hum Pathol. 2010 Mar;41(3):352–7. PMID:19913281

1610. Hoffmann C, Schmid H, Müller M, et al. Improved outcome with rituximab in patients with HIV-associated multicentric Castleman disease. Blood. 2011 Sep 29;118(13):3499–503. PMID:21778341

1611. Hoffmann T, De Libero G, Colonna M, et al. Natural killer-type receptors for HLA class I antigens are clonally expressed in lymphoproliferative disorders of natural killer and T-cell type. Br J Haematol. 2000 Sep;110(3):525–36. PMID:10997961

1612. Hofscheier A, Ponciano A, Bonzheim I, et al. Geographic variation in the prevalence of Epstein-Barr virus-positive diffuse large B-cell lymphoma of the elderly: a comparative analysis of a Mexican and a German population. Mod Pathol. 2011 Aug;24(8):1046–54. PMID:21499229

1613. Höglund M, Sehn L, Connors JM, et al. Identification of cytogenetic subgroups and karyotypic pathways of clonal evolution in follicular lymphomas. Genes Chromosomes Cancer. 2004 Mar;39(3):195–204. PMID:14732921

1614. Hollender A, Kvaloy S, Nome O, et al. Central nervous system involvement following diagnosis of non-Hodgkin's lymphoma: a risk model. Ann Oncol. 2002 Jul;13(7):1099–107. PMID:12176790

1615. Hollingsworth HC, Longo DL, Jaffe ES. Small noncleaved cell lymphoma associated with florid epithelioid granulomatous response. A clinicopathologic study of seven patients. Am J Surg Pathol. 1993 Jan;17(1):51–9. PMID:8447509

1616. Hollingsworth HC, Stetler-Stevenson M, Gagneten D, et al. Immunodeficiency-associated malignant lymphoma. Three cases showing genotypic evidence of both T- and

B-cell lineages. Am J Surg Pathol. 1994 Nov;18(11):1092–101. PMID:7943530
1617. Holm AM, Tjønnfjord G, Yndestad A, et al. Polyclonal expansion of large granular lymphocytes in common variable immunodeficiency - association with neutropenia. Clin Exp Immunol. 2006 Jun;144(3):418–24. PMID:16734610
1618. Holmes AB, Corinaldesi C, Shen Q, et al. Single-cell analysis of germinal-center B cells informs on lymphoma cell of origin and outcome. J Exp Med. 2020 Oct 5;217(10):e20200483. PMID:32603407
1619. Holmes GK, Prior P, Lane MR, et al. Malignancy in coeliac disease–effect of a gluten free diet. Gut. 1989 Mar;30(3):333–8. PMID:2707633
1620. Holmfeldt L, Wei L, Diaz-Flores E, et al. The genomic landscape of hypodiploid acute lymphoblastic leukemia. Nat Genet. 2013 Mar;45(3):242–52. PMID:23334668
1621. Holzelova E, Vonarbourg C, Stolzenberg MC, et al. Autoimmune lymphoproliferative syndrome with somatic Fas mutations. N Engl J Med. 2004 Sep 30;351(14):1409–18. PMID:15459302
1622. Homminga I, Pieters R, Langerak AW, et al. Integrated transcript and genome analyses reveal NKX2-1 and MEF2C as potential oncogenes in T cell acute lymphoblastic leukemia. Cancer Cell. 2011 Apr 12;19(4):484–97. PMID:21481790
1623. Hong M, Ko YH, Yoo KH, et al. EBV-positive T/NK-cell lymphoproliferative disease of childhood. Korean J Pathol. 2013 Apr;47(2):137–47. PMID:23667373
1624. Hong M, Lee T, Young Kang S, et al. Nasal-type NK/T-cell lymphomas are more frequently T rather than NK lineage based on T-cell receptor gene, RNA, and protein studies: lineage does not predict clinical behavior. Mod Pathol. 2016 May;29(5):430–43. PMID:27015135
1625. Hongyo T, Kurooka M, Taniguchi E, et al. Frequent p53 mutations at dipyrimidine sites in patients with pyothorax-associated lymphoma. Cancer Res. 1998 Mar 15;58(6):1105–7. PMID:9515788
1626. Honma K, Tsuzuki S, Nakagawa M, et al. TNFAIP3/A20 functions as a novel tumor suppressor gene in several subtypes of non-Hodgkin lymphomas. Blood. 2009 Sep 17;114(12):2467–75. PMID:19608751
1627. Horie A, Ishii N, Matsumoto M, et al. Leiomyomatosis in the pelvic lymph node and peritoneum. Acta Pathol Jpn. 1984 Jul;34(4):813–9. PMID:6485798
1628. Horiguchi H, Matsui-Horiguchi M, Sakata H, et al. Inflammatory pseudotumor-like follicular dendritic cell tumor of the spleen. Pathol Int. 2004 Feb;54(2):124–31. PMID:14720144
1629. Hormann FM, Hoogkamer AQ, Beverloo HB, et al. NUTM1 is a recurrent fusion gene partner in B-cell precursor acute lymphoblastic leukemia associated with increased expression of genes on chromosome band 10p12.31-12.2. Haematologica. 2019 Oct;104(10):e455–9. PMID:30872366
1630. Horn H, Kalmbach S, Wagener R, et al. A diagnostic approach to the identification of Burkitt-like lymphoma with 11q aberration in aggressive B-cell lymphomas. Am J Surg Pathol. 2021 Mar 1;45(3):356–64. PMID:33136583
1631. Horn H, Kohler C, Witzig R, et al. Gene expression profiling reveals a close relationship between follicular lymphoma grade 3A and 3B, but distinct profiles of follicular lymphoma grade 1 and 2. Haematologica. 2018 Jul;103(7):1182–90. PMID:29567771
1632. Horn H, Schmelter C, Leich E, et al. Follicular lymphoma grade 3B is a distinct neoplasm according to cytogenetic and immunohistochemical profiles. Haematologica. 2011 Sep;96(9):1327–34. PMID:21659362
1633. Horn H, Staiger AM, Vöhringer M, et al. Diffuse large B-cell lymphomas of immunoblastic type are a major reservoir for MYC-IGH translocations. Am J Surg Pathol. 2015 Jan;39(1):61–6. PMID:25229766
1634. Horn H, Ziepert M, Becher C, et al. MYC status in concert with BCL2 and BCL6 expression predicts outcome in diffuse large B-cell lymphoma. Blood. 2013 Mar 21;121(12):2253–63. PMID:23335369
1635. Horna P, Olteanu H, Jevremovic D, et al. Single-antibody evaluation of T-cell receptor β constant chain monotypia by flow cytometry facilitates the diagnosis of T-cell large granular lymphocytic leukemia. Am J Clin Pathol. 2021 Jun 17;156(1):139–48. PMID:33438036
1636. Horwitz SM, Advani RH, Bartlett NL, et al. Objective responses in relapsed T-cell lymphomas with single-agent brentuximab vedotin. Blood. 2014 May 15;123(20):3095–100. PMID:24652992
1637. Hoshida Y, Li T, Dong Z, et al. Lymphoproliferative disorders in renal transplant patients in Japan. Int J Cancer. 2001 Mar 15;91(6):869–75. PMID:11275994
1638. Hoshida Y, Xu JX, Fujita S, et al. Lymphoproliferative disorders in rheumatoid arthritis: clinicopathological analysis of 76 cases in relation to methotrexate medication. J Rheumatol. 2007 Feb;34(2):322–31. PMID:17117491
1639. Hosoya T, Kuroha T, Moriguchi T, et al. GATA-3 is required for early T lineage progenitor development. J Exp Med. 2009 Dec 21;206(13):2987–3000. PMID:19934022
1640. Hoster E, Dreyling M, Klapper W, et al. A new prognostic index (MIPI) for patients with advanced-stage mantle cell lymphoma. Blood. 2008 Jan 15;111(2):558–65. PMID:17962512
1641. Hoster E, Klapper W, Hermine O, et al. Confirmation of the mantle-cell lymphoma International Prognostic Index in randomized trials of the European Mantle-Cell Lymphoma Network. J Clin Oncol. 2014 May 1;32(13):1338–46. PMID:24687837
1642. Hoster E, Rosenwald A, Berger F, et al. Prognostic value of Ki-67 index, cytology, and growth pattern in mantle-cell lymphoma: results from randomized trials of the European Mantle Cell Lymphoma Network. J Clin Oncol. 2016 Apr 20;34(12):1386–94. PMID:26926679
1643. Houillier C, Soussain C, Ghesquières H, et al. Management and outcome of primary CNS lymphoma in the modern era: an LOC network study. Neurology. 2020 Mar 10;94(10):e1027–39. PMID:31907289
1644. Hovorkova L, Zaliova M, Venn NC, et al. Monitoring of childhood ALL using BCR-ABL1 genomic breakpoints identifies a subgroup with CML-like biology. Blood. 2017 May 18;129(20):2771–81. PMID:28331056
1645. Howard MT, Bejanyan N, Maciejewski JP, et al. T/NK large granular lymphocyte leukemia and coexisting monoclonal B-cell lymphocytosis-like proliferations. An unrecognized and frequent association. Am J Clin Pathol. 2010 Jun;133(6):936–41. PMID:20472852
1646. Howard MT, Hodnefield J, Morice WG. Immunohistochemical phenotyping of plasma cells in lymphoplasmacytic lymphoma/ Waldenström's macroglobulinemia is comparable to flow cytometric techniques. Clin Lymphoma Myeloma Leuk. 2011 Feb;11(1):96–8. PMID:21454202
1647. Howell WM, Leung ST, Jones DB, et al. HLA-DRB, -DQA, and -DQB polymorphism in celiac disease and enteropathy-associated T-cell lymphoma. Common features and additional risk factors for malignancy. Hum Immunol. 1995 May;43(1):29–37. PMID:7558926
1648. Hrusák O, Porwit-MacDonald A. Antigen expression patterns reflecting genotype of acute leukemias. Leukemia. 2002 Jul;16(7):1233–58. PMID:12094248
1649. Hsi AC, Robirds DH, Luo J, et al. T-cell prolymphocytic leukemia frequently shows cutaneous involvement and is associated with gains of MYC, loss of ATM, and TCL1A rearrangement. Am J Surg Pathol. 2014 Nov;38(11):1468–83. PMID:25310835
1650. Hsiao SC, Cortada IR, Colomo L, et al. SOX11 is useful in differentiating cyclin D1-positive diffuse large B-cell lymphoma from mantle cell lymphoma. Histopathology. 2012 Oct;61(4):685–93. PMID:22642745
1651. Hsu P, Yang T, Sheikh-Fayyaz S, et al. Mantle cell lymphoma with in situ or mantle zone growth pattern: a study of five cases and review of literature. Int J Clin Exp Pathol. 2014 Feb 15;7(3):1042–50. PMID:24696721
1652. Hsu SM, Jaffe ES. Leu M1 and peanut agglutinin stain the neoplastic cells of Hodgkin's disease. Am J Clin Pathol. 1984 Jul;82(1):29–32. PMID:6741873
1653. Hsu YK, Rosenshein NB, Parmley TH, et al. Leiomyomatosis in pelvic lymph nodes. Obstet Gynecol. 1981 Jun;57(6 Suppl):91S–93S. PMID:7243134
1654. Hu H, Johani K, Almatroudi A, et al. Bacterial biofilm infection detected in breast implant-associated anaplastic large-cell lymphoma. Plast Reconstr Surg. 2016 Jun;137(6):1659–69. PMID:26890506
1655. Hu J, Tipps AMP, Hasteh F, et al. Intranodal palisaded myofibroblastoma of para-esophageal lymph node: case report with cytologic and histologic findings. Diagn Cytopathol. 2019 Dec;47(12):1306–9. PMID:31400261
1656. Hu S, Xu-Monette ZY, Balasubramanyam A, et al. CD30 expression defines a novel subgroup of diffuse large B-cell lymphoma with favorable prognosis and distinct gene expression signature: a report from the International DLBCL Rituximab-CHOP Consortium Program Study. Blood. 2013 Apr 4;121(14):2715–24. PMID:23343832
1657. Hu S, Young KH, Konoplev SN, et al. Follicular T-cell lymphoma: a member of an emerging family of follicular helper T-cell derived T-cell lymphomas. Hum Pathol. 2012 Nov;43(11):1789–98. PMID:22959759
1658. Hu Z, Pan Z, Chen W, et al. Primary effusion lymphoma: a clinicopathological study of 70 cases. Cancers (Basel). 2021 Feb 19;13(4):878. PMID:33669719
1659. Huang AH, Kwatra SG, Khanna R, et al. Racial disparities in the clinical presentation and prognosis of patients with mycosis fungoides. J Natl Med Assoc. 2019 Dec;111(6):633–9. PMID:31623818
1660. Huang C, Geng H, Boss I, et al. Cooperative transcriptional repression by BCL6 and BACH2 in germinal center B-cell differentiation. Blood. 2014 Feb 13;123(7):1012–20. PMID:24277074
1661. Huang D, Lim JQ, Cheah DMZ, et al. Whole-genome sequencing reveals potent therapeutic strategy for monomorphic epitheliotropic intestinal T-cell lymphoma. Blood Adv. 2020 Oct 13;4(19):4769–74. PMID:33017466
1662. Huang FL, Liao EC, Li CL, et al. Pathogenesis of pediatric B-cell acute lymphoblastic leukemia: molecular pathways and disease treatments. Oncol Lett. 2020 Jul;20(1):448–54. PMID:32565969
1663. Huang JZ, Weisenburger DD, Vose JM, et al. Diffuse large B-cell lymphoma arising in nodular lymphocyte predominant Hodgkin lymphoma: a report of 21 cases from the Nebraska Lymphoma Study Group. Leuk Lymphoma. 2004 Aug;45(8):1551–7. PMID:15370206
1664. Huang KP, Weinstock MA, Clarke CA, et al. Second lymphomas and other malignant neoplasms in patients with mycosis fungoides and Sezary syndrome: evidence from population-based and clinical cohorts. Arch Dermatol. 2007 Jan;143(1):45–50. PMID:17224541
1665. Huang L, Liu D, Wang N, et al. Integrated genomic analysis identifies deregulated JAK/STAT-MYC-biosynthesis axis in aggressive NK-cell leukemia. Cell Res. 2018 Feb;28(2):172–86. PMID:29148541
1666. Huang W, Medeiros LJ, Lin P, et al. MYC/ BCL2/BCL6 triple hit lymphoma: a study of 40 patients with a comparison to MYC/BCL2 and MYC/BCL6 double hit lymphomas. Mod Pathol. 2018 Sep;31(9):1470–8. PMID:29785017
1667. Huang Y, Chen S, Wei R, et al. CD20-positive extranodal NK/T cell lymphoma: clinicopathologic and prognostic features. Virchows Arch. 2020 Dec;477(6):873–83. PMID:32314054
1668. Huang Y, de Reyniès A, de Leval L, et al. Gene expression profiling identifies emerging oncogenic pathways operating in extranodal NK/T-cell lymphoma, nasal type. Blood. 2010 Feb 11;115(6):1226–37. PMID:19965620
1669. Huang Y, Moreau A, Dupuis J, et al. Peripheral T-cell lymphomas with a follicular growth pattern are derived from follicular helper T cells (TFH) and may show overlapping features with angioimmunoblastic T-cell lymphomas. Am J Surg Pathol. 2009 May;33(5):682–90. PMID:19295409
1670. Huang Y, Shi X, Zhong P, et al. De novo testicular extranodal NK/T-cell lymphoma: a clinicopathologic study of 21 cases with review of additional 18 cases in the literature. Am J Surg Pathol. 2019 Apr;43(4):549–58. PMID:30589649
1671. Hübel K. The changing landscape of lymphoma associated with HIV infection. Curr Oncol Rep. 2020 Aug 15;22(11):111. PMID:32803474
1672. Hubers LM, Vos H, Schuurman AR, et al. Annexin A11 is targeted by IgG4 and IgG1 autoantibodies in IgG4-related disease. Gut. 2018 Apr;67(4):728–35. PMID:28765476
1673. Hübschmann D, Kleinheinz K, Wagener R, et al. Mutational mechanisms shaping the coding and noncoding genome of germinal center derived B-cell lymphomas. Leukemia. 2021 Jul;35(7):2002–16. PMID:33953289
1674. Huck K, Feyen O, Niehues T, et al. Girls homozygous for an IL-2-inducible T cell kinase mutation that leads to protein deficiency develop fatal EBV-associated lymphoproliferation. J Clin Invest. 2009 May;119(5):1350–8. PMID:19425169
1675. Hudnall SD, Betancourt E, Barnhart E, et al. Comparative flow immunophenotypic features of the inflammatory infiltrates of Hodgkin lymphoma and lymphoid hyperplasia. Cytometry B Clin Cytom. 2008 Jan;74(1):1–8. PMID:18061945
1676. Hudnall SD, Chen T, Amr S, et al. Detection of human herpesvirus DNA in Kikuchi-Fujimoto disease and reactive lymphoid hyperplasia. Int J Clin Exp Pathol. 2008 Jan 1;1(4):362–8. PMID:18787614
1677. Hue SS, Oon ML, Wang S, et al. Epstein-Barr virus-associated T- and NK-cell lymphoproliferative diseases: an update and diagnostic approach. Pathology. 2020 Jan;52(1):111–27. PMID:31767131
1678. Huet S, Sujobert P, Salles G. From genetics to the clinic: a translational perspective on follicular lymphoma. Nat Rev Cancer. 2018 Apr;18(4):224–39. PMID:29422597
1679. Huet S, Szafer-Glusman E, Tesson B, et al. BCL2 mutations do not confer adverse prognosis in follicular lymphoma patients treated with rituximab. Am J Hematol. 2017 Jun;92(6):515–9. PMID:28247997
1680. Huet S, Tesson B, Jais JP, et al. A

gene-expression profiling score for prediction of outcome in patients with follicular lymphoma: a retrospective training and validation analysis in three international cohorts. Lancet Oncol. 2018 Apr;19(4):549–61. PMID:29475724
1681. Huettl KS, Staiger AM, Horn H, et al. Cytokeratin expression in plasmablastic lymphoma - a possible diagnostic pitfall in the routine work-up of tumours. Histopathology. 2021 May;78(6):831–7. PMID:33165992
1682. Huggett MT, Culver EL, Kumar M, et al. Type 1 autoimmune pancreatitis and IgG4-related sclerosing cholangitis is associated with extrapancreatic organ failure, malignancy, and mortality in a prospective UK cohort. Am J Gastroenterol. 2014 Oct;109(10):1675–83. PMID:25155229
1683. Hummel M, Bentink S, Berger H, et al. A biologic definition of Burkitt's lymphoma from transcriptional and genomic profiling. N Engl J Med. 2006 Jun 8;354(23):2419–30. PMID:16760442
1684. Hunger SP, Devaraj PE, Foroni L, et al. Two types of genomic rearrangements create alternative E2A-HLF fusion proteins in t(17;19)-ALL. Blood. 1994 May 15;83(10):2970–7. PMID:8180393
1685. Hunter ZR, Xu L, Tsakmaklis N, et al. Insights into the genomic landscape of MYD88 wild-type Waldenström macroglobulinemia. Blood Adv. 2018 Nov 13;2(21):2937–46. PMID:30401751
1686. Hunter ZR, Xu L, Yang G, et al. The genomic landscape of Waldenstrom macroglobulinemia is characterized by highly recurring MYD88 and WHIM-like CXCR4 mutations, and small somatic deletions associated with B-cell lymphomagenesis. Blood. 2014 Mar 13;123(11):1637–46. PMID:24366360
1687. Hunter ZR, Xu L, Yang G, et al. Transcriptome sequencing reveals a profile that corresponds to genomic variants in Waldenström macroglobulinemia. Blood. 2016 Aug 11;128(6):827–38. PMID:27301862
1688. Huppmann AR, Nicolae A, Slack GW, et al. EBV may be expressed in the LP cells of nodular lymphocyte-predominant Hodgkin lymphoma (NLPHL) in both children and adults. Am J Surg Pathol. 2014 Mar;38(3):316–24. PMID:24525501
1689. Huppmann AR, Roullet MR, Raffeld M, et al. Angioimmunoblastic T-cell lymphoma partially obscured by an Epstein-Barr virus-negative clonal plasma cell proliferation. J Clin Oncol. 2013 Jan 10;31(2):e28–30. PMID:23213091
1690. Huppmann AR, Xi L, Raffeld M, et al. Subcutaneous panniculitis-like T-cell lymphoma in the pediatric age group: a lymphoma of low malignant potential. Pediatr Blood Cancer. 2013 Jul;60(7):1165–70. PMID:23382035
1691. Hussein HAM, Alfhili MA, Pakala P, et al. miRNAs and their roles in KSHV pathogenesis. Virus Res. 2019 Jun;266:15–24. PMID:30951791
1692. Hussein S, Gindin T, Lagana SM, et al. Clonal T cell receptor gene rearrangements in coeliac disease: implications for diagnosing refractory coeliac disease. J Clin Pathol. 2018 Sep;71(9):825–31. PMID:29703761
1693. Hussell T, Isaacson PG, Crabtree JE, et al. The response of cells from low-grade B-cell gastric lymphomas of mucosa-associated lymphoid tissue to Helicobacter pylori. Lancet. 1993 Sep 4;342(8871):571–4. PMID:8102718
1694. Hüttl KS, Staiger AM, Richter J, et al. The "Burkitt-like" immunophenotype and genotype is rarely encountered in diffuse large B cell lymphoma and high-grade B cell lymphoma, NOS. Virchows Arch. 2021 Sep;479(3):575–83. PMID:33655392
1695. Hwang J, Suh CH, Won Kim K, et al. The incidence of Epstein-Barr virus-positive diffuse large B-cell lymphoma: a systematic review and meta-analysis. Cancers (Basel). 2021 Apr 8;13(8):1785. PMID:33917961
1696. Hwang SM, Paik JH, Lee JY. Immunoglobulin G4-related disease mimicking lymphoma. Ann Hematol. 2019 Sep;98(9):2239–41. PMID:31154475
1697. Hyjek E, Isaacson PG. Primary B cell lymphoma of the thyroid and its relationship to Hashimoto's thyroiditis. Hum Pathol. 1988 Nov;19(11):1315–26. PMID:3141260
1698. Hyjek E, Smith WJ, Isaacson PG. Primary B-cell lymphoma of salivary glands and its relationship to myoepithelial sialadenitis. Hum Pathol. 1988 Jul;19(7):766–76. PMID:3136072
1699. Iaccarino I, Afify L, Aukema SM, et al. t(11;14)-positive mantle cell lymphomas lacking cyclin D1 (CCND1) immunostaining because of a CCND1 mutation or exclusive expression of the CCND1b isoform. Haematologica. 2018 Sep;103(9):e432–5. PMID:29773591
1700. Iacobucci I, Kimura S, Mullighan CG. Biologic and therapeutic implications of genomic alterations in acute lymphoblastic leukemia. J Clin Med. 2021 Aug 25;10(17):3792. PMID:34501239
1701. Iacobucci I, Li Y, Roberts KG, et al. Truncating erythropoietin receptor rearrangements in acute lymphoblastic leukemia. Cancer Cell. 2016 Feb 8;29(2):186–200. PMID:26859458
1702. Iacobucci I, Lonetti A, Messa F, et al. Expression of spliced oncogenic Ikaros isoforms in Philadelphia-positive acute lymphoblastic leukemia patients treated with tyrosine kinase inhibitors: implications for a new mechanism of resistance. Blood. 2008 Nov 1;112(9):3847–55. PMID:18650450
1703. Iacobucci I, Lonetti A, Paoloni F, et al. The PAX5 gene is frequently rearranged in BCR-ABL1-positive acute lymphoblastic leukemia but is not associated with outcome. A report on behalf of the GIMEMA Acute Leukemia Working Party. Haematologica. 2010 Oct;95(10):1683–90. PMID:20534699
1704. Iacobucci I, Mullighan CG. Genetic basis of acute lymphoblastic leukemia. J Clin Oncol. 2017 Mar 20;35(9):975–83. PMID:28297628
1705. Iacobucci I, Roberts KG. Genetic alterations and therapeutic targeting of Philadelphia-like acute lymphoblastic leukemia. Genes (Basel). 2021 May 1;12(5):687. PMID:34062932
1706. Ibrahim HA, Balachandran K, Bower M, et al. Bone marrow manifestations in multicentric Castleman disease. Br J Haematol. 2016 Mar;172(6):923–9. PMID:26817834
1707. Ibrahim HA, Menasce LP, Pomplun S, et al. Presence of monoclonal T-cell populations in B-cell post-transplant lymphoproliferative disorders. Mod Pathol. 2011 Feb;24(2):232–40. PMID:20834235
1708. Ichikawa A, Arakawa F, Kiyasu J, et al. Methotrexate/iatrogenic lymphoproliferative disorders in rheumatoid arthritis: histology, Epstein-Barr virus, and clonality are important predictors of disease progression and regression. Eur J Haematol. 2013 Jul;91(1):20–8. PMID:23560463
1709. Ichikawa K, Noguchi M, Koike M, et al. Rituximab plus a CHOP-like regimen, central nervous system prophylaxis, and contralateral testicular irradiation for localized primary testicular diffuse large B-cell lymphoma lead to prolonged progression-free survival. Int J Hematol. 2014 Oct;100(4):370–8. PMID:25085255
1710. Ichiki A, Hashimoto N, Ueda T, et al. IgG4-related disease with bone marrow involvement. Intern Med. 2016;55(16):2295–9. PMID:27523012
1711. Igawa T, Sato Y. TAFRO syndrome. Hematol Oncol Clin North Am. 2018 Feb;32(1):107–18. PMID:29157612
1712. Ikeda S, Kobayashi T, Saito M, et al. Multiparameter flow cytometry for the identification of neoplastic plasma cells in POEMS syndrome with IgG-kappa gammopathy: successful treatment using lenalidomide and dexamethasone. Intern Med. 2019 Dec 1;58(23):3461–8. PMID:31391391
1713. Ikeda T, Gion Y, Sakamoto M, et al. Clinicopathological analysis of 34 Japanese patients with EBV-positive mucocutaneous ulcer. Mod Pathol. 2020 Dec;33(12):2437–48. PMID:32561847
1714. Illerhaus G, Marks R, Ihorst G, et al. High-dose chemotherapy with autologous stem-cell transplantation and hyperfractionated radiotherapy as first-line treatment of primary CNS lymphoma. J Clin Oncol. 2006 Aug 20;24(24):3865–70. PMID:16864853
1715. Ilus T, Kaukinen K, Virta LJ, et al. Refractory coeliac disease in a country with a high prevalence of clinically-diagnosed coeliac disease. Aliment Pharmacol Ther. 2014 Feb;39(4):418–25. PMID:24387637
1716. Imamura M, Ueno H, Matsuura A, et al. An ultrastructural study of subacute necrotizing lymphadenitis. Am J Pathol. 1982 Jun;107(3):292–9. PMID:6282130
1717. Imamura N, Kusunoki Y, Kawa-Ha K, et al. Aggressive natural killer cell leukaemia/lymphoma: report of four cases and review of the literature. Possible existence of a new clinical entity originating from the third lineage of lymphoid cells. Br J Haematol. 1990 May;75(1):49–59. PMID:2375924
1718. Inaba H, Mullighan CG. Pediatric acute lymphoblastic leukemia. Haematologica. 2020 Nov 1;105(11):2524–39. PMID:33054110
1719. Inagaki H, Chan JK, Ng JW, et al. Primary thymic extranodal marginal-zone B-cell lymphoma of mucosa-associated lymphoid tissue type exhibits distinctive clinicopathological and molecular features. Am J Pathol. 2002 Apr;160(4):1435–43. PMID:11943727
1720. Inamdar KV, Medeiros LJ, Jorgensen JL, et al. Bone marrow involvement by marginal zone B-cell lymphomas of different types. Am J Clin Pathol. 2008 May;129(5):714–22. PMID:18426730
1721. Inghirami G, Foitl DR, Sabichi A, et al. Autoantibody-associated cross-reactive idiotype-bearing human B lymphocytes: distribution and characterization, including Ig VH gene and CD5 antigen expression. Blood. 1991 Sep 15;78(6):1503–15. PMID:1715792
1722. Inghirami G, Pileri SA, European T-Cell Lymphoma Study Group. Anaplastic large-cell lymphoma. Semin Diagn Pathol. 2011 Aug;28(3):190–201. PMID:21850985
1723. Inhorn RC, Aster JC, Roach SA, et al. A syndrome of lymphoblastic lymphoma, eosinophilia, and myeloid hyperplasia/malignancy associated with t(8;13)(p11;q11): description of a distinctive clinicopathologic entity. Blood. 1995 Apr 1;85(7):1881–7. PMID:7661940
1724. Inoue D, Yoshida K, Yoneda N, et al. IgG4-related disease: dataset of 235 consecutive patients. Medicine (Baltimore). 2015 Apr;94(15):e680. PMID:25881845
1725. International Association of Cancer Registries (IACR) [Internet]. Lyon (France): International Agency for Research on Cancer; 2021. International Classification of Diseases for Oncology (ICD-O) – ICD-O-3.2; updated 2021 Jan 25. Available from: http://www.iacr.com.fr/index.php?option=com_content&view=category&layout=blog&id=100&Itemid=577.
1726. International CLL-IPI working group. An international prognostic index for patients with chronic lymphocytic leukaemia (CLL-IPI): a meta-analysis of individual patient data. Lancet Oncol. 2016 Jun;17(6):779–90. PMID:27185642
1727. International Non-Hodgkin's Lymphoma Prognostic Factors Project. A predictive model for aggressive non-Hodgkin's lymphoma. N Engl J Med. 1993 Sep 30;329(14):987–94. PMID:8141877
1728. Inukai T, Hirose K, Inaba T, et al. Hypercalcemia in childhood acute lymphoblastic leukemia: frequent implication of parathyroid hormone-related peptide and E2A-HLF from translocation 17;19. Leukemia. 2007 Feb;21(2):288–96. PMID:17183364
1729. Inukai T, Kiyokawa N, Campana D, et al. Clinical significance of early T-cell precursor acute lymphoblastic leukaemia: results of the Tokyo Children's Cancer Study Group Study L99-15. Br J Haematol. 2012 Feb;156(3):358–65. PMID:22128890
1730. Ioannidis I, Kahn AG. Splenic lymphangioma. Arch Pathol Lab Med. 2015 Feb;139(2):278–82. PMID:25611113
1731. Ionescu P, Vibert F, Amé S, et al. New data on the epidemiology of breast implant-associated anaplastic large cell lymphoma. Eur J Breast Health. 2021 Oct 4;17(4):302–7. PMID:34651107
1732. Iqbal J, Greiner TC, Patel K, et al. Distinctive patterns of BCL6 molecular alterations and their functional consequences in different subgroups of diffuse large B-cell lymphoma. Leukemia. 2007 Nov;21(11):2332–43. PMID:17625604
1733. Iqbal J, Kucuk C, Deleeuw RJ, et al. Genomic analyses reveal global functional alterations that promote tumor growth and novel tumor suppressor genes in natural killer-cell malignancies. Leukemia. 2009 Jun;23(6):1139–51. PMID:19194464
1734. Iqbal J, Weisenburger DD, Chowdhury A, et al. Natural killer cell lymphoma shares strikingly similar molecular features with a group of non-hepatosplenic γδ T-cell lymphoma and is highly sensitive to a novel aurora kinase A inhibitor in vitro. Leukemia. 2011 Feb;25(2):348–58. PMID:21052088
1735. Iqbal J, Weisenburger DD, Greiner TC, et al. Molecular signatures to improve diagnosis in peripheral T-cell lymphoma and prognostication in angioimmunoblastic T-cell lymphoma. Blood. 2010 Feb 4;115(5):1026–36. PMID:19965671
1736. Iqbal J, Wright G, Wang C, et al. Gene expression signatures delineate biological and prognostic subgroups in peripheral T-cell lymphoma. Blood. 2014 May 8;123(19):2915–23. PMID:24632715
1737. Isaacson PG, Du MQ. Gastrointestinal lymphoma: where morphology meets molecular biology. J Pathol. 2005 Jan;205(2):255–74. PMID:15643667
1738. Isaacson PG, Matutes E, Burke M, et al. The histopathology of splenic lymphoma with villous lymphocytes. Blood. 1994 Dec 1;84(11):3828–34. PMID:7949139
1739. Ise M, Kageyama H, Araki A, et al. Identification of a novel GORASP2-ALK fusion in an ALK-positive large B-cell lymphoma. Leuk Lymphoma. 2019 Feb;60(2):493–7. PMID:30187817
1740. Ishibashi H, Nimura S, Kayashima Y, et al. Endoscopic and clinicopathological characteristics of gastrointestinal adult T-cell leukemia/lymphoma. J Gastrointest Oncol. 2019 Aug;10(4):723–33. PMID:31392053
1741. Ishibashi H, Nimura S, Kayashima Y, et al. Multiple lesions of gastrointestinal tract invasion by monomorphic epitheliotropic intestinal T-cell lymphoma, accompanied by duodenal and intestinal enteropathy-like lesions and microscopic lymphocytic proctocolitis: a case series. Diagn Pathol. 2016 Jul 25;11(1):66. PMID:27457239
1742. Ishida F, Ko YH, Kim WS, et al. Aggressive

natural killer cell leukemia: therapeutic potential of L-asparaginase and allogeneic hematopoietic stem cell transplantation. Cancer Sci. 2012 Jun;103(6):1079–83. PMID:22360679

1743. Ishiguro T, Takayanagi N, Katoh N, et al. Waldenström's macroglobulinemia accompanying systemic amyloidosis: the usefulness of endobronchial ultrasound-guided transbronchial needle aspiration for detecting amyloid deposits. Intern Med. 2014;53(24):2789–93. PMID:25500440

1744. Ishihara S, Ohshima K, Tokura Y, et al. Hypersensitivity to mosquito bites conceals clonal lymphoproliferation of Epstein-Barr viral DNA-positive natural killer cells. Jpn J Cancer Res. 1997 Jan;88(1):82–7. PMID:9045900

1745. Ishihara S, Okada S, Wakiguchi H, et al. Clonal lymphoproliferation following chronic active Epstein-Barr virus infection and hypersensitivity to mosquito bites. Am J Hematol. 1997 Apr;54(4):276–81. PMID:9092681

1746. Ishikawa Y, Terao C. Genetic analysis of IgG4-related disease. Mod Rheumatol. 2020 Jan;30(1):17–23. PMID:31104539

1747. Ishimura M, Eguchi K, Shiraishi A, et al. Systemic Epstein-Barr virus-positive T/NK lymphoproliferative diseases with SH2D1A/XIAP hypomorphic gene variants. Front Pediatr. 2019 May 21;7:183. PMID:31231620

1747A. Isobe Y, Aritaka N, Setoguchi Y, et al. T/NK cell type chronic active Epstein-Barr virus disease in adults: an underlying condition for Epstein-Barr virus-associated T/NK-cell lymphoma. J Clin Pathol. 2012 Mar;65(3):278–82. PMID:22247563

1748. Isomoto H, Maeda T, Akashi T, et al. Multiple lymphomatous polyposis of the colon originating from T-cells: a case report. Dig Liver Dis. 2004 Mar;36(3):218–21. PMID:15046193

1749. Isufi I, Seropian S, Gowda L, et al. Outcomes for allogeneic stem cell transplantation in refractory mycosis fungoides and primary cutaneous gamma delta T cell lymphomas. Leuk Lymphoma. 2020 Dec;61(12):2955–61. PMID:32643494

1750. Ito S, Iwanaga M, Nosaka K, et al. Epidemiology of adult T-cell leukemia-lymphoma in Japan: an updated analysis, 2012-2013. Cancer Sci. 2021 Oct;112(10):4346–54. PMID:34355480

1751. Ito Y, Kimura H, Maeda Y, et al. Pretreatment EBV-DNA copy number is predictive of response and toxicities to SMILE chemotherapy for extranodal NK/T-cell lymphoma, nasal type. Clin Cancer Res. 2012 Aug 1;18(15):4183–90. PMID:22675173

1752. Iwafuchi H. The histopathology of bone marrow failure in children. J Clin Exp Hematop. 2018;58(2):68–86. PMID:29998978

1753. Iwaki N, Fajgenbaum DC, Nabel CS, et al. Clinicopathologic analysis of TAFRO syndrome demonstrates a distinct subtype of HHV-8-negative multicentric Castleman disease. Am J Hematol. 2016 Feb;91(2):220–6. PMID:26805758

1754. Iwanaga M, Watanabe T, Yamaguchi K. Adult T-cell leukemia: a review of epidemiological evidence. Front Microbiol. 2012 Sep 10;3:322. PMID:22973265

1755. Iwatsuki K, Miyake T, Hirai Y, et al. Hydroa vacciniforme: a distinctive form of Epstein-Barr virus-associated T-cell lymphoproliferative disorders. Eur J Dermatol. 2019 Feb 1;29(1):21–8. PMID:30998212

1756. Izumi M, Mochizuki M, Kuroda M, et al. Angiomyoid proliferative lesion: an unusual stroma-rich variant of Castleman's disease of hyaline-vascular type. Virchows Arch. 2002 Oct;441(4):400–5. PMID:12404066

1757. Jabbour MN, Fedda FA, Tawil AN, et al. Follicular dendritic cell sarcoma of the head and neck expressing thyroid transcription factor-1: a case report with clinicopathologic and immunohistochemical literature review. Appl Immunohistochem Mol Morphol. 2014 Oct;22(9):705–12. PMID:21836499

1758. Jachimowicz RD, Pieper L, Reinke S, et al. Whole-slide image analysis of the tumor microenvironment identifies low B-cell content as a predictor of adverse outcome in patients with advanced-stage classical Hodgkin lymphoma treated with BEACOPP. Haematologica. 2021 Jun 1;106(6):1684–92. PMID:32381573

1759. Jacks T, Shih TS, Schmitt EM, et al. Tumour predisposition in mice heterozygous for a targeted mutation in Nf1. Nat Genet. 1994 Jul;7(3):353–61. PMID:7920653

1760. Jackson C, Sirohi B, Cunningham D, et al. Lymphocyte-predominant Hodgkin lymphoma–clinical features and treatment outcomes from a 30-year experience. Ann Oncol. 2010 Oct;21(10):2061–8. PMID:20332141

1761. Jaffe ES. Nasal and nasal-type T/NK cell lymphoma: a unique form of lymphoma associated with the Epstein-Barr virus. Histopathology. 1995 Dec;27(6):581–3. PMID:8838342

1762. Jaffe ES. Pathobiology of peripheral T-cell lymphomas. Hematology Am Soc Hematol Educ Program. 2006:317–22. PMID:17124078

1763. Jaffe ES, Ashar BS, Clemens MW, et al. Best practices guideline for the pathologic diagnosis of breast implant-associated anaplastic large-cell lymphoma. J Clin Oncol. 2020 Apr 1;38(10):1102–11. PMID:32045544

1764. Jaffe ES, Blattner WA, Blayney DW, et al. The pathologic spectrum of adult T-cell leukemia/lymphoma in the United States. Human T-cell leukemia/lymphoma virus-associated lymphoid malignancies. Am J Surg Pathol. 1984 Apr;8(4):263–75. PMID:6324600

1765. Jaffe ES, Chan JK, Su IJ, et al. Report of the workshop on nasal and related extranodal angiocentric T/natural killer cell lymphomas. Definitions, differential diagnosis, and epidemiology. Am J Surg Pathol. 1996 Jan;20(1):103–11. PMID:8540601

1766. Jaffe ES, Diebold J, Harris NL, et al. Burkitt's lymphoma: a single disease with multiple variants. The World Health Organization classification of neoplastic diseases of the hematopoietic and lymphoid tissues. Blood. 1999 Feb 1;93(3):1124. PMID:10025990

1767. Jäger U, Barcellini W, Broome CM, et al. Diagnosis and treatment of autoimmune hemolytic anemia in adults: recommendations from the First International Consensus Meeting. Blood Rev. 2020 May;41:100648. PMID:31839434

1768. Jahnke K, Coupland SE, Na IK, et al. Expression of the chemokine receptors CXCR4, CXCR5, and CCR7 in primary central nervous system lymphoma. Blood. 2005 Jul 1;106(1):384–5. PMID:15967804

1769. Jain AG, Chang CC, Ahmad S, et al. Leukemic non-nodal mantle cell lymphoma: diagnosis and treatment. Curr Treat Options Oncol. 2019 Nov 27;20(12):85. PMID:31776787

1770. Jain D, Dorwal P, Gajendra S, et al. CD5 positive hairy cell leukemia: a rare case report with brief review of literature. Cytometry B Clin Cytom. 2016 Sep;90(5):467–72. PMID:27129891

1771. Jain H, Sengar M, Goli VB, et al. Bortezomib and rituximab in de novo adolescent/adult CD20-positive, Ph-negative pre-B-cell acute lymphoblastic leukemia. Blood Adv. 2021 Sep 14;5(17):3436–44. PMID:34461632

1772. Jain N, Keating MJ. Richter transformation of CLL. Expert Rev Hematol. 2016 Aug;9(8):793–801. PMID:27351634

1773. Jain N, Lamb AV, O'Brien S, et al. Early T-cell precursor acute lymphoblastic leukemia/lymphoma (ETP-ALL/LBL) in adolescents and adults: a high-risk subtype. Blood. 2016 Apr 14;127(15):1863–9. PMID:26747249

1774. Jain N, Roberts KG, Jabbour E, et al. Ph-like acute lymphoblastic leukemia: a high-risk subtype in adults. Blood. 2017 Feb 2;129(5):572–81. PMID:27919910

1775. Jain P, Aoki E, Keating M, et al. Characteristics, outcomes, prognostic factors and treatment of patients with T-cell prolymphocytic leukemia (T-PLL). Ann Oncol. 2017 Jul 1;28(7):1554–9. PMID:28379307

1776. Jain P, Kanagal-Shamanna R, Zhang S, et al. Long-term outcomes and mutation profiling of patients with mantle cell lymphoma (MCL) who discontinued ibrutinib. Br J Haematol. 2018 Nov;183(4):578–87. PMID:30175400

1777. Jain S, Lone MR, Goswami A, et al. Lymphoma subtypes in India: a tertiary care center review. Clin Exp Med. 2021 May;21(2):315–21. PMID:33481141

1778. Jaiswal S, Ebert BL. Clonal hematopoiesis in human aging and disease. Science. 2019 Nov 1;366(6465):eaan4673. PMID:31672865

1779. Jakobczyk H, Jiang Y, Debaize L, et al. ETV6-RUNX1 and RUNX1 directly regulate RAG1 expression: one more step in the understanding of childhood B-cell acute lymphoblastic leukemia leukemogenesis. Leukemia. 2022 Feb;36(2):549–54. PMID:34535762

1780. Jallades L, Baseggio L, Sujobert P, et al. Exome sequencing identifies recurrent BCOR alterations and the absence of KLF2, TNFAIP3 and MYD88 mutations in splenic diffuse red pulp small B-cell lymphoma. Haematologica. 2017 Oct;102(10):1758–66. PMID:28751561

1781. Jamee M, Moniri S, Zaki-Dizaji M, et al. Clinical, immunological, and genetic features in patients with activated PI3Kδ syndrome (APDS): a systematic review. Clin Rev Allergy Immunol. 2020 Dec;59(3):323–33. PMID:31111319

1782. James E, Sokhn JG, Gibson JF, et al. CD4 + primary cutaneous small/medium-sized pleomorphic T-cell lymphoma: a retrospective case series and review of literature. Leuk Lymphoma. 2015 Apr;56(4):951–7. PMID:24996443

1783. James WD, Odom RB, Katzenstein AL. Cutaneous manifestations of lymphomatoid granulomatosis. Report of 44 cases and a review of the literature. Arch Dermatol. 1981 Apr;117(4):196–202. PMID:7212740

1784. Janssen JW, Ludwig WD, Sterry W, et al. SIL-TAL1 deletion in T-cell acute lymphoblastic leukemia. Leukemia. 1993 Aug;7(8):1204–10. PMID:8350619

1785. Jantunen E, Boumendil A, Finel H, et al. Autologous stem cell transplantation for enteropathy-associated T-cell lymphoma: a retrospective study by the EBMT. Blood. 2013 Mar 28;121(13):2529–32. PMID:23361910

1786. Jaramillo S, Agathangelidis A, Schneider C, et al. Prognostic impact of prevalent chronic lymphocytic leukemia stereotyped subsets: analysis within prospective clinical trials of the German CLL Study Group (GCLLSG). Haematologica. 2020 Nov 1;105(11):2598–607. PMID:33131249

1787. Jares P, Campo E, Pinyol M, et al. Expression of retinoblastoma gene product (pRb) in mantle cell lymphomas. Correlation with cyclin D1 (PRAD1/CCND1) mRNA levels and proliferative activity. Am J Pathol. 1996 May;148(5):1591–600. PMID:8623927

1788. Jares P, Colomer D, Campo E. Molecular pathogenesis of mantle cell lymphoma. J Clin Invest. 2012 Oct;122(10):3416–23. PMID:23023712

1789. Jarjour M, Jorquera A, Mondor I, et al. Fate mapping reveals origin and dynamics of lymph node follicular dendritic cells. J Exp Med. 2014 Jun 2;211(6):1109–22. PMID:24863064

1790. Jaso J, Chen L, Li S, et al. CD5-positive mucosa-associated lymphoid tissue (MALT) lymphoma: a clinicopathologic study of 14 cases. Hum Pathol. 2012 Sep;43(9):1436–43. PMID:22406370

1791. Jaso JM, Yin CC, Wang SA, et al. Clinicopathologic features of CD5-positive nodal marginal zone lymphoma. Am J Clin Pathol. 2013 Nov;140(5):693–700. PMID:24124149

1792. Jawed SI, Myskowski PL, Horwitz S, et al. Primary cutaneous T-cell lymphoma (mycosis fungoides and Sézary syndrome): part I. Diagnosis: clinical and histopathologic features and new molecular and biologic markers. J Am Acad Dermatol. 2014 Feb;70(2):205.e1–216. PMID:24438969

1793. Jegalian AG, Eberle FC, Pack SD, et al. Follicular lymphoma in situ: clinical implications and comparisons with partial involvement by follicular lymphoma. Blood. 2011 Sep 15;118(11):2976–84. PMID:21768298

1794. Jeha S, Choi J, Roberts KG, et al. Clinical significance of novel subtypes of acute lymphoblastic leukemia in the context of minimal residual disease-directed therapy. Blood Cancer Discov. 2021 Jul;2(4):326–37. PMID:34250504

1795. Jeha S, Pei D, Raimondi SC, et al. Increased risk for CNS relapse in pre-B cell leukemia with the t(1;19)/TCF3-PBX1. Leukemia. 2009 Aug;23(8):1406–9. PMID:19282835

1796. Jelinek T, Bezdekova R, Zatopkova M, et al. Current applications of multiparameter flow cytometry in plasma cell disorders. Blood Cancer J. 2018 Jan 19;8(1):e621. PMID:29351272

1797. Jeon YK, Kim JH, Sung JY, et al. Epstein-Barr virus-positive nodal T/NK-cell lymphoma: an analysis of 15 cases with distinct clinicopathological features. Hum Pathol. 2015 Jul;46(7):981–90. PMID:25907865

1798. Jerez A, Clemente MJ, Makishima H, et al. STAT3 mutations unify the pathogenesis of chronic lymphoproliferative disorders of NK cells and T-cell large granular lymphocyte leukemia. Blood. 2012 Oct 11;120(15):3048–57. PMID:22859607

1799. Jessen B, Maul-Pavicic A, Ufheil H, et al. Subtle differences in CTL cytotoxicity determine susceptibility to hemophagocytic lymphohistiocytosis in mice and humans with Chediak-Higashi syndrome. Blood. 2011 Oct 27;118(17):4620–9. PMID:21878672

1800. Jhala DN, Medeiros LJ, Lopez-Terrada D, et al. Neutrophil-rich anaplastic large cell lymphoma of T-cell lineage. A report of two cases arising in HIV-positive patients. Am J Clin Pathol. 2000 Sep;114(3):478–82. PMID:10989649

1801. Jhavar S, Agarwal JP, Naresh KN, et al. Primary extranodal mucosa associated lymphoid tissue (MALT) lymphoma of the prostate. Leuk Lymphoma. 2001 Apr;41(3-4):445–9. PMID:11378561

1802. Jhuang JY, Chang ST, Weng SF, et al. Extranodal natural killer/T-cell lymphoma, nasal type in Taiwan: a relatively higher frequency of T-cell lineage and poor survival for extranasal tumors. Hum Pathol. 2015 Feb;46(2):313–21. PMID:25554090

1803. Jiang L, Gu ZH, Yan ZX, et al. Exome sequencing identifies somatic mutations of DDX3X in natural killer/T-cell lymphoma. Nat Genet. 2015 Sep;47(9):1061–6. PMID:26192917

1804. Jiang XN, Yu BH, Wang WG, et al. Anaplastic lymphoma kinase-positive large B-cell lymphoma: clinico-pathological study of 17 cases with review of literature. PLoS One. 2017 Jun 30;12(6):e0178416. PMID:28665943

1805. Jiang XN, Zhang Y, Xue T, et al. New clinicopathologic scenarios of EBV+ inflammatory follicular dendritic cell sarcoma: report of 9 extrahepatosplenic cases. Am J Surg Pathol. 2021 Jun 1;45(6):765–72. PMID:33264138

1806. Jianlan X, Yuhua H, Yuanyuan Z, et al.

Acute Epstein-Barr virus-positive cytotoxic T cell lymphoid hyperplasia in the upper aerodigestive tract, mimicking extranodal natural killer/T cell lymphoma, nasal type. Virchows Arch. 2019 Feb;474(2):219–26. PMID:30488123
1807. Jiménez-Heffernan JA, Díaz Del Arco C, Adrados M. A cytological review of follicular dendritic cell-derived tumors with emphasis on follicular dendritic cell sarcoma and unicentric Castleman disease. Diagnostics (Basel). 2022 Feb 4;12(2):406. PMID:35204497
1808. Jin MK, Hoster E, Dreyling M, et al. Follicular dendritic cells in follicular lymphoma and types of non-Hodgkin lymphoma show reduced expression of CD23, CD35 and CD54 but no association with clinical outcome. Histopathology. 2011 Mar;58(4):586–92. PMID:21401698
1809. Jin Y, Hu H, Regmi P, et al. Treatment options for sclerosing angiomatoid nodular transformation of spleen. HPB (Oxford). 2020 Nov;22(11):1577–82. PMID:32063479
1810. Jo JC, Kim M, Choi Y, et al. Expression of programmed cell death 1 and programmed cell death ligand 1 in extranodal NK/T-cell lymphoma, nasal type. Ann Hematol. 2017 Jan;96(1):25–31. PMID:27696202
1811. Johansson J, Björnsson B, Ignatova S, et al. Littoral cell angioma in a patient with Crohn's disease. Case Rep Gastrointest Med. 2015;2015:474969. PMID:25705528
1812. Johnson AO, Stevens BP, Lam JT, et al. Two cases of rare subglottic MALT lymphoma of the larynx. Am J Otolaryngol. 2020 Nov-Dec;41(6):102736. PMID:33198051
1813. Johnson NA, Slack GW, Savage KJ, et al. Concurrent expression of MYC and BCL2 in diffuse large B-cell lymphoma treated with rituximab plus cyclophosphamide, doxorubicin, vincristine, and prednisone. J Clin Oncol. 2012 Oct 1;30(28):3452–9. PMID:22851565
1814. Johnson RC, Weinberg OK, Cascio MJ, et al. Cytogenetic variation of B-lymphoblastic leukemia with intrachromosomal amplification of chromosome 21 (iAMP21): a multi-institutional series review. Am J Clin Pathol. 2015 Jul;144(1):103–12. PMID:26071468
1815. Johnson SM, Umakanthan JM, Yuan J, et al. Lymphomas with pseudo-double-hit BCL6-MYC translocations due to t(3;8)(q27;q24) are associated with a germinal center immunophenotype, extranodal involvement, and frequent BCL2 translocations. Hum Pathol. 2018 Oct;80:192–200. PMID:29902576
1816. Johnston WT, Erdmann F, Newton R, et al. Childhood cancer: estimating regional and global incidence. Cancer Epidemiol. 2021 Apr;71 Pt B:101662. PMID:31924557
1817. Johnston WT, Mutalima N, Sun D, et al. Relationship between Plasmodium falciparum malaria prevalence, genetic diversity and endemic Burkitt lymphoma in Malawi. Sci Rep. 2014 Jan 17;4:3741. PMID:24434689
1818. Jöhrens K, Stein H, Anagnostopoulos I. T-bet transcription factor detection facilitates the diagnosis of minimal hairy cell leukemia infiltrates in bone marrow trephines. Am J Surg Pathol. 2007 Aug;31(8):1181–5. PMID:17667540
1819. Joly F, Cohen C, Javaugue V, et al. Randall-type monoclonal immunoglobulin deposition disease: novel insights from a nationwide cohort study. Blood. 2019 Feb 7;133(6):576–87. PMID:30578255
1820. Jondreville L, Krzisch D, Chapiro E, et al. The complex karyotype and chronic lymphocytic leukemia: prognostic value and diagnostic recommendations. Am J Hematol. 2020 Nov;95(11):1361–7. PMID:32777106
1821. Jones CL, Degasperi A, Grandi V, et al. Spectrum of mutational signatures in T-cell lymphoma reveals a key role for UV radiation in cutaneous T-cell lymphoma. Sci Rep. 2021 Feb 17;11(1):3962. PMID:33597573
1822. Jones D. Dismantling the germinal center: comparing the processes of transformation, regression, and fragmentation of the lymphoid follicle. Adv Anat Pathol. 2002 Mar;9(2):129–38. PMID:11917166
1823. Jones D, Amin M, Ordonez NG, et al. Reticulum cell sarcoma of lymph node with mixed dendritic and fibroblastic features. Mod Pathol. 2001 Oct;14(10):1059–67. PMID:11598178
1824. Jones D, Woyach JA, Zhao W, et al. PLCG2 C2 domain mutations co-occur with BTK and PLCG2 resistance mutations in chronic lymphocytic leukemia undergoing ibrutinib treatment. Leukemia. 2017 Jul;31(7):1645–7. PMID:28366935
1825. Jones JF, Shurin S, Abramowsky C, et al. T-cell lymphomas containing Epstein-Barr viral DNA in patients with chronic Epstein-Barr virus infections. N Engl J Med. 1988 Mar 24;318(12):733–41. PMID:2831453
1826. Joos S, Menz CK, Wrobel G, et al. Classical Hodgkin lymphoma is characterized by recurrent copy number gains of the short arm of chromosome 2. Blood. 2002 Feb 15;99(4):1381–7. PMID:11830490
1827. Jordan MB, Allen CE, Weitzman S, et al. How I treat hemophagocytic lymphohistiocytosis. Blood. 2011 Oct 13;118(15):4041–52. PMID:21828139
1828. Jordanova ES, Philippo K, Giphart MJ, et al. Mutations in the HLA class II genes leading to loss of expression of HLA-DR and HLA-DQ in diffuse large B-cell lymphoma. Immunogenetics. 2003 Jul;55(4):203–9. PMID:12756506
1829. Jordanova ES, Riemersma SA, Philippo K, et al. Beta2-microglobulin aberrations in diffuse large B-cell lymphoma of the testis and the central nervous system. Int J Cancer. 2003 Jan 20;103(3):393–8. PMID:12471623
1830. Jordanova ES, Riemersma SA, Philippo K, et al. Hemizygous deletions in the HLA region account for loss of heterozygosity in the majority of diffuse large B-cell lymphomas of the testis and the central nervous system. Genes Chromosomes Cancer. 2002 Sep;35(1):38–48. PMID:12203788
1831. Joyon N, Kanaan C, Cotteret S, et al. Multifocal in situ mantle cell neoplasia of the ileocecal region: a case report with simultaneous nodal and extranodal involvement. Virchows Arch. 2021 Nov;479(5):1037–40. PMID:33650040
1832. Ju JY, Stelow EB, Mahadevan MS, et al. Atypical lymphoid proliferations and clonality in Helicobacter-associated inflammatory infiltrates in children. Am J Surg Pathol. 2019 Oct;43(10):1361–7. PMID:31261290
1833. Juin Hsien BL, Shelat VG. Spleen angiosarcoma: a world review. Expert Rev Gastroenterol Hepatol. 2021 Oct;15(10):1115–41. PMID:34160346
1834. Juliusson G, Samuelsson H, Swedish Lymphoma Registry. Hairy cell leukemia: epidemiology, pharmacokinetics of cladribine, and long-term follow-up of subcutaneous therapy. Leuk Lymphoma. 2011 Jun;52 Suppl 2:46–9. PMID:21599605
1835. Jung JM, Lim DJ, Won CH, et al. Mycosis fungoides in children and adolescents: a systematic review. JAMA Dermatol. 2021 Apr 1;157(4):431–8. PMID:33656521
1836. Jung KS, Cho SH, Kim SJ, et al. Clinical features and treatment outcome of Epstein-Barr virus-positive nodal T-cell lymphoma. Int J Hematol. 2016 Nov;104(5):591–5. PMID:27456462
1837. Junlén HR, Peterson S, Kimby E, et al. Follicular lymphoma in Sweden: nationwide improved survival in the rituximab era, particularly in elderly women: a Swedish Lymphoma Registry study. Leukemia. 2015 Mar;29(3):668–76. PMID:25151959
1838. Jurinovic V, Kridel R, Staiger AM, et al. Clinicogenetic risk models predict early progression of follicular lymphoma after first-line immunochemotherapy. Blood. 2016 Aug 25;128(8):1112–20. PMID:27418643
1839. Juskevicius D, Dirnhofer S, Tzankov A. Genetic background and evolution of relapses in aggressive B-cell lymphomas. Haematologica. 2017 Jul;102(7):1139–49. PMID:28554945
1840. Juskevicius D, Lorber T, Gsponer J, et al. Distinct genetic evolution patterns of relapsing diffuse large B-cell lymphoma revealed by genome-wide copy number aberration and targeted sequencing analysis. Leukemia. 2016 Dec;30(12):2385–95. PMID:27198204
1841. Kaasinen E, Kuismin O, Rajamäki K, et al. Impact of constitutional TET2 haploinsufficiency on molecular and clinical phenotype in humans. Nat Commun. 2019 Mar 19;10(1):1252. PMID:30890702
1842. Kadin ME, Deva A, Xu H, et al. Biomarkers provide clues to early events in the pathogenesis of breast implant-associated anaplastic large cell lymphoma. Aesthet Surg J. 2016 Jul;36(7):773–81. PMID:26979456
1843. Kadin ME, Hamilton RG, Vonderheid EC. Evidence linking atopy and staphylococcal superantigens to the pathogenesis of lymphomatoid papulosis, a recurrent CD30+ cutaneous lymphoproliferative disorder. PLoS One. 2020 Feb 12;15(2):e0228751. PMID:32049976
1844. Kadin ME, Morgan J, Xu H, et al. IL-13 is produced by tumor cells in breast implant-associated anaplastic large cell lymphoma: implications for pathogenesis. Hum Pathol. 2018 Aug;78:54–62. PMID:29689246
1845. Kadin ME, Pinkus JL, Pinkus GS, et al. Primary cutaneous ALCL with phosphorylated/activated cytoplasmic ALK and novel phenotype: EMA/MUC1+, cutaneous lymphocyte antigen negative. Am J Surg Pathol. 2008 Sep;32(9):1421–6. PMID:18670345
1846. Kadin ME, Vonderheid EC, Weiss LM. Absence of Epstein-Barr viral RNA in lymphomatoid papulosis. J Pathol. 1993 Jun;170(2):145–8. PMID:8393923
1847. Kadri S, Lee J, Fitzpatrick C, et al. Clonal evolution underlying leukemia progression and Richter transformation in patients with ibrutinib-relapsed CLL. Blood Adv. 2017 May 2;1(12):715–27. PMID:29296715
1848. Kaffenberger B, Haverkos B, Tyler K, et al. Extranodal marginal zone lymphoma-like presentations of angioimmunoblastic T-cell lymphoma: a T-cell lymphoma masquerading as a B-cell lymphoproliferative disorder. Am J Dermatopathol. 2015 Aug;37(8):604–13. PMID:25839892
1849. Kagdi HH, Demontis MA, Fields PA, et al. Risk stratification of adult T-cell leukemia/lymphoma using immunophenotyping. Cancer Med. 2017 Jan;6(1):298–309. PMID:28035765
1850. Kaji D, Ota Y, Sato Y, et al. Primary human herpesvirus 8-negative effusion-based lymphoma: a large B-cell lymphoma with favorable prognosis. Blood Adv. 2020 Sep 22;4(18):4442–50. PMID:32936906
1851. Kaji S, Hiruta N, Sasai D, et al. Cytokeratin-positive interstitial reticulum cell (CIRC) tumor in the lymph node: a case report of the transformation from the epithelioid cell type to the spindle cell type. Diagn Pathol. 2020 Sep 26;15(1):121. PMID:32979929
1852. Kalisz K, Alessandrino F, Beck R, et al. An update on Burkitt lymphoma: a review of pathogenesis and multimodality imaging assessment of disease presentation, treatment response, and recurrence. Insights Imaging. 2019 May 21;10(1):56. PMID:31115699
1853. Kallemeijn MJ, de Ridder D, Schilperoord-Vermeulen J, et al. Dysregulated signaling, proliferation and apoptosis impact on the pathogenesis of TCRγδ+ T cell large granular lymphocyte leukemia. PLoS One. 2017 Apr 13;12(4):e0175670. PMID:28407008
1854. Kallinich T, Muche JM, Qin S, et al. Chemokine receptor expression on neoplastic and reactive T cells in the skin at different stages of mycosis fungoides. J Invest Dermatol. 2003 Nov;121(5):1045–52. PMID:14708605
1855. Kalpadakis C, Pangalis GA, Vassilakopoulos TP, et al. Detection of L265P MYD-88 mutation in a series of clonal B-cell lymphocytosis of marginal zone origin (CBL-MZ). Hematol Oncol. 2017 Dec;35(4):542–7. PMID:27734522
1856. Kamani NR, Kumar S, Hassebroek A, et al. Malignancies after hematopoietic cell transplantation for primary immune deficiencies: a report from the Center for International Blood and Marrow Transplant Research. Biol Blood Marrow Transplant. 2011 Dec;17(12):1783–9. PMID:21658461
1857. Kamijo H, Miyagaki T, Norimatsu Y, et al. Primary cutaneous γδ T-cell lymphoma with unusual immunophenotype: a case report and review of published work. J Dermatol. 2020 Mar;47(3):300–5. PMID:31912565
1858. Kamisawa T, Funata N, Hayashi Y, et al. A new clinicopathological entity of IgG4-related autoimmune disease. J Gastroenterol. 2003;38(10):982–4. PMID:14614606
1859. Kamisawa T, Nakazawa T, Tazuma S, et al. Clinical practice guidelines for IgG4-related sclerosing cholangitis. J Hepatobiliary Pancreat Sci. 2019 Jan;26(1):9–42. PMID:30575336
1860. Kampitak T. Fatal Kikuchi-Fujimoto disease associated with SLE and hemophagocytic syndrome: a case report. Clin Rheumatol. 2008 Aug;27(8):1073–5. PMID:18465190
1861. Kanagal-Shamanna R, Jain P, Patel KP, et al. Targeted multigene deep sequencing of Bruton tyrosine kinase inhibitor-resistant chronic lymphocytic leukemia with disease progression and Richter transformation. Cancer. 2019 Feb 15;125(4):559–74. PMID:30508305
1862. Kanagal-Shamanna R, Medeiros LJ, Lu G, et al. High-grade B cell lymphoma, unclassifiable, with blastoid features: an unusual morphological subgroup associated frequently with BCL2 and/or MYC gene rearrangements and a poor prognosis. Histopathology. 2012 Nov;61(5):945–54. PMID:22804688
1863. Kanagal-Shamanna R, Xu-Monette ZY, Miranda RN, et al. Crystal-storing histiocytosis: a clinicopathological study of 13 cases. Histopathology. 2016 Mar;68(4):482–91. PMID:26118455
1864. Kanakry JA, Hegde AM, Durand CM, et al. The clinical significance of EBV DNA in the plasma and peripheral blood mononuclear cells of patients with or without EBV diseases. Blood. 2016 Apr 21;127(16):2007–17. PMID:26744460
1865. Kanavaros P, Gaulard P, Charlotte F, et al. Discordant expression of immunoglobulin and its associated molecule mb-1/CD79a is frequently found in mediastinal large B cell lymphomas. Am J Pathol. 1995 Mar;146(3):735–41. PMID:7887454
1866. Kanavaros P, Lescs MC, Brière J, et al. Nasal T-cell lymphoma: a clinicopathologic entity associated with peculiar phenotype and with Epstein-Barr virus. Blood. 1993 May 15;81(10):2688–95. PMID:8387835
1867. Kandemir NO, Barut F, Ekinci T, et al. Intranodal palisaded myofibroblastoma (intranodal hemorrhagic spindle cell tumor with amianthoid fibers): a case report and literature review. Diagn Pathol. 2010 Feb 9;5:12. PMID:20181136
1868. Kanegane H, Bhatia K, Gutierrez M, et al. A syndrome of peripheral blood T-cell

infection with Epstein-Barr virus (EBV) followed by EBV-positive T-cell lymphoma. Blood. 1998 Mar 15;91(6):2085–91. PMID:9490694

1869. Kanellis G, Mollejo M, Montes-Moreno S, et al. Splenic diffuse red pulp small B-cell lymphoma: revision of a series of cases reveals characteristic clinico-pathological features. Haematologica. 2010 Jul;95(7):1122–9. PMID:20220064

1870. Kanellis G, Roncador G, Arribas A, et al. Identification of MNDA as a new marker for nodal marginal zone lymphoma. Leukemia. 2009 Oct;23(10):1847–57. PMID:19474799

1871. Kanemitsu N, Isobe Y, Masuda A, et al. Expression of Epstein-Barr virus-encoded proteins in extranodal NK/T-cell Lymphoma, nasal type (ENKL): differences in biologic and clinical behaviors of LMP1-positive and -negative ENKL. Clin Cancer Res. 2012 Apr 15;18(8):2164–72. PMID:22371452

1872. Kang H, Wilson CS, Harvey RC, et al. Gene expression profiles predictive of outcome and age in infant acute lymphoblastic leukemia: a Children's Oncology Group study. Blood. 2012 Feb 23;119(8):1872–81. PMID:22210879

1873. Kang J, Hong JY, Suh C. Clinical features and survival outcomes of patients with lymphoplasmacytic lymphoma, including non-IgM type, in Korea: a single-center experience. Blood Res. 2018 Sep;53(3):189–97. PMID:30310784

1874. Kang WY, Shen KN, Duan MH, et al. 14q32 translocations and 13q14 dclctions are common cytogenetic abnormalities in POEMS syndrome. Eur J Haematol. 2013 Dec;91(6):490–6. PMID:23957213

1875. Kanno H, Aozasa K. Mechanism for the development of pyothorax-associated lymphoma. Pathol Int. 1998 Sep;48(9):653–64. PMID:9778104

1876. Kanno H, Kojya S, Li T, et al. Low frequency of HLA-A*0201 allele in patients with Epstein-Barr virus-positive nasal lymphomas with polymorphic reticulosis morphology. Int J Cancer. 2000 Jul 15;87(2):195–9. PMID:10861473

1877. Kanno H, Naka N, Yasunaga Y, et al. Role of an immunosuppressive cytokine, interleukin-10, in the development of pyothorax-associated lymphoma. Leukemia. 1997 Apr;11 Suppl 3:525–6. PMID:9209445

1878. Kanno H, Nakatsuka S, Iuchi K, et al. Sequences of cytotoxic T-lymphocyte epitopes in the Epstein-Barr virus (EBV) nuclear antigen-3B gene in a Japanese population with or without EBV-positive lymphoid malignancies. Int J Cancer. 2000 Nov 15;88(4):626–32. PMID:11058881

1879. Kanno H, Ohsawa M, Hashimoto M, et al. HLA-A alleles of patients with pyothorax-associated lymphoma: anti-Epstein-Barr virus (EBV) host immune responses during the development of EBV latent antigen-positive lymphomas. Int J Cancer. 1999 Aug 27;82(5):630–4. PMID:10417757

1880. Kanno H, Yasunaga Y, Iuchi K, et al. Interleukin-6-mediated growth enhancement of cell lines derived from pyothorax-associated lymphoma. Lab Invest. 1996 Aug;75(2):167–73. PMID:8765317

1881. Kansal R, Nathwani BN, Yiakoumis X, et al. Exuberant cortical thymocyte proliferation mimicking T-lymphoblastic lymphoma within recurrent large inguinal lymph node masses of localized Castleman disease. Hum Pathol. 2015 Jul;46(7):1057–61. PMID:25953658

1882. Kanungo A, Medeiros LJ, Abruzzo LV, et al. Lymphoid neoplasms associated with concurrent t(14;18) and 8q24/c-MYC translocation generally have a poor prognosis. Mod Pathol. 2006 Jan;19(1):25–33. PMID:16258503

1883. Kanzler H, Küppers R, Hansmann ML, et al. Hodgkin and Reed-Sternberg cells in Hodgkin's disease represent the outgrowth of a dominant tumor clone derived from (crippled) germinal center B cells. J Exp Med. 1996 Oct 1;184(4):1495–505. PMID:8879220

1884. Kapatai G, Murray P. Contribution of the Epstein Barr virus to the molecular pathogenesis of Hodgkin lymphoma. J Clin Pathol. 2007 Dec;60(12):1342–9. PMID:18042690

1885. Kaplan JE, Osame M, Kubota H, et al. The risk of development of HTLV-I-associated myelopathy/tropical spastic paraparesis among persons infected with HTLV-I. J Acquir Immune Defic Syndr. 1988;19903(11):1096–101. PMID:2213510

1886. Karabulut YY, Kara T, Berkeşoğlu M. Intranodal palisaded myofibroblastoma - a rare case report and literature review. APMIS. 2016 Oct;124(10):905–10. PMID:27500890

1887. Karai LJ, Kadin ME, Hsi ED, et al. Chromosomal rearrangements of 6p25.3 define a new subtype of lymphomatoid papulosis. Am J Surg Pathol. 2013 Aug;37(8):1173–81. PMID:23648461

1888. Karam M, Novak L, Cyriac J, et al. Role of fluorine-18 fluoro-deoxyglucose positron emission tomography scan in the evaluation and follow-up of patients with low-grade lymphomas. Cancer. 2006 Jul 1;107(1):175–83. PMID:16721817

1889. Karim F, Loeffen J, Bramer W, et al. IgG4-related disease: a systematic review of this unrecognized disease in pediatrics. Pediatr Rheumatol Online J. 2016 Mar 25;14(1):18. PMID:27012661

1890. Karim Z, Saravana R, Shenjere P, et al. Fibroblastic reticulum cell tumor of spleen: a case report. Int J Surg Pathol. 2014 Aug;22(5):447–50. PMID:24220998

1891. Karligkiotis A, Contis D, Bella M, et al. Pediatric follicular dendritic cell sarcoma of the head and neck: a case report and review of the literature. Int J Pediatr Otorhinolaryngol. 2013 Jul;77(7):1059–64. PMID:23684177

1892. Karpate A, Barcena C, Hohl D, et al. Cutaneous presentation of hepatosplenic T-cell lymphoma-a potential mimicker of primary cutaneous gamma-delta T-cell lymphoma. Virchows Arch. 2016 Nov;469(5):591–6. PMID:27562705

1893. Karube K, Guo Y, Suzumiya J, et al. CD10-MUM1+ follicular lymphoma lacks BCL2 gene translocation and shows characteristic biologic and clinical features. Blood. 2007 Apr 1;109(7):3076–9. PMID:17138820

1894. Karube K, Nakagawa M, Tsuzuki S, et al. Identification of FOXO3 and PRDM1 as tumor-suppressor gene candidates in NK-cell neoplasms by genomic and functional analyses. Blood. 2011 Sep 22;118(12):3195–204. PMID:21690554

1895. Karube K, Ohshima K, Tsuchiya T, et al. A "floral" variant of nodal marginal zone lymphoma. Hum Pathol. 2005 Feb;36(2):202–6. PMID:15754298

1896. Karube K, Ohshima K, Tsuchiya T, et al. Expression of FoxP3, a key molecule in CD4CD25 regulatory T cells, in adult T-cell leukaemia/lymphoma cells. Br J Haematol. 2004 Jul;126(1):81–4. PMID:15198736

1897. Karube K, Scarfò L, Campo E, et al. Monoclonal B cell lymphocytosis and "in situ" lymphoma. Semin Cancer Biol. 2014 Feb;24:3–14. PMID:23999128

1898. Karube K, Suzumiya J, Okamoto M, et al. Adult T-cell lymphoma/leukemia with angioimmunoblastic T-cell lymphomalike features: report of 11 cases. Am J Surg Pathol. 2007 Feb;31(2):216–23. PMID:17255766

1899. Karube K, Takatori M, Sakihama S, et al. Clinicopathological features of adult T-cell leukemia/lymphoma with HTLV-1-infected Hodgkin and Reed-Sternberg-like cells. Blood Adv. 2021 Jan 12;5(1):198–206. PMID:33570645

1900. Karube K, Ying G, Tagawa H, et al. BCL6 gene amplification/3q27 gain is associated with unique clinicopathological characteristics among follicular lymphoma without BCL2 gene translocation. Mod Pathol. 2008 Aug;21(8):973–8. PMID:18500267

1901. Karvonen H, Perttilä R, Niininen W, et al. Wnt5a and ROR1 activate non-canonical Wnt signaling via RhoA in TCF3-PBX1 acute lymphoblastic leukemia and highlight new treatment strategies via Bcl-2 co-targeting. Oncogene. 2019 Apr;38(17):3288–300. PMID:30631148

1902. Kasahara Y, Yachie A, Takei K, et al. Differential cellular targets of Epstein-Barr virus (EBV) infection between acute EBV-associated hemophagocytic lymphohistiocytosis and chronic active EBV infection. Blood. 2001 Sep 15;98(6):1882–8. PMID:11535525

1903. Kasashima S, Kawashima A, Kasashima F, et al. Inflammatory features, including symptoms, increased serum interleukin-6, and C-reactive protein, in IgG4-related vascular diseases. Heart Vessels. 2018 Dec;33(12):1471–81. PMID:29931542

1904. Kasenda B, Schorb E, Fritsch K, et al. Prognosis after high-dose chemotherapy followed by autologous stem-cell transplantation as first-line treatment in primary CNS lymphoma–a long-term follow-up study. Ann Oncol. 2012 Oct;23(10):2670–5. PMID:22473593

1905. Kastenhuber ER, Lowe SW. Putting p53 in context. Cell. 2017 Sep 7;170(6):1062–78. PMID:28886379

1906. Kasuya A, Fujiyama T, Shirahama S, et al. Decreased expression of homeostatic chemokine receptors in intravascular large B-cell lymphoma. Eur J Dermatol. 2012 Mar-Apr;22(2):272–3. PMID:22381519

1907. Katano H, Sato Y, Itoh H, et al. Expression of human herpesvirus 8 (HHV-8)-encoded immediate early protein, open reading frame 50, in HHV-8-associated diseases. J Hum Virol. 2001 Mar-Apr;4(2):96–102. PMID:11437319

1908. Kataoka K, Iwanaga M, Yasunaga JI, et al. Prognostic relevance of integrated genetic profiling in adult T-cell leukemia/lymphoma. Blood. 2018 Jan 11;131(2):215–25. PMID:29084771

1909. Kataoka K, Miyoshi H, Sakata S, et al. Frequent structural variations involving programmed death ligands in Epstein-Barr virus-associated lymphomas. Leukemia. 2019 Jul;33(7):1687–99. PMID:30683910

1910. Kataoka K, Nagata Y, Kitanaka A, et al. Integrated molecular analysis of adult T cell leukemia/lymphoma. Nat Genet. 2015 Nov;47(11):1304–15. PMID:26437031

1911. Kataoka K, Ogawa S. Variegated RHOA mutations in human cancers. Exp Hematol. 2016 Dec;44(12):1123–9. PMID:27693615

1912. Kataoka K, Shiraishi Y, Takeda Y, et al. Aberrant PD-L1 expression through 3'-UTR disruption in multiple cancers. Nature. 2016 Jun 16;534(7607):402–6. PMID:27281199

1913. Kato I, Tajima K, Suchi T, et al. Chronic thyroiditis as a risk factor of B-cell lymphoma in the thyroid gland. Jpn J Cancer Res. 1985 Nov;76(11):1085–90. PMID:3936828

1914. Kato K, Ohshima K, Anzai K, et al. Elevated serum-soluble Fas ligand in histiocytic necrotizing lymphadenitis. Int J Hematol. 2001 Jan;73(1):84–6. PMID:11372760

1915. Kato K, Ohshima K, Ishihara S, et al. Elevated serum soluble Fas ligand in natural killer cell proliferative disorders. Br J Haematol. 1998 Dec;103(4):1164–6. PMID:9886336

1916. Kato S, Asano N, Miyata-Takata T, et al. T-cell receptor (TCR) phenotype of nodal Epstein-Barr virus (EBV)-positive cytotoxic T-cell lymphoma (CTL): a clinicopathologic study of 39 cases. Am J Surg Pathol. 2015 Apr;39(4):462–71. PMID:25634749

1917. Kato S, Takahashi E, Asano N, et al. Nodal cytotoxic molecule (CM)-positive Epstein-Barr virus (EBV)-associated peripheral T cell lymphoma (PTCL): a clinicopathological study of 26 cases. Histopathology. 2012 Aug;61(2):186–99. PMID:22690710

1918. Katsuya H, Ishitsuka K, Utsunomiya A, et al. Treatment and survival among 1594 patients with ATL. Blood. 2015 Dec 10;126(24):2570–7. PMID:26361794

1919. Katsuya H, Shimokawa M, Ishitsuka K, et al. Prognostic index for chronic- and smoldering-type adult T-cell leukemia-lymphoma. Blood. 2017 Jul 6;130(1):39–47. PMID:28515095

1920. Katsuya H, Yamanaka T, Ishitsuka K, et al. Prognostic index for acute- and lymphoma-type adult T-cell leukemia/lymphoma. J Clin Oncol. 2012 May 10;30(14):1635–40. PMID:22473153

1921. Katz RL. Modern approach to lymphoma diagnosis by fine-needle aspiration: restoring respect to a valuable procedure. Cancer. 2005 Dec 25;105(6):429–31. PMID:16222689

1922. Katzenberger T, Kalla J, Leich E, et al. A distinctive subtype of t(14;18)-negative nodal follicular non-Hodgkin lymphoma characterized by a predominantly diffuse growth pattern and deletions in the chromosomal region 1p36. Blood. 2009 Jan 29;113(5):1053–61. PMID:18978208

1923. Katzenberger T, Ott G, Klein T, et al. Cytogenetic alterations affecting BCL6 are predominantly found in follicular lymphomas grade 3B with a diffuse large B-cell component. Am J Pathol. 2004 Aug;165(2):481–90. PMID:15277222

1924. Katzenstein AL, Carrington CB, Liebow AA. Lymphomatoid granulomatosis: a clinicopathologic study of 152 cases. Cancer. 1979 Jan;43(1):360–73. PMID:761171

1925. Katzenstein AL, Doxtader E, Narendra S. Lymphomatoid granulomatosis: insights gained over 4 decades. Am J Surg Pathol. 2010 Dec;34(12):e35–48. PMID:21107080

1926. Kaufman AE, Patel K, Goyal K, et al. Mycosis fungoides: developments in incidence, treatment and survival. J Eur Acad Dermatol Venereol. 2020 Oct;34(10):2288–94. PMID:32141115

1927. Kaur R, Mehta J, Borges A. Extranodal follicular dendritic cell sarcoma-a review: "What the mind does not know the eye does not see". Adv Anat Pathol. 2021 Jan;28(1):21–9. PMID:32991350

1928. Kaur R, Mitra S, Rajwanshi A, et al. Fine needle aspiration cytology of IgG4-related disease: a potential diagnostic pitfall? Diagn Cytopathol. 2017 Jan;45(1):14–21. PMID:27666423

1929. Kawa K, Sawada A, Sato M, et al. Excellent outcome of allogeneic hematopoietic SCT with reduced-intensity conditioning for the treatment of chronic active EBV infection. Bone Marrow Transplant. 2011 Jan;46(1):77–83. PMID:20498651

1930. Kawada JI, Kamiya Y, Sawada A, et al. Viral DNA loads in various blood components of patients with Epstein-Barr virus-positive T-cell/natural killer cell lymphoproliferative diseases. J Infect Dis. 2019 Sep 13;220(8):1307–11. PMID:31240305

1931. Kawaguchi M, Kato H, Kito Y, et al. Imaging findings of primary immunoglobulin G4-related cervical lymphadenopathy. Neuroradiology. 2017 Nov;59(11):1111–9. PMID:28918513

1932. Kawa-Ha K, Ishihara S, Ninomiya T, et al. CD3-negative lymphoproliferative disease of granular lymphocytes containing Epstein-Barr viral DNA. J Clin Invest. 1989 Jul;84(1):51–5. PMID:2544630

1933. Kawamata N, Inagaki N, Mizumura S, et al. Methylation status analysis of cell cycle regulatory genes (p16INK4A, p15INK4B, p21Waf1/Cip1, p27Kip1 and p73) in natural killer cell disorders. Eur J Haematol. 2005 May;74(5):424–9. PMID:15813917

1934. Kawamoto K, Miyoshi H, Suzuki T, et al. A distinct subtype of Epstein-Barr virus-positive T/NK-cell lymphoproliferative disorder: adult patients with chronic active Epstein-Barr virus infection-like features. Haematologica. 2018 Jun;103(6):1018–28. PMID:29242302

1935. Kawamoto K, Miyoshi H, Suzuki T, et al. Frequent expression of CD30 in extranodal NK/T-cell lymphoma: potential therapeutic target for anti-CD30 antibody-based therapy. Hematol Oncol. 2018 Feb;36(1):166–73. PMID:29052238

1936. Kawamoto K, Miyoshi H, Yanagida E, et al. Comparison of clinicopathological characteristics between T-cell prolymphocytic leukemia and peripheral T-cell lymphoma, not otherwise specified. Eur J Haematol. 2017 May;98(5):459–66. PMID:28129454

1937. Kawamoto K, Nakamura S, Iwashita A, et al. Clinicopathological characteristics of primary gastric T-cell lymphoma. Histopathology. 2009 Dec;55(6):641–53. PMID:20002766

1938. Kaymaz Y, Oduor CI, Yu H, et al. Comprehensive transcriptome and mutational profiling of endemic Burkitt lymphoma reveals EBV type-specific differences. Mol Cancer Res. 2017 May;15(5):563–76. PMID:28465297

1939. Ke X, He H, Zhang Q, et al. Epstein-Barr virus-positive inflammatory follicular dendritic cell sarcoma presenting as a solitary colonic mass: two rare cases and a literature review. Histopathology. 2020 Nov;77(5):832–40. PMID:32506505

1940. Kebir S, Kuchelmeister K, Niehusmann P, et al. Intravascular CNS lymphoma: successful therapy using high-dose methotrexate-based polychemotherapy. Exp Hematol Oncol. 2012 Dec 5;1(1):37. PMID:23217063

1941. Kedra J, Seror R, Dieudé P, et al. Lymphoma complicating rheumatoid arthritis: results from a French case-control study. RMD Open. 2021 Sep;7(3):e001698. PMID:34470830

1942. Kelly GL, Long HM, Stylianou J, et al. An Epstein-Barr virus anti-apoptotic protein constitutively expressed in transformed cells and implicated in Burkitt lymphomagenesis: the Wp/BHRF1 link. PLoS Pathog. 2009 Mar;5(3):e1000341. PMID:19283066

1943. Kelly GL, Milner AE, Tierney RJ, et al. Epstein-Barr virus nuclear antigen 2 (EBNA2) gene deletion is consistently linked with EBNA3A, -3B, and -3C expression in Burkitt's lymphoma cells and with increased resistance to apoptosis. J Virol. 2005 Aug;79(16):10709–17. PMID:16051863

1944. Kelly LM, Pereira JP, Yi T, et al. EBI2 guides serial movements of activated B cells and ligand activity is detectable in lymphoid and nonlymphoid tissues. J Immunol. 2011 Sep 15;187(6):3026–32. PMID:21844396

1945. Kempf W. CD30+ lymphoproliferative disorders: histopathology, differential diagnosis, new variants, and simulators. J Cutan Pathol. 2006 Feb;33 Suppl 1:58–70. PMID:16412214

1946. Kempf W, Kadin ME, Dvorak AM, et al. Endogenous retroviral elements, but not exogenous retroviruses, are detected in CD30-positive lymphoproliferative disorders of the skin. Carcinogenesis. 2003 Feb;24(2):301–6. PMID:12584181

1947. Kempf W, Kadin ME, Kutzner H, et al. Lymphomatoid papulosis and human herpesviruses–a PCR-based evaluation for the presence of human herpesvirus 6, 7 and 8 related herpesviruses. J Cutan Pathol. 2001 Jan;28(1):29–33. PMID:11168749

1948. Kempf W, Kazakov DV, Baumgartner HP, et al. Follicular lymphomatoid papulosis revisited: a study of 11 cases, with new histopathological findings. J Am Acad Dermatol. 2013 May;68(5):809–16. PMID:23375516

1949. Kempf W, Kazakov DV, Buechner SA, et al. Primary cutaneous marginal zone lymphoma in children: a report of 3 cases and review of the literature. Am J Dermatopathol. 2014 Aug;36(8):661–6. PMID:24698939

1950. Kempf W, Kazakov DV, Cozzio A, et al. Primary cutaneous CD8(+) small- to medium-sized lymphoproliferative disorder in extrafacial sites: clinicopathologic features and concept on their classification. Am J Dermatopathol. 2013 Apr;35(2):159–66. PMID:22885550

1951. Kempf W, Kazakov DV, Mitteldorf C. Cutaneous lymphomas: an update. Part 2: B-cell lymphomas and related conditions. Am J Dermatopathol. 2014 Mar;36(3):197–208. PMID:24658377

1952. Kempf W, Kazakov DV, Schärer L, et al. Angioinvasive lymphomatoid papulosis: a new variant simulating aggressive lymphomas. Am J Surg Pathol. 2013 Jan;37(1):1–13. PMID:23026936

1953. Kempf W, Kerl K, Mitteldorf C. Cutaneous CD30-positive T-cell lymphoproliferative disorders-clinical and histopathologic features, differential diagnosis, and treatment. Semin Cutan Med Surg. 2018 Mar;37(1):24–9. PMID:29719017

1954. Kempf W, Levi E, Kamarashev J, et al. Fascin expression in CD30-positive cutaneous lymphoproliferative disorders. J Cutan Pathol. 2002 May;29(5):295–300. PMID:12100631

1955. Kempf W, Mitteldorf C. Cutaneous T-cell lymphomas-an update 2021. Hematol Oncol. 2021 Jun;39 Suppl 1:46–51. PMID:34105822

1956. Kempf W, Mitteldorf C, Battistella M, et al. Primary cutaneous peripheral T-cell lymphoma, not otherwise specified: results of a multicentre European Organization for Research and Treatment of Cancer (EORTC) cutaneous lymphoma taskforce study on the clinico-pathological and prognostic features. J Eur Acad Dermatol Venereol. 2021 Mar;35(3):658–68. PMID:32997839

1957. Kempf W, Ostheeren-Michaelis S, Paulli M, et al. Granulomatous mycosis fungoides and granulomatous slack skin: a multicenter study of the Cutaneous Lymphoma Histopathology Task Force Group of the European Organization For Research and Treatment of Cancer (EORTC). Arch Dermatol. 2008 Dec;144(12):1609–17. PMID:19075143

1958. Kempf W, Petrella T, Willemze R, et al. Clinical, histopathological and prognostic features of primary cutaneous acral CD8+ T-cell lymphoma and other dermal CD8+ cutaneous lymphoproliferations: results of an EORTC Cutaneous Lymphoma Group workshop. Br J Dermatol. 2022 May;186(5):887–97. PMID:34988968

1959. Kempf W, Pfaltz K, Vermeer MH, et al. EORTC, ISCL, and USCLC consensus recommendations for the treatment of primary cutaneous CD30-positive lymphoproliferative disorders: lymphomatoid papulosis and primary cutaneous anaplastic large-cell lymphoma. Blood. 2011 Oct 13;118(15):4024–35. PMID:21841159

1960. Kenderian SS, Habermann TM, Macon WR, et al. Large B-cell transformation in nodular lymphocyte-predominant Hodgkin lymphoma: 40-year experience from a single institution. Blood. 2016 Apr 21;127(16):1960–6. PMID:26837698

1961. Kennedy DE, Okoreeh MK, Maienschein-Cline M, et al. Novel specialized cell state and spatial compartments within the germinal center. Nat Immunol. 2020 Jun;21(6):660–70. PMID:32341509

1962. Kennedy R, Klein U. A T cell-B cell tumor-suppressive axis in the germinal center. Immunity. 2019 Aug 20;51(2):204–6. PMID:31433965

1963. Keto J, Hahtola S, Linna M, et al. Mycosis fungoides and Sézary syndrome: a population-wide study on prevalence and health care use in Finland in 1998-2016. BMC Health Serv Res. 2021 Feb 22;21(1):166. PMID:33618714

1964. Kezlarian B, Alhyari M, Venkataraman G, et al. GATA3 immunohistochemical staining in Hodgkin lymphoma: diagnostic utility in differentiating classic Hodgkin lymphoma from nodular lymphocyte predominant Hodgkin lymphoma and other mimicking entities. Appl Immunohistochem Mol Morphol. 2019 Mar;27(3):180–4. PMID:28877074

1965. Khalaf WF, Caldwell ME, Reddy N. Brentuximab in the treatment of CD30-positive enteropathy-associated T-cell lymphoma. J Natl Compr Canc Netw. 2013 Feb 1;11(2):137–40. PMID:23411380

1966. Khalidi HS, Chang KL, Medeiros LJ, et al. Acute lymphoblastic leukemia. Survey of immunophenotype, French-American-British classification, frequency of myeloid antigen expression, and karyotypic abnormalities in 210 pediatric and adult cases. Am J Clin Pathol. 1999 Apr;111(4):467–76. PMID:10191766

1967. Khalil MO, Morton LM, Devesa SS, et al. Incidence of marginal zone lymphoma in the United States, 2001-2009 with a focus on primary anatomic site. Br J Haematol. 2014 Apr;165(1):67–77. PMID:24417667

1968. Khamaysi Z, Ben-Arieh Y, Epelbaum R, et al. Pleomorphic CD8+ small/medium size cutaneous T-cell lymphoma. Am J Dermatopathol. 2006 Oct;28(5):434–7. PMID:17012921

1969. Khan J, Sykes DB. Case report: a 37-year-old male with telangiectasias, polycythemia vera, perinephric fluid collections, and intrapulmonary shunting. BMC Hematol. 2014 Jul 22;14(1):11. PMID:25143825

1970. Khanam T, Sandmann S, Seggewiss J, et al. Integrative genomic analysis of pediatric T-cell lymphoblastic lymphoma reveals candidates of clinical significance. Blood. 2021 Apr 29;137(17):2347–59. PMID:33152759

1971. Khanlari M, Li S, Miranda RN, et al. Small cell/lymphohistiocytic morphology is associated with peripheral blood involvement, CD8 positivity and retained T-cell antigens, but not outcome in adults with ALK+ anaplastic large cell lymphoma. Mod Pathol. 2022 Mar;35(3):412–8. PMID:34628481

1972. Khanlari M, Medeiros LJ, Lin P, et al. Blastoid high-grade B-cell lymphoma initially presenting in bone marrow: a diagnostic challenge. Mod Pathol. 2022 Mar;35(3):419–26. PMID:34608246

1973. Khanmohammadi S, Shabani M, Tabary M, et al. Lymphoma in the setting of autoimmune diseases: a review of association and mechanisms. Crit Rev Oncol Hematol. 2020 Jun;150:102945. PMID:32353704

1974. Kharazmi E, Fallah M, Pukkala E, et al. Risk of familial classical Hodgkin lymphoma by relationship, histology, age, and sex: a joint study from five Nordic countries. Blood. 2015 Oct 22;126(17):1990–5. PMID:26311361

1975. Khieu ML, Broadwater DR, Aden JK, et al. The utility of phosphohistone H3 (PHH3) in follicular lymphoma grading: a comparative study with Ki-67 and H&E mitotic count. Am J Clin Pathol. 2019 May 3;151(6):542–50. PMID:30788495

1976. Khogeer H, Rahman H, Jain N, et al. Early T precursor acute lymphoblastic leukaemia/lymphoma shows differential immunophenotypic characteristics including frequent CD33 expression and in vitro response to targeted CD33 therapy. Br J Haematol. 2019 Aug;186(4):538–48. PMID:31115909

1977. Khokhar FA, Payne WD, Talwalkar SS, et al. Angioimmunoblastic T-cell lymphoma in bone marrow: a morphologic and immunophenotypic study. Hum Pathol. 2010 Jan;41(1):79–87. PMID:19740519

1978. Khong PL, Huang B, Lee EY, et al. Midtreatment 18F-FDG PET/CT scan for early response assessment of SMILE therapy in natural killer/T-cell lymphoma: a prospective study from a single center. J Nucl Med. 2014 Jun;55(6):911–6. PMID:24819420

1979. Khong PL, Pang CB, Liang R, et al. Fluorine-18 fluorodeoxyglucose positron emission tomography in mature T-cell and natural killer cell malignancies. Ann Hematol. 2008 Aug;87(8):613–21. PMID:18509641

1980. Khoor A, Myers JL, Tazelaar HD, et al. Amyloid-like pulmonary nodules, including localized light-chain deposition: clinicopathologic analysis of three cases. Am J Clin Pathol. 2004 Feb;121(2):200–4. PMID:14983932

1981. Kiel MJ, Sahasrabuddhe AA, Rolland DCM, et al. Genomic analyses reveal recurrent mutations in epigenetic modifiers and the JAK-STAT pathway in Sézary syndrome. Nat Commun. 2015 Sep 29;6:8470. PMID:26415585

1982. Kiel MJ, Velusamy T, Rolland D, et al. Integrated genomic sequencing reveals mutational landscape of T-cell prolymphocytic leukemia. Blood. 2014 Aug 28;124(9):1460–72. PMID:24825865

1983. Kienle D, Kröber A, Katzenberger T, et al. VH mutation status and VDJ rearrangement structure in mantle cell lymphoma: correlation with genomic aberrations, clinical characteristics, and outcome. Blood. 2003 Oct 15;102(8):3003–9. PMID:12842981

1984. Kiesewetter B, Copie-Bergman C, Levy M, et al. Genetic characterization and clinical features of Helicobacter pylori negative gastric mucosa-associated lymphoid tissue lymphoma. Cancers (Basel). 2021 Jun 15;13(12):2993. PMID:34203889

1985. Kiesewetter B, Lamm W, Dolak W, et al. Transformed mucosa-associated lymphoid tissue lymphomas: a single institution retrospective study including polymerase chain reaction-based clonality analysis. Br J Haematol. 2019 Aug;186(3):448–59. PMID:31124124

1986. Kiesewetter B, Raderer M. How can we assess and measure prognosis for MALT lymphoma? A review of current findings and strategies. Expert Rev Hematol. 2021 Apr;14(4):391–9. PMID:33764848

1987. Kiessling MK, Oberholzer PA, Mondal C, et al. High-throughput mutation profiling of CTCL samples reveals KRAS and NRAS mutations sensitizing tumors toward inhibition of the RAS/RAF/MEK signaling cascade. Blood. 2011 Feb 24;117(8):2433–40. PMID:21209378

1988. Kiil K, Bein J, Schuhmacher B, et al. A high number of IgG4-positive plasma cells rules out nodular lymphocyte predominant Hodgkin lymphoma. Virchows Arch. 2018 Dec;473(6):759–64. PMID:30259184

1989. Kiiskilä J, Uotila P, Haapasaari KM, et al. Incidence and clinicopathological features of follicular T-cell lymphoma in Finland: a population-based immunohistochemical study. Hum Pathol. 2021 Nov;117:79–87. PMID:34364921

1990. Kikuchi M. Histiocytic necrotizing lymphadenitis (Kikuchi-Fujimoto disease) in Japan. Am J Surg Pathol. 1991;15(2):197–8.

1991. Kikuchi M. Lymphadenitis showing focal reticulum cells hyperplasia with nuclear debris and phagocytosis: a clinicopathological study. Nippon Ketsueki Gakkai Zasshi. 1972;35:379–80.

1992. Kikuta H, Sakiyama Y, Matsumoto S, et al. Fatal Epstein-Barr virus-associated hemophagocytic syndrome. Blood. 1993 Dec 1;82(11):3259–64. PMID:8241498

1993. Kilciksiz S, Celik OK, Pak Y, et al. Clinical and prognostic features of plasmacytomas: a multicenter study of Turkish Oncology Group-Sarcoma Working Party. Am J Hematol. 2008 Sep;83(9):702–7. PMID:18543343
1994. Kilciksiz S, Karakoyun-Celik O, Agaoglu FY, et al. A review for solitary plasmacytoma of bone and extramedullary plasmacytoma. ScientificWorldJournal. 2012;2012:895765. PMID:22654647
1995. Kilger E, Kieser A, Baumann M, et al. Epstein-Barr virus-mediated B-cell proliferation is dependent upon latent membrane protein 1, which simulates an activated CD40 receptor. EMBO J. 1998 Mar 16;17(6):1700–9. PMID:9501091
1996. Kim CH, Lim HW, Kim JR, et al. Unique gene expression program of human germinal center T helper cells. Blood. 2004 Oct 1;104(7):1952–60. PMID:15213097
1997. Kim DH, Medeiros LJ, Aung PP, et al. Mantle cell lymphoma involving skin: a clinicopathologic study of 37 cases. Am J Surg Pathol. 2019 Oct;43(10):1421–8. PMID:31219818
1998. Kim EK, Jang M, Yang WI, et al. Primary gastrointestinal T/NK cell lymphoma. Cancers (Basel). 2021 May 29;13(11):2679. PMID:34072328
1999. Kim H, Jeong H, Yamaguchi M, et al. Prediction and prevention of central nervous system relapse in patients with extranodal natural killer/T-cell lymphoma. Blood. 2020 Nov 26;136(22):2548–56. PMID:32584959
2000. Kim HJ, You E, Hong S, et al. A case of IgG4-related disease with bone marrow involvement: bone marrow findings and flow cytometric immunophenotyping of plasma cells. Ann Lab Med. 2021 Mar 1;41(2):243–6. PMID:33063688
2001. Kim JE, Lee EK, Lee JM, et al. Kikuchi-Fujimoto disease mimicking malignant lymphoma with 2-[(18)F]fluoro-2-deoxy-D-glucose PET/CT in children. Korean J Pediatr. 2014 May;57(5):226–31. PMID:25045365
2002. Kim JH, Kim YB, In SI, et al. The cutaneous lesions of Kikuchi's disease: a comprehensive analysis of 16 cases based on the clinicopathologic, immunohistochemical, and immunofluorescence studies with an emphasis on the differential diagnosis. Hum Pathol. 2010 Sep;41(9):1245–54. PMID:20434191
2003. Kim SJ, Choi CW, Mun YC, et al. Multicenter retrospective analysis of 581 patients with primary intestinal non-Hodgkin lymphoma from the Consortium for Improving Survival of Lymphoma (CISL). BMC Cancer. 2011 Jul 29;11:321. PMID:21798075
2004. Kim SJ, Choi JY, Hyun SH, et al. Risk stratification on the basis of Deauville score on PET-CT and the presence of Epstein-Barr virus DNA after completion of primary treatment for extranodal natural killer/T-cell lymphoma, nasal type: a multicentre, retrospective analysis. Lancet Haematol. 2015 Feb;2(2):e66–74. PMID:26687611
2005. Kim SJ, Lee SU, Kang MS, et al. IgG4-related disease presenting as recurrent scleritis combined with optic neuropathy. BMC Ophthalmol. 2021 Jan 5;21(1):5. PMID:33402162
2006. Kim SJ, Lim JQ, Laurensia Y, et al. Avelumab for the treatment of relapsed or refractory extranodal NK/T-cell lymphoma: an open-label phase 2 study. Blood. 2020 Dec 10;136(24):2754–63. PMID:32766875
2007. Kim SJ, Oh SY, Hong JY, et al. When do we need central nervous system prophylaxis in patients with extranodal NK/T-cell lymphoma, nasal type? Ann Oncol. 2010 May;21(5):1058–63. PMID:19850636
2008. Kim SJ, Yang DH, Kim JS, et al. Concurrent chemoradiotherapy followed by L-asparaginase-containing chemotherapy, VIDL, for localized nasal extranodal NK/T cell lymphoma: CISL08-01 phase II study. Ann Hematol. 2014 Nov;93(11):1895–901. PMID:24947798
2009. Kim SJ, Yoon DH, Jaccard A, et al. A prognostic index for natural killer cell lymphoma after non-anthracycline-based treatment: a multicentre, retrospective analysis. Lancet Oncol. 2016 Mar;17(3):389–400. PMID:26873565
2010. Kim TM, Lee SY, Jeon YK, et al. Clinical heterogeneity of extranodal NK/T-cell lymphoma, nasal type: a national survey of the Korean Cancer Study Group. Ann Oncol. 2008 Aug;19(8):1477–84. PMID:18385201
2011. Kim TY, Ha KS, Kim Y, et al. Characteristics of Kikuchi-Fujimoto disease in children compared with adults. Eur J Pediatr. 2014 Jan;173(1):111–6. PMID:23955486
2012. Kim WY, Kim H, Jeon YK, et al. Follicular dendritic cell sarcoma with immature T-cell proliferation. Hum Pathol. 2010 Jan;41(1):129–33. PMID:19740517
2013. Kim WY, Montes-Mojarro IA, Fend F, et al. Epstein-Barr virus-associated T and NK-cell lymphoproliferative diseases. Front Pediatr. 2019 Mar 15;7:71. PMID:30931288
2014. Kim WY, Nam SJ, Kim S, et al. Prognostic implications of CD30 expression in extranodal natural killer/T-cell lymphoma according to treatment modalities. Leuk Lymphoma. 2015 Jun;56(6):1778–86. PMID:25288491
2015. Kim YH, Willemze R, Pimpinelli N, et al. TNM classification system for primary cutaneous lymphomas other than mycosis fungoides and Sezary syndrome: a proposal of the International Society for Cutaneous Lymphomas (ISCL) and the Cutaneous Lymphoma Task Force of the European Organization of Research and Treatment of Cancer (EORTC). Blood. 2007 Jul 15;110(2):479–84. PMID:17339420
2016. Kimani SM, Painschab MS, Horner MJ, et al. Epidemiology of haematological malignancies in people living with HIV. Lancet HIV. 2020 Sep;7(9):e641–51. PMID:32791045
2017. Kimura H. EBV in T-/NK-cell tumorigenesis. Adv Exp Med Biol. 2018;1045:459–75. PMID:29896680
2018. Kimura H. Pathogenesis of chronic active Epstein-Barr virus infection: Is this an infectious disease, lymphoproliferative disorder, or immunodeficiency? Rev Med Virol. 2006 Jul-Aug;16(4):251–61. PMID:16791843
2019. Kimura H, Hoshino Y, Hara S, et al. Differences between T cell-type and natural killer cell-type chronic active Epstein-Barr virus infection. J Infect Dis. 2005 Feb 15;191(4):531–9. PMID:15655776
2020. Kimura H, Hoshino Y, Kanegane H, et al. Clinical and virologic characteristics of chronic active Epstein-Barr virus infection. Blood. 2001 Jul 15;98(2):280–6. PMID:11435294
2021. Kimura H, Ito Y, Kawabe S, et al. EBV-associated T/NK-cell lymphoproliferative diseases in nonimmunocompromised hosts: prospective analysis of 108 cases. Blood. 2012 Jan 19;119(3):673–86. PMID:22096243
2022. Kimura H, Morishima T, Kanegane H, et al. Prognostic factors for chronic active Epstein-Barr virus infection. J Infect Dis. 2003 Feb 15;187(4):527–33. PMID:12599068
2023. Kimura S, Mullighan CG. Molecular markers in ALL: clinical implications. Best Pract Res Clin Haematol. 2020 Sep;33(3):101193. PMID:33038982
2024. Kinch A, Baecklund E, Backlin C, et al. A population-based study of 135 lymphomas after solid organ transplantation: the role of Epstein-Barr virus, hepatitis C and diffuse large B-cell lymphoma subtype in clinical presentation and survival. Acta Oncol. 2014 May;53(5):669–79. PMID:24164103
2025. King RL, Dao LN, McPhail ED, et al. Morphologic features of ALK-negative anaplastic large cell lymphomas with DUSP22 rearrangements. Am J Surg Pathol. 2016 Jan;40(1):36–43. PMID:26379151
2026. King RL, Gonsalves WI, Ansell SM, et al. Lymphoplasmacytic lymphoma with a non-IgM paraprotein shows clinical and pathologic heterogeneity and may harbor MYD88 L265P mutations. Am J Clin Pathol. 2016 Jun;145(6):843–51. PMID:27329639
2027. King RL, Goodlad JR, Calaminici M, et al. Lymphomas arising in immune-privileged sites: insights into biology, diagnosis, and pathogenesis. Virchows Arch. 2020 May;476(5):647–65. PMID:31863183
2028. King RL, Gupta A, Kurtin PJ, et al. Chronic lymphocytic leukemia (CLL) with Reed-Sternberg-like cells vs Classic Hodgkin lymphoma transformation of CLL: Does this distinction matter? Blood Cancer J. 2022 Jan 28;12(1):18. PMID:35091549
2029. King RL, Khurana A, Mwangi R, et al. Clinicopathologic characteristics, treatment, and outcomes of post-transplant lymphoproliferative disorders: a single-institution experience using 2017 WHO diagnostic criteria. Hemasphere. 2021 Sep 6;5(10):e640. PMID:34514344
2030. King RL, McPhail ED, Meyer RG, et al. False-negative rates for MYC fluorescence in situ hybridization probes in B-cell neoplasms. Haematologica. 2019 Jun;104(6):e248–51. PMID:30523057
2031. Kinney MC, Collins RD, Greer JP, et al. A small-cell-predominant variant of primary Ki-1 (CD30)+ T-cell lymphoma. Am J Surg Pathol. 1993 Sep;17(9):859–68. PMID:8394652
2032. Kinoshita M, Izumoto S, Hashimoto N, et al. Immunohistochemical analysis of adhesion molecules and matrix metalloproteinases in malignant CNS lymphomas: a study comparing primary CNS malignant and CNS intravascular lymphomas. Brain Tumor Pathol. 2008;25(2):73–8. PMID:18987832
2033. Kipps TJ. The CD5 B cell. Adv Immunol. 1989;47:117–85. PMID:2479233
2034. Kirsch IR, Watanabe R, O'Malley JT, et al. TCR sequencing facilitates diagnosis and identifies mature T cells as the cell of origin in CTCL. Sci Transl Med. 2015 Oct 7;7(308):308ra158. PMID:26446955
2035. Kittai AS, Miller C, Goldstein D, et al. The impact of increasing karyotypic complexity and evolution on survival in patients with CLL treated with ibrutinib. Blood. 2021 Dec 9;138(23):2372–82. PMID:34314481
2036. Kiyokawa N, Iijima K, Tomita O, et al. Significance of CD66c expression in childhood acute lymphoblastic leukemia. Leuk Res. 2014 Jan;38(1):42–8. PMID:24231528
2037. Klairmont MM, Zhou Y, Cheng C, et al. Clinicopathologic and prognostic features of TdT-negative pediatric B-lymphoblastic leukemia. Mod Pathol. 2021 Nov;34(11):2050–4. PMID:34148065
2038. Klapper W, Hoster E, Determann O, et al. Ki-67 as a prognostic marker in mantle cell lymphoma-consensus guidelines of the pathology panel of the European MCL Network. J Hematop. 2009 Jul;2(2):103–11. PMID:19669190
2039. Klapper W, Hoster E, Rölver L, et al. Tumor sclerosis but not cell proliferation or malignancy grade is a prognostic marker in advanced-stage follicular lymphoma: the German Low Grade Lymphoma Study Group. J Clin Oncol. 2007 Aug 1;25(22):3330–6. PMID:17664481
2040. Klapper W, Kreuz M, Kohler CW, et al. Patient age at diagnosis is associated with the molecular characteristics of diffuse large B-cell lymphoma. Blood. 2012 Feb 23;119(8):1882–7. PMID:22238326
2041. Klapper W, Szczepanowski M, Burkhardt B, et al. Molecular profiling of pediatric mature B-cell lymphoma treated in population-based prospective clinical trials. Blood. 2008 Aug 15;112(4):1374–81. PMID:18509088
2042. Klein JL, Nguyen TT, Bien-Willner GA, et al. CD163 immunohistochemistry is superior to CD68 in predicting outcome in classical Hodgkin lymphoma. Am J Clin Pathol. 2014 Mar;141(3):381–7. PMID:24515766
2043. Klein U, Dalla-Favera R. Germinal centres: role in B-cell physiology and malignancy. Nat Rev Immunol. 2008 Jan;8(1):22–33. PMID:18097447
2044. Klein U, Heise N. Unexpected functions of nuclear factor-κB during germinal center B-cell development: implications for lymphomagenesis. Curr Opin Hematol. 2015 Jul;22(4):379–87. PMID:26049760
2045. Klein U, Lia M, Crespo M, et al. The DLEU2/miR-15a/16-1 cluster controls B cell proliferation and its deletion leads to chronic lymphocytic leukemia. Cancer Cell. 2010 Jan 19;17(1):28–40. PMID:20060366
2046. Kleinstern G, Camp NJ, Goldin LR, et al. Association of polygenic risk score with the risk of chronic lymphocytic leukemia and monoclonal B-cell lymphocytosis. Blood. 2018 Jun 7;131(23):2541–51. PMID:29674426
2047. Kleinstern G, Weinberg JB, Parikh SA, et al. Polygenic risk score and risk of monoclonal B-cell lymphocytosis in caucasians and risk of chronic lymphocytic leukemia (CLL) in African Americans. Leukemia. 2022 Jan;36(1):119–25. PMID:34285341
2048. Kleist B, Poetsch M, Schmoll J. Intranodal palisaded myofibroblastoma with overexpression of cyclin D1. Arch Pathol Lab Med. 2003 Aug;127(8):1040–3. PMID:12873184
2049. Klekawka T, Balwierz W, Brozyna A, et al. Nodular lymphocyte predominant Hodgkin lymphoma: experience of Polish Pediatric Leukemia/Lymphoma Study Group. Pediatr Hematol Oncol. 2021 Oct;38(7):609–19. PMID:33734010
2050. Klemke CD, Booken N, Weiss C, et al. Histopathological and immunophenotypical criteria for the diagnosis of Sézary syndrome in differentiation from other erythrodermic skin diseases: a European Organisation for Research and Treatment of Cancer (EORTC) Cutaneous Lymphoma Task Force Study of 97 cases. Br J Dermatol. 2015 Jul;173(1):93–105. PMID:25864856
2051. Klimm B, Goergen H, Fuchs M, et al. Impact of risk factors on outcomes in early-stage Hodgkin's lymphoma: an analysis of international staging definitions. Ann Oncol. 2013 Dec;24(12):3070–6. PMID:24148816
2052. Klintman J, Appleby N, Stamatopoulos B, et al. Genomic and transcriptomic correlates of Richter transformation in chronic lymphocytic leukemia. Blood. 2021 May 20;137(20):2800–16. PMID:33206936
2053. Klintman J, Barmpouti K, Knight SJL, et al. Clinical-grade validation of whole genome sequencing reveals robust detection of low-frequency variants and copy number alterations in CLL. Br J Haematol. 2018 Aug;182(3):412–7. PMID:29808933
2054. Klomjit N, Leung N, Fervenza F, et al. Rate and predictors of finding monoclonal gammopathy of renal significance (MGRS) lesions on kidney biopsy in patients with monoclonal gammopathy. J Am Soc Nephrol. 2020 Oct;31(10):2400–11. PMID:32747354
2055. Kluin PM, Langerak AW, Beverdam-Vincent J, et al. Paediatric nodal marginal zone B-cell lymphadenopathy of the neck: a Haemophilus influenzae-driven immune disorder? J Pathol. 2015 Jul;236(3):302–14. PMID:25722108

2056. Kluin-Nelemans HC, Coenen JL, Boers JE, et al. EBV-positive immunodeficiency lymphoma after alemtuzumab-CHOP therapy for peripheral T-cell lymphoma. Blood. 2008 Aug 15;112(4):1039–41. PMID:18502831
2057. Kluin-Nelemans HC, Krouwels MM, Jansen JH, et al. Hairy cell leukemia preferentially expresses the IgG3-subclass. Blood. 1990 Feb 15;75(4):972–5. PMID:2137355
2058. Kluk J, Kai A, Koch D, et al. Indolent CD8-positive lymphoid proliferation of acral sites: three further cases of a rare entity and an update on a unique patient. J Cutan Pathol. 2016 Feb;43(2):125–36. PMID:26423705
2059. Kluk MJ, Chapuy B, Sinha P, et al. Immunohistochemical detection of MYC-driven diffuse large B-cell lymphomas. PLoS One. 2012;7(4):e33813. PMID:22511926
2060. Knobel D, Zouhair A, Tsang RW, et al. Prognostic factors in solitary plasmacytoma of the bone: a multicenter Rare Cancer Network study. BMC Cancer. 2006 May 5;6:118. PMID:16677383
2061. Knowles DM, Cesarman E, Chadburn A, et al. Correlative morphologic and molecular genetic analysis demonstrates three distinct categories of posttransplantation lymphoproliferative disorders. Blood. 1995 Jan 15;85(2):552–65. PMID:7812011
2062. Knowles DM, Inghirami G, Ubriaco A, et al. Molecular genetic analysis of three AIDS-associated neoplasms of uncertain lineage demonstrates their B-cell derivation and the possible pathogenetic role of the Epstein-Barr virus. Blood. 1989 Feb 15;73(3):792–9. PMID:2537119
2063. Knowling MA, Harwood AR, Bergsagel DE. Comparison of extramedullary plasmacytomas with solitary and multiple plasma cell tumors of bone. J Clin Oncol. 1983 Apr;1(4):255–62. PMID:6668499
2064. Knuutila S, Alitalo R, Ruutu T. Power of the MAC (morphology-antibody-chromosomes) method in distinguishing reactive and clonal cells: report of a patient with acute lymphatic leukemia, eosinophilia, and t(5;14). Genes Chromosomes Cancer. 1993 Dec;8(4):219–23. PMID:7512364
2065. Ko BS, Chen LJ, Huang HH, et al. Epidemiology, treatment patterns and survival of chronic lymphocytic leukaemia/small lymphocytic lymphoma (CLL/SLL) in Taiwan, 2006-2015. Int J Clin Pract. 2021 Aug;75(8):e14258. PMID:33884738
2066. Ko M, An J, Pastor WA, et al. TET proteins and 5-methylcytosine oxidation in hematological cancers. Immunol Rev. 2015 Jan;263(1):6–21. PMID:25510268
2067. Ko YH, Karnan S, Kim KM, et al. Enteropathy-associated T-cell lymphoma–a clinicopathologic and array comparative genomic hybridization study. Hum Pathol. 2010 Sep;41(9):1231–7. PMID:20399483
2068. Ko YH, Park S, Kim K, et al. Aggressive natural killer cell leukemia: Is Epstein-Barr virus negativity an indicator of a favorable prognosis? Acta Haematol. 2008;120(4):199–206. PMID:19153474
2069. Kobayashi K, Mizuta S, Yamane N, et al. Paraneoplastic hypereosinophilic syndrome associated with IL3-IgH positive acute lymphoblastic leukemia. Pediatr Blood Cancer. 2019 Jan;66(1):e27449. PMID:30207070
2070. Kobayashi S, Nakano K, Watanabe E, et al. CADM1 expression and stepwise downregulation of CD7 are closely associated with clonal expansion of HTLV-I-infected cells in adult T-cell leukemia/lymphoma. Clin Cancer Res. 2014 Jun 1;20(11):2851–61. PMID:24727323
2071. Kobayashi Y, Kamitsuji Y, Kuroda J, et al. Comparison of human herpes virus 8 related primary effusion lymphoma with human herpes virus 8 unrelated primary effusion lymphoma-like lymphoma on the basis of HIV: report of 2 cases and review of 212 cases in the literature. Acta Haematol. 2007;117(3):132–44. PMID:17135726
2072. Koch K, Hoster E, Ziepert M, et al. Clinical, pathological and genetic features of follicular lymphoma grade 3A: a joint analysis of the German low-grade and high-grade lymphoma study groups GLSG and DSHNHL. Ann Oncol. 2016 Jul;27(7):1323–9. PMID:27117536
2073. Koch K, Richter J, Hanel C, et al. Follicular lymphoma grade 3B and diffuse large B-cell lymphoma present a histopathological and molecular continuum lacking features of progression/ transformation. Haematologica. 2022 Sep 1;107(9):2144–53. PMID:35021600
2074. Kodama K, Massone C, Chott A, et al. Primary cutaneous large B-cell lymphomas: clinicopathologic features, classification, and prognostic factors in a large series of patients. Blood. 2005 Oct 1;106(7):2491–7. PMID:15947086
2075. Kodama T, Ohshima K, Nomura K, et al. Lymphomatous polyposis of the gastrointestinal tract, including mantle cell lymphoma, follicular lymphoma and mucosa-associated lymphoid tissue lymphoma. Histopathology. 2005 Nov;47(5):467–78. PMID:16241994
2076. Koens L, Senff NJ, Vermeer MH, et al. Methotrexate-associated B-cell lymphoproliferative disorders presenting in the skin: a clinicopathologic and immunophenotypical study of 10 cases. Am J Surg Pathol. 2014 Jul;38(7):999–1006. PMID:24805861
2077. Koens L, Vermeer MH, Willemze R, et al. IgM expression on paraffin sections distinguishes primary cutaneous large B-cell lymphoma, leg type from primary cutaneous follicle center lymphoma. Am J Surg Pathol. 2010 Jul;34(7):1043–8. PMID:20551823
2078. Koens L, Zoutman WH, Ngarmlertsirichai P, et al. Nuclear factor-κB pathway-activating gene aberrancies in primary cutaneous large B-cell lymphoma, leg type. J Invest Dermatol. 2014 Jan;134(1):290–2. PMID:23863863
2079. Kofides A, Hunter ZR, Xu L, et al. Diagnostic next-generation sequencing frequently fails to detect MYD88L265P in Waldenström macroglobulinemia. Hemasphere. 2021 Jul 19;5(8):e624. PMID:34291197
2080. Kogawa R, Okumura Y, Watanabe I, et al. Difference between dormant conduction sites revealed by adenosine triphosphate provocation and unipolar pace-capture sites along the ablation line after pulmonary vein isolation. Int Heart J. 2016;57(1):25–9. PMID:26673441
2081. Kogure Y, Kameda T, Koya J, et al. Whole-genome landscape of adult T-cell leukemia/lymphoma. Blood. 2022 Feb 17;139(7):967–82. PMID:34695199
2082. Koh J, Jang I, Mun S, et al. Genetic profiles of subcutaneous panniculitis-like T-cell lymphoma and clinicopathological impact of HAVCR2 mutations. Blood Adv. 2021 Oct 26;5(20):3919–30. PMID:34535012
2083. Koh YW, Hwang HS, Park CS, et al. Prognostic effect of Ki-67 expression in rituximab, cyclophosphamide, doxorubicin, vincristine and prednisone-treated diffuse large B-cell lymphoma is limited to non-germinal center B-cell-like subtype in late-elderly patients. Leuk Lymphoma. 2015;56(9):2630–6. PMID:25573205
2084. Kohno K, Suzuki Y, Elsayed AA, et al. Immunohistochemical assessment of the diagnostic utility of PD-L1 (Clone SP142) for methotrexate-associated lymphoproliferative disorders with an emphasis of neoplastic PD-L1 (Clone SP142)-positive classic Hodgkin lymphoma type. Am J Clin Pathol. 2020 Apr 15;153(5):571–82. PMID:31977037
2085. Kojima M, Carreras J, Kikuti YY, et al. A case of diffuse large B-cell lymphoma with MYC gene cluster amplification related to chromothripsis. Leuk Lymphoma. 2018 Oct;59(10):2460–4. PMID:29345169
2086. Kojima M, Inagaki H, Motoori T, et al. Clinical implications of nodal marginal zone B-cell lymphoma among Japanese: study of 65 cases. Cancer Sci. 2007 Jan;98(1):44–9. PMID:17052258
2087. Kojima M, Motoori T, Asano S, et al. Histological diversity of reactive and atypical proliferative lymph node lesions in systemic lupus erythematosus patients. Pathol Res Pract. 2007;203(6):423–31. PMID:17540509
2088. Kojima M, Nakamura N, Shimizu K, et al. Histopathological variation of primary mucosa-associated lymphoid tissue lymphoma of the oral cavity. Pathol Oncol Res. 2007;13(4):345–9. PMID:18158571
2089. Kojima M, Nakamura S, Morishita Y, et al. Reactive follicular hyperplasia in the lymph node lesions from systemic lupus erythematosus patients: a clinicopathological and immunohistological study of 21 cases. Pathol Int. 2000 Apr;50(4):304–12. PMID:10849316
2090. Kojima M, Nakamura S, Oyama T, et al. Autoimmune disease-associated lymphadenopathy with histological appearance of T-zone dysplasia with hyperplastic follicles. A clinicopathological analysis of nine cases. Pathol Res Pract. 2001;197(4):237–44. PMID:11358009
2091. Kojima M, Nakamura S, Shimizu K, et al. Inflammatory pseudotumor of lymph nodes: clinicopathologic and immunohistological study of 11 Japanese cases. Int J Surg Pathol. 2001 Jul;9(3):207–14. PMID:11584317
2092. Kojima M, Sato E, Oshimi K, et al. Characteristics of CD5-positive splenic marginal zone lymphoma with leukemic manifestation; clinical, flow cytometry, and histopathological findings of 11 cases. J Clin Exp Hematop. 2010;50(2):107–12. PMID:21123968
2093. Koletsa T, Markou K, Ouzounidou S, et al. In situ mantle cell lymphoma in the nasopharynx. Head Neck. 2013 Nov;35(11):E333–7. PMID:23280758
2094. Kolhatkar NS, Brahmandam A, Thouvenel CD, et al. Altered BCR and TLR signals promote enhanced positive selection of autoreactive transitional B cells in Wiskott-Aldrich syndrome. J Exp Med. 2015 Sep 21;212(10):1663–77. PMID:26371186
2095. Komorowski L, Fidyt K, Patkowska E, et al. Philadelphia chromosome-positive leukemia in the lymphoid lineage-similarities and differences with the myeloid lineage and specific vulnerabilities. Int J Mol Sci. 2020 Aug 12;21(16):5776. PMID:32806528
2096. Kondo T, Kono H, Miyamoto N, et al. Age- and sex-specific cumulative rate and risk of ATLL for HTLV-I carriers. Int J Cancer. 1989 Jun 15;43(6):1061–4. PMID:2732000
2097. Kondratiev S, Duraisamy S, Unitt CL, et al. Aberrant expression of the dendritic cell marker TNFAIP2 by the malignant cells of Hodgkin lymphoma and primary mediastinal large B-cell lymphoma distinguishes these tumor types from morphologically and phenotypically similar lymphomas. Am J Surg Pathol. 2011 Oct;35(10):1531–9. PMID:21921781
2098. Kong E, Chun K, Hong Y, et al. 18F-FDG PET/CT findings in patients with Kikuchi disease. Nuklearmedizin. 2013;52(3):101–6. PMID:23681151
2099. Kong M, Wang Z, Teng X, et al. Hepatic carcinoma with indolent T-lymphoblastic proliferation (iT-LBP). Int J Clin Exp Pathol. 2018 Mar 1;11(3):1674–8. PMID:31938268
2100. Koning MT, Quinten E, Zoutman WH, et al. Acquired N-linked glycosylation motifs in B-cell receptors of primary cutaneous B-cell lymphoma and the normal B-cell repertoire. J Invest Dermatol. 2019 Oct;139(10):2195–203. PMID:31042459
2101. Konoplev S, Lu X, Konopleva M, et al. CRLF2-positive B-cell acute lymphoblastic leukemia in adult patients: a single-institution experience. Am J Clin Pathol. 2017 Apr 1;147(4):357–63. PMID:28340183
2102. Koo GC, Tan SY, Tang T, et al. Janus kinase 3-activating mutations identified in natural killer/T-cell lymphoma. Cancer Discov. 2012 Jul;2(7):591–7. PMID:22705984
2103. Koo M, Ohgami RS. Pediatric-type follicular lymphoma and pediatric nodal marginal zone lymphoma: recent clinical, morphologic, immunophenotypic, and genetic insights. Adv Anat Pathol. 2017 May;24(3):128–35. PMID:28277421
2104. Kooy-Winkelaar YM, Bouwer D, Janssen GM, et al. CD4 T-cell cytokines synergize to induce proliferation of malignant and nonmalignant innate intraepithelial lymphocytes. Proc Natl Acad Sci U S A. 2017 Feb 7;114(6):E980–9. PMID:28049849
2105. Korfel A, Schlegel U. Diagnosis and treatment of primary CNS lymphoma. Nat Rev Neurol. 2013 Jun;9(6):317–27. PMID:23670107
2106. Korona B, Korona D, Zhao W, et al. CCR6 activation links innate immune responses to mucosa-associated lymphoid tissue lymphoma development. Haematologica. 2022 Jun 1;107(6):1384–96. PMID:35142152
2107. Korona B, Korona D, Zhao W, et al. GPR34 activation potentially bridges lymphoepithelial lesions to genesis of salivary gland MALT lymphoma. Blood. 2022 Apr 7;139(14):2186–97. PMID:34086889
2108. Koskela HL, Eldfors S, Ellonen P, et al. Somatic STAT3 mutations in large granular lymphocytic leukemia. N Engl J Med. 2012 May 17;366(20):1905–13. PMID:22591296
2109. Kosmidis P, Bonzheim I, Dufke C, et al. Next generation sequencing of the clonal IGH rearrangement detects ongoing mutations and interfollicular trafficking in in situ follicular neoplasia. PLoS One. 2017 Jun 22;12(6):e0178503. PMID:28640838
2110. Koss MN, Hochholzer L, Langloss JM, et al. Lymphomatoid granulomatosis: a clinicopathologic study of 42 patients. Pathology. 1986 Jul;18(3):283–8. PMID:3785978
2111. Kotler E, Segal E, Oren M. Functional characterization of the p53 "mutome". Mol Cell Oncol. 2018 Sep 25;5(6):e1511207. PMID:30525089
2112. Kotlyar DS, Osterman MT, Diamond RH, et al. A systematic review of factors that contribute to hepatosplenic T-cell lymphoma in patients with inflammatory bowel disease. Clin Gastroenterol Hepatol. 2011 Jan;9(1):36–41.e1. PMID:20888436
2113. Kotrova M, Novakova M, Oberbeck S, et al. Next-generation amplicon TRB locus sequencing can overcome limitations of flow-cytometric Vβ expression analysis and confirms clonality in all T-cell prolymphocytic leukemia cases. Cytometry A. 2018 Nov;93(11):1118–24. PMID:30414304
2114. Koulis A, Trivedi P, Ibrahim H, et al. The role of the microenvironment in human immunodeficiency virus-associated classical Hodgkin lymphoma. Histopathology. 2014 Dec;65(6):749–56. PMID:24809535
2115. Kourelis TV, Buadi FK, Kumar SK, et al. Long-term outcome of patients with POEMS syndrome: an update of the Mayo Clinic experience. Am J Hematol. 2016 Jun;91(6):585–9. PMID:26972803
2116. Kourelis TV, Nasr SH, Dispenzieri A, et al. Outcomes of patients with renal monoclonal immunoglobulin deposition disease. Am J Hematol. 2016 Nov;91(11):1123–8.

PMID:27501122
2117. Koutros S, Harris SA, Spinelli JJ, et al. Non-Hodgkin lymphoma risk and organophosphate and carbamate insecticide use in the north American pooled project. Environ Int. 2019 Jun;127:199–205. PMID:30928843
2118. Kovalchuk AL, Ansarah-Sobrinho C, Hakim O, et al. Mouse model of endemic Burkitt translocations reveals the long-range boundaries of Ig-mediated oncogene deregulation. Proc Natl Acad Sci U S A. 2012 Jul 3;109(27):10972–7. PMID:22711821
2119. Kraus TS, Sillings CN, Saxe DF, et al. The role of CD11c expression in the diagnosis of mantle cell lymphoma. Am J Clin Pathol. 2010 Aug;134(2):271–7. PMID:20660331
2120. Krautler NJ, Kana V, Kranich J, et al. Follicular dendritic cells emerge from ubiquitous perivascular precursors. Cell. 2012 Jul 6;150(1):194–206. PMID:22770220
2121. Kreft A, Weber A, Springer E, et al. Bone marrow findings in multicentric Castleman disease in HIV-negative patients. Am J Surg Pathol. 2007 Mar;31(3):398–402. PMID:17325481
2122. Kreitman RJ, Arons E. Diagnosis and treatment of hairy cell leukemia as the COVID-19 pandemic continues. Blood Rev. 2022 Jan;51:100888. PMID:34535326
2123. Kreitman RJ, Dearden C, Zinzani PL, et al. Moxetumomab pasudotox in heavily pretreated patients with relapsed/refractory hairy cell leukemia (HCL): long-term follow-up from the pivotal trial. J Hematol Oncol. 2021 Feb 24;14(1):35. PMID:33627164
2124. Krejsgaard T, Lindahl LM, Mongan NP, et al. Malignant inflammation in cutaneous T-cell lymphoma-a hostile takeover. Semin Immunopathol. 2017 Apr;39(3):269–82. PMID:27717961
2125. Kremer M, Ott G, Nathrath M, et al. Primary extramedullary plasmacytoma and multiple myeloma: phenotypic differences revealed by immunohistochemical analysis. J Pathol. 2005 Jan;205(1):92–101. PMID:15586381
2126. Kretzmer H, Biran A, Purroy N, et al. Preneoplastic alterations define CLL DNA methylome and persist through disease progression and therapy. Blood Cancer Discov. 2021 Jan;2(1):54–69. PMID:33604581
2127. Kridel R, Chan FC, Mottok A, et al. Histological transformation and progression in follicular lymphoma: a clonal evolution study. PLoS Med. 2016 Dec 13;13(12):e1002197. PMID:27959929
2128. Kridel R, Mottok A, Farinha P, et al. Cell of origin of transformed follicular lymphoma. Blood. 2015 Oct 29;126(18):2118–27. PMID:26307535
2129. Kriekard P, Garcia JA, Nardi-Korver L, et al. Tumor melt: primary effusion lymphoma of the heart. Am J Med. 2012 Sep;125(9):e5–6. PMID:22682793
2130. Krijgsman O, Gonzalez P, Ponz OB, et al. Dissecting the gray zone between follicular lymphoma and marginal zone lymphoma using morphological and genetic features. Haematologica. 2013 Dec;98(12):1921–9. PMID:23850804
2131. Krishnan C, Warnke RA, Arber DA, et al. PD-1 expression in T-cell lymphomas and reactive lymphoid entities: potential overlap in staining patterns between lymphoma and viral lymphadenitis. Am J Surg Pathol. 2010 Feb;34(2):178–89. PMID:20087161
2132. Krishnan R, Ring K, Williams E, et al. An enteropathy-like indolent NK-cell proliferation presenting in the female genital tract. Am J Surg Pathol. 2020 Apr;44(4):561–5. PMID:31609783
2133. Kroft SH. Stratification of follicular lymphoma: time for a paradigm shift? Am J Clin Pathol. 2019 May 3;151(6):539–41. PMID:30918966
2134. Kroft SH, Sever CE, Bagg A, et al. Laboratory workup of lymphoma in adults. Am J Clin Pathol. 2021 Jan 4;155(1):12–37. PMID:33219376
2135. Krull JE, Wenzl K, Hartert KT, et al. Somatic copy number gains in MYC, BCL2, and BCL6 identifies a subset of aggressive alternative-DH/TH DLBCL patients. Blood Cancer J. 2020 Nov 9;10(11):117. PMID:33168821
2136. Kubota M, Tsukamoto R, Kurokawa K, et al. Elevated serum interferon gamma and interleukin-6 in patients with necrotizing lymphadenitis (Kikuchi's disease). Br J Haematol. 1996 Dec;95(4):613–5. PMID:8982035
2137. Kubota T, Sasaki Y, Shiozawa E, et al. Age and CD20 expression are significant prognostic factors in human herpes virus-8-negative effusion-based lymphoma. Am J Surg Pathol. 2018 Dec;42(12):1607–16. PMID:30273194
2138. Kubota Y, Kusaba K. Monomorphic epitheliotropic intestinal T-cell lymphoma involving the central nervous system. Blood. 2018 Apr 12;131(15):1765. PMID:29650734
2139. Küçük C, Hu X, Jiang B, et al. Global promoter methylation analysis reveals novel candidate tumor suppressor genes in natural killer cell lymphoma. Clin Cancer Res. 2015 Apr 1;21(7):1699–711. PMID:25614448
2140. Küçük C, Iqbal J, Hu X, et al. PRDM1 is a tumor suppressor gene in natural killer cell malignancies. Proc Natl Acad Sci U S A. 2011 Dec 13;108(50):20119–24. PMID:22143801
2141. Küçük C, Jiang B, Hu X, et al. Activating mutations of STAT5B and STAT3 in lymphomas derived from γδ-T or NK cells. Nat Commun. 2015 Jan 14;6:6025. PMID:25586472
2142. Kuehl WM, Bergsagel PL. Molecular pathogenesis of multiple myeloma and its premalignant precursor. J Clin Invest. 2012 Oct;122(10):3456–63. PMID:23023717
2143. Kuiper R, Broyl A, de Knegt Y, et al. A gene expression signature for high-risk multiple myeloma. Leukemia. 2012 Nov;26(11):2406–13. PMID:22722715
2144. Küker W, Nägele T, Korfel A, et al. Primary central nervous system lymphomas (PCNSL): MRI features at presentation in 100 patients. J Neurooncol. 2005 Apr;72(2):169–77. PMID:15925998
2145. Kulis M, Heath S, Bibikova M, et al. Epigenomic analysis detects widespread gene-body DNA hypomethylation in chronic lymphocytic leukemia. Nat Genet. 2012 Nov;44(11):1236–42. PMID:23064414
2146. Kulis M, Merkel A, Heath S, et al. Whole-genome fingerprint of the DNA methylome during human B cell differentiation. Nat Genet. 2015 Jul;47(7):746–56. PMID:26053498
2147. Kulkarni GB, Mahadevan A, Taly AB, et al. Clinicopathological profile of polyneuropathy, organomegaly, endocrinopathy, M protein and skin changes (POEMS) syndrome. J Clin Neurosci. 2011 Mar;18(3):356–60. PMID:21256753
2148. Kumánovics A, Perkins SL, Gilbert H, et al. Diffuse large B cell lymphoma in hyper-IgE syndrome due to STAT3 mutation. J Clin Immunol. 2010 Nov;30(6):886–93. PMID:20859667
2149. Kumar E, Pickard L, Okosun J. Pathogenesis of follicular lymphoma: genetics to the microenvironment to clinical translation. Br J Haematol. 2021 Sep;194(5):810–21. PMID:33694181
2149A. Kumar S, Dispenzieri A, Lacy MQ, et al. Revised prognostic staging system for light chain amyloidosis incorporating cardiac biomarkers and serum free light chain measurements. J Clin Oncol. 2012 Mar 20;30(9):989–95. PMID:22331953
2150. Kumar S, Kaufman JL, Gasparetto C, et al. Efficacy of venetoclax as targeted therapy for relapsed/refractory t(11;14) multiple myeloma. Blood. 2017 Nov 30;130(22):2401–9. PMID:29018077
2151. Kumar SK, Callander NS, Adekola K, et al. Multiple myeloma, Version 3.2021, NCCN Clinical Practice Guidelines in Oncology. J Natl Compr Canc Netw. 2020 Dec 2;18(12):1685–717. PMID:33285522
2152. Kumar SK, Gertz MA, Dispenzieri A. Validation of Mayo Clinic staging system for light chain amyloidosis with high-sensitivity troponin. J Clin Oncol. 2019 Jan 10;37(2):171–3. PMID:30433848
2153. Kumar SK, Rajkumar SV. The multiple myelomas - current concepts in cytogenetic classification and therapy. Nat Rev Clin Oncol. 2018 Jul;15(7):409–21. PMID:29686421
2154. Kummer JA, Vermeer MH, Dukers D, et al. Most primary cutaneous CD30-positive lymphoproliferative disorders have a CD4-positive cytotoxic T-cell phenotype. J Invest Dermatol. 1997 Nov;109(5):636–40. PMID:9347791
2155. Kunder C, Cascio MJ, Bakke A, et al. Predominance of CD4+ T cells in T-cell/histiocyte-rich large B-cell lymphoma and identification of a subset of patients with peripheral B-cell lymphopenia. Am J Clin Pathol. 2017 Jun 1;147(6):596–603. PMID:28575178
2156. Kuo SH, Tsai HJ, Lin CW, et al. The B-cell-activating factor signalling pathway is associated with Helicobacter pylori independence in gastric mucosa-associated lymphoid tissue lymphoma without t(11;18)(q21;q21). J Pathol. 2017 Feb;241(3):420–33. PMID:27873317
2157. Kuo TT. Kikuchi's disease (histiocytic necrotizing lymphadenitis). A clinicopathologic study of 79 cases with an analysis of histologic subtypes, immunohistology, and DNA ploidy. Am J Surg Pathol. 1995 Jul;19(7):798–809. PMID:7793478
2158. Kuo TT, Chen MJ, Kuo MC. Cutaneous intravascular NK-cell lymphoma: report of a rare variant associated with Epstein-Barr virus. Am J Surg Pathol. 2006 Sep;30(9):1197–201. PMID:16931967
2159. Küppers R, Rajewsky K, Zhao M, et al. Hodgkin disease: Hodgkin and Reed-Sternberg cells picked from histological sections show clonal immunoglobulin gene rearrangements and appear to be derived from B cells at various stages of development. Proc Natl Acad Sci U S A. 1994 Nov 8;91(23):10962–6. PMID:7971992
2160. Kurita D, Miyoshi H, Ichikawa A, et al. Methotrexate-associated lymphoproliferative disorders in patients with rheumatoid arthritis: clinicopathologic features and prognostic factors. Am J Surg Pathol. 2019 Jul;43(7):869–84. PMID:31116708
2161. Kurita D, Miyoshi H, Yoshida N, et al. A clinicopathologic study of Lennert lymphoma and possible prognostic factors: the importance of follicular helper T-cell markers and the association with angioimmunoblastic T-cell lymphoma. Am J Surg Pathol. 2016 Sep;40(9):1249–60. PMID:27428734
2162. Kurt H, Jorgensen JL, Amin HM, et al. Chronic lymphoproliferative disorder of NK-cells: a single-institution review with emphasis on relative utility of multimodality diagnostic tools. Eur J Haematol. 2018 May;100(5):444–54. PMID:29385279
2163. Kurtin PJ, Myers JL, Adlakha H, et al. Pathologic and clinical features of primary pulmonary extranodal marginal zone B-cell lymphoma of MALT type. Am J Surg Pathol. 2001 Aug;25(8):997–1008. PMID:11474283
2164. Kussick SJ, Kalnoski M, Braziel RM, et al. Prominent clonal B-cell populations identified by flow cytometry in histologically reactive lymphoid proliferations. Am J Clin Pathol. 2004 Apr;121(4):464–72. PMID:15080297
2165. Kutok JL, Pinkus GS, Dorfman DM, et al. Inflammatory pseudotumor of lymph node and spleen: an entity biologically distinct from inflammatory myofibroblastic tumor. Hum Pathol. 2001 Dec;32(12):1382–7. PMID:11774173
2166. Kütting B, Bonsmann G, Metze D, et al. Borrelia burgdorferi-associated primary cutaneous B cell lymphoma: complete clearing of skin lesions after antibiotic pulse therapy or intralesional injection of interferon alfa-2a. J Am Acad Dermatol. 1997 Feb;36(2 Pt 2):311–4. PMID:9039207
2167. Kutzner H, Kerl H, Pfaltz MC, et al. CD123-positive plasmacytoid dendritic cells in primary cutaneous marginal zone B-cell lymphoma: diagnostic and pathogenetic implications. Am J Surg Pathol. 2009 Sep;33(9):1307–13. PMID:19718787
2168. Kuybulu A, Sipahi T, Topal I, et al. Splenic angiomatoid nodular transformation in a child with increased erythrocyte sedimentation rate. Pediatr Hematol Oncol. 2009 Oct-Nov;26(7):533–7. PMID:19863210
2169. Kwok M, Korde N, Landgren O. Bortezomib to treat the TEMPI syndrome. N Engl J Med. 2012 May 10;366(19):1843–5. PMID:22571216
2170. Kwong YL. Natural killer-cell malignancies: diagnosis and treatment. Leukemia. 2005 Dec;19(12):2186–94. PMID:16179910
2171. Kwong YL, Au WY, Leung AY, et al. T-cell large granular lymphocyte leukemia: an Asian perspective. Ann Hematol. 2010 Apr;89(4):331–9. PMID:20084380
2172. Kwong YL, Chan AC, Liang RH. Natural killer cell lymphoma/leukemia: pathology and treatment. Hematol Oncol. 1997 May;15(2):71–9. PMID:9375032
2173. Kwong YL, Chan TSY, Tan D, et al. PD1 blockade with pembrolizumab is highly effective in relapsed or refractory NK/T-cell lymphoma failing L-asparaginase. Blood. 2017 Apr 27;129(17):2437–42. PMID:28188133
2174. Kwong YL, Kim SJ, Tse E, et al. Sequential chemotherapy/radiotherapy was comparable with concurrent chemoradiotherapy for stage I/II NK/T-cell lymphoma. Ann Oncol. 2018 Jan 1;29(1):256–63. PMID:29077846
2175. Kwong YL, Kim WS, Lim ST, et al. SMILE for natural killer/T-cell lymphoma: analysis of safety and efficacy from the Asia Lymphoma Study Group. Blood. 2012 Oct 11;120(15):2973–80. PMID:22919026
2176. Kwong YL, Lam CC, Chan TM. Post-transplantation lymphoproliferative disease of natural killer cell lineage: a clinicopathological and molecular analysis. Br J Haematol. 2000 Jul;110(1):197–202. PMID:10930998
2177. Kwong YL, Pang AW, Leung AY, et al. Quantification of circulating Epstein-Barr virus DNA in NK/T-cell lymphoma treated with the SMILE protocol: diagnostic and prognostic significance. Leukemia. 2014 Apr;28(4):865–70. PMID:23842425
2178. Kwong YL, Wong KF, Chan LC, et al. Large granular lymphocyte leukemia. A study of nine cases in a Chinese population. Am J Clin Pathol. 1995 Jan;103(1):76–81. PMID:7817949
2179. Kyle RA, Dispenzieri A, Kumar S, et al. IgM monoclonal gammopathy of undetermined significance (MGUS) and smoldering Waldenström's macroglobulinemia (SWM). Clin Lymphoma Myeloma Leuk. 2011 Feb;11(1):74–6. PMID:21454195
2180. Kyle RA, Durie BG, Rajkumar SV, et al. Monoclonal gammopathy of undetermined significance (MGUS) and smoldering (asymptomatic) multiple myeloma: IMWG consensus perspectives risk factors for progression and guidelines for monitoring and management. Leukemia. 2010 Jun;24(6):1121–7. PMID:20410922

2181. Kyle RA, Gertz MA. Primary systemic amyloidosis: clinical and laboratory features in 474 cases. Semin Hematol. 1995 Jan;32(1):45–59. PMID:7878478
2182. Kyle RA, Larson DR, Kurtin PJ, et al. Incidence of AL amyloidosis in Olmsted County, Minnesota, 1990 through 2015. Mayo Clin Proc. 2019 Mar;94(3):465–71. PMID:30713046
2183. Kyle RA, Larson DR, Therneau TM, et al. Long-term follow-up of monoclonal gammopathy of undetermined significance. N Engl J Med. 2018 Jan 18;378(3):241–9. PMID:29342381
2184. Kyle RA, Remstein ED, Therneau TM, et al. Clinical course and prognosis of smoldering (asymptomatic) multiple myeloma. N Engl J Med. 2007 Jun 21;356(25):2582–90. PMID:17582068
2185. Kyle RA, Therneau TM, Rajkumar SV, et al. Prevalence of monoclonal gammopathy of undetermined significance. N Engl J Med. 2006 Mar 30;354(13):1362–9. PMID:16571879
2186. Kyrtsonis MC, Vassilakopoulos TP, Angelopoulou MK, et al. Waldenström's macroglobulinemia: clinical course and prognostic factors in 60 patients. Experience from a single hematology unit. Ann Hematol. 2001 Dec;80(12):722–7. PMID:11797112
2187. La Rocca G, Auricchio AM, Mazzucchi E, et al. Intracranial dural based marginal zone MALT-type B-cell lymphoma: a case - based update and literature review. Br J Neurosurg. 2023 Dec;37(6):1480–6. PMID:34180316
2188. Laban KG, Tobon-Morales RE, Hodge JA, et al. Single benign metastasising leiomyoma of an inguinal lymph node. BMJ Case Rep. 2016 Aug 10;2016:bcr2016216546. PMID:27511755
2189. Lachenal F, Berger F, Ghesquières H, et al. Angioimmunoblastic T-cell lymphoma: clinical and laboratory features at diagnosis in 77 patients. Medicine (Baltimore). 2007 Sep;86(5):282–92. PMID:17873758
2190. Lachmann HJ, Booth DR, Booth SE, et al. Misdiagnosis of hereditary amyloidosis as AL (primary) amyloidosis. N Engl J Med. 2002 Jun 6;346(23):1786–91. PMID:12050338
2191. Lacy SE, Barrans SL, Beer PA, et al. Targeted sequencing in DLBCL, molecular subtypes, and outcomes: a Haematological Malignancy Research Network report. Blood. 2020 May 14;135(20):1759–71. PMID:32187361
2192. Lae ME, Ahmed I, Macon WR. Clusterin is widely expressed in systemic anaplastic large cell lymphoma but fails to differentiate primary from secondary cutaneous anaplastic large cell lymphoma. Am J Clin Pathol. 2002 Nov;118(5):773–9. PMID:12428799
2193. Laginestra MA, Tripodo C, Agostinelli C, et al. Distinctive histogenesis and immunological microenvironment based on transcriptional profiles of follicular dendritic cell sarcomas. Mol Cancer Res. 2017 May;15(5):541–52. PMID:28130401
2194. Laharanne E, Oumouhou N, Bonnet F, et al. Genome-wide analysis of cutaneous T-cell lymphomas identifies three clinically relevant classes. J Invest Dermatol. 2010 Jun;130(6):1707–18. PMID:20130593
2195. Lahuerta JJ, Paiva B, Vidriales MB, et al. Depth of response in multiple myeloma: a pooled analysis of three PETHEMA/GEM clinical trials. J Clin Oncol. 2017 Sep 1;35(25):2900–10. PMID:28498784
2196. Lai R, Medeiros LJ, Dabbagh L, et al. Sinusoidal CD30-positive large B-cell lymphoma: a morphologic mimic of anaplastic large cell lymphoma. Mod Pathol. 2000 Mar;13(3):223–8. PMID:10757332
2197. Lai R, Weiss LM, Chang KL, et al. Frequency of CD43 expression in non-Hodgkin lymphoma. A survey of 742 cases and further characterization of rare CD43+ follicular lymphomas. Am J Clin Pathol. 1999 Apr;111(4):488–94. PMID:10191768
2198. Laidlaw BJ, Cyster JG. Transcriptional regulation of memory B cell differentiation. Nat Rev Immunol. 2021 Apr;21(4):209–20. PMID:33024284
2199. Lam KY, Yip KH, Peh WC. Splenic vascular lesions: unusual features and a review of the literature. Aust N Z J Surg. 1999 Jun;69(6):422–5. PMID:10392884
2200. Lamant L, Dastugue N, Pulford K, et al. A new fusion gene TPM3-ALK in anaplastic large cell lymphoma created by a (1;2)(q25;p23) translocation. Blood. 1999 May 1;93(9):3088–95. PMID:10216106
2201. Lamant L, Gascoyne RD, Duplantier MM, et al. Non-muscle myosin heavy chain (MYH9): a new partner fused to ALK in anaplastic large cell lymphoma. Genes Chromosomes Cancer. 2003 Aug;37(4):427–32. PMID:12800156
2202. Lamant L, McCarthy K, d'Amore E, et al. Prognostic impact of morphologic and phenotypic features of childhood ALK-positive anaplastic large-cell lymphoma: results of the ALCL99 study. J Clin Oncol. 2011 Dec 10;29(35):4669–76. PMID:22084369
2203. Lamb MJ, Smith A, Painter D, et al. Health impact of monoclonal gammopathy of undetermined significance (MGUS) and monoclonal B-cell lymphocytosis (MBL): findings from a UK population-based cohort. BMJ Open. 2021 Feb 22;11(2):e041296. PMID:33619185
2204. Lamovec J, Jancar J. Primary malignant lymphoma of the breast. Lymphoma of the mucosa-associated lymphoid tissue. Cancer. 1987 Dec 15;60(12):3033–41. PMID:3315180
2205. Lampert IA, Wotherspoon A, Van Noorden S, et al. High expression of CD23 in the proliferation centers of chronic lymphocytic leukemia in lymph nodes and spleen. Hum Pathol. 1999 Jun;30(6):648–54. PMID:10374772
2206. Lamy T, Liu JH, Landowski TH, et al. Dysregulation of CD95/CD95 ligand-apoptotic pathway in CD3(+) large granular lymphocyte leukemia. Blood. 1998 Dec 15;92(12):4771–7. PMID:9845544
2207. Lamy T, Loughran TP Jr. Clinical features of large granular lymphocyte leukemia. Semin Hematol. 2003 Jul;40(3):185–95. PMID:12876667
2208. Lamy T, Loughran TP Jr. How I treat LGL leukemia. Blood. 2011 Mar 10;117(10):2764–74. PMID:21190991
2209. Landau DA, Sun C, Rosebrock D, et al. The evolutionary landscape of chronic lymphocytic leukemia treated with ibrutinib targeted therapy. Nat Commun. 2017 Dec 19;8(1):2185. PMID:29259203
2210. Landau DA, Tausch E, Taylor-Weiner AN, et al. Mutations driving CLL and their evolution in progression and relapse. Nature. 2015 Oct 22;526(7574):525–30. PMID:26466571
2211. Landgren O, Gilbert ES, Rizzo JD, et al. Risk factors for lymphoproliferative disorders after allogeneic hematopoietic cell transplantation. Blood. 2009 May 14;113(20):4992–5001. PMID:19264919
2212. Landgren O, Kristinsson SY, Goldin LR, et al. Risk of plasma cell and lymphoproliferative disorders among 14621 first-degree relatives of 4458 patients with monoclonal gammopathy of undetermined significance in Sweden. Blood. 2009 Jul 23;114(4):791–5. PMID:19182202
2213. Landgren O, Kyle RA, Pfeiffer RM, et al. Monoclonal gammopathy of undetermined significance (MGUS) consistently precedes multiple myeloma: a prospective study. Blood. 2009 May 28;113(22):5412–7. PMID:19179464
2214. Landsburg DJ, Falkiewicz MK, Maly J, et al. Outcomes of patients with double-hit lymphoma who achieve first complete remission. J Clin Oncol. 2017 Jul 10;35(20):2260–7. PMID:28475457
2215. Landsburg DJ, Falkiewicz MK, Petrich AM, et al. Sole rearrangement but not amplification of MYC is associated with a poor prognosis in patients with diffuse large B cell lymphoma and B cell lymphoma unclassifiable. Br J Haematol. 2016 Nov;175(4):631–40. PMID:27469075
2216. Landsburg DJ, Petrich AM, Abramson JS, et al. Impact of oncogene rearrangement patterns on outcomes in patients with double-hit non-Hodgkin lymphoma. Cancer. 2016 Feb 15;122(4):559–64. PMID:26565895
2217. Lanemo Myhrinder A, Hellqvist E, Sidorova E, et al. A new perspective: molecular motifs on oxidized LDL, apoptotic cells, and bacteria are targets for chronic lymphocytic leukemia antibodies. Blood. 2008 Apr 1;111(7):3838–48. PMID:18223168
2218. Langabeer SE. Variant BCR-ABL1 fusion genes in adult Philadelphia chromosome-positive B-cell acute lymphoblastic leukemia. EXCLI J. 2017 Oct 18;16:1144–7. PMID:29285010
2219. Langerak AW, Groenen PJ, Brüggemann M, et al. EuroClonality/BIOMED-2 guidelines for interpretation and reporting of Ig/TCR clonality testing in suspected lymphoproliferations. Leukemia. 2012 Oct;26(10):2159–71. PMID:22918122
2220. Lanoy E, Rosenberg PS, Fily F, et al. HIV-associated Hodgkin lymphoma during the first months on combination antiretroviral therapy. Blood. 2011 Jul 7;118(1):44–9. PMID:21551234
2221. Lanzillotta M, Fernàndez-Codina A, Culver E, et al. Emerging therapy options for IgG4-related disease. Expert Rev Clin Immunol. 2021 May;17(5):471–83. PMID:33689549
2222. Lanzillotta M, Mancuso G, Della-Torre E. Advances in the diagnosis and management of IgG4 related disease. BMJ. 2020 Jun 16;369:m1067. PMID:32546500
2223. Lardelli P, Bookman MA, Sundeen J, et al. Lymphocytic lymphoma of intermediate differentiation. Morphologic and immunophenotypic spectrum and clinical correlations. Am J Surg Pathol. 1990 Aug;14(8):752–63. PMID:2198813
2224. Larsen BT, Bishop MC, Hunter GC, et al. Low-grade, metastasizing splenic littoral cell angiosarcoma presenting with hepatic cirrhosis and splenic artery aneurysm. Int J Surg Pathol. 2013 Dec;21(6):618–26. PMID:23426963
2225. Laskin WB, Alasadi R, Variakojis D. Splenic hamartoma. Am J Surg Pathol. 2005 Aug;29(8):1114–5. PMID:16006808
2226. Laskin WB, Lasota JP, Fetsch JF, et al. Intranodal palisaded myofibroblastoma: another mesenchymal neoplasm with CTNNB1 (β-catenin gene) mutations: clinicopathologic, immunohistochemical, and molecular genetic study of 18 cases. Am J Surg Pathol. 2015 Feb;39(2):197–205. PMID:25025452
2227. Latour S, Fischer A. Signaling pathways involved in the T-cell-mediated immunity against Epstein-Barr virus: lessons from genetic diseases. Immunol Rev. 2019 Sep;291(1):174–89. PMID:31402499
2228. Laude MC, Lebras L, Sesques P, et al. First-line treatment of double-hit and triple-hit lymphomas: survival and tolerance data from a retrospective multicenter French study. Am J Hematol. 2021 Mar 1;96(3):302–11. PMID:33306213
2229. Laukkanen K, Saarinen M, Mallet F, et al. Cutaneous T-cell lymphoma (CTCL) cell line-derived extracellular vesicles contain HERV-W-encoded fusogenic syncytin-1. J Invest Dermatol. 2020 Jul;140(7):1466–1469.e4. PMID:31883959
2230. Launay E, Pangault C, Bertrand P, et al. High rate of TNFRSF14 gene alterations related to 1p36 region in de novo follicular lymphoma and impact on prognosis. Leukemia. 2012 Mar;26(3):559–62. PMID:21941365
2231. Laurent C, Adélaïde J, Guille A, et al. High-grade follicular lymphomas exhibit clinicopathologic, cytogenetic, and molecular diversity extending beyond grades 3A and 3B. Am J Surg Pathol. 2021 Oct 1;45(10):1324–36. PMID:34334687
2232. Laurent C, Baron M, Amara N, et al. Impact of expert pathologic review of lymphoma diagnosis: study of patients from the French Lymphopath Network. J Clin Oncol. 2017 Jun 20;35(18):2008–17. PMID:28459613
2233. Laurent C, Delas A, Gaulard P, et al. Breast implant-associated anaplastic large cell lymphoma: two distinct clinicopathological variants with different outcomes. Ann Oncol. 2016 Feb;27(2):306–14. PMID:26598546
2234. Laurent C, Do C, Gascoyne RD, et al. Anaplastic lymphoma kinase-positive diffuse large B-cell lymphoma: a rare clinicopathologic entity with poor prognosis. J Clin Oncol. 2009 Sep 1;27(25):4211–6. PMID:19636007
2235. Laurent C, Do C, Gourraud PA, et al. Prevalence of common non-Hodgkin lymphomas and subtypes of Hodgkin lymphoma by nodal site of involvement: a systematic retrospective review of 938 cases. Medicine (Baltimore). 2015 Jun;94(25):e987. PMID:26107683
2236. Laurent C, Fabiani B, Do C, et al. Immune-checkpoint expression in Epstein-Barr virus positive and negative plasmablastic lymphoma: a clinical and pathological study in 82 patients. Haematologica. 2016 Aug;101(8):976–84. PMID:27175027
2237. Laurent C, Nicolae A, Laurent C, et al. Gene alterations in epigenetic modifiers and JAK-STAT signaling are frequent in breast implant-associated ALCL. Blood. 2020 Jan 30;135(5):360–70. PMID:31774495
2238. Laurini JA, Aoun P, Iqbal J, et al. Investigation of the BRAF V600E mutation by pyrosequencing in lymphoproliferative disorders. Am J Clin Pathol. 2012 Dec;138(6):877–83. PMID:23161722
2239. Laurini JA, Perry AM, Boilesen E, et al. Classification of non-Hodgkin lymphoma in Central and South America: a review of 1028 cases. Blood. 2012 Dec 6;120(24):4795–801. PMID:23086753
2240. Le Deley MC, Reiter A, Williams D, et al. Prognostic factors in childhood anaplastic large cell lymphoma: results of a large European intergroup study. Blood. 2008 Feb 1;111(3):1560–6. PMID:17957029
2241. Le Gouill S, Talmant P, Touzeau C, et al. The clinical presentation and prognosis of diffuse large B-cell lymphoma with t(14;18) and 8q24/c-MYC rearrangement. Haematologica. 2007 Oct;92(10):1335–42. PMID:18024371
2242. Le M, Ghazawi FM, Alakel A, et al. Incidence and mortality trends and geographic patterns of follicular lymphoma in Canada. Curr Oncol. 2019 Aug;26(4):e473–81. PMID:31548815
2243. LeBlanc FR, Liu X, Hengst J, et al. Sphingosine kinase inhibitors decrease viability and induce cell death in natural killer-large granular lymphocyte leukemia. Cancer Biol Ther. 2015;16(12):1830–40. PMID:26252351
2244. LeBlanc FR, Pearson JM, Tan SF, et al. Sphingosine kinase-2 is overexpressed in large granular lymphocyte leukaemia and promotes survival through Mcl-1. Br J Haematol. 2020 Aug;190(3):405–17. PMID:32124438
2245. Leblond V, Choquet S. Lymphoproliferative disorders after liver transplantation. J Hepatol. 2004 May;40(5):728–35. PMID:15094218
2246. LeBrun DP. E2A basic helix-loop-helix transcription factors in human leukemia. Front

Biosci. 2003 May 1;8:s206–22. PMID:12700034
2246A. Lechner MG, Megiel C, Church CH, et al. Survival signals and targets for therapy in breast implant-associated ALK–anaplastic large cell lymphoma. Clin Cancer Res. 2012 Sep 1;18(17):4549–59. PMID:22791880
2247. Lecluse Y, Lebailly P, Roulland S, et al. t(11;14)-positive clones can persist over a long period of time in the peripheral blood of healthy individuals. Leukemia. 2009 Jun;23(6):1190–3. PMID:19242498
2248. Lecuit M, Abachin E, Martin A, et al. Immunoproliferative small intestinal disease associated with Campylobacter jejuni. N Engl J Med. 2004 Jan 15;350(3):239–48. PMID:14724303
2249. Lee H, Maeda K. Hamartoma of the spleen. Arch Pathol Lab Med. 2009 Jan;133(1):147–51. PMID:19123729
2250. Lee H, Oh D, Yang K, et al. Radiation therapy outcome and clinical features of duodenal-type follicular lymphoma. Cancer Res Treat. 2019 Apr;51(2):547–55. PMID:29986575
2251. Lee H, Park HJ, Park EH, et al. Nationwide statistical analysis of lymphoid malignancies in Korea. Cancer Res Treat. 2018 Jan;50(1):222–38. PMID:28361523
2252. Lee HE, Zhang L. Immunoglobulin G4-related hepatobiliary disease. Semin Diagn Pathol. 2019 Nov;36(6):423–33. PMID:31358425
2253. Lee HS, Suh KS, Lee DY, et al. Cutaneous lymphoma in Korea: a nationwide retrospective study. Acta Derm Venereol. 2016 May;96(4):535–9. PMID:26560051
2254. Lee IJ, Kim SC, Kim HS, et al. Paraneoplastic pemphigus associated with follicular dendritic cell sarcoma arising from Castleman's tumor. J Am Acad Dermatol. 1999 Feb;40(2 Pt 2):294–7. PMID:10025851
2255. Lee JW, Kim Y, Cho B, et al. High incidence of RAS pathway mutations among sentinel genetic lesions of Korean pediatric BCR-ABL1-like acute lymphoblastic leukemia. Cancer Med. 2020 Jul;9(13):4632–9. PMID:32378810
2256. Lee K, Evans MG, Yang L, et al. Primary cytotoxic T-cell lymphomas harbor recurrent targetable alterations in the JAK-STAT pathway. Blood. 2021 Dec 9;138(23):2435–40. PMID:34432866
2257. Lee KY, Yeon YH, Lee BC. Kikuchi-Fujimoto disease with prolonged fever in children. Pediatrics. 2004 Dec;114(6):e752–6. PMID:15545615
2258. Lee MH, Choi ME, Won CH, et al. Comparative clinicopathologic analysis of cutaneous peripheral T-cell lymphoma, not otherwise specified, according to primary tumor site. J Am Acad Dermatol. 2019 Jun;80(6):1771–4. PMID:30296539
2259. Lee S, Park HY, Kang SY, et al. Genetic alterations of JAK/STAT cascade and histone modification in extranodal NK/T-cell lymphoma nasal type. Oncotarget. 2015 Jul 10;6(19):17764–76. PMID:25980440
2260. Lee SC, Berg KD, Racke FK, et al. Pseudo-spikes are common in histologically benign lymphoid tissues. J Mol Diagn. 2000 Aug;2(3):145–52. PMID:11229519
2261. Lee SE, Kang SY, Takeuchi K, et al. Identification of RANBP2-ALK fusion in ALK positive diffuse large B-cell lymphoma. Hematol Oncol. 2014 Dec;32(4):221–4. PMID:24470379
2262. Lee SH, Kim JS, Kim J, et al. A highly recurrent novel missense mutation in CD28 among angioimmunoblastic T-cell lymphoma patients. Haematologica. 2015 Dec;100(12):e505–7. PMID:26405154
2263. Lee SJ, Tien HF, Park HJ, et al. Gradual increase of chronic lymphocytic leukemia incidence in Korea, 1999-2010: comparison to plasma cell myeloma. Leuk Lymphoma. 2016;57(3):585–9. PMID:26133722
2264. Lee W, Shin E, Kim BH, et al. Diagnostic accuracy of SOX11 immunohistochemistry in mantle cell lymphoma: a meta-analysis. PLoS One. 2019 Nov 12;14(11):e0225096. PMID:31714947
2265. Lee YS, Filie A, Arthur D, et al. Breast implant-associated anaplastic large cell lymphoma in a patient with Li-Fraumeni syndrome. Histopathology. 2015 Dec;67(6):925–7. PMID:25974645
2266. Leeksma AC, Baliakas P, Moysiadis T, et al. Genomic arrays identify high-risk chronic lymphocytic leukemia with genomic complexity: a multi-center study. Haematologica. 2021 Jan 1;106(1):87–97. PMID:31974198
2267. Leich E, Hoster E, Wartenberg M, et al. Similar clinical features in follicular lymphomas with and without breaks in the BCL2 locus. Leukemia. 2016 Apr;30(4):854–60. PMID:26621338
2268. Leich E, Salaverria I, Bea S, et al. Follicular lymphomas with and without translocation t(14;18) differ in gene expression profiles and genetic alterations. Blood. 2009 Jul 23;114(4):826–34. PMID:19471018
2269. Leithäuser F, Bäuerle M, Huynh MQ, et al. Isotype-switched immunoglobulin genes with a high load of somatic hypermutation and lack of ongoing mutational activity are prevalent in mediastinal B-cell lymphoma. Blood. 2001 Nov 1;98(9):2762–70. PMID:11675349
2270. Lejman M, Włodarczyk M, Zawitkowska J, et al. Comprehensive chromosomal aberrations in a case of a patient with TCF3-HLF-positive BCP-ALL. BMC Med Genomics. 2020 Apr 3;13(1):58. PMID:32245383
2271. Leleu X, O'Connor K, Ho AW, et al. Hepatitis C viral infection is not associated with Waldenström's macroglobulinemia. Am J Hematol. 2007 Jan;82(1):83–4. PMID:16955461
2272. Lemonnier F, Cairns RA, Inoue S, et al. The IDH2 R172K mutation associated with angioimmunoblastic T-cell lymphoma produces 2HG in T cells and impacts lymphoid development. Proc Natl Acad Sci U S A. 2016 Dec 27;113(52):15084–9. PMID:27956631
2273. Lemonnier F, Safar V, Beldi-Ferchiou A, et al. Integrative analysis of a phase 2 trial combining lenalidomide with CHOP in angioimmunoblastic T-cell lymphoma. Blood Adv. 2021 Jan 26;5(2):539–48. PMID:33496747
2274. Lennert K, editor. Malignant lymphomas other than Hodgkin's disease. New York (NY): Springer Verlag; 1978.
2275. Lennert K, Stein H, Kaiserling E. Cytological and functional criteria for the classification of malignant lymphomata. Br J Cancer Suppl. 1975 Mar;2:29–43. PMID:52366
2276. Lenti MV, Biagi F, Lucioni M, et al. Two cases of monomorphic epitheliotropic intestinal T-cell lymphoma associated with coeliac disease. Scand J Gastroenterol. 2019 Aug;54(8):965–8. PMID:31361171
2277. Lenz G, Wright G, Dave SS, et al. Stromal gene signatures in large-B-cell lymphomas. N Engl J Med. 2008 Nov 27;359(22):2313–23. PMID:19038878
2278. Lenze D, Leoncini L, Hummel M, et al. The different epidemiologic subtypes of Burkitt lymphoma share a homogenous micro RNA profile distinct from diffuse large B-cell lymphoma. Leukemia. 2011 Dec;25(12):1869–76. PMID:21701491
2279. Leon ME, Schinasi LH, Lebailly P, et al. Pesticide use and risk of non-Hodgkin lymphoid malignancies in agricultural cohorts from France, Norway and the USA: a pooled analysis from the AGRICOH consortium. Int J Epidemiol. 2019 Oct 1;48(5):1519–35. PMID:30880337
2280. Leonard JP, Kolibaba KS, Reeves JA, et al. Randomized phase II study of R-CHOP with or without bortezomib in previously untreated patients with non-germinal center B-cell-like diffuse large B-cell lymphoma. J Clin Oncol. 2017 Nov 1;35(31):3538–46. PMID:28862883
2281. Leoncini L. Epstein-Barr virus positivity as a defining pathogenetic feature of Burkitt lymphoma subtypes. Br J Haematol. 2022 Feb;196(3):468–70. PMID:34725813
2282. Letourneau A, Maerevoet M, Milowich D, et al. Dual JAK1 and STAT3 mutations in a breast implant-associated anaplastic large cell lymphoma. Virchows Arch. 2018 Oct;473(4):505–11. PMID:29637270
2283. Leucci E, Cocco M, Onnis A, et al. MYC translocation-negative classical Burkitt lymphoma cases: an alternative pathogenetic mechanism involving miRNA deregulation. J Pathol. 2008 Dec;216(4):440–50. PMID:18802929
2284. Leung N, Bridoux F, Batuman V, et al. The evaluation of monoclonal gammopathy of renal significance: a consensus report of the International Kidney and Monoclonal Gammopathy Research Group. Nat Rev Nephrol. 2019 Jan;15(1):45–59. PMID:30510265
2285. Leung N, Bridoux F, Nasr SH. Monoclonal gammopathy of renal significance. N Engl J Med. 2021 May 20;384(20):1931–41. PMID:34010532
2286. Leventaki V, Bhattacharyya S, Lim MS. Pathology and genetics of anaplastic large cell lymphoma. Semin Diagn Pathol. 2020 Jan;37(1):57–71. PMID:31882178
2287. Leventaki V, Drakos E, Medeiros LJ, et al. NPM-ALK oncogenic kinase promotes cell-cycle progression through activation of JNK/cJun signaling in anaplastic large-cell lymphoma. Blood. 2007 Sep 1;110(5):1621–30. PMID:17416736
2288. Levine AM. AIDS-related malignancies: the emerging epidemic. J Natl Cancer Inst. 1993 Sep 1;85(17):1382–97. PMID:8350362
2289. Levine EG, Arthur DC, Machnicki J, et al. Four new recurring translocations in non-Hodgkin lymphoma. Blood. 1989 Oct;74(5):1796–800. PMID:2506953
2290. Levine PH, Kamaraju LS, Connelly RR, et al. The American Burkitt's Lymphoma Registry: eight years' experience. Cancer. 1982 Mar 1;49(5):1016–22. PMID:7059918
2291. Levy M, Copie-Bergman C, Traulle C, et al. Conservative treatment of primary gastric low-grade B-cell lymphoma of mucosa-associated lymphoid tissue: predictive factors of response and outcome. Am J Gastroenterol. 2002 Feb;97(2):292–7. PMID:11866264
2292. Lewinsky H, Gunes EG, David K, et al. CD84 is a regulator of the immunosuppressive microenvironment in multiple myeloma. JCI Insight. 2021 Feb 22;6(4):e141683. PMID:33465053
2293. Lewis JT, Gaffney RL, Casey MB, et al. Inflammatory pseudotumor of the spleen associated with a clonal Epstein-Barr virus genome. Case report and review of the literature. Am J Clin Pathol. 2003 Jul;120(1):56–61. PMID:12866373
2294. Li A, Swift M. Mutations at the ataxia-telangiectasia locus and clinical phenotypes of A-T patients. Am J Med Genet. 2000 May 29;92(3):170–7. PMID:10817650
2295. Li C, Tian Y, Wang J, et al. Abnormal immunophenotype provides a key diagnostic marker: a report of 29 cases of de novo aggressive natural killer cell leukemia. Transl Res. 2014 Jun;163(6):565–77. PMID:24524877
2296. Li D, Xie P, Mi C. Primary testicular diffuse large B-cell lymphoma shows an activated B-cell-like phenotype. Pathol Res Pract. 2010 Sep 15;206(9):611–5. PMID:20627604
2297. Li H, Shen P, Liang Y, et al. Fibroblastic reticular cell tumor of the breast: a case report and review of the literature. Exp Ther Med. 2016 Feb;11(2):561–4. PMID:26893647
2298. Li J, Dai Y, Wu L, et al. Emerging molecular subtypes and therapeutic targets in B-cell precursor acute lymphoblastic leukemia. Front Med. 2021 Jun;15(3):347–71. PMID:33400146
2299. Li J, Liu X, Yao Z, et al. High-grade B-cell lymphomas, not otherwise specified: a study of 41 cases. Cancer Manag Res. 2020 Mar 13;12:1903–12. PMID:32214848
2300. Li J, Zhang W, Wang W, et al. Forty-nine cases of acute lymphoblastic leukaemia/lymphoma in pleural and pericardial effusions: a cytological-histological correlation. Cytopathology. 2018 Apr;29(2):172–8. PMID:29575419
2301. Li JF, Dai YT, Lilljebjörn H, et al. Transcriptional landscape of B cell precursor acute lymphoblastic leukemia based on an international study of 1,223 cases. Proc Natl Acad Sci U S A. 2018 Dec 11;115(50):E11711–20. PMID:30487223
2302. Li JY, Gaillard F, Moreau A, et al. Detection of translocation t(11;14)(q13;q32) in mantle cell lymphoma by fluorescence in situ hybridization. Am J Pathol. 1999 May;154(5):1449–52. PMID:10329598
2303. Li JY, Guitart J, Pulitzer MP, et al. Multicenter case series of indolent small/medium-sized CD8+ lymphoid proliferations with predilection for the ear and face. Am J Dermatopathol. 2014 May;36(5):402–8. PMID:24394306
2304. Li L, Shi YH, Guo ZJ, et al. Clinicopathological features and prognosis assessment of extranodal follicular dendritic cell sarcoma. World J Gastroenterol. 2010 May 28;16(20):2504–19. PMID:20503450
2305. Li M, Liu Y, Wang Y, et al. Anaplastic variant of diffuse large B-cell lymphoma displays intricate genetic alterations and distinct biological features. Am J Surg Pathol. 2017 Oct;41(10):1322–32. PMID:28319526
2306. Li N, Jiang M, Wu WC, et al. How to identify patients at high risk of developing nasal-type, extranodal nature killer/T-cell lymphoma-associated hemophagocytic syndrome. Front Oncol. 2021 Aug 18;11:704962. PMID:34490105
2307. Li S, Desai P, Lin P, et al. MYC/BCL6 double-hit lymphoma (DHL): a tumour associated with an aggressive clinical course and poor prognosis. Histopathology. 2016 Jun;68(7):1090–8. PMID:26426741
2308. Li S, Feng X, Li T, et al. Extranodal NK/T-cell lymphoma, nasal type: a report of 73 cases at MD Anderson Cancer Center. Am J Surg Pathol. 2013 Jan;37(1):14–23. PMID:23232851
2309. Li S, Juco J, Mann KP, et al. Flow cytometry in the differential diagnosis of lymphocyte-rich thymoma from precursor T-cell acute lymphoblastic leukemia/lymphoblastic lymphoma. Am J Clin Pathol. 2004 Feb;121(2):268–74. PMID:14983942
2310. Li S, Lin P, Fayad LE, et al. B-cell lymphomas with MYC/8q24 rearrangements and IGH@BCL2/t(14;18)(q32;q21): an aggressive disease with heterogeneous histology, germinal center B-cell immunophenotype and poor outcome. Mod Pathol. 2012 Jan;25(1):145–56. PMID:22002575
2311. Li S, Lin P, Medeiros LJ. Advances in pathological understanding of high-grade B cell lymphomas. Expert Rev Hematol. 2018 Aug;11(8):637–48. PMID:29989509
2312. Li S, Qiu L, Xu J, et al. High-grade B-cell lymphoma (HGBL)-NOS is clinicopathologically and genetically more similar to DLBCL/HGBL-DH than DLBCL. Leukemia. 2023 Feb;37(2):422–32. PMID:36513804
2313. Li S, Saksena A, Desai P, et al. Prognostic

impact of history of follicular lymphoma, induction regimen and stem cell transplant in patients with MYC/BCL2 double hit lymphoma. Oncotarget. 2016 Jun 21;7(25):38122–32. PMID:27203548

2314. Li S, Seegmiller AC, Lin P, et al. B-cell lymphomas with concurrent MYC and BCL2 abnormalities other than translocations behave similarly to MYC/BCL2 double-hit lymphomas. Mod Pathol. 2015 Feb;28(2):208–17. PMID:25103070

2315. Li S, Xu J, You MJ. The pathologic diagnosis of mantle cell lymphoma. Histol Histopathol. 2021 Oct;36(10):1037–51. PMID:34114641

2316. Li S, Young KH, Medeiros LJ. Diffuse large B-cell lymphoma. Pathology. 2018 Jan;50(1):74–87. PMID:29167021

2317. Li W. Histone methyltransferase SETD2 in lymphoid malignancy. In: Gallamini A, Juweid M, editors. Lymphoma. Brisbane (Australia): Exon Publications; 2021 Dec 28. Chapter 3. PMID:35226431

2318. Li W, Chen Y, Sun ZP, et al. Clinicopathological characteristics of immunoglobulin G4-related sialadenitis. Arthritis Res Ther. 2015 Jul 21;17(1):186. PMID:26194097

2319. Li WW, Liang P, Zhao HP, et al. Composite hemangioendothelioma of the spleen with multiple metastases: CT findings and review of the literature. Medicine (Baltimore). 2021 May 28;100(21):e25846. PMID:34032697

2320. Li X, Ma X, Hao J, et al. Primary splenic epithelioid hemangioendothelioma with diffuse metastases revealed by FDG PET/CT imaging: a case report. Medicine (Baltimore). 2021 Apr 2;100(13):e25065. PMID:33787588

2321. Li X, Shi Z, You R, et al. Inflammatory pseudotumor-like follicular dendritic cell sarcoma of the spleen: computed tomography imaging characteristics in 5 patients. J Comput Assist Tomogr. 2018 May/Jun;42(3):399–404. PMID:29287022

2322. Li XQ, Cheuk W, Lam PW, et al. Inflammatory pseudotumor-like follicular dendritic cell tumor of liver and spleen: granulomatous and eosinophil-rich variants mimicking inflammatory or infective lesions. Am J Surg Pathol. 2014 May;38(5):646–53. PMID:24503752

2323. Li Y, Gao H, Li Z, et al. Clinical characteristics of 76 patients with IgG4-related hypophysitis: a systematic literature review. Int J Endocrinol. 2019 Dec 18;2019:5382640. PMID:31929792

2324. Li Y, Gordon MW, Xu-Monette ZY, et al. Single nucleotide variation in the TP53 3' untranslated region in diffuse large B-cell lymphoma treated with rituximab-CHOP: a report from the International DLBCL Rituximab-CHOP Consortium Program. Blood. 2013 May 30;121(22):4529–40. PMID:23515929

2325. Li Y, Gupta G, Molofsky A, et al. B lymphoblastic leukemia/lymphoma with Burkitt-like morphology and IGH/MYC rearrangement: report of 3 cases in adult patients. Am J Surg Pathol. 2018 Feb;42(2):269–76. PMID:29112016

2326. Li Y, Schwab C, Ryan S, et al. Constitutional and somatic rearrangement of chromosome 21 in acute lymphoblastic leukaemia. Nature. 2014 Apr 3;508(7494):98–102. PMID:24670643

2327. Li Y, Yang W, Devidas M, et al. Germline RUNX1 variation and predisposition to childhood acute lymphoblastic leukemia. J Clin Invest. 2021 Jun 24;131(17):e147898. PMID:34166225

2328. Li Z, Lan X, Li C, et al. Recurrent PDGFRB mutations in unicentric Castleman disease. Leukemia. 2019 Apr;33(4):1035–8. PMID:30607019

2329. Li Z, Lee SHR, Chin WHN, et al. Distinct clinical characteristics of DUX4- and PAX5-altered childhood B-lymphoblastic leukemia. Blood Adv. 2021 Dec 14;5(23):5226–38. PMID:34547766

2330. Li Z, Lu L, Zhou Z, et al. Recurrent mutations in epigenetic modifiers and the PI3K/AKT/mTOR pathway in subcutaneous panniculitis-like T-cell lymphoma. Br J Haematol. 2018 May;181(3):406–10. PMID:28294301

2331. Li Z, Xia Y, Feng LN, et al. Genetic risk of extranodal natural killer T-cell lymphoma: a genome-wide association study. Lancet Oncol. 2016 Sep;17(9):1240–7. PMID:27470079

2332. Liang HC, Costanza M, Prutsch N, et al. Super-enhancer-based identification of a BATF3/IL-2R-module reveals vulnerabilities in anaplastic large cell lymphoma. Nat Commun. 2021 Sep 22;12(1):5577. PMID:34552066

2333. Liang J, Chen Y, Zhang F, et al. Genomic variation of Epstein-Barr virus in inflammatory pseudotumour-like follicular dendritic cell tumour. Histopathology. 2016 Nov;69(5):883–4. PMID:27146079

2334. Liang JH, Lu TX, Tian T, et al. Epstein-Barr virus (EBV) DNA in whole blood as a superior prognostic and monitoring factor than EBV-encoded small RNA in situ hybridization in diffuse large B-cell lymphoma. Clin Microbiol Infect. 2015 Jun;21(6):596–602. PMID:25743579

2335. Liang Y, Yang Z, Qin B, et al. Primary Sjogren's syndrome and malignancy risk: a systematic review and meta-analysis. Ann Rheum Dis. 2014 Jun;73(6):1151–6. PMID:23687261

2336. Liao J, Wang Z, Li Q, et al. CT and MRI features of sclerosing angiomatoid nodular transformation of the spleen: a report of 18 patients with pathologic correlation. Diagn Interv Imaging. 2021 Jun;102(6):389–96. PMID:33495124

2337. Liapis K, Clear A, Owen A, et al. The microenvironment of AIDS-related diffuse large B-cell lymphoma provides insight into the pathophysiology and indicates possible therapeutic strategies. Blood. 2013 Jul 18;122(3):424–33. PMID:23652804

2338. Lieber MR. Mechanisms of human lymphoid chromosomal translocations. Nat Rev Cancer. 2016 May 25;16(6):387–98. PMID:27220482

2339. Liebers N, Roider T, Bohn JP, et al. BRAF inhibitor treatment in classic hairy cell leukemia: a long-term follow-up study of patients treated outside clinical trials. Leukemia. 2020 May;34(5):1454–7. PMID:31740808

2340. Liebowitz D. Epstein-Barr virus and a cellular signaling pathway in lymphomas from immunosuppressed patients. N Engl J Med. 1998 May 14;338(20):1413–21. PMID:9580648

2341. Liebross RH, Ha CS, Cox JD, et al. Clinical course of solitary extramedullary plasmacytoma. Radiother Oncol. 1999 Sep;52(3):245–9. PMID:10580871

2341A. Lilleness B, Ruberg FL, Mussinelli R, et al. Development and validation of a survival staging system incorporating BNP in patients with light chain amyloidosis. Blood. 2019 Jan 17;133(3):215–23. PMID:30333122

2342. Lilljebjörn H, Henningsson R, Hyrenius-Wittsten A, et al. Identification of ETV6-RUNX1-like and DUX4-rearranged subtypes in paediatric B-cell precursor acute lymphoblastic leukaemia. Nat Commun. 2016 Jun 6;7:11790. PMID:27265895

2343. Lilly AJ, Fedoriw Y. Human immunodeficiency virus-associated lymphoproliferative disorders. Surg Pathol Clin. 2019 Sep;12(3):771–82. PMID:31352987

2344. Lim JQ, Huang D, Tang T, et al. Whole-genome sequencing identifies responders to pembrolizumab in relapse/refractory natural-killer/T cell lymphoma. Leukemia. 2020 Dec;34(12):3413–9. PMID:32753688

2345. Lim MS, Beaty M, Sorbara L, et al. T-cell/histiocyte-rich large B-cell lymphoma: a heterogeneous entity with derivation from germinal center B cells. Am J Surg Pathol. 2002 Nov;26(11):1458–66. PMID:12409722

2346. Lim MS, Carlson ML, Crockett DK, et al. The proteomic signature of NPM/ALK reveals deregulation of multiple cellular pathways. Blood. 2009 Aug 20;114(8):1585–95. PMID:19531656

2347. Lim MS, Straus SE, Dale JK, et al. Pathological findings in human autoimmune lymphoproliferative syndrome. Am J Pathol. 1998 Nov;153(5):1541–50. PMID:9811346

2348. Lim ST, Karim R, Tulpule A, et al. Prognostic factors in HIV-related diffuse large-cell lymphoma: before versus after highly active antiretroviral therapy. J Clin Oncol. 2005 Nov 20;23(33):8477–82. PMID:16230675

2349. Lim T, Kim SJ, Kim K, et al. Primary CNS lymphoma other than DLBCL: a descriptive analysis of clinical features and treatment outcomes. Ann Hematol. 2011 Dec;90(12):1391–8. PMID:21479535

2350. Lima M, Almeida J, Dos Anjos Teixeira M, et al. TCRalphabeta+/CD4+ large granular lymphocytosis: a new clonal T-cell lymphoproliferative disorder. Am J Pathol. 2003 Aug;163(2):763–71. PMID:12875995

2351. Limpens J, de Jong D, van Krieken JH, et al. Bcl-2/JH rearrangements in benign lymphoid tissues with follicular hyperplasia. Oncogene. 1991 Dec;6(12):2271–6. PMID:1766674

2352. Lin A, Cheng FWT, Chiang AKS, et al. Excellent outcome of acute lymphoblastic leukaemia with TCF3-PBX1 rearrangement in Hong Kong. Pediatr Blood Cancer. 2018 Dec;65(12):e27346. PMID:30051646

2353. Lin CW, Chang CL, Li CC, et al. Spontaneous regression of Kikuchi lymphadenopathy with oligoclonal T-cell populations favors a benign immune reaction over a T-cell lymphoma. Am J Clin Pathol. 2002 Apr;117(4):627–35. PMID:11939739

2354. Lin GW, Xu C, Chen K, et al. Genetic risk of extranodal natural killer T-cell lymphoma: a genome-wide association study in multiple populations. Lancet Oncol. 2020 Feb;21(2):306–16. PMID:31879220

2355. Lin J, Markowitz GS, Valeri AM, et al. Renal monoclonal immunoglobulin deposition disease: the disease spectrum. J Am Soc Nephrol. 2001 Jul;12(7):1482–92. PMID:11423577

2356. Lin O, Frizzera G. Angiomyoid and follicular dendritic cell proliferative lesions in Castleman's disease of hyaline-vascular type: a study of 10 cases. Am J Surg Pathol. 1997 Nov;21(11):1295–306. PMID:9351567

2357. Lin P, Jones D, Dorfman DM, et al. Precursor B-cell lymphoblastic lymphoma: a predominantly extranodal tumor with low propensity for leukemic involvement. Am J Surg Pathol. 2000 Nov;24(11):1480–90. PMID:11075849

2358. Lin P, Mansoor A, Bueso-Ramos C, et al. Diffuse large B-cell lymphoma occurring in patients with lymphoplasmacytic lymphoma/Waldenström macroglobulinemia. Clinicopathologic features of 12 cases. Am J Clin Pathol. 2003 Aug;120(2):246–53. PMID:12931555

2359. Lin P, Molina TJ, Cook JR, et al. Lymphoplasmacytic lymphoma and other non-marginal zone lymphomas with plasmacytic differentiation. Am J Clin Pathol. 2011 Aug;136(2):195–210. PMID:21757593

2360. Lin YC, Jhunjhunwala S, Benner C, et al. A global network of transcription factors, involving E2A, EBF1 and Foxo1, that orchestrates B cell fate. Nat Immunol. 2010 Jul;11(7):635–43. PMID:20543837

2361. Lindahl LM, Willerslev-Olsen A, Gjerdrum LMR, et al. Antibiotics inhibit tumor and disease activity in cutaneous T-cell lymphoma. Blood. 2019 Sep 26;134(13):1072–83. PMID:31331920

2362. Lindmark K, Pilebro B, Sundström T, et al. Prevalence of wild type transtyrethin cardiac amyloidosis in a heart failure clinic. ESC Heart Fail. 2021 Feb;8(1):745–9. PMID:33205581

2363. Linet MS, Vajdic CM, Morton LM, et al. Medical history, lifestyle, family history, and occupational risk factors for follicular lymphoma: the InterLymph Non-Hodgkin Lymphoma Subtypes Project. J Natl Cancer Inst Monogr. 2014 Aug;2014(48):26–40. PMID:25174024

2364. Ling YH, Zhu CM, Wen SH, et al. Pseudoepitheliomatous hyperplasia mimicking invasive squamous cell carcinoma in extranodal natural killer/T-cell lymphoma: a report of 34 cases. Histopathology. 2015 Sep;67(3):404–9. PMID:25619876

2365. Link BK, Maurer MJ, Nowakowski GS, et al. Rates and outcomes of follicular lymphoma transformation in the immunochemotherapy era: a report from the University of Iowa/MayoClinic Specialized Program of Research Excellence Molecular Epidemiology Resource. J Clin Oncol. 2013 Sep 10;31(26):3272–8. PMID:23897955

2366. Linke-Serinsöz E, Fend F, Quintanilla-Martinez L. Human immunodeficiency virus (HIV) and Epstein-Barr virus (EBV) related lymphomas, pathology view point. Semin Diagn Pathol. 2017 Jul;34(4):352–63. PMID:28506687

2367. Linnebank M, Moskau S, Kowoll A, et al. Association of transcobalamin c. 776C>G with overall survival in patients with primary central nervous system lymphoma. Br J Cancer. 2012 Nov 20;107(11):1840–3. PMID:23099805

2368. Liso A, Capello D, Marafioti T, et al. Aberrant somatic hypermutation in tumor cells of nodular-lymphocyte-predominant and classic Hodgkin lymphoma. Blood. 2006 Aug 1;108(3):1013–20. PMID:16614247

2369. Lister TA, Crowther D, Sutcliffe SB, et al. Report of a committee convened to discuss the evaluation and staging of patients with Hodgkin's disease: Cotswolds meeting. J Clin Oncol. 1989 Nov;7(11):1630–6. PMID:2809679

2370. Litzow MR, Ferrando AA. How I treat T-cell acute lymphoblastic leukemia in adults. Blood. 2015 Aug 13;126(7):833–41. PMID:25966987

2371. Liu AY, Nabel CS, Finkelman BS, et al. Idiopathic multicentric Castleman's disease: a systematic literature review. Lancet Haematol. 2016 Apr;3(4):e163–75. PMID:27063975

2372. Liu CY, Chen BJ, Chuang SS. Primary effusion lymphoma: a timely review on the association with HIV, HHV8, and EBV. Diagnostics (Basel). 2022 Mar 15;12(3):713. PMID:35328266

2373. Liu CY, Chen BJ, Chuang SS. Malignant effusions from extranodal NK/T-cell lymphomas are frequently of anaplastic morphology with azurophilic granules and of T-cell lineage. Diagn Cytopathol. 2020 May;48(5):453–63. PMID:32020785

2374. Liu F, Asano N, Tatematsu A, et al. Plasmablastic lymphoma of the elderly: a clinicopathological comparison with age-related Epstein-Barr virus-associated B cell lymphoproliferative disorder. Histopathology. 2012 Dec;61(6):1183–97. PMID:22958176

2375. Liu H, Brais R, Lavergne-Slove A, et al. Continual monitoring of intraepithelial lymphocyte immunophenotype and clonality is more important than snapshot analysis in the surveillance of refractory coeliac disease. Gut. 2010 Apr;59(4):452–60. PMID:19996326

2376. Liu H, Xiang C, Wu M, et al. Follicular dendritic cell sarcoma with co-expression of CD4 and CD30 mimics anaplastic large cell lymphoma. Front Oncol. 2020 May 29;10:876.

PMID:32547956
2377. Liu H, Xu-Monette ZY, Tang G, et al. EBV+ high-grade B cell lymphoma with MYC and BCL2 and/or BCL6 rearrangements: a multi-institutional study. Histopathology. 2022 Feb;80(3):575–88. PMID:34637146
2378. Liu H, Ye H, Ruskone-Fourmestraux A, et al. T(11;18) is a marker for all stage gastric MALT lymphomas that will not respond to H. pylori eradication. Gastroenterology. 2002 May;122(5):1286–94. PMID:11984515
2379. Liu HL, Hoppe RT, Kohler S, et al. CD30+ cutaneous lymphoproliferative disorders: the Stanford experience in lymphomatoid papulosis and primary cutaneous anaplastic large cell lymphoma. J Am Acad Dermatol. 2003 Dec;49(6):1049–58. PMID:14639383
2380. Liu Q, Salaverria I, Pittaluga S, et al. Follicular lymphomas in children and young adults: a comparison of the pediatric variant with usual follicular lymphoma. Am J Surg Pathol. 2013 Mar;37(3):333–43. PMID:23108024
2381. Liu W, Hu S, Konopleva M, et al. De novo MYC and BCL2 double-hit B-cell precursor acute lymphoblastic leukemia (BCP-ALL) in pediatric and young adult patients associated with poor prognosis. Pediatr Hematol Oncol. 2015;32(8):535–47. PMID:26558423
2382. Liu X, Loughran TP Jr. The spectrum of large granular lymphocyte leukemia and Felty's syndrome. Curr Opin Hematol. 2011 Jul;18(4):254–9. PMID:21546829
2383. Liu Y, Easton J, Shao Y, et al. The genomic landscape of pediatric and young adult T-lineage acute lymphoblastic leukemia. Nat Genet. 2017 Aug;49(8):1211–8. PMID:28671688
2384. Liu Y, Jelloul F, Zhang Y, et al. Genetic basis of extramedullary plasmablastic transformation of multiple myeloma. Am J Surg Pathol. 2020 Jun;44(6):838–48. PMID:32118627
2385. Liu Y, Ma C, Wang G, et al. Hydroa vacciniforme-like lymphoproliferative disorder: clinicopathologic study of 41 cases. J Am Acad Dermatol. 2019 Aug;81(2):534–40. PMID:30654082
2386. Liu Y, Sattarzadeh A, Diepstra A, et al. The microenvironment in classical Hodgkin lymphoma: an actively shaped and essential tumor component. Semin Cancer Biol. 2014 Feb;24:15–22. PMID:23867303
2387. Liu Y, Zhang W, An J, et al. Cutaneous intravascular natural killer-cell lymphoma: a case report and review of the literature. Am J Clin Pathol. 2014 Aug;142(2):243–7. PMID:25015867
2388. Liu YF, Wang BY, Zhang WN, et al. Genomic profiling of adult and pediatric B-cell acute lymphoblastic leukemia. EBioMedicine. 2016 Jun;8:173–83. PMID:27428428
2389. Liu YJ, Zhang J, Lane PJ, et al. Sites of specific B cell activation in primary and secondary responses to T cell-dependent and T cell-independent antigens. Eur J Immunol. 1991 Dec;21(12):2951–62. PMID:1748148
2390. Liu Z, Filip I, Gomez K, et al. Genomic characterization of HIV-associated plasmablastic lymphoma identifies pervasive mutations in the JAK-STAT pathway. Blood Cancer Discov. 2020 Jul;1(1):112–25. PMID:33225311
2391. Liu Z, Zhang Y, Zhu Y, et al. Prognosis of intravascular large B cell lymphoma (IVLBCL): analysis of 182 patients from global case series. Cancer Manag Res. 2020 Oct 23;12:10531–40. PMID:33122951
2392. Livingston B, Bonner A, Pope J. Differences in clinical manifestations between childhood-onset lupus and adult-onset lupus: a meta-analysis. Lupus. 2011 Nov;20(13):1345–55. PMID:21951943
2393. Lobello C, Tichy B, Bystry V, et al. STAT3 and TP53 mutations associate with poor prognosis in anaplastic large cell lymphoma. Leukemia. 2021 May;35(5):1500–5. PMID:33247178
2394. Locatelli F, Zugmaier G, Mergen N, et al. Blinatumomab in pediatric patients with relapsed/refractory acute lymphoblastic leukemia: results of the RIALTO trial, an expanded access study. Blood Cancer J. 2020 Jul 24;10(7):77. PMID:32709851
2395. Locke FL, Ghobadi A, Jacobson CA, et al. Long-term safety and activity of axicabtagene ciloleucel in refractory large B-cell lymphoma (ZUMA-1): a single-arm, multicentre, phase 1-2 trial. Lancet Oncol. 2019 Jan;20(1):31–42. PMID:30518502
2396. Loddenkemper C, Anagnostopoulos I, Hummel M, et al. Differential Emu enhancer activity and expression of BOB.1/OBF.1, Oct2, PU.1, and immunoglobulin in reactive B-cell populations, B-cell non-Hodgkin lymphomas, and Hodgkin lymphomas. J Pathol. 2004 Jan;202(1):60–9. PMID:14694522
2397. Loghavi S, Alayed K, Aladily TN, et al. Stage, age, and EBV status impact outcomes of plasmablastic lymphoma patients: a clinicopathologic analysis of 61 patients. J Hematol Oncol. 2015 Jun 10;8:65. PMID:26055271
2398. Loghavi S, Khoury JD, Medeiros LJ. Epstein-Barr virus-positive plasmacytoma in immunocompetent patients. Histopathology. 2015 Aug;67(2):225–34. PMID:25556356
2399. Loghavi S, Wang SA, Medeiros LJ, et al. Immunophenotypic and diagnostic characterization of angioimmunoblastic T-cell lymphoma by advanced flow cytometric technology. Leuk Lymphoma. 2016 Dec;57(12):2804–12. PMID:27105079
2400. Loh ML, Sakai DS, Flotho C, et al. Mutations in CBL occur frequently in juvenile myelomonocytic leukemia. Blood. 2009 Aug 27;114(9):1859–63. PMID:19571318
2401. Loh ML, Vattikuti S, Schubbert S, et al. Mutations in PTPN11 implicate the SHP-2 phosphatase in leukemogenesis. Blood. 2004 Mar 15;103(6):2325–31. PMID:14644997
2402. Lohneis P, Wienert S, Klauschen F, et al. Marginal zone lymphomas with monocytoid morphology express T-bet and are associated with a low number of T cells in extranodal locations. Leuk Lymphoma. 2014 Jan;55(1):143–8. PMID:23607257
2403. Löhr JM, Beuers U, Vujasinovic M, et al. European Guideline on IgG4-related digestive disease - UEG and SGF evidence-based recommendations. United European Gastroenterol J. 2020 Jul;8(6):637–66. PMID:32552502
2404. Lones MA, Cairo MS, Perkins SL. T-cell-rich large B-cell lymphoma in children and adolescents: a clinicopathologic report of six cases from the Children's Cancer Group study CCG-5961. Cancer. 2000 May 15;88(10):2378–86. PMID:10820362
2405. Lones MA, Raphael M, McCarthy K, et al. Primary follicular lymphoma of the testis in children and adolescents. J Pediatr Hematol Oncol. 2012 Jan;34(1):68–71. PMID:22215099
2406. Lo Nigro L. Biology of childhood acute lymphoblastic leukemia. J Pediatr Hematol Oncol. 2013 May;35(4):245–52. PMID:23612374
2407. Loo EY, Medeiros LJ, Aladily TN, et al. Classical Hodgkin lymphoma arising in the setting of iatrogenic immunodeficiency: a clinicopathologic study of 10 cases. Am J Surg Pathol. 2013 Aug;37(8):1290–7. PMID:23774171
2408. Loong F, Chan AC, Ho BC, et al. Diffuse large B-cell lymphoma associated with chronic inflammation as an incidental finding and new clinical scenarios. Mod Pathol. 2010 Apr;23(4):493–501. PMID:20062008
2409. Lopes JP, Ho HE, Cunningham-Rundles C. Interstitial lung disease in common variable immunodeficiency. Front Immunol. 2021 Mar 11;12:605945. PMID:33776995
2410. López C, Bergmann AK, Paul U, et al. Genes encoding members of the JAK-STAT pathway or epigenetic regulators are recurrently mutated in T-cell prolymphocytic leukaemia. Br J Haematol. 2016 Apr;173(2):265–73. PMID:26917488
2411. López C, Kleinheinz K, Aukema SM, et al. Genomic and transcriptomic changes complement each other in the pathogenesis of sporadic Burkitt lymphoma. Nat Commun. 2019 Mar 29;10(1):1459. PMID:30926794
2412. López-Corral L, Gutiérrez NC, Vidriales MB, et al. The progression from MGUS to smoldering myeloma and eventually to multiple myeloma involves a clonal expansion of genetically abnormal plasma cells. Clin Cancer Res. 2011 Apr 1;17(7):1692–700. PMID:21325290
2413. López-Corral L, Sarasquete ME, Beà S, et al. SNP-based mapping arrays reveal high genomic complexity in monoclonal gammopathies, from MGUS to myeloma status. Leukemia. 2012 Dec;26(12):2521–9. PMID:22565645
2414. Lopez-Hisijos N, Omman R, Pambuccian S, et al. Follicular dendritic cell sarcoma or not? A series of 5 diagnostically challenging cases. Clin Med Insights Oncol. 2019 May 23;13:1179554919844531. PMID:31205436
2415. López-Lerma I, Peñate Y, Gallardo F, et al. Subcutaneous panniculitis-like T-cell lymphoma: clinical features, therapeutic approach, and outcome in a case series of 16 patients. J Am Acad Dermatol. 2018 Nov;79(5):892–8. PMID:30126736
2416. López-Nevado M, Docampo-Cordeiro J, Ramos JT, et al. Next generation sequencing for detecting somatic FAS mutations in patients with autoimmune lymphoproliferative syndrome. Front Immunol. 2021 Apr 29;12:656356. PMID:33995372
2417. López-Nevado M, González-Granado LI, Ruiz-García R, et al. Primary immune regulatory disorders with an autoimmune lymphoproliferative syndrome-like phenotype: immunologic evaluation, early diagnosis and management. Front Immunol. 2021 Aug 10;12:671755. PMID:34447369
2418. Lopez-Olivo MA, Tayar JH, Martinez-Lopez JA, et al. Risk of malignancies in patients with rheumatoid arthritis treated with biologic therapy: a meta-analysis. JAMA. 2012 Sep 5;308(9):898–908. PMID:22948700
2419. Lorenzi L, Döring C, Rausch T, et al. Identification of novel follicular dendritic cell sarcoma markers, FDCSP and SRGN, by whole transcriptome sequencing. Oncotarget. 2017 Mar 7;8(10):16463–72. PMID:28145886
2420. Lorenzi L, Lonardi S, Essatari MH, et al. Intrafollicular Epstein-Barr virus-positive large B cell lymphoma. A variant of "germinotropic" lymphoproliferative disorder. Virchows Arch. 2016 Apr;468(4):441–50. PMID:26762526
2421. Lorenzi L, Tabellini G, Vermi W, et al. Occurrence of nodular lymphocyte-predominant Hodgkin lymphoma in Hermansky-Pudlak type 2 syndrome is associated to natural killer and natural killer T cell defects. PLoS One. 2013 Nov 26;8(11):e80131. PMID:24302998
2422. Lorsbach RB, Shay-Seymore D, Moore J, et al. Clinicopathologic analysis of follicular lymphoma occurring in children. Blood. 2002 Mar 15;99(6):1959–64. PMID:11877266
2423. Los-de Vries GT, de Boer M, van Dijk E, et al. Chromosome 20 loss is characteristic of breast implant-associated anaplastic large cell lymphoma. Blood. 2020 Dec 17;136(25):2927–32. PMID:33331925
2424. Los-de Vries GT, Stathi P, Rutkens R, et al. Large B-cell lymphomas of immune-privileged sites relapse via parallel clonal evolution from a common progenitor B cell. Cancer Res. 2023 Jun 2;83(11):1917–27. PMID:36971477
2425. Los-de Vries GT, Stevens WBC, van Dijk E, et al. Genomic and microenvironmental landscape of stage I follicular lymphoma, compared with stage III/IV. Blood Adv. 2022 Sep 27;6(18):5482–93. PMID:35816682
2426. Lossos IS, Alizadeh AA, Diehn M, et al. Transformation of follicular lymphoma to diffuse large-cell lymphoma: alternative patterns with increased or decreased expression of c-myc and its regulated genes. Proc Natl Acad Sci U S A. 2002 Jun 25;99(13):8886–91. PMID:12077300
2427. Lossos IS, Gascoyne RD. Transformation of follicular lymphoma. Best Pract Res Clin Haematol. 2011 Jun;24(2):147–63. PMID:21658615
2428. Loughran TP Jr. Clonal diseases of large granular lymphocytes. Blood. 1993 Jul 1;82(1):1–14. PMID:8324214
2429. Loughran TP Jr, Hadlock KG, Perzova R, et al. Epitope mapping of HTLV envelope seroreactivity in LGL leukaemia. Br J Haematol. 1998 May;101(2):318–24. PMID:9609528
2430. Louissaint A Jr, Ackerman AM, Dias-Santagata D, et al. Pediatric-type nodal follicular lymphoma: an indolent clonal proliferation in children and adults with high proliferation index and no BCL2 rearrangement. Blood. 2012 Sep 20;120(12):2395–404. PMID:22855608
2431. Louissaint A Jr, Ferry JA, Soupir CP, et al. Infectious mononucleosis mimicking lymphoma: distinguishing morphological and immunophenotypic features. Mod Pathol. 2012 Aug;25(8):1149–59. PMID:22627742
2432. Louissaint A Jr, Schafernak KT, Geyer JT, et al. Pediatric-type nodal follicular lymphoma: a biologically distinct lymphoma with frequent MAPK pathway mutations. Blood. 2016 Aug 25;128(8):1093–100. PMID:27325104
2433. Lousada I, Boedicker M. The impact of AL amyloidosis: the patient experience. Hematol Oncol Clin North Am. 2020 Dec;34(6):1193–203. PMID:33099433
2434. Love C, Sun Z, Jima D, et al. The genetic landscape of mutations in Burkitt lymphoma. Nat Genet. 2012 Dec;44(12):1321–5. PMID:23143597
2435. Lovec H, Grzeschiczek A, Kowalski MB, et al. Cyclin D1/bcl-1 cooperates with myc genes in the generation of B-cell lymphoma in transgenic mice. EMBO J. 1994 Aug 1;13(15):3487–95. PMID:8062825
2436. Lowe EJ, Reilly AF, Lim MS, et al. Brentuximab vedotin in combination with chemotherapy for pediatric patients with ALK+ ALCL: results of COG trial ANHL12P1. Blood. 2021 Jul 1;137(26):3595–603. PMID:33684925
2437. Lu CL, Tang Y, Yang QP, et al. Hepatosplenic T-cell lymphoma: clinicopathologic, immunophenotypic, and molecular characterization of 17 Chinese cases. Hum Pathol. 2011 Dec;42(12):1965–78. PMID:21683978
2438. Lu TX, Liang JH, Miao Y, et al. Epstein-Barr virus positive diffuse large B-cell lymphoma predict poor outcome, regardless of the age. Sci Rep. 2015 Jul 23;5:12168. PMID:26202875
2439. Lucas CL, Kuehn HS, Zhao F, et al. Dominant-activating germline mutations in the gene encoding the PI(3)K catalytic subunit p110δ result in T cell senescence and human immunodeficiency. Nat Immunol. 2014 Jan;15(1):88–97. PMID:24165795
2440. Lucas F, Larkin K, Gregory CT, et al. Novel BCL2 mutations in venetoclax-resistant, ibrutinib-resistant CLL patients with BTK/PLCG2 mutations. Blood. 2020 Jun 11;135(24):2192–5. PMID:32232486
2441. Luchtel RA, Dasari S, Oishi N, et al. Molecular profiling reveals immunogenic cues in anaplastic large cell lymphomas with

DUSP22 rearrangements. Blood. 2018 Sep 27;132(13):1386–98. PMID:30093402
2442. Luchtel RA, Zimmermann MT, Hu G, et al. Recurrent MSC E116K mutations in ALK-negative anaplastic large cell lymphoma. Blood. 2019 Jun 27;133(26):2776–89. PMID:31101622
2443. Lucioni M, Pescia C, Bonometti A, et al. Double expressor and double/triple hit status among primary cutaneous diffuse large B-cell lymphoma: a comparison between leg type and not otherwise specified subtypes. Hum Pathol. 2021 May;111:1–9. PMID:33548250
2444. Ludvigsson JF, Bai JC, Biagi F, et al. Diagnosis and management of adult coeliac disease: guidelines from the British Society of Gastroenterology. Gut. 2014 Aug;63(8):1210–28. PMID:24917550
2445. Lukes RJ, Butler JJ. The pathology and nomenclature of Hodgkin's disease. Cancer Res. 1966 Jun;26(6):1063–83. PMID:5947336
2446. Luminari S, Cesaretti M, Marcheselli L, et al. Decreasing incidence of gastric MALT lymphomas in the era of anti-Helicobacter pylori interventions: results from a population-based study on extranodal marginal zone lymphomas. Ann Oncol. 2010 Apr;21(4):855–9. PMID:19850642
2447. Luminari S, Merli M, Rattotti S, et al. Early progression as a predictor of survival in marginal zone lymphomas: an analysis from the FIL-NF10 study. Blood. 2019 Sep 5;134(10):798–801. PMID:31292118
2448. Lundell R, Hartung L, Hill S, et al. T-cell large granular lymphocyte leukemias have multiple phenotypic abnormalities involving pan-T-cell antigens and receptors for MHC molecules. Am J Clin Pathol. 2005 Dec;124(6):937–46. PMID:16416744
2449. Luo Y, Liu Z, Liu J, et al. Mycosis fungoides and variants of mycosis fungoides: a retrospective study of 93 patients in a Chinese population at a single center. Ann Dermatol. 2020 Feb;32(1):14–20. PMID:33911704
2450. Lurain K, Polizzotto MN, Aleman K, et al. Viral, immunologic, and clinical features of primary effusion lymphoma. Blood. 2019 Apr 18;133(16):1753–61. PMID:30782610
2451. Lyapichev KA, Piña-Oviedo S, Medeiros LJ, et al. A proposal for pathologic processing of breast implant capsules in patients with suspected breast implant anaplastic large cell lymphoma. Mod Pathol. 2020 Mar;33(3):367–79. PMID:31383966
2452. Lynch DT, Koya S, Acharya U, et al. Mantle cell lymphoma. 2023 Jul 28. In: StatPearls. Treasure Island (FL): StatPearls Publishing; 2024 Jan–. PMID:30725670
2453. Ma H, Tao W, Zhu S. T lymphocytes in the intestinal mucosa: defense and tolerance. Cell Mol Immunol. 2019 Mar;16(3):216–24. PMID:30787416
2454. Ma M, Wang X, Tang J, et al. Early T-cell precursor leukemia: a subtype of high risk childhood acute lymphoblastic leukemia. Front Med. 2012 Dec;6(4):416–20. PMID:23065427
2455. Ma RZ, Tian L, Tao LY, et al. The survival and prognostic factors of primary testicular lymphoma: two-decade single-center experience. Asian J Androl. 2018 Nov-Dec;20(6):615–20. PMID:30246707
2456. Ma Y, Visser L, Blokzijl T, et al. The CD4+CD26- T-cell population in classical Hodgkin's lymphoma displays a distinctive regulatory T-cell profile. Lab Invest. 2008 May;88(5):482–90. PMID:18362907
2457. Macaulay WL. Lymphomatoid papulosis. A continuing self-healing eruption, clinically benign–histologically malignant. Arch Dermatol. 1968 Jan;97(1):23–30. PMID:5634442
2458. Maccari ME, Fuchs S, Kury P, et al. A distinct CD38+CD45RA+ population of CD4+, CD8+, and double-negative T cells is controlled by FAS. J Exp Med. 2021 Feb 1;218(2):e20192191. PMID:33170215
2459. Macgrogan G, Vergier B, Dubus P, et al. CD30-positive cutaneous large cell lymphomas. A comparative study of clinicopathologic and molecular features of 16 cases. Am J Clin Pathol. 1996 Apr;105(4):440–50. PMID:8604686
2460. Machan S, Rodríguez M, Alonso-Alonso R, et al. Subcutaneous panniculitis-like T-cell lymphoma, lupus erythematosus profundus, and overlapping cases: molecular characterization through the study of 208 genes. Leuk Lymphoma. 2021 Sep;62(9):2130–40. PMID:33966586
2461. Maciocia N, O'Brien A, Ardeshna K. Remission of follicular lymphoma after treatment for hepatitis C virus infection. N Engl J Med. 2016 Oct 27;375(17):1699–701. PMID:27783921
2462. Mackrides N, Campuzano-Zuluaga G, Maque-Acosta Y, et al. Epstein-Barr virus-positive follicular lymphoma. Mod Pathol. 2017 Apr;30(4):519–29. PMID:27982024
2463. MacLennan IC. Germinal centers. Annu Rev Immunol. 1994;12:117–39. PMID:8011279
2464. MacLennan IC, Liu YJ, Oldfield S, et al. The evolution of B-cell clones. Curr Top Microbiol Immunol. 1990;159:37–63. PMID:2189692
2465. MacLennan KA, Bennett MH, Tu A, et al. Relationship of histopathologic features to survival and relapse in nodular sclerosing Hodgkin's disease. A study of 1659 patients. Cancer. 1989 Oct 15;64(8):1686–93. PMID:2790683
2466. Macon WR, Cousar JB, Waldron JA Jr, et al. Interleukin-4 may contribute to the abundant T-cell reaction and paucity of neoplastic B cells in T-cell-rich B-cell lymphomas. Am J Pathol. 1992 Nov;141(5):1031–6. PMID:1443042
2467. Macon WR, Levy NB, Kurtin PJ, et al. Hepatosplenic alphabeta T-cell lymphomas: a report of 14 cases and comparison with hepatosplenic gammadelta T-cell lymphomas. Am J Surg Pathol. 2001 Mar;25(3):285–96. PMID:11224598
2468. Madden SK, de Araujo AD, Gerhardt M, et al. Taking the Myc out of cancer: toward therapeutic strategies to directly inhibit c-Myc. Mol Cancer. 2021 Jan 4;20(1):3. PMID:33397405
2469. Maddocks KJ, Ruppert AS, Lozanski G, et al. Etiology of ibrutinib therapy discontinuation and outcomes in patients with chronic lymphocytic leukemia. JAMA Oncol. 2015 Apr;1(1):80–7. PMID:26182309
2470. Madero S, Oñate JM, Garzón A. Giant lymph node hyperplasia in an angiolipomatous mediastinal mass. Arch Pathol Lab Med. 1986 Sep;110(9):853–5. PMID:3755897
2471. Maekawa F, Kishimori C, Nakagawa M, et al. Truncation of 3' CCND1 by t(11;22) leads to negative SP4 CCND1 immunohistochemistry in blastoid mantle cell lymphoma. Blood Adv. 2021 Jan 12;5(1):61–5. PMID:33570637
2472. Maeshima AM, Taniguchi H, Suzuki T, et al. Comparison of clinicopathologic characteristics of gastric follicular lymphomas and duodenal follicular lymphomas. Hum Pathol. 2017 Jul;65:201–8. PMID:28504205
2473. Maeshima AM, Taniguchi H, Toyoda K, et al. Clinicopathological features of histological transformation from extranodal marginal zone B-cell lymphoma of mucosa-associated lymphoid tissue to diffuse large B-cell lymphoma: an analysis of 467 patients. Br J Haematol. 2016 Sep;174(6):923–31. PMID:27460179
2474. Magaña M, Massone C, Magaña P, et al. Clinicopathologic features of hydroa vacciniforme-like lymphoma: a series of 9 patients. Am J Dermatopathol. 2016 Jan;38(1):20–5. PMID:26368647
2475. Magaña M, Sangüeza P, Gil-Beristain J, et al. Angiocentric cutaneous T-cell lymphoma of childhood (hydroa-like lymphoma): a distinctive type of cutaneous T-cell lymphoma. J Am Acad Dermatol. 1998 Apr;38(4):574–9. PMID:9580256
2476. Maghsoudi R, Shakiba B, Panahi M, et al. Castleman disease mimicking an adrenal tumor: a case report. Urol Case Rep. 2021 Oct 1;40:101876. PMID:34646746
2477. Magnusson M, Beath K, Cooter R, et al. The epidemiology of breast implant-associated anaplastic large cell lymphoma in Australia and New Zealand confirms the highest risk for grade 4 surface breast implants. Plast Reconstr Surg. 2019 May;143(5):1285–92. PMID:30789476
2478. Magrath IT, Janus C, Edwards BK, et al. An effective therapy for both undifferentiated (including Burkitt's) lymphomas and lymphoblastic lymphomas in children and young adults. Blood. 1984 May;63(5):1102–11. PMID:6546890
2479. Magrath IT, Sariban E. Clinical features of Burkitt's lymphoma in the USA. IARC Sci Publ. 1985; (60):119–27. PMID:2998986
2480. Magro CM, Olson LC, Fulmer CG. CD30+ T cell enriched primary cutaneous CD4+ small/medium sized pleomorphic T cell lymphoma: a distinct variant of indolent CD4+ T cell lymphoproliferative disease. Ann Diagn Pathol. 2017 Oct;30:52–8. PMID:28965629
2481. Maguire A, Chen X, Wisner L, et al. Enhanced DNA repair and genomic stability identify a novel HIV-related diffuse large B-cell lymphoma signature. Int J Cancer. 2019 Dec 1;145(11):3078–88. PMID:31044434
2482. Mahajan VS, Mattoo H, Deshpande V, et al. IgG4-related disease. Annu Rev Pathol. 2014;9:315–47. PMID:24111912
2483. Mahmoud AZ, George TI, Czuchlewski DR, et al. Scoring of MYC protein expression in diffuse large B-cell lymphomas: concordance rate among hematopathologists. Mod Pathol. 2015 Apr;28(4):545–51. PMID:25431238
2484. Maia C, Puig N, Cedena MT, et al. Biological and clinical significance of dysplastic hematopoiesis in patients with newly diagnosed multiple myeloma. Blood. 2020 Jun 25;135(26):2375–87. PMID:32299093
2485. Maisnar V, Tichy M, Stulik J, et al. Capillary immunotyping electrophoresis and high resolution two-dimensional electrophoresis for the detection of mu-heavy chain disease. Clin Chim Acta. 2008 Mar;389(1-2):171–3. PMID:18036562
2486. Maisonobe L, Bertinchamp R, Damian L, et al. Characteristics of thrombocytopenia, anasarca, fever, reticulin fibrosis and organomegaly syndrome: a retrospective study from a large western cohort. Br J Haematol. 2022 Feb;196(3):599–605. PMID:34585382
2487. Maitra A, McKenna RW, Weinberg AG, et al. Precursor B-cell lymphoblastic lymphoma. A study of nine cases lacking blood and bone marrow involvement and review of the literature. Am J Clin Pathol. 2001 Jun;115(6):868–75. PMID:11392884
2488. Maitre E, Bertrand P, Maingonnat C, et al. New generation sequencing of targeted genes in the classical and the variant form of hairy cell leukemia highlights mutations in epigenetic regulation genes. Oncotarget. 2018 Jun 22;9(48):28866–76. PMID:29989027
2489. Maitre E, Tomowiak C, Lebecque B, et al. Deciphering genetic alterations of hairy cell leukemia and hairy cell leukemia-like disorders in 98 patients. Cancers (Basel). 2022 Apr 10;14(8):1904. PMID:35454811
2490. Makarova O, Oschlies I, Müller S, et al. Excellent outcome with limited treatment in paediatric patients with marginal zone lymphoma. Br J Haematol. 2018 Sep;182(5):735–9. PMID:28771659
2491. Mäkinen A, Nikkilä A, Haapaniemi T, et al. IGF2BP3 associates with proliferative phenotype and prognostic features in B-cell acute lymphoblastic leukemia. Cancers (Basel). 2021 Mar 25;13(7):1505. PMID:33805930
2492. Makishima H, Ito T, Momose K, et al. Chemokine system and tissue infiltration in aggressive NK-cell leukemia. Leuk Res. 2007 Sep;31(9):1237–45. PMID:17123604
2493. Makker J, Wotherspoon A, Tzioni MM, et al. Relapses in early-stage follicular lymphoma frequently develop via a divergent evolution from their clonally related precursor cells. J Pathol. 2024 Mar;262(3):289–95. PMID:38156368
2494. Maksten EF, Vase MØ, Kampmann J, et al. Post-transplant lymphoproliferative disorder following kidney transplantation: a population-based cohort study. Transpl Int. 2016 Apr;29(4):483–93. PMID:26749337
2495. Malamut G, Afchain P, Verkarre V, et al. Presentation and long-term follow-up of refractory celiac disease: comparison of type I with type II. Gastroenterology. 2009 Jan;136(1):81–90. PMID:19014942
2496. Malamut G, Chandesris O, Verkarre V, et al. Enteropathy associated T cell lymphoma in celiac disease: a large retrospective study. Dig Liver Dis. 2013 May;45(5):377–84. PMID:23313469
2497. Malamut G, El Machhour R, Montcuquet N, et al. IL-15 triggers an antiapoptotic pathway in human intraepithelial lymphocytes that is a potential new target in celiac disease-associated inflammation and lymphomagenesis. J Clin Invest. 2010 Jun;120(6):2131–43. PMID:20440074
2498. Malamut G, Meresse B, Cellier C, et al. Refractory celiac disease: from bench to bedside. Semin Immunopathol. 2012 Jul;34(4):601–13. PMID:22810901
2499. Malamut G, Meresse B, Kaltenbach S, et al. Small intestinal CD4+ T-cell lymphoma is a heterogenous entity with common pathology features. Clin Gastroenterol Hepatol. 2014 Apr;12(4):599–608.e1. PMID:24316103
2500. Malamut G, Verkarre V, Suarez F, et al. The enteropathy associated with common variable immunodeficiency: the delineated frontiers with celiac disease. Am J Gastroenterol. 2010 Oct;105(10):2262–75. PMID:20551941
2501. Malard F, Mohty M. Acute lymphoblastic leukaemia. Lancet. 2020 Apr 4;395(10230):1146–62. PMID:32247396
2502. Malavasi F, Deaglio S, Damle R, et al. CD38 and chronic lymphocytic leukemia: a decade later. Blood. 2011 Sep 29;118(13):3470–8. PMID:21765022
2503. Malcikova J, Tausch E, Rossi D, et al. ERIC recommendations for TP53 mutation analysis in chronic lymphocytic leukemia-update on methodological approaches and results interpretation. Leukemia. 2018 May;32(5):1070–80. PMID:29467486
2504. Małecka A, Delabie J, Østlie I, et al. Cold agglutinin-associated B-cell lymphoproliferative disease shows highly recurrent gains of chromosome 3 and 12 or 18. Blood Adv. 2020 Mar 24;4(6):993–6. PMID:32168377
2505. Małecka A, Trøen G, Tierens A, et al. Frequent somatic mutations of KMT2D (MLL2) and CARD11 genes in primary cold agglutinin disease. Br J Haematol. 2018 Dec;183(5):838–42. PMID:29265349
2506. Małecka A, Trøen G, Tierens A, et al. Immunoglobulin heavy and light chain gene features are correlated with primary cold agglutinin disease onset and activity. Haematologica. 2016 Sep;101(9):e361–4. PMID:27198717
2507. Maljaei SH, Brito-Babapulle V, Hiorns LR, et al. Abnormalities of chromosomes 8, 11, 14, and X in T-prolymphocytic leukemia studied

by fluorescence in situ hybridization. Cancer Genet Cytogenet. 1998 Jun;103(2):110–6. PMID:9614908
2508. Mallett RB, Matutes E, Catovsky D, et al. Cutaneous infiltration in T-cell prolymphocytic leukaemia. Br J Dermatol. 1995 Feb;132(2):263–6. PMID:7888364
2509. Malpica L, Enriquez DJ, Castro DA, et al. Real-world data on adult T-cell leukemia/lymphoma in Latin America: a study from the Grupo de Estudio Latinoamericano de Linfoproliferativos. JCO Glob Oncol. 2021 Jul;7:1151–66. PMID:34270330
2510. Malyukova A, Dohda T, von der Lehr N, et al. The tumor suppressor gene hCDC4 is frequently mutated in human T-cell acute lymphoblastic leukemia with functional consequences for Notch signaling. Cancer Res. 2007 Jun 15;67(12):5611–6. PMID:17575125
2511. Mamessier E, Broussais-Guillaumot F, Chetaille B, et al. Nature and importance of follicular lymphoma precursors. Haematologica. 2014 May;99(5):802–10. PMID:24790058
2512. Mamessier E, Drevet C, Broussais-Guillaumot F, et al. Contiguous follicular lymphoma and follicular lymphoma in situ harboring N-glycosylated sites. Haematologica. 2015 Apr;100(4):e155–7. PMID:25527563
2513. Mamessier E, Song JY, Eberle FC, et al. Early lesions of follicular lymphoma: a genetic perspective. Haematologica. 2014 Mar;99(3):481–8. PMID:24162788
2514. Mancao C, Hammerschmidt W. Epstein-Barr virus latent membrane protein 2A is a B-cell receptor mimic and essential for B-cell survival. Blood. 2007 Nov 15;110(10):3715–21. PMID:17682125
2515. Mandava A, Koppula V, Wortsman X, et al. The clinical value of imaging in primary cutaneous lymphomas: role of high resolution ultrasound and PET-CT. Br J Radiol. 2019 Mar;92(1095):20180904. PMID:30608186
2516. Mandelker DL, Dorfman DM, Li B, et al. Antigen expression patterns of MYC-rearranged versus non-MYC-rearranged B-cell lymphomas by flow cytometry. Leuk Lymphoma. 2014 Nov;55(11):2592–6. PMID:24397618
2517. Mani H, Jaffe ES. Hodgkin lymphoma: an update on its biology with new insights into classification. Clin Lymphoma Myeloma. 2009 Jun;9(3):206–16. PMID:19525189
2518. Manier S, Salem KZ, Park J, et al. Genomic complexity of multiple myeloma and its clinical implications. Nat Rev Clin Oncol. 2017 Feb;14(2):100–13. PMID:27531699
2519. Mann RB, Berard CW. Criteria for the cytologic subclassification of follicular lymphomas: a proposed alternative method. Hematol Oncol. 1983 Apr-Jun;1(2):187–92. PMID:6376315
2520. Manoukian SB, Kowal DJ. Comprehensive imaging manifestations of tuberous sclerosis. AJR Am J Roentgenol. 2015 May;204(5):933–43. PMID:25905927
2521. Manso R, González-Rincón J, Rodríguez-Justo M, et al. Overlap at the molecular and immunohistochemical levels between angioimmunoblastic T-cell lymphoma and a subgroup of peripheral T-cell lymphomas without specific morphological features. Oncotarget. 2018 Mar 1;9(22):16124–33. PMID:29662631
2522. Mansoor A, Pittaluga S, Beck PL, et al. NK-cell enteropathy: a benign NK-cell lymphoproliferative disease mimicking intestinal lymphoma: clinicopathologic features and follow-up in a unique case series. Blood. 2011 Feb 3;117(5):1447–52. PMID:20966166
2523. Mansouri L, Wierzbinska JA, Plass C, et al. Epigenetic deregulation in chronic lymphocytic leukemia: clinical and biological impact. Semin Cancer Biol. 2018 Aug;51:1–11. PMID:29427646
2524. Manzano M, Patil A, Waldrop A, et al. Gene essentiality landscape and druggable oncogenic dependencies in herpesviral primary effusion lymphoma. Nat Commun. 2018 Aug 15;9(1):3263. PMID:30111820
2525. Mao X, Lillington DM, Czepulkowski B, et al. Molecular cytogenetic characterization of Sézary syndrome. Genes Chromosomes Cancer. 2003 Mar;36(3):250–60. PMID:12557225
2526. Mao Z, Quintanilla-Martinez L, Raffeld M, et al. IgVH mutational status and clonality analysis of Richter's transformation: diffuse large B-cell lymphoma and Hodgkin lymphoma in association with B-cell chronic lymphocytic leukemia (B-CLL) represent 2 different pathways of disease evolution. Am J Surg Pathol. 2007 Oct;31(10):1605–14. PMID:17895764
2527. Marafioti T, Copie-Bergman C, Calaminici M, et al. Another look at follicular lymphoma: immunophenotypic and molecular analyses identify distinct follicular lymphoma subgroups. Histopathology. 2013 May;62(6):860–75. PMID:23509938
2528. Marafioti T, Mancini C, Ascani S, et al. Leukocyte-specific phosphoprotein-1 and PU.1: two useful markers for distinguishing T-cell-rich B-cell lymphoma from lymphocyte-predominant Hodgkin's disease. Haematologica. 2004 Aug;89(8):957–64. PMID:15339679
2529. Marafioti T, Paterson JC, Ballabio E, et al. Novel markers of normal and neoplastic human plasmacytoid dendritic cells. Blood. 2008 Apr 1;111(7):3778–92. PMID:18218851
2530. Marafioti T, Paterson JC, Ballabio E, et al. The inducible T-cell co-stimulator molecule is expressed on subsets of T cells and is a new marker of lymphomas of T follicular helper cell-derivation. Haematologica. 2010 Mar;95(3):432–9. PMID:20207847
2531. Marcel V, Dichtel-Danjoy ML, Sagne C, et al. Biological functions of p53 isoforms through evolution: lessons from animal and cellular models. Cell Death Differ. 2011 Dec;18(12):1815–24. PMID:21941372
2532. Marcelis L, Berghen C, De Zutter A, et al. Other immunomodulatory agent-related lymphoproliferative diseases: a single-center series of 72 biopsy-confirmed cases. Mod Pathol. 2018 Sep;31(9):1457–69. PMID:29765143
2533. Marcus A, Sadimin E, Richardson M, et al. Fluorescence microscopy is superior to polarized microscopy for detecting amyloid deposits in Congo red-stained trephine bone marrow biopsy specimens. Am J Clin Pathol. 2012 Oct;138(4):590–3. PMID:23010714
2534. Marcus R, Davies A, Ando K, et al. Obinutuzumab for the first-line treatment of follicular lymphoma. N Engl J Med. 2017 Oct 5;377(14):1331–44. PMID:28976863
2535. Mareschal S, Dubois S, Viailly PJ, et al. Whole exome sequencing of relapsed/refractory patients expands the repertoire of somatic mutations in diffuse large B-cell lymphoma. Genes Chromosomes Cancer. 2016 Mar;55(3):251–67. PMID:26608593
2536. Mareschal S, Pham-Ledard A, Viailly PJ, et al. Identification of somatic mutations in primary cutaneous diffuse large B-cell lymphoma, leg type by massive parallel sequencing. J Invest Dermatol. 2017 Sep;137(9):1984–94. PMID:28479318
2537. Margolskee E, Jobanputra V, Lewis SK, et al. Indolent small intestinal CD4+ T-cell lymphoma is a distinct entity with unique biologic and clinical features. PLoS One. 2013 Jul 4;8(7):e68343. PMID:23861889
2537A. Maric I, Pittaluga S, Dale JK, et al. Histologic features of sinus histiocytosis with massive lymphadenopathy in patients with autoimmune lymphoproliferative syndrome. Am J Surg Pathol. 2005 Jul;29(7):903–11. PMID:15958855
2538. Márkus B, Kántor E, Pintér G, et al. Adjuvant chemotherapy in the treatment of the breast. Acta Chir Hung. 1994;34(1-2):161–9. PMID:7604619
2539. Marques-Piubelli ML, Salas YI, Pachas C, et al. Epstein-Barr virus-associated B-cell lymphoproliferative disorders and lymphomas: a review. Pathology. 2020 Jan;52(1):40–52. PMID:31706670
2540. Marschalek R. Mechanisms of leukemogenesis by MLL fusion proteins. Br J Haematol. 2011 Jan;152(2):141–54. PMID:21118195
2541. Marshall NA, Christie LE, Munro LR, et al. Immunosuppressive regulatory T cells are abundant in the reactive lymphocytes of Hodgkin lymphoma. Blood. 2004 Mar 1;103(5):1755–62. PMID:14604957
2542. Martel M, Cheuk W, Lombardi L, et al. Sclerosing angiomatoid nodular transformation (SANT): report of 25 cases of a distinctive benign splenic lesion. Am J Surg Pathol. 2004 Oct;28(10):1268–79. PMID:15371942
2543. Marti GE, Rawstron AC, Ghia P, et al. Diagnostic criteria for monoclonal B-cell lymphocytosis. Br J Haematol. 2005 Aug;130(3):325–32. PMID:16042682
2544. Martin A, Capron F, Liguory-Brunaud MD, et al. Epstein-Barr virus-associated primary malignant lymphomas of the pleural cavity occurring in longstanding pleural chronic inflammation. Hum Pathol. 1994 Dec;25(12):1314–8. PMID:8001926
2545. Martin P, Chadburn A, Christos P, et al. Outcome of deferred initial therapy in mantle-cell lymphoma. J Clin Oncol. 2009 Mar 10;27(8):1209–13. PMID:19188674
2546. Martinelli G, Ryan G, Seymour JF, et al. Primary follicular and marginal-zone lymphoma of the breast: clinical features, prognostic factors and outcome: a study by the International Extranodal Lymphoma Study Group. Ann Oncol. 2009 Dec;20(12):1993–9. PMID:19570964
2547. Martinez A, Pittaluga S, Villamor N, et al. Clonal T-cell populations and increased risk for cytotoxic T-cell lymphomas in B-CLL patients: clinicopathologic observations and molecular analysis. Am J Surg Pathol. 2004 Jul;28(7):849–58. PMID:15223953
2548. Martinez D, Navarro A, Martinez-Trillos A, et al. NOTCH1, TP53, and MAP2K1 mutations in splenic diffuse red pulp small B-cell lymphoma are associated with progressive disease. Am J Surg Pathol. 2016 Feb;40(2):192–201. PMID:26426381
2549. Martinez D, Valera A, Perez NS, et al. Plasmablastic transformation of low-grade B-cell lymphomas: report on 6 cases. Am J Surg Pathol. 2013 Feb;37(2):272–81. PMID:23282972
2550. Martinez LL, Friedländer E, van der Laak JA, et al. Abundance of IgG4+ plasma cells in isolated reactive lymphadenopathy is no indication of IgG4-related disease. Am J Clin Pathol. 2014 Oct;142(4):459–66. PMID:25239412
2551. Martinez OM, Krams SM. The immune response to Epstein Barr virus and implications for posttransplant lymphoproliferative disorder. Transplantation. 2017 Sep;101(9):2009–16. PMID:28376031
2552. Martinez-Escala ME, Kantor RW, Cices A, et al. CD8+ mycosis fungoides: a low-grade lymphoproliferative disorder. J Am Acad Dermatol. 2017 Sep;77(3):489–96. PMID:28676328
2553. Martínez-Feito A, Melero J, Mora-Díaz S, et al. Autoimmune lymphoproliferative syndrome due to somatic FAS mutation (ALPS-sFAS) combined with a germline caspase-10 (CASP10) variation. Immunobiology. 2016 Jan;221(1):40–7. PMID:26323380
2554. Martinez-Lopez A, Curiel-Olmo S, Mollejo M, et al. MYD88 (L265P) somatic mutation in marginal zone B-cell lymphoma. Am J Surg Pathol. 2015 May;39(5):644–51. PMID:25723115
2555. Martínez-Onsurbe P, Jiménez-Heffernan JA, Guadalix-Hidalgo G. Fine needle aspiration cytology of intranodal myofibroblastoma. A case report. Acta Cytol. 2002 Nov-Dec;46(6):1143–7. PMID:12462097
2556. Martínez-Trillos A, Pinyol M, Delgado J, et al. The mutational landscape of small lymphocytic lymphoma compared to non-early stage chronic lymphocytic leukemia. Leuk Lymphoma. 2018 Oct;59(10):2318–26. PMID:29115891
2557. Martín-Garcia D, Navarro A, Valdés-Mas R, et al. CCND2 and CCND3 hijack immunoglobulin light-chain enhancers in cyclin D1- mantle cell lymphoma. Blood. 2019 Feb 28;133(9):940–51. PMID:30538135
2558. Martin-Guerrero I, Salaverria I, Burkhardt B, et al. Recurrent loss of heterozygosity in 1p36 associated with TNFRSF14 mutations in IRF4 translocation negative pediatric follicular lymphomas. Haematologica. 2013 Aug;98(8):1237–41. PMID:23445872
2559. Martín-Jiménez P, García-Sanz R, González D, et al. Molecular characterization of complete and incomplete immunoglobulin heavy chain gene rearrangements in hairy cell leukemia. Clin Lymphoma Myeloma. 2007 Nov;7(9):573–9. PMID:18186965
2560. Martín-Moro F, Marquet-Palomanes J, Piris-Villaespesa M, et al. Diffuse follicular lymphoma variant with a typical diagnostic pattern and an unusually aggressive clinical presentation. Int J Hematol. 2020 Aug;112(2):136–8. PMID:32506320
2561. Martino G, Ascani S. Atypical intrasinusoidal bone marrow involvement by hairy cell leukemia. Blood. 2020 Jan 30;135(5):392. PMID:31999816
2562. Martín-Subero JI, Gesk S, Harder L, et al. Recurrent involvement of the REL and BCL11A loci in classical Hodgkin lymphoma. Blood. 2002 Feb 15;99(4):1474–7. PMID:11830502
2563. Martín-Subero JI, Ibbotson R, Klapper W, et al. A comprehensive genetic and histopathologic analysis identifies two subgroups of B-cell malignancies carrying a t(14;19)(q32;q13) or variant BCL3-translocation. Leukemia. 2007 Jul;21(7):1532–44. PMID:17495977
2564. Martorana D, Márquez A, Carmona FD, et al. A large-scale genetic analysis reveals an autoimmune origin of idiopathic retroperitoneal fibrosis. J Allergy Clin Immunol. 2018 Nov;142(5):1662–5. PMID:30081155
2565. Marzano AV, Berti E, Alessi E, et al. Clonal CD8 infiltration of the skin in common variable immunodeficiency: a prelymphomatous stage? J Am Acad Dermatol. 2001 Apr;44(4):710–3. PMID:11260556
2566. Marzano AV, Vezzoli P, Mariotti F, et al. Paraneoplastic pemphigus associated with follicular dendritic cell sarcoma and Castleman disease. Br J Dermatol. 2005 Jul;153(1):214–5. PMID:16029358
2567. Masaki Y, Kawabata H, Fujimoto S, et al. Epidemiological analysis of multicentric and unicentric Castleman disease and TAFRO syndrome in Japan. J Clin Exp Hematop. 2019 Dec 22;59(4):175–8. PMID:31708515
2568. Masaki Y, Kawabata H, Takai K, et al. 2019 Updated diagnostic criteria and disease severity classification for TAFRO syndrome. Int J Hematol. 2020 Jan;111(1):155–8. PMID:31782045
2569. Masaki Y, Kawabata H, Takai K, et al. Proposed diagnostic criteria, disease severity classification and treatment strategy for TAFRO syndrome, 2015 version. Int J Hematol. 2016 Jun;103(6):686–92. PMID:27084250
2570. Masamune A, Kikuta K, Hamada S, et al.

Nationwide epidemiological survey of autoimmune pancreatitis in Japan in 2016. J Gastroenterol. 2020 Apr;55(4):462–70. PMID:31872350
2571. Maserati E, Ottolini A, Veggiotti P, et al. Ataxia-without-telangiectasia in two sisters with rearrangements of chromosomes 7 and 14. Clin Genet. 1988 Nov;34(5):283–7. PMID:3228996
2572. Masir N, Marafioti T, Jones M, et al. Loss of CD19 expression in B-cell neoplasms. Histopathology. 2006 Feb;48(3):239–46. PMID:16430470
2573. Mason EF, Brown RD, Szeto DP, et al. Detection of activating MAP2K1 mutations in atypical hairy cell leukemia and hairy cell leukemia variant. Leuk Lymphoma. 2017 Jan;58(1):233–6. PMID:27241017
2574. Mass J, Park DC. Posttransplant T lymphoblastic lymphoma mimicking Burkitt lymphoma. Blood. 2021 May 27;137(21):3002. PMID:34042977
2575. Massone C, Cerroni L. Phenotypic variability in primary cutaneous anaplastic large T-cell lymphoma: a study on 35 patients. Am J Dermatopathol. 2014 Feb;36(2):153–7. PMID:24394302
2576. Massone C, El-Shabrawi-Caelen L, Kerl H, et al. The morphologic spectrum of primary cutaneous anaplastic large T-cell lymphoma: a histopathologic study on 66 biopsy specimens from 47 patients with report of rare variants. J Cutan Pathol. 2008 Jan;35(1):46–53. PMID:18095994
2577. Massone C, Fink-Puches R, Cerroni L. Atypical clinical presentation of primary and secondary cutaneous follicle center lymphoma (FCL) on the head characterized by macular lesions. J Am Acad Dermatol. 2016 Nov;75(5):1000–6. PMID:27380773
2578. Massone C, Fink-Puches R, Laimer M, et al. Miliary and agminated-type primary cutaneous follicle center lymphoma: report of 18 cases. J Am Acad Dermatol. 2011 Oct;65(4):749–55. PMID:21601947
2579. Massone C, Kodama K, Kerl H, et al. Histopathologic features of early (patch) lesions of mycosis fungoides: a morphologic study on 745 biopsy specimens from 427 patients. Am J Surg Pathol. 2005 Apr;29(4):550–60. PMID:15767812
2580. Massoth LR, Hung YP, Ferry JA, et al. Histiocytic and dendritic cell sarcomas of hematopoietic origin share targetable genomic alterations distinct from follicular dendritic cell sarcoma. Oncologist. 2021 Jul;26(7):e1263–72. PMID:33904632
2581. Mata E, Fernández S, Astudillo A, et al. Genomic analyses of microdissected Hodgkin and Reed-Sternberg cells: mutations in epigenetic regulators and p53 are frequent in refractory classic Hodgkin lymphoma. Blood Cancer J. 2019 Mar 11;9(3):34. PMID:30858359
2582. Mateo M, Mollejo M, Villuendas R, et al. 7q31-32 allelic loss is a frequent finding in splenic marginal zone lymphoma. Am J Pathol. 1999 May;154(5):1583–9. PMID:10329610
2583. Mateo V, Ménager M, de Saint-Basile G, et al. Perforin-dependent apoptosis functionally compensates Fas deficiency in activation-induced cell death of human T lymphocytes. Blood. 2007 Dec 15;110(13):4285–92. PMID:17724145
2584. Matnani R, Ganapathi KA, Lewis SK, et al. Indolent T- and NK-cell lymphoproliferative disorders of the gastrointestinal tract: a review and update. Hematol Oncol. 2017 Mar;35(1):3–16. PMID:27353398
2585. Matsue K, Abe Y, Kitadate A, et al. Sensitivity and specificity of incisional random skin biopsy for diagnosis of intravascular large B-cell lymphoma. Blood. 2019 Mar 14;133(11):1257–9. PMID:30647028
2586. Matsue K, Abe Y, Narita K, et al. Diagnosis of intravascular large B cell lymphoma: novel insights into clinicopathological features from 42 patients at a single institution over 20 years. Br J Haematol. 2019 Nov;187(3):328–36. PMID:31267524
2587. Matsui S, Yamamoto H, Minamoto S, et al. Proposed diagnostic criteria for IgG4-related respiratory disease. Respir Investig. 2016 Mar;54(2):130–2. PMID:26879484
2588. Matsuoka R, Sakamoto N, Sakata-Yanagimoto M, et al. An overlapping case of in situ mantle cell neoplasia and leukemic non-nodal mantle cell lymphoma. J Clin Exp Hematop. 2020 Dec 15;60(4):169–73. PMID:33028761
2589. Mattano LA Jr, Devidas M, Maloney KW, et al. Favorable trisomies and ETV6-RUNX1 predict cure in low-risk B-cell acute lymphoblastic leukemia: results from Children's Oncology Group trial AALL0331. J Clin Oncol. 2021 May 10;39(14):1540–52. PMID:33739852
2590. Matthias P, Rolink AG. Transcriptional networks in developing and mature B cells. Nat Rev Immunol. 2005 Jun;5(6):497–508. PMID:15928681
2591. Mattia AR, Ferry JA, Harris NL. Breast lymphoma. A B-cell spectrum including the low grade B-cell lymphoma of mucosa associated lymphoid tissue. Am J Surg Pathol. 1993 Jun;17(6):574–87. PMID:8333556
2592. Mattoo H, Mahajan VS, Della-Torre E, et al. De novo oligoclonal expansions of circulating plasmablasts in active and relapsing IgG4-related disease. J Allergy Clin Immunol. 2014 Sep;134(3):679–87. PMID:24815737
2593. Mattoo H, Stone JH, Pillai S. Clonally expanded cytotoxic CD4+ T cells and the pathogenesis of IgG4-related disease. Autoimmunity. 2017 Feb;50(1):19–24. PMID:28166682
2594. Matutes E. Diagnostic and therapeutic challenges in hairy cell leukemia-variant: Where are we in 2021? Expert Rev Hematol. 2021 Apr;14(4):355–63. PMID:33759673
2595. Matutes E. Immunophenotyping and differential diagnosis of hairy cell leukemia. Hematol Oncol Clin North Am. 2006 Oct;20(5):1051–63. PMID:16990106
2596. Matutes E, Brito-Babapulle V, Swansbury J, et al. Clinical and laboratory features of 78 cases of T-prolymphocytic leukemia. Blood. 1991 Dec 15;78(12):3269–74. PMID:1742486
2597. Matutes E, Martínez-Trillos A, Campo E. Hairy cell leukaemia-variant: disease features and treatment. Best Pract Res Clin Haematol. 2015 Dec;28(4):253–63. PMID:26614904
2598. Matutes E, Morilla R, Owusu-Ankomah K, et al. The immunophenotype of splenic lymphoma with villous lymphocytes and its relevance to the differential diagnosis with other B-cell disorders. Blood. 1994 Mar 15;83(6):1558–62. PMID:8123845
2599. Matutes E, Oscier D, Garcia-Marco J, et al. Trisomy 12 defines a group of CLL with atypical morphology: correlation between cytogenetic, clinical and laboratory features in 544 patients. Br J Haematol. 1996 Feb;92(2):382–8. PMID:8603004
2600. Matutes E, Oscier D, Montalban C, et al. Splenic marginal zone lymphoma proposals for a revision of diagnostic, staging and therapeutic criteria. Leukemia. 2008 Mar;22(3):487–95. PMID:18094718
2601. Matutes E, Wotherspoon A, Brito-Babapulle V, et al. The natural history and clinico-pathological features of the variant form of hairy cell leukemia. Leukemia. 2001 Jan;15(1):184–6. PMID:11243388
2602. Matutes E, Wotherspoon A, Catovsky D. Differential diagnosis in chronic lymphocytic leukaemia. Best Pract Res Clin Haematol. 2007 Sep;20(3):367–84. PMID:17707827
2603. Matutes E, Wotherspoon A, Catovsky D. The variant form of hairy-cell leukaemia. Best Pract Res Clin Haematol. 2003 Mar;16(1):41–56. PMID:12670464
2604. Matutes E, Wotherspoon AC, Parker NE, et al. Transformation of T-cell large granular lymphocyte leukaemia into a high-grade large T-cell lymphoma. Br J Haematol. 2001 Dec;115(4):801–6. PMID:11843812
2605. Maubec E, Marinho E, Laroche L, et al. Primary cutaneous acral CD8+ T-cell lymphomas relapse more frequently in younger patients. Br J Haematol. 2019 May;185(3):598–601. PMID:30351475
2606. Maura F, Bolli N, Angelopoulos N, et al. Genomic landscape and chronological reconstruction of driver events in multiple myeloma. Nat Commun. 2019 Aug 23;10(1):3835. PMID:31444325
2607. Maura F, Dodero A, Carniti C, et al. CDKN2A deletion is a frequent event associated with poor outcome in patients with peripheral T-cell lymphoma not otherwise specified (PTCL-NOS). Haematologica. 2021 Nov 1;106(11):2918–26. PMID:33054126
2608. Maurus K, Appenzeller S, Roth S, et al. Panel sequencing shows recurrent genetic FAS alterations in primary cutaneous marginal zone lymphoma. J Invest Dermatol. 2018 Jul;138(7):1573–81. PMID:29481902
2609. Maurus K, Appenzeller S, Roth S, et al. Recurrent oncogenic JAK and STAT alterations in cutaneous CD30-positive lymphoproliferative disorders. J Invest Dermatol. 2020 Oct;140(10):2023–2031.e1. PMID:32147503
2610. Mauz-Körholz C, Gorde-Grosjean S, Hasenclever D, et al. Resection alone in 58 children with limited stage, lymphocyte-predominant Hodgkin lymphoma-experience from the European network group on pediatric Hodgkin lymphoma. Cancer. 2007 Jul 1;110(1):179–85. PMID:17526010
2611. Mayor PC, Eng KH, Singel KL, et al. Cancer in primary immunodeficiency diseases: cancer incidence in the United States Immune Deficiency Network Registry. J Allergy Clin Immunol. 2018 Mar;141(3):1028–35. PMID:28606585
2612. Mazloom A, Medeiros LJ, McLaughlin PW, et al. Marginal zone lymphomas: factors that affect the final outcome. Cancer. 2010 Sep 15;116(18):4291–8. PMID:20549822
2613. Mbulaiteye SM, Anderson WF, Bhatia K, et al. Trimodal age-specific incidence patterns for Burkitt lymphoma in the United States, 1973-2005. Int J Cancer. 2010 Apr 1;126(7):1732–9. PMID:19810101
2614. Mbulaiteye SM, Anderson WF, Ferlay J, et al. Pediatric, elderly, and emerging adult-onset peaks in Burkitt's lymphoma incidence diagnosed in four continents, excluding Africa. Am J Hematol. 2012 Jun;87(6):573–8. PMID:22488262
2615. Mbulaiteye SM, Biggar RJ, Bhatia K, et al. Sporadic childhood Burkitt lymphoma incidence in the United States during 1992-2005. Pediatr Blood Cancer. 2009 Sep;53(3):366–70. PMID:19434731
2616. McClory S, Hughes T, Freud AG, et al. Evidence for a stepwise program of extrathymic T cell development within the human tonsil. J Clin Invest. 2012 Apr;122(4):1403–15. PMID:22378041
2617. McDaniel LD, Schultz RA. Elevated sister chromatid exchange phenotype of Bloom syndrome cells is complemented by human chromosome 15. Proc Natl Acad Sci U S A. 1992 Sep 1;89(17):7968–72. PMID:1518822
2618. McKenzie RC, Jones CL, Tosi I, et al. Constitutive activation of STAT3 in Sézary syndrome is independent of SHP-1. Leukemia. 2012 Feb;26(2):323–31. PMID:21818116
2619. McKinney M, Moffitt AB, Gaulard P, et al. The genetic basis of hepatosplenic T-cell lymphoma. Cancer Discov. 2017 Apr;7(4):369–79. PMID:28122867
2620. McLean TW, Ringold S, Neuberg D, et al. TEL/AML-1 dimerizes and is associated with a favorable outcome in childhood acute lymphoblastic leukemia. Blood. 1996 Dec 1;88(11):4252–8. PMID:8943861
2621. McNamara C, Davies J, Dyer M, et al. Guidelines on the investigation and management of follicular lymphoma. Br J Haematol. 2012 Feb;156(4):446–67. PMID:22211428
2622. McNamara C, Montoto S, Eyre TA, et al. The investigation and management of follicular lymphoma. Br J Haematol. 2020 Nov;191(3):363–81. PMID:32579717
2623. McNeer JL, Devidas M, Dai Y, et al. Hematopoietic stem-cell transplantation does not improve the poor outcome of children with hypodiploid acute lymphoblastic leukemia: a report from Children's Oncology Group. J Clin Oncol. 2019 Apr 1;37(10):780–9. PMID:30742559
2624. McPhail ED, Maurer MJ, Macon WR, et al. Inferior survival in high-grade B-cell lymphoma with MYC and BCL2 and/or BCL6 rearrangements is not associated with MYC/IG gene rearrangements. Haematologica. 2018 Nov;103(11):1899–907. PMID:29903764
2625. Medeiros LJ, Marques-Piubelli ML, Sangiorgio VFI, et al. Epstein-Barr-virus-positive large B-cell lymphoma associated with breast implants: an analysis of eight patients suggesting a possible pathogenetic relationship. Mod Pathol. 2021 Dec;34(12):2154–67. PMID:34226673
2626. Meech SJ, McGavran L, Odom LF, et al. Unusual childhood extramedullary hematologic malignancy with natural killer cell properties that contains tropomyosin 4–anaplastic lymphoma kinase gene fusion. Blood. 2001 Aug 15;98(4):1209–16. PMID:11493472
2627. Meeker TC, Hardy D, Willman C, et al. Activation of the interleukin-3 gene by chromosome translocation in acute lymphocytic leukemia with eosinophilia. Blood. 1990 Jul 15;76(2):285–9. PMID:2114933
2628. Megahed NA, Kohno K, Sakakibara A, et al. Anaplastic variant of diffuse large B-cell lymphoma: reappraisal as a nodal disease with sinusoidal involvement. Pathol Int. 2019 Dec;69(12):697–705. PMID:31872533
2629. Mehta SH, Switzer JA, Biddinger P, et al. IgG4-related leptomeningitis: a reversible cause of rapidly progressive cognitive decline. Neurology. 2014 Feb 11;82(6):540–2. PMID:24384648
2630. Meijerink JP. Genetic rearrangements in relation to immunophenotype and outcome in T-cell acute lymphoblastic leukaemia. Best Pract Res Clin Haematol. 2010 Sep;23(3):307–18. PMID:21112032
2631. Meister A, Hentrich M, Wyen C, et al. Malignant lymphoma in the HIV-positive patient. Eur J Haematol. 2018 Jul;101(1):119–26. PMID:29663523
2632. Melani C, Jaffe ES, Wilson WH. Pathobiology and treatment of lymphomatoid granulomatosis, a rare EBV-driven disorder. Blood. 2020 Apr 16;135(16):1344–52. PMID:32107539
2633. Melchers RC, Willemze R, Bekkenk MW, et al. Frequency and prognosis of associated malignancies in 504 patients with lymphomatoid papulosis. J Eur Acad Dermatol Venereol. 2020 Feb;34(2):260–6. PMID:31715046
2634. Melchers RC, Willemze R, van de Loo M, et al. Clinical, histologic, and molecular characteristics of anaplastic lymphoma kinase-positive primary cutaneous anaplastic large cell lymphoma. Am J Surg Pathol. 2020 Jun;44(6):776–81. PMID:32412717
2635. Mele A, Pulsoni A, Bianco E, et al. Hepatitis C virus and B-cell non-Hodgkin lymphomas:

an Italian multicenter case-control study. Blood. 2003 Aug 1;102(3):996–9. PMID:12714514
2636. Mellors PW, Binder M, Ketterling RP, et al. Metaphase cytogenetics and plasma cell proliferation index for risk stratification in newly diagnosed multiple myeloma. Blood Adv. 2020 May 26;4(10):2236–44. PMID:32442300
2637. Melo JV, Catovsky D, Galton DA. The relationship between chronic lymphocytic leukaemia and prolymphocytic leukaemia. II. Patterns of evolution of 'prolymphocytoid' transformation. Br J Haematol. 1986 Sep;64(1):77–86. PMID:3463362
2638. Melo JV, Hegde U, Parreira A, et al. Splenic B cell lymphoma with circulating villous lymphocytes: differential diagnosis of B cell leukaemias with large spleens. J Clin Pathol. 1987 Jun;40(6):642–51. PMID:3497180
2639. Mena-Durán A, Muñoz Vicente E, Pareja Llorens G, et al. Liver failure caused by light chain deposition disease associated with multiple myeloma. Intern Med. 2012;51(7):773–6. PMID:22466837
2640. Mendenhall WM, Mendenhall CM, Mendenhall NP. Solitary plasmacytoma of bone and soft tissues. Am J Otolaryngol. 2003 Nov-Dec;24(6):395–9. PMID:14608572
2641. Mendeville M, Roemer MGM, van den Hout MFCM, et al. Aggressive genomic features in clinically indolent primary HHV8-negative effusion-based lymphoma. Blood. 2019 Jan 24;133(4):377–80. PMID:30510084
2642. Menguy S, Beylot-Barry M, Parrens M, et al. Primary cutaneous large B-cell lymphomas: relevance of the 2017 World Health Organization classification: clinicopathological and molecular analyses of 64 cases. Histopathology. 2019 Jun;74(7):1067–80. PMID:30715765
2643. Menguy S, Frison E, Prochazkova-Carlotti M, et al. Double-hit or dual expression of MYC and BCL2 in primary cutaneous large B-cell lymphomas. Mod Pathol. 2018 Aug;31(8):1332–42. PMID:29581544
2644. Menguy S, Gros A, Pham-Ledard A, et al. MYD88 somatic mutation is a diagnostic criterion in primary cutaneous large B-cell lymphoma. J Invest Dermatol. 2016 Aug;136(8):1741–4. PMID:27189828
2645. Menguy S, Laharanne E, Prochazkova-Carlotti M, et al. Challenges in assessing MYC rearrangement in primary cutaneous diffuse large B-cell lymphoma, leg-type. Am J Surg Pathol. 2020 Mar;44(3):424–7. PMID:31764222
2646. Menke DM, Horny HP, Griesser H, et al. Primary lymph node plasmacytomas (plasmacytic lymphomas). Am J Clin Pathol. 2001 Jan;115(1):119–26. PMID:11190797
2647. Menke JR, Spinner MA, Natkunam Y, et al. CD20-negative nodular lymphocyte-predominant Hodgkin lymphoma: a 20-year consecutive case series from a tertiary cancer center. Arch Pathol Lab Med. 2021 Jun 1;145(6):753–8. PMID:32991677
2648. Menon MP, Nicolae A, Meeker H, et al. Primary CNS T-cell lymphomas: a clinical, morphologic, immunophenotypic, and molecular analysis. Am J Surg Pathol. 2015 Dec;39(12):1719–29. PMID:26379152
2649. Menter T, Dirnhofer S, Tzankov A. LEF1: a highly specific marker for the diagnosis of chronic lymphocytic B cell leukaemia/small lymphocytic B cell lymphoma. J Clin Pathol. 2015 Jun;68(6):473–8. PMID:25713417
2650. Menter T, Ernst M, Drachneris J, et al. Phenotype profiling of primary testicular diffuse large B-cell lymphomas. Hematol Oncol. 2014 Jun;32(2):72–81. PMID:23949965
2651. Menter T, Gasser A, Juskevicius D, et al. Diagnostic utility of the germinal center-associated markers GCET1, HGAL, and LMO2 in hematolymphoid neoplasms. Appl Immunohistochem Mol Morphol. 2015 Aug;23(7):491–8. PMID:25203428
2652. Menter T, Juskevicius D, Alikian M, et al. Mutational landscape of B-cell post-transplant lymphoproliferative disorders. Br J Haematol. 2017 Jul;178(1):48–56. PMID:28419429
2653. Menter T, Medani H, Ahmad R, et al. MYC and BCL2 evaluation in routine diagnostics of aggressive B-cell lymphomas - presentation of a work-flow and the experience with 248 cases. Br J Haematol. 2017 Nov;179(4):681–4. PMID:27447126
2654. Menter T, Trivedi P, Ahmad R, et al. Diagnostic utility of lymphoid enhancer binding factor 1 immunohistochemistry in small B-cell lymphomas. Am J Clin Pathol. 2017 Mar 1;147(3):292–300. PMID:28395058
2655. Mention JJ, Ben Ahmed M, Bègue B, et al. Interleukin 15: a key to disrupted intraepithelial lymphocyte homeostasis and lymphomagenesis in celiac disease. Gastroenterology. 2003 Sep;125(3):730–45. PMID:12949719
2656. Mentz M, Keay W, Strobl CD, et al. PARP14 is a novel target in STAT6 mutant follicular lymphoma. Leukemia. 2022 Sep;36(9):2281–92. PMID:35851155
2657. Mercer LK, Davies R, Galloway JB, et al. Risk of cancer in patients receiving non-biologic disease-modifying therapy for rheumatoid arthritis compared with the UK general population. Rheumatology (Oxford). 2013 Jan;52(1):91–8. PMID:23238979
2658. Mercer LK, Regierer AC, Mariette X, et al. Spectrum of lymphomas across different drug treatment groups in rheumatoid arthritis: a European registries collaborative project. Ann Rheum Dis. 2017 Dec;76(12):2025–30. PMID:28822981
2659. Meriranta L, Pasanen A, Alkodsi A, et al. Molecular background delineates outcome of double protein expressor diffuse large B-cell lymphoma. Blood Adv. 2020 Aug 11;4(15):3742–53. PMID:32780847
2660. Merli M, Maffioli M, Ferrario A, et al. Looking for familial nodular lymphocyte-predominant Hodgkin lymphoma. Am J Hematol. 2013 Aug;88(8):719–20. PMID:23686933
2661. Merlini G. AL amyloidosis: from molecular mechanisms to targeted therapies. Hematology Am Soc Hematol Educ Program. 2017 Dec 8;2017(1):1–12. PMID:29222231
2662. Merlini G, Palladini G. Differential diagnosis of monoclonal gammopathy of undetermined significance. Hematology Am Soc Hematol Educ Program. 2012;2012:595–603. PMID:23233640
2663. Merlini G, Seldin DC, Gertz MA. Amyloidosis: pathogenesis and new therapeutic options. J Clin Oncol. 2011 May 10;29(14):1924–33. PMID:21483018
2664. Merlio JP, Kadin ME. Cytokines, genetic lesions and signaling pathways in anaplastic large cell lymphomas. Cancers (Basel). 2021 Aug 24;13(17):4256. PMID:34503066
2665. Merrill ED, Agbay R, Miranda RN, et al. Primary cutaneous T-cell lymphomas showing gamma-delta (γδ) phenotype and predominantly epidermotropic pattern are clinicopathologically distinct from classic primary cutaneous γδ T-cell lymphomas. Am J Surg Pathol. 2017 Feb;41(2):204–15. PMID:27879514
2666. Mescam L, Camus V, Schiano JM, et al. EBV+ diffuse large B-cell lymphoma associated with chronic inflammation expands the spectrum of breast implant-related lymphomas. Blood. 2020 May 28;135(22):2004–9. PMID:32110798
2667. Messmer BT, Albesiano E, Efremov DG, et al. Multiple distinct sets of stereotyped antigen receptors indicate a role for antigen in promoting chronic lymphocytic leukemia. J Exp Med. 2004 Aug 16;200(4):519–25. PMID:15314077
2668. Metcalf RA, Monabati A, Vyas M, et al. Myeloid cell nuclear differentiation antigen is expressed in a subset of marginal zone lymphomas and is useful in the differential diagnosis with follicular lymphoma. Hum Pathol. 2014 Aug;45(8):1730–6. PMID:24925224
2669. Metcalf RA, Zhao S, Anderson MW, et al. Characterization of D-cyclin proteins in hematolymphoid neoplasms: lack of specificity of cyclin-D2 and D3 expression in lymphoma subtypes. Mod Pathol. 2010 Mar;23(3):420–33. PMID:20062012
2670. Metter GE, Nathwani BN, Burke JS, et al. Morphological subclassification of follicular lymphoma: variability of diagnoses among hematopathologists, a collaborative study between the Repository Center and Pathology Panel for Lymphoma Clinical Studies. J Clin Oncol. 1985 Jan;3(1):25–38. PMID:3965631
2671. Meyer AH, Stroux A, Lerch K, et al. Transformation and additional malignancies are leading risk factors for an adverse course of disease in marginal zone lymphoma. Ann Oncol. 2014 Jan;25(1):210–5. PMID:24356632
2672. Meyer C, Burmeister T, Gröger D, et al. The MLL recombinome of acute leukemias in 2017. Leukemia. 2018 Feb;32(2):273–84. PMID:28701730
2673. Meyer C, Hofmann J, Burmeister T, et al. The MLL recombinome of acute leukemias in 2013. Leukemia. 2013 Nov;27(11):2165–76. PMID:23628958
2674. Meyerson HJ, Awadallah A, Pavlidakey P, et al. Follicular center helper T-cell (TFH) marker positive mycosis fungoides/Sezary syndrome. Mod Pathol. 2013 Jan;26(1):32–43. PMID:22918164
2675. Meznarich J, Miles R, Paxton CN, et al. Pediatric B-cell lymphoma with lymphoblastic morphology, TdT expression, MYC rearrangement, and features overlapping with Burkitt lymphoma. Pediatr Blood Cancer. 2016 May;63(5):938–40. PMID:26785246
2676. Mhawech-Fauceglia P, Oberholzer M, Aschenafi S, et al. Potential predictive patterns of minimal residual disease detected by immunohistochemistry on bone marrow biopsy specimens during a long-term follow-up in patients treated with cladribine for hairy cell leukemia. Arch Pathol Lab Med. 2006 Mar;130(3):374–7. PMID:16519567
2677. Miao Y, Hu S, Lu X, et al. Double-hit follicular lymphoma with MYC and BCL2 translocations: a study of 7 cases with a review of literature. Hum Pathol. 2016 Dec;58:72–7. PMID:27544800
2678. Michal M, Chlumská A, Povýsilová V. Intranodal "amianthoid" myofibroblastoma. Report of six cases immunohistochemical and electron microscopical study. Pathol Res Pract. 1992 Feb;188(1-2):199–204. PMID:1594491
2679. Michal M, Skálová A, Fakan F, et al. Littoral cell angioma of the spleen. A case report with ultrastructural and immunohistochemical observations. Zentralbl Pathol. 1993 Nov;139(4-5):361–5. PMID:7510515
2680. Michonneau D, Petrella T, Ortonne N, et al. Subcutaneous panniculitis-like T-cell lymphoma: immunosuppressive drugs induce better response than polychemotherapy. Acta Derm Venereol. 2017 Mar 10;97(3):358–64. PMID:27722764
2681. Miest RY, Comfere NI, Dispenzieri A, et al. Cutaneous manifestations in patients with POEMS syndrome. Int J Dermatol. 2013 Nov;52(11):1349–56. PMID:23557151
2682. Mignot F, Schernberg A, Arsène-Henry A, et al. Solitary plasmacytoma treated by lenalidomide-dexamethasone in combination with radiation therapy: clinical outcomes. Int J Radiat Oncol Biol Phys. 2020 Mar 1;106(3):589–96. PMID:31707123
2683. Miguet L, Lennon S, Baseggio L, et al. Cell-surface expression of the TLR homolog CD180 in circulating cells from splenic and nodal marginal zone lymphomas. Leukemia. 2013 Aug;27(8):1748–50. PMID:23302770
2684. Mikulasova A, Wardell CP, Murison A, et al. The spectrum of somatic mutations in monoclonal gammopathy of undetermined significance indicates a less complex genomic landscape than that in multiple myeloma. Haematologica. 2017 Sep;102(9):1617–25. PMID:28550183
2685. Miller DV, Firchau DJ, McClure RF, et al. Epstein-Barr virus-associated diffuse large B-cell lymphoma arising on cardiac prostheses. Am J Surg Pathol. 2010 Mar;34(3):377–84. PMID:20139760
2686. Mills SE. Decidua and squamous metaplasia in abdominopelvic lymph nodes. Int J Gynecol Pathol. 1983;2(2):209–15. PMID:6629633
2687. Milpied P, Gandhi AK, Cartron G, et al. Follicular lymphoma dynamics. Adv Immunol. 2021;150:43–103. PMID:34176559
2688. Minard-Colin V, Brugières L, Reiter A, et al. Non-Hodgkin lymphoma in children and adolescents: progress through effective collaboration, current knowledge, and challenges ahead. J Clin Oncol. 2015 Sep 20;33(27):2963–74. PMID:26304908
2689. Minici C, Gounari M, Übelhart R, et al. Distinct homotypic B-cell receptor interactions shape the outcome of chronic lymphocytic leukaemia. Nat Commun. 2017 Jun 9;8:15746. PMID:28598442
2690. Minnema MC, Kimby E, D'Sa S, et al. Guideline for the diagnosis, treatment and response criteria for Bing-Neel syndrome. Haematologica. 2017 Jan;102(1):43–51. PMID:27758817
2690A. Miranda RN, Aladily TN, Prince HM, et al. Breast implant-associated anaplastic large-cell lymphoma: long-term follow-up of 60 patients. J Clin Oncol. 2014 Jan 10;32(2):114–20. PMID:24323027
2691. Miranda RN, Briggs RC, Kinney MC, et al. Immunohistochemical detection of cyclin D1 using optimized conditions is highly specific for mantle cell lymphoma and hairy cell leukemia. Mod Pathol. 2000 Dec;13(12):1308–14. PMID:11144927
2692. Miranda RN, Cousar JB, Hammer RD, et al. Somatic mutation analysis of IgH variable regions reveals that tumor cells of most parafollicular (monocytoid) B-cell lymphoma, splenic marginal zone B-cell lymphoma, and some hairy cell leukemia are composed of memory B lymphocytes. Hum Pathol. 1999 Mar;30(3):306–12. PMID:10088550
2693. Miranda RN, Loo E, Medeiros LJ. Iatrogenic immunodeficiency-associated classical Hodgkin lymphoma: clinicopathologic features of 54 cases reported in the literature. Am J Surg Pathol. 2013 Dec;37(12):1895–7. PMID:24145656
2694. Miranda-Filho A, Piñeros M, Ferlay J, et al. Epidemiological patterns of leukaemia in 184 countries: a population-based study. Lancet Haematol. 2018 Jan;5(1):e14–24. PMID:29304322
2695. Mirels L, Ball WD. Neonatal rat submandibular gland protein SMG-A and parotid secretory protein are alternatively regulated members of a salivary protein multigene family. J Biol Chem. 1992 Feb 5;267(4):2679–87. PMID:1370829
2696. Mirza I, Macpherson N, Paproski S, et al. Primary cutaneous follicular lymphoma: an assessment of clinical, histopathologic, immunophenotypic, and molecular features. J Clin Oncol. 2002 Feb 1;20(3):647–55.

PMID:11821444
2697. Misawa S, Sato Y, Katayama K, et al. Vascular endothelial growth factor as a predictive marker for POEMS syndrome treatment response: retrospective cohort study. BMJ Open. 2015 Nov 11;5(11):e009157. PMID:26560063
2698. Misund K, Keane N, Stein CK, et al. MYC dysregulation in the progression of multiple myeloma. Leukemia. 2020 Jan;34(1):322–6. PMID:31439946
2699. Mitteldorf C, Stadler R, Sander CA, et al. Folliculotropic mycosis fungoides. J Dtsch Dermatol Ges. 2018 May;16(5):543–57. PMID:29726638
2700. Miwa H, Takakuwa T, Nakatsuka S, et al. DNA sequences of the immunoglobulin heavy chain variable region gene in pyothorax-associated lymphoma. Oncology. 2002;62(3):241–50. PMID:12065872
2701. Miyake T, Yamamoto T, Hirai Y, et al. Survival rates and prognostic factors of Epstein-Barr virus-associated hydroa vacciniforme and hypersensitivity to mosquito bites. Br J Dermatol. 2015 Jan;172(1):56–63. PMID:25234411
2702. Miyaoka M, Kikuti YY, Carreras J, et al. Clinicopathological and genomic analysis of double-hit follicular lymphoma: comparison with high-grade B-cell lymphoma with MYC and BCL2 and/or BCL6 rearrangements. Mod Pathol. 2018 Feb;31(2):313–26. PMID:28984304
2703. Miyoshi H, Sakata-Yanagimoto M, Shimono J, et al. RHOA mutation in follicular T-cell lymphoma: clinicopathological analysis of 16 cases. Pathol Int. 2020 Sep;70(9):653–60. PMID:32648273
2704. Miyoshi H, Sato K, Niino D, et al. Clinicopathologic analysis of peripheral T-cell lymphoma, follicular variant, and comparison with angioimmunoblastic T-cell lymphoma: Bcl-6 expression might affect progression between these disorders. Am J Clin Pathol. 2012 Jun;137(6):879–89. PMID:22586046
2705. Mizushima I, Kasashima S, Fujinaga Y, et al. Clinical and pathological characteristics of IgG4-related periaortitis/periarteritis and retroperitoneal fibrosis diagnosed based on experts' diagnosis. Ann Vasc Dis. 2019 Dec 25;12(4):460–72. PMID:31942203
2706. Mneimneh WS, Vyas SG, Cheng L, et al. Is ALK-gene rearrangement overlooked in primary gastrointestinal T-cell lymphomas? About two cases. Pathol Int. 2015 Dec;65(12):666–70. PMID:26531107
2707. Moccia AA, Donaldson J, Chhanabhai M, et al. International Prognostic Score in advanced-stage Hodgkin's lymphoma: altered utility in the modern era. J Clin Oncol. 2012 Sep 20;30(27):3383–8. PMID:22869887
2708. Modkharkar S, Navale P, Amare PK, et al. Applicability of 2008 World Health Organization classification system of hematolymphoid neoplasms: learning experiences. Indian J Pathol Microbiol. 2018 Jan-Mar;61(1):58–65. PMID:29567885
2709. Moffitt AB, Ondrejka SL, McKinney M, et al. Enteropathy-associated T cell lymphoma subtypes are characterized by loss of function of SETD2. J Exp Med. 2017 May 1;214(5):1371–86. PMID:28424246
2710. Mograbi M, Stump MS, Luyimbazi DT, et al. Pancreatic inflammatory pseudotumor-like follicular dendritic cell tumor. Case Rep Pathol. 2019 Dec 5;2019:2648123. PMID:31885993
2711. Moh M, Sangoi AR, Rabban JT. Angiomyomatous hamartoma of lymph nodes, revisited: clinicopathologic study of 21 cases, emphasizing its distinction from lymphangioleiomyomatosis of lymph nodes. Hum Pathol. 2017 Oct;68:175–83. PMID:28899739
2712. Mohammadi F, Wolverson MK, Bastani B. A new case of TEMPI syndrome. Clin Kidney J. 2012 Dec;5(6):556–8. PMID:26069800
2713. Mohan M, Buros A, Mathur P, et al. Clinical characteristics and prognostic factors in multiple myeloma patients with light chain deposition disease. Am J Hematol. 2017 Aug;92(8):739–45. PMID:28383130
2714. Mohseni M, Uludag H, Brandwein JM. Advances in biology of acute lymphoblastic leukemia (ALL) and therapeutic implications. Am J Blood Res. 2018 Dec 10;8(4):29–56. PMID:30697448
2715. Molica S, Baumann TS, Lentini M, et al. The BALL prognostic score identifies relapsed/refractory CLL patients who benefit the most from single-agent ibrutinib therapy. Leuk Res. 2020 Aug;95:106401. PMID:32562875
2716. Molica S, Tucci L, Levato D, et al. Clinical and prognostic evaluation of bone marrow infiltration (biopsy versus aspirate) in early chronic lymphocytic leukemia. A single center study. Haematologica. 1997 May-Jun;82(3):286–90. PMID:9234573
2717. Molin D, Linderoth J, Wahlin BE. Nodular lymphocyte predominant Hodgkin lymphoma in Sweden between 2000 and 2014: an analysis of the Swedish Lymphoma Registry. Br J Haematol. 2017 May;177(3):449–56. PMID:28233899
2718. Mollejo M, Algara P, Mateo MS, et al. Splenic small B-cell lymphoma with predominant red pulp involvement: a diffuse variant of splenic marginal zone lymphoma? Histopathology. 2002 Jan;40(1):22–30. PMID:11903595
2719. Mollejo M, Menárguez J, Lloret E, et al. Splenic marginal zone lymphoma: a distinctive type of low-grade B-cell lymphoma. A clinicopathological study of 13 cases. Am J Surg Pathol. 1995 Oct;19(10):1146–57. PMID:7573673
2720. Möller P, Lämmler B, Herrmann B, et al. The primary mediastinal clear cell lymphoma of B-cell type has variable defects in MHC antigen expression. Immunology. 1986 Nov;59(3):411–7. PMID:3491784
2721. Möller P, Moldenhauer G, Momburg F, et al. Mediastinal lymphoma of clear cell type is a tumor corresponding to terminal steps of B cell differentiation. Blood. 1987 Apr;69(4):1087–95. PMID:3103712
2722. Molyneux EM, Rochford R, Griffin B, et al. Burkitt's lymphoma. Lancet. 2012 Mar 31;379(9822):1234–44. PMID:22333947
2723. Momose S, Tamaru JI. Iatrogenic immunodeficiency-associated lymphoproliferative disorders of B-cell type that develop in patients receiving immunosuppressive drugs other than in the post-transplant setting. J Clin Exp Hematop. 2019;59(2):48–55. PMID:31257345
2724. Momose S, Weißbach S, Pischimarov J, et al. The diagnostic gray zone between Burkitt lymphoma and diffuse large B-cell lymphoma is also a gray zone of the mutational spectrum. Leukemia. 2015 Aug;29(8):1789–91. PMID:25673238
2725. Momota H, Narita Y, Maeshima AM, et al. Prognostic value of immunohistochemical profile and response to high-dose methotrexate therapy in primary CNS lymphoma. J Neurooncol. 2010 Jul;98(3):341–8. PMID:20012911
2726. Momotow J, Borchmann S, Eichenauer DA, et al. Hodgkin lymphoma-review on pathogenesis, diagnosis, current and future treatment approaches for adult patients. J Clin Med. 2021 Mar 8;10(5):1125. PMID:33800409
2727. Monabati A, Safaei A, Noori S, et al. Subtype distribution of lymphomas in South of Iran, analysis of 1085 cases based on World Health Organization classification. Ann Hematol. 2016 Mar;95(4):613–8. PMID:26754635
2728. Monda L, Warnke R, Rosai J. A primary lymph node malignancy with features suggestive of dendritic reticulum cell differentiation. A report of 4 cases. Am J Pathol. 1986 Mar;122(3):562–72. PMID:2420185
2729. Monforte-Muñoz H, Ro JY, Manning JT Jr, et al. Inflammatory pseudotumor of the spleen. Report of two cases with a review of the literature. Am J Clin Pathol. 1991 Oct;96(4):491–5. PMID:1892124
2730. Monga N, Nastoupil L, Garside J, et al. Burden of illness of follicular lymphoma and marginal zone lymphoma. Ann Hematol. 2019 Jan;98(1):175–83. PMID:30315345
2731. Monnereau A, Slager SL, Hughes AM, et al. Medical history, lifestyle, and occupational risk factors for hairy cell leukemia: the InterLymph Non-Hodgkin Lymphoma Subtypes Project. J Natl Cancer Inst Monogr. 2014 Aug;2014(48):115–24. PMID:25174032
2732. Montalbán C, Abraira V, Arcaini L, et al. Risk stratification for splenic marginal zone lymphoma based on haemoglobin concentration, platelet count, high lactate dehydrogenase level and extrahilar lymphadenopathy: development and validation on 593 cases. Br J Haematol. 2012 Oct;159(2):164–71. PMID:22924582
2733. Montanari F, O'Connor OA, Savage DG, et al. Bone marrow involvement in patients with posttransplant lymphoproliferative disorders: incidence and prognostic factors. Hum Pathol. 2010 Aug;41(8):1150–8. PMID:20381113
2734. Montanari F, Radeski D, Seshan V, et al. Recursive partitioning analysis of prognostic factors in post-transplant lymphoproliferative disorders (PTLD): a 120 case single institution series. Br J Haematol. 2015 Nov;171(4):491–500. PMID:26250758
2735. Montes de Jesus F, Vergote V, Noordzij W, et al. Semi-quantitative characterization of post-transplant lymphoproliferative disorder morphological subtypes with [18F]FDG PET/CT. J Clin Med. 2021 Jan 19;10(2):361. PMID:33477971
2736. Montesinos-Rongen M, Akasaka T, Zühlke-Jenisch R, et al. Molecular characterization of BCL6 breakpoints in primary diffuse large B-cell lymphomas of the central nervous system identifies GAPD as novel translocation partner. Brain Pathol. 2003 Oct;13(4):534–8. PMID:14655758
2737. Montesinos-Rongen M, Brunn A, Bentink S, et al. Gene expression profiling suggests primary central nervous system lymphomas to be derived from a late germinal center B cell. Leukemia. 2008 Feb;22(2):400–5. PMID:17989719
2738. Montesinos-Rongen M, Brunn A, Tuchscherer A, et al. Analysis of driver mutational hot spots in blood-derived cell-free DNA of patients with primary central nervous system lymphoma obtained before intracerebral biopsy. J Mol Diagn. 2020 Oct;22(10):1300–7. PMID:32745612
2739. Montesinos-Rongen M, Godlewska E, Brunn A, et al. Activating L265P mutations of the MYD88 gene are common in primary central nervous system lymphoma. Acta Neuropathol. 2011 Dec;122(6):791–2. PMID:22020631
2740. Montesinos-Rongen M, Küppers R, Schlüter D, et al. Primary central nervous system lymphomas are derived from germinal-center B cells and show a preferential usage of the V4-34 gene segment. Am J Pathol. 1999 Dec;155(6):2077–86. PMID:10595937
2741. Montesinos-Rongen M, Purschke F, Brunn A, et al. Response to comment on "Primary central nervous system (CNS) lymphoma B cell receptors recognize CNS proteins". J Immunol. 2015 Nov 15;195(10):4550–1. PMID:26546684
2742. Montesinos-Rongen M, Purschke F, Küppers R, et al. Immunoglobulin repertoire of primary lymphomas of the central nervous system. J Neuropathol Exp Neurol. 2014 Dec;73(12):1116–25. PMID:25383641
2743. Montesinos-Rongen M, Purschke FG, Brunn A, et al. Primary central nervous system (CNS) lymphoma B cell receptors recognize CNS proteins. J Immunol. 2015 Aug 1;195(3):1312–9. PMID:26116512
2744. Montesinos-Rongen M, Schäfer E, Siebert R, et al. Genes regulating the B cell receptor pathway are recurrently mutated in primary central nervous system lymphoma. Acta Neuropathol. 2012 Dec;124(6):905–6. PMID:23138649
2745. Montesinos-Rongen M, Terrao M, May C, et al. The process of somatic hypermutation increases polyreactivity for central nervous system antigens in primary central nervous system lymphoma. Haematologica. 2021 Mar 1;106(3):708–17. PMID:32193251
2746. Montesinos-Rongen M, Van Roost D, Schaller C, et al. Primary diffuse large B-cell lymphomas of the central nervous system are targeted by aberrant somatic hypermutation. Blood. 2004 Mar 1;103(5):1869–75. PMID:14592832
2747. Montesinos-Rongen M, Zühlke-Jenisch R, Gesk S, et al. Interphase cytogenetic analysis of lymphoma-associated chromosomal breakpoints in primary diffuse large B-cell lymphomas of the central nervous system. J Neuropathol Exp Neurol. 2002 Oct;61(10):926–33. PMID:12387458
2748. Montes-Mojarro IA, Chen BJ, Ramirez-Ibarguen AF, et al. Mutational profile and EBV strains of extranodal NK/T-cell lymphoma, nasal type in Latin America. Mod Pathol. 2020 May;33(5):781–91. PMID:31822801
2749. Montes-Mojarro IA, Kim WY, Fend F, et al. Epstein - Barr virus positive T and NK-cell lymphoproliferations: morphological features and differential diagnosis. Semin Diagn Pathol. 2020 Jan;37(1):32–46. PMID:31889602
2750. Montes-Mojarro IA, Steinhilber J, Bonzheim I, et al. The pathological spectrum of systemic anaplastic large cell lymphoma (ALCL). Cancers (Basel). 2018 Apr 4;10(4):107. PMID:29617304
2751. Montes-Moreno S, Castro Y, Rodríguez-Pinilla SM, et al. Intrafollicular neoplasia/in situ follicular lymphoma: review of a series of 13 cases. Histopathology. 2010 Apr;56(5):658–62. PMID:20459579
2752. Montes-Moreno S, Gonzalez-Medina AR, Rodriguez-Pinilla SM, et al. Aggressive large B-cell lymphoma with plasma cell differentiation: immunohistochemical characterization of plasmablastic lymphoma and diffuse large B-cell lymphoma with partial plasmablastic phenotype. Haematologica. 2010 Aug;95(8):1342–9. PMID:20418245
2753. Montes-Moreno S, King RL, Oschlies I, et al. Update on lymphoproliferative disorders of the gastrointestinal tract: disease spectrum from indolent lymphoproliferations to aggressive lymphomas. Virchows Arch. 2020 May;476(5):667–81. PMID:31773249
2754. Montes-Moreno S, Martinez-Magunacelaya N, Zecchini-Barrese T, et al. Plasmablastic lymphoma phenotype is determined by genetic alterations in MYC and PRDM1. Mod Pathol. 2017 Jan;30(1):85–94. PMID:27687004
2755. Montes-Moreno S, Odqvist L, Diaz-Perez JA, et al. EBV-positive diffuse large B-cell lymphoma of the elderly is an aggressive post-germinal center B-cell neoplasm characterized by prominent nuclear factor-kB activation. Mod Pathol. 2012 Jul;25(7):968–82. PMID:22538516
2756. Montes-Moreno S, Roncador G, Maestre L, et al. Gcet1 (centerin), a highly restricted marker for a subset of germinal center-derived lymphomas. Blood. 2008 Jan 1;111(1):351–8. PMID:17898315
2757. Monti G, Pioltelli P, Saccardo F, et al.

Incidence and characteristics of non-Hodgkin lymphomas in a multicenter case file of patients with hepatitis C virus-related symptomatic mixed cryoglobulinemias. Arch Intern Med. 2005 Jan 10;165(1):101–5. PMID:15642884
2758. Montoto S, Davies AJ, Matthews J, et al. Risk and clinical implications of transformation of follicular lymphoma to diffuse large B-cell lymphoma. J Clin Oncol. 2007 Jun 10;25(17):2426–33. PMID:17485708
2759. Montoto S, Shaw K, Okosun J, et al. HIV status does not influence outcome in patients with classical Hodgkin lymphoma treated with chemotherapy using doxorubicin, bleomycin, vinblastine, and dacarbazine in the highly active antiretroviral therapy era. J Clin Oncol. 2012 Nov 20;30(33):4111–6. PMID:23045581
2760. Montserrat E, Villamor N, Reverter JC, et al. Bone marrow assessment in B-cell chronic lymphocytic leukaemia: aspirate or biopsy? A comparative study in 258 patients. Br J Haematol. 1996 Apr;93(1):111–6. PMID:8611442
2761. Moody S, Escudero-Ibarz L, Wang M, et al. Significant association between TNFAIP3 inactivation and biased immunoglobulin heavy chain variable region 4-34 usage in mucosa-associated lymphoid tissue lymphoma. J Pathol. 2017 Sep;243(1):3–8. PMID:28682481
2762. Moody S, Thompson JS, Chuang SS, et al. Novel GPR34 and CCR6 mutation and distinct genetic profiles in MALT lymphomas of different sites. Haematologica. 2018 Aug;103(8):1329–36. PMID:29674500
2763. Moore EM, Aggarwal N, Surti U, et al. Further exploration of the complexities of large B-cell lymphomas with MYC abnormalities and the importance of a blastoid morphology. Am J Surg Pathol. 2017 Sep;41(9):1155–66. PMID:28614202
2764. Moore EM, Swerdlow SH, Gibson SE. Comparison of myocyte enhancer factor 2B versus other germinal center-associated antigens in the differential diagnosis of B-cell non-Hodgkin lymphomas. Am J Surg Pathol. 2018 Mar;42(3):342–50. PMID:29309299
2765. Moore EM, Swerdlow SH, Gibson SE. J chain and myocyte enhancer factor 2B are useful in differentiating classical Hodgkin lymphoma from nodular lymphocyte predominant Hodgkin lymphoma and primary mediastinal large B-cell lymphoma. Hum Pathol. 2017 Oct;68:47–53. PMID:28851661
2766. Moorman AV, Chilton L, Wilkinson J, et al. A population-based cytogenetic study of adults with acute lymphoblastic leukemia. Blood. 2010 Jan 14;115(2):206–14. PMID:19897583
2767. Moorman AV, Harrison CJ, Buck GA, et al. Karyotype is an independent prognostic factor in adult acute lymphoblastic leukemia (ALL): analysis of cytogenetic data from patients treated on the Medical Research Council (MRC) UKALLXII/Eastern Cooperative Oncology Group (ECOG) 2993 trial. Blood. 2007 Apr 15;109(8):3189–97. PMID:17170120
2768. Moorman AV, Richards SM, Martineau M, et al. Outcome heterogeneity in childhood high-hyperdiploid acute lymphoblastic leukemia. Blood. 2003 Oct 15;102(8):2756–62. PMID:12829593
2769. Moorman AV, Richards SM, Robinson HM, et al. Prognosis of children with acute lymphoblastic leukemia (ALL) and intrachromosomal amplification of chromosome 21 (iAMP21). Blood. 2007 Mar 15;109(6):2327–30. PMID:17095619
2770. Moorman AV, Robinson H, Schwab C, et al. Risk-directed treatment intensification significantly reduces the risk of relapse among children and adolescents with acute lymphoblastic leukemia and intrachromosomal amplification of chromosome 21: a comparison of the MRC ALL97/99 and UKALL2003 trials. J Clin Oncol. 2013 Sep 20;31(27):3389–96. PMID:23940220
2771. Moormann AM, Heller KN, Chelimo K, et al. Children with endemic Burkitt lymphoma are deficient in EBNA1-specific IFN-gamma T cell responses. Int J Cancer. 2009 Apr 1;124(7):1721–6. PMID:19089927
2772. Moormeier JA, Neilly ME, Vardiman JW, et al. Familial lymphoproliferative disorders with chromosomal fragile site analysis. Leuk Lymphoma. 1991;5(5-6):311–6. PMID:27463340
2773. Morabito F, Mosca L, Cutrona G, et al. Clinical monoclonal B lymphocytosis versus Rai 0 chronic lymphocytic leukemia: a comparison of cellular, cytogenetic, molecular, and clinical features. Clin Cancer Res. 2013 Nov 1;19(21):5890–900. PMID:24036852
2774. Morak M, Attarbaschi A, Fischer S, et al. Small sizes and indolent evolutionary dynamics challenge the potential role of P2RY8-CRLF2-harboring clones as main relapse-driving force in childhood ALL. Blood. 2012 Dec 20;120(26):5134–42. PMID:23091296
2775. Morales AT, Cignarella AG, Jabeen IS, et al. An update on IgG4-related lung disease. Eur J Intern Med. 2019 Aug;66:18–24. PMID:31227290
2776. Morales AV, Arber DA, Seo K, et al. Evaluation of B-cell clonality using the BIOMED-2 PCR method effectively distinguishes cutaneous B-cell lymphoma from benign lymphoid infiltrates. Am J Dermatopathol. 2008 Oct;30(5):425–30. PMID:18806482
2777. Morales-Vargas B, Deeb K, Peker D. Clinicopathologic and molecular analysis of inflammatory pseudotumor-like follicular/fibroblastic dendritic cell sarcoma: a case report and review of literature. Turk Patoloji Derg. 2021;37(3):266–72. PMID:34514557
2778. Moreira J, Rabe KG, Cerhan JR, et al. Infectious complications among individuals with clinical monoclonal B-cell lymphocytosis (MBL): a cohort study of newly diagnosed cases compared to controls. Leukemia. 2013 Jan;27(1):136–41. PMID:22781591
2779. Morel P, Duhamel A, Gobbi P, et al. International prognostic scoring system for Waldenstrom macroglobulinemia. Blood. 2009 Apr 30;113(18):4163–70. PMID:19196866
2780. Morel P, Lepage E, Brice P, et al. Prognosis and treatment of lymphoblastic lymphoma in adults: a report on 80 patients. J Clin Oncol. 1992 Jul;10(7):1078–85. PMID:1607914
2781. Morello L, Rattotti S, Giordano L, et al. Mantle cell lymphoma of mucosa-associated lymphoid tissue: a European Mantle Cell Lymphoma Network study. Hemasphere. 2019 Dec 16;4(1):e302. PMID:32072136
2782. Moreno C, Hodgson K, Ferrer G, et al. Autoimmune cytopenia in chronic lymphocytic leukemia: prevalence, clinical associations, and prognostic significance. Blood. 2010 Dec 2;116(23):4771–6. PMID:20736453
2783. Moretta A, Bottino C, Vitale M, et al. Activating receptors and coreceptors involved in human natural killer cell-mediated cytolysis. Annu Rev Immunol. 2001;19:197–223. PMID:11244035
2784. Mori H, Colman SM, Xiao Z, et al. Chromosome translocations and covert leukemic clones are generated during normal fetal development. Proc Natl Acad Sci U S A. 2002 Jun 11;99(12):8242–7. PMID:12048236
2785. Mori N, Yamashita Y, Tsuzuki T, et al. Lymphomatous features of aggressive NK cell leukaemia/lymphoma with massive necrosis, haemophagocytosis and EB virus infection. Histopathology. 2000 Oct;37(4):363–71. PMID:11012744
2786. Morice WG. The immunophenotypic attributes of NK cells and NK-cell lineage lymphoproliferative disorders. Am J Clin Pathol. 2007 Jun;127(6):881–6. PMID:17509985
2787. Morice WG, Jevremovic D, Hanson CA. The expression of the novel cytotoxic protein granzyme M by large granular lymphocytic leukaemias of both T-cell and NK-cell lineage: an unexpected finding with implications regarding the pathobiology of these disorders. Br J Haematol. 2007 May;137(3):237–9. PMID:17408463
2788. Morice WG, Kurtin PJ, Leibson PJ, et al. Demonstration of aberrant T-cell and natural killer-cell antigen expression in all cases of granular lymphocytic leukaemia. Br J Haematol. 2003 Mar;120(6):1026–36. PMID:12648073
2789. Morice WG, Kurtin PJ, Tefferi A, et al. Distinct bone marrow findings in T-cell granular lymphocytic leukemia revealed by paraffin section immunoperoxidase stains for CD8, TIA-1, and granzyme B. Blood. 2002 Jan 1;99(1):268–74. PMID:11756181
2790. Morice WG, Leibson PJ, Tefferi A. Natural killer cells and the syndrome of chronic natural killer cell lymphocytosis. Leuk Lymphoma. 2001 Apr;41(3-4):277–84. PMID:11378540
2791. Möricke A, Zimmermann M, Valsecchi MG, et al. Dexamethasone vs prednisone in induction treatment of pediatric ALL: results of the randomized trial AIEOP-BFM ALL 2000. Blood. 2016 Apr 28;127(17):2101–12. PMID:26888258
2792. Morimoto A, Fujioka Y, Ushiku T, et al. Monomorphic epitheliotropic intestinal T-cell lymphoma invades brain. Intern Med. 2021 Mar 1;60(5):815–6. PMID:33028779
2793. Morin RD, Arthur SE, Hodson DJ. Molecular profiling in diffuse large B-cell lymphoma: Why so many types of subtypes? Br J Haematol. 2022 Feb;196(4):814–29. PMID:34467527
2794. Morita K, Jain N, Kantarjian H, et al. Outcome of T-cell acute lymphoblastic leukemia/lymphoma: focus on near-ETP phenotype and differential impact of nelarabine. Am J Hematol. 2021 May 1;96(5):589–98. PMID:33639000
2795. Moroch J, Copie-Bergman C, de Leval L, et al. Follicular peripheral T-cell lymphoma expands the spectrum of classical Hodgkin lymphoma mimics. Am J Surg Pathol. 2012 Nov;36(11):1636–46. PMID:23073322
2796. Morrell D, Cromartie E, Swift M. Mortality and cancer incidence in 263 patients with ataxia-telangiectasia. J Natl Cancer Inst. 1986 Jul;77(1):89–92. PMID:3459930
2797. Morris EC. Allogeneic hematopoietic stem cell transplantation in adults with primary immunodeficiency. Hematology Am Soc Hematol Educ Program. 2020 Dec 4;2020(1):649–60. PMID:33275750
2798. Morris PG, Correa DD, Yahalom J, et al. Rituximab, methotrexate, procarbazine, and vincristine followed by consolidation reduced-dose whole-brain radiotherapy and cytarabine in newly diagnosed primary CNS lymphoma: final results and long-term outcome. J Clin Oncol. 2013 Nov 1;31(31):3971–9. PMID:24101038
2799. Morris RW, Kumar V, Saad AG. Anaplastic plasmacytoma: a rare tumor presenting as a pathological fracture in a younger adult. Skeletal Radiol. 2018 Jul;47(7):995–1001. PMID:29388036
2800. Morris SW, Kirstein MN, Valentine MB, et al. Fusion of a kinase gene, ALK, to a nucleolar protein gene, NPM, in non-Hodgkin's lymphoma. Science. 1994 Mar 4;263(5151):1281–4. PMID:8122112
2801. Morrow M, Samanta A, Kioussis D, et al. TEL-AML1 preleukemic activity requires the DNA binding domain of AML1 and the dimerization and corepressor binding domains of TEL. Oncogene. 2007 Jun 28;26(30):4404–14. PMID:17237815
2802. Morschhauser F, Fowler NH, Feugier P, et al. Rituximab plus lenalidomide in advanced untreated follicular lymphoma. N Engl J Med. 2018 Sep 6;379(10):934–47. PMID:30184451
2803. Morschhauser F, Tilly H, Chaidos A, et al. Tazemetostat for patients with relapsed or refractory follicular lymphoma: an open-label, single-arm, multicentre, phase 2 trial. Lancet Oncol. 2020 Nov;21(11):1433–42. PMID:33035457
2804. Morscio J, Bittoun E, Volders N, et al. Secondary B-cell lymphoma associated with the Epstein-Barr virus in chronic lymphocytic leukemia patients. J Hematop. 2016 May 21;9:113–20. PMID:29861791
2805. Morscio J, Dierickx D, Ferreiro JF, et al. Gene expression profiling reveals clear differences between EBV-positive and EBV-negative posttransplant lymphoproliferative disorders. Am J Transplant. 2013 May;13(5):1305–16. PMID:23489474
2806. Morscio J, Dierickx D, Nijs J, et al. Clinicopathologic comparison of plasmablastic lymphoma in HIV-positive, immunocompetent, and posttransplant patients: single-center series of 25 cases and meta-analysis of 277 reported cases. Am J Surg Pathol. 2014 Jul;38(7):875–86. PMID:24832164
2807. Morscio J, Finalet Ferreiro J, Vander Borght S, et al. Identification of distinct subgroups of EBV-positive post-transplant diffuse large B-cell lymphoma. Mod Pathol. 2017 Mar;30(3):370–81. PMID:28059091
2808. Moshous D, Callebaut I, de Chasseval R, et al. Artemis, a novel DNA double-strand break repair/V(D)J recombination protein, is mutated in human severe combined immune deficiency. Cell. 2001 Apr 20;105(2):177–86. PMID:11336668
2809. Moshynska OV, Saxena A. Clonal relationship between Hashimoto thyroiditis and thyroid lymphoma. J Clin Pathol. 2008 Apr;61(4):438–44. PMID:18006670
2810. Mossé YP, Voss SD, Lim MS, et al. Targeting ALK with crizotinib in pediatric anaplastic large cell lymphoma and inflammatory myofibroblastic tumor: a Children's Oncology Group study. J Clin Oncol. 2017 Oct 1;35(28):3215–21. PMID:28787259
2811. Mottok A, Hung SS, Chavez EA, et al. Integrative genomic analysis identifies key pathogenic mechanisms in primary mediastinal large B-cell lymphoma. Blood. 2019 Sep 5;134(10):802–13. PMID:31292115
2812. Mottok A, Renné C, Willenbrock K, et al. Somatic hypermutation of SOCS1 in lymphocyte-predominant Hodgkin lymphoma is accompanied by high JAK2 expression and activation of STAT6. Blood. 2007 Nov 1;110(9):3387–90. PMID:17652621
2813. Mottok A, Woolcock B, Chan FC, et al. Genomic alterations in CIITA are frequent in primary mediastinal large B cell lymphoma and are associated with diminished MHC class II expression. Cell Rep. 2015 Nov 17;13(7):1418–31. PMID:26549456
2814. Mottok A, Wright G, Rosenwald A, et al. Molecular classification of primary mediastinal large B-cell lymphoma using routinely available tissue specimens. Blood. 2018 Nov 29;132(22):2401–5. PMID:30257882
2815. Mourad A, Gniadecki R. Overall survival in mycosis fungoides: a systematic review and meta-analysis. J Invest Dermatol. 2020 Feb;140(2):495–497.e5. PMID:31465745
2816. Mourad N, Mounier N, Brière J, et al. Clinical, biologic, and pathologic features in 157 patients with angioimmunoblastic T-cell lymphoma treated within the Groupe d'Etude des Lymphomes de l'Adulte (GELA) trials. Blood. 2008 May 1;111(9):4463–70. PMID:18292286
2817. Mouttet B, Vinti L, Ancliff P, et al. Durable remissions in TCF3-HLF positive acute

lymphoblastic leukemia with blinatumomab and stem cell transplantation. Haematologica. 2019 Jun;104(6):e244–7. PMID:30765470
2818. Mozas P, Nadeu F, Rivas-Delgado A, et al. Patterns of change in treatment, response, and outcome in patients with follicular lymphoma over the last four decades: a single-center experience. Blood Cancer J. 2020 Mar 5;10(3):31. PMID:32139690
2819. Mozas P, Rivero A, Rivas-Delgado A, et al. A low lymphocyte-to-monocyte ratio is an independent predictor of poorer survival and higher risk of histological transformation in follicular lymphoma. Leuk Lymphoma. 2021 Jan;62(1):104–11. PMID:32954916
2820. Mozos A, Royo C, Hartmann E, et al. SOX11 expression is highly specific for mantle cell lymphoma and identifies the cyclin D1-negative subtype. Haematologica. 2009 Nov;94(11):1555–62. PMID:19880778
2821. Mroczek A, Zawitkowska J, Kowalczyk J, et al. Comprehensive overview of gene rearrangements in childhood T-cell acute lymphoblastic leukaemia. Int J Mol Sci. 2021 Jan 15;22(2):808. PMID:33467425
2822. Mrózek K, Harper DP, Aplan PD. Cytogenetics and molecular genetics of acute lymphoblastic leukemia. Hematol Oncol Clin North Am. 2009 Oct;23(5):991–1010, v. PMID:19825449
2823. Muccio VE, Saraci E, Gilestro M, et al. Multiple myeloma: new surface antigens for the characterization of plasma cells in the era of novel agents. Cytometry B Clin Cytom. 2016 Jan;90(1):81–90. PMID:26287276
2824. Muchtar E, Gertz MA, Kumar SK, et al. Improved outcomes for newly diagnosed AL amyloidosis between 2000 and 2014: cracking the glass ceiling of early death. Blood. 2017 Apr 13;129(15):2111–9. PMID:28126928
2825. Muchtar E, Gertz MA, Kyle RA, et al. A modern primer on light chain amyloidosis in 592 patients with mass spectrometry-verified typing. Mayo Clin Proc. 2019 Mar;94(3):472–83. PMID:30770096
2826. Muchtar E, Jevremovic D, Dispenzieri A, et al. The prognostic value of multiparametric flow cytometry in AL amyloidosis at diagnosis and at the end of first-line treatment. Blood. 2017 Jan 5;129(1):82–7. PMID:27729322
2827. Muchtar E, Koehler AB, Johnson MJ, et al. Humoral and cellular immune responses to recombinant herpes zoster vaccine in patients with chronic lymphocytic leukemia and monoclonal B cell lymphocytosis. Am J Hematol. 2022 Jan 1;97(1):90–8. PMID:34699616
2828. Mueller NE, Grufferman S, Chang ET. The epidemiology of Hodgkin lymphoma. In: Hoppe RT, Mauch PM, Armitage JO, et al, editors. Hodgkin lymphoma. 2nd ed. Philadelphia (PA): Lippincott Williams & Wilkins; 2007. pp. 7–23.
2829. Mueller NE, Grufferman S, Chang ET. The epidemiology of Hodgkin lymphoma. In: Hoppe RT, Mauch PM, Armitage JO, et al, editors. Hodgkin lymphoma. 2nd ed. Philadelphia (PA): Lippincott Williams & Wilkins; 2007. pp. 7–23.
2830. Mühlbacher V, Zenger M, Schnittger S, et al. Acute lymphoblastic leukemia with low hypodiploid/near triploid karyotype is a specific clinical entity and exhibits a very high TP53 mutation frequency of 93%. Genes Chromosomes Cancer. 2014 Jun;53(6):524–36. PMID:24619868
2831. Mukherjee S, Martin R, Sande B, et al. Epidemiology and treatment patterns of idiopathic multicentric Castleman disease in the era of IL-6-directed therapy. Blood Adv. 2022 Jan 25;6(2):359–67. PMID:34535010
2832. Müller-Hermelink HK, Zettl A, Pfeifer W, et al. Pathology of lymphoma progression. Histopathology. 2001 Apr;38(4):285–306. PMID:11318894
2833. Mullighan CG, Collins-Underwood JR, Phillips LA, et al. Rearrangement of CRLF2 in B-progenitor- and Down syndrome-associated acute lymphoblastic leukemia. Nat Genet. 2009 Nov;41(11):1243–6. PMID:19838194
2834. Mullighan CG, Miller CB, Radtke I, et al. BCR-ABL1 lymphoblastic leukaemia is characterized by the deletion of Ikaros. Nature. 2008 May 1;453(7191):110–4. PMID:18408710
2835. Mullighan CG, Su X, Zhang J, et al. Deletion of IKZF1 and prognosis in acute lymphoblastic leukemia. N Engl J Med. 2009 Jan 29;360(5):470–80. PMID:19129520
2836. Mullighan CG, Williams RT, Downing JR, et al. Failure of CDKN2A/B (INK4A/B-ARF)-mediated tumor suppression and resistance to targeted therapy in acute lymphoblastic leukemia induced by BCR-ABL. Genes Dev. 2008 Jun 1;22(11):1411–5. PMID:18519632
2837. Mundo L, Ambrosio MR, Raimondi F, et al. Molecular switch from MYC to MYCN expression in MYC protein negative Burkitt lymphoma cases. Blood Cancer J. 2019 Nov 20;9(12):91. PMID:31748534
2838. Mundo L, Del Porro L, Granai M, et al. Correction: Frequent traces of EBV infection in Hodgkin and non-Hodgkin lymphomas classified as EBV-negative by routine methods: expanding the landscape of EBV-related lymphomas. Mod Pathol. 2020 Dec;33(12):2637. PMID:32601381
2839. Mundo L, Del Porro L, Granai M, et al. Frequent traces of EBV infection in Hodgkin and non-Hodgkin lymphomas classified as EBV-negative by routine methods: expanding the landscape of EBV-related lymphomas. Mod Pathol. 2020 Dec;33(12):2407–21. PMID:32483241
2840. Muniesa C, Estrach T, Pujol RM, et al. Folliculotropic mycosis fungoides: clinicopathological features and outcome in a series of 20 cases. J Am Acad Dermatol. 2010 Mar;62(3):418–26. PMID:20079954
2841. Muñoz-Mármol AM, Sanz C, Tapia G, et al. MYC status determination in aggressive B-cell lymphoma: the impact of FISH probe selection. Histopathology. 2013 Sep;63(3):418–24. PMID:23795946
2842. Munshi N, Mehra M, van de Velde H, et al. Use of a claims database to characterize and estimate the incidence rate for Castleman disease. Leuk Lymphoma. 2015 May;56(5):1252–60. PMID:25120049
2843. Munshi NC, Avet-Loiseau H, Rawstron AC, et al. Association of minimal residual disease with superior survival outcomes in patients with multiple myeloma: a meta-analysis. JAMA Oncol. 2017 Jan 1;3(1):28–35. PMID:27632282
2844. Munshi NC, Digumarthy S, Rahemtullah A. Case records of the Massachusetts General Hospital. Case 13-2008. A 46-year-old man with rheumatoid arthritis and lymphadenopathy. N Engl J Med. 2008 Apr 24;358(17):1838–48. PMID:18434654
2845. Münz C. Latency and lytic replication in Epstein-Barr virus-associated oncogenesis. Nat Rev Microbiol. 2019 Nov;17(11):691–700. PMID:31477887
2846. Murakami YI, Yatabe Y, Sakaguchi T, et al. c-Maf expression in angioimmunoblastic T-cell lymphoma. Am J Surg Pathol. 2007 Nov;31(11):1695–702. PMID:18059226
2847. Murase T, Nakamura S, Kawauchi K, et al. An Asian variant of intravascular large B-cell lymphoma: clinical, pathological and cytogenetic approaches to diffuse large B-cell lymphoma associated with haemophagocytic syndrome. Br J Haematol. 2000 Dec;111(3):826–34. PMID:11122144
2848. Murase T, Yamaguchi M, Suzuki R, et al. Intravascular large B-cell lymphoma (IVLBCL): a clinicopathologic study of 96 cases with special reference to the immunophenotypic heterogeneity of CD5. Blood. 2007 Jan 15;109(2):478–85. PMID:16985183
2849. Muretto P, Lungarotti F, Lemma E. Giant lymph node hyperplasia in angiohamartomatous soft tissues. Tumori. 1981 Aug;67(4):383–90. PMID:7314265
2850. Muris JJ, Meijer CJ, Vos W, et al. Immunohistochemical profiling based on Bcl-2, CD10 and MUM1 expression improves risk stratification in patients with primary nodal diffuse large B cell lymphoma. J Pathol. 2006 Apr;208(5):714–23. PMID:16400625
2851. Murphy BA, Meda BA, Buss DH, et al. Marginal zone and mantle cell lymphomas: assessment of cytomorphology in subtyping small B-cell lymphomas. Diagn Cytopathol. 2003 Mar;28(3):126–30. PMID:12619092
2852. Murray A, Cuevas EC, Jones DB, et al. Study of the immunohistochemistry and T cell clonality of enteropathy-associated T cell lymphoma. Am J Pathol. 1995 Feb;146(2):509–19. PMID:7856760
2853. Murray DL, Willrich MAV. Evolution of myeloma testing in clinical chemistry with mass spectrometry. J Appl Lab Med. 2019 Nov;4(3):474–6. PMID:31659091
2854. Murro D, Agab M, Brickman A, et al. Cytological features of Castleman disease: a review. J Am Soc Cytopathol. 2016 Mar-Apr;5(2):100–6. PMID:31042489
2855. Musto P, Engelhardt M, Caers J, et al. 2021 European Myeloma Network review and consensus statement on smoldering multiple myeloma: how to distinguish (and manage) Dr. Jekyll and Mr. Hyde. Haematologica. 2021 Nov 1;106(11):2799–812. PMID:34261295
2856. Muthukrishnan S, Amudhan A, Rajendran S. Primary Hodgkin's lymphoma of liver in HIV-a case report and review of literature. AME Case Rep. 2018 May 10;2:21. PMID:30264017
2857. Muto H, Sakata-Yanagimoto M, Nagae G, et al. Reduced TET2 function leads to T-cell lymphoma with follicular helper T-cell-like features in mice. Blood Cancer J. 2014 Dec 12;4(12):e264. PMID:25501021
2858. Muto R, Miyoshi H, Sato K, et al. Epidemiology and secular trends of malignant lymphoma in Japan: analysis of 9426 cases according to the World Health Organization classification. Cancer Med. 2018 Nov;7(11):5843–58. PMID:30311404
2859. Mutzbauer G, Maurus K, Buszello C, et al. SYK expression in monomorphic epitheliotropic intestinal T-cell lymphoma. Mod Pathol. 2018 Mar;31(3):505–16. PMID:29052597
2860. Mylona EE, Baraboutis IG, Lekakis LJ, et al. Multicentric Castleman's disease in HIV infection: a systematic review of the literature. AIDS Rev. 2008 Jan-Mar;10(1):25–35. PMID:18385778
2861. Nabel CS, Sameroff S, Shilling D, et al. Virome capture sequencing does not identify active viral infection in unicentric and idiopathic multicentric Castleman disease. PLoS One. 2019 Jun 26;14(6):e0218660. PMID:31242229
2862. Nachman JB, Heerema NA, Sather H, et al. Outcome of treatment in children with hypodiploid acute lymphoblastic leukemia. Blood. 2007 Aug 15;110(4):1112–5. PMID:17473063
2863. Naddaf E, Dispenzieri A, Mandrekar J, et al. Clinical spectrum of Castleman disease-associated neuropathy. Neurology. 2016 Dec 6;87(23):2457–62. PMID:27807187
2864. Nadeu F, Martin-Garcia D, Clot G, et al. Genomic and epigenomic insights into the origin, pathogenesis, and clinical behavior of mantle cell lymphoma subtypes. Blood. 2020 Sep 17;136(12):1419–32. PMID:32584970
2865. Nadeu F, Royo R, Clot G, et al. IGLV3-21R110 identifies an aggressive biological subtype of chronic lymphocytic leukemia with intermediate epigenetics. Blood. 2021 May 27;137(21):2935–46. PMID:33211804
2866. Nador RG, Cesarman E, Chadburn A, et al. Primary effusion lymphoma: a distinct clinicopathologic entity associated with the Kaposi's sarcoma-associated herpes virus. Blood. 1996 Jul 15;88(2):645–56. PMID:8695812
2867. Nador RG, Chadburn A, Gundappa G, et al. Human immunodeficiency virus (HIV)-associated polymorphic lymphoproliferative disorders. Am J Surg Pathol. 2003 Mar;27(3):293–302. PMID:12604885
2868. Naeini YB, Wu A, O'Malley DP. Aggressive B-cell lymphomas: frequency, immunophenotype, and genetics in a reference laboratory population. Ann Diagn Pathol. 2016 Dec;25:7–14. PMID:27806850
2869. Nagafuchi S, Ishibashi H, Anzai K, et al. Budd-Chiari syndrome and Epstein-Barr virus (EBV) associated plasmacytoma in a patient with chronic active EBV infection. Clin Investig. 1994 Nov;72(11):883–6. PMID:7894217
2870. Nagao Y, Mimura N, Takeda J, et al. Genetic and transcriptional landscape of plasma cells in POEMS syndrome. Leukemia. 2019 Jul;33(7):1723–35. PMID:30635632
2871. Nagarajan P, Cai G, Padda MS, et al. Littoral cell angioma of the spleen diagnosed by endoscopic ultrasound-guided fine-needle aspiration biopsy. Diagn Cytopathol. 2011 May;39(5):318–22. PMID:21488173
2872. Nagato T, Ohkuri T, Ohara K, et al. Programmed death-ligand 1 and its soluble form are highly expressed in nasal natural killer/T-cell lymphoma: a potential rationale for immunotherapy. Cancer Immunol Immunother. 2017 Jul;66(7):877–90. PMID:28349165
2873. Nagel I, Bartels M, Duell J, et al. Hematopoietic stem cell involvement in BCR-ABL1-positive ALL as a potential mechanism of resistance to blinatumomab therapy. Blood. 2017 Nov 2;130(18):2027–31. PMID:28827408
2874. Nagel S, Leich E, Quentmeier H, et al. Amplification at 7q22 targets cyclin-dependent kinase 6 in T-cell lymphoma. Leukemia. 2008 Feb;22(2):387–92. PMID:17989712
2875. Nagy A, Bhaduri A, Shahmarvand N, et al. Next-generation sequencing of idiopathic multicentric and unicentric Castleman disease and follicular dendritic cell sarcomas. Blood Adv. 2018 Mar 13;2(5):481–91. PMID:29496669
2876. Nagy N, Klein G, Klein E. To the genesis of Burkitt lymphoma: regulation of apoptosis by EBNA-1 and SAP may determine the fate of Ig-myc translocation carrying B lymphocytes. Semin Cancer Biol. 2009 Dec;19(6):407–10. PMID:19874894
2877. Nair S, Branagan AR, Liu J, et al. Clonal immunoglobulin against lysolipids in the origin of myeloma. N Engl J Med. 2016 Feb 11;374(6):555–61. PMID:26863356
2878. Nairismägi M, Gerritsen ME, Li ZM, et al. Oncogenic activation of JAK3-STAT signaling confers clinical sensitivity to PRN371, a novel selective and potent JAK3 inhibitor, in natural killer/T-cell lymphoma. Leukemia. 2018 May;32(5):1147–56. PMID:29434279
2879. Nairismägi ML, Tan J, Lim JQ, et al. JAK-STAT and G-protein-coupled receptor signaling pathways are frequently altered in epitheliotropic intestinal T-cell lymphoma. Leukemia. 2016 Jun;30(6):1311–9. PMID:26854024
2880. Nakagawa M, Schmitz R, Xiao W, et al. Gain-of-function CCR4 mutations in adult T cell leukemia/lymphoma. J Exp Med. 2014 Dec 15;211(13):2497–505. PMID:25488980
2881. Nakajima M, Shimoda M, Takeuchi K, et al. Lymphomatoid gastropathy/NK-cell enteropathy involving the stomach and intestine. J Clin Exp Hematop. 2022 Jun 28;62(2):114–8. PMID:35474034

2882. Nakamoto T, Yamagata T, Sakai R, et al. CIZ, a zinc finger protein that interacts with p130(cas) and activates the expression of matrix metalloproteinases. Mol Cell Biol. 2000 Mar;20(5):1649–58. PMID:10669742

2883. Nakamura M, Øverby A, Michimae H, et al. PCR analysis and specific immunohistochemistry revealing a high prevalence of non-Helicobacter pylori Helicobacters in Helicobacter pylori-negative gastric disease patients in Japan: high susceptibility to an Hp eradication regimen. Helicobacter. 2020 Oct;25(5):e12700. PMID:32790220

2884. Nakamura S, Akazawa K, Yao T, et al. A clinicopathologic study of 233 cases with special reference to evaluation with the MIB-1 index. Cancer. 1995 Oct 15;76(8):1313–24. PMID:8620403

2885. Nakamura S, Ponzoni M. Marginal zone B-cell lymphoma: lessons from western and eastern diagnostic approaches. Pathology. 2020 Jan;52(1):15–29. PMID:31757436

2886. Nakamura S, Shiota M, Nakagawa A, et al. Anaplastic large cell lymphoma: a distinct molecular pathologic entity: a reappraisal with special reference to p80(NPM/ALK) expression. Am J Surg Pathol. 1997 Dec;21(12):1420–32. PMID:9414185

2887. Nakase K, Kita K, Miwa H, et al. Clinical and prognostic significance of cytokine receptor expression in adult acute lymphoblastic leukemia: interleukin-2 receptor alpha-chain predicts a poor prognosis. Leukemia. 2007 Feb;21(2):326–32. PMID:17205058

2888. Nakashima Y, Tagawa H, Suzuki R, et al. Genome-wide array-based comparative genomic hybridization of natural killer cell lymphoma/leukemia: different genomic alteration patterns of aggressive NK-cell leukemia and extranodal NK/T-cell lymphoma, nasal type. Genes Chromosomes Cancer. 2005 Nov;44(3):247–55. PMID:16049916

2889. Nakatsuka S, Yao M, Hoshida Y, et al. Pyothorax-associated lymphoma: a review of 106 cases. J Clin Oncol. 2002 Oct 15;20(20):4255–60. PMID:12377970

2890. Nakayama-Ichiyama S, Yokote T, Hirata Y, et al. Multiple cytokine-producing plasmablastic solitary plasmacytoma of bone with polyneuropathy, organomegaly, endocrinology, monoclonal protein, and skin changes syndrome. J Clin Oncol. 2012 Mar 1;30(7):e91–4. PMID:22231043

2891. Nam-Cha SH, Montes-Moreno S, Salcedo MT, et al. Lymphocyte-rich classical Hodgkin's lymphoma: distinctive tumor and microenvironment markers. Mod Pathol. 2009 Aug;22(8):1006–15. PMID:19465900

2892. Nam-Cha SH, Roncador G, Sanchez-Verde L, et al. PD-1, a follicular T-cell marker useful for recognizing nodular lymphocyte-predominant Hodgkin lymphoma. Am J Surg Pathol. 2008 Aug;32(8):1252–7. PMID:18594468

2893. Nan FF, Zhang L, Li L, et al. Clinical features and survival impact of EBV-positive diffuse large B-cell lymphoma with different age cutoffs. Eur Rev Med Pharmacol Sci. 2020 Jan;24(17):8947–56. PMID:32964985

2894. Nann D, Bonzheim I, Müller I, et al. Clonally related duodenal-type follicular lymphoma and in situ follicular neoplasia. Haematologica. 2019 Nov;104(11):e537–9. PMID:31371415

2895. Nann D, Ramis-Zaldivar JE, Müller I, et al. Follicular lymphoma t(14;18)-negative is genetically a heterogeneous disease. Blood Adv. 2020 Nov 24;4(22):5652–65. PMID:33211828

2896. Napaki S, Stirling JW. Spindle and epithelioid (histiocytoid) haemangioendothelioma of cervical lymph nodes. Pathology. 2004 Dec;36(6):587–9. PMID:15841699

2897. Nappi L, Sorrentino F, Angioni S, et al. Leiomyomatosis peritonealis disseminata (LPD) ten years after laparoscopic myomectomy associated with ascites and lymph nodes enlargement: a case report. Int J Surg Case Rep. 2016;25:1–3. PMID:27280492

2898. Naresh KN. MUM1 expression dichotomises follicular lymphoma into predominantly, MUM1-negative low-grade and MUM1-positive high-grade subtypes. Haematologica. 2007 Feb;92(2):267–8. PMID:17296585

2899. Naresh KN. Nodal marginal zone B-cell lymphoma with prominent follicular colonization - difficulties in diagnosis: a study of 15 cases. Histopathology. 2008 Feb;52(3):331–9. PMID:18269584

2900. Naresh KN. Proliferation center cells in the lymph nodes of B-cell chronic lymphatic leukemia express relatively higher levels of CD20. Hum Pathol. 2000 Jun;31(6):775. PMID:10872678

2901. Naresh KN, Ibrahim HA, Lazzi S, et al. Diagnosis of Burkitt lymphoma using an algorithmic approach–applicable in both resource-poor and resource-rich countries. Br J Haematol. 2011 Sep;154(6):770–6. PMID:21718280

2902. Naresh KN, Johnson J, Srinivas V, et al. Epstein-Barr virus association in classical Hodgkin's disease provides survival advantage to patients and correlates with higher expression of proliferation markers in Reed-Sternberg cells. Ann Oncol. 2000 Jan;11(1):91–6. PMID:10690394

2903. Naresh KN, Lazzi S, Santi R, et al. A refined approach to the diagnosis of Burkitt lymphoma in a resource-poor setting. Histopathology. 2022 Mar;80(4):743–5. PMID:34725849

2904. Naresh KN, Menasce LP, Shenjere P, et al. 'Precursors' of classical Hodgkin lymphoma in samples of angioimmunoblastic T-cell lymphoma. Br J Haematol. 2008 Apr;141(1):124–6. PMID:18324974

2905. Narimatsu H, Ota Y, Kami M, et al. Clinicopathological features of pyothorax-associated lymphoma; a retrospective survey involving 98 patients. Ann Oncol. 2007 Jan;18(1):122–8. PMID:17043091

2906. Nascimento AF, Pinkus JL, Pinkus GS. Clusterin, a marker for anaplastic large cell lymphoma immunohistochemical profile in hematopoietic and nonhematopoietic malignant neoplasms. Am J Clin Pathol. 2004 May;121(5):709–17. PMID:15151211

2907. Nascimento AG, Keeney GL, Sciot R, et al. Polymorphous hemangioendothelioma: a report of two cases, one affecting extranodal soft tissues, and review of the literature. Am J Surg Pathol. 1997 Sep;21(9):1083–9. PMID:9298885

2908. Nasr SH, Kudose SS, Said SM, et al. Immunotactoid glomerulopathy is a rare entity with monoclonal and polyclonal variants. Kidney Int. 2021 Feb;99(2):410–20. PMID:32818517

2909. Nasr SH, Satoskar A, Markowitz GS, et al. Proliferative glomerulonephritis with monoclonal IgG deposits. J Am Soc Nephrol. 2009 Sep;20(9):2055–64. PMID:19470674

2910. Nasr SH, Valeri AM, Cornell LD, et al. Renal monoclonal immunoglobulin deposition disease: a report of 64 patients from a single institution. Clin J Am Soc Nephrol. 2012 Feb;7(2):231–9. PMID:22156754

2911. Nassif S, Ozdemirli M. EBV-positive low-grade marginal zone lymphoma in the breast with massive amyloid deposition arising in a heart transplant patient: a report of an unusual case. Pediatr Transplant. 2013 Sep;17(6):E141–5. PMID:23773403

2912. Nastoupil LJ, Sinha R, Byrtek M, et al. Outcomes following watchful waiting for stage II-IV follicular lymphoma patients in the modern era. Br J Haematol. 2016 Mar;172(5):724–34. PMID:26729445

2913. Nasu S, Misawa S, Sekiguchi Y, et al. Different neurological and physiological profiles in POEMS syndrome and chronic inflammatory demyelinating polyneuropathy. J Neurol Neurosurg Psychiatry. 2012 May;83(5):476–9. PMID:22338030

2914. Nathwani BN, Anderson JR, Armitage JO, et al. Marginal zone B-cell lymphoma: a clinical comparison of nodal and mucosa-associated lymphoid tissue types. Non-Hodgkin's Lymphoma Classification Project. J Clin Oncol. 1999 Aug;17(8):2486–92. PMID:10561313

2915. Nathwani BN, Metter GE, Miller TP, et al. What should be the morphologic criteria for the subdivision of follicular lymphomas? Blood. 1986 Oct;68(4):837–45. PMID:3530348

2916. Nathwani BN, Vornanen M, Winkelmann R, et al. Intranodular clusters of activated cells with T follicular helper phenotype in nodular lymphocyte predominant Hodgkin lymphoma: a pilot study of 32 cases from Finland. Hum Pathol. 2013 Sep;44(9):1737–46. PMID:23684509

2917. Natkunam Y, Farinha P, Hsi ED, et al. LMO2 protein expression predicts survival in patients with diffuse large B-cell lymphoma treated with anthracycline-based chemotherapy with and without rituximab. J Clin Oncol. 2008 Jan 20;26(3):447–54. PMID:18086797

2918. Natkunam Y, Goodlad JR, Chadburn A, et al. EBV-positive B-cell proliferations of varied malignant potential: 2015 SH/EAHP Workshop Report-Part 1. Am J Clin Pathol. 2017 Feb 1;147(2):129–52. PMID:28395107

2919. Natkunam Y, Gratzinger D, Chadburn A, et al. Immunodeficiency-associated lymphoproliferative disorders: time for reappraisal? Blood. 2018 Nov 1;132(18):1871–8. PMID:30082493

2920. Natkunam Y, Gratzinger D, de Jong D, et al. Immunodeficiency and dysregulation: report of the 2015 workshop of the Society for Hematopathology/European Association for Haematopathology. Am J Clin Pathol. 2017 Feb 1;147(2):124–8. PMID:28395103

2921. Natkunam Y, Warnke RA, Haghighi B, et al. Co-expression of CD56 and CD30 in lymphomas with primary presentation in the skin: clinicopathologic, immunohistochemical and molecular analyses of seven cases. J Cutan Pathol. 2000 Sep;27(8):392–9. PMID:10955685

2922. Nato Y, Miyazaki K, Imai H, et al. Early central nervous system relapse of monomorphic epitheliotropic intestinal T-cell lymphoma after cord blood transplantation. Int J Hematol. 2021 Jul;114(1):129–35. PMID:33646526

2923. Navari M, Etebari M, De Falco G, et al. The presence of Epstein-Barr virus significantly impacts the transcriptional profile in immunodeficiency-associated Burkitt lymphoma. Front Microbiol. 2015 Jun 10;6:556. PMID:26113842

2924. Navarro A, Clot G, Royo C, et al. Molecular subsets of mantle cell lymphoma defined by the IGHV mutational status and SOX11 expression have distinct biologic and clinical features. Cancer Res. 2012 Oct 15;72(20):5307–16. PMID:22915760

2925. Navid F, Mosijczuk AD, Head DR, et al. Acute lymphoblastic leukemia with the (8;14) (q24;q32) translocation and FAB L3 morphology associated with a B-precursor immunophenotype: the Pediatric Oncology Group experience. Leukemia. 1999 Jan;13(1):135–41. PMID:10049049

2926. Neben MA, Morice WG, Tefferi A. Clinical features in T-cell vs. natural killer-cell variants of large granular lymphocyte leukemia. Eur J Haematol. 2003 Oct;71(4):263–5. PMID:12950235

2927. Neelapu SS, Locke FL, Bartlett NL, et al. Axicabtagene ciloleucel CAR T-cell therapy in refractory large B-cell lymphoma. N Engl J Med. 2017 Dec 28;377(26):2531–44. PMID:29226797

2928. Nelson AM, Manabe YC, Lucas SB. Immune reconstitution inflammatory syndrome (IRIS): what pathologists should know. Semin Diagn Pathol. 2017 Jul;34(4):340–51. PMID:28552210

2929. Nelson BP, Wolniak KL, Evens A, et al. Early posttransplant lymphoproliferative disease: clinicopathologic features and correlation with mTOR signaling pathway activation. Am J Clin Pathol. 2012 Oct;138(4):568–78. PMID:23010712

2930. Nelson JA, Dabic S, Mehrara BJ, et al. Breast implant-associated anaplastic large cell lymphoma incidence: determining an accurate risk. Ann Surg. 2020 Sep 1;272(3):403–9. PMID:32694446

2931. Nelson M, Horsman DE, Weisenburger DD, et al. Cytogenetic abnormalities and clinical correlations in peripheral T-cell lymphoma. Br J Haematol. 2008 May;141(4):461–9. PMID:18341637

2932. Neubauer A, Thiede C, Morgner A, et al. Cure of Helicobacter pylori infection and duration of remission of low-grade gastric mucosa-associated lymphoid tissue lymphoma. J Natl Cancer Inst. 1997 Sep 17;89(18):1350–5. PMID:9308704

2933. Neuhauser TS, Derringer GA, Thompson LD, et al. Splenic angiosarcoma: a clinicopathologic and immunophenotypic study of 28 cases. Mod Pathol. 2000 Sep;13(9):978–87. PMID:11007038

2934. Neumann M, Coskun E, Fransecky L, et al. FLT3 mutations in early T-cell precursor ALL characterize a stem cell like leukemia and imply the clinical use of tyrosine kinase inhibitors. PLoS One. 2013;8(1):e53190. PMID:23359050

2935. Neumann M, Heesch S, Gökbuget N, et al. Clinical and molecular characterization of early T-cell precursor leukemia: a high-risk subgroup in adult T-ALL with a high frequency of FLT3 mutations. Blood Cancer J. 2012 Jan;2(1):e55. PMID:22829239

2936. Neumann M, Heesch S, Schlee C, et al. Whole-exome sequencing in adult ETP-ALL reveals a high rate of DNMT3A mutations. Blood. 2013 Jun 6;121(23):4749–52. PMID:23603912

2937. Neven B, Magerus-Chatinet A, Florkin B, et al. A survey of 90 patients with autoimmune lymphoproliferative syndrome related to TNFRSF6 mutation. Blood. 2011 Nov 3;118(18):4798–807. PMID:21885602

2938. Neven Q, Boulanger C, Bruwier A, et al. Clinical spectrum of Ras-associated autoimmune leukoproliferative disorder (RALD). J Clin Immunol. 2021 Jan;41(1):51–8. PMID:33011939

2939. Newman AM, Zaka M, Zhou P, et al. Genomic abnormalities of TP53 define distinct risk groups of paediatric B-cell non-Hodgkin lymphoma. Leukemia. 2022 Mar;36(3):781–9. PMID:34675373

2940. Ney Garcia DR, de Souza MT, de Figueiredo AF, et al. Molecular characterization of KMT2A fusion partner genes in 13 cases of pediatric leukemia with complex or cryptic karyotypes. Hematol Oncol. 2017 Dec;35(4):760–8. PMID:27282883

2941. Ng A, Chiorazzi N. Potential relevance of B-cell maturation pathways in defining the cell(s) of origin for chronic lymphocytic leukemia. Hematol Oncol Clin North Am. 2021 Aug;35(4):665–85. PMID:34174979

2942. Ng CS, Lo ST, Chan JK, et al. CD56+ putative natural killer cell lymphomas: production of cytolytic effectors and related proteins mediating tumor cell apoptosis? Hum Pathol. 1997 Nov;28(11):1276–82. PMID:9385933

2943. Ng SB, Chung TH, Kato S, et al. Epstein-Barr virus-associated primary nodal T/NK-cell lymphoma shows a distinct molecular signature

and copy number changes. Haematologica. 2018 Feb;103(2):278–87. PMID:29097495
2944. Ng SB, Ohshima K, Selvarajan V, et al. Epstein-Barr virus-associated T/natural killer-cell lymphoproliferative disorder in children and young adults has similar molecular signature to extranodal nasal natural killer/T-cell lymphoma but shows distinctive stem cell-like phenotype. Leuk Lymphoma. 2015;56(8):2408–15. PMID:25382618
2945. Ng SB, Ohshima K, Selvarajan V, et al. Prognostic implication of morphology, cyclinE2 and proliferation in EBV-associated T/NK lymphoproliferative disease in non-immunocompromised hosts. Orphanet J Rare Dis. 2014 Dec 5;9:165. PMID:25475054
2946. Ng SB, Selvarajan V, Huang G, et al. Activated oncogenic pathways and therapeutic targets in extranodal nasal-type NK/T cell lymphoma revealed by gene expression profiling. J Pathol. 2011 Mar;223(4):496–510. PMID:21294123
2947. Ng SB, Yan J, Huang G, et al. Dysregulated microRNAs affect pathways and targets of biologic relevance in nasal-type natural killer/T-cell lymphoma. Blood. 2011 Nov 3;118(18):4919–29. PMID:21921041
2948. Ng WK, Ip P, Choy C, et al. Cytologic findings of angioimmunoblastic T-cell lymphoma: analysis of 16 fine-needle aspirates over 9-year period. Cancer. 2002 Jun 25;96(3):166–73. PMID:12115305
2949. Ngo VN, Young RM, Schmitz R, et al. Oncogenically active MYD88 mutations in human lymphoma. Nature. 2011 Feb 3;470(7332):115–9. PMID:21179087
2950. Nguyen T, Eltorky MA. Intranodal palisaded myofibroblastoma. Arch Pathol Lab Med. 2007 Feb;131(2):306–10. PMID:17284119
2951. Nguyen TB, Sakata-Yanagimoto M, Fujisawa M, et al. Dasatinib is an effective treatment for angioimmunoblastic T-cell lymphoma. Cancer Res. 2020 May 1;80(9):1875–84. PMID:32107212
2952. Nicol I, Boye T, Carsuzaa F, et al. Post-transplant plasmablastic lymphoma of the skin. Br J Dermatol. 2003 Oct;149(4):889–91. PMID:14616390
2953. Nicolae A, Ganapathi KA, Pham TH, et al. EBV-negative aggressive NK-cell leukemia/lymphoma: clinical, pathologic, and genetic features. Am J Surg Pathol. 2017 Jan;41(1):67–74. PMID:27631517
2954. Nicolae A, Pittaluga S, Abdullah S, et al. EBV-positive large B-cell lymphomas in young patients: a nodal lymphoma with evidence for a tolerogenic immune environment. Blood. 2015 Aug 13;126(7):863–72. PMID:25999451
2955. Nicolae A, Pittaluga S, Venkataraman G, et al. Peripheral T-cell lymphomas of follicular T-helper cell derivation with Hodgkin/Reed-Sternberg cells of B-cell lineage: both EBV-positive and EBV-negative variants exist. Am J Surg Pathol. 2013 Jun;37(6):816–26. PMID:23598959
2956. Nicolae A, Xi L, Pham TH, et al. Mutations in the JAK/STAT and RAS signaling pathways are common in intestinal T-cell lymphomas. Leukemia. 2016 Nov;30(11):2245–7. PMID:27389054
2957. Nieborowska-Skorska M, Slupianek A, Xue L, et al. Role of signal transducer and activator of transcription 5 in nucleophosmin/anaplastic lymphoma kinase-mediated malignant transformation of lymphoid cells. Cancer Res. 2001 Sep 1;61(17):6517–23. PMID:11522649
2958. Niemeyer CM, Arico M, Basso G, et al. Chronic myelomonocytic leukemia in childhood: a retrospective analysis of 110 cases. Blood. 1997 May 15;89(10):3534–43. PMID:9160658
2959. Niens M, Jarrett RF, Hepkema B, et al. HLA-A*02 is associated with a reduced risk and HLA-A*01 with an increased risk of developing EBV+ Hodgkin lymphoma. Blood. 2007 Nov 1;110(9):3310–5. PMID:17630352
2960. Nieto WG, Almeida J, Romero A, et al. Increased frequency (12%) of circulating chronic lymphocytic leukemia-like B-cell clones in healthy subjects using a highly sensitive multicolor flow cytometry approach. Blood. 2009 Jul 2;114(1):33–7. PMID:19420353
2961. Niitsu N, Okamoto M, Nakamine H, et al. Clinicopathologic correlations of diffuse large B-cell lymphoma in rheumatoid arthritis patients treated with methotrexate. Cancer Sci. 2010 May;101(5):1309–13. PMID:20210795
2962. Niitsu N, Okamoto M, Tamaru JI, et al. Clinicopathologic characteristics and treatment outcome of the addition of rituximab to chemotherapy for CD5-positive in comparison with CD5-negative diffuse large B-cell lymphoma. Ann Oncol. 2010 Oct;21(10):2069–74. PMID:20231297
2963. Nikiphorou E, Galloway J, Fragoulis GE. Overview of IgG4-related aortitis and periaortitis. A decade since their first description. Autoimmun Rev. 2020 Dec;19(12):102694. PMID:33121641
2964. Niller HH, Wolf H, Minarovits J. Viral hit and run-oncogenesis: genetic and epigenetic scenarios. Cancer Lett. 2011 Jun 28;305(2):200–17. PMID:20813452
2965. Nishii R, Baskin-Doerfler R, Yang W, et al. Molecular basis of ETV6-mediated predisposition to childhood acute lymphoblastic leukemia. Blood. 2021 Jan 21;137(3):364–73. PMID:32693409
2966. Nishimura MF, Igawa T, Gion Y, et al. Pulmonary manifestations of plasma cell type idiopathic multicentric Castleman disease: a clinicopathological study in comparison with IgG4-related disease. J Pers Med. 2020 Dec 10;10(4):269. PMID:33321725
2967. Nishimura Y, Fajgenbaum DC, Pierson SK, et al. Validated international definition of the thrombocytopenia, anasarca, fever, reticulin fibrosis, renal insufficiency, and organomegaly clinical subtype (TAFRO) of idiopathic multicentric Castleman disease. Am J Hematol. 2021 Oct 1;96(10):1241–52. PMID:34265103
2968. Nishishinya MB, Pereda CA, Muñoz-Fernández S, et al. Identification of lymphoma predictors in patients with primary Sjögren's syndrome: a systematic literature review and meta-analysis. Rheumatol Int. 2015 Jan;35(1):17–26. PMID:24899571
2969. Nishiu M, Tomita Y, Nakatsuka S, et al. Distinct pattern of gene expression in pyothorax-associated lymphoma (PAL), a lymphoma developing in long-standing inflammation. Cancer Sci. 2004 Oct;95(10):828–34. PMID:15504251
2970. Nishizawa S, Sakata-Yanagimoto M, Hattori K, et al. BCL6 locus is hypermethylated in angioimmunoblastic T-cell lymphoma. Int J Hematol. 2017 Apr;105(4):465–9. PMID:27921272
2971. Nitta Y, Iwatsuki K, Kimura H, et al. Fatal natural killer cell lymphoma arising in a patient with a crop of Epstein-Barr virus-associated disorders. Eur J Dermatol. 2005 Nov-Dec;15(6):503–6. PMID:16280311
2972. Nizze H, Cogliatti SB, von Schilling C, et al. Monocytoid B-cell lymphoma: morphological variants and relationship to low-grade B-cell lymphoma of the mucosa-associated lymphoid tissue. Histopathology. 1991 May;18(5):403–14. PMID:1885166
2973. Nofal A, Abdel-Mawla MY, Assaf M, et al. Primary cutaneous aggressive epidermotropic CD8+ T-cell lymphoma: proposed diagnostic criteria and therapeutic evaluation. J Am Acad Dermatol. 2012 Oct;67(4):748–59. PMID:22226429
2974. Nomani L, Cotta CV, Hsi ED, et al. Extranodal marginal zone lymphoma of the central nervous system includes parenchymal-based cases with characteristic features. Am J Clin Pathol. 2020 Jun 8;154(1):124–32. PMID:32318699
2975. Nomura R, Tokumura H, Katayose Y, et al. Sclerosing angiomatoid nodular transformation of the spleen: lessons from a rare case and review of the literature. Intern Med. 2019 May 15;58(10):1433–41. PMID:30626827
2976. Non-Hodgkin's Lymphoma Classification Project. A clinical evaluation of the International Lymphoma Study Group classification of non-Hodgkin's lymphoma. The Non-Hodgkin's Lymphoma Classification Project. Blood. 1997 Jun 1;89(11):3909–18. PMID:9166827
2977. Non-Hodgkin's Lymphoma Classification Project. A clinical evaluation of the International Lymphoma Study Group classification of non-Hodgkin's lymphoma. The Non-Hodgkin's Lymphoma Classification Project. Blood. 1997 Jun 1;89(11):3909–18. PMID:9166827
2978. Nooka AK, Nabhan C, Zhou X, et al. Examination of the follicular lymphoma international prognostic index (FLIPI) in the National LymphoCare study (NLCS): a prospective US patient cohort treated predominantly in community practices. Ann Oncol. 2013 Feb;24(2):441–8. PMID:23041589
2979. Norton AJ, Matthews J, Pappa V, et al. Mantle cell lymphoma: natural history defined in a serially biopsied population over a 20-year period. Ann Oncol. 1995 Mar;6(3):249–56. PMID:7612490
2980. Nosaka K, Iwanaga M, Imaizumi Y, et al. Epidemiological and clinical features of adult T-cell leukemia-lymphoma in Japan, 2010-2011: a nationwide survey. Cancer Sci. 2017 Dec;108(12):2478–86. PMID:28905463
2981. Nosrati A, Monabati A, Sadeghipour A, et al. MYC, BCL2, and BCL6 rearrangements in primary central nervous system lymphoma of large B cell type. Ann Hematol. 2019 Jan;98(1):169–73. PMID:30306208
2982. Novakova M, Zaliova M, Fiser K, et al. DUX4r, ZNF384r and PAX5-P80R mutated B-cell precursor acute lymphoblastic leukemia frequently undergo monocytic switch. Haematologica. 2021 Aug 1;106(8):2066–75. PMID:32646889
2983. Novelli S, Briones J, Flotats A, et al. PET/CT assessment of follicular lymphoma and high grade B cell lymphoma - good correlation with clinical and histological features at diagnosis. Adv Clin Exp Med. 2015 Mar-Apr;24(2):325–30. PMID:25931367
2984. Nowak D, Le Toriellec E, Stern MH, et al. Molecular allelokaryotyping of T-cell prolymphocytic leukemia cells with high density single nucleotide polymorphism arrays identifies novel common genomic lesions and acquired uniparental disomy. Haematologica. 2009 Apr;94(4):518–27. PMID:19278963
2985. Nowakowski GS, Chiappella A, Gascoyne RD, et al. ROBUST: a phase III study of lenalidomide plus R-CHOP versus placebo plus R-CHOP in previously untreated patients with ABC-type diffuse large B-cell lymphoma. J Clin Oncol. 2021 Apr 20;39(12):1317–28. PMID:33621109
2986. Noy A. Optimizing treatment of HIV-associated lymphoma. Blood. 2019 Oct 24;134(17):1385–94. PMID:30992269
2987. Noy A, Lee JY, Cesarman E, et al. AMC 048: modified CODOX-M/IVAC-rituximab is safe and effective for HIV-associated Burkitt lymphoma. Blood. 2015 Jul 9;126(2):160–6. PMID:25957391
2988. Noy A, Schöder H, Gönen M, et al. The majority of transformed lymphomas have high standardized uptake values (SUVs) on positron emission tomography (PET) scanning similar to diffuse large B-cell lymphoma (DLBCL). Ann Oncol. 2009 Mar;20(3):508–12. PMID:19139176
2989. Núñez-García B, Rodriguez-Pertierra M, Sequero S, et al. Long-term follow-up of patients with nodular lymphocyte predominant Hodgkin lymphoma: a report from the Spanish Lymphoma Oncology Group. Hematol Oncol. 2021 Oct;39(4):506–12. PMID:33528063
2990. Nyland SB, Feith DJ, Poss M, et al. Retroviral sero-reactivity in LGL leukaemia patients and family members. Br J Haematol. 2020 Feb;188(4):522–7. PMID:31608437
2991. Oakes CC, Claus R, Gu L, et al. Evolution of DNA methylation is linked to genetic aberrations in chronic lymphocytic leukemia. Cancer Discov. 2014 Mar;4(3):348–61. PMID:24356097
2992. Oakes CC, Seifert M, Assenov Y, et al. DNA methylation dynamics during B cell maturation underlie a continuum of disease phenotypes in chronic lymphocytic leukemia. Nat Genet. 2016 Mar;48(3):253–64. PMID:26780610
2993. Oberbeck S, Schrader A, Warner K, et al. Noncanonical effector functions of the T-memory-like T-PLL cell are shaped by cooperative TCL1A and TCR signaling. Blood. 2020 Dec 10;136(24):2786–802. PMID:33301031
2994. O'Connell KM. Kaposi's sarcoma in lymph nodes: histological study of lesions from 16 cases in Malawi. J Clin Pathol. 1977 Aug;30(8):696–703. PMID:579631
2995. Odabashian M, Carlotti E, Araf S, et al. IGHV sequencing reveals acquired N-glycosylation sites as a clonal and stable event during follicular lymphoma evolution. Blood. 2020 Mar 12;135(11):834–44. PMID:31932843
2996. Odejide O, Weigert O, Lane AA, et al. A targeted mutational landscape of angioimmunoblastic T-cell lymphoma. Blood. 2014 Feb 27;123(9):1293–6. PMID:24345752
2997. Oertel SH, Verschuuren E, Reinke P, et al. Effect of anti-CD 20 antibody rituximab in patients with post-transplant lymphoproliferative disorder (PTLD). Am J Transplant. 2005 Dec;5(12):2901–6. PMID:16303003
2998. O'Farrelly C, Feighery C, O'Briain DS, et al. Humoral response to wheat protein in patients with coeliac disease and enteropathy associated T cell lymphoma. Br Med J (Clin Res Ed). 1986 Oct 11;293(6552):908–10. PMID:3094712
2999. Offit K, Parsa NZ, Gaidano G, et al. 6q deletions define distinct clinico-pathologic subsets of non-Hodgkin's lymphoma. Blood. 1993 Oct 1;82(7):2157–62. PMID:8104536
3000. Ogata S, Miyoshi H, Arakawa F, et al. Clinicopathological features of in situ follicular neoplasm and relations with follicular lymphoma in Japan. Ann Hematol. 2020 Feb;99(2):241–53. PMID:31897674
3001. Ogembo JG, Milner DA Jr, Mansfield KG, et al. SIRPα/CD172a and FHOD1 are unique markers of littoral cells, a recently evolved major cell population of red pulp of human spleen. J Immunol. 2012 May 1;188(9):4496–505. PMID:22490440
3002. Ogwang MD, Bhatia K, Biggar RJ, et al. Incidence and geographic distribution of endemic Burkitt lymphoma in northern Uganda revisited. Int J Cancer. 2008 Dec 1;123(11):2658–63. PMID:18767045
3003. Oh J, Yoon H, Shin DK, et al. A case of successful management of HHV-8+, EBV+ germinotropic lymphoproliferative disorder (GLD). Int J Hematol. 2012 Jan;95(1):107–11. PMID:22167655
3004. Oh SY, Ryoo BY, Kim WS, et al. Nodal marginal zone B-cell lymphoma: analysis of 36 cases. Clinical presentation and treatment

outcomes of nodal marginal zone B-cell lymphoma. Ann Hematol. 2006 Nov;85(11):781–6. PMID:16847665
3005. O'Hara CJ, Said JW, Pinkus GS. Non-Hodgkin's lymphoma, multilobated B-cell type: report of nine cases with immunohistochemical and immunoultrastructural evidence for a follicular center cell derivation. Hum Pathol. 1986 Jun;17(6):593–9. PMID:3486810
3006. Ohashi A, Kato S, Okamoto A, et al. Reappraisal of Epstein-Barr virus (EBV) in diffuse large B-cell lymphoma (DLBCL): comparative analysis between EBV-positive and EBV-negative DLBCL with EBV-positive bystander cells. Histopathology. 2017 Jul;71(1):89–97. PMID:28231401
3007. Ohga S, Ishimura M, Yoshimoto G, et al. Clonal origin of Epstein-Barr virus (EBV)-infected T/NK-cell subpopulations in EBV-positive T/NK-cell lymphoproliferative disorders of childhood. J Clin Virol. 2011 May;51(1):31–7. PMID:21377409
3008. Ohgami RS, Arber DA, Zehnder JL, et al. Indolent T-lymphoblastic proliferation (iT-LBP): a review of clinical and pathologic features and distinction from malignant T-lymphoblastic lymphoma. Adv Anat Pathol. 2013 May;20(3):137–40. PMID:23574769
3009. Ohgami RS, Ohgami JK, Pereira IT, et al. Refining the diagnosis of T-cell large granular lymphocytic leukemia by combining distinct patterns of antigen expression with T-cell clonality studies. Leukemia. 2011 Sep;25(9):1439–43. PMID:21617700
3010. Ohgami RS, Sendamarai AK, Atwater SK, et al. Indolent T-lymphoblastic proliferation with disseminated multinodal involvement and partial CD33 expression. Am J Surg Pathol. 2014 Sep;38(9):1298–304. PMID:24618611
3011. Ohgami RS, Zhao S, Natkunam Y. Large B-cell lymphomas poor in B cells and rich in PD-1+ T cells can mimic T-cell lymphomas. Am J Clin Pathol. 2014 Aug;142(2):150–6. PMID:25015854
3012. Ohgami RS, Zhao S, Ohgami JK, et al. TdT+ T-lymphoblastic populations are increased in Castleman disease, in Castleman disease in association with follicular dendritic cell tumors, and in angioimmunoblastic T-cell lymphoma. Am J Surg Pathol. 2012 Nov;36(11):1619–28. PMID:23060347
3013. Ohki K, Kiyokawa N, Saito Y, et al. Clinical and molecular characteristics of MEF2D fusion-positive B-cell precursor acute lymphoblastic leukemia in childhood, including a novel translocation resulting in MEF2D-HN-RNPH1 gene fusion. Haematologica. 2019 Jan;104(1):128–37. PMID:30171027
3014. Ohki K, Takahashi H, Fukushima T, et al. Impact of immunophenotypic characteristics on genetic subgrouping in childhood acute lymphoblastic leukemia: Tokyo Children's Cancer Study Group (TCCSG) study L04-16. Genes Chromosomes Cancer. 2020 Oct;59(10):551–61. PMID:32368831
3015. Ohno T, Kanoh T, Arita Y, et al. Fulminant clonal expansion of large granular lymphocytes. Characterization of their morphology, phenotype, genotype, and function. Cancer. 1988 Nov 1;62(9):1918–27. PMID:3262409
3016. Ohno Y, Amakawa R, Fukuhara S, et al. Acute transformation of chronic large granular lymphocyte leukemia associated with additional chromosome abnormality. Cancer. 1989 Jul 1;64(1):63–7. PMID:2731121
3017. Ohshima K. Pathological features of diseases associated with human T-cell leukemia virus type I. Cancer Sci. 2007 Jun;98(6):772–8. PMID:17388788
3018. Ohshima K, Haraoka S, Takahata Y, et al. Interferon-gamma, interleukin-18, monokine induced by interferon-gamma and interferon-gamma-inducible protein-10 in histiocytic necrotizing lymphadenitis. Leuk Lymphoma. 2002 May;43(5):1115–20. PMID:12148894
3019. Ohshima K, Ishiguro M, Yamasaki S, et al. Chromosomal and comparative genomic analyses of HHV-8-negative primary effusion lymphoma in five HIV-negative Japanese patients. Leuk Lymphoma. 2002 Mar;43(3):595–601. PMID:12002764
3020. Ohshima K, Karube K, Hamasaki M, et al. Apoptosis- and cell cycle-associated gene expression profiling of histiocytic necrotising lymphadenitis. Eur J Haematol. 2004 May;72(5):322–9. PMID:15059066
3021. Ohshima K, Kimura H, Yoshino T, et al. Proposed categorization of pathological states of EBV-associated T/natural killer-cell lymphoproliferative disorder (LPD) in children and young adults: overlap with chronic active EBV infection and infantile fulminant EBV T-LPD. Pathol Int. 2008 Apr;58(4):209–17. PMID:18324913
3022. Ohshima K, Shimazaki K, Kume T, et al. Perforin and Fas pathways of cytotoxic T-cells in histiocytic necrotizing lymphadenitis. Histopathology. 1998 Nov;33(5):471–8. PMID:9839173
3023. Ohshima K, Suzumiya J, Kato A, et al. Clonal HTLV-I-infected CD4+ T-lymphocytes and non-clonal non-HTLV-I-infected giant cells in incipient ATLL with Hodgkin-like histologic features. Int J Cancer. 1997 Aug 7;72(4):592–8. PMID:9259396
3024. Ohshima K, Suzumiya J, Shimazaki K, et al. Nasal T/NK cell lymphomas commonly express perforin and Fas ligand: important mediators of tissue damage. Histopathology. 1997 Nov;31(5):444–50. PMID:9416485
3025. Oishi N, Brody GS, Ketterling RP, et al. Genetic subtyping of breast implant-associated anaplastic large cell lymphoma. Blood. 2018 Aug 2;132(5):544–7. PMID:29921615
3026. Oishi N, Hundal T, Phillips JL, et al. Molecular profiling reveals a hypoxia signature in breast implant-associated anaplastic large cell lymphoma. Haematologica. 2021 Jun 1;106(6):1714–24. PMID:32414854
3027. Oishi N, Miranda RN, Feldman AL. Genetics of breast implant-associated anaplastic large cell lymphoma (BIA-ALCL). Aesthet Surg J. 2019 Jan 31;39 Suppl_1:S14–20. PMID:30715169
3028. Oishi N, Montes-Moreno S, Feldman AL. In situ neoplasia in lymph node pathology. Semin Diagn Pathol. 2018 Jan;35(1):76–83. PMID:29129357
3029. Oishi N, Segawa T, Miyake K, et al. Incidence, clinicopathological features and genetics of in-situ follicular neoplasia: a comprehensive screening study in a Japanese cohort. Histopathology. 2022 Apr;80(5):820–6. PMID:35038193
3030. Ojha SS, Jain R, Meenai F, et al. Cytomorphological findings of follicular dendritic cell sarcoma on fine-needle aspiration cytology. Acta Cytol. 2018;62(2):145–50. PMID:29275417
3031. Ok CY, Li L, Xu-Monette ZY, et al. Prevalence and clinical implications of Epstein-Barr virus infection in de novo diffuse large B-cell lymphoma in western countries. Clin Cancer Res. 2014 May 1;20(9):2338–49. PMID:24583797
3032. Ok CY, Medeiros LJ. High-grade B-cell lymphoma: a term re-purposed in the revised WHO classification. Pathology. 2020 Jan;52(1):68–77. PMID:31735344
3033. Ok CY, Medeiros LJ, Thakral B, et al. High-grade B-cell lymphomas with TdT expression: a diagnostic and classification dilemma. Mod Pathol. 2019 Jan;32(1):48–58. PMID:30181564
3034. Ok CY, Papathomas TG, Medeiros LJ, et al. EBV-positive diffuse large B-cell lymphoma of the elderly. Blood. 2013 Jul 18;122(3):328–40. PMID:23649469
3035. Okada T, Miller MJ, Parker I, et al. Antigen-engaged B cells undergo chemotaxis toward the T zone and form motile conjugates with helper T cells. PLoS Biol. 2005 Jun;3(6):e150. PMID:15857154
3036. Okada Y, Feng Q, Lin Y, et al. hDOT1L links histone methylation to leukemogenesis. Cell. 2005 Apr 22;121(2):167–78. PMID:15851025
3037. Okamoto A, Yanada M, Miura H, et al. Prognostic significance of Epstein-Barr virus DNA detection in pretreatment serum in diffuse large B-cell lymphoma. Cancer Sci. 2015 Nov;106(11):1576–81. PMID:26353084
3038. Okano M, Kawa K, Kimura H, et al. Proposed guidelines for diagnosing chronic active Epstein-Barr virus infection. Am J Hematol. 2005 Sep;80(1):64–9. PMID:16138335
3039. Okano M, Thiele GM, Davis JR, et al. Epstein-Barr virus and human diseases: recent advances in diagnosis. Clin Microbiol Rev. 1988 Jul;1(3):300–12. PMID:2848624
3040. Okosun J, Bödör C, Wang J, et al. Integrated genomic analysis identifies recurrent mutations and evolution patterns driving the initiation and progression of follicular lymphoma. Nat Genet. 2014 Feb;46(2):176–81. PMID:24362818
3041. Okosun J, Montoto S, Fitzgibbon J. The routes for transformation of follicular lymphoma. Curr Opin Hematol. 2016 Jul;23(4):385–91. PMID:27135979
3042. Oksenhendler E, Boulanger E, Galicier L, et al. High incidence of Kaposi sarcoma-associated herpesvirus-related non-Hodgkin lymphoma in patients with HIV infection and multicentric Castleman disease. Blood. 2002 Apr 1;99(7):2331–6. PMID:11895764
3043. Oksenhendler E, Boutboul D, Fajgenbaum D, et al. The full spectrum of Castleman disease: 273 patients studied over 20 years. Br J Haematol. 2018 Jan;180(2):206–16. PMID:29143319
3044. Oksenhendler E, Carcelain G, Aoki Y, et al. High levels of human herpesvirus 8 viral load, human interleukin-6, interleukin-10, and C reactive protein correlate with exacerbation of multicentric Castleman disease in HIV-infected patients. Blood. 2000 Sep 15;96(6):2069–73. PMID:10979949
3045. Oksenhendler E, Duarte M, Soulier J, et al. Multicentric Castleman's disease in HIV infection: a clinical and pathological study of 20 patients. AIDS. 1996 Jan;10(1):61–7. PMID:8924253
3046. Okuda T, Sakamoto S, Deguchi T, et al. Hemophagocytic syndrome associated with aggressive natural killer cell leukemia. Am J Hematol. 1991 Dec;38(4):321–3. PMID:1746541
3047. Okudolo JO, Bagg A, Meghpara BB, et al. Conjunctival pediatric-type follicular lymphoma. Ophthalmic Plast Reconstr Surg. 2020 Mar/Apr;36(2):e46–9. PMID:31868792
3048. Okuma K, Kuramitsu M, Niwa T, et al. Establishment of a novel diagnostic test algorithm for human T-cell leukemia virus type 1 infection with line immunoassay replacement of western blotting: a collaborative study for performance evaluation of diagnostic assays in Japan. Retrovirology. 2020 Aug 24;17(1):26. PMID:32831150
3049. Okumura K, Ikebe M, Shimokama T, et al. An unusual enteropathy-associated T-cell lymphoma with MYC translocation arising in a Japanese patient: a case report. World J Gastroenterol. 2012 May 21;18(19):2434–7. PMID:22654438
3050. Okuno Y, Murata T, Sato Y, et al. Defective Epstein-Barr virus in chronic active infection and haematological malignancy. Nat Microbiol. 2019 Mar;4(3):404–13. PMID:30664667
3051. Okuyama K, Strid T, Kuruvilla J, et al. PAX5 is part of a functional transcription factor network targeted in lymphoid leukemia. PLoS Genet. 2019 Aug 5;15(8):e1008280. PMID:31381561
3052. Oliveira JB, Bleesing JJ, Dianzani U, et al. Revised diagnostic criteria and classification for the autoimmune lymphoproliferative syndrome (ALPS): report from the 2009 NIH International Workshop. Blood. 2010 Oct 7;116(14):e35–40. PMID:20538792
3053. Ollila TA, Reagan JL, Olszewski AJ. Clinical features and survival of patients with T-cell/histiocyte-rich large B-cell lymphoma: analysis of the National Cancer Data Base. Leuk Lymphoma. 2019 Dec;60(14):3426–33. PMID:31287335
3054. Olsen E, Vonderheid E, Pimpinelli N, et al. Revisions to the staging and classification of mycosis fungoides and Sezary syndrome: a proposal of the International Society for Cutaneous Lymphomas (ISCL) and the cutaneous lymphoma task force of the European Organization of Research and Treatment of Cancer (EORTC). Blood. 2007 Sep 15;110(6):1713–22. PMID:17540844
3055. Olsson L, Castor A, Behrendtz M, et al. Deletions of IKZF1 and SPRED1 are associated with poor prognosis in a population-based series of pediatric B-cell precursor acute lymphoblastic leukemia diagnosed between 1992 and 2011. Leukemia. 2014 Feb;28(2):302–10. PMID:23823658
3056. Olszewski AJ, Castillo JJ. Outcomes of HIV-associated Hodgkin lymphoma in the era of antiretroviral therapy. AIDS. 2016 Mar 13;30(5):787–96. PMID:26730566
3057. Olszewski AJ, Chorzalska AD, Petersen M, et al. Detection of clonotypic DNA in the cerebrospinal fluid as a marker of central nervous system invasion in lymphoma. Blood Adv. 2021 Dec 28;5(24):5525–35. PMID:34551072
3058. Olszewski AJ, Jakobsen LH, Collins GP, et al. Burkitt Lymphoma International Prognostic Index. J Clin Oncol. 2021 Apr 1;39(10):1129–38. PMID:33502927
3059. Olszewski AJ, Kurt H, Evens AM. Defining and treating high-grade B-cell lymphoma, NOS. Blood. 2022 Sep 1;140(9):943–54. PMID:34525177
3060. O'Malley DP, Kim YS, Weiss LM. Distinctive immunohistochemical staining in littoral cell angioma using ERG and WT-1. Ann Diagn Pathol. 2015 Jun;19(3):143–5. PMID:25792460
3061. O'Malley DP, Orazi A. Terminal deoxynucleotidyl transferase-positive cells in spleen, appendix and branchial cleft cysts in pediatric patients. Haematologica. 2006 Aug;91(8):1139–40. PMID:16885057
3062. Onaindia A, Martínez N, Montes-Moreno S, et al. CD30 expression by B and T cells: a frequent finding in angioimmunoblastic T-cell lymphoma and peripheral T-cell lymphoma-not otherwise specified. Am J Surg Pathol. 2016 Mar;40(3):378–85. PMID:26574847
3063. Onaindia A, Montes-Moreno S, Rodríguez-Pinilla SM, et al. Primary cutaneous anaplastic large cell lymphomas with 6p25.3 rearrangement exhibit particular histological features. Histopathology. 2015 May;66(6):846–55. PMID:25131361
3064. Onciu M, Behm FG, Downing JR, et al. ALK-positive plasmablastic B-cell lymphoma with expression of the NPM-ALK fusion transcript: report of 2 cases. Blood. 2003 Oct 1;102(7):2642–4. PMID:12816858
3065. Onciu M, Lorsbach RB, Henry EC, et

al. Terminal deoxynucleotidyl transferase-positive lymphoid cells in reactive lymph nodes from children with malignant tumors: incidence, distribution pattern, and immunophenotype in 26 patients. Am J Clin Pathol. 2002 Aug;118(2):248–54. PMID:12162686
3066. Ondrejka SL, Grzywacz B, Bodo J, et al. Angioimmunoblastic T-cell lymphomas with the RHOA p.Gly17Val mutation have classic clinical and pathologic features. Am J Surg Pathol. 2016 Mar;40(3):335–41. PMID:26574844
3067. Ondrejka SL, Lai R, Smith SD, et al. Indolent mantle cell leukemia: a clinicopathological variant characterized by isolated lymphocytosis, interstitial bone marrow involvement, kappa light chain restriction, and good prognosis. Haematologica. 2011 Aug;96(8):1121–7. PMID:21508124
3068. O'Neil J, Grim J, Strack P, et al. FBW7 mutations in leukemic cells mediate NOTCH pathway activation and resistance to gamma-secretase inhibitors. J Exp Med. 2007 Aug 6;204(8):1813–24. PMID:17646409
3069. Opatrny V, Treska V, Waloschek T, et al. Littoral cell angioma of the spleen: a case report. SAGE Open Med Case Rep. 2020 Oct 4;8:X20959874. PMID:33088569
3070. Opie J, Antel K, Koller A, et al. In the South African setting, HIV-associated Burkitt lymphoma is associated with frequent leukaemic presentation, complex cytogenetic karyotypes, and adverse clinical outcomes. Ann Hematol. 2020 Mar;99(3):571–8. PMID:31955214
3071. Orchard J, Garand R, Davis Z, et al. A subset of t(11;14) lymphoma with mantle cell features displays mutated IgVH genes and includes patients with good prognosis, nonnodal disease. Blood. 2003 Jun 15;101(12):4975–81. PMID:12609845
3072. Ortonne N, Huet D, Gaudez C, et al. Significance of circulating T-cell clones in Sezary syndrome. Blood. 2006 May 15;107(10):4030–8. PMID:16418328
3073. Ortonne N, Le Gouvello S, Mansour H, et al. CD158K/KIR3DL2 transcript detection in lesional skin of patients with erythroderma is a tool for the diagnosis of Sézary syndrome. J Invest Dermatol. 2008 Feb;128(2):465–72. PMID:17703174
3074. Oschlies I, Burkhardt B, Salaverria I, et al. Clinical, pathological and genetic features of primary mediastinal large B-cell lymphomas and mediastinal gray zone lymphomas in children. Haematologica. 2011 Feb;96(2):262–8. PMID:20971819
3075. Oschlies I, Kohler CW, Szczepanowski M, et al. Spindle-cell variants of primary cutaneous follicle center B-cell lymphomas are germinal center B-cell lymphomas by gene expression profiling using a formalin-fixed paraffin-embedded specimen. J Invest Dermatol. 2017 Nov;137(11):2450–3. PMID:28684330
3076. Oschlies I, Lisfeld J, Lamant L, et al. ALK-positive anaplastic large cell lymphoma limited to the skin: clinical, histopathological and molecular analysis of 6 pediatric cases. A report from the ALCL99 study. Haematologica. 2013 Jan;98(1):50–6. PMID:22773605
3077. Oschlies I, Salaverria I, Mahn F, et al. Pediatric follicular lymphoma–a clinico-pathological study of a population-based series of patients treated within the Non-Hodgkin's Lymphoma–Berlin-Frankfurt-Munster (NHL-BFM) multicenter trials. Haematologica. 2010 Feb;95(2):253–9. PMID:19679882
3078. O'Shea D, O'Riain C, Taylor C, et al. The presence of TP53 mutation at diagnosis of follicular lymphoma identifies a high-risk group of patients with shortened time to disease progression and poorer overall survival. Blood. 2008 Oct 15;112(8):3126–9. PMID:18628487
3079. Oshimi K, Yamada O, Kaneko T, et al. Laboratory findings and clinical courses of 33 patients with granular lymphocyte-proliferative disorders. Leukemia. 1993 Jun;7(6):782–8. PMID:8388971
3080. Ostrom QT, Gittleman H, Truitt G, et al. CBTRUS statistical report: primary brain and other central nervous system tumors diagnosed in the United States in 2011-2015. Neuro Oncol. 2018 Oct 1;20 suppl_4:iv1–86. PMID:30445539
3081. Osuji N, Beiske K, Randen U, et al. Characteristic appearances of the bone marrow in T-cell large granular lymphocyte leukaemia. Histopathology. 2007 Apr;50(5):547–54. PMID:17394489
3082. Osuji N, Matutes E, Catovsky D, et al. Histopathology of the spleen in T-cell large granular lymphocyte leukemia and T-cell prolymphocytic leukemia: a comparative review. Am J Surg Pathol. 2005 Jul;29(7):935–41. PMID:15958859
3083. O'Suoji C, Welch JJ, Perkins SL, et al. Rare pediatric non-Hodgkin lymphomas: a report from Children's Oncology Group study ANHL 04B1. Pediatr Blood Cancer. 2016 May;63(5):794–800. PMID:26728447
3084. Otani K, Inoue D, Fujikura K, et al. Idiopathic multicentric Castleman's disease: a clinicopathologic study in comparison with IgG4-related disease. Oncotarget. 2018 Jan 9;9(6):6691–706. PMID:29467920
3085. Ott G. Aggressive B-cell lymphomas in the update of the 4th edition of the World Health Organization classification of haematopoietic and lymphatic tissues: refinements of the classification, new entities and genetic findings. Br J Haematol. 2017 Sep;178(6):871–87. PMID:28748558
3086. Ott G, Kalla J, Ott MM, et al. Blastoid variants of mantle cell lymphoma: frequent bcl-1 rearrangements at the major translocation cluster region and tetraploid chromosome clones. Blood. 1997 Feb 15;89(4):1421–9. PMID:9028966
3087. Ott G, Katzenberger T, Lohr A, et al. Cytomorphologic, immunohistochemical, and cytogenetic profiles of follicular lymphoma: 2 types of follicular lymphoma grade 3. Blood. 2002 May 15;99(10):3806–12. PMID:11986240
3088. Ott G, Ziepert M, Klapper W, et al. Immunoblastic morphology but not the immunohistochemical GCB/nonGCB classifier predicts outcome in diffuse large B-cell lymphoma in the RICOVER-60 trial of the DSHNHL. Blood. 2010 Dec 2;116(23):4916–25. PMID:20736456
3089. Ouansafi I, He B, Fraser C, et al. Transformation of follicular lymphoma to plasmablastic lymphoma with c-myc gene rearrangement. Am J Clin Pathol. 2010 Dec;134(6):972–81. PMID:21088162
3090. Owaidah TM, Rawas FI, Al Khayatt MF, et al. Expression of CD66c and CD25 in acute lymphoblastic leukemia as a predictor of the presence of BCR/ABL rearrangement. Hematol Oncol Stem Cell Ther. 2008 Jan-Mar;1(1):34–7. PMID:20063526
3091. Oyama T, Ichimura K, Suzuki R, et al. Senile EBV+ B-cell lymphoproliferative disorders: a clinicopathologic study of 22 patients. Am J Surg Pathol. 2003 Jan;27(1):16–26. PMID:12502924
3092. Oyama T, Yamamoto K, Asano N, et al. Age-related EBV-associated B-cell lymphoproliferative disorders constitute a distinct clinicopathologic group: a study of 96 patients. Clin Cancer Res. 2007 Sep 1;13(17):5124–32. PMID:17785567
3093. Ozawa MG, Bhaduri A, Chisholm KM, et al. A study of the mutational landscape of pediatric-type follicular lymphoma and pediatric nodal marginal zone lymphoma. Mod Pathol. 2016 Oct;29(10):1212–20. PMID:27338637
3094. Ozawa MG, Ewalt MD, Gratzinger D. Dasatinib-related follicular hyperplasia: an underrecognized entity with characteristic morphology. Am J Surg Pathol. 2015 Oct;39(10):1363–9. PMID:26360368
3095. Ozsahin M, Tsang RW, Poortmans P, et al. Outcomes and patterns of failure in solitary plasmacytoma: a multicenter Rare Cancer Network study of 258 patients. Int J Radiat Oncol Biol Phys. 2006 Jan 1;64(1):210–7. PMID:16229966
3096. Ozuah NW, Lubega J, Allen CE, et al. Five decades of low intensity and low survival: adapting intensified regimens to cure pediatric Burkitt lymphoma in Africa. Blood Adv. 2020 Aug 25;4(16):4007–19. PMID:32841337
3097. Pacheco SE, Gottschalk SM, Gresik MV, et al. Chronic active Epstein-Barr virus infection of natural killer cells presenting as severe skin reaction to mosquito bites. J Allergy Clin Immunol. 2005 Aug;116(2):470–2. PMID:16083813
3098. Pae J, Ersching J, Castro TBR, et al. Cyclin D3 drives inertial cell cycling in dark zone germinal center B cells. J Exp Med. 2021 Apr 5;218(4):e20201699. PMID:33332554
3099. Pai RK, Mullins FM, Kim YH, et al. Cytologic evaluation of lymphadenopathy associated with mycosis fungoides and Sezary syndrome: role of immunophenotypic and molecular ancillary studies. Cancer. 2008 Oct 25;114(5):323–32. PMID:18798522
3100. Paietta E, Ferrando AA, Neuberg D, et al. Activating FLT3 mutations in CD117/KIT(+) T-cell acute lymphoblastic leukemias. Blood. 2004 Jul 15;104(2):558–60. PMID:15044257
3101. Paietta E, Racevskis J, Neuberg D, et al. Expression of CD25 (interleukin-2 receptor alpha chain) in adult acute lymphoblastic leukemia predicts for the presence of BCR/ABL fusion transcripts: results of a preliminary laboratory analysis of ECOG/MRC Intergroup Study E2993. Leukemia. 1997 Nov;11(11):1887–90. PMID:9369422
3102. Paietta E, Roberts KG, Wang V, et al. Molecular classification improves risk assessment in adult BCR-ABL1-negative B-ALL. Blood. 2021 Sep 16;138(11):948–58. PMID:33895809
3103. Paik JH, Jang JY, Jeon YK, et al. MicroRNA-146a downregulates NFκB activity via targeting TRAF6 and functions as a tumor suppressor having strong prognostic implications in NK/T cell lymphoma. Clin Cancer Res. 2011 Jul 15;17(14):4761–71. PMID:21610143
3104. Paiva B, Almeida J, Pérez-Andrés M, et al. Utility of flow cytometry immunophenotyping in multiple myeloma and other clonal plasma cell-related disorders. Cytometry B Clin Cytom. 2010 Jul;78(4):239–52. PMID:20155853
3105. Paiva B, Chandia M, Vidriales MB, et al. Multiparameter flow cytometry for staging of solitary bone plasmacytoma: new criteria for risk of progression to myeloma. Blood. 2014 Aug 21;124(8):1300–3. PMID:24876564
3106. Paiva B, Pérez-Andrés M, Vidriales MB, et al. Competition between clonal plasma cells and normal cells for potentially overlapping bone marrow niches is associated with a progressively altered cellular distribution in MGUS vs myeloma. Leukemia. 2011 Apr;25(4):697–706. PMID:21252988
3107. Paiva B, Puig N, Cedena MT, et al. Measurable residual disease by next-generation flow cytometry in multiple myeloma. J Clin Oncol. 2020 Mar 10;38(8):784–92. PMID:31770060
3108. Paiva B, Vidriales MB, Mateo G, et al. The persistence of immunophenotypically normal residual bone marrow plasma cells at diagnosis identifies a good prognostic subgroup of symptomatic multiple myeloma patients. Blood. 2009 Nov 12;114(20):4369–72. PMID:19755674
3109. Paiva B, Vidriales MB, Pérez JJ, et al. The clinical utility and prognostic value of multiparameter flow cytometry immunophenotyping in light-chain amyloidosis. Blood. 2011 Mar 31;117(13):3613–6. PMID:21266717
3110. Paiva B, Vídriales MB, Rosiñol L, et al. A multiparameter flow cytometry immunophenotypic algorithm for the identification of newly diagnosed symptomatic myeloma with an MGUS-like signature and long-term disease control. Leukemia. 2013 Oct;27(10):2056–61. PMID:23743858
3111. Palacios G, Shaw TI, Li Y, et al. Novel ALK fusion in anaplastic large cell lymphoma involving EEF1G, a subunit of the eukaryotic elongation factor-1 complex. Leukemia. 2017 Mar;31(3):743–7. PMID:27840423
3111A. Palladini G, Campana C, Klersy C, et al. Serum N-terminal pro-brain natriuretic peptide is a sensitive marker of myocardial dysfunction in AL amyloidosis. Circulation. 2003 May 20;107(19):2440–5. PMID:12719281
3112. Palladini G, Dispenzieri A, Gertz MA, et al. New criteria for response to treatment in immunoglobulin light chain amyloidosis based on free light chain measurement and cardiac biomarkers: impact on survival outcomes. J Clin Oncol. 2012 Dec 20;30(36):4541–9. PMID:23091105
3113. Palladini G, Schönland SO, Sanchorawala V, et al. Clarification on the definition of complete haematologic response in light-chain (AL) amyloidosis. Amyloid. 2021 Mar;28(1):1–2. PMID:33410355
3114. Palomero J, Vegliante MC, Eguileor A, et al. SOX11 defines two different subtypes of mantle cell lymphoma through transcriptional regulation of BCL6. Leukemia. 2016 Jul;30(7):1596–9. PMID:26710884
3115. Palomero T, Couronné L, Khiabanian H, et al. Recurrent mutations in epigenetic regulators, RHOA and FYN kinase in peripheral T cell lymphomas. Nat Genet. 2014 Feb;46(2):166–70. PMID:24413734
3116. Palumbo A, Avet-Loiseau H, Oliva S, et al. Revised International Staging System for multiple myeloma: a report from International Myeloma Working Group. J Clin Oncol. 2015 Sep 10;33(26):2863–9. PMID:26240224
3117. Pan Q, Li J, Li F, et al. Characterizing POEMS Syndrome with 18F-FDG PET/CT. J Nucl Med. 2015 Sep;56(9):1334–7. PMID:26182964
3118. Pan ST, Cheng CY, Lee NS, et al. Follicular dendritic cell sarcoma of the inflammatory pseudotumor-like variant presenting as a colonic polyp. Korean J Pathol. 2014 Apr;48(2):140–5. PMID:24868227
3119. Pan ST, Wang RC, Su YZ, et al. Lymphomatous effusion of monomorphic epitheliotropic intestinal T-cell lymphoma is characterized by azurophilic granules and is a dismal sign: report of two new cases with literature review. Diagn Cytopathol. 2021 Jul;49(7):E247–52. PMID:33387400
3120. Pan Z, Chen M, Zhang Q, et al. CD3-positive plasmablastic B-cell neoplasms: a diagnostic pitfall. Mod Pathol. 2018 May;31(5):718–31. PMID:29327711
3121. Pan Z, Hu S, Li M, et al. ALK-positive large B-cell lymphoma: a clinicopathologic study of 26 cases with review of additional 108 cases in the literature. Am J Surg Pathol. 2017 Jan;41(1):25–38. PMID:27740969
3122. Pan Z, Xie Q, Repertinger S, et al. Plasmablastic transformation of low-grade CD5+ B-cell lymphoproliferative disorder with MYC gene rearrangements. Hum Pathol. 2013 Oct;44(10):2139–48. PMID:23791008
3123. Panagopoulos I, Micci F, Thorsen J, et al. A novel TCF3-HLF fusion transcript in acute lymphoblastic leukemia with a t(17;19)(q22;p13). Cancer Genet. 2012 Dec;205(12):669–72. PMID:23181981

3124. Pandolfi F, Loughran TP Jr, Starkebaum G, et al. Clinical course and prognosis of the lymphoproliferative disease of granular lymphocytes. A multicenter study. Cancer. 1990 Jan 15;65(2):341–8. PMID:2403836

3125. Panea RI, Love CL, Shingleton JR, et al. The whole-genome landscape of Burkitt lymphoma subtypes. Blood. 2019 Nov 7;134(19):1598–607. PMID:31558468

3126. Pang J, Mydlarz WK, Gooi Z, et al. Follicular dendritic cell sarcoma of the head and neck: case report, literature review, and pooled analysis of 97 cases. Head Neck. 2016 Apr;38 Suppl 1(Suppl 1):E2241–9. PMID:25917851

3127. Panjwani PK, Charu V, DeLisser M, et al. Programmed death-1 ligands PD-L1 and PD-L2 show distinctive and restricted patterns of expression in lymphoma subtypes. Hum Pathol. 2018 Jan;71:91–9. PMID:29122656

3128. Pantziarka P. Li Fraumeni syndrome, cancer and senescence: a new hypothesis. Cancer Cell Int. 2013 Apr 15;13(1):35. PMID:23587008

3129. Papadaki L, Wotherspoon AC, Isaacson PG. The lymphoepithelial lesion of gastric low-grade B-cell lymphoma of mucosa-associated lymphoid tissue (MALT): an ultrastructural study. Histopathology. 1992 Nov;21(5):415–21. PMID:1452124

3130. Papadaki T, Stamatopoulos K, Belessi C, et al. Splenic marginal-zone lymphoma: one or more entities? A histologic, immunohistochemical, and molecular study of 42 cases. Am J Surg Pathol. 2007 Mar;31(3):438–46. PMID:17325486

3131. Papaemmanuil E, Hosking FJ, Vijayakrishnan J, et al. Loci on 7p12.2, 10q21.2 and 14q11.2 are associated with risk of childhood acute lymphoblastic leukemia. Nat Genet. 2009 Sep;41(9):1006–10. PMID:19684604

3132. Papanicolau-Sengos A, Wang-Rodriguez J, Wang HY, et al. Rare case of a primary non-dural central nervous system low grade B-cell lymphoma and literature review. Int J Clin Exp Pathol. 2012;5(1):89–95. PMID:22295152

3133. Parihar M, Singh MK, Islam R, et al. A triple-probe FISH screening strategy for risk-stratified therapy of acute lymphoblastic leukaemia in low-resource settings. Pediatr Blood Cancer. 2018 Dec;65(12):e27366. PMID:30168245

3134. Parikh PM, Desai S, Naresh KN, et al. Incidence of 5' bcl-2 rearrangement in patients with B cell chronic lymphocytic leukemia from India. Leuk Res. 1996 Sep;20(9):791–3. PMID:8947590

3135. Parikh SA, Leis JF, Chaffee KG, et al. Hypogammaglobulinemia in newly diagnosed chronic lymphocytic leukemia: natural history, clinical correlates, and outcomes. Cancer. 2015 Sep 1;121(17):2883–91. PMID:25931291

3136. Parikh SA, Rabe KG, Kay NE, et al. The CLL International Prognostic Index predicts outcomes in monoclonal B-cell lymphocytosis and Rai 0 CLL. Blood. 2021 Jul 15;138(2):149–59. PMID:33876228

3137. Park J, Daniels J, Wartewig T, et al. Integrated genomic analyses of cutaneous T-cell lymphomas reveal the molecular bases for disease heterogeneity. Blood. 2021 Oct 7;138(14):1225–36. PMID:34115827

3138. Park J, Yang J, Wenzel AT, et al. Genomic analysis of 220 CTCLs identifies a novel recurrent gain-of-function alteration in RLTPR (p.Q575E). Blood. 2017 Sep 21;130(12):1430–40. PMID:28694326

3139. Park JH, Shin HT, Lee DY, et al. World Health Organization-European Organization for Research and Treatment of Cancer classification of cutaneous lymphoma in Korea: a retrospective study at a single tertiary institution. J Am Acad Dermatol. 2012 Dec;67(6):1200–9. PMID:22521781

3140. Park MJ, Park SH, Park PW, et al. Prognostic impact of concordant and discordant bone marrow involvement and cell-of-origin in Korean patients with diffuse large B-cell lymphoma treated with R-CHOP. J Clin Pathol. 2015 Sep;68(9):733–8. PMID:25998512

3141. Park S, Ko YH. Epstein-Barr virus-associated T/natural killer-cell lymphoproliferative disorders. J Dermatol. 2014 Jan;41(1):29–39. PMID:24438142

3142. Park S, Lee J, Ko YH, et al. The impact of Epstein-Barr virus status on clinical outcome in diffuse large B-cell lymphoma. Blood. 2007 Aug 1;110(3):972–8. PMID:17400912

3143. Parkin JL, Arthur DC, Abramson CS, et al. Acute leukemia associated with the t(4;11) chromosome rearrangement: ultrastructural and immunologic characteristics. Blood. 1982 Dec;60(6):1321–31. PMID:6958337

3144. Parravicini C, Chandran B, Corbellino M, et al. Differential viral protein expression in Kaposi's sarcoma-associated herpesvirus-infected diseases: Kaposi's sarcoma, primary effusion lymphoma, and multicentric Castleman's disease. Am J Pathol. 2000 Mar;156(3):743–9. PMID:10702388

3145. Parravicini C, Corbellino M, Paulli M, et al. Expression of a virus-derived cytokine, KSHV vIL-6, in HIV-seronegative Castleman's disease. Am J Pathol. 1997 Dec;151(6):1517–22. PMID:9403701

3146. Parrilla Castellar ER, Jaffe ES, Said JW, et al. ALK-negative anaplastic large cell lymphoma is a genetically heterogeneous disease with widely disparate clinical outcomes. Blood. 2014 Aug 28;124(9):1473–80. PMID:24894770

3147. Parsonnet J, Hansen S, Rodriguez L, et al. Helicobacter pylori infection and gastric lymphoma. N Engl J Med. 1994 May 5;330(18):1267–71. PMID:8145781

3148. Pascal V, Schleinitz N, Brunet C, et al. Comparative analysis of NK cell subset distribution in normal and lymphoproliferative disease of granular lymphocyte conditions. Eur J Immunol. 2004 Oct;34(10):2930–40. PMID:15368309

3149. Pascart T, Herbaux C, Lemaire A, et al. Coexistence of rheumatoid arthritis and TEMPI syndrome: new insight in microangiogenic-related diseases. Joint Bone Spine. 2016 Oct;83(5):587–8. PMID:26639219

3150. Paschold L, Willscher E, Bein J, et al. Evolutionary clonal trajectories in nodular lymphocyte-predominant Hodgkin lymphoma with high risk of transformation. Haematologica. 2021 Oct 1;106(10):2654–66. PMID:33882641

3151. Pasqualucci L, Dalla-Favera R. The genetic landscape of diffuse large B-cell lymphoma. Semin Hematol. 2015 Apr;52(2):67–76. PMID:25805586

3152. Pasqualucci L, Khiabanian H, Fangazio M, et al. Genetics of follicular lymphoma transformation. Cell Rep. 2014 Jan 16;6(1):130–40. PMID:24388756

3153. Passet M, Boissel N, Sigaux F, et al. PAX5 P80R mutation identifies a novel subtype of B-cell precursor acute lymphoblastic leukemia with favorable outcome. Blood. 2019 Jan 17;133(3):280–4. PMID:30510083

3154. Pastore A, Jurinovic V, Kridel R, et al. Integration of gene mutations in risk prognostication for patients receiving first-line immunochemotherapy for follicular lymphoma: a retrospective analysis of a prospective clinical trial and validation in a population-based registry. Lancet Oncol. 2015 Sep;16(9):1111–22. PMID:26256760

3155. Pastorello RG, D'Almeida Costa F, Osório CABT, et al. Breast implant-associated anaplastic large cell lymphoma in a Li-Fraumeni patient: a case report. Diagn Pathol. 2018 Jan 25;13(1):10. PMID:29370815

3156. Pastoret C, Desmots F, Drillet G, et al. Linking the KIR phenotype with STAT3 and TET2 mutations to identify chronic lymphoproliferative disorders of NK cells. Blood. 2021 Jun 10;137(23):3237–50. PMID:33512451

3157. Patel JL, Smith LM, Anderson J, et al. The immunophenotype of T-lymphoblastic lymphoma in children and adolescents: a Children's Oncology Group report. Br J Haematol. 2012 Nov;159(4):454–61. PMID:22994934

3158. Patel MP, Kirkpatrick JP, Johnson MO, et al. Patterns of relapse after successful completion of initial therapy in primary central nervous system lymphoma: a case series. J Neurooncol. 2020 Apr;147(2):477–83. PMID:32140975

3159. Patel N, Durkin L, Bodo J, et al. Immunohistochemical expression of lymphoid enhancer binding factor 1 in CD5-positive marginal zone, lymphoplasmacytic, and follicular lymphomas. Am J Clin Pathol. 2020 Apr 15;153(5):646–55. PMID:31953940

3160. Patel VM, Flanagan CE, Martins M, et al. Frequent and persistent PLCG1 mutations in Sézary cells directly enhance PLCγ1 activity and stimulate NFκB, AP-1, and NFAT signaling. J Invest Dermatol. 2020 Feb;140(2):380–389.e4. PMID:31376383

3161. Patil P, Cieslak A, Bernhart SH, et al. Reconstruction of rearranged T-cell receptor loci by whole genome and transcriptome sequencing gives insights into the initial steps of T-cell prolymphocytic leukemia. Genes Chromosomes Cancer. 2020 Apr;59(4):261–7. PMID:31677197

3162. Patkar N, Bhanshe P, Rajpal S, et al. NARASIMHA: novel assay based on targeted RNA sequencing to identify chimeric gene fusions in hematological malignancies. Blood Cancer J. 2020 May 5;10(5):50. PMID:32372024

3163. Patrick K, Wade R, Goulden N, et al. Outcome for children and young people with Early T-cell precursor acute lymphoblastic leukaemia treated on a contemporary protocol, UKALL 2003. Br J Haematol. 2014 Aug;166(3):421–4. PMID:24708207

3164. Patsalides AD, Atac G, Hedge U, et al. Lymphomatoid granulomatosis: abnormalities of the brain at MR imaging. Radiology. 2005 Oct;237(1):265–73. PMID:16100084

3165. Patzelt M, Zarubova L, Klener P, et al. Anaplastic large-cell lymphoma associated with breast implants: a case report of a transgender female. Aesthetic Plast Surg. 2018 Apr;42(2):451–5. PMID:29101436

3166. Paul S, Kantarjian H, Jabbour EJ. Adult acute lymphoblastic leukemia. Mayo Clin Proc. 2016 Nov;91(11):1645–66. PMID:27814839

3167. Paulli M, Berti E. Cutaneous T-cell lymphomas (including rare subtypes). Current concepts. II. Haematologica. 2004 Nov;89(11):1372–88. PMID:15531460

3168. Paulli M, Berti E, Rosso R, et al. CD30/Ki-1-positive lymphoproliferative disorders of the skin–clinicopathologic correlation and statistical analysis of 86 cases: a multicentric study from the European Organization for Research and Treatment of Cancer Cutaneous Lymphoma Project Group. J Clin Oncol. 1995 Jun;13(6):1343–54. PMID:7751878

3169. Paulli M, Sträter J, Gianelli U, et al. Mediastinal B-cell lymphoma: a study of its histomorphologic spectrum based on 109 cases. Hum Pathol. 1999 Feb;30(2):178–87. PMID:10029446

3170. Paulsson K, Forestier E, Andersen MK, et al. High modal number and triple trisomies are highly correlated favorable factors in childhood B-cell precursor high hyperdiploid acute lymphoblastic leukemia treated according to the NOPHO ALL 1992/2000 protocols. Haematologica. 2013 Sep;98(9):1424–32. PMID:23645689

3171. Paulsson K, Johansson B. High hyperdiploid childhood acute lymphoblastic leukemia. Genes Chromosomes Cancer. 2009 Aug;48(8):637–60. PMID:19415723

3172. Paulsson K, Lilljebjörn H, Biloglav A, et al. The genomic landscape of high hyperdiploid childhood acute lymphoblastic leukemia. Nat Genet. 2015 Jun;47(6):672–6. PMID:25961940

3173. Payne K, Wright P, Grant JW, et al. BIOMED-2 PCR assays for IGK gene rearrangements are essential for B-cell clonality analysis in follicular lymphoma. Br J Haematol. 2011 Oct;155(1):84–92. PMID:21790530

3174. Peckova K, Michal M, Hadravsky L, et al. Littoral cell angioma of the spleen: a study of 25 cases with confirmation of frequent association with visceral malignancies. Histopathology. 2016 Nov;69(5):762–74. PMID:27374010

3175. Pedersen MB, Hamilton-Dutoit SJ, Bendix K, et al. DUSP22 and TP63 rearrangements predict outcome of ALK-negative anaplastic large cell lymphoma: a Danish cohort study. Blood. 2017 Jul 27;130(4):554–7. PMID:28522440

3176. Pedersen MØ, Gang AO, Clasen-Linde E, et al. Stratification by MYC expression has prognostic impact in MYC translocated B-cell lymphoma-Identifies a subgroup of patients with poor outcome. Eur J Haematol. 2019 May;102(5):395–406. PMID:30737994

3177. Pedersen MØ, Gang AO, Poulsen TS, et al. Double-hit BCL2/MYC translocations in a consecutive cohort of patients with large B-cell lymphoma - a single centre's experience. Eur J Haematol. 2012 Jul;89(1):63–71. PMID:22510149

3178. Pedersen RK, Pedersen NT. Primary non-Hodgkin's lymphoma of the thyroid gland: a population based study. Histopathology. 1996 Jan;28(1):25–32. PMID:8838117

3179. Peffault de Latour R, Soulier J. How I treat MDS and AML in Fanconi anemia. Blood. 2016 Jun 16;127(24):2971–9. PMID:27020090

3180. Pekarsky Y, Hallas C, Isobe M, et al. Abnormalities at 14q32.1 in T cell malignancies involve two oncogenes. Proc Natl Acad Sci U S A. 1999 Mar 16;96(6):2949–51. PMID:10077617

3181. Pelicci PG, Knowles DM 2nd, Magrath I, et al. Chromosomal breakpoints and structural alterations of the c-myc locus differ in endemic and sporadic forms of Burkitt lymphoma. Proc Natl Acad Sci U S A. 1986 May;83(9):2984–8. PMID:3458257

3182. Pelizzo G, Villanacci V, Lorenzi L, et al. Sclerosing angiomatoid nodular transformation presenting with abdominal hemorrhage: first report in infancy. Pediatr Rep. 2019 May 23;11(2):7848. PMID:31214299

3183. Pellicci DG, Koay HF, Berzins SP. Thymic development of unconventional T cells: how NKT cells, MAIT cells and γδ T cells emerge. Nat Rev Immunol. 2020 Dec;20(12):756–70. PMID:32581346

3184. Pemov A, Pathak A, Jones SJ, et al. In search of genetic factors predisposing to familial hairy cell leukemia (HCL): exome-sequencing of four multiplex HCL pedigrees. Leukemia. 2020 Jul;34(7):1934–8. PMID:31992839

3185. Peng RJ, Han BW, Cai QQ, et al. Genomic and transcriptomic landscapes of Epstein-Barr virus in extranodal natural killer T-cell lymphoma. Leukemia. 2019 Jun;33(6):1451–62. PMID:30546078

3186. Pepe F, Disma S, Teodoro C, et al. Kikuchi-Fujimoto disease: a clinicopathologic update. Pathologica. 2016 Sep;108(3):120–9. PMID:28195263

3187. Pérez C, Mondéjar R, García-Díaz N, et al. Advanced-stage mycosis fungoides: role of the signal transducer and activator of

transcription 3, nuclear factor-κB and nuclear factor of activated T cells pathways. Br J Dermatol. 2020 Jan;182(1):147–55. PMID:31049933
3188. Pérez González YC, Llamas Velasco MDM, Díaz Recuero JL, et al. Adnexotropism as a histopathological clue for the diagnosis of primary cutaneous CD4+ small/medium-sized T-cell lymphoproliferative disorder. Am J Dermatopathol. 2020 May;42(5):383–4. PMID:31313694
3189. Perez-Andreu V, Roberts KG, Harvey RC, et al. Inherited GATA3 variants are associated with Ph-like childhood acute lymphoblastic leukemia and risk of relapse. Nat Genet. 2013 Dec;45(12):1494–8. PMID:24141364
3190. Perez-Ordonez B, Erlandson RA, Rosai J. Follicular dendritic cell tumor: report of 13 additional cases of a distinctive entity. Am J Surg Pathol. 1996 Aug;20(8):944–55. PMID:8712294
3191. Perez-Ordoñez B, Rosai J. Follicular dendritic cell tumor: review of the entity. Semin Diagn Pathol. 1998 May;15(2):144–54. PMID:9606805
3192. Perkins SL, Gross TG. Pediatric indolent lymphoma–Would less be better? Pediatr Blood Cancer. 2011 Aug;57(2):189–90. PMID:21495166
3193. Perkins SM, Shinohara ET. Interdigitating and follicular dendritic cell sarcomas: a SEER analysis. Am J Clin Oncol. 2013 Aug;36(4):395–8. PMID:22772431
3194. Perrone S, D'Elia GM, Annechini G, et al. Infectious aetiology of marginal zone lymphoma and role of anti-infective therapy. Mediterr J Hematol Infect Dis. 2016 Jan 1;8(1):e2016006. PMID:26740867
3195. Perrone T, De Wolf-Peeters C, Frizzera G. Inflammatory pseudotumor of lymph nodes. A distinctive pattern of nodal reaction. Am J Surg Pathol. 1988 May;12(5):351–61. PMID:3364619
3196. Perrot A, Lauwers-Cances V, Corre J, et al. Minimal residual disease negativity using deep sequencing is a major prognostic factor in multiple myeloma. Blood. 2018 Dec 6;132(23):2456–64. PMID:30249784
3197. Perry AM, Bailey NG, Bonnett M, et al. Disease progression in a patient with indolent T-cell lymphoproliferative disease of the gastrointestinal tract. Int J Surg Pathol. 2019 Feb;27(1):102–7. PMID:29986618
3198. Perry AM, Diebold J, Nathwani BN, et al. Non-Hodgkin lymphoma in the developing world: review of 4539 cases from the International Non-Hodgkin Lymphoma Classification Project. Haematologica. 2016 Oct;101(10):1244–50. PMID:27354024
3199. Perry AM, Matsuda K, Wadhwa V, et al. Multifocal brain involvement in a patient with hairy cell leukemia successfully treated with rituximab and cladribine. Blood Adv. 2017 May 30;1(14):899–902. PMID:29296733
3200. Perry AM, Nelson M, Sanger WG, et al. Cytogenetic abnormalities in follicular dendritic cell sarcoma: report of two cases and literature review. In Vivo. 2013 Mar-Apr;27(2):211–4. PMID:23422480
3201. Perry AM, Warnke RA, Hu Q, et al. Indolent T-cell lymphoproliferative disease of the gastrointestinal tract. Blood. 2013 Nov 21;122(22):3599–606. PMID:24009234
3202. Pertesi M, Went M, Hansson M, et al. Genetic predisposition for multiple myeloma. Leukemia. 2020 Mar;34(3):697–708. PMID:31913320
3203. Perugino CA, AlSalem SB, Mattoo H, et al. Identification of galectin-3 as an autoantigen in patients with IgG4-related disease. J Allergy Clin Immunol. 2019 Feb;143(2):736–745.e6. PMID:29852256
3204. Perugino CA, Stone JH. IgG4-related disease: an update on pathophysiology and implications for clinical care. Nat Rev Rheumatol. 2020 Dec;16(12):702–14. PMID:32939060
3205. Pervez S, Mumtaz K, Ullah SS, et al. Immunoproliferative small intestinal disease (IPSID). J Coll Physicians Surg Pak. 2011 Jan;21(1):57–8. PMID:21276391
3206. Pesin N, Lam C, Margolin E. Central nervous system Burkitt lymphoma presenting as atypical Guillain-Barre syndrome. Can J Neurol Sci. 2020 Jan;47(1):145–7. PMID:31685043
3207. Peterson JF, Baughn LB, Ketterling RP, et al. Characterization of a cryptic IGH/CCND1 rearrangement in a case of mantle cell lymphoma with negative CCND1 FISH studies. Blood Adv. 2019 Apr 23;3(8):1298–302. PMID:31015206
3208. Peterson JF, Baughn LB, Pearce KE, et al. KMT2A (MLL) rearrangements observed in pediatric/young adult T-lymphoblastic leukemia/lymphoma: a 10-year review from a single cytogenetic laboratory. Genes Chromosomes Cancer. 2018 Nov;57(11):541–6. PMID:30203571
3209. Petit B, Le Meur Y, Jaccard A, et al. Influence of host-recipient origin on clinical aspects of posttransplantation lymphoproliferative disorders in kidney transplantation. Transplantation. 2002 Jan 27;73(2):265–71. PMID:11821742
3210. Petitjean B, Jardin F, Joly B, et al. Pyothorax-associated lymphoma: a peculiar clinicopathologic entity derived from B cells at late stage of differentiation and with occasional aberrant dual B- and T-cell phenotype. Am J Surg Pathol. 2002 Jun;26(6):724–32. PMID:12023576
3211. Petrella T, Maubec E, Cornillet-Lefebvre P, et al. Indolent CD8-positive lymphoid proliferation of the ear: a distinct primary cutaneous T-cell lymphoma? Am J Surg Pathol. 2007 Dec;31(12):1887–92. PMID:18043044
3212. Petri M, Orbai AM, Alarcón GS, et al. Derivation and validation of the Systemic Lupus International Collaborating Clinics classification criteria for systemic lupus erythematosus. Arthritis Rheum. 2012 Aug;64(8):2677–86. PMID:22553077
3213. Petrich AM, Gandhi M, Jovanovic B, et al. Impact of induction regimen and stem cell transplantation on outcomes in double-hit lymphoma: a multicenter retrospective analysis. Blood. 2014 Oct 9;124(15):2354–61. PMID:25161267
3214. Petrich AM, Helenowski IB, Bryan LJ, et al. Factors predicting survival in peripheral T-cell lymphoma in the USA: a population-based analysis of 8802 patients in the modern era. Br J Haematol. 2015 Mar;168(5):708–18. PMID:25382108
3215. Petruzziello F, Zeppa P, Catalano L, et al. Amyloid in bone marrow smears of patients affected by multiple myeloma. Ann Hematol. 2010 May;89(5):469–74. PMID:19894050
3216. Pettirossi V, Santi A, Imperi E, et al. BRAF inhibitors reverse the unique molecular signature and phenotype of hairy cell leukemia and exert potent antileukemic activity. Blood. 2015 Feb 19;125(8):1207–16. PMID:25480661
3217. Pham-Ledard A, Beylot-Barry M, Barbe C, et al. High frequency and clinical prognostic value of MYD88 L265P mutation in primary cutaneous diffuse large B-cell lymphoma, leg-type. JAMA Dermatol. 2014 Nov;150(11):1173–9. PMID:25055137
3218. Pham-Ledard A, Cappellen D, Martinez F, et al. MYD88 somatic mutation is a genetic feature of primary cutaneous diffuse large B-cell lymphoma, leg type. J Invest Dermatol. 2012 Aug;132(8):2118–20. PMID:22495176
3219. Pham-Ledard A, Cowppli-Bony A, Doussau A, et al. Diagnostic and prognostic value of BCL2 rearrangement in 53 patients with follicular lymphoma presenting as primary skin lesions. Am J Clin Pathol. 2015 Mar;143(3):362–73. PMID:25696794
3220. Pham-Ledard A, Prochazkova-Carlotti M, Andrique L, et al. Multiple genetic alterations in primary cutaneous large B-cell lymphoma, leg type support a common lymphomagenesis with activated B-cell-like diffuse large B-cell lymphoma. Mod Pathol. 2014 Mar;27(3):402–11. PMID:24030746
3221. Pham-Ledard A, Prochazkova-Carlotti M, Deveza M, et al. Molecular analysis of immunoglobulin variable genes supports a germinal center experienced normal counterpart in primary cutaneous diffuse large B-cell lymphoma, leg-type. J Dermatol Sci. 2017 Nov;88(2):238–46. PMID:28838616
3222. Pham-Ledard A, Prochazkova-Carlotti M, Laharanne E, et al. IRF4 gene rearrangements define a subgroup of CD30-positive cutaneous T-cell lymphoma: a study of 54 cases. J Invest Dermatol. 2010 Mar;130(3):816–25. PMID:19812605
3223. Phan TG, Green JA, Gray EE, et al. Immune complex relay by subcapsular sinus macrophages and noncognate B cells drives antibody affinity maturation. Nat Immunol. 2009 Jul;10(7):786–93. PMID:19503106
3224. Phang KC, Akhter A, Tizen NMS, et al. Comparison of protein-based cell-of-origin classification to the Lymph2Cx RNA assay in a cohort of diffuse large B-cell lymphomas in Malaysia. J Clin Pathol. 2018 Mar;71(3):215–20. PMID:28775174
3225. Philipone E, Bhagat G, Alobeid B. Oral cavity lymphoid neoplasms. A fifteen-year single institution review. N Y State Dent J. 2015 Apr;81(3):44–7. PMID:26094364
3226. Phillips AA, Shapira I, Willim RD, et al. A critical analysis of prognostic factors in North American patients with human T-cell lymphotropic virus type-1-associated adult T-cell leukemia/lymphoma: a multicenter clinicopathologic experience and new prognostic score. Cancer. 2010 Jul 15;116(14):3438–46. PMID:20564100
3227. Phillips AA, Smith DA. Health disparities and the global landscape of lymphoma care today. Am Soc Clin Oncol Educ Book. 2017;37:526–34. PMID:28561692
3228. Phyo ZH, Shanbhag S, Rozati S. Update on biology of cutaneous T-cell lymphoma. Front Oncol. 2020 May 12;10:765. PMID:32477957
3229. Piccaluga PP, De Falco G, Kustagi M, et al. Gene expression analysis uncovers similarity and differences among Burkitt lymphoma subtypes. Blood. 2011 Mar 31;117(13):3596–608. PMID:21245480
3230. Piccaluga PP, Fuligni F, De Leo A, et al. Molecular profiling improves classification and prognostication of nodal peripheral T-cell lymphomas: results of a phase III diagnostic accuracy study. J Clin Oncol. 2013 Aug 20;31(24):3019–25. PMID:23857971
3231. Pierson SK, Shenoy S, Oromendia AB, et al. Discovery and validation of a novel subgroup and therapeutic target in idiopathic multicentric Castleman disease. Blood Adv. 2021 Sep 14;5(17):3445–56. PMID:34438448
3232. Pieters R, De Lorenzo P, Ancliffe P, et al. Outcome of infants younger than 1 year with acute lymphoblastic leukemia treated with the Interfant-06 protocol: results from an international phase III randomized study. J Clin Oncol. 2019 Sep 1;37(25):2246–56. PMID:31283407
3233. Pileri A, Agostinelli C, Fuligni F, et al. Primary cutaneous peripheral T-cell lymphoma not otherwise specified a rare and aggressive lymphoma. J Eur Acad Dermatol Venereol. 2018 Oct;32(10):e373–6. PMID:29573477
3234. Pileri S, Kikuchi M, Helbron D, et al. Histiocytic necrotizing lymphadenitis without granulocytic infiltration. Virchows Arch A Pathol Anat Histol. 1982;395(3):257–71. PMID:7112935
3235. Pileri SA, Facchetti F, Ascani S, et al. Myeloperoxidase expression by histiocytes in Kikuchi's and Kikuchi-like lymphadenopathy. Am J Pathol. 2001 Sep;159(3):915–24. PMID:11549584
3236. Pileri SA, Gaidano G, Zinzani PL, et al. Primary mediastinal B-cell lymphoma: high frequency of BCL-6 mutations and consistent expression of the transcription factors OCT-2, BOB.1, and PU.1 in the absence of immunoglobulins. Am J Pathol. 2003 Jan;162(1):243–53. PMID:12507907
3237. Pileri SA, Grogan TM, Harris NL, et al. Tumours of histiocytes and accessory dendritic cells: an immunohistochemical approach to classification from the International Lymphoma Study Group based on 61 cases. Histopathology. 2002 Jul;41(1):1–29. PMID:12121233
3238. Pileri SA, Sabattini E, Rosito P, et al. Primary follicular lymphoma of the testis in childhood: an entity with peculiar clinical and molecular characteristics. J Clin Pathol. 2002 Sep;55(9):684–8. PMID:12194999
3239. Pilichowska M, Pittaluga S, Ferry JA, et al. Clinicopathologic consensus study of gray zone lymphoma with features intermediate between DLBCL and classical HL. Blood Adv. 2017 Dec 11;1(26):2600–9. PMID:29296913
3240. Pilichowska M, Shariftabrizi A, Mukand-Cerro I, et al. Primary hairy cell leukemia/lymphoma of the breast: a case report and review of the literature. Case Rep Pathol. 2014;2014:497027. PMID:25133005
3241. Pillai RK, Sathanoori M, Van Oss SB, et al. Double-hit B-cell lymphomas with BCL6 and MYC translocations are aggressive, frequently extranodal lymphomas distinct from BCL2 double-hit B-cell lymphomas. Am J Surg Pathol. 2013 Mar;37(3):323–32. PMID:23348205
3242. Pillai RK, Surti U, Swerdlow SH. Follicular lymphoma-like B cells of uncertain significance (in situ follicular lymphoma) may infrequently progress, but precedes follicular lymphoma, is associated with other overt lymphomas and mimics follicular lymphoma in flow cytometric studies. Haematologica. 2013 Oct;98(10):1571–80. PMID:23831923
3243. Pillonel V, Juskevicius D, Ng CKY, et al. High-throughput sequencing of nodal marginal zone lymphomas identifies recurrent BRAF mutations. Leukemia. 2018 Nov;32(11):2412–26. PMID:29556019
3244. Pilozzi E, Müller-Hermelink HK, Falini B, et al. Gene rearrangements in T-cell lymphoblastic lymphoma. J Pathol. 1999 Jul;188(3):267–70. PMID:10419594
3245. Pilozzi E, Pulford K, Jones M, et al. Co-expression of CD79a (JCB117) and CD3 by lymphoblastic lymphoma. J Pathol. 1998 Oct;186(2):140–3. PMID:9924428
3246. Pimpinelli N, Olsen EA, Santucci M, et al. Defining early mycosis fungoides. J Am Acad Dermatol. 2005 Dec;53(6):1053–63. PMID:16310068
3247. Pina-Oviedo S, Miranda RN, Lin P, et al. Follicular lymphoma with hyaline-vascular Castleman-like features: analysis of 6 cases and review of the literature. Hum Pathol. 2017 Oct;68:136–46. PMID:28873356
3248. Pina-Oviedo S, Miranda RN, Medeiros LJ. Cancer therapy-associated lymphoproliferative disorders: an under-recognized type of immunodeficiency-associated lymphoproliferative disorder. Am J Surg Pathol. 2018 Jan;42(1):116–29. PMID:29112013
3249. Piña-Oviedo S, Moran CA. Primary mediastinal nodal and extranodal non-Hodgkin lymphomas: current concepts, historical evolution, and useful diagnostic approach: part

1. Adv Anat Pathol. 2019 Nov;26(6):346–70. PMID:31567132
3250. Pina-Oviedo S, Ortiz-Hidalgo C, Carballo-Zarate AA, et al. ALK-negative anaplastic large cell lymphoma: current concepts and molecular pathogenesis of a heterogeneous group of large T-cell lymphomas. Cancers (Basel). 2021 Sep 17;13(18):4667. PMID:34572893
3251. Pincus LB, LeBoit PE, McCalmont TH, et al. Subcutaneous panniculitis-like T-cell lymphoma with overlapping clinicopathologic features of lupus erythematosus: coexistence of 2 entities? Am J Dermatopathol. 2009 Aug;31(6):520–6. PMID:19590424
3252. Pinkerton R, Cairo MS, Cotter FE. Childhood, adolescent and young adult non-Hodgkin lymphoma: state of the science. Br J Haematol. 2016 May;173(4):503–4. PMID:27098994
3253. Pinnix CC, Shah JJ, Chuang H, et al. Doxorubicin-based chemotherapy and radiation therapy produces favorable outcomes in limited-stage plasmablastic lymphoma: a single-institution review. Clin Lymphoma Myeloma Leuk. 2016 Mar;16(3):122–8. PMID:26795083
3254. Pinto A, Hutchison RE, Grant LH, et al. Follicular lymphomas in pediatric patients. Mod Pathol. 1990 May;3(3):308–13. PMID:2194214
3255. Pinyol M, Cobo F, Bea S, et al. p16(INK4a) gene inactivation by deletions, mutations, and hypermethylation is associated with transformed and aggressive variants of non-Hodgkin's lymphomas. Blood. 1998 Apr 15;91(8):2977–84. PMID:9531609
3256. Pircher C, Schneeberger S, Boesmueller C, et al. A rare case of Epstein-Barr virus-associated hepatosplenic smooth muscle tumors after kidney transplantation. Transpl Infect Dis. 2018 Jun;20(3):e12860. PMID:29427352
3257. Piriou E, Asito AS, Sumba PO, et al. Early age at time of primary Epstein-Barr virus infection results in poorly controlled viral infection in infants from western Kenya: clues to the etiology of endemic Burkitt lymphoma. J Infect Dis. 2012 Mar 15;205(6):906–13. PMID:22301635
3258. Piris MA, Medeiros LJ, Chang KC. Hodgkin lymphoma: a review of pathological features and recent advances in pathogenesis. Pathology. 2020 Jan;52(1):154–65. PMID:31699300
3259. Pittaluga S, Nicolae A, Wright GW, et al. Gene expression profiling of mediastinal gray zone lymphoma and its relationship to primary mediastinal B-cell lymphoma and classical Hodgkin lymphoma. Blood Cancer Discov. 2020 Sep 1;1(2):155–61. PMID:32914098
3260. Pittaluga S, Tierens A, Dodoo YL, et al. How reliable is histologic examination of bone marrow trephine biopsy specimens for the staging of non-Hodgkin lymphoma? A study of hairy cell leukemia and mantle cell lymphoma involvement of the bone marrow trephine specimen by histologic, immunohistochemical, and polymerase chain reaction techniques. Am J Clin Pathol. 1999 Feb;111(2):179–84. PMID:9930138
3261. Pittaluga S, Wlodarska I, Pulford K, et al. The monoclonal antibody ALK1 identifies a distinct morphological subtype of anaplastic large cell lymphoma associated with 2p23/ALK rearrangements. Am J Pathol. 1997 Aug;151(2):343–51. PMID:9250148
3262. Piubelli MLM, Ferrufino-Schmidt MC, Miranda RN. Gluteal implant-associated anaplastic large cell lymphoma (ALCL) is distinct from systemic ALCL ALK negative in a patient with gluteal implants. Aesthet Surg J. 2019 Sep 13;39(10):NP441–2. PMID:31504160
3263. Piva R, Agnelli L, Pellegrino E, et al. Gene expression profiling uncovers molecular classifiers for the recognition of anaplastic large-cell lymphoma within peripheral T-cell neoplasms. J Clin Oncol. 2010 Mar 20;28(9):1583–90. PMID:20159827
3264. Piva R, Deaglio S, Famà R, et al. The Krüppel-like factor 2 transcription factor gene is recurrently mutated in splenic marginal zone lymphoma. Leukemia. 2015 Feb;29(2):503–7. PMID:25283840
3265. Pizzi M, Brignola S, Righi S, et al. Benign TdT-positive cells in pediatric and adult lymph nodes: a potential diagnostic pitfall. Hum Pathol. 2018 Nov;81:131–7. PMID:29969607
3266. Pizzi M, Covey S, Mathew S, et al. Hepatosplenic T-cell lymphoma mimicking acute myeloid leukemia. Clin Lymphoma Myeloma Leuk. 2016 Mar;16(3):e47–50. PMID:26708981
3267. Plaza JA, Sangueza M. Hydroa vacciniforme-like lymphoma with primarily periorbital swelling: 7 cases of an atypical clinical manifestation of this rare cutaneous T-cell lymphoma. Am J Dermatopathol. 2015 Jan;37(1):20–5. PMID:25162933
3268. Podar K, Anderson KC. Emerging therapies targeting tumor vasculature in multiple myeloma and other hematologic and solid malignancies. Curr Cancer Drug Targets. 2011 Nov;11(9):1005–24. PMID:21933109
3269. Poirel HA, Bernheim A, Schneider A, et al. Characteristic pattern of chromosomal imbalances in posttransplantation lymphoproliferative disorders: correlation with histopathological subcategories and EBV status. Transplantation. 2005 Jul 27;80(2):176–84. PMID:16041261
3270. Pojero F, Flores-Montero J, Sanoja L, et al. Utility of CD54, CD229, and CD319 for the identification of plasma cells in patients with clonal plasma cell diseases. Cytometry B Clin Cytom. 2016 Jan;90(1):91–100. PMID:26130131
3271. Polizzotto MN, Uldrick TS, Hu D, et al. Clinical manifestations of Kaposi sarcoma herpesvirus lytic activation: multicentric Castleman disease (KSHV-MCD) and the KSHV inflammatory cytokine syndrome. Front Microbiol. 2012 Mar 2;3:73. PMID:22403576
3272. Polizzotto MN, Uldrick TS, Wang V, et al. Human and viral interleukin-6 and other cytokines in Kaposi sarcoma herpesvirus-associated multicentric Castleman disease. Blood. 2013 Dec 19;122(26):4189–98. PMID:24174627
3273. Polonis K, Schultz MJ, Olteanu H, et al. Detection of cryptic CCND1 rearrangements in mantle cell lymphoma by next generation sequencing. Ann Diagn Pathol. 2020 Jun;46:151533. PMID:32408254
3274. Polprasert C, Takeuchi Y, Kakiuchi N, et al. Frequent germline mutations of HAVCR2 in sporadic subcutaneous panniculitis-like T-cell lymphoma. Blood Adv. 2019 Feb 26;3(4):588–95. PMID:30792187
3275. Pongpruttipan T, Sukpanichnant S, Assanasen T, et al. Extranodal NK/T-cell lymphoma, nasal type, includes cases of natural killer cell and αβ, γδ, and αβ/γδ T-cell origin: a comprehensive clinicopathologic and phenotypic study. Am J Surg Pathol. 2012 Apr;36(4):481–99. PMID:22314189
3276. Ponti R, Quaglino P, Novelli M, et al. T-cell receptor gamma gene rearrangement by multiplex polymerase chain reaction/heteroduplex analysis in patients with cutaneous T-cell lymphoma (mycosis fungoides/Sézary syndrome) and benign inflammatory disease: correlation with clinical, histological and immunophenotypical findings. Br J Dermatol. 2005 Sep;153(3):565–73. PMID:16120144
3277. Ponzoni M, Arrigoni G, Gould VE, et al. Lack of CD 29 (beta1 integrin) and CD 54 (ICAM-1) adhesion molecules in intravascular lymphomatosis. Hum Pathol. 2000 Feb;31(2):220–6. PMID:10685637
3278. Ponzoni M, Berger F, Chassagne-Clement C, et al. Reactive perivascular T-cell infiltrate predicts survival in primary central nervous system B-cell lymphomas. Br J Haematol. 2007 Aug;138(3):316–23. PMID:17555470
3279. Ponzoni M, Campo E, Nakamura S. Intravascular large B-cell lymphoma: a chameleon with multiple faces and many masks. Blood. 2018 Oct 11;132(15):1561–7. PMID:30111607
3280. Ponzoni M, Ferreri AJ. Bacteria associated with marginal zone lymphomas. Best Pract Res Clin Haematol. 2017 Mar-Jun;30(1-2):32–40. PMID:28288714
3281. Pophali PA, Marinelli LM, Ketterling RP, et al. High level MYC amplification in B-cell lymphomas: Is it a marker of aggressive disease? Blood Cancer J. 2020 Jan 13;10(1):5. PMID:31932576
3282. Popov SW, Moldenhauer G, Wotschke B, et al. Target sequence accessibility limits activation-induced cytidine deaminase activity in primary mediastinal B-cell lymphoma. Cancer Res. 2007 Jul 15;67(14):6555–64. PMID:17638864
3283. Poppe B, De Paepe P, Michaux L, et al. PAX5/IGH rearrangement is a recurrent finding in a subset of aggressive B-NHL with complex chromosomal rearrangements. Genes Chromosomes Cancer. 2005 Oct;44(2):218–23. PMID:15942942
3284. Posnett DN, Sinha R, Kabak S, et al. Clonal populations of T cells in normal elderly humans: the T cell equivalent to "benign monoclonal gammapathy". J Exp Med. 1994 Feb 1;179(2):609–18. PMID:8294871
3285. Pouliou E, Xochelli A, Kanellis G, et al. Numerous ontogenetic roads to mantle cell lymphoma: immunogenetic and immunohistochemical evidence. Am J Pathol. 2017 Jul;187(7):1454–8. PMID:28457696
3286. Poullot E, Zambello R, Leblanc F, et al. Chronic natural killer lymphoproliferative disorders: characteristics of an international cohort of 70 patients. Ann Oncol. 2014 Oct;25(10):2030–5. PMID:25096606
3287. Poveda J, Cassidy DP, Zhou Y, et al. Expression of germinal center cell markers by extranodal marginal zone lymphomas of MALT type within colonized follicles, a diagnostic pitfall with follicular lymphoma. Leuk Lymphoma. 2021 May;62(5):1116–22. PMID:33283568
3288. Powell BC, Jiang L, Muzny DM, et al. Identification of TP53 as an acute lymphocytic leukemia susceptibility gene through exome sequencing. Pediatr Blood Cancer. 2013 Jun;60(6):E1–3. PMID:23255406
3289. Powles T, Stebbing J, Bazeos A, et al. The role of immune suppression and HHV-8 in the increasing incidence of HIV-associated multicentric Castleman's disease. Ann Oncol. 2009 Apr;20(4):775–9. PMID:19179554
3290. Pozdnyakova O, Orazi A, Kelemen K, et al. Myeloid/lymphoid neoplasms associated with eosinophilia and rearrangements of PDGFRA, PDGFRB, or FGFR1 or with PCM1-JAK2. Am J Clin Pathol. 2021 Feb 4;155(2):160–78. PMID:33367495
3291. Pozzi C, D'Amico M, Fogazzi GB, et al. Light chain deposition disease with renal involvement: clinical characteristics and prognostic factors. Am J Kidney Dis. 2003 Dec;42(6):1154–63. PMID:14655186
3292. Prakash S, Fountaine T, Raffeld M, et al. IgD positive L&H cells identify a unique subset of nodular lymphocyte predominant Hodgkin lymphoma. Am J Surg Pathol. 2006 May;30(5):585–92. PMID:16699312
3293. Prasad A, Rabionet R, Espinet B, et al. Identification of gene mutations and fusion genes in patients with Sézary syndrome. J Invest Dermatol. 2016 Jul;136(7):1490–9. PMID:27039262
3294. Preusser M, Woehrer A, Koperek O, et al. Primary central nervous system lymphoma: a clinicopathological study of 75 cases. Pathology. 2010;42(6):547–52. PMID:20854073
3295. Prevot S, Hamilton-Dutoit S, Audouin J, et al. Analysis of African Burkitt's and high-grade B cell non-Burkitt's lymphoma for Epstein-Barr virus genomes using in situ hybridization. Br J Haematol. 1992 Jan;80(1):27–32. PMID:1311194
3296. Pria AD, Pinato D, Roe J, et al. Relapse of HHV8-positive multicentric Castleman disease following rituximab-based therapy in HIV-positive patients. Blood. 2017 Apr 13;129(15):2143–7. PMID:28143881
3297. Pribyl K, Vakayil V, Farooqi N, et al. Castleman disease: a single-center case series. Int J Surg Case Rep. 2021 Mar;80:105650. PMID:33631648
3298. Price S, Shaw PA, Seitz A, et al. Natural history of autoimmune lymphoproliferative syndrome associated with FAS gene mutations. Blood. 2014 Mar 27;123(13):1989–99. PMID:24398331
3299. Price SK. Immunoproliferative small intestinal disease: a study of 13 cases with alpha heavy-chain disease. Histopathology. 1990 Jul;17(1):7–17. PMID:2227833
3300. Prieto-Torres L, Eraña I, Gil-Redondo R, et al. The spectrum of EBV-positive mucocutaneous ulcer: a study of 9 cases. Am J Surg Pathol. 2019 Feb;43(2):201–10. PMID:30418184
3301. Pritchett JC, Yang ZZ, Kim HJ, et al. High-dimensional and single-cell transcriptome analysis of the tumor microenvironment in angioimmunoblastic T cell lymphoma (AITL). Leukemia. 2022 Jan;36(1):165–76. PMID:34230608
3302. Pro B, Allen P, Behdad A. Hepatosplenic T-cell lymphoma: a rare but challenging entity. Blood. 2020 Oct 29;136(18):2018–26. PMID:32756940
3303. Prudent E, La Scola B, Drancourt M, et al. Molecular strategy for the diagnosis of infectious lymphadenitis. Eur J Clin Microbiol Infect Dis. 2018 Jun;37(6):1179–86. PMID:29594802
3304. Pruksaeakanan C, Teyateeti P, Pathamalai P, et al. Primary cutaneous lymphomas in Thailand: a 10-year retrospective study. Biomed Res Int. 2021 Jun 11;2021:4057661. PMID:34235215
3305. Pruneri G, Valentini S, Bertolini F, et al. SP4, a novel anti-cyclin D1 rabbit monoclonal antibody, is a highly sensitive probe for identifying mantle cell lymphomas bearing the t(11;14)(q13;q32) translocation. Appl Immunohistochem Mol Morphol. 2005 Dec;13(4):318–22. PMID:16280660
3306. Przybylski GK, Wu H, Macon WR, et al. Hepatosplenic and subcutaneous panniculitis-like gamma/delta T cell lymphomas are derived from different Vdelta subsets of gamma/delta T lymphocytes. J Mol Diagn. 2000 Feb;2(1):11–9. PMID:11272897
3307. Puente XS, Beà S, Valdés-Mas R, et al. Non-coding recurrent mutations in chronic lymphocytic leukaemia. Nature. 2015 Oct 22;526(7574):519–24. PMID:26200345
3308. Pugh TJ, Fink JM, Lu X, et al. Assessing genome-wide copy number aberrations and copy-neutral loss-of-heterozygosity as best practice: an evidence-based review from the Cancer Genomics Consortium working group for plasma cell disorders. Cancer Genet. 2018 Dec;228-229:184–96. PMID:30393007
3309. Pui CH, Chessells JM, Camitta B, et al. Clinical heterogeneity in childhood acute lymphoblastic leukemia with 11q23 rearrangements. Leukemia. 2003 Apr;17(4):700–6. PMID:12682627
3310. Pui CH, Rebora P, Schrappe M, et al. Outcome of children with hypodiploid acute

lymphoblastic leukemia: a retrospective multinational study. J Clin Oncol. 2019 Apr 1;37(10):770–9. PMID:30657737
3311. Pui CH, Robison LL, Look AT. Acute lymphoblastic leukaemia. Lancet. 2008 Mar 22;371(9617):1030–43. PMID:18358930
3312. Pujol RM, Muret MP, Bergua P, et al. Oral involvement in lymphomatoid papulosis. Report of two cases and review of the literature. Dermatology. 2005;210(1):53–7. PMID:15604547
3313. Pulido JS, Johnston PB, Nowakowski GS, et al. The diagnosis and treatment of primary vitreoretinal lymphoma: a review. Int J Retina Vitreous. 2018 May 7;4:18. PMID:29760948
3314. Pullarkat VA, Lacayo NJ, Jabbour E, et al. Venetoclax and navitoclax in combination with chemotherapy in patients with relapsed or refractory acute lymphoblastic leukemia and lymphoblastic lymphoma. Cancer Discov. 2021 Jun;11(6):1440–53. PMID:33593877
3315. Qi S, Yahalom J, Hsu M, et al. Encouraging experience in the treatment of nasal type extra-nodal NK/T-cell lymphoma in a non-Asian population. Leuk Lymphoma. 2016 Nov;57(11):2575–83. PMID:27183991
3316. Qian M, Zhang H, Kham SK, et al. Whole-transcriptome sequencing identifies a distinct subtype of acute lymphoblastic leukemia with predominant genomic abnormalities of EP300 and CREBBP. Genome Res. 2017 Feb;27(2):185–95. PMID:27903646
3317. Qian YW, Weissmann D, Goodell L, et al. Indolent T-lymphoblastic proliferation in Castleman lymphadenopathy. Leuk Lymphoma. 2009 Feb;50(2):306–8. PMID:19197736
3318. Qin YZ, Jiang Q, Jiang H, et al. Prevalence and outcomes of uncommon BCR-ABL1 fusion transcripts in patients with chronic myeloid leukaemia: data from a single centre. Br J Haematol. 2018 Sep;182(5):693–700. PMID:29974949
3319. Qiu L, Tang G, Li S, et al. DUSP22 rearrangement is associated with a distinctive immunophenotype but not outcome in patients with systemic ALK-negative anaplastic large cell lymphoma. Haematologica. 2023 Jun 1;108(6):1604–15. PMID:36453104
3320. Qiu ZY, Fan L, Wang R, et al. Methotrexate therapy of T-cell large granular lymphocytic leukemia impact of STAT3 mutation. Oncotarget. 2016 Sep 20;7(38):61419–25. PMID:27542218
3321. Qu X, Li H, Braziel RM, et al. Genomic alterations important for the prognosis in patients with follicular lymphoma treated in SWOG study S0016. Blood. 2019 Jan 3;133(1):81–93. PMID:30446494
3322. Quaglino P, Fava P, Pileri A, et al. Phenotypical markers, molecular mutations, and immune microenvironment as targets for new treatments in patients with mycosis fungoides and/or Sézary syndrome. J Invest Dermatol. 2021 Mar;141(3):484–95. PMID:33162051
3323. Queirós AC, Villamor N, Clot G, et al. A B-cell epigenetic signature defines three biologic subgroups of chronic lymphocytic leukemia with clinical impact. Leukemia. 2015 Mar;29(3):598–605. PMID:25151957
3324. Quesada AE, Liu H, Miranda RN, et al. Burkitt lymphoma presenting as a mass in the thyroid gland: a clinicopathologic study of 7 cases and review of the literature. Hum Pathol. 2016 Oct;56:101–8. PMID:27257042
3325. Quesada AE, Medeiros LJ, Clemens MW, et al. Breast implant-associated anaplastic large cell lymphoma: a review. Mod Pathol. 2019 Feb;32(2):166–88. PMID:30206414
3326. Quesada AE, Medeiros LJ, Desai PA, et al. Increased MYC copy number is an independent prognostic factor in patients with diffuse large B-cell lymphoma. Mod Pathol. 2017 Dec;30(12):1688–97. PMID:28776574
3327. Quesada AE, Zhang Y, Ptashkin R, et al. Next generation sequencing of breast implant-associated anaplastic large cell lymphomas reveals a novel STAT3-JAK2 fusion among other activating genetic alterations within the JAK-STAT pathway. Breast J. 2021 Apr;27(4):314–21. PMID:33660353
3328. Quest GR, Johnston JB. Clinical features and diagnosis of hairy cell leukemia. Best Pract Res Clin Haematol. 2015 Dec;28(4):180–92. PMID:26614896
3329. Quinquenel A, Fornecker LM, Letestu R, et al. Prevalence of BTK and PLCG2 mutations in a real-life CLL cohort still on ibrutinib after 3 years: a FILO group study. Blood. 2019 Aug 15;134(7):641–4. PMID:31243043
3330. Quintanilla-Martinez L, Davies-Hill T, Fend F, et al. Sequestration of p27Kip1 protein by cyclin D1 in typical and blastic variants of mantle cell lymphoma (MCL): implications for pathogenesis. Blood. 2003 Apr 15;101(8):3181–7. PMID:12515730
3331. Quintanilla-Martinez L, de Jong D, de Mascarel A, et al. Gray zones around diffuse large B cell lymphoma. Conclusions based on the workshop of the XIV meeting of the European Association for Hematopathology and the Society of Hematopathology in Bordeaux, France. J Hematop. 2009 Dec 22;2(4):211–36. PMID:20309430
3332. Quintanilla-Martinez L, Fend F, Moguel LR, et al. Peripheral T-cell lymphoma with Reed-Sternberg-like cells of B-cell phenotype and genotype associated with Epstein-Barr virus infection. Am J Surg Pathol. 1999 Oct;23(10):1233–40. PMID:10524524
3333. Quintanilla-Martinez L, Franklin JL, Guerrero I, et al. Histological and immunophenotypic profile of nasal NK/T cell lymphomas from Peru: high prevalence of p53 overexpression. Hum Pathol. 1999 Jul;30(7):849–55. PMID:10414505
3334. Quintanilla-Martinez L, Jansen PM, Kinney MC, et al. Non-mycosis fungoides cutaneous T-cell lymphomas: report of the 2011 Society for Hematopathology/European Association for Haematopathology workshop. Am J Clin Pathol. 2013 Apr;139(4):491–514. PMID:23525618
3335. Quintanilla-Martinez L, Kremer M, Keller G, et al. p53 Mutations in nasal natural killer/T-cell lymphoma from Mexico: association with large cell morphology and advanced disease. Am J Pathol. 2001 Dec;159(6):2095–105. PMID:11733360
3336. Quintanilla-Martinez L, Kumar S, Fend F, et al. Fulminant EBV(+) T-cell lymphoproliferative disorder following acute/chronic EBV infection: a distinct clinicopathologic syndrome. Blood. 2000 Jul 15;96(2):443–51. PMID:10887104
3337. Quintanilla-Martinez L, Ridaura C, Nagl F, et al. Hydroa vacciniforme-like lymphoma: a chronic EBV+ lymphoproliferative disorder with risk to develop a systemic lymphoma. Blood. 2013 Oct 31;122(18):3101–10. PMID:23982171
3338. Quintanilla-Martinez L, Sander B, Chan JK, et al. Indolent lymphomas in the pediatric population: follicular lymphoma, IRF4/MUM1+ lymphoma, nodal marginal zone lymphoma and chronic lymphocytic leukemia. Virchows Arch. 2016 Feb;468(2):141–57. PMID:26416032
3339. Qunaj L, Castillo JJ, Olszewski AJ. Survival of patients with CD20-negative variants of large B-cell lymphoma: an analysis of the National Cancer Data Base. Leuk Lymphoma. 2018 Jun;59(6):1375–83. PMID:29019447
3340. Raanani P, Trakhtenbrot L, Rechavi G, et al. Philadelphia-chromosome-positive T-lymphoblastic leukemia: acute leukemia or chronic myelogenous leukemia blastic crisis. Acta Haematol. 2005;113(3):181–9. PMID:15870488
3341. Rabban JT, Firetag B, Sangoi AR, et al. Incidental pelvic and para-aortic lymph node lymphangioleiomyomatosis detected during surgical staging of pelvic cancer in women without symptomatic pulmonary lymphangioleiomyomatosis or tuberous sclerosis complex. Am J Surg Pathol. 2015 Aug;39(8):1015–25. PMID:25786086
3342. Raderer M, Kiesewetter B. What you always wanted to know about gastric MALT-lymphoma: a focus on recent developments. Ther Adv Med Oncol. 2021 Jul 23;13:17588359211033825. PMID:34621332
3343. Raderer M, Kiesewetter B, Ferreri AJ. Clinicopathologic characteristics and treatment of marginal zone lymphoma of mucosa-associated lymphoid tissue (MALT lymphoma). CA Cancer J Clin. 2016 Mar-Apr;66(2):153–71. PMID:26773441
3344. Raetz EA, Teachey DT. T-cell acute lymphoblastic leukemia. Hematology Am Soc Hematol Educ Program. 2016 Dec 2;2016(1):580–8. PMID:27913532
3345. Ragg S, Zehentner BK, Loken MR, et al. Evidence for BCR/ABL1-positive T-cell acute lymphoblastic leukemia arising in an early lymphoid progenitor cell. Pediatr Blood Cancer. 2019 Sep;66(9):e27829. PMID:31136068
3346. Rahemtullah A, Longtine JA, Harris NL, et al. CD20+ T-cell lymphoma: clinicopathologic analysis of 9 cases and a review of the literature. Am J Surg Pathol. 2008 Nov;32(11):1593–607. PMID:18753947
3347. Rahemtullah A, Reichard KK, Preffer FI, et al. A double-positive CD4+CD8+ T-cell population is commonly found in nodular lymphocyte predominant Hodgkin lymphoma. Am J Clin Pathol. 2006 Nov;126(5):805–14. PMID:17050078
3348. Raine JI, Dowse R, Attygalle AD. Paratrabecular bone marrow involvement in autoimmune lymphoproliferative syndrome: a potential diagnostic pitfall as a lymphoma mimic. Histopathology. 2022 Mar;80(4):740–2. PMID:34492736
3349. Raja KR, Kovarova L, Hajek R. Review of phenotypic markers used in flow cytometric analysis of MGUS and MM, and applicability of flow cytometry in other plasma cell disorders. Br J Haematol. 2010 May;149(3):334–51. PMID:20201947
3350. Rajala HL, Eldfors S, Kuusanmäki H, et al. Discovery of somatic STAT5b mutations in large granular lymphocytic leukemia. Blood. 2013 May 30;121(22):4541–50. PMID:23596048
3351. Rajkumar SV. Multiple myeloma: 2016 update on diagnosis, risk-stratification, and management. Am J Hematol. 2016 Jul;91(7):719–34. PMID:27291302
3352. Rajkumar SV, Dimopoulos MA, Palumbo A, et al. International Myeloma Working Group updated criteria for the diagnosis of multiple myeloma. Lancet Oncol. 2014 Nov;15(12):e538–48. PMID:25439696
3353. Rajkumar SV, Kyle RA, Therneau TM, et al. Serum free light chain ratio is an independent risk factor for progression in monoclonal gammopathy of undetermined significance. Blood. 2005 Aug 1;106(3):812–7. PMID:15855274
3354. Rajyaguru DJ, Bhaskar C, Borgert AJ, et al. Intravascular large B-cell lymphoma in the United States (US): a population-based study using Surveillance, Epidemiology, and End Results Program and National Cancer Database. Leuk Lymphoma. 2017 Sep;58(9):1–9. PMID:28278725
3355. Ramael M, Schoeters P, De Pooter K, et al. Multi-focal splenic tumour in a Belgian patient and a brief review of the literature on littoral cell angioma. Eur J Case Rep Intern Med. 2020 Aug 29;7(11):001863. PMID:33194866
3356. Ramalingam P, Zoroquiain P, Valbuena JR, et al. Florid reactive lymphoid hyperplasia (lymphoma-like lesion) of the uterine cervix. Ann Diagn Pathol. 2012 Jan;16(1):21–8. PMID:22056039
3357. Ramaswami R, Chia G, Dalla Pria A, et al. Evolution of HIV-associated lymphoma over 3 decades. J Acquir Immune Defic Syndr. 2016 Jun 1;72(2):177–83. PMID:26859827
3358. Ramaswami R, Lurain K, Polizzotto MN, et al. Characteristics and outcomes of KSHV-associated multicentric Castleman disease with or without other KSHV diseases. Blood Adv. 2021 Mar 23;5(6):1660–70. PMID:33720337
3359. Ramdall RB, Alasio TM, Cai G, et al. Primary vascular neoplasms unique to the spleen: littoral cell angioma and splenic hamartoma diagnosis by fine-needle aspiration biopsy. Diagn Cytopathol. 2007 Mar;35(3):137–42. PMID:17304535
3360. Ramezani-Rad P, Chen C, Zhu Z, et al. Cyclin D3 governs clonal expansion of dark zone germinal center B cells. Cell Rep. 2020 Nov 17;33(7):108403. PMID:33207194
3361. Ramis-Zaldivar JE, Gonzalez-Farré B, Balagué O, et al. Distinct molecular profile of IRF4-rearranged large B-cell lymphoma. Blood. 2020 Jan 23;135(4):274–86. PMID:31738823
3362. Ramis-Zaldivar JE, Gonzalez-Farre B, Nicolae A, et al. MAPK and JAK-STAT pathways dysregulation in plasmablastic lymphoma. Haematologica. 2021 Oct 1;106(10):2682–93. PMID:33951889
3363. Ramot B, Shahin N, Bubis JJ. Malabsorption syndrome in lymphoma of small intestine. A study of 13 cases. Isr J Med Sci. 1965 Mar;1:221–6. PMID:14279068
3364. Rana I, Dahlberg S, Steinmaus C, et al. Benzene exposure and non-Hodgkin lymphoma: a systematic review and meta-analysis of human studies. Lancet Planet Health. 2021 Sep;5(9):e633–43. PMID:34450064
3365. Randen U, Tierens AM, Tjønnfjord GE, et al. Bone marrow histology in monoclonal B-cell lymphocytosis shows various B-cell infiltration patterns. Am J Clin Pathol. 2013 Mar;139(3):390–5. PMID:23429376
3366. Randen U, Trøen G, Tierens A, et al. Primary cold agglutinin-associated lymphoproliferative disease: a B-cell lymphoma of the bone marrow distinct from lymphoplasmacytic lymphoma. Haematologica. 2014 Mar;99(3):497–504. PMID:24143001
3367. Ranjan P, Naresh KN. CD30 expression in L&H cells of Hodgkin's disease, nodular lymphocyte predominant type. Histopathology. 2003 Apr;42(4):406–7. PMID:12653955
3368. Raoux D, Duband S, Forest F, et al. Primary central nervous system lymphoma: immunohistochemical profile and prognostic significance. Neuropathology. 2010 Jun;30(3):232–40. PMID:19925562
3369. Rasche L, Chavan SS, Stephens OW, et al. Spatial genomic heterogeneity in multiple myeloma revealed by multi-region sequencing. Nat Commun. 2017 Aug 16;8(1):268. PMID:28814763
3370. Rasche L, Kapp M, Einsele H, et al. EBV-induced post transplant lymphoproliferative disorders: a persisting challenge in allogeneic hematopoetic SCT. Bone Marrow Transplant. 2014 Feb;49(2):163–7. PMID:23832092
3371. Ratterman M, Kruczek K, Sulo S, et al. Extramedullary chronic lymphocytic leukemia: systematic analysis of cases reported between 1975 and 2012. Leuk Res. 2014 Mar;38(3):299–303. PMID:24064196
3372. Ravell JC, Chauvin SD, He T, et al. An update on XMEN disease. J Clin Immunol. 2020 Jul;40(5):671–81. PMID:32451662
3373. Ravichandran S, Cohen OC, Law S, et

al. Impact of early response on outcomes in AL amyloidosis following treatment with front-line bortezomib. Blood Cancer J. 2021 Jun 21;11(6):118. PMID:34155191
3374. Ravichandran S, Lachmann HJ, Wechalekar AD. Epidemiologic and survival trends in amyloidosis, 1987-2019. N Engl J Med. 2020 Apr 16;382(16):1567–8. PMID:32294353
3375. Ravindran A, Feldman AL, Ketterling RP, et al. Striking association of lymphoid enhancing factor (LEF1) overexpression and DUSP22 rearrangements in anaplastic large cell lymphoma. Am J Surg Pathol. 2021 Apr 1;45(4):550–7. PMID:33165091
3376. Rawat A, Jindal AK, Suri D, et al. Clinical and genetic profile of X-linked agammaglobulinemia: a multicenter experience from India. Front Immunol. 2021 Jan 15;11:612323. PMID:33584693
3377. Rawstron AC, Bennett FL, O'Connor SJ, et al. Monoclonal B-cell lymphocytosis and chronic lymphocytic leukemia. N Engl J Med. 2008 Aug 7;359(6):575–83. PMID:18687638
3378. Rawstron AC, Green MJ, Kuzmicki A, et al. Monoclonal B lymphocytes with the characteristics of "indolent" chronic lymphocytic leukemia are present in 3.5% of adults with normal blood counts. Blood. 2002 Jul 15;100(2):635–9. PMID:12091358
3379. Rawstron AC, Kreuzer KA, Soosapilla A, et al. Reproducible diagnosis of chronic lymphocytic leukemia by flow cytometry: an European Research Initiative on CLL (ERIC) & European Society for Clinical Cell Analysis (ESCCA) Harmonisation project. Cytometry B Clin Cytom. 2018 Jan;94(1):121–8. PMID:29024461
3380. Rawstron AC, Shanafelt T, Lanasa MC, et al. Different biology and clinical outcome according to the absolute numbers of clonal B-cells in monoclonal B-cell lymphocytosis (MBL). Cytometry B Clin Cytom. 2010;78 Suppl 1(Suppl 1):S19–23. PMID:20839333
3381. Rawstron AC, Ssemaganda A, de Tute R, et al. Monoclonal B-cell lymphocytosis in a hospital-based UK population and a rural Ugandan population: a cross-sectional study. Lancet Haematol. 2017 Jul;4(7):e334–40. PMID:28668191
3382. Razzaghi R, Agarwal S, Kotlov N, et al. Compromised counterselection by FAS creates an aggressive subtype of germinal center lymphoma. J Exp Med. 2021 Mar 1;218(3):e20201173. PMID:33237303
3383. Rea B, Haun P, Emerson R, et al. Role of high-throughput sequencing in the diagnosis of cutaneous T-cell lymphoma. J Clin Pathol. 2018 Sep;71(9):814–20. PMID:29636372
3384. Reckel S, Gehin C, Tardivon D, et al. Structural and functional dissection of the DH and PH domains of oncogenic Bcr-Abl tyrosine kinase. Nat Commun. 2017 Dec 13;8(1):2101. PMID:29235475
3385. Redaelli A, Laskin BL, Stephens JM, et al. A systematic literature review of the clinical and epidemiological burden of acute lymphoblastic leukaemia (ALL). Eur J Cancer Care (Engl). 2005 Mar;14(1):53–62. PMID:15698386
3386. Reddy A, Zhang J, Davis NS, et al. Genetic and functional drivers of diffuse large B cell lymphoma. Cell. 2017 Oct 5;171(2):481–494.e15. PMID:28985567
3387. Ree HJ, Kadin ME, Kikuchi M, et al. Bcl-6 expression in reactive follicular hyperplasia, follicular lymphoma, and angioimmunoblastic T-cell lymphoma with hyperplastic germinal centers: heterogeneity of intrafollicular T-cells and their altered distribution in the pathogenesis of angioimmunoblastic T-cell lymphoma. Hum Pathol. 1999 Apr;30(4):403–11. PMID:10208461
3388. Reed JC. Bcl-2-family proteins and hematologic malignancies: history and future prospects. Blood. 2008 Apr 1;111(7):3322–30. PMID:18362212
3389. Reed V, Shah J, Medeiros LJ, et al. Solitary plasmacytomas: outcome and prognostic factors after definitive radiation therapy. Cancer. 2011 Oct 1;117(19):4468–74. PMID:21437886
3390. Reichel J, Chadburn A, Rubinstein PG, et al. Flow sorting and exome sequencing reveal the oncogenome of primary Hodgkin and Reed-Sternberg cells. Blood. 2015 Feb 12;125(7):1061–72. PMID:25488972
3391. Reid A, Naresh K, Wagner S, et al. Interphase FISH using a BCL3 probe to diagnose the t(14;19)(q32;q13)-positive small B-cell leukemia. Leuk Lymphoma. 2008 Feb;49(2):356–8. PMID:18231927
3392. Remstein ED, James CD, Kurtin PJ. Incidence and subtype specificity of API2-MALT1 fusion translocations in extranodal, nodal, and splenic marginal zone lymphomas. Am J Pathol. 2000 Apr;156(4):1183–8. PMID:10751343
3393. Ren R, Sun X, Staerkel G, et al. Fine-needle aspiration cytology of a liver metastasis of follicular dendritic cell sarcoma. Diagn Cytopathol. 2005 Jan;32(1):38–43. PMID:15584048
3394. Rengstl B, Newrzela S, Heinrich T, et al. Incomplete cytokinesis and re-fusion of small mononucleated Hodgkin cells lead to giant multinucleated Reed-Sternberg cells. Proc Natl Acad Sci U S A. 2013 Dec 17;110(51):20729–34. PMID:24302766
3395. Renné C, Martín-Subero JI, Hansmann ML, et al. Molecular cytogenetic analyses of immunoglobulin loci in nodular lymphocyte predominant Hodgkin's lymphoma reveal a recurrent IGH-BCL6 juxtaposition. J Mol Diagn. 2005 Aug;7(3):352–6. PMID:16049307
3396. Resende de Paiva C, Grønhøj C, Feldt-Rasmussen U, et al. Association between Hashimoto's thyroiditis and thyroid cancer in 64,628 patients. Front Oncol. 2017 Apr 10;7:53. PMID:28443243
3397. Reshmi SC, Harvey RC, Roberts KG, et al. Targetable kinase gene fusions in high-risk B-ALL: a study from the Children's Oncology Group. Blood. 2017 Jun 22;129(25):3352–61. PMID:28408464
3398. Retamozo S, Brito-Zerón P, Ramos-Casals M. Prognostic markers of lymphoma development in primary Sjögren syndrome. Lupus. 2019 Jul;28(8):923–36. PMID:31215845
3399. Rezk SA, Weiss LM. Epstein-Barr virus-associated lymphoproliferative disorders. Hum Pathol. 2007 Sep;38(9):1293–304. PMID:17707260
3400. Riaz IB, Faridi W, Patnaik MM, et al. A systematic review on predisposition to lymphoid (B and T cell) neoplasias in patients with primary immunodeficiencies and immune dysregulatory disorders (inborn errors of immunity). Front Immunol. 2019 Apr 16;10:777. PMID:31057537
3401. Ribera J, Granada I, Morgades M, et al. Prognostic heterogeneity of adult B-cell precursor acute lymphoblastic leukaemia patients with t(1;19)(q23;p13)/TCF3-PBX1 treated with measurable residual disease-oriented protocols. Br J Haematol. 2022 Feb;196(3):670–5. PMID:34549416
3402. Richard P, Vassallo J, Valmary S, et al. "In situ-like" mantle cell lymphoma: a report of two cases. J Clin Pathol. 2006 Sep;59(9):995–6. PMID:16935977
3403. Richard-Carpentier G, Kantarjian HM, Tang G, et al. Outcomes of acute lymphoblastic leukemia with KMT2A (MLL) rearrangement: the MD Anderson experience. Blood Adv. 2021 Dec 14;5(23):5415–9. PMID:34525185
3404. Richardson AI, Yin CC, Cui W, et al. p53 and β-catenin expression predict poorer prognosis in patients with anaplastic large-cell lymphoma. Clin Lymphoma Myeloma Leuk. 2019 Jul;19(7):e385–92. PMID:31078446
3405. Richter J, John K, Staiger AM, et al. Epstein-Barr virus status of sporadic Burkitt lymphoma is associated with patient age and mutational features. Br J Haematol. 2022 Feb;196(3):681–9. PMID:34617271
3406. Richter J, Schlesner M, Hoffmann S, et al. Recurrent mutation of the ID3 gene in Burkitt lymphoma identified by integrated genome, exome and transcriptome sequencing. Nat Genet. 2012 Dec;44(12):1316–20. PMID:23143595
3407. Riemersma SA, Jordanova ES, Schop RF, et al. Extensive genetic alterations of the HLA region, including homozygous deletions of HLA class II genes in B-cell lymphomas arising in immune-privileged sites. Blood. 2000 Nov 15;96(10):3569–77. PMID:11071656
3408. Rigaud C, Bogomoletz WV. Leiomyomatosis in pelvic lymph node. Arch Pathol Lab Med. 1983 Mar;107(3):153–4. PMID:6687533
3409. Rigaud G, Moore PS, Taruscio D, et al. Alteration of chromosome arm 6p is characteristic of primary mediastinal B-cell lymphoma, as identified by genome-wide allelotyping. Genes Chromosomes Cancer. 2001 Jun;31(2):191–5. PMID:11319807
3410. Riller Q, Rieux-Laucat F. RASopathies: from germline mutations to somatic and multigenic diseases. Biomed J. 2021 Aug;44(4):422–32. PMID:34175492
3411. Rimsza L, Pittaluga S, Dirnhofer S, et al. The clinicopathologic spectrum of mature aggressive B cell lymphomas. Virchows Arch. 2017 Oct;471(4):453–66. PMID:28844114
3412. Rimsza LM, Day WA, McGinn S, et al. Kappa and lambda light chain mRNA in situ hybridization compared to flow cytometry and immunohistochemistry in B cell lymphomas. Diagn Pathol. 2014 Jul 21;9:144. PMID:25047073
3413. Rimsza LM, Li H, Braziel RM, et al. Impact of histological grading on survival in the SWOG S0016 follicular lymphoma cohort. Haematologica. 2018 Apr;103(4):e151–3. PMID:29472351
3414. Rinaldi A, Mian M, Chigrinova E, et al. Genome-wide DNA profiling of marginal zone lymphomas identifies subtype-specific lesions with an impact on the clinical outcome. Blood. 2011 Feb 3;117(5):1595–604. PMID:21115979
3415. Ripamonti D, Marini B, Rambaldi A, et al. Treatment of primary effusion lymphoma with highly active antiviral therapy in the setting of HIV infection. AIDS. 2008 Jun 19;22(10):1236–7. PMID:18525275
3416. Rizvi MA, Evens AM, Tallman MS, et al. T-cell non-Hodgkin lymphoma. Blood. 2006 Feb 15;107(4):1255–64. PMID:16210342
3417. Rizvi S, Raza ST, Mahdi F. Telomere length variations in aging and age-related diseases. Curr Aging Sci. 2014;7(3):161–7. PMID:25612739
3418. Rizzi R, Curci P, Delia M, et al. Spontaneous remission of "methotrexate-associated lymphoproliferative disorders" after discontinuation of immunosuppressive treatment for autoimmune disease. Review of the literature. Med Oncol. 2009;26(1):1–9. PMID:18461290
3419. Rizzo KA, Streubel B, Pittaluga S, et al. Marginal zone lymphomas in children and the young adult population; characterization of genetic aberrations by FISH and RT-PCR. Mod Pathol. 2010 Jun;23(6):866–73. PMID:20305621
3420. Robak T. Current treatment options in hairy cell leukemia and hairy cell leukemia variant. Cancer Treat Rev. 2006 Aug;32(5):365–76. PMID:16781083
3421. Robak T. Hairy-cell leukemia variant: recent view on diagnosis, biology and treatment. Cancer Treat Rev. 2011 Feb;37(1):3–10. PMID:20558005
3422. Robak T, Janus A, Jamroziak K, et al. Vemurafenib and rituximab in patients with hairy cell leukemia previously treated with moxetumomab pasudotox. J Clin Med. 2021 Jun 25;10(13):2800. PMID:34202156
3423. Robak T, Matutes E, Catovsky D, et al. Hairy cell leukaemia: ESMO Clinical Practice Guidelines for diagnosis, treatment and follow-up. Ann Oncol. 2015 Sep;26 Suppl 5:v100–7. PMID:26269205
3424. Robbiani DF, Deroubaix S, Feldhahn N, et al. Plasmodium infection promotes genomic instability and AID-dependent B cell lymphoma. Cell. 2015 Aug 13;162(4):727–37. PMID:26276629
3425. Roberti A, Dobay MP, Bisig B, et al. Type II enteropathy-associated T-cell lymphoma features a unique genomic profile with highly recurrent SETD2 alterations. Nat Commun. 2016 Sep 7;7:12602. PMID:27600764
3426. Roberts KG, Gu Z, Payne-Turner D, et al. High frequency and poor outcome of Philadelphia chromosome-like acute lymphoblastic leukemia in adults. J Clin Oncol. 2017 Feb;35(4):394–401. PMID:27870571
3427. Roberts KG, Li Y, Payne-Turner D, et al. Targetable kinase-activating lesions in Ph-like acute lymphoblastic leukemia. N Engl J Med. 2014 Sep 11;371(11):1005–15. PMID:25207766
3428. Roberts KG, Morin RD, Zhang J, et al. Genetic alterations activating kinase and cytokine receptor signaling in high-risk acute lymphoblastic leukemia. Cancer Cell. 2012 Aug 14;22(2):153–66. PMID:22897847
3429. Roberts RA, Wright G, Rosenwald AR, et al. Loss of major histocompatibility class II gene and protein expression in primary mediastinal large B-cell lymphoma is highly coordinated and related to poor patient survival. Blood. 2006 Jul 1;108(1):311–8. PMID:16543468
3430. Robertson PB, Neiman RS, Worapongpaiboon S, et al. 013 (CD99) positivity in hematologic proliferations correlates with TdT positivity. Mod Pathol. 1997 Apr;10(4):277–82. PMID:9110287
3431. Robinson HM, Broadfield ZJ, Cheung KL, et al. Amplification of AML1 in acute lymphoblastic leukemia is associated with a poor outcome. Leukemia. 2003 Nov;17(11):2249–50. PMID:14523475
3432. Robson A, Assaf C, Bagot M, et al. Aggressive epidermotropic cutaneous CD8+ lymphoma: a cutaneous lymphoma with distinct clinical and pathological features. Report of an EORTC Cutaneous Lymphoma Task Force Workshop. Histopathology. 2015 Oct;67(4):425–41. PMID:24438036
3433. Roccaro AM, Sacco A, Shi J, et al. Exome sequencing reveals recurrent germ line variants in patients with familial Waldenström macroglobulinemia. Blood. 2016 May 26;127(21):2598–606. PMID:26903547
3434. Rochford R. Reframing Burkitt lymphoma: virology not epidemiology defines clinical variants. Ann Lymphoma. 2021 Sep;5(Sep):5. PMID:34888589
3435. Rodig SJ, Savage KJ, LaCasce AS, et al. Expression of TRAF1 and nuclear c-Rel distinguishes primary mediastinal large cell lymphoma from other types of diffuse large B-cell lymphoma. Am J Surg Pathol. 2007 Jan;31(1):106–12. PMID:17197926
3436. Rodig SJ, Vergilio JA, Shahsafaei A, et al. Characteristic expression patterns of TCL1, CD38, and CD44 identify aggressive lymphomas harboring a MYC translocation. Am J Surg Pathol. 2008 Jan;32(1):113–22. PMID:18162778
3437. Rodrigues CD, Peixeiro RP, Viegas D, et al. Clinical characteristics, treatment and

evolution of splenic and nodal marginal zone lymphomas-retrospective and multicentric analysis of Portuguese centers. Clin Lymphoma Myeloma Leuk. 2021 Nov;21(11):e839–44. PMID:34326035

3438. Rodríguez Pinilla SM, Roncador G, Rodríguez-Peralto JL, et al. Primary cutaneous CD4+ small/medium-sized pleomorphic T-cell lymphoma expresses follicular T-cell markers. Am J Surg Pathol. 2009 Jan;33(1):81–90. PMID:18987541

3439. Rodriguez-Justo M, Attygalle AD, Munson P, et al. Angioimmunoblastic T-cell lymphoma with hyperplastic germinal centres: a neoplasia with origin in the outer zone of the germinal centre? Clinicopathological and immunohistochemical study of 10 cases with follicular T-cell markers. Mod Pathol. 2009 Jun;22(6):753–61. PMID:19329936

3440. Rodriguez-Justo M, Huang Y, Ye H, et al. Cyclin D1-positive diffuse large B-cell lymphoma. Histopathology. 2008 Jun;52(7):900–3. PMID:18494615

3441. Rodríguez-Otero P, Mateos MV, Martínez-López J, et al. Predicting long-term disease control in transplant-ineligible patients with multiple myeloma: impact of an MGUS-like signature. Blood Cancer J. 2019 Mar 18;9(4):36. PMID:30886139

3442. Rodríguez-Pinilla SM, Barrionuevo C, García J, et al. Epstein-Barr virus-positive systemic NK/T-cell lymphomas in children: report of six cases. Histopathology. 2011 Dec;59(6):1183–93. PMID:22175898

3443. Rodríguez-Pinilla SM, García FJS, Balagué O, et al. Breast implant-associated Epstein-Barr virus-positive large B-cell lymphomas: a report of three cases. Haematologica. 2020 Aug;105(8):e412–4. PMID:31753922

3444. Rodríguez-Pinilla SM, Ortiz-Romero PL, Monsalvez V, et al. TCR-γ expression in primary cutaneous T-cell lymphomas. Am J Surg Pathol. 2013 Mar;37(3):375–84. PMID:23348211

3445. Roelandt PR, Maertens J, Vandenberghe P, et al. Hepatosplenic gammadelta T-cell lymphoma after liver transplantation: report of the first 2 cases and review of the literature. Liver Transpl. 2009 Jul;15(7):686–92. PMID:19562701

3446. Roemer MG, Advani RH, Ligon AH, et al. PD-L1 and PD-L2 genetic alterations define classical Hodgkin lymphoma and predict outcome. J Clin Oncol. 2016 Aug 10;34(23):2690–7. PMID:27069084

3447. Roemer MGM, Redd RA, Cader FZ, et al. Major histocompatibility complex class II and programmed death ligand 1 expression predict outcome after programmed death 1 blockade in classic Hodgkin lymphoma. J Clin Oncol. 2018 Apr 1;36(10):942–50. PMID:29394125

3448. Rohr J, Guo S, Huo J, et al. Recurrent activating mutations of CD28 in peripheral T-cell lymphomas. Leukemia. 2016 May;30(5):1062–70. PMID:26719098

3449. Roithmann S, Toledano M, Tourani JM, et al. HIV-associated non-Hodgkin's lymphomas: clinical characteristics and outcome. The experience of the French Registry of HIV-associated tumors. Ann Oncol. 1991 Apr;2(4):289–95. PMID:1868025

3450. Rokx C, Rijnders BJ, van Laar JA. Treatment of multicentric Castleman's disease in HIV-1 infected and uninfected patients: a systematic review. Neth J Med. 2015 Jun;73(5):202–10. PMID:26087799

3451. Roldan-Vasquez E, Roldan-Vasquez A, Jarrin-Estupiñan X, et al. Case report: infrequent littoral cell angioma of the spleen. Int J Surg Case Rep. 2021 Aug;85:106242. PMID:34333257

3452. Rollins-Raval MA, Marafioti T, Swerdlow SH, et al. The number and growth pattern of plasmacytoid dendritic cells vary in different types of reactive lymph nodes: an immunohistochemical study. Hum Pathol. 2013 Jun;44(6):1003–10. PMID:23260330

3453. Roman E, Smith AG. Epidemiology of lymphomas. Histopathology. 2011 Jan;58(1):4–14. PMID:21261679

3454. Ronaghy A, Wang HY, Thorson JA, et al. PD-L1 and Notch1 expression in KSHV/HHV-8 and EBV associated germinotropic lymphoproliferative disorder: case report and review of the literature. Pathology. 2017 Jun;49(4):430–5. PMID:28450091

3455. Roncador G, Garcia JF, Garcia JF, et al. FOXP3, a selective marker for a subset of adult T-cell leukaemia/lymphoma. Leukemia. 2005 Dec;19(12):2247–53. PMID:16193085

3456. Roncador G, García Verdes-Montenegro JF, Tedoldi S, et al. Expression of two markers of germinal center T cells (SAP and PD-1) in angioimmunoblastic T-cell lymphoma. Haematologica. 2007 Aug;92(8):1059–66. PMID:17640856

3457. Ronceray L, Abla O, Barzilai-Birenboim S, et al. Children and adolescents with marginal zone lymphoma have an excellent prognosis with limited chemotherapy or a watch-and-wait strategy after complete resection. Pediatr Blood Cancer. 2018 Apr;65(4). PMID:29286565

3458. Rongioletti F, Romanelli P, Rebora A. Cutaneous mucinous angiomatosis as a presenting sign of bone plasmacytoma: a new case of (A)ESOP syndrome. J Am Acad Dermatol. 2006 Nov;55(5):909–10. PMID:17052506

3459. Ros PR, Moser RP Jr, Dachman AH, et al. Hemangioma of the spleen: radiologic-pathologic correlation in ten cases. Radiology. 1987 Jan;162(1 Pt 1):73–7. PMID:3538155

3460. Rosado FG, Oliveira JL, Sohani AR, et al. Bone marrow findings of the newly described TEMPI syndrome: when erythrocytosis and plasma cell dyscrasia coexist. Mod Pathol. 2015 Mar;28(3):367–72. PMID:25216227

3461. Rosado FG, Tang YW, Hasserjian RP, et al. Kikuchi-Fujimoto lymphadenitis: role of parvovirus B-19, Epstein-Barr virus, human herpesvirus 6, and human herpesvirus 8. Hum Pathol. 2013 Feb;44(2):255–9. PMID:22939574

3462. Roschewski M, Dunleavy K, Abramson JS, et al. Multicenter study of risk-adapted therapy with dose-adjusted EPOCH-R in adults with untreated Burkitt lymphoma. J Clin Oncol. 2020 Aug 1;38(22):2519–29. PMID:32453640

3463. Roschewski M, Wilson WH. Lymphomatoid granulomatosis. Cancer J. 2012 Sep-Oct;18(5):469–74. PMID:23006954

3464. Rosebeck S, Madden L, Jin X, et al. Cleavage of NIK by the API2-MALT1 fusion oncoprotein leads to noncanonical NF-kappaB activation. Science. 2011 Jan 28;331(6016):468–72. PMID:21273489

3465. Rosen DS, Smith S, Gurbuxani S, et al. Extranodal hairy cell leukemia presenting in the lumbar spine. J Neurosurg Spine. 2008 Oct;9(4):374–6. PMID:18939925

3466. Rosenberg PS, Tamary H, Alter BP. How high are carrier frequencies of rare recessive syndromes? Contemporary estimates for Fanconi anemia in the United States and Israel. Am J Med Genet A. 2011 Aug;155A(8):1877–83. PMID:21739583

3467. Rosenbloom BE, Weinreb NJ, Zimran A, et al. Gaucher disease and cancer incidence: a study from the Gaucher Registry. Blood. 2005 Jun 15;105(12):4569–72. PMID:15718419

3468. Rosenquist R, Beà S, Du MQ, et al. Genetic landscape and deregulated pathways in B-cell lymphoid malignancies. J Intern Med. 2017 Nov;282(5):371–94. PMID:28631441

3469. Rosenquist R, Ghia P, Hadzidimitriou A, et al. Immunoglobulin gene sequence analysis in chronic lymphocytic leukemia: updated ERIC recommendations. Leukemia. 2017 Jul;31(7):1477–81. PMID:28439111

3470. Rosenquist R, Rosenwald A, Du MQ, et al. Clinical impact of recurrently mutated genes on lymphoma diagnostics: state-of-the-art and beyond. Haematologica. 2016 Sep;101(9):1002–9. PMID:27582569

3471. Rosenwald A, Bens S, Advani R, et al. Prognostic significance of MYC rearrangement and translocation partner in diffuse large B-cell lymphoma: a study by the Lunenburg Lymphoma Biomarker Consortium. J Clin Oncol. 2019 Dec 10;37(35):3359–68. PMID:31498031

3472. Rosenwald A, Wright G, Chan WC, et al. The use of molecular profiling to predict survival after chemotherapy for diffuse large-B-cell lymphoma. N Engl J Med. 2002 Jun 20;346(25):1937–47. PMID:12075054

3473. Rosenwald A, Wright G, Leroy K, et al. Molecular diagnosis of primary mediastinal B cell lymphoma identifies a clinically favorable subgroup of diffuse large B cell lymphoma related to Hodgkin lymphoma. J Exp Med. 2003 Sep 15;198(6):851–62. PMID:12975453

3474. Rosenwald A, Wright G, Wiestner A, et al. The proliferation gene expression signature is a quantitative integrator of oncogenic events that predicts survival in mantle cell lymphoma. Cancer Cell. 2003 Feb;3(2):185–97. PMID:12620412

3475. Roskin KM, Simchoni N, Liu Y, et al. IgH sequences in common variable immune deficiency reveal altered B cell development and selection. Sci Transl Med. 2015 Aug 26;7(302):302ra135. PMID:26311730

3476. Rosolen A, Perkins SL, Pinkerton CR, et al. Revised International Pediatric Non-Hodgkin Lymphoma Staging System. J Clin Oncol. 2015 Jun 20;33(18):2112–8. PMID:25940716

3477. Rossi A, Bulgarini A, Rondanelli E, et al. Intranodal palisaded myofibroblastoma: report of three new cases. Tumori. 1995 Nov-Dec;81(6):464–8. PMID:8804479

3478. Rossi D, Rasi S, Fabbri G, et al. Mutations of NOTCH1 are an independent predictor of survival in chronic lymphocytic leukemia. Blood. 2012 Jan 12;119(2):521–9. PMID:22077063

3479. Rossi D, Sozzi E, Puma A, et al. The prognosis of clinical monoclonal B cell lymphocytosis differs from prognosis of Rai 0 chronic lymphocytic leukaemia and is recapitulated by biological risk factors. Br J Haematol. 2009 Jun;146(1):64–75. PMID:19438485

3480. Rossi D, Spina V, Deambrogi C, et al. The genetics of Richter syndrome reveals disease heterogeneity and predicts survival after transformation. Blood. 2011 Mar 24;117(12):3391–401. PMID:21266718

3481. Rossi D, Spina V, Gaidano G. Biology and treatment of Richter syndrome. Blood. 2018 Jun 21;131(25):2761–72. PMID:29692342

3482. Rossi ED, Pantanowitz L, Hornick JL. Cytologic and histological features of rare nonepithelial and nonlymphoid tumors of the thyroid. Cancer Cytopathol. 2021 Aug;129(8):583–602. PMID:33493367

3483. Rossi G, Cozzi I, Della Starza I, et al. Human herpesvirus-8-positive primary effusion lymphoma in HIV-negative patients: single institution case series with a multidisciplinary characterization. Cancer Cytopathol. 2021 Jan;129(1):62–74. PMID:32975904

3484. Rossi JG, Bernasconi AR, Alonso CN, et al. Lineage switch in childhood acute leukemia: an unusual event with poor outcome. Am J Hematol. 2012 Sep;87(9):890–7. PMID:22685031

3485. Rossky PJ, Walker GC. Retrospective. Paul F. Barbara (1953-2010). Science. 2010 Nov 26;330(6008):1191. PMID:21109661

3486. Rosso R, Paulli M, Gianelli U, et al. Littoral cell angiosarcoma of the spleen. Case report with immunohistochemical and ultrastructural analysis. Am J Surg Pathol. 1995 Oct;19(10):1203–8. PMID:7573679

3487. Roulland S, Kelly RS, Morgado E, et al. t(14;18) Translocation: a predictive blood biomarker for follicular lymphoma. J Clin Oncol. 2014 May 1;32(13):1347–55. PMID:24687831

3488. Roulland S, Navarro JM, Grenot P, et al. Follicular lymphoma-like B cells in healthy individuals: a novel intermediate step in early lymphomagenesis. J Exp Med. 2006 Oct 30;203(11):2425–31. PMID:17043145

3489. Roullet MR, Martinez D, Ma L, et al. Coexisting follicular and mantle cell lymphoma with each having an in situ component: a novel, curious, and complex consultation case of coincidental, composite, colonizing lymphoma. Am J Clin Pathol. 2010 Apr;133(4):584–91. PMID:20231612

3490. Roux C, Nicolini FE, Rea D, et al. Reversible lymph node follicular hyperplasia associated with dasatinib treatment of chronic myeloid leukemia in chronic phase. Blood. 2013 Oct 24;122(17):3082–4. PMID:24159167

3491. Rowczenio DM, Noor I, Gillmore JD, et al. Online registry for mutations in hereditary amyloidosis including nomenclature recommendations. Hum Mutat. 2014 Sep;35(9):E2403–12. PMID:25044787

3492. Rowe M, Rowe DT, Gregory CD, et al. Differences in B cell growth phenotype reflect novel patterns of Epstein-Barr virus latent gene expression in Burkitt's lymphoma cells. EMBO J. 1987 Sep;6(9):2743–51. PMID:2824192

3493. Rowley JD. Chromosome studies in the non-Hodgkin's lymphomas: the role of the 14;18 translocation. J Clin Oncol. 1988 May;6(5):919–25. PMID:3284977

3494. Rowsey RA, Smoley SA, Williamson CM, et al. Characterization of TCF3 rearrangements in pediatric B-lymphoblastic leukemia/lymphoma by mate-pair sequencing (MPseq) identifies complex genomic rearrangements and a novel TCF3/TEF gene fusion. Blood Cancer J. 2019 Oct 1;9(10):81. PMID:31575852

3495. Royo C, Navarro A, Clot G, et al. Non-nodal type of mantle cell lymphoma is a specific biological and clinical subgroup of the disease. Leukemia. 2012 Aug;26(8):1895–8. PMID:22425896

3496. Royo C, Salaverria I, Hartmann EM, et al. The complex landscape of genetic alterations in mantle cell lymphoma. Semin Cancer Biol. 2011 Nov;21(5):322–34. PMID:21945515

3497. Ruan Y, Shen X, Shi R, et al. Hydroa vacciniforme-like lymphoproliferative disorder treated with intravenous immunoglobulin: long-term remission without haematopoietic stem cell transplantation or chemotherapy. Acta Derm Venereol. 2020 Jun 18;100(13):adv00192. PMID:32516422

3498. Rubio MA, Cabranes JA, Schally AV, et al. Prolactin-lowering effect of luteinizing hormone-releasing hormone agonist administration in prolactinoma patients. J Clin Endocrinol Metab. 1989 Aug;69(2):444–7. PMID:2526819

3499. Rubio-Tapia A, Kelly DG, Lahr BD, et al. Clinical staging and survival in refractory celiac disease: a single center experience. Gastroenterology. 2009 Jan;136(1):99–107. PMID:18996383

3500. Rüdiger T, Gascoyne RD, Jaffe ES, et al. Workshop on the relationship between nodular lymphocyte predominant Hodgkin's lymphoma and T cell/histiocyte-rich B cell lymphoma. Ann Oncol. 2002;13 Suppl 1:44-51. PMID:12078902

3501. Ruiz A, Reischl U, Swerdlow SH, et al. Extranodal marginal zone B-cell lymphomas of the ocular adnexa: multiparameter analysis of 34 cases including interphase molecular cytogenetics and PCR for Chlamydia psittaci.

Am J Surg Pathol. 2007 May;31(5):792–802. PMID:17460465
3502. Ruiz-Ballesteros E, Mollejo M, Mateo M, et al. MicroRNA losses in the frequently deleted region of 7q in SMZL. Leukemia. 2007 Dec;21(12):2547–9. PMID:17625607
3503. Rumi E, Passamonti F, Zibellini S, et al. HLA typing and VH gene rearrangement analysis in a family with hairy cell leukaemia. Leuk Lymphoma. 2007 Apr;48(4):805–7. PMID:17454641
3504. Ruminy P, Marchand V, Buchbinder N, et al. Multiplexed targeted sequencing of recurrent fusion genes in acute leukaemia. Leukemia. 2016 Mar;30(3):757–60. PMID:26139430
3505. Runge HFP, Lacy S, Barrans S, et al. Application of the LymphGen classification tool to 928 clinically and genetically-characterised cases of diffuse large B cell lymphoma (DLBCL). Br J Haematol. 2021 Jan;192(1):216–20. PMID:33010029
3506. Ruskoné-Fourmestraux A, Fischbach W, Aleman BM, et al. EGILS consensus report. Gastric extranodal marginal zone B-cell lymphoma of MALT. Gut. 2011 Jun;60(6):747–58. PMID:21317175
3507. Rustad EH, Yellapantula VD, Glodzik D, et al. Revealing the impact of structural variants in multiple myeloma. Blood Cancer Discov. 2020 Nov;1(3):258–73. PMID:33392515
3508. Ryan RJ, Sloan JM, Collins AB, et al. Extranodal marginal zone lymphoma of mucosa-associated lymphoid tissue with amyloid deposition: a clinicopathologic case series. Am J Clin Pathol. 2012 Jan;137(1):51–64. PMID:22180478
3509. Ryder J, Wang X, Bao L, et al. Aggressive natural killer cell leukemia: report of a Chinese series and review of the literature. Int J Hematol. 2007 Jan;85(1):18–25. PMID:17261497
3510. Rymkiewicz G, Grygalewicz B, Chechlinska M, et al. A comprehensive flow-cytometry-based immunophenotypic characterization of Burkitt-like lymphoma with 11q aberration. Mod Pathol. 2018 May;31(5):732–43. PMID:29327714
3511. Saarinen S, Aavikko M, Aittomäki K, et al. Exome sequencing reveals germline NPAT mutation as a candidate risk factor for Hodgkin lymphoma. Blood. 2011 Jul 21;118(3):493–8. PMID:21562039
3512. Saarinen S, Kaasinen E, Karjalainen-Lindsberg ML, et al. Primary mediastinal large B-cell lymphoma segregating in a family: exome sequencing identifies MLL as a candidate predisposition gene. Blood. 2013 Apr 25;121(17):3428–30. PMID:23457195
3513. Saarinen S, Pukkala E, Vahteristo P, et al. High familial risk in nodular lymphocyte-predominant Hodgkin lymphoma. J Clin Oncol. 2013 Mar 1;31(7):938–43. PMID:23284040
3514. Sabattini E, Pizzi M, Tabanelli V, et al. CD30 expression in peripheral T-cell lymphomas. Haematologica. 2013 Aug;98(8):e81–2. PMID:23716537
3515. Sadasivam N, Johnson RJ, Owen RG. Resolution of methotrexate-induced Epstein-Barr virus-associated mucocutaneous ulcer. Br J Haematol. 2014 Jun;165(5):584. PMID:24456137
3516. Sadeghi Shoreh Deli A, Scharf S, Steiner Y, et al. 3D analyses reveal T cells with activated nuclear features in T-cell/histiocyte-rich large B-cell lymphoma. Mod Pathol. 2022 Oct;35(10):1431–8. PMID:35173297
3517. Sadighi Akha AA. Aging and the immune system: an overview. J Immunol Methods. 2018 Dec;463:21–6. PMID:30114401
3518. Sadras T, Müschen M. MEF2D fusions drive oncogenic pre-BCR signaling in B-ALL. Blood Cancer Discov. 2020 Jun 22;1(1):18–20. PMID:34661138
3519. Saeki T, Kawano M, Nagasawa T, et al. Validation of the diagnostic criteria for IgG4-related kidney disease (IgG4-RKD) 2011, and proposal of a new 2020 version. Clin Exp Nephrol. 2021 Feb;25(2):99–109. PMID:33398598
3520. Saffer H, Wahed A, Rassidakis GZ, et al. Clusterin expression in malignant lymphomas: a survey of 266 cases. Mod Pathol. 2002 Nov;15(11):1221–6. PMID:12429802
3521. Sagar J, Vargiamidou A, Manikkapurath H. Intranodal palisaded myofibroblastoma originating from retroperitoneum: an unusual origin. BMC Clin Pathol. 2011 Jun 30;11:7. PMID:21718465
3522. Saggini A, Gulia A, Argenyi Z, et al. A variant of lymphomatoid papulosis simulating primary cutaneous aggressive epidermotropic CD8+ cytotoxic T-cell lymphoma. Description of 9 cases. Am J Surg Pathol. 2010 Aug;34(8):1168–75. PMID:20661014
3523. Saglam A, Singh K, Gollapudi S, et al. Indolent T-lymphoblastic proliferation: a systematic review of the literature analyzing the epidemiologic, clinical, and pathologic features of 45 cases. Int J Lab Hematol. 2022 Aug;44(4):700–11. PMID:35577551
3524. Saha A, Robertson ES. Mechanisms of B-cell oncogenesis induced by Epstein-Barr virus. J Virol. 2019 Jun 14;93(13):e00238-19. PMID:30971472
3525. Sahar N, Schiby G, Davidson T, et al. Hairy cell leukemia presenting as multiple discrete hepatic lesions. World J Gastroenterol. 2009 Sep 21;15(35):4453–6. PMID:19764101
3526. Said J, Smart C. Severe mosquito bite allergy: an unusual EBV+ NK cell lymphoproliferative disorder. Blood. 2019 Feb 28;133(9):999. PMID:30819780
3527. Said JW, Shintaku IP, Asou H, et al. Herpesvirus 8 inclusions in primary effusion lymphoma: report of a unique case with T-cell phenotype. Arch Pathol Lab Med. 1999 Mar;123(3):257–60. PMID:10086517
3528. Sainati L, Matutes E, Mulligan S, et al. A variant form of hairy cell leukemia resistant to alpha-interferon: clinical and phenotypic characteristics of 17 patients. Blood. 1990 Jul 1;76(1):157–62. PMID:2364167
3529. Saito M, Morioka M, Izumiyama K, et al. Epstein-Barr virus-positive ileal extraosseous plasmacytoma containing plasmablastic lymphoma components with CD20-positive lymph node involvement. Int J Gen Med. 2012;5:715–8. PMID:22969303
3530. Sakai M, Higashi M, Fujiwara T, et al. MRI imaging features of HIV-related central nervous system diseases: diagnosis by pattern recognition in daily practice. Jpn J Radiol. 2021 Nov;39(11):1023–38. PMID:34125369
3531. Sakakibara A, Inagaki Y, Imaoka E, et al. Divergence and heterogeneity of neoplastic PD-L1 expression: two autopsy case reports of intravascular large B-cell lymphoma. Pathol Int. 2019 Mar;69(3):148–54. PMID:30688388
3532. Sakakibara Y, Wada T, Muraoka M, et al. Basophil activation by mosquito extracts in patients with hypersensitivity to mosquito bites. Cancer Sci. 2015 Aug;106(8):965–71. PMID:25990049
3533. Sakamoto K, Nakasone H, Togashi Y, et al. ALK-positive large B-cell lymphoma: identification of EML4-ALK and a review of the literature focusing on the ALK immunohistochemical staining pattern. Int J Hematol. 2016 Apr;103(4):399–408. PMID:26781614
3534. Sakata-Yanagimoto M, Enami T, Yoshida K, et al. Somatic RHOA mutation in angioimmunoblastic T cell lymphoma. Nat Genet. 2014 Feb;46(2):171–5. PMID:24413737
3535. Sakemi H, Okada H. An autopsy case of Crow-Fukase syndrome which developed 18 years after the first manifestation of plasmacytoma. Intern Med. 1992 Jan;31(1):50–4. PMID:1568043
3536. Sakhdari A, Ok CY, Patel KP, et al. TP53 mutations are common in mantle cell lymphoma, including the indolent leukemic non-nodal variant. Ann Diagn Pathol. 2019 Aug;41:38–42. PMID:31132650
3537. Sakr H, Cruise M, Chahal P, et al. Anaplastic lymphoma kinase positive large B-cell lymphoma: literature review and report of an endoscopic fine needle aspiration case with tigroid backgrounds mimicking seminoma. Diagn Cytopathol. 2017 Feb;45(2):148–55. PMID:27686567
3538. Salama ME, Lossos IS, Warnke RA, et al. Immunoarchitectural patterns in nodal marginal zone B-cell lymphoma: a study of 51 cases. Am J Clin Pathol. 2009 Jul;132(1):39–49. PMID:19864232
3539. Salama ME, Rajan Mariappan M, Inamdar K, et al. The value of CD23 expression as an additional marker in distinguishing mediastinal (thymic) large B-cell lymphoma from Hodgkin lymphoma. Int J Surg Pathol. 2010 Apr;18(2):121–8. PMID:19223373
3540. Salas MQ, Climent F, Tapia G, et al. Clinicopathologic features and prognostic significance of CD30 expression in de novo diffuse large B-cell lymphoma (DLBCL): results in a homogeneous series from a single institution. Biomarkers. 2020 Feb;25(1):69–75. PMID:31752540
3541. Salaverria I, Beà S, Lopez-Guillermo A, et al. Genomic profiling reveals different genetic aberrations in systemic ALK-positive and ALK-negative anaplastic large cell lymphomas. Br J Haematol. 2008 Mar;140(5):516–26. PMID:18275429
3542. Salaverria I, Martin-Guerrero I, Burkhardt B, et al. High resolution copy number analysis of IRF4 translocation-positive diffuse large B-cell and follicular lymphomas. Genes Chromosomes Cancer. 2013 Feb;52(2):150–5. PMID:23073988
3543. Salaverria I, Martin-Guerrero I, Wagener R, et al. A recurrent 11q aberration pattern characterizes a subset of MYC-negative high-grade B-cell lymphomas resembling Burkitt lymphoma. Blood. 2014 Feb 20;123(8):1187–98. PMID:24398325
3544. Salaverria I, Philipp C, Oschlies I, et al. Translocations activating IRF4 identify a subtype of germinal center-derived B-cell lymphoma affecting predominantly children and young adults. Blood. 2011 Jul 7;118(1):139–47. PMID:21487109
3545. Salaverria I, Royo C, Carvajal-Cuenca A, et al. CCND2 rearrangements are the most frequent genetic events in cyclin D1(-) mantle cell lymphoma. Blood. 2013 Feb 21;121(8):1394–402. PMID:23255553
3546. Salaverria I, Siebert R. Follicular lymphoma grade 3B. Best Pract Res Clin Haematol. 2011 Jun;24(2):111–9. PMID:21658612
3547. Saleh K, Michot JM, Camara-Clayette V, et al. Burkitt and Burkitt-like lymphomas: a systematic review. Curr Oncol Rep. 2020 Mar 6;22(4):33. PMID:32144513
3548. Salhany KE, Macon WR, Choi JK, et al. Subcutaneous panniculitis-like T-cell lymphoma: clinicopathologic, immunophenotypic, and genotypic analysis of alpha/beta and gamma/delta subtypes. Am J Surg Pathol. 1998 Jul;22(7):881–93. PMID:9669350
3549. Salido M, Baró C, Oscier D, et al. Cytogenetic aberrations and their prognostic value in a series of 330 splenic marginal zone B-cell lymphomas: a multicenter study of the Splenic B-Cell Lymphoma Group. Blood. 2010 Sep 2;116(9):1479–88. PMID:20479288
3550. Salim M, Heldt F, Thomay K, et al. Cryptic TCF3 fusions in childhood leukemia: detection by RNA sequencing. Genes Chromosomes Cancer. 2022 Jan;61(1):22–6. PMID:34460133
3551. Sallah S, Wan JY, Hanrahan LR. Future development of lymphoproliferative disorders in patients with autoimmune hemolytic anemia. Clin Cancer Res. 2001 Apr;7(4):791–4. PMID:11309323
3552. Salles G, de Jong D, Xie W, et al. Prognostic significance of immunohistochemical biomarkers in diffuse large B-cell lymphoma: a study from the Lunenburg Lymphoma Biomarker Consortium. Blood. 2011 Jun 30;117(26):7070–8. PMID:21536860
3553. Salloum E, Cooper DL, Howe G, et al. Spontaneous regression of lymphoproliferative disorders in patients treated with methotrexate for rheumatoid arthritis and other rheumatic diseases. J Clin Oncol. 1996 Jun;14(6):1943–9. PMID:8656264
3554. Salmeron-Villalobos J, Egan C, Borgmann V, et al. A unifying hypothesis for PNMZL and PTFL: morphological variants with a common molecular profile. Blood Adv. 2022 Aug 23;6(16):4661–74. PMID:35609565
3555. Salzburg J, Burkhardt B, Zimmermann M, et al. Prevalence, clinical pattern, and outcome of CNS involvement in childhood and adolescent non-Hodgkin's lymphoma differ by non-Hodgkin's lymphoma subtype: a Berlin-Frankfurt-Munster Group report. J Clin Oncol. 2007 Sep 1;25(25):3915–22. PMID:17761975
3556. Samols MA, Su A, Ra S, et al. Intralymphatic cutaneous anaplastic large cell lymphoma/lymphomatoid papulosis: expanding the spectrum of CD30-positive lymphoproliferative disorders. Am J Surg Pathol. 2014 Sep;38(9):1203–11. PMID:24805854
3557. Samra B, Jabbour E, Ravandi F, et al. Evolving therapy of adult acute lymphoblastic leukemia: state-of-the-art treatment and future directions. J Hematol Oncol. 2020 Jun 5;13(1):70. PMID:32503572
3558. San Miguel JF, Vidriales MB, Ocio E, et al. Immunophenotypic analysis of Waldenstrom's macroglobulinemia. Semin Oncol. 2003 Apr;30(2):187–95. PMID:12720134
3559. Sanchez S, Veloza L, Wang L, et al. HHV8-positive, EBV-positive Hodgkin lymphoma-like large B cell lymphoma: expanding the spectrum of HHV8 and EBV-associated lymphoproliferative disorders. Int J Hematol. 2020 Nov;112(5):734–40. PMID:32529584
3560. Sánchez-Aguilera A, Montalbán C, de la Cueva P, et al. Tumor microenvironment and mitotic checkpoint are key factors in the outcome of classic Hodgkin lymphoma. Blood. 2006 Jul 15;108(2):662–8. PMID:16551964
3561. Sandell RF, Boddicker RL, Feldman AL. Genetic landscape and classification of peripheral T cell lymphomas. Curr Oncol Rep. 2017 Apr;19(4):28. PMID:28303495
3562. Sander B, Quintanilla-Martinez L, Ott G, et al. Mantle cell lymphoma–a spectrum from indolent to aggressive disease. Virchows Arch. 2016 Mar;468(3):245–57. PMID:26298543
3563. Sander CA, Jaffe ES, Gebhardt FC, et al. Mediastinal lymphoblastic lymphoma with an immature B-cell immunophenotype. Am J Surg Pathol. 1992 Mar;16(3):300–5. PMID:1317999
3564. Sandoval N, Platzer M, Rosenthal A, et al. Characterization of ATM gene mutations in 66 ataxia telangiectasia families. Hum Mol Genet. 1999 Jan;8(1):69–79. PMID:9887333
3565. Sangiorgio VFI, Arber DA. Non-hematopoietic neoplastic and pseudoneoplastic lesions of the spleen. Semin Diagn Pathol. 2021 Mar;38(2):159–64. PMID:32600744
3566. Sangiorgio VFI, Arber DA. Vascular neoplasms and non-neoplastic vascular lesions of the spleen. Semin Diagn Pathol. 2021 Mar;38(2):154–8. PMID:32674844

3567. Sangueza M, Plaza JA. Hydroa vacciniforme-like cutaneous T-cell lymphoma: clinicopathologic and immunohistochemical study of 12 cases. J Am Acad Dermatol. 2013 Jul;69(1):112–9. PMID:23541598
3568. Sanikommu SR, Clemente MJ, Chomczynski P, et al. Clinical features and treatment outcomes in large granular lymphocytic leukemia (LGLL). Leuk Lymphoma. 2018 Feb;59(2):416–22. PMID:28633612
3569. Sanoja-Flores L, Flores-Montero J, Garcés JJ, et al. Next generation flow for minimally-invasive blood characterization of MGUS and multiple myeloma at diagnosis based on circulating tumor plasma cells (CTPC). Blood Cancer J. 2018 Nov 19;8(12):117. PMID:30455467
3570. Santanelli di Pompeo F, Clemens MW, Atlan M, et al. 2022 practice recommendation updates from the World Consensus Conference on BIA-ALCL. Aesthet Surg J. 2022 Oct 13;42(11):1262–78. PMID:35639805
3571. Santonja C, Soto C, Manso R, et al. Primary cutaneous follicular helper T-cell lymphoma. J Cutan Pathol. 2016 Feb;43(2):164–70. PMID:26282465
3572. Santos FP, O'Brien S. Small lymphocytic lymphoma and chronic lymphocytic leukemia: Are they the same disease? Cancer J. 2012 Sep-Oct;18(5):396–403. PMID:23006943
3573. Santos GdaC, Saieg MA, Ko HM, et al. Multiplex sequencing for EZH2, CD79B, and MYD88 mutations using archival cytospin preparations from B-cell non-Hodgkin lymphoma aspirates previously tested for MYC rearrangement and IGH/BCL2 translocation. Cancer Cytopathol. 2015 Jul;123(7):413–20. PMID:25807917
3574. Santucci M, Pimpinelli N, Arganini L. Primary cutaneous B-cell lymphoma: a unique type of low-grade lymphoma. Clinicopathologic and immunologic study of 83 cases. Cancer. 1991 May 1;67(9):2311–26. PMID:2013039
3575. Santucci M, Pimpinelli N, Massi D, et al. Cytotoxic/natural killer cell cutaneous lymphomas. Report of EORTC Cutaneous Lymphoma Task Force Workshop. Cancer. 2003 Feb 1;97(3):610–27. PMID:12548603
3576. Sarfraz H, Gentille C, Ensor J, et al. Primary cutaneous anaplastic large-cell lymphoma: a review of the SEER database from 2005 to 2016. Clin Exp Dermatol. 2021 Dec;46(8):1420–6. PMID:34081802
3577. Sarkozy C, Chong L, Takata K, et al. Gene expression profiling of gray zone lymphoma. Blood Adv. 2020 Jun 9;4(11):2523–35. PMID:32516416
3578. Sarkozy C, Copie-Bergman C, Damotte D, et al. Gray-zone lymphoma between cHL and large B-cell lymphoma: a histopathologic series from the LYSA. Am J Surg Pathol. 2019 Mar;43(3):341–51. PMID:30540571
3579. Sarkozy C, Hung SS, Chavez EA, et al. Mutational landscape of gray zone lymphoma. Blood. 2021 Apr 1;137(13):1765–76. PMID:32961552
3580. Sarkozy C, Molina T, Ghesquières H, et al. Mediastinal gray zone lymphoma: clinico-pathological characteristics and outcomes of 99 patients from the Lymphoma Study Association. Haematologica. 2017 Jan;102(1):150–9. PMID:27758822
3581. Saruta H, Ohata C, Muto I, et al. Hematopoietic stem cell transplantation in advanced cutaneous T-cell lymphoma. J Dermatol. 2017 Sep;44(9):1038–42. PMID:28391645
3582. Sasajima Y, Yamabe H, Kobashi Y, et al. High expression of the Epstein-Barr virus latent protein EB nuclear antigen-2 on pyothorax-associated lymphomas. Am J Pathol. 1993 Nov;143(5):1280–5. PMID:8238246
3583. Sato A, Nakamura N, Kojima M, et al. Clinical outcome of Epstein-Barr virus-positive diffuse large B-cell lymphoma of the elderly in the rituximab era. Cancer Sci. 2014 Sep;105(9):1170–5. PMID:24974976
3584. Sato Y, Ichimura K, Tanaka T, et al. Duodenal follicular lymphomas share common characteristics with mucosa-associated lymphoid tissue lymphomas. J Clin Pathol. 2008 Mar;61(3):377–81. PMID:17601964
3585. Sato Y, Notohara K, Kojima M, et al. IgG4-related disease: historical overview and pathology of hematological disorders. Pathol Int. 2010 Apr;60(4):247–58. PMID:20403026
3586. Satou A, Banno S, Hanamura I, et al. EBV-positive mucocutaneous ulcer arising in rheumatoid arthritis patients treated with methotrexate: single center series of nine cases. Pathol Int. 2019 Jan;69(1):21–8. PMID:30615240
3587. Satou A, Notohara K, Zen Y, et al. Clinicopathological differential diagnosis of IgG4-related disease: a historical overview and a proposal of the criteria for excluding mimickers of IgG4-related disease. Pathol Int. 2020 Jul;70(7):391–402. PMID:32314497
3588. Satou A, Tabata T, Miyoshi H, et al. Methotrexate-associated lymphoproliferative disorders of T-cell phenotype: clinicopathological analysis of 28 cases. Mod Pathol. 2019 Jul;32(8):1135–46. PMID:30952973
3589. Satou A, Tabata T, Suzuki Y, et al. Nodal EBV-positive polymorphic B cell lymphoproliferative disorder with plasma cell differentiation: clinicopathological analysis of five cases. Virchows Arch. 2021 May;478(5):969–76. PMID:33169195
3590. Satou A, Tsuzuki T, Nakamura S. Other iatrogenic immunodeficiency-associated lymphoproliferative disorders with a T- or NK-cell phenotype. J Clin Exp Hematop. 2019;59(2):56–63. PMID:31257346
3591. Sausville EA, Worsham GF, Matthews MJ, et al. Histologic assessment of lymph nodes in mycosis fungoides/Sézary syndrome (cutaneous T-cell lymphoma): clinical correlations and prognostic import of a new classification system. Hum Pathol. 1985 Nov;16(11):1098–109. PMID:3876976
3592. Savage KJ. Primary mediastinal large B-cell lymphoma. Blood. 2022 Sep 1;140(9):955–70. PMID:34496020
3593. Savage KJ, Harris NL, Vose JM, et al. ALK- anaplastic large-cell lymphoma is clinically and immunophenotypically different from both ALK+ ALCL and peripheral T-cell lymphoma, not otherwise specified: report from the International Peripheral T-Cell Lymphoma Project. Blood. 2008 Jun 15;111(12):5496–504. PMID:18385450
3594. Savage KJ, Monti S, Kutok JL, et al. The molecular signature of mediastinal large B-cell lymphoma differs from that of other diffuse large B-cell lymphomas and shares features with classical Hodgkin lymphoma. Blood. 2003 Dec 1;102(12):3871–9. PMID:12933571
3595. Savilo E, Campo E, Mollejo M, et al. Absence of cyclin D1 protein expression in splenic marginal zone lymphoma. Mod Pathol. 1998 Jul;11(7):601–6. PMID:9688179
3596. Savitsky K, Bar-Shira A, Gilad S, et al. A single ataxia telangiectasia gene with a product similar to PI-3 kinase. Science. 1995 Jun 23;268(5218):1749–53. PMID:7792600
3597. Savola P, Martelius T, Kankainen M, et al. Somatic mutations and T-cell clonality in patients with immunodeficiency. Haematologica. 2020 Dec 1;105(12):2757–68. PMID:33256375
3598. Sawada Y, Hino R, Hama K, et al. Type of skin eruption is an independent prognostic indicator for adult T-cell leukemia/lymphoma. Blood. 2011 Apr 14;117(15):3961–7. PMID:21325600
3599. Sawyer JR. The prognostic significance of cytogenetics and molecular profiling in multiple myeloma. Cancer Genet. 2011 Jan;204(1):3–12. PMID:21356186
3600. Sayed RH, Wechalekar AD, Gilbertson JA, et al. Natural history and outcome of light chain deposition disease. Blood. 2015 Dec 24;126(26):2805–10. PMID:26392598
3601. Saygin C, Uzunaslan D, Ozguroglu M, et al. Dendritic cell sarcoma: a pooled analysis including 462 cases with presentation of our case series. Crit Rev Oncol Hematol. 2013 Nov;88(2):253–71. PMID:23755890
3602. Sbihi Z, Dossier A, Boutboul D, et al. iNKT and memory B-cell alterations in HHV-8 multicentric Castleman disease. Blood. 2017 Feb 16;129(7):855–65. PMID:28060720
3603. Scarfò I, Pellegrino E, Mereu E, et al. Identification of a new subclass of ALK-negative ALCL expressing aberrant levels of ERBB4 transcripts. Blood. 2016 Jan 14;127(2):221–32. PMID:26463425
3604. Scarisbrick JJ, Prince HM, Vermeer MH, et al. Cutaneous Lymphoma International Consortium study of outcome in advanced stages of mycosis fungoides and Sézary syndrome: effect of specific prognostic markers on survival and development of a prognostic model. J Clin Oncol. 2015 Nov 10;33(32):3766–73. PMID:26438120
3605. Scarisbrick JJ, Woolford AJ, Calonje E, et al. Frequent abnormalities of the p15 and p16 genes in mycosis fungoides and Sezary syndrome. J Invest Dermatol. 2002 Mar;118(3):493–9. PMID:11874489
3606. Schade AE, Powers JJ, Wlodarski MW, et al. Phosphatidylinositol-3-phosphate kinase pathway activation protects leukemic large granular lymphocytes from undergoing homeostatic apoptosis. Blood. 2006 Jun 15;107(12):4834–40. PMID:16484592
3607. Schäfer D, Olsen M, Lähnemann D, et al. Five percent of healthy newborns have an ETV6-RUNX1 fusion as revealed by DNA-based GIPFEL screening. Blood. 2018 Feb 15;131(7):821–6. PMID:29311095
3608. Schebesta A, McManus S, Salvagiotto G, et al. Transcription factor Pax5 activates the chromatin of key genes involved in B cell signaling, adhesion, migration, and immune function. Immunity. 2007 Jul;27(1):49–63. PMID:17658281
3609. Scheffer E, Meijer CJ, van Vloten WA, et al. A histologic study of lymph nodes from patients with the Sézary syndrome. Cancer. 1986 Jun 15;57(12):2375–80. PMID:2938724
3610. Scheffer E, Meijer CJ, Van Vloten WA. Dermatopathic lymphadenopathy and lymph node involvement in mycosis fungoides. Cancer. 1980 Jan 1;45(1):137–48. PMID:7350998
3611. Scheubeck G, Jiang L, Hermine O, et al. Clinical outcome of mantle cell lymphoma patients with high-risk disease (high-risk MIPI-c or high p53 expression). Leukemia. 2023 Sep;37(9):1887–94. PMID:37495776
3612. Schinasi L, Leon ME. Non-Hodgkin lymphoma and occupational exposure to agricultural pesticide chemical groups and active ingredients: a systematic review and meta-analysis. Int J Environ Res Public Health. 2014 Apr 23;11(4):4449–527. PMID:24762670
3613. Schinnerl D, Mejstrikova E, Schumich A, et al. CD371 cell surface expression: a unique feature of DUX4-rearranged acute lymphoblastic leukemia. Haematologica. 2019 Aug;104(8):e352–5. PMID:30705095
3614. Schlegel U. Primary CNS lymphoma. Ther Adv Neurol Disord. 2009 Mar;2(2):93–104. PMID:21180644
3615. Schmatz AI, Streubel B, Kretschmer-Chott E, et al. Primary follicular lymphoma of the duodenum is a distinct mucosal/submucosal variant of follicular lymphoma: a retrospective study of 63 cases. J Clin Oncol. 2011 Apr 10;29(11):1445–51. PMID:21383289
3616. Schmelz M, Montes-Moreno S, Piris M, et al. Lack and/or aberrant localization of major histocompatibility class II (MHCII) protein in plasmablastic lymphoma. Haematologica. 2012 Oct;97(10):1614–6. PMID:22689685
3617. Schmid C, Pan L, Diss T, et al. Expression of B-cell antigens by Hodgkin's and Reed-Sternberg cells. Am J Pathol. 1991 Oct;139(4):701–7. PMID:1656757
3618. Schmid S, Tinguely M, Cione P, et al. Flow cytometry as an accurate tool to complement fine needle aspiration cytology in the diagnosis of low grade malignant lymphomas. Cytopathology. 2011 Dec;22(6):397–406. PMID:20735454
3619. Schmidt J, Gong S, Marafioti T, et al. Genome-wide analysis of pediatric-type follicular lymphoma reveals low genetic complexity and recurrent alterations of TNFRSF14 gene. Blood. 2016 Aug 25;128(8):1101–11. PMID:27257180
3620. Schmidt J, Ramis-Zaldivar JE, Bonzheim I, et al. CREBBP gene mutations are frequently detected in in situ follicular neoplasia. Blood. 2018 Dec 20;132(25):2687–90. PMID:30401710
3621. Schmidt J, Ramis-Zaldivar JE, Nadeu F, et al. Mutations of MAP2K1 are frequent in pediatric-type follicular lymphoma and result in ERK pathway activation. Blood. 2017 Jul 20;130(3):323–7. PMID:28533310
3622. Schmidt J, Salaverria I, Haake A, et al. Increasing genomic and epigenomic complexity in the clonal evolution from in situ to manifest t(14;18)-positive follicular lymphoma. Leukemia. 2014 May;28(5):1103–12. PMID:24153014
3623. Schmidt TM, Barwick BG, Joseph N, et al. Gain of chromosome 1q is associated with early progression in multiple myeloma patients treated with lenalidomide, bortezomib, and dexamethasone. Blood Cancer J. 2019 Nov 25;9(12):94. PMID:31767829
3624. Schmidt TM, Fonseca R, Usmani SZ. Chromosome 1q21 abnormalities in multiple myeloma. Blood Cancer J. 2021 Apr 29;11(4):83. PMID:33927196
3625. Schmitz C, Rekowski J, Reinke S, et al. Metabolic tumor volume, cancer cell fraction, and prognosis - the case of T-cell/histiocyte-rich large B-cell lymphoma. Leuk Lymphoma. 2020 Jun;61(6):1372–9. PMID:32022621
3626. Schmitz F, Tjon JM, Lai Y, et al. Identification of a potential physiological precursor of aberrant cells in refractory coeliac disease type II. Gut. 2013 Apr;62(4):509–19. PMID:22760007
3627. Schmitz N, Trümper L, Ziepert M, et al. Treatment and prognosis of mature T-cell and NK-cell lymphoma: an analysis of patients with T-cell lymphoma treated in studies of the German High-Grade Non-Hodgkin Lymphoma Study Group. Blood. 2010 Nov 4;116(18):3418–25. PMID:20660290
3628. Schmitz R, Hansmann ML, Bohle V, et al. TNFAIP3 (A20) is a tumor suppressor gene in Hodgkin lymphoma and primary mediastinal B cell lymphoma. J Exp Med. 2009 May 11;206(5):981–9. PMID:19380639
3629. Schmitz R, Wright GW, Huang DW, et al. Genetics and pathogenesis of diffuse large B-cell lymphoma. N Engl J Med. 2018 Apr 12;378(15):1396–407. PMID:29641966
3630. Schmitz R, Young RM, Ceribelli M, et al. Burkitt lymphoma pathogenesis and therapeutic targets from structural and functional genomics. Nature. 2012 Oct 4;490(7418):116–20. PMID:22885699

3631. Schnaidt U, Thiele J, Georgii A. Angioimmunoblastic lymphadenopathy. Fine structure of the lymph nodes by correction of light and electron microscopical findings. Virchows Arch A Pathol Anat Histol. 1980;389(3):381–95. PMID:7456329
3632. Schnaiter A, Paschka P, Rossi M, et al. NOTCH1, SF3B1, and TP53 mutations in fludarabine-refractory CLL patients treated with alemtuzumab: results from the CLL2H trial of the GCLLSG. Blood. 2013 Aug 15;122(7):1266–70. PMID:23821658
3633. Schnittger S, Bacher U, Haferlach T, et al. Development and validation of a real-time quantification assay to detect and monitor BRAFV600E mutations in hairy cell leukemia. Blood. 2012 Mar 29;119(13):3151–4. PMID:22331186
3634. Scholtysik R, Kreuz M, Klapper W, et al. Detection of genomic aberrations in molecularly defined Burkitt's lymphoma by array-based, high resolution, single nucleotide polymorphism analysis. Haematologica. 2010 Dec;95(12):2047–55. PMID:20823134
3635. Schommers P, Hentrich M, Hoffmann C, et al. Survival of AIDS-related diffuse large B-cell lymphoma, Burkitt lymphoma, and plasmablastic lymphoma in the German HIV Lymphoma Cohort. Br J Haematol. 2015 Mar;168(6):806–10. PMID:25403997
3636. Schoolmeester JK, Park KJ. Incidental nodal lymphangioleiomyomatosis is not a harbinger of pulmonary lymphangioleiomyomatosis: a study of 19 cases with evaluation of diagnostic immunohistochemistry. Am J Surg Pathol. 2015 Oct;39(10):1404–10. PMID:26135558
3637. Schrader A, Crispatzu G, Oberbeck S, et al. Actionable perturbations of damage responses by TCL1/ATM and epigenetic lesions form the basis of T-PLL. Nat Commun. 2018 Feb 15;9(1):697. PMID:29449575
3638. Schrader AM, Chung YY, Jansen PM, et al. No TP63 rearrangements in a selected group of primary cutaneous CD30+ lymphoproliferative disorders with aggressive clinical course. Blood. 2016 Jul 7;128(1):141–3. PMID:27146432
3639. Schrader AMR, de Groen RAL, Willemze R, et al. Cell-of-origin classification using the Hans and Lymph2Cx algorithms in primary cutaneous large B-cell lymphomas. Virchows Arch. 2022 Mar;480(3):667–75. PMID:35028710
3640. Schrader AMR, Jansen PM, Vermeer MH, et al. High incidence and clinical significance of MYC rearrangements in primary cutaneous diffuse large B-cell lymphoma, leg type. Am J Surg Pathol. 2018 Nov;42(11):1488–94. PMID:30113335
3641. Schrader AMR, Jansen PM, Willemze R, et al. High prevalence of MYD88 and CD79B mutations in intravascular large B-cell lymphoma. Blood. 2018 May 3;131(18):2086–9. PMID:29514783
3642. Schrader C, Meusers P, Brittinger G, et al. Growth pattern and distribution of follicular dendritic cells in mantle cell lymphoma: a clinicopathological study of 96 patients. Virchows Arch. 2006 Feb;448(2):151–9. PMID:16133361
3643. Schrappe M, Valsecchi MG, Bartram CR, et al. Late MRD response determines relapse risk overall and in subsets of childhood T-cell ALL: results of the AIEOP-BFM-ALL 2000 study. Blood. 2011 Aug 25;118(8):2077–84. PMID:21719599
3644. Schroers R, Baraniskin A, Heute C, et al. Diagnosis of leptomeningeal disease in diffuse large B-cell lymphomas of the central nervous system by flow cytometry and cytopathology. Eur J Haematol. 2010 Dec;85(6):520–8. PMID:20727005
3645. Schubert D, Bode C, Kenefeck R, et al. Autosomal dominant immune dysregulation syndrome in humans with CTLA4 mutations. Nat Med. 2014 Dec;20(12):1410–6. PMID:25329329
3646. Schuh A, Becq J, Humphray S, et al. Monitoring chronic lymphocytic leukemia progression by whole genome sequencing reveals heterogeneous clonal evolution patterns. Blood. 2012 Nov 15;120(20):4191–6. PMID:22915640
3647. Schuhmacher B, Bein J, Rausch T, et al. JUNB, DUSP2, SGK1, SOCS1 and CREBBP are frequently mutated in T-cell/histiocyte-rich large B-cell lymphoma. Haematologica. 2019 Feb;104(2):330–7. PMID:30213827
3648. Schultz KR, Pullen DJ, Sather HN, et al. Risk- and response-based classification of childhood B-precursor acute lymphoblastic leukemia: a combined analysis of prognostic markers from the Pediatric Oncology Group (POG) and Children's Cancer Group (CCG). Blood. 2007 Feb 1;109(3):926–35. PMID:17003380
3649. Schwarting R, Gerdes J, Dürkop H, et al. BER-H2: a new anti-Ki-1 (CD30) monoclonal antibody directed at a formol-resistant epitope. Blood. 1989 Oct;74(5):1678–89. PMID:2477085
3650. Schwarzmann F, von Baehr R, Jäger M, et al. A case of severe chronic active infection with Epstein-Barr virus: immunologic deficiencies associated with a lytic virus strain. Clin Infect Dis. 1999 Sep;29(3):626–31. PMID:10530459
3651. Schwering I, Bräuninger A, Klein U, et al. Loss of the B-lineage-specific gene expression program in Hodgkin and Reed-Sternberg cells of Hodgkin lymphoma. Blood. 2003 Feb 15;101(4):1505–12. PMID:12393731
3652. Schwindt H, Akasaka T, Zühlke-Jenisch R, et al. Chromosomal translocations fusing the BCL6 gene to different partner loci are recurrent in primary central nervous system lymphoma and may be associated with aberrant somatic hypermutation or defective class switch recombination. J Neuropathol Exp Neurol. 2006 Aug;65(8):776–82. PMID:16896311
3653. Schwindt H, Vater I, Kreuz M, et al. Chromosomal imbalances and partial uniparental disomies in primary central nervous system lymphoma. Leukemia. 2009 Oct;23(10):1875–84. PMID:19494841
3654. Schwock J, Geddie WR. Diagnosis of B-cell non-Hodgkin lymphomas with small-/intermediate-sized cells in cytopathology. Patholog Res Int. 2012;2012:164934. PMID:22693682
3655. Sciallis AP, Law ME, Inwards DJ, et al. Mucosal CD30-positive T-cell lymphoproliferations of the head and neck show a clinicopathologic spectrum similar to cutaneous CD30-positive T-cell lymphoproliferative disorders. Mod Pathol. 2012 Jul;25(7):983–92. PMID:22388754
3656. Scott DW, Chan FC, Hong F, et al. Gene expression-based model using formalin-fixed paraffin-embedded biopsies predicts overall survival in advanced-stage classical Hodgkin lymphoma. J Clin Oncol. 2013 Feb 20;31(6):692–700. PMID:23182984
3657. Scott DW, King RL, Staiger AM, et al. High-grade B-cell lymphoma with MYC and BCL2 and/or BCL6 rearrangements with diffuse large B-cell lymphoma morphology. Blood. 2018 May 3;131(18):2060–4. PMID:29475959
3658. Scott DW, Mottok A, Ennishi D, et al. Prognostic significance of diffuse large B-cell lymphoma cell of origin determined by digital gene expression in formalin-fixed paraffin-embedded tissue biopsies. J Clin Oncol. 2015 Sep 10;33(26):2848–56. PMID:26240231
3659. Scott GD, Kumar J, Oak JS, et al. Histology-independent signature distinguishes Kikuchi-Fujimoto disease/systemic lupus erythematosus-associated lymphadenitis from benign and malignant lymphadenopathies. Am J Clin Pathol. 2020 Jul 7;154(2):215–24. PMID:32367142
3660. Sculier D, Doco-Lecompte T, Rougemont M, et al. Haemophagocytic syndrome and elevated EBV load as initial manifestation of Hodgkin lymphoma in a HIV patient: case report and review of the literature. J Int AIDS Soc. 2014 Nov 2;17(4 Suppl 3):19650. PMID:25394154
3661. Sebire NJ, Haselden S, Malone M, et al. Isolated EBV lymphoproliferative disease in a child with Wiskott-Aldrich syndrome manifesting as cutaneous lymphomatoid granulomatosis and responsive to anti-CD20 immunotherapy. J Clin Pathol. 2003 Jul;56(7):555–7. PMID:12835306
3662. Seçkin D. Cutaneous lymphoproliferative disorders in organ transplant recipients: update 2014. G Ital Dermatol Venereol. 2014 Aug;149(4):401–8. PMID:25068227
3663. Seçkin D, Barete S, Euvrard S, et al. Primary cutaneous posttransplant lymphoproliferative disorders in solid organ transplant recipients: a multicenter European case series. Am J Transplant. 2013 Aug;13(8):2146–53. PMID:23718915
3664. Seegmiller AC, Kroft SH, Karandikar NJ, et al. Characterization of immunophenotypic aberrancies in 200 cases of B acute lymphoblastic leukemia. Am J Clin Pathol. 2009 Dec;132(6):940–9. PMID:19926587
3665. Seesaghur A, Petruski-Ivleva N, Banks VL, et al. Clinical features and diagnosis of multiple myeloma: a population-based cohort study in primary care. BMJ Open. 2021 Oct 6;11(10):e052759. PMID:34615682
3666. Sehn LH, Salles G. Diffuse large B-cell lymphoma. N Engl J Med. 2021 Mar 4;384(9):842–58. PMID:33657296
3667. Sehn LH, Scott DW, Chhanabhai M, et al. Impact of concordant and discordant bone marrow involvement on outcome in diffuse large B-cell lymphoma treated with R-CHOP. J Clin Oncol. 2011 Apr 10;29(11):1452–7. PMID:21383296
3668. Seibel NL. Treatment of acute lymphoblastic leukemia in children and adolescents: peaks and pitfalls. Hematology Am Soc Hematol Educ Program. 2008:374–80. PMID:19074113
3669. Seidel MG, Kindle G, Gathmann B, et al. The European Society for Immunodeficiencies (ESID) Registry working definitions for the clinical diagnosis of inborn errors of immunity. J Allergy Clin Immunol Pract. 2019 Jul-Aug;7(6):1763–70. PMID:30776527
3670. Sekhar J, Sanfilippo K, Zhang Q, et al. Waldenström macroglobulinemia: a Surveillance, Epidemiology, and End Results database review from 1988 to 2005. Leuk Lymphoma. 2012 Aug;53(8):1625–6. PMID:22239669
3671. Sekiguchi S, Yamamoto Y, Hatakeyama S, et al. Recurrent aseptic meningitis associated with Kikuchi's disease (histiocytic necrotizing lymphadenitis): a case report and literature review. Intern Med. 2021 Jun 1;60(11):1779–84. PMID:33431735
3672. Seliem RM, Ferry JA, Hasserjian RP, et al. Nodular lymphocyte-predominant Hodgkin lymphoma (NLPHL) with CD30-positive lymphocyte-predominant (LP) cells. J Hematop. 2011 Jul 23;4(3):175. PMID:32288859
3673. Selove W, Picarsic J, Swerdlow SH. Langerin staining identifies most littoral cell angiomas but not most other splenic angiomatous lesions. Hum Pathol. 2019 Jan;83:43–9. PMID:30130631
3674. Selvanathan SN, Suhumaran S, Sahu VK, et al. Kikuchi-Fujimoto disease in children. J Paediatr Child Health. 2020 Mar;56(3):389–93. PMID:31576642
3675. Selvarajan V, Osato M, Nah GSS, et al. RUNX3 is oncogenic in natural killer/T-cell lymphoma and is transcriptionally regulated by MYC. Leukemia. 2017 Oct;31(10):2219–27. PMID:28119527
3676. Selves J, Meggetto F, Brousset P, et al. Inflammatory pseudotumor of the liver. Evidence for follicular dendritic reticulum cell proliferation associated with clonal Epstein-Barr virus. Am J Surg Pathol. 1996 Jun;20(6):747–53. PMID:8651355
3677. Semenzato G, Calabretto G, Barilà G, et al. Not all LGL leukemias are created equal. Blood Rev. 2023 Jul;60:101058. PMID:36870881
3678. Semenzato G, Zambello R, Starkebaum G, et al. The lymphoproliferative disease of granular lymphocytes: updated criteria for diagnosis. Blood. 1997 Jan 1;89(1):256–60. PMID:8978299
3679. Senff NJ, Hoefnagel JJ, Jansen PM, et al. Reclassification of 300 primary cutaneous B-cell lymphomas according to the new WHO-EORTC classification for cutaneous lymphomas: comparison with previous classifications and identification of prognostic markers. J Clin Oncol. 2007 Apr 20;25(12):1581–7. PMID:17353548
3680. Senff NJ, Noordijk EM, Kim YH, et al. European Organization for Research and Treatment of Cancer and International Society for Cutaneous Lymphoma consensus recommendations for the management of cutaneous B-cell lymphomas. Blood. 2008 Sep 1;112(5):1600–9. PMID:18567836
3681. Senff NJ, Zoutman WH, Vermeer MH, et al. Fine-mapping chromosomal loss at 9p21: correlation with prognosis in primary cutaneous diffuse large B-cell lymphoma, leg type. J Invest Dermatol. 2009 May;129(5):1149–55. PMID:19020554
3682. Seong H, Jeong YH, Lee WJ, et al. Splenic uptake on FDG PET/CT correlates with Kikuchi-Fujimoto disease severity. Sci Rep. 2021 May 25;11(1):10836. PMID:34035381
3683. Servitje O, Muniesa C, Benavente Y, et al. Primary cutaneous marginal zone B-cell lymphoma: response to treatment and disease-free survival in a series of 137 patients. J Am Acad Dermatol. 2013 Sep;69(3):357–65. PMID:23796549
3684. Sevilla DW, Murty VV, Sun XL, et al. Cytogenetic abnormalities in reactive lymphoid hyperplasia: byproducts of the germinal centre reaction or indicators of lymphoma? Hematol Oncol. 2011 Jun;29(2):81–90. PMID:20687199
3685. Seymour EK, Ruterbusch JJ, Beebe-Dimmer JL, et al. Real-world testing and treatment patterns in chronic lymphocytic leukemia: a SEER patterns of care analysis. Cancer. 2019 Jan 1;125(1):135–43. PMID:30343488
3686. Sha C, Barrans S, Cucco F, et al. Molecular high-grade B-cell lymphoma: defining a poor-risk group that requires different approaches to therapy. J Clin Oncol. 2019 Jan 20;37(3):202–12. PMID:30523719
3687. Shago M, Abla O, Hitzler J, et al. Frequency and outcome of pediatric acute lymphoblastic leukemia with ZNF384 gene rearrangements including a novel translocation resulting in an ARID1B/ZNF384 gene fusion. Pediatr Blood Cancer. 2016 Nov;63(11):1915–21. PMID:27392123
3688. Shah A, Safaya A. Granulomatous slack skin disease: a review, in comparison with mycosis fungoides. J Eur Acad Dermatol Venereol. 2012 Dec;26(12):1472–8. PMID:22435618
3689. Shah MV, Hook CC, Call TG, et al. A population-based study of large granular lymphocyte leukemia. Blood Cancer J. 2016 Aug

5;6(8):e455. PMID:27494824
3690. Shah S, Schrader KA, Waanders E, et al. A recurrent germline PAX5 mutation confers susceptibility to pre-B cell acute lymphoblastic leukemia. Nat Genet. 2013 Oct;45(10):1226–31. PMID:24013638
3691. Shah UA, Chung EY, Giricz O, et al. North American ATLL has a distinct mutational and transcriptional profile and responds to epigenetic therapies. Blood. 2018 Oct 4;132(14):1507–18. PMID:30104217
3692. Shahrabani-Gargir L, Shomrat R, Yaron Y, et al. High frequency of a common Bloom syndrome Ashkenazi mutation among Jews of Polish origin. Genet Test. 1998;2(4):293–6. PMID:10464606
3693. Shanafelt TD, Kay NE, Parikh SA, et al. Risk of serious infection among individuals with and without low count monoclonal B-cell lymphocytosis (MBL). Leukemia. 2021 Jan;35(1):239–44. PMID:32203143
3694. Shanafelt TD, Kay NE, Rabe KG, et al. Brief report: natural history of individuals with clinically recognized monoclonal B-cell lymphocytosis compared with patients with Rai 0 chronic lymphocytic leukemia. J Clin Oncol. 2009 Aug 20;27(24):3959–63. PMID:19620484
3695. Shankar AG, Kirkwood AA, Hall GW, et al. Childhood and adolescent nodular lymphocyte predominant Hodgkin lymphoma - a review of clinical outcome based on the histological variants. Br J Haematol. 2015 Oct;171(2):254–62. PMID:26115355
3696. Shao H, Xi L, Raffeld M, et al. Clonally related histiocytic/dendritic cell sarcoma and chronic lymphocytic leukemia/small lymphocytic lymphoma: a study of seven cases. Mod Pathol. 2011 Nov;24(11):1421–32. PMID:21666687
3697. Shao H, Xi L, Raffeld M, et al. Nodal and extranodal plasmacytomas expressing immunoglobulin a: an indolent lymphoproliferative disorder with a low risk of clinical progression. Am J Surg Pathol. 2010 Oct;34(10):1425–35. PMID:20871216
3698. Shapira Y, Weinberger A, Wysenbeek AJ. Lymphadenopathy in systemic lupus erythematosus. Prevalence and relation to disease manifestations. Clin Rheumatol. 1996 Jul;15(4):335–8. PMID:8853165
3699. Shapiro NL, Strocker AM, Bhattacharyya N. Risk factors for adenotonsillar hypertrophy in children following solid organ transplantation. Int J Pediatr Otorhinolaryngol. 2003 Feb;67(2):151–5. PMID:12623151
3700. Shapiro-Shelef M, Lin KI, McHeyzer-Williams LJ, et al. Blimp-1 is required for the formation of immunoglobulin secreting plasma cells and pre-plasma memory B cells. Immunity. 2003 Oct;19(4):607–20. PMID:14563324
3701. Sharaiha RZ, Lebwohl B, Reimers L, et al. Increasing incidence of enteropathy-associated T-cell lymphoma in the United States, 1973-2008. Cancer. 2012 Aug 1;118(15):3786–92. PMID:22169928
3702. Sharapova SO, Pashchenko OE, Bondarenko AV, et al. Geographical distribution, incidence, malignancies, and outcome of 136 Eastern Slavic patients with Nijmegen breakage syndrome and NBN founder variant c.657_661del5. Front Immunol. 2021 Jan 8;11:602482. PMID:33488600
3703. Sharma A, Oishi N, Boddicker RL, et al. Recurrent STAT3-JAK2 fusions in indolent T-cell lymphoproliferative disorder of the gastrointestinal tract. Blood. 2018 May 17;131(20):2262–6. PMID:29592893
3704. Sharma N, Smadbeck JB, Abdallah N, et al. The prognostic role of MYC structural variants identified by NGS and FISH in multiple myeloma. Clin Cancer Res. 2021 Oct 1;27(19):5430–9. PMID:34233962
3705. Sharpe RW, Bethel KJ. Hairy cell leukemia: diagnostic pathology. Hematol Oncol Clin North Am. 2006 Oct;20(5):1023–49. PMID:16990105
3706. Shastri A, Janakiram M, Mantzaris I, et al. Sites of extranodal involvement are prognostic in patients with stage 1 follicular lymphoma. Oncotarget. 2017 Jul 14;8(45):78410–8. PMID:29108238
3707. Shauly O, Gould DJ, Siddiqi I, et al. The first reported case of gluteal implant-associated anaplastic large cell lymphoma (ALCL). Aesthet Surg J. 2019 Jun 21;39(7):NP253–8. PMID:30768141
3708. Shen J, Medeiros LJ, Li S, et al. CD8 expression in anaplastic large cell lymphoma correlates with noncommon morphologic variants and T-cell antigen expression suggesting biological differences with CD8-negative anaplastic large cell lymphoma. Hum Pathol. 2020 Apr;98:1–9. PMID:32032618
3709. Shen X, Liu S, Wu C, et al. Survival trends and prognostic factors in patients with solitary plasmacytoma of bone: a population-based study. Cancer Med. 2021 Jan;10(2):462–70. PMID:33145987
3710. Shenkier TN, Blay JY, O'Neill BP, et al. Primary CNS lymphoma of T-cell origin: a descriptive analysis from the international primary CNS lymphoma collaborative group. J Clin Oncol. 2005 Apr 1;23(10):2233–9. PMID:15800313
3711. Shenoy P, Maggioncalda A, Malik N, et al. Incidence patterns and outcomes for Hodgkin lymphoma patients in the United States. Adv Hematol. 2011;2011:725219. PMID:21197477
3712. Sherman MJ, Hanson CA, Hoyer JD. An assessment of the usefulness of immunohistochemical stains in the diagnosis of hairy cell leukemia. Am J Clin Pathol. 2011 Sep;136(3):390–9. PMID:21846914
3713. Sherouse GW, Novins K, Chaney EL. Computation of digitally reconstructed radiographs for use in radiotherapy treatment design. Int J Radiat Oncol Biol Phys. 1990 Mar;18(3):651–8. PMID:2318699
3714. Shi M, He R, Feldman AL, et al. STAT3 mutation and its clinical and histopathologic correlation in T-cell large granular lymphocytic leukemia. Hum Pathol. 2018 Mar;73:74–81. PMID:29288042
3715. Shi M, Olteanu H, Jevremovic D, et al. T-cell clones of uncertain significance are highly prevalent and show close resemblance to T-cell large granular lymphocytic leukemia. Implications for laboratory diagnostics. Mod Pathol. 2020 Oct;33(10):2046–57. PMID:32404954
3716. Shi M, Roemer MG, Chapuy B, et al. Expression of programmed cell death 1 ligand 2 (PD-L2) is a distinguishing feature of primary mediastinal (thymic) large B-cell lymphoma and associated with PDCD1LG2 copy gain. Am J Surg Pathol. 2014 Dec;38(12):1715–23. PMID:25025450
3717. Shi X, Hu S, Luo X, et al. CT characteristics in 24 patients with POEMS syndrome. Acta Radiol. 2016 Jan;57(1):51–7. PMID:25571895
3718. Shibuya K, Misawa S, Horikoshi T, et al. Detection of bone lesions by CT in POEMS syndrome. Intern Med. 2011;50(13):1393–6. PMID:21720058
3719. Shiels MS, Pfeiffer RM, Besson C, et al. Trends in primary central nervous system lymphoma incidence and survival in the U.S. Br J Haematol. 2016 Aug;174(3):417–24. PMID:27018254
3720. Shih YH, Yang Y, Chang KH, et al. Clinical features and outcome of lymphoma patients with pre-existing autoimmune diseases. Int J Rheum Dis. 2018 Jan;21(1):93–101. PMID:29205866
3721. Shimada K, Kinoshita T, Naoe T, et al. Presentation and management of intravascular large B-cell lymphoma. Lancet Oncol. 2009 Sep;10(9):895–902. PMID:19717091
3722. Shimada K, Kiyoi H. Current progress and future perspectives of research on intravascular large B-cell lymphoma. Cancer Sci. 2021 Oct;112(10):3953–61. PMID:34327781
3723. Shimada K, Matsue K, Yamamoto K, et al. Retrospective analysis of intravascular large B-cell lymphoma treated with rituximab-containing chemotherapy as reported by the IVL study group in Japan. J Clin Oncol. 2008 Jul 1;26(19):3189–95. PMID:18506023
3724. Shimada K, Murase T, Matsue K, et al. Central nervous system involvement in intravascular large B-cell lymphoma: a retrospective analysis of 109 patients. Cancer Sci. 2010 Jun;101(6):1480–6. PMID:20412122
3725. Shimada K, Shimada S, Sugimoto K, et al. Development and analysis of patient-derived xenograft mouse models in intravascular large B-cell lymphoma. Leukemia. 2016 Jul;30(7):1568–79. PMID:27001523
3726. Shimada K, Yamaguchi M, Atsuta Y, et al. Rituximab, cyclophosphamide, doxorubicin, vincristine, and prednisolone combined with high-dose methotrexate plus intrathecal chemotherapy for newly diagnosed intravascular large B-cell lymphoma (PRIMEUR-IVL): a multicentre, single-arm, phase 2 trial. Lancet Oncol. 2020 Apr;21(4):593–602. PMID:32171071
3727. Shimada K, Yoshida K, Suzuki Y, et al. Frequent genetic alterations in immune checkpoint-related genes in intravascular large B-cell lymphoma. Blood. 2021 Mar 18;137(11):1491–502. PMID:33512416
3728. Shimoyama M. Diagnostic criteria and classification of clinical subtypes of adult T-cell leukaemia-lymphoma. A report from the Lymphoma Study Group (1984-87). Br J Haematol. 1991 Nov;79(3):428–37. PMID:1751370
3729. Shiokawa M, Kodama Y, Sekiguchi K, et al. Laminin 511 is a target antigen in autoimmune pancreatitis. Sci Transl Med. 2018 Aug 8;10(453):eaaq0997. PMID:30089633
3730. Shiota H, Barral S, Buchou T, et al. Nut directs p300-dependent, genome-wide H4 hyperacetylation in male germ cells. Cell Rep. 2018 Sep 25;24(13):3477–3487.e6. PMID:30257209
3731. Shiota M, Nakamura S, Ichinohasama R, et al. Anaplastic large cell lymphomas expressing the novel chimeric protein p80NPM/ALK: a distinct clinicopathologic entity. Blood. 1995 Sep 1;86(5):1954–60. PMID:7655022
3732. Shivarov V, Ivanova M. Nodular lymphocyte predominant Hodgkin lymphoma in USA between 2000 and 2014: an updated analysis based on the SEER data. Br J Haematol. 2018 Sep;182(5):727–30. PMID:28737250
3733. Shlush LI. Age-related clonal hematopoiesis. Blood. 2018 Feb 1;131(5):496–504. PMID:29141946
3734. Short NJ, Jabbour E, Sasaki K, et al. Impact of complete molecular response on survival in patients with Philadelphia chromosome-positive acute lymphoblastic leukemia. Blood. 2016 Jul 28;128(4):504–7. PMID:27235138
3735. Shurtleff SA, Buijs A, Behm FG, et al. TEL/AML1 fusion resulting from a cryptic t(12;21) is the most common genetic lesion in pediatric ALL and defines a subgroup of patients with an excellent prognosis. Leukemia. 1995 Dec;9(12):1985–9. PMID:8609706
3736. Shustov A, Cabrera ME, Civallero M, et al. ALK-negative anaplastic large cell lymphoma: features and outcomes of 235 patients from the International T-Cell Project. Blood Adv. 2021 Feb 9;5(3):640–8. PMID:33560375
3737. Sibaud V, Beylot-Barry M, Thiébaut R, et al. Bone marrow histopathologic and molecular staging in epidermotropic T-cell lymphomas. Am J Clin Pathol. 2003 Mar;119(3):414–23. PMID:12645344
3738. Sibon D, Fournier M, Brière J, et al. Long-term outcome of adults with systemic anaplastic large-cell lymphoma treated within the Groupe d'Etude des Lymphomes de l'Adulte trials. J Clin Oncol. 2012 Nov 10;30(32):3939–46. PMID:23045585
3739. Sibon D, Nguyen DP, Schmitz N, et al. ALK-positive anaplastic large-cell lymphoma in adults: an individual patient data pooled analysis of 263 patients. Haematologica. 2019 Dec;104(12):e562–5. PMID:31004022
3739A. Sidana S, Larson DP, Greipp PT, et al. IgM AL amyloidosis: delineating disease biology and outcomes with clinical, genomic and bone marrow morphological features. Leukemia. 2020 May;34(5):1373–82. PMID:31780812
3740. Siddiqi IN, Friedman J, Barry-Holson KQ, et al. Characterization of a variant of t(14;18) negative nodal diffuse follicular lymphoma with CD23 expression, 1p36/TNFRSF14 abnormalities, and STAT6 mutations. Mod Pathol. 2016 Jun;29(6):570–81. PMID:26965583
3741. Side L, Taylor B, Cayouette M, et al. Homozygous inactivation of the NF1 gene in bone marrow cells from children with neurofibromatosis type 1 and malignant myeloid disorders. N Engl J Med. 1997 Jun 12;336(24):1713–20. PMID:9180088
3742. Siegel RL, Miller KD, Fuchs HE, et al. Cancer statistics, 2021. CA Cancer J Clin. 2021 Jan;71(1):7–33. PMID:33433946
3743. Sieniawski M, Angamuthu N, Boyd K, et al. Evaluation of enteropathy-associated T-cell lymphoma comparing standard therapies with a novel regimen including autologous stem cell transplantation. Blood. 2010 May 6;115(18):3664–70. PMID:20197551
3744. Sigurdardottir EE, Turesson I, Lund SH, et al. The role of diagnosis and clinical follow-up of monoclonal gammopathy of undetermined significance on survival in multiple myeloma. JAMA Oncol. 2015 May;1(2):168–74. PMID:26181017
3745. Sigvardsson M. Molecular regulation of differentiation in early B-lymphocyte development. Int J Mol Sci. 2018 Jun 30;19(7):1928. PMID:29966360
3746. Silkenstedt E, Dreyling M. Mantle cell lymphoma-advances in molecular biology, prognostication and treatment approaches. Hematol Oncol. 2021 Jun;39 Suppl 1:31–8. PMID:34105823
3747. Silva EG, Phillips MJ, Langer B, et al. Spindle and histiocytoid (epithelioid) hemangioendothelioma. Primary in lymph node. Am J Clin Pathol. 1986 Jun;85(6):731–5. PMID:3706210
3748. Silverman LB, Sallan SE. Newly diagnosed childhood acute lymphoblastic leukemia: update on prognostic factors and treatment. Curr Opin Hematol. 2003 Jul;10(4):290–6. PMID:12799535
3749. Silverman ML, LiVolsi VA. Splenic hamartoma. Am J Clin Pathol. 1978 Aug;70(2):224–9. PMID:696681
3750. Sim J, Ahn HI, Han H, et al. Splenic hamartoma: a case report and review of the literature. World J Clin Cases. 2013 Oct 16;1(7):217–9. PMID:24340270
3751. Sima A, Hollander P, Baecklund E, et al. Superior outcome for splenectomised patients in a population-based study of splenic marginal zone lymphoma in Sweden. Br J Haematol. 2021 Aug;194(3):568–79. PMID:34109612
3752. Simeone FJ, Harvey JP, Yee AJ, et al. Value of low-dose whole-body CT in the management of patients with multiple myeloma and precursor states. Skeletal Radiol. 2019 May;48(5):773–9. PMID:30218303
3753. Simon TA, Thompson A, Gandhi KK, et

al. Incidence of malignancy in adult patients with rheumatoid arthritis: a meta-analysis. Arthritis Res Ther. 2015 Aug 15;17(1):212. PMID:26271620

3754. Singer S, Efebera Y, Bumma N, et al. Heavy lifting: nomenclature and novel therapy for gamma heavy chain disease and other heavy chain disorders. Clin Lymphoma Myeloma Leuk. 2020 Aug;20(8):493–8. PMID:32245744

3755. Singh A, Joshi V, Jindal AK, et al. An updated review on activated PI3 kinase delta syndrome (APDS). Genes Dis. 2019 Oct 14;7(1):67–74. PMID:32181277

3756. Singh N, Chowdhury N, Pal S, et al. Hyaline vascular type of Castleman disease: diagnostic pitfalls on cytology and its clinical relevance. Cureus. 2021 Aug 14;13(8):e17174. PMID:34532195

3757. Skacel M, Ross CW, Hsi ED. A reassessment of primary thyroid lymphoma: high-grade MALT-type lymphoma as a distinct subtype of diffuse large B-cell lymphoma. Histopathology. 2000 Jul;37(1):10–8. PMID:10931213

3758. Slack GW, Ferry JA, Hasserjian RP, et al. Lymphocyte depleted Hodgkin lymphoma: an evaluation with immunophenotyping and genetic analysis. Leuk Lymphoma. 2009 Jun;50(6):937–43. PMID:19455461

3759. Slack GW, Steidl C, Sehn LH, et al. CD30 expression in de novo diffuse large B-cell lymphoma: a population-based study from British Columbia. Br J Haematol. 2014 Dec;167(5):608–17. PMID:25135752

3760. Slager SL, Lanasa MC, Marti GE, et al. Natural history of monoclonal B-cell lymphocytosis among relatives in CLL families. Blood. 2021 Apr 15;137(15):2046–56. PMID:33512457

3761. Slany RK. MLL fusion proteins and transcriptional control. Biochim Biophys Acta Gene Regul Mech. 2020 Mar;1863(3):194503. PMID:32061883

3762. Slayton WB, Schultz KR, Kairalla JA, et al. Dasatinib plus intensive chemotherapy in children, adolescents, and young adults with Philadelphia chromosome-positive acute lymphoblastic leukemia: results of Children's Oncology Group trial AALL0622. J Clin Oncol. 2018 Aug 1;36(22):2306–14. PMID:29812996

3763. Sloan C, Xiong QB, Crivaro A, et al. Multifocal mantle cell lymphoma in situ in the setting of a composite lymphoma. Am J Clin Pathol. 2015 Feb;143(2):274–82. PMID:25596254

3764. Slovak ML, Weiss LM, Nathwani BN, et al. Cytogenetic studies of composite lymphomas: monocytoid B-cell lymphoma and other B-cell non-Hodgkin's lymphomas. Hum Pathol. 1993 Oct;24(10):1086–94. PMID:7691710

3765. Slupianek A, Nieborowska-Skorska M, Hoser G, et al. Role of phosphatidylinositol 3-kinase-Akt pathway in nucleophosmin/anaplastic lymphoma kinase-mediated lymphomagenesis. Cancer Res. 2001 Mar 1;61(5):2194–9. PMID:11280786

3765A. Smith BK, Gray SS. Large B-cell lymphoma occurring in a breast implant capsule. Plast Reconstr Surg. 2014 Oct;134(4):670e–1e. PMID:25357072

3766. Smith MC, Cohen DN, Greig B, et al. The ambiguous boundary between EBV-related hemophagocytic lymphohistiocytosis and systemic EBV-driven T cell lymphoproliferative disorder. Int J Clin Exp Pathol. 2014 Aug 15;7(9):5738–49. PMID:25337215

3767. Smith T, Cunningham-Rundles C. Lymphoid malignancy in common variable immunodeficiency in a single-center cohort. Eur J Haematol. 2021 Nov;107(5):503–16. PMID:34255892

3768. Sneller MC, Wang J, Dale JK, et al. Clincal, immunologic, and genetic features of an autoimmune lymphoproliferative syndrome associated with abnormal lymphocyte apoptosis. Blood. 1997 Feb 15;89(4):1341–8. PMID:9028957

3769. Snuderl M, Kolman OK, Chen YB, et al. B-cell lymphomas with concurrent IGH-BCL2 and MYC rearrangements are aggressive neoplasms with clinical and pathologic features distinct from Burkitt lymphoma and diffuse large B-cell lymphoma. Am J Surg Pathol. 2010 Mar;34(3):327–40. PMID:20118770

3770. Soderquist CR, Bhagat G. Cellular and molecular bases of refractory celiac disease. Int Rev Cell Mol Biol. 2021;358:207–40. PMID:33707055

3771. Soderquist CR, Bhagat G. Gastrointestinal T- and NK-cell lymphomas and indolent lymphoproliferative disorders. Semin Diagn Pathol. 2020 Jan;37(1):11–23. PMID:31522873

3772. Soderquist CR, Lewis SK, Gru AA, et al. Immunophenotypic spectrum and genomic landscape of refractory celiac disease type II. Am J Surg Pathol. 2021 Jul 1;45(7):905–16. PMID:33544565

3773. Soderquist CR, Patel N, Murty VV, et al. Genetic and phenotypic characterization of indolent T-cell lymphoproliferative disorders of the gastrointestinal tract. Haematologica. 2020 Jul;105(7):1895–906. PMID:31558678

3774. Sohani AR, Jaffe ES, Harris NL, et al. Nodular lymphocyte-predominant Hodgkin lymphoma with atypical T cells: a morphologic variant mimicking peripheral T-cell lymphoma. Am J Surg Pathol. 2011 Nov;35(11):1666–78. PMID:21997687

3775. Soilleux EJ, Wotherspoon A, Eyre TA, et al. Diagnostic dilemmas of high-grade transformation (Richter's syndrome) of chronic lymphocytic leukaemia: results of the phase II National Cancer Research Institute CHOP-OR clinical trial specialist haemato-pathology central review. Histopathology. 2016 Dec;69(6):1066–76. PMID:27345622

3776. Sokol L, Agrawal D, Loughran TP Jr. Characterization of HTLV envelope seroreactivity in large granular lymphocyte leukemia. Leuk Res. 2005 Apr;29(4):381–7. PMID:15725471

3777. Solal-Céligny P, Roy P, Colombat P, et al. Follicular lymphoma international prognostic index. Blood. 2004 Sep 1;104(5):1258–65. PMID:15126323

3778. Soma LA, Craig FE, Swerdlow SH. The proliferation center microenvironment and prognostic markers in chronic lymphocytic leukemia/small lymphocytic lymphoma. Hum Pathol. 2006 Feb;37(2):152–9. PMID:16426914

3779. Somekh I, Thian M, Medgyesi D, et al. CD137 deficiency causes immune dysregulation with predisposition to lymphomagenesis. Blood. 2019 Oct 31;134(18):1510–6. PMID:31501153

3780. Somja J, Bisig B, Bonnet C, et al. Peripheral T-cell lymphoma with t(6;14)(p25;q11.2) translocation presenting with massive splenomegaly. Virchows Arch. 2014 Jun;464(6):735–41. PMID:24604141

3781. Sommer VH, Clemmensen OJ, Nielsen O, et al. In vivo activation of STAT3 in cutaneous T-cell lymphoma. Evidence for an antiapoptotic function of STAT3. Leukemia. 2004 Jul;18(7):1288–95. PMID:15141228

3782. Song JY, Lee J, Park DW, et al. Clinical outcome and predictive factors of recurrence among patients with Kikuchi's disease. Int J Infect Dis. 2009 May;13(3):322–6. PMID:19208493

3783. Song JY, Pittaluga S, Dunleavy K, et al. Lymphomatoid granulomatosis–a single institute experience: pathologic findings and clinical correlations. Am J Surg Pathol. 2015 Feb;39(2):141–56. PMID:25321327

3784. Song JY, Song L, Herrera AF, et al. Cyclin D1 expression in peripheral T-cell lymphomas. Mod Pathol. 2016 Nov;29(11):1306–12. PMID:27469326

3785. Song MK, Chung JS, Joo YD, et al. Clinical importance of Bcl-6-positive non-deep-site involvement in non-HIV-related primary central nervous system diffuse large B-cell lymphoma. J Neurooncol. 2011 Sep;104(3):825–31. PMID:21380743

3786. Song S, Matthias PD. The transcriptional regulation of germinal center formation. Front Immunol. 2018 Sep 5;9:2026. PMID:30233601

3787. Song SY, Kim WS, Ko YH, et al. Aggressive natural killer cell leukemia: clinical features and treatment outcome. Haematologica. 2002 Dec;87(12):1343–5. PMID:12495907

3788. Song TL, Nairismägi ML, Laurensia Y, et al. Oncogenic activation of the STAT3 pathway drives PD-L1 expression in natural killer/T-cell lymphoma. Blood. 2018 Sep 13;132(11):1146–58. PMID:30054295

3789. Sonigo G, Battistella M, Beylot-Barry M, et al. HAVCR2 mutations are associated with severe hemophagocytic syndrome in subcutaneous panniculitis-like T-cell lymphoma. Blood. 2020 Mar 26;135(13):1058–61. PMID:32005988

3789A. Sonke GS, Ludwig I, van Oosten H, et al. Poor outcomes of chronic active Epstein-Barr virus infection and hemophagocytic lymphohistiocytosis in non-Japanese adult patients. Clin Infect Dis. 2008 Jul 1;47(1):105–8. PMID:18491961

3790. Sonneveld P, Avet-Loiseau H, Lonial S, et al. Treatment of multiple myeloma with high-risk cytogenetics: a consensus of the International Myeloma Working Group. Blood. 2016 Jun 16;127(24):2955–62. PMID:27002115

3791. Sonneveld P, Goldschmidt H, Rosiñol L, et al. Bortezomib-based versus nonbortezomib-based induction treatment before autologous stem-cell transplantation in patients with previously untreated multiple myeloma: a meta-analysis of phase III randomized, controlled trials. J Clin Oncol. 2013 Sep 10;31(26):3279–87. PMID:23897961

3792. Sonneveld P, Schmidt-Wolf IG, van der Holt B, et al. Bortezomib induction and maintenance treatment in patients with newly diagnosed multiple myeloma: results of the randomized phase III HOVON-65/ GMMG-HD4 trial. J Clin Oncol. 2012 Aug 20;30(24):2946–55. PMID:22802322

3793. Sood N. Diagnostic clues for FNA diagnosis of intranodal palisaded myofibroblastoma, a rare benign lesion, an introspective case report. Diagn Cytopathol. 2016 Apr;44(4):317–23. PMID:26799943

3794. Sopeña B, Rivera A, Vázquez-Triñanes C, et al. Autoimmune manifestations of Kikuchi disease. Semin Arthritis Rheum. 2012 Jun;41(6):900–6. PMID:22192931

3795. Sordillo PP, Epremian B, Koziner B, et al. Lymphomatoid granulomatosis: an analysis of clinical and immunologic characteristics. Cancer. 1982 May 15;49(10):2070–6. PMID:6978760

3796. Sorge C, Costa LJ, Taub JW, et al. Incidence and outcomes of rare paediatric non-Hodgkin lymphomas. Br J Haematol. 2019 Mar;184(5):864–7. PMID:29611181

3797. Soriano AO, Thompson MA, Admirand JH, et al. Follicular dendritic cell sarcoma: a report of 14 cases and a review of the literature. Am J Hematol. 2007 Aug;82(8):725–8. PMID:17373675

3798. Sorigué M, García O, Tapia G, et al. HIV-infection has no prognostic impact on advanced-stage Hodgkin lymphoma. AIDS. 2017 Jun 19;31(10):1445–9. PMID:28574963

3799. Sorolla A, Wang E, Golden E, et al. Precision medicine by designer interference peptides: applications in oncology and molecular therapeutics. Oncogene. 2020 Feb;39(6):1167–84. PMID:31636382

3800. Souabni A, Cobaleda C, Schebesta M, et al. Pax5 promotes B lymphopoiesis and blocks T cell development by repressing Notch1. Immunity. 2002 Dec;17(6):781–93. PMID:12479824

3801. Soulier J, Grollet L, Oksenhendler E, et al. Kaposi's sarcoma-associated herpesvirus-like DNA sequences in multicentric Castleman's disease. Blood. 1995 Aug 15;86(4):1276–80. PMID:7632932

3802. Soussain C, Patte C, Ostronoff M, et al. Small noncleaved cell lymphoma and leukemia in adults. A retrospective study of 65 adults treated with the LMB pediatric protocols. Blood. 1995 Feb 1;85(3):664–74. PMID:7833470

3803. Soverini S, Albano F, Bassan R, et al. Next-generation sequencing for BCR-ABL1 kinase domain mutations in adult patients with Philadelphia chromosome-positive acute lymphoblastic leukemia: a position paper. Cancer Med. 2020 May;9(9):2960–70. PMID:32154668

3804. Sozzi E, Amato T, Sahota SS, et al. Lack of allelic exclusion by secondary rearrangements of tumour B-cell receptor light chains in hairy cell leukaemia. Hematol Oncol. 2011 Mar;29(1):31–7. PMID:20658474

3805. Spencer J, Cerf-Bensussan N, Jarry A, et al. Enteropathy-associated T cell lymphoma (malignant histiocytosis of the intestine) is recognized by a monoclonal antibody (HML-1) that defines a membrane molecule on human mucosal lymphocytes. Am J Pathol. 1988 Jul;132(1):1–5. PMID:3260750

3806. Spies J, Foucar K, Thompson CT, et al. The histopathology of cutaneous lesions of Kikuchi's disease (necrotizing lymphadenitis): a report of five cases. Am J Surg Pathol. 1999 Sep;23(9):1040–7. PMID:10478663

3807. Spina M, Vaccher E, Nasti G, et al. Human immunodeficiency virus-associated Hodgkin's disease. Semin Oncol. 2000 Aug;27(4):480–8. PMID:10950375

3808. Spina V, Khiabanian H, Messina M, et al. The genetics of nodal marginal zone lymphoma. Blood. 2016 Sep 8;128(10):1362–73. PMID:27335277

3809. Spina V, Rossi D. Molecular pathogenesis of splenic and nodal marginal zone lymphoma. Best Pract Res Clin Haematol. 2017 Mar-Jun;30(1-2):5–12. PMID:28288716

3810. Srinivas SK, Sample JT, Sixbey JW. Spontaneous loss of viral episomes accompanying Epstein-Barr virus reactivation in a Burkitt's lymphoma cell line. J Infect Dis. 1998 Jun;177(6):1705–9. PMID:9607853

3811. Sriskandarajah P, Dearden CE. Epidemiology and environmental aspects of marginal zone lymphomas. Best Pract Res Clin Haematol. 2017 Mar-Jun;30(1-2):84–91. PMID:28288721

3812. Staber PB, Herling M, Bellido M, et al. Consensus criteria for diagnosis, staging, and treatment response assessment of T-cell prolymphocytic leukemia. Blood. 2019 Oct 3;134(14):1132–43. PMID:31292114

3813. Staber PB, Kersten MJ. EHA endorsement of ESMO clinical practice guidelines for diagnosis, treatment, and follow-up for Waldenström's macroglobulinemia. Hemasphere. 2021 Sep 10;5(10):e634. PMID:34522842

3814. Stachurski D, Miron PM, Al-Homsi S, et al. Anaplastic lymphoma kinase-positive diffuse large B-cell lymphoma with a complex karyotype and cryptic 3' ALK gene insertion to chromosome 4 q22-24. Hum Pathol. 2007 Jun;38(6):940–5. PMID:17509395

3815. Staiger AM, Ziepert M, Horn H, et al. Clinical impact of the cell-of-origin classification and the MYC/ BCL2 dual expresser status in diffuse large B-cell lymphoma treated within prospective clinical trials of the German High-Grade Non-Hodgkin's Lymphoma Study Group. J Clin Oncol. 2017 Aug 1;35(22):2515–26. PMID:28525305

3816. Stamatopoulos K, Agathangelidis A, Rosenquist R, et al. Antigen receptor stereotypy in chronic lymphocytic leukemia. Leukemia. 2017 Feb;31(2):282–91. PMID:27811850

3817. Stanley CC, Westmoreland KD, Heimlich BJ, et al. Outcomes for paediatric Burkitt lymphoma treated with anthracycline-based therapy in Malawi. Br J Haematol. 2016 Jun;173(5):705–12. PMID:26914979

3818. Starasoler L, Vuitch F, Albores-Saavedra J. Intranodal leiomyoma. Another distinctive primary spindle cell neoplasm of lymph node. Am J Clin Pathol. 1991 Jun;95(6):858–62. PMID:2042595

3819. Starr AG, Caimi PF, Fu P, et al. Dual institution experience of nodal marginal zone lymphoma reveals excellent long-term outcomes in the rituximab era. Br J Haematol. 2016 Oct;175(2):275–80. PMID:27443247

3820. Stebbing J, Ngan S, Ibrahim H, et al. The successful treatment of haemophagocytic syndrome in patients with human immunodeficiency virus-associated multi-centric Castleman's disease. Clin Exp Immunol. 2008 Dec;154(3):399–405. PMID:19222502

3821. Stebegg M, Kumar SD, Silva-Cayetano A, et al. Regulation of the germinal center response. Front Immunol. 2018 Oct 25;9:2469. PMID:30410492

3822. Stefanovic A, Morgensztern D, Fong T, et al. Pulmonary marginal zone lymphoma: a single centre experience and review of the SEER database. Leuk Lymphoma. 2008 Jul;49(7):1311–20. PMID:18604720

3823. Steidl C, Lee T, Shah SP, et al. Tumor-associated macrophages and survival in classic Hodgkin's lymphoma. N Engl J Med. 2010 Mar 11;362(10):875–85. PMID:20220182

3824. Steidl C, Shah SP, Woolcock BW, et al. MHC class II transactivator CIITA is a recurrent gene fusion partner in lymphoid cancers. Nature. 2011 Mar 17;471(7338):377–81. PMID:21368758

3825. Steidl C, Telenius A, Shah SP, et al. Genome-wide copy number analysis of Hodgkin Reed-Sternberg cells identifies recurrent imbalances with correlations to treatment outcome. Blood. 2010 Jul 22;116(3):418–27. PMID:20339089

3826. Stein H, Foss HD, Dürkop H, et al. CD30(+) anaplastic large cell lymphoma: a review of its histopathologic, genetic, and clinical features. Blood. 2000 Dec 1;96(12):3681–95. PMID:11090048

3827. Stein H, Gerdes J, Kirchner H, et al. Hodgkin and Sternberg-Reed cell antigen(s) detected by an antiserum to a cell line (L428) derived from Hodgkin's disease. Int J Cancer. 1981 Oct 15;28(4):425–9. PMID:6946981

3828. Stein H, Marafioti T, Foss HD, et al. Down-regulation of BOB.1/OBF.1 and Oct2 in classical Hodgkin disease but not in lymphocyte predominant Hodgkin disease correlates with immunoglobulin transcription. Blood. 2001 Jan 15;97(2):496–501. PMID:11154228

3829. Stein H, Mason DY, Gerdes J, et al. The expression of the Hodgkin's disease associated antigen Ki-1 in reactive and neoplastic lymphoid tissue: evidence that Reed-Sternberg cells and histiocytic malignancies are derived from activated lymphoid cells. Blood. 1985 Oct;66(4):848–58. PMID:3876124

3830. Stein H, Uchánska-Ziegler B, Gerdes J, et al. Hodgkin and Sternberg-Reed cells contain antigens specific to late cells of granulopoiesis. Int J Cancer. 1982 Mar 15;29(3):283–90. PMID:6175588

3831. Steiner N, Göbel G, Suchecki P, et al. Monoclonal gammopathy of renal significance (MGRS) increases the risk for progression to multiple myeloma: an observational study of 2935 MGUS patients. Oncotarget. 2017 Dec 18;9(2):2344–56. PMID:29416776

3832. Steinhilber J, Mederake M, Bonzheim I, et al. The pathological features of angioimmunoblastic T-cell lymphomas with IDH2R172 mutations. Mod Pathol. 2019 Jul;32(8):1123–34. PMID:30952970

3833. Steinhoff M, Hummel M, Anagnostopoulos I, et al. Single-cell analysis of CD30+ cells in lymphomatoid papulosis demonstrates a common clonal T-cell origin. Blood. 2002 Jul 15;100(2):578–84. PMID:12091351

3834. Steininger H, Pfofe D, Marquardt L, et al. Isolated diffuse hemangiomatosis of the spleen: case report and review of literature. Pathol Res Pract. 2004;200(6):479–85. PMID:15310152

3835. Stevens TM, Morlote D, Xiu J, et al. NUTM1-rearranged neoplasia: a multi-institution experience yields novel fusion partners and expands the histologic spectrum. Mod Pathol. 2019 Jun;32(6):764–73. PMID:30723300

3836. Stevens WBC, Mendeville M, Redd R, et al. Prognostic relevance of CD163 and CD8 combined with EZH2 and gain of chromosome 18 in follicular lymphoma: a study by the Lunenburg Lymphoma Biomarker Consortium. Haematologica. 2017 Aug;102(8):1413–23. PMID:28411252

3837. Stewart JP, Gazdova J, Darzentas N, et al. Validation of the EuroClonality-NGS DNA capture panel as an integrated genomic tool for lymphoproliferative disorders. Blood Adv. 2021 Aug 24;5(16):3188–98. PMID:34424321

3838. Stilgenbauer S, Schnaiter A, Paschka P, et al. Gene mutations and treatment outcome in chronic lymphocytic leukemia: results from the CLL8 trial. Blood. 2014 May 22;123(21):3247–54. PMID:24652989

3839. Stiller CA, Parkin DM. International variations in the incidence of childhood lymphomas. Paediatr Perinat Epidemiol. 1990 Jul;4(3):303–24. PMID:2374749

3840. Stokes MB, Valeri AM, Herlitz L, et al. Light chain proximal tubulopathy: clinical and pathologic characteristics in the modern treatment era. J Am Soc Nephrol. 2016 May;27(5):1555–65. PMID:26374607

3841. Stoll JR, Willner J, Oh Y, et al. Primary cutaneous T-cell lymphomas other than mycosis fungoides and Sézary syndrome. Part I: clinical and histologic features and diagnosis. J Am Acad Dermatol. 2021 Nov;85(5):1073–90. PMID:33940098

3842. Stong N, Ortiz-Estévez M, Towfic F, et al. The location of the t(4;14) translocation breakpoint within the NSD2 gene identifies a subset of patients with high-risk NDMM. Blood. 2023 Mar 30;141(13):1574–83. PMID:35984902

3843. Strati P, Nasr SH, Leung N, et al. Renal complications in chronic lymphocytic leukemia and monoclonal B-cell lymphocytosis: the Mayo Clinic experience. Haematologica. 2015 Sep;100(9):1180–8. PMID:26088927

3844. Stratmann JA, von Rose AB, Koschade S, et al. Clinical and genetic characterization of de novo double-hit B cell precursor leukemia/lymphoma. Ann Hematol. 2019 Mar;98(3):647–56. PMID:30613837

3845. Stratta P, Gravellone L, Cena T, et al. Renal outcome and monoclonal immunoglobulin deposition disease in 289 old patients with blood cell dyscrasias: a single center experience. Crit Rev Oncol Hematol. 2011 Jul;79(1):31–42. PMID:20570173

3846. Strauchen JA. Indolent T-lymphoblastic proliferation: report of a case with an 11-year history and association with myasthenia gravis. Am J Surg Pathol. 2001 Mar;25(3):411–5. PMID:11224614

3847. Strauchen JA, Miller LK. Terminal deoxynucleotidyl transferase-positive cells in human tonsils. Am J Clin Pathol. 2001 Jul;116(1):12–6. PMID:11447741

3848. Straus SE, Jaffe ES, Puck JM, et al. The development of lymphomas in families with autoimmune lymphoproliferative syndrome with germline Fas mutations and defective lymphocyte apoptosis. Blood. 2001 Jul 1;98(1):194–200. PMID:11418480

3849. Streubel B, Huber D, Wöhrer S, et al. Frequency of chromosomal aberrations involving MALT1 in mucosa-associated lymphoid tissue lymphoma in patients with Sjögren's syndrome. Clin Cancer Res. 2004 Jan 15;10(2):476–80. PMID:14760068

3850. Streubel B, Lamprecht A, Dierlamm J, et al. T(14;18)(q32;q21) involving IGH and MALT1 is a frequent chromosomal aberration in MALT lymphoma. Blood. 2003 Mar 15;101(6):2335–9. PMID:12406890

3851. Streubel B, Simonitsch-Klupp I, Müllauer L, et al. Variable frequencies of MALT lymphoma-associated genetic aberrations in MALT lymphomas of different sites. Leukemia. 2004 Oct;18(10):1722–6. PMID:15356642

3852. Streubel B, Vinatzer U, Lamprecht A, et al. T(3;14)(p14.1;q32) involving IGH and FOXP1 is a novel recurrent chromosomal aberration in MALT lymphoma. Leukemia. 2005 Apr;19(4):652–8. PMID:15703784

3853. Streubel B, Vinatzer U, Willheim M, et al. Novel t(5;9)(q33;q22) fuses ITK to SYK in unspecified peripheral T-cell lymphoma. Leukemia. 2006 Feb;20(2):313–8. PMID:16341044

3854. Strobbe L, Valke LL, Diets IJ, et al. A 20-year population-based study on the epidemiology, clinical features, treatment, and outcome of nodular lymphocyte predominant Hodgkin lymphoma. Ann Hematol. 2016 Feb;95(3):417–23. PMID:26732883

3855. Strocchio L, Pagliara D, Algeri M, et al. HLA-haploidentical TCRαβ+/CD19+-depleted stem cell transplantation in children and young adults with Fanconi anemia. Blood Adv. 2021 Mar 9;5(5):1333–9. PMID:33656536

3856. Stuhlmann-Laeisz C, Borchert A, Quintanilla-Martinez L, et al. In Europe expression of EBNA2 is associated with poor survival in EBV-positive diffuse large B-cell lymphoma of the elderly. Leuk Lymphoma. 2016;57(1):39–44. PMID:25899404

3857. Stuhlmann-Laeisz C, Szczepanowski M, Borchert A, et al. Epstein-Barr virus-negative diffuse large B-cell lymphoma hosts intra- and peritumoral B-cells with activated Epstein-Barr virus. Virchows Arch. 2015 Jan;466(1):85–92. PMID:25339301

3858. Styczynski J, Gil L, Tridello G, et al. Response to rituximab-based therapy and risk factor analysis in Epstein Barr virus-related lymphoproliferative disorder after hematopoietic stem cell transplant in children and adults: a study from the Infectious Diseases Working Party of the European Group for Blood and Marrow Transplantation. Clin Infect Dis. 2013 Sep;57(6):794–802. PMID:23771985

3859. Su C, Nguyen KA, Bai HX, et al. Racial disparity in mycosis fungoides: an analysis of 4495 cases from the US National Cancer Database. J Am Acad Dermatol. 2017 Sep;77(3):497–502.e2. PMID:28645647

3860. Su IJ, Chen RL, Lin DT, et al. Epstein-Barr virus (EBV) infects T lymphocytes in childhood EBV-associated hemophagocytic syndrome in Taiwan. Am J Pathol. 1994 Jun;144(6):1219–25. PMID:8203462

3861. Suárez D, Izquierdo FM, Méndez JR, et al. Tumor of fibroblastic reticular cells of lymph node coincidental with an undifferentiated endometrial stromal sarcoma. Report of a case with distinctive immunophenotype and Kikuchi-like necro-inflammatory response. APMIS. 2011 Mar;119(3):216–20. PMID:21284739

3862. Suarez F, Lortholary O, Hermine O, et al. Infection-associated lymphomas derived from marginal zone B cells: a model of antigen-driven lymphoproliferation. Blood. 2006 Apr 15;107(8):3034–44. PMID:16397126

3863. Suarez F, Mahlaoui N, Canioni D, et al. Incidence, presentation, and prognosis of malignancies in ataxia-telangiectasia: a report from the French national registry of primary immune deficiencies. J Clin Oncol. 2015 Jan 10;33(2):202–8. PMID:25488969

3864. Subhawong AP, Subhawong TK, Ali SZ. Large cell transformation of mycosis fungoides on fine needle aspiration: an unusual case mimicking classical Hodgkin lymphoma. Acta Cytol. 2012;56(3):321–4. PMID:22555537

3865. Subramaniam K, Yeung D, Grimpen F, et al. Hepatosplenic T-cell lymphoma, immunosuppressive agents and biologicals: What are the risks? Intern Med J. 2014 Mar;44(3):287–90. PMID:24621284

3866. Subtil A, Xu Z. Follicular lymphoma with composite in situ mantle cell neoplasia. Blood. 2019 May 30;133(22):2460. PMID:31147376

3867. Sud A, Chattopadhyay S, Thomsen H, et al. Analysis of 153 115 patients with hematological malignancies refines the spectrum of familial risk. Blood. 2019 Sep 19;134(12):960–9. PMID:31395603

3868. Sud A, Thomsen H, Orlando G, et al. Genome-wide association study implicates immune dysfunction in the development of Hodgkin lymphoma. Blood. 2018 Nov 8;132(19):2040–52. PMID:30194254

3869. Suehara Y, Sakata-Yanagimoto M, Hattori K, et al. Liquid biopsy for the identification of intravascular large B-cell lymphoma. Haematologica. 2018 Jun;103(6):e241–4. PMID:29472348

3870. Sufficool KE, Lockwood CM, Abel HJ, et al. T-cell clonality assessment by next-generation sequencing improves detection sensitivity in mycosis fungoides. J Am Acad Dermatol. 2015 Aug;73(2):228–36.e2. PMID:26048061

3871. Sugimoto KJ, Shimada A, Wakabayashi M, et al. A probable identical Epstein-Barr virus clone-positive composite lymphoma with aggressive natural killer-cell leukemia and cytotoxic T-cell lymphoma. Int J Clin Exp Pathol. 2013 Dec 15;7(1):411–7. PMID:24427365

3872. Suh C, Huh J, Roh JL. Extranodal marginal zone B-cell lymphoma of mucosa-associated lymphoid tissue arising in the extracranial head and neck region: a high rate of dissemination and disease recurrence. Oral Oncol. 2008 Oct;44(10):949–55. PMID:18234544

3873. Suh YG, Suh CO, Kim JS, et al. Radiotherapy for solitary plasmacytoma of bone and soft tissue: outcomes and prognostic factors. Ann Hematol. 2012 Nov;91(11):1785–93. PMID:22752147

3874. Suichi T, Misawa S, Beppu M, et al. Prevalence, clinical profiles, and prognosis of POEMS syndrome in Japanese nationwide survey. Neurology. 2019 Sep 3;93(10):e975–83. PMID:31371568

3875. Sukswai N, Jung HR, Amr SS, et al. Immunopathology of Kikuchi-Fujimoto disease: a reappraisal using novel immunohistochemistry markers. Histopathology. 2020 Aug;77(2):262–74. PMID:31854007

3876. Sukswai N, Lyapichev K, Khoury JD, et al. Diffuse large B-cell lymphoma variants: an update. Pathology. 2020 Jan;52(1):53–67. PMID:31735345

3877. Sun C, Xu J, Zhang B, et al. Whole-genome sequencing suggests a role of MIF in the pathophysiology of TEMPI syndrome. Blood Adv. 2021 Jun 22;5(12):2563–8.

PMID:34129019
3878. Sun DP, Chen WM, Wang L, et al. Clinical characteristics and immunological abnormalities of Castleman disease complicated with autoimmune diseases. J Cancer Res Clin Oncol. 2021 Jul;147(7):2107–15. PMID:33544201
3879. Sun J, Lu Z, Yang D, et al. Primary intestinal T-cell and NK-cell lymphomas: a clinicopathological and molecular study from China focused on type II enteropathy-associated T-cell lymphoma and primary intestinal NK-cell lymphoma. Mod Pathol. 2011 Jul;24(7):983–92. PMID:21423155
3880. Sun J, Yang Q, Lu Z, et al. Distribution of lymphoid neoplasms in China: analysis of 4,638 cases according to the World Health Organization classification. Am J Clin Pathol. 2012 Sep;138(3):429–34. PMID:22912361
3881. Sun J, Yi S, Qiu L, et al. SATB1 defines a subtype of cutaneous CD30+ lymphoproliferative disorders associated with a T-helper 17 cytokine profile. J Invest Dermatol. 2018 Aug;138(8):1795–804. PMID:29510190
3882. Sun L, Zhao Y, Shi H, et al. LMP-1 induces survivin expression to inhibit cell apoptosis through the NF-κB and PI3K/Akt signaling pathways in nasal NK/T-cell lymphoma. Oncol Rep. 2015 May;33(5):2253–60. PMID:25760809
3883. Sun X, Chang KC, Abruzzo LV, et al. Epidermal growth factor receptor expression in follicular dendritic cells: a shared feature of follicular dendritic cell sarcoma and Castleman's disease. Hum Pathol. 2003 Sep;34(9):835–40. PMID:14562277
3884. Sun X, Du Y, Zhang Y, et al. Unicentric Castleman disease: multidetector computed tomography classification with surgical and pathologic correlation. Quant Imaging Med Surg. 2021 Aug;11(8):3562–8. PMID:34341731
3885. Sundeen JT, Cossman J, Jaffe ES. Lymphocyte predominant Hodgkin's disease nodular subtype with coexistent "large cell lymphoma". Histological progression or composite malignancy? Am J Surg Pathol. 1988 Aug;12(8):599–606. PMID:3041849
3886. Sungalee S, Mamessier E, Morgado E, et al. Germinal center reentries of BCL2-overexpressing B cells drive follicular lymphoma progression. J Clin Invest. 2014 Dec;124(12):5337–51. PMID:25384217
3887. Surmanowicz P, Doherty S, Sivanand A, et al. The clinical spectrum of primary cutaneous CD4+ small/medium-sized pleomorphic T-cell lymphoproliferative disorder: an updated systematic literature review and case series. Dermatology. 2021;237(4):618–28. PMID:33326960
3888. Surveillance, Epidemiology, and End Results (SEER) Program [Internet]. Bethesda (MD): National Cancer Institute; 2020. Cancer Stat Facts: myeloma. Available from: https://seer.cancer.gov/statfacts/html/mulmy.html.
3889. Suster S, Rosai J. Intranodal hemorrhagic spindle-cell tumor with "amianthoid" fibers. Report of six cases of a distinctive mesenchymal neoplasm of the inguinal region that simulates Kaposi's sarcoma. Am J Surg Pathol. 1989 May;13(5):347–57. PMID:2712187
3890. Sutton LA, Young E, Baliakas P, et al. Different spectra of recurrent gene mutations in subsets of chronic lymphocytic leukemia harboring stereotyped B-cell receptors. Haematologica. 2016 Aug;101(8):959–67. PMID:27198719
3891. Suzuki K, Ohshima K, Karube K, et al. Clinicopathological states of Epstein-Barr virus-associated T/NK-cell lymphoproliferative disorders (severe chronic active EBV infection) of children and young adults. Int J Oncol. 2004 May;24(5):1165–74. PMID:15067338
3892. Suzuki K, Okuno Y, Kawashima N, et al. MEF2D-BCL9 fusion gene is associated with high-risk acute B-cell precursor lymphoblastic leukemia in adolescents. J Clin Oncol. 2016 Oct 1;34(28):3451–9. PMID:27507882
3893. Suzuki R. Treatment of advanced extranodal NK/T cell lymphoma, nasal-type and aggressive NK-cell leukemia. Int J Hematol. 2010 Dec;92(5):697–701. PMID:21116747
3894. Suzuki R, Suzumiya J, Nakamura S, et al. Aggressive natural killer-cell leukemia revisited: large granular lymphocyte leukemia of cytotoxic NK cells. Leukemia. 2004 Apr;18(4):763–70. PMID:14961041
3895. Suzuki R, Suzumiya J, Yamaguchi M, et al. Prognostic factors for mature natural killer (NK) cell neoplasms: aggressive NK cell leukemia and extranodal NK cell lymphoma, nasal type. Ann Oncol. 2010 May;21(5):1032–40. PMID:19850638
3896. Suzuki R, Yamaguchi M, Izutsu K, et al. Prospective measurement of Epstein-Barr virus-DNA in plasma and peripheral blood mononuclear cells of extranodal NK/T-cell lymphoma, nasal type. Blood. 2011 Dec 1;118(23):6018–22. PMID:21984805
3897. Suzuki Y, Kohno K, Matsue K, et al. PD-L1 (SP142) expression in neoplastic cells predicts a poor prognosis for patients with intravascular large B-cell lymphoma treated with rituximab-based multi-agent chemotherapy. Cancer Med. 2020 Jul;9(13):4768–76. PMID:32367674
3898. Suzuki Y, Minemura H, Tomita H, et al. Monomorphic epitheliotropic intestinal T-cell lymphoma involving the lung and brain: a rare case study. Intern Med. 2020 Oct 15;59(20):2559–63. PMID:32641648
3899. Suzumiya J, Marutsuka K, Nabeshima K, et al. Autopsy findings in 47 cases of adult T-cell leukemia/lymphoma in Miyazaki prefecture, Japan. Leuk Lymphoma. 1993 Oct;11(3-4):281–6. PMID:8260899
3900. Swan N, Skinner M, O'Hara CJ. Bone marrow core biopsy specimens in AL (primary) amyloidosis. A morphologic and immunohistochemical study of 100 cases. Am J Clin Pathol. 2003 Oct;120(4):610–6. PMID:14560572
3901. Sweet RA, Lee SK, Vinuesa CG. Developing connections amongst key cytokines and dysregulated germinal centers in autoimmunity. Curr Opin Immunol. 2012 Dec;24(6):658–64. PMID:23123277
3902. Swerdlow SH. Cutaneous marginal zone lymphomas. Semin Diagn Pathol. 2017 Jan;34(1):76–84. PMID:27986434
3903. Swerdlow SH. Pediatric follicular lymphomas, marginal zone lymphomas, and marginal zone hyperplasia. Am J Clin Pathol. 2004 Dec;122 Suppl:S98–109. PMID:15690646
3904. Swerdlow SH, Campo E, Harris NL, et al., editors. WHO classification of tumours of haematopoietic and lymphoid tissues. Lyon (France): International Agency for Research on Cancer; 2008. (WHO classification of tumours series, 4th ed.; vol. 2). https://publications.iarc.who.int/12.
3905. Swerdlow SH, Campo E, Harris NL, et al., editors. WHO classification of tumours of haematopoietic and lymphoid tissues. Lyon (France): International Agency for Research on Cancer; 2017. (WHO classification of tumours series, 4th rev. ed.; vol. 2). https://publications.iarc.who.int/556.
3906. Swerdlow SH, Campo E, Pileri SA, et al. The 2016 revision of the World Health Organization classification of lymphoid neoplasms. Blood. 2016 May 19;127(20):2375–90. PMID:26980727
3907. Swerdlow SH, Kuzu I, Dogan A, et al. The many faces of small B cell lymphomas with plasmacytic differentiation and the contribution of MYD88 testing. Virchows Arch. 2016 Mar;468(3):259–75. PMID:26454445
3908. Swerdlow SH, Zukerberg LR, Yang WI, et al. The morphologic spectrum of non-Hodgkin's lymphomas with BCL1/cyclin D1 gene rearrangements. Am J Surg Pathol. 1996 May;20(5):627–40. PMID:8619427
3909. Swick BL, Baum CL, Venkat AP, et al. Indolent CD8+ lymphoid proliferation of the ear: report of two cases and review of the literature. J Cutan Pathol. 2011 Feb;38(2):209–15. PMID:21083681
3910. Swiecicki PL, Hegerova LT, Gertz MA. Cold agglutinin disease. Blood. 2013 Aug 15;122(7):1114–21. PMID:23757733
3911. Swift M, Morrell D, Cromartie E, et al. The incidence and gene frequency of ataxia-telangiectasia in the United States. Am J Hum Genet. 1986 Nov;39(5):573–83. PMID:3788973
3912. Sykes DB, O'Connell C, Schroyens W. The TEMPI syndrome. Blood. 2020 Apr 9;135(15):1199–203. PMID:32108223
3913. Sykes DB, Schroyens W, O'Connell C. The TEMPI syndrome–a novel multisystem disease. N Engl J Med. 2011 Aug 4;365(5):475–7. PMID:21812700
3914. Szablewski V, René C, Costes V. Indolent cytotoxic T cell lymphoproliferation associated with nodular regenerative hyperplasia: a common liver lesion in the context of common variable immunodeficiency disorder. Virchows Arch. 2015 Oct 22. PMID:26493984
3915. Szczepański T, Pongers-Willemse MJ, Langerak AW, et al. Ig heavy chain gene rearrangements in T-cell acute lymphoblastic leukemia exhibit predominant DH6-19 and DH7-27 gene usage, can result in complete V-D-J rearrangements, and are rare in T-cell receptor alpha beta lineage. Blood. 1999 Jun 15;93(12):4079–85. PMID:10361104
3916. Tabanelli V, Corsini C, Fiori S, et al. Recurrent PDL1 expression and PDL1 (CD274) copy number alterations in breast implant-associated anaplastic large cell lymphomas. Hum Pathol. 2019 Aug;90:60–9. PMID:31125630
3917. Tabata T, Takata K, Miyata-Takata T, et al. Characteristic distribution pattern of CD30-positive cytotoxic T cells aids diagnosis of Kikuchi-Fujimoto disease. Appl Immunohistochem Mol Morphol. 2018 Apr;26(4):274–82. PMID:27389558
3918. Tack GJ, van Wanrooij RL, Langerak AW, et al. Origin and immunophenotype of aberrant IEL in RCDII patients. Mol Immunol. 2012 Apr;50(4):262–70. PMID:22364936
3919. Taddesse-Heath L, Meloni-Ehrig A, Scheerle J, et al. Plasmablastic lymphoma with MYC translocation: evidence for a common pathway in the generation of plasmablastic features. Mod Pathol. 2010 Jul;23(7):991–9. PMID:20348882
3920. Taddesse-Heath L, Pittaluga S, Sorbara L, et al. Marginal zone B-cell lymphoma in children and young adults. Am J Surg Pathol. 2003 Apr;27(4):522–31. PMID:12657939
3921. Tadmor T, Polliack A. Epidemiology and environmental risk in hairy cell leukemia. Best Pract Res Clin Haematol. 2015 Dec;28(4):175–9. PMID:26614895
3922. Tadmor T, Polliack A. Hairy cell leukemia: uncommon clinical features, unusual sites of involvement and some rare associations. Best Pract Res Clin Haematol. 2015 Dec;28(4):193–9. PMID:26614897
3923. Tajan M, Paccoud R, Branka S, et al. The RASopathy family: consequences of germline activation of the RAS/MAPK pathway. Endocr Rev. 2018 Oct 1;39(5):676–700. PMID:29924299
3924. Takagi M, Shinoda K, Piao J, et al. Autoimmune lymphoproliferative syndrome-like disease with somatic KRAS mutation. Blood. 2011 Mar 10;117(10):2887–90. PMID:21063026
3925. Takahara T, Satou A, Ishikawa E, et al. Clinicopathological analysis of neoplastic PD-L1-positive EBV+ diffuse large B cell lymphoma, not otherwise specified, in a Japanese cohort. Virchows Arch. 2021 Mar;478(3):541–52. PMID:32803453
3926. Takahashi E, Asano N, Li C, et al. Nodal T/NK-cell lymphoma of nasal type: a clinicopathological study of six cases. Histopathology. 2008 Apr;52(5):585–96. PMID:18370955
3927. Takahashi H, Sakai R, Hattori Y, et al. Successful disease control with L-asparaginase monotherapy for aggressive natural killer cell leukemia with severe hepatic failure. Leuk Lymphoma. 2013 Mar;54(3):662–4. PMID:22891745
3928. Takahashi K, Wang F, Morita K, et al. Integrative genomic analysis of adult mixed phenotype acute leukemia delineates lineage associated molecular subtypes. Nat Commun. 2018 Jul 10;9(1):2670. PMID:29991687
3929. Takakuwa T, Ham MF, Luo WJ, et al. Loss of expression of Epstein-Barr virus nuclear antigen-2 correlates with a poor prognosis in cases of pyothorax-associated lymphoma. Int J Cancer. 2006 Jun 1;118(11):2782–9. PMID:16385574
3930. Takakuwa T, Luo WJ, Ham MF, et al. Establishment and characterization of unique cell lines derived from pyothorax-associated lymphoma which develops in long-standing pyothorax and is strongly associated with Epstein-Barr virus infection. Cancer Sci. 2003 Oct;94(10):858–63. PMID:14556658
3931. Takakuwa T, Ohnuma S, Koike J, et al. Involvement of cell-mediated killing in apoptosis in histiocytic necrotizing lymphadenitis (Kikuchi-Fujimoto disease). Histopathology. 1996 Jan;28(1):41–8. PMID:8838119
3932. Takakuwa T, Tresnasari K, Rahadiani N, et al. Cell origin of pyothorax-associated lymphoma: a lymphoma strongly associated with Epstein-Barr virus infection. Leukemia. 2008 Mar;22(3):620–7. PMID:18079737
3933. Takanashi S, Akiyama M, Suzuki K, et al. IgG4-related fibrosing mediastinitis diagnosed with computed tomography-guided percutaneous needle biopsy: two case reports and a review of the literature. Medicine (Baltimore). 2018 Jun;97(22):e10935. PMID:29851832
3934. Takata K, Hong ME, Sitthinamsuwan P, et al. Primary cutaneous NK/T-cell lymphoma, nasal type and CD56-positive peripheral T-cell lymphoma: a cellular lineage and clinicopathologic study of 60 patients from Asia. Am J Surg Pathol. 2015 Jan;39(1):1–12. PMID:25188863
3935. Takata K, Noujima-Harada M, Miyata-Takata T, et al. Clinicopathologic analysis of 6 lymphomatoid gastropathy cases: expanding the disease spectrum to CD4-CD8+ cases. Am J Surg Pathol. 2015 Sep;39(9):1259–66. PMID:25929350
3936. Takata K, Okada H, Ohmiya N, et al. Primary gastrointestinal follicular lymphoma involving the duodenal second portion is a distinct entity: a multicenter, retrospective analysis in Japan. Cancer Sci. 2011 Aug;102(8):1532–6. PMID:21561531
3937. Takata K, Sato Y, Nakamura N, et al. Duodenal follicular lymphoma lacks AID but expresses BACH2 and has memory B-cell characteristics. Mod Pathol. 2013 Jan;26(1):22–31. PMID:22899287
3938. Takata K, Tanino M, Ennishi D, et al. Duodenal follicular lymphoma: comprehensive gene expression analysis with insights into pathogenesis. Cancer Sci. 2014 May;105(5):608–15. PMID:24602001
3939. Takatori M, Sakihama S, Miyara M, et al. A new diagnostic algorithm using biopsy specimens in adult T-cell leukemia/lymphoma:

combination of RNA in situ hybridization and quantitative PCR for HTLV-1. Mod Pathol. 2021 Jan;34(1):51–8. PMID:32801340
3940. Takeda R, Yokoyama K, Ogawa M, et al. The first case of elderly TCF3-HLF-positive B-cell acute lymphoblastic leukemia. Leuk Lymphoma. 2019 Nov;60(11):2821–4. PMID:31058556
3941. Takei I, Kawai K, Nakajima M, et al. Primary cutaneous CD4+ small/medium T-cell lymphoproliferative disorder with high Ki-67 proliferation index. J Dermatol. 2021 May;48(5):e212–4. PMID:33624292
3942. Takeshima K, Li Y, Kakudo K, et al. Proposal of diagnostic criteria for IgG4-related thyroid disease. Endocr J. 2021 Jan 28;68(1):1–6. PMID:33311000
3943. Takeshita M, Akamatsu M, Ohshima K, et al. CD30 (Ki-1) expression in adult T-cell leukaemia/lymphoma is associated with distinctive immunohistological and clinical characteristics. Histopathology. 1995 Jun;26(6):539–46. PMID:7665144
3944. Takeshita M, Nakamura S, Kikuma K, et al. Pathological and immunohistological findings and genetic aberrations of intestinal enteropathy-associated T cell lymphoma in Japan. Histopathology. 2011 Feb;58(3):395–407. PMID:21323966
3945. Takeuchi K, Soda M, Togashi Y, et al. Identification of a novel fusion, SQSTM1-ALK, in ALK-positive large B-cell lymphoma. Haematologica. 2011 Mar;96(3):464–7. PMID:21134980
3946. Takeuchi K, Yokoyama M, Ishizawa S, et al. Lymphomatoid gastropathy: a distinct clinicopathologic entity of self-limited pseudomalignant NK-cell proliferation. Blood. 2010 Dec 16;116(25):5631–7. PMID:20829373
3947. Takigawa H, Yuge R, Masaki S, et al. Involvement of non-Helicobacter pylori helicobacter infections in Helicobacter pylori-negative gastric MALT lymphoma pathogenesis and efficacy of eradication therapy. Gastric Cancer. 2021 Jul;24(4):937–45. PMID:33638751
3948. Takino H, Li C, Hu S, et al. Primary cutaneous marginal zone B-cell lymphoma: a molecular and clinicopathological study of cases from Asia, Germany, and the United States. Mod Pathol. 2008 Dec;21(12):1517–26. PMID:18820662
3949. Talat N, Belgaumkar AP, Schulte KM. Surgery in Castleman's disease: a systematic review of 404 published cases. Ann Surg. 2012 Apr;255(4):677–84. PMID:22367441
3950. Talluri S, Samur MK, Buon L, et al. Dysregulated APOBEC3G causes DNA damage and promotes genomic instability in multiple myeloma. Blood Cancer J. 2021 Oct 8;11(10):166. PMID:34625538
3951. Talwalkar SS, Miranda RN, Valbuena JR, et al. Lymphomas involving the breast: a study of 106 cases comparing localized and disseminated neoplasms. Am J Surg Pathol. 2008 Sep;32(9):1299–309. PMID:18636016
3952. Tamaru J, Tokuhira M, Nittsu N, et al. Hodgkin-like anaplastic large cell lymphoma (previously designated in the REAL classification) has same immunophenotypic features to classical Hodgkin lymphoma. Leuk Lymphoma. 2007 Jun;48(6):1127–38. PMID:17577776
3953. Tamber GS, Chévarie-Davis M, Warner M, et al. In-situ follicular neoplasia: a clinicopathological spectrum. Histopathology. 2021 Dec;79(6):1072–86. PMID:34333806
3954. Tan SH, Bertulfo FC, Sanda T. Leukemia-initiating cells in T-cell acute lymphoblastic leukemia. Front Oncol. 2017 Sep 25;7:218. PMID:29034206
3955. Tan SY, Chuang SS, Tang T, et al. Type II EATL (epitheliotropic intestinal T-cell lymphoma): a neoplasm of intra-epithelial T-cells with predominant CD8αα phenotype. Leukemia. 2013 Aug;27(8):1688–96. PMID:23399895
3956. Tan SY, Nakamura S, Tan HC, et al. Diagnosis of type II enteropathy-associated T-cell lymphoma should be limited to EBER-cases. Am J Hematol. 2012 Nov;87(11):E129–30. PMID:22965422
3957. Tan SY, Ooi AS, Ang MK, et al. Nuclear expression of MATK is a novel marker of type II enteropathy-associated T-cell lymphoma. Leukemia. 2011 Mar;25(3):555–7. PMID:21233830
3958. Tanaka M, Suda T, Haze K, et al. Fas ligand in human serum. Nat Med. 1996 Mar;2(3):317–22. PMID:8612231
3959. Tanaka R, Kaburaki T, Taoka K, et al. More accurate diagnosis of vitreoretinal lymphoma using a combination of diagnostic test results: a prospective observational study. Ocul Immunol Inflamm. 2022 Aug;30(6):1354–60. PMID:33793360
3960. Tanaka T, Ohmori M, Yasunaga S, et al. DNA typing of HLA class II genes (HLA-DR, -DQ and -DP) in Japanese patients with histiocytic necrotizing lymphadenitis (Kikuchi's disease). Tissue Antigens. 1999 Sep;54(3):246–53. PMID:10519361
3961. Tanase A, Schmitz N, Stein H, et al. Allogeneic and autologous stem cell transplantation for hepatosplenic T-cell lymphoma: a retrospective study of the EBMT Lymphoma Working Party. Leukemia. 2015 Mar;29(3):686–8. PMID:25234166
3962. Tanasi I, Ba I, Sirvent N, et al. Efficacy of tyrosine kinase inhibitors in Ph-like acute lymphoblastic leukemia harboring ABL-class rearrangements. Blood. 2019 Oct 17;134(16):1351–5. PMID:31434701
3963. Tanda F, Massarelli G, Cossu A, et al. Primary spindle cell tumor of lymph node with "amianthoid" fibers: a histological, immunohistochemical and ultrastructural study. Ultrastruct Pathol. 1993 Mar-Apr;17(2):195–205. PMID:8316966
3964. Tandon B, Peterson L, Gao J, et al. Nuclear overexpression of lymphoid-enhancer-binding factor 1 identifies chronic lymphocytic leukemia/small lymphocytic lymphoma in small B-cell lymphomas. Mod Pathol. 2011 Nov;24(11):1433–43. PMID:21685909
3965. Tang H, Yang H, Zhang P, et al. Malignancy and IgG4-related disease: the incidence, related factors and prognosis from a prospective cohort study in China. Sci Rep. 2020 Mar 18;10(1):4910. PMID:32188869
3966. Tang YT, Wang D, Luo H, et al. Aggressive NK-cell leukemia: clinical subtypes, molecular features, and treatment outcomes. Blood Cancer J. 2017 Dec 21;7(12):660. PMID:29263371
3967. Tangye SG, Al-Herz W, Bousfiha A, et al. Human inborn errors of immunity: 2019 update on the classification from the International Union of Immunological Societies Expert Committee. J Clin Immunol. 2020 Jan;40(1):24–64. PMID:31953710
3968. Tangye SG, Al-Herz W, Bousfiha A, et al. Human inborn errors of immunity: 2022 update on the classification from the International Union of Immunological Societies Expert Committee. J Clin Immunol. 2022 Oct;42(7):1473–507. PMID:35748970
3969. Tangye SG, Al-Herz W, Bousfiha A, et al. The ever-increasing array of novel inborn errors of immunity: an interim update by the IUIS Committee. J Clin Immunol. 2021 Apr;41(3):666–79. PMID:33598806
3970. Taniguchi N, Mukai M, Nagaoki T, et al. Impaired B-cell differentiation and T-cell regulatory function in four patients with Bloom's syndrome. Clin Immunol Immunopathol. 1982 Feb;22(2):247–58. PMID:6980748
3971. Tao LL, Huang YH, Chen YL, et al. SSTR2a is a useful diagnostic marker for follicular dendritic cells and their related tumors. Am J Surg Pathol. 2019 Mar;43(3):374–81. PMID:30585825
3972. Tapia G, Lopez R, Muñoz-Mármol AM, et al. Immunohistochemical detection of MYC protein correlates with MYC gene status in aggressive B cell lymphomas. Histopathology. 2011 Oct;59(4):672–8. PMID:22014048
3973. Tari A, Kitadai Y, Mouri R, et al. Watch-and-wait policy versus rituximab-combined chemotherapy in Japanese patients with intestinal follicular lymphoma. J Gastroenterol Hepatol. 2018 Aug;33(8):1461–8. PMID:29377265
3974. Tartaglia M, Niemeyer CM, Fragale A, et al. Somatic mutations in PTPN11 in juvenile myelomonocytic leukemia, myelodysplastic syndromes and acute myeloid leukemia. Nat Genet. 2003 Jun;34(2):148–50. PMID:12717436
3975. Tasian SK, Doral MY, Borowitz MJ, et al. Aberrant STAT5 and PI3K/mTOR pathway signaling occurs in human CRLF2-rearranged B-precursor acute lymphoblastic leukemia. Blood. 2012 Jul 26;120(4):833–42. PMID:22685175
3976. Tasian SK, Loh ML, Hunger SP. Philadelphia chromosome-like acute lymphoblastic leukemia. Blood. 2017 Nov 9;130(19):2064–72. PMID:28972016
3977. Tatsuno K, Fujiyama T, Matsuoka H, et al. Clinical categories of exaggerated skin reactions to mosquito bites and their pathophysiology. J Dermatol Sci. 2016 Jun;82(3):145–52. PMID:27177994
3978. Tausch E, Close W, Dolnik A, et al. Venetoclax resistance and acquired BCL2 mutations in chronic lymphocytic leukemia. Haematologica. 2019 Sep;104(9):e434–7. PMID:31004028
3979. Tausch E, Schneider C, Robrecht S, et al. Prognostic and predictive impact of genetic markers in patients with CLL treated with obinutuzumab and venetoclax. Blood. 2020 Jun 25;135(26):2402–12. PMID:32206772
3980. Taverna J, Nair A, Yun S, et al. A rare presentation of in situ mantle cell lymphoma and follicular lymphoma: a case report and review of the literature. Case Rep Hematol. 2014;2014:145129. PMID:25478252
3981. Taylor AM, Harnden DG, Arlett CF, et al. Ataxia telangiectasia: a human mutation with abnormal radiation sensitivity. Nature. 1975 Dec 4;258(5534):427–9. PMID:1196376
3982. Taylor AM, Metcalfe JA, Thick J, et al. Leukemia and lymphoma in ataxia telangiectasia. Blood. 1996 Jan 15;87(2):423–38. PMID:8555463
3983. Tedoldi S, Mottok A, Ying J, et al. Selective loss of B-cell phenotype in lymphocyte predominant Hodgkin lymphoma. J Pathol. 2007 Dec;213(4):429–40. PMID:17935142
3984. Tellier J, Menard C, Roulland S, et al. Human t(14;18)positive germinal center B cells: a new step in follicular lymphoma pathogenesis? Blood. 2014 May 29;123(22):3462–5. PMID:24677543
3985. Tembhare PR, Chatterjee G, Khanka T, et al. Eleven-marker 10-color flow cytometric assessment of measurable residual disease for T-cell acute lymphoblastic leukemia using an approach of exclusion. Cytometry B Clin Cytom. 2021 Jul;100(4):421–33. PMID:32812702
3986. Tembhare PR, Ghogale S, Ghatwai N, et al. Evaluation of new markers for minimal residual disease monitoring in B-cell precursor acute lymphoblastic leukemia: CD73 and CD86 are the most relevant new markers to increase the efficacy of MRD 2016; 00B: 000-000. Cytometry B Clin Cytom. 2018 Jan;94(1):100–11. PMID:27718302
3987. Tembhare PR, Ghogale S, Tauro W, et al. Evaluation of CD229 as a new alternative plasma cell gating marker in the flow cytometric immunophenotyping of monoclonal gammopathies. Cytometry B Clin Cytom. 2018 May;94(3):509–19. PMID:29316178
3988. Tembhare PR, Subramanian Pg PG, Ghogale S, et al. A high-sensitivity 10-color flow cytometric minimal residual disease assay in B-lymphoblastic leukemia/lymphoma can easily achieve the sensitivity of 2-in-106 and is superior to standard minimal residual disease assay: a study of 622 patients. Cytometry B Clin Cytom. 2020 Jan;98(1):57–67. PMID:31197916
3989. Tembhare PR, Yuan CM, Venzon D, et al. Flow cytometric differentiation of abnormal and normal plasma cells in the bone marrow in patients with multiple myeloma and its precursor diseases. Leuk Res. 2014 Mar;38(3):371–6. PMID:24462038
3990. Teramo A, Barilà G, Calabretto G, et al. Insights into genetic landscape of large granular lymphocyte leukemia. Front Oncol. 2020 Feb 18;10:152. PMID:32133291
3991. Teramo A, Barilà G, Calabretto G, et al. STAT3 mutation impacts biological and clinical features of T-LGL leukemia. Oncotarget. 2017 Jun 27;8(37):61876–89. PMID:28977911
3992. Teramo A, Binatti A, Ciabatti E, et al. Defining TCRγδ lymphoproliferative disorders by combined immunophenotypic and molecular evaluation. Nat Commun. 2022 Jun 8;13(1):3298. PMID:35676278
3993. Teras LR, DeSantis CE, Cerhan JR, et al. 2016 US lymphoid malignancy statistics by World Health Organization subtypes. CA Cancer J Clin. 2016 Nov 12;66(6):443–59. PMID:27618563
3994. Teruya-Feldstein J, Jaffe ES, Burd PR, et al. The role of Mig, the monokine induced by interferon-gamma, and IP-10, the interferon-gamma-inducible protein-10, in tissue necrosis and vascular damage associated with Epstein-Barr virus-positive lymphoproliferative disease. Blood. 1997 Nov 15;90(10):4099–105. PMID:9354680
3995. Tesher MS, Esteban Y, Henderson TO, et al. Mucosal-associated lymphoid tissue (MALT) lymphoma in association with pediatric primary Sjogren syndrome: 2 cases and review. J Pediatr Hematol Oncol. 2019 Jul;41(5):413–6. PMID:30371536
3996. Teshima T, Akashi K, Shibuya T, et al. Central nervous system involvement in adult T-cell leukemia/lymphoma. Cancer. 1990 Jan 15;65(2):327–32. PMID:2295055
3997. Thakurta A, Ortiz M, Blecua P, et al. High subclonal fraction of 17p deletion is associated with poor prognosis in multiple myeloma. Blood. 2019 Mar 14;133(11):1217–21. PMID:30692124
3998. Thanendrarajan S, Tian E, Qu P, et al. The level of deletion 17p and bi-allelic inactivation of TP53 has a significant impact on clinical outcome in multiple myeloma. Haematologica. 2017 Sep;102(9):e364–7. PMID:28550191
3999. Thieblemont C, Cascione L, Conconi A, et al. A MALT lymphoma prognostic index. Blood. 2017 Sep 21;130(12):1409–17. PMID:28720586
4000. Thiede C, Alpen B, Morgner A, et al. Ongoing somatic mutations and clonal expansions after cure of Helicobacter pylori infection in gastric mucosa-associated lymphoid tissue B-cell lymphoma. J Clin Oncol. 1998 Dec;16(12):3822–31. PMID:9850027
4001. Thiel CT, Mortier G, Kaitila I, et al. Type and level of RMRP functional impairment predicts phenotype in the cartilage hair hypoplasia-anauxetic dysplasia spectrum. Am J Hum Genet. 2007 Sep;81(3):519–29. PMID:17701897
4002. Thol F. ALL is not the same in the era of

genetics. Blood. 2021 Sep 16;138(11):915–6. PMID:34529020
4003. Thomas RM, Jaffe ES, Zarate-Osorno A, et al. Inflammatory pseudotumor of the spleen. A clinicopathologic and immunophenotypic study of eight cases. Arch Pathol Lab Med. 1993 Sep;117(9):921–6. PMID:8368906
4004. Thompsett AR, Ellison DW, Stevenson FK, et al. V(H) gene sequences from primary central nervous system lymphomas indicate derivation from highly mutated germinal center B cells with ongoing mutational activity. Blood. 1999 Sep 1;94(5):1738–46. PMID:10477699
4005. Thompson ER, Lim KJC, Kuzich JA, et al. Detection of an IGH-BRAF fusion in a patient with BRAF Val600Glu negative hairy cell leukemia. Leuk Lymphoma. 2020 Aug;61(8):2024–6. PMID:32319330
4006. Thordardottir M, Lindqvist EK, Lund SH, et al. Obesity and risk of monoclonal gammopathy of undetermined significance and progression to multiple myeloma: a population-based study. Blood Adv. 2017 Nov 1;1(24):2186–92. PMID:29296866
4007. Thorley-Lawson DA, Gross A. Persistence of the Epstein-Barr virus and the origins of associated lymphomas. N Engl J Med. 2004 Mar 25;350(13):1328–37. PMID:15044644
4008. Thorns C, Bastian B, Pinkel D, et al. Chromosomal aberrations in angioimmunoblastic T-cell lymphoma and peripheral T-cell lymphoma unspecified: a matrix-based CGH approach. Genes Chromosomes Cancer. 2007 Jan;46(1):37–44. PMID:17044049
4009. Thorsélius M, Walsh SH, Thunberg U, et al. Heterogeneous somatic hypermutation status confounds the cell of origin in hairy cell leukemia. Leuk Res. 2005 Feb;29(2):153–8. PMID:15607363
4010. Thumallapally N, Meshref A, Mousa M, et al. Solitary plasmacytoma: population-based analysis of survival trends and effect of various treatment modalities in the USA. BMC Cancer. 2017 Jan 5;17(1):13. PMID:28056880
4011. Thurner L, Hartmann S, Fadle N, et al. Lymphocyte predominant cells detect Moraxella catarrhalis-derived antigens in nodular lymphocyte-predominant Hodgkin lymphoma. Nat Commun. 2020 May 18;11(1):2465. PMID:32424289
4012. Thurner L, Preuss KD, Bewarder M, et al. Hyper-N-glycosylated SAMD14 and neurabin-I as driver autoantigens of primary central nervous system lymphoma. Blood. 2018 Dec 27;132(26):2744–53. PMID:30249786
4013. Tiacci E, De Carolis L, Simonetti E, et al. Safety and efficacy of the BRAF inhibitor dabrafenib in relapsed or refractory hairy cell leukemia: a pilot phase-2 clinical trial. Leukemia. 2021 Nov;35(11):3314–8. PMID:33731847
4014. Tiacci E, Ladewig E, Schiavoni G, et al. Pervasive mutations of JAK-STAT pathway genes in classical Hodgkin lymphoma. Blood. 2018 May 31;131(22):2454–65. PMID:29650799
4015. Tiacci E, Park JH, De Carolis L, et al. Targeting mutant BRAF in relapsed or refractory hairy-cell leukemia. N Engl J Med. 2015 Oct 29;373(18):1733–47. PMID:26352686
4016. Tiacci E, Pettirossi V, Schiavoni G, et al. Genomics of hairy cell leukemia. J Clin Oncol. 2017 Mar 20;35(9):1002–10. PMID:28297625
4017. Tiacci E, Schiavoni G, Forconi F, et al. Simple genetic diagnosis of hairy cell leukemia by sensitive detection of the BRAF-V600E mutation. Blood. 2012 Jan 5;119(1):192–5. PMID:22028477
4018. Tiacci E, Schiavoni G, Martelli MP, et al. Constant activation of the RAF-MEK-ERK pathway as a diagnostic and therapeutic target in hairy cell leukemia. Haematologica. 2013 Apr;98(4):635–9. PMID:23349307
4019. Tiemann M, Riener MO, Claviez A, et al. Proliferation rate and outcome in children with T-cell rich B-cell lymphoma: a clinicopathologic study from the NHL-BFM-study group. Leuk Lymphoma. 2005 Sep;46(9):1295–300. PMID:16109606
4020. Tiemann M, Schrader C, Klapper W, et al. Histopathology, cell proliferation indices and clinical outcome in 304 patients with mantle cell lymphoma (MCL): a clinicopathological study from the European MCL Network. Br J Haematol. 2005 Oct;131(1):29–38. PMID:16173960
4021. Tilly H, Rossi A, Stamatoullas A, et al. Prognostic value of chromosomal abnormalities in follicular lymphoma. Blood. 1994 Aug 15;84(4):1043–9. PMID:8049424
4022. Timár B, Fülöp Z, Csernus B, et al. Relationship between the mutational status of VH genes and pathogenesis of diffuse large B-cell lymphoma in Richter's syndrome. Leukemia. 2004 Feb;18(2):326–30. PMID:14671632
4023. Timeus F, Crescenzio N, Baldassarre G, et al. Functional evaluation of circulating hematopoietic progenitors in Noonan syndrome. Oncol Rep. 2013 Aug;30(2):553–9. PMID:23756559
4024. Tirelli U, Vaccher E, Zagonel V, et al. CD30 (Ki-1)-positive anaplastic large-cell lymphomas in 13 patients with and 27 patients without human immunodeficiency virus infection: the first comparative clinicopathologic study from a single institution that also includes 80 patients with other human immunodeficiency virus-related systemic lymphomas. J Clin Oncol. 1995 Feb;13(2):373–80. PMID:7844598
4025. Tjahjono LA, Davis MDP, Witzig TE, et al. Primary cutaneous acral CD8+ T-cell lymphoma-a single center review of 3 cases and recent literature review. Am J Dermatopathol. 2019 Sep;41(9):644–8. PMID:31433793
4026. Tjon JM, Verbeek WH, Kooy-Winkelaar YM, et al. Defective synthesis or association of T-cell receptor chains underlies loss of surface T-cell receptor-CD3 expression in enteropathy-associated T-cell lymphoma. Blood. 2008 Dec 15;112(13):5103–10. PMID:18815285
4027. Toberer F, Christopoulos P, Lasitschka F, et al. Double-positive CD8/CD4 primary cutaneous acral T-cell lymphoma. J Cutan Pathol. 2019 Mar;46(3):231–3. PMID:30552698
4028. Tobin JWD, Keane C, Gunawardana J, et al. Progression of disease within 24 months in follicular lymphoma is associated with reduced intratumoral immune infiltration. J Clin Oncol. 2019 Dec 1;37(34):3300–9. PMID:31461379
4029. Toboso DG, Campos CB. Peripheral eosinophilia as the first manifestation of B-cell acute lymphoblastic leukemia with t(5;14)(q31;q32). Blood. 2017 Jul 20;130(3):380. PMID:28729339
4030. Todd DJ, McHeyzer-Williams LJ, Kowal C, et al. XBP1 governs late events in plasma cell differentiation and is not required for antigen-specific memory B cell development. J Exp Med. 2009 Sep 28;206(10):2151–9. PMID:19752183
4031. Todd WU, Drabick JJ, Benninghoff MG, et al. Pulmonary crystal-storing histiocytosis diagnosed by computed tomography-guided fine-needle aspiration. Diagn Cytopathol. 2010 Apr;38(4):274–8. PMID:19845034
4032. Todorovic Balint M, Jelicic J, Mihaljevic B, et al. Gene mutation profiles in primary diffuse large B cell lymphoma of central nervous system: next generation sequencing analyses. Int J Mol Sci. 2016 May 6;17(5):683. PMID:27164089
4033. Tokuhira M, Saito S, Okuyama A, et al. Clinicopathologic investigation of methotrexate-induced lymphoproliferative disorders, with a focus on regression. Leuk Lymphoma. 2018 May;59(5):1143–52. PMID:28877615
4034. Tokuhira M, Tamaru JI, Kizaki M. Clinical management for other iatrogenic immunodeficiency-associated lymphoproliferative disorders. J Clin Exp Hematop. 2019;59(2):72–92. PMID:31257348
4035. Tokunaga T, Shimada K, Yamamoto K, et al. Retrospective analysis of prognostic factors for angioimmunoblastic T-cell lymphoma: a multicenter cooperative study in Japan. Blood. 2012 Mar 22;119(12):2837–43. PMID:22308294
4036. Tokura Y, Ishihara S, Tagawa S, et al. Hypersensitivity to mosquito bites as the primary clinical manifestation of a juvenile type of Epstein-Barr virus-associated natural killer cell leukemia/lymphoma. J Am Acad Dermatol. 2001 Oct;45(4):569–78. PMID:11568749
4037. Tokura Y, Tamura Y, Takigawa M, et al. Severe hypersensitivity to mosquito bites associated with natural killer cell lymphocytosis. Arch Dermatol. 1990 Mar;126(3):362–8. PMID:1689990
4038. Tolkachjov SN, Weenig RH, Comfere NI. Cutaneous peripheral T-cell lymphoma, not otherwise specified: a single-center prognostic analysis. J Am Acad Dermatol. 2016 Nov;75(5):992–9. PMID:27498959
4039. Tomita S, Kikuti YY, Carreras J, et al. Genomic and immunohistochemical profiles of enteropathy-associated T-cell lymphoma in Japan. Mod Pathol. 2015 Oct;28(10):1286–96. PMID:26226842
4040. Tomita S, Kikuti YY, Carreras J, et al. Monomorphic epitheliotropic intestinal T-cell lymphoma in Asia frequently shows SETD2 alterations. Cancers (Basel). 2020 Nov 27;12(12):3539. PMID:33260897
4041. Tomita S, Kikuti YY, Carreras J, et al. Monomorphic epitheliotropic intestinal T-cell lymphoma with T-cell receptor (TCR) of silent phenotype shows rearrangement of TCRβ or TCRγ gene. Pathol Int. 2019 Feb;69(2):117–8. PMID:30576040
4042. Tomita Y, Ohsawa M, Hashimoto M, et al. Plasmacytoma of the gastrointestinal tract in Korea: higher incidence than in Japan and Epstein-Barr virus association. Oncology. 1998 Jan-Feb;55(1):27–32. PMID:9428372
4043. Tomoka T, Painschab MS, Montgomery ND, et al. A prospective description of HIV-associated multicentric Castleman disease in Malawi. Haematologica. 2019 May;104(5):e215–7. PMID:30442726
4044. Tono-oka T, Sato Y, Matsumoto T, et al. Hypereosinophilic syndrome in acute lymphoblastic leukemia with a chromosome translocation [t(5q;14q)]. Med Pediatr Oncol. 1984;12(1):33–7. PMID:6583469
4045. Topar G, Zelger B, Schmuth M, et al. Granulomatous slack skin: a distinct disorder or a variant of mycosis fungoides? Acta Derm Venereol. 2001 Jan-Feb;81(1):42–4. PMID:11411914
4046. Torka P, Kothari SK, Sundaram S, et al. Outcomes of patients with limited-stage aggressive large B-cell lymphoma with high-risk cytogenetics. Blood Adv. 2020 Jan 28;4(2):253–62. PMID:31945157
4047. Torlakovic E, Nielsen S, Vyberg M. Antibody selection in immunohistochemical detection of cyclin D1 in mantle cell lymphoma. Am J Clin Pathol. 2005 Nov;124(5):782–9. PMID:16203276
4048. Torlakovic E, Tierens A, Dang HD, et al. The transcription factor PU.1, necessary for B-cell development is expressed in lymphocyte predominance, but not classical Hodgkin's disease. Am J Pathol. 2001 Nov;159(5):1807–14. PMID:11696441
4049. Torlakovic E, Torlakovic G, Nguyen PL, et al. The value of anti-pax-5 immunostaining in routinely fixed and paraffin-embedded sections: a novel pan pre-B and B-cell marker. Am J Surg Pathol. 2002 Oct;26(10):1343–50. PMID:12360049
4050. Toro JR, Beaty M, Sorbara L, et al. Gamma delta T-cell lymphoma of the skin: a clinical, microscopic, and molecular study. Arch Dermatol. 2000 Aug;136(8):1024–32. PMID:10926739
4051. Toro JR, Liewehr DJ, Pabby N, et al. Gamma-delta T-cell phenotype is associated with significantly decreased survival in cutaneous T-cell lymphoma. Blood. 2003 May 1;101(9):3407–12. PMID:12522013
4052. Tort F, Camacho E, Bosch F, et al. Familial lymphoid neoplasms in patients with mantle cell lymphoma. Haematologica. 2004 Mar;89(3):314–9. PMID:15020270
4053. Tousseyn T, De Wolf-Peeters C. T cell/histiocyte-rich large B-cell lymphoma: an update on its biology and classification. Virchows Arch. 2011 Dec;459(6):557–63. PMID:22081105
4054. Toyoda K, Maeshima AM, Nomoto J, et al. Mucosa-associated lymphoid tissue lymphoma with t(11;18)(q21;q21) translocation: long-term follow-up results. Ann Hematol. 2019 Jul;98(7):1675–87. PMID:30923996
4055. Tracy SI, Habermann TM, Feldman AL, et al. Outcomes among North American patients with diffuse large B-cell lymphoma are independent of tumor Epstein-Barr virus positivity or immunosuppression. Haematologica. 2018 Feb;103(2):297–303. PMID:29170255
4056. Tran J, Duvic M, Torres-Cabala CA. Lymphomatoid papulosis with a unique T follicular helper-like phenotype. Am J Dermatopathol. 2020 Oct;42(10):776–9. PMID:32568843
4057. Trappe RU, Choquet S, Dierickx D, et al. International prognostic index, type of transplant and response to rituximab are key parameters to tailor treatment in adults with CD20-positive B cell PTLD: clues from the PTLD-1 trial. Am J Transplant. 2015 Apr;15(4):1091–100. PMID:25736912
4058. Trappe RU, Dierickx D, Zimmermann H, et al. Response to rituximab induction is a predictive marker in B-cell post-transplant lymphoproliferative disorder and allows successful stratification into rituximab or R-CHOP consolidation in an international, prospective, multicenter phase II trial. J Clin Oncol. 2017 Feb 10;35(5):536–43. PMID:27992268
4059. Travaglino A, Giordano C, Pace M, et al. Sjögren syndrome in primary salivary gland lymphoma. Am J Clin Pathol. 2020 May 5;153(6):719–24. PMID:32076706
4060. Travassos DC, Silveira HA, Silva EV, et al. Primary cutaneous CD8+ cytotoxic T-cell lymphoma of the face with intraoral involvement, resulting in facial nerve palsy after chemotherapy. J Cutan Pathol. 2022 Jun;49(6):560–4. PMID:35001425
4061. Traverse-Glehen A, Bachy E, Baseggio L, et al. Immunoarchitectural patterns in splenic marginal zone lymphoma: correlations with chromosomal aberrations, IGHV mutations, and survival. A study of 76 cases. Histopathology. 2013 May;62(6):876–93. PMID:23611359
4062. Traverse-Glehen A, Baseggio L, Bauchu EC, et al. Splenic red pulp lymphoma with numerous basophilic villous lymphocytes: a distinct clinicopathologic and molecular entity? Blood. 2008 Feb 15;111(4):2253–60. PMID:18042795
4063. Traverse-Glehen A, Baseggio L, Salles G, et al. Splenic diffuse red pulp small-B cell lymphoma: toward the emergence of a new lymphoma entity. Discov Med. 2012 Apr;13(71):253–65. PMID:22541613
4064. Traverse-Glehen A, Davi F, Ben Simon E, et al. Analysis of VH genes in marginal zone lymphoma reveals marked heterogeneity between splenic and nodal tumors

and suggests the existence of clonal selection. Haematologica. 2005 Apr;90(4):470–8. PMID:15820942
4065. Traverse-Glehen A, Felman P, Callet-Bauchu E, et al. A clinicopathological study of nodal marginal zone B-cell lymphoma. A report on 21 cases. Histopathology. 2006 Jan;48(2):162–73. PMID:16405665
4066. Traverse-Glehen A, Pittaluga S, Gaulard P, et al. Mediastinal gray zone lymphoma: the missing link between classic Hodgkin's lymphoma and mediastinal large B-cell lymphoma. Am J Surg Pathol. 2005 Nov;29(11):1411–21. PMID:16224207
4067. Traverse-Glehen A, Verney A, Gazzo S, et al. Splenic diffuse red pulp lymphoma has a distinct pattern of somatic mutations amongst B-cell malignancies. Leuk Lymphoma. 2017 Mar;58(3):666–75. PMID:27347751
4068. Travert M, Huang Y, de Leval L, et al. Molecular features of hepatosplenic T-cell lymphoma unravels potential novel therapeutic targets. Blood. 2012 Jun 14;119(24):5795–806. PMID:22510872
4069. Trecourt A, Mauduit C, Szablewski V, et al. Plasticity of mature B cells between follicular and classic Hodgkin lymphomas: a series of 22 cases expanding the spectrum of transdifferentiation. Am J Surg Pathol. 2022 Jan 1;46(1):58–70. PMID:34265801
4070. Treetipsatit J, Metcalf RA, Warnke RA, et al. Large B-cell lymphoma with T-cell-rich background and nodules lacking follicular dendritic cell meshworks: description of an insufficiently recognized variant. Hum Pathol. 2015 Jan;46(1):74–83. PMID:25456392
4071. Treon SP, Gustine J, Xu L, et al. MYD88 wild-type Waldenstrom macroglobulinaemia: differential diagnosis, risk of histological transformation, and overall survival. Br J Haematol. 2018 Feb;180(3):374–80. PMID:29181840
4072. Treon SP, Hunter ZR, Aggarwal A, et al. Characterization of familial Waldenstrom's macroglobulinemia. Ann Oncol. 2006 Mar;17(3):488–94. PMID:16357024
4073. Treon SP, Tripsas C, Hanzis C, et al. Familial disease predisposition impacts treatment outcome in patients with Waldenström macroglobulinemia. Clin Lymphoma Myeloma Leuk. 2012 Dec;12(6):433–7. PMID:23084402
4074. Treon SP, Xu L, Guerrera ML, et al. Genomic landscape of Waldenström macroglobulinemia and its impact on treatment strategies. J Clin Oncol. 2020 Apr 10;38(11):1198–208. PMID:32083995
4075. Treon SP, Xu L, Yang G, et al. MYD88 L265P somatic mutation in Waldenström's macroglobulinemia. N Engl J Med. 2012 Aug 30;367(9):826–33. PMID:22931316
4076. Trimech M, Letourneau A, Missiaglia E, et al. Angioimmunoblastic T-cell lymphoma and chronic lymphocytic leukemia/small lymphocytic lymphoma: a novel form of composite lymphoma potentially mimicking Richter syndrome. Am J Surg Pathol. 2021 Jun 1;45(6):773–86. PMID:33739791
4077. Tripodo C, Zanardi F, Iannelli F, et al. A spatially resolved dark- versus light-zone microenvironment signature subdivides germinal center-related aggressive B cell lymphomas. iScience. 2020 Sep 16;23(10):101562. PMID:33083730
4078. Trotter MJ, Whittaker SJ, Orchard GE, et al. Cutaneous histopathology of Sézary syndrome: a study of 41 cases with a proven circulating T-cell clone. J Cutan Pathol. 1997 May;24(5):286–91. PMID:9194581
4079. Troxell ML, Schwartz EJ, van de Rijn M, et al. Follicular dendritic cell immunohistochemical markers in angioimmunoblastic T-cell lymphoma. Appl Immunohistochem Mol Morphol. 2005 Dec;13(4):297–303. PMID:16280657
4080. Tsagarakis NJ, Papadhimitriou SI, Pavlidis D, et al. Contribution of immunophenotype to the investigation and differential diagnosis of Burkitt lymphoma, double-hit high-grade B-cell lymphoma, and single-hit MYC-rearranged diffuse large B-cell lymphoma. Cytometry B Clin Cytom. 2020 Sep;98(5):412–20. PMID:32497402
4081. Tsagarakis NJ, Papadhimitriou SI, Pavlidis D, et al. Flow cytometric predictive scoring systems for common fusions ETV6/RUNX1, BCR/ABL1, TCF3/PBX1 and rearrangements of the KMT2A gene, proposed for the initial cytogenetic approach in cases of B-acute lymphoblastic leukemia. Int J Lab Hematol. 2019 Jun;41(3):364–72. PMID:30730614
4082. Tsagiopoulou M, Papakonstantinou N, Moysiadis T, et al. DNA methylation profiles in chronic lymphocytic leukemia patients treated with chemoimmunotherapy. Clin Epigenetics. 2019 Dec 2;11(1):177. PMID:31791414
4083. Tsai CC, Su YC, Bamodu OA, et al. High-grade B-cell lymphoma (HGBL) with MYC and BCL2 and/or BCL6 rearrangements is predominantly BCL6-rearranged and BCL6-expressing in Taiwan. Cancers (Basel). 2021 Mar 31;13(7):1620. PMID:33807449
4084. Tsai HT, Caporaso NE, Kyle RA, et al. Evidence of serum immunoglobulin abnormalities up to 9.8 years before diagnosis of chronic lymphocytic leukemia: a prospective study. Blood. 2009 Dec 3;114(24):4928–32. PMID:19828698
4085. Tsang M, Parikh SA. A concise review of autoimmune cytopenias in chronic lymphocytic leukemia. Curr Hematol Malig Rep. 2017 Feb;12(1):29–38. PMID:28197963
4086. Tsang RW, Campbell BA, Goda JS, et al. Radiation therapy for solitary plasmacytoma and multiple myeloma: guidelines from the International Lymphoma Radiation Oncology Group. Int J Radiat Oncol Biol Phys. 2018 Jul 15;101(4):794–808. PMID:29976492
4087. Tsang WY, Chan JK. Bacillary angiomatosis. A "new" disease with a broadening clinicopathologic spectrum. Histol Histopathol. 1992 Jan;7(1):143–52. PMID:1576430
4088. Tsang WY, Chan JK. Fine-needle aspiration cytologic diagnosis of Kikuchi's lymphadenitis. A report of 27 cases. Am J Clin Pathol. 1994 Oct;102(4):454–8. PMID:7524300
4089. Tsang WY, Chan JK, Dorfman RF, et al. Vasoproliferative lesions of the lymph node. Pathol Annu. 1994;29(Pt 1):63–133. PMID:8127627
4090. Tsang WY, Chan JK, Ng CS. Kikuchi's lymphadenitis. A morphologic analysis of 75 cases with special reference to unusual features. Am J Surg Pathol. 1994 Mar;18(3):219–31. PMID:8116791
4091. Tsao L, Draoua HY, Mansukhani M, et al. EBV-associated, extranodal NK-cell lymphoma, nasal type of the breast, after heart transplantation. Mod Pathol. 2004 Jan;17(1):125–30. PMID:14631361
4092. Tschernitz S, Flossbach L, Bonengel M, et al. Alternative BRAF mutations in BRAF V600E-negative hairy cell leukaemias. Br J Haematol. 2014 May;165(4):529–33. PMID:24433452
4093. Tse E, Au-Yeung R, Kwong YL. Recent advances in the diagnosis and treatment of natural killer/T-cell lymphomas. Expert Rev Hematol. 2019 Nov;12(11):927–35. PMID:31487202
4094. Tse E, Gill H, Loong F, et al. Type II enteropathy-associated T-cell lymphoma: a multicenter analysis from the Asia Lymphoma Study Group. Am J Hematol. 2012 Jul;87(7):663–8. PMID:22641357
4095. Tse E, Kwong YL. The diagnosis and management of NK/T-cell lymphomas. J Hematol Oncol. 2017 Apr 14;10(1):85. PMID:28410601
4096. Tse E, Leung R, Khong PL, et al. Non-nasal natural killer cell lymphoma: not non-nasal after all. Ann Hematol. 2009 Feb;88(2):185–7. PMID:18677482
4097. Tseng H, Ho CM, Tien YW. Reappraisal of surgical decision-making in patients with splenic sclerosing angiomatoid nodular transformation: case series and literature review. World J Gastrointest Surg. 2021 Aug 27;13(8):848–58. PMID:34512908
4098. Tsujikawa T, Tsuchida T, Imamura Y, et al. Kikuchi-Fujimoto disease: PET/CT assessment of a rare cause of cervical lymphadenopathy. Clin Nucl Med. 2011 Aug;36(8):661–4. PMID:21716016
4099. Tsukamoto T, Tokuda Y, Nakano M, et al. Expression of activated B-cell gene signature is predictive of the outcome of follicular lymphoma. Blood Adv. 2022 Mar 22;6(6):1932–6. PMID:34991156
4100. Tsukasaki K, Hermine O, Bazarbachi A, et al. Definition, prognostic factors, treatment, and response criteria of adult T-cell leukemia-lymphoma: a proposal from an international consensus meeting. J Clin Oncol. 2009 Jan 20;27(3):453–9. PMID:19064971
4101. Tsukasaki K, Imaizumi Y, Tawara M, et al. Diversity of leukaemic cell morphology in ATL correlates with prognostic factors, aberrant immunophenotype and defective HTLV-1 genotype. Br J Haematol. 1999 May;105(2):369–75. PMID:10233406
4102. Tsuyama N, Yokoyama M, Fujisaki J, et al. Villous colonization (glove balloon sign): a histopathological diagnostic marker for follicular lymphomas with duodenal involvement including duodenal-type follicular lymphoma. Pathol Int. 2019 Jan;69(1):48–50. PMID:30582768
4103. Tu PH, Giannini C, Judkins AR, et al. Clinicopathologic and genetic profile of intracranial marginal zone lymphoma: a primary low-grade CNS lymphoma that mimics meningioma. J Clin Oncol. 2005 Aug 20;23(24):5718–27. PMID:16009945
4104. Tumwine LK, Orem J, Kerchan P, et al. EBV, HHV8 and HIV in B cell non Hodgkin lymphoma in Kampala, Uganda. Infect Agent Cancer. 2010 Jun 30;5:12. PMID:20591151
4105. Turakhia S, Lanigan C, Hamadeh F, et al. Immunohistochemistry for BRAF V600E in the differential diagnosis of hairy cell leukemia vs other splenic B-cell lymphomas. Am J Clin Pathol. 2015 Jul;144(1):87–93. PMID:26071465
4106. Turesson I, Kovalchik SA, Pfeiffer RM, et al. Monoclonal gammopathy of undetermined significance and risk of lymphoid and myeloid malignancies: 728 cases followed up to 30 years in Sweden. Blood. 2014 Jan 16;123(3):338–45. PMID:24222331
4107. Turner RR, Martin J, Dorfman RF. Necrotizing lymphadenitis. A study of 30 cases. Am J Surg Pathol. 1983 Mar;7(2):115–23. PMID:6859386
4108. Turner SD, Inghirami G, Miranda RN, et al. Cell of origin and immunologic events in the pathogenesis of breast implant-associated anaplastic large-cell lymphoma. Am J Pathol. 2020 Jan;190(1):2–10. PMID:31610171
4109. Tursz T, Brouet JC, Flandrin G, et al. Clinical and pathologic features of Waldenström's macroglobulinemia in seven patients with serum monoclonal IgG or IgA. Am J Med. 1977 Oct;63(4):499–502. PMID:410294
4110. Twa DD, Chan FC, Ben-Neriah S, et al. Genomic rearrangements involving programmed death ligands are recurrent in primary mediastinal large B-cell lymphoma. Blood. 2014 Mar 27;123(13):2062–5. PMID:24497532
4111. Tzankov A, Bourgau C, Kaiser A, et al. Rare expression of T-cell markers in classical Hodgkin's lymphoma. Mod Pathol. 2005 Dec;18(12):1542–9. PMID:16056244
4112. Uccini S, Al-Jadiry MF, Scarpino S, et al. Epstein-Barr virus-positive diffuse large B-cell lymphoma in children: a disease reminiscent of Epstein-Barr virus-positive diffuse large B-cell lymphoma of the elderly. Hum Pathol. 2015 May;46(5):716–24. PMID:25704629
4113. Uckun FM, Sather HN, Gaynon PS, et al. Clinical features and treatment outcome of children with myeloid antigen positive acute lymphoblastic leukemia: a report from the Children's Cancer Group. Blood. 1997 Jul 1;90(1):28–35. PMID:9207434
4114. Uehara T, Masumoto J, Yoshizawa A, et al. IgG4-related disease-like fibrosis as an indicator of IgG4-related lymphadenopathy. Ann Diagn Pathol. 2013 Oct;17(5):416–20. PMID:23702322
4115. Ueno H. T follicular helper cells in human autoimmunity. Curr Opin Immunol. 2016 Dec;43:24–31. PMID:27588918
4116. Ueno H, Yoshida K, Shiozawa Y, et al. Landscape of driver mutations and their clinical impacts in pediatric B-cell precursor acute lymphoblastic leukemia. Blood Adv. 2020 Oct 27;4(20):5165–73. PMID:33095873
4117. Uhrmacher S, Schmidt C, Erdfelder F, et al. Use of the receptor tyrosine kinase-like orphan receptor 1 (ROR1) as a diagnostic tool in chronic lymphocytic leukemia (CLL). Leuk Res. 2011 Oct;35(10):1360–6. PMID:21531460
4118. UICC [Internet]. Geneva (Switzerland): Union for International Cancer Control; 2022. TNM Publications and Resources – Errata; updated 2022 Jan 25. Available from: https://www.uicc.org/resources/tnm/publications-resources.
4119. Uldrick TS, Little RF. How I treat classical Hodgkin lymphoma in patients infected with human immunodeficiency virus. Blood. 2015 Feb 19;125(8):1226–35. PMID:25499453
4120. Uldrick TS, Polizzotto MN, Aleman K, et al. High-dose zidovudine plus valganciclovir for Kaposi sarcoma herpesvirus-associated multicentric Castleman disease: a pilot study of virus-activated cytotoxic therapy. Blood. 2011 Jun 30;117(26):6977–86. PMID:21487108
4121. Uldrick TS, Polizzotto MN, Aleman K, et al. Rituximab plus liposomal doxorubicin in HIV-infected patients with KSHV-associated multicentric Castleman disease. Blood. 2014 Dec 4;124(24):3544–52. PMID:25331113
4122. Umehara H, Okazaki K, Kawa S, et al. The 2020 revised comprehensive diagnostic (RCD) criteria for IgG4-RD. Mod Rheumatol. 2021 May;31(3):529–33. PMID:33274670
4123. Umeki K, Umekita K, Hashikura Y, et al. Evaluation of line immunoassay to detect HTLV-1 infection in an endemic area, southwestern Japan; comparison with polymerase chain reaction and western blot. Clin Lab. 2017 Feb 1;63(2):227–33. PMID:28182361
4124. Unger S, Seidl M, Schmitt-Graeff A, et al. Ill-defined germinal centers and severely reduced plasma cells are histological hallmarks of lymphadenopathy in patients with common variable immunodeficiency. J Clin Immunol. 2014 Aug;34(6):615–26. PMID:24789743
4125. Ungewickell A, Bhaduri A, Rios E, et al. Genomic analysis of mycosis fungoides and Sézary syndrome identifies recurrent alterations in TNFR2. Nat Genet. 2015 Sep;47(9):1056–60. PMID:26258847
4126. Untanu RV, Back J, Appel B, et al. Variant histology, IgD and CD30 expression in low-risk pediatric nodular lymphocyte predominant Hodgkin lymphoma: a report from the Children's Oncology Group. Pediatr Blood Cancer. 2018 Jan;65(1). PMID:28802087
4127. Uppal G, Ly V, Wang ZX, et al. The utility of BRAF V600E mutation-specific antibody

VE1 for the diagnosis of hairy cell leukemia. Am J Clin Pathol. 2015 Jan;143(1):120–5. PMID:25511150
4128. Urayama KY, Jarrett RF, Hjalgrim H, et al. Genome-wide association study of classical Hodgkin lymphoma and Epstein-Barr virus status-defined subgroups. J Natl Cancer Inst. 2012 Feb 8;104(3):240–53. PMID:22286212
4129. Usmani SZ, Mitchell A, Waheed S, et al. Prognostic implications of serial 18-fluoro-deoxyglucose emission tomography in multiple myeloma treated with total therapy 3. Blood. 2013 Mar 7;121(10):1819–23. PMID:23305732
4130. Uzun S, Özcan Ö, Işık A, et al. Loss of CTNNB1 exon 3 in sclerosing angiomatoid nodular transformation of the spleen. Virchows Arch. 2021 Oct;479(4):747–54. PMID:33650044
4131. Vacca A, Ribatti D. Bone marrow angiogenesis in multiple myeloma. Leukemia. 2006 Feb;20(2):193–9. PMID:16357836
4132. Vachon CM, Kyle RA, Therneau TM, et al. Increased risk of monoclonal gammopathy in first-degree relatives of patients with multiple myeloma or monoclonal gammopathy of undetermined significance. Blood. 2009 Jul 23;114(4):785–90. PMID:19179466
4133. Vacquier VD, O'Dell DS. Concanavalin A inhibits the dispersion of the cortical granule contents of sand dollar eggs. Exp Cell Res. 1975 Feb;90(2):465–8. PMID:1112284
4134. Vaghefi P, Martin A, Prévot S, et al. Genomic imbalances in AIDS-related lymphomas: relation with tumoral Epstein-Barr virus status. AIDS. 2006 Nov 28;20(18):2285–91. PMID:17117014
4135. Vakiani E, Basso K, Klein U, et al. Genetic and phenotypic analysis of B-cell post-transplant lymphoproliferative disorders provides insights into disease biology. Hematol Oncol. 2008 Dec;26(4):199–211. PMID:18457340
4136. Vakiani E, Nandula SV, Subramaniyam S, et al. Cytogenetic analysis of B-cell post-transplant lymphoproliferations validates the World Health Organization classification and suggests inclusion of florid follicular hyperplasia as a precursor lesion. Hum Pathol. 2007 Feb;38(2):315–25. PMID:17134734
4137. Valbuena JR, Herling M, Admirand JH, et al. T-cell prolymphocytic leukemia involving extramedullary sites. Am J Clin Pathol. 2005 Mar;123(3):456–64. PMID:15716243
4138. Valera A, Colomo L, Martínez A, et al. ALK-positive large B-cell lymphomas express a terminal B-cell differentiation program and activated STAT3 but lack MYC rearrangements. Mod Pathol. 2013 Oct;26(10):1329–37. PMID:23599149
4139. Valera A, López-Guillermo A, Cardesa-Salzmann T, et al. MYC protein expression and genetic alterations have prognostic impact in patients with diffuse large B-cell lymphoma treated with immunochemotherapy. Haematologica. 2013 Oct;98(10):1554–62. PMID:23716551
4140. Vallianatou K, Brito-Babapulle V, Matutes E, et al. p53 gene deletion and trisomy 12 in hairy cell leukemia and its variant. Leuk Res. 1999 Nov;23(11):1041–5. PMID:10576509
4141. Vallois D, Dobay MP, Morin RD, et al. Activating mutations in genes related to TCR signaling in angioimmunoblastic and other follicular helper T-cell-derived lymphomas. Blood. 2016 Sep 15;128(11):1490–502. PMID:27369867
4142. van de Ven AAJM, Seidl M, Drendel V, et al. IgG4-related disease in autoimmune lymphoproliferative syndrome. Clin Immunol. 2017 Jul;180:97–9. PMID:28478106
4143. van den Berg A, Maggio E, Diepstra A, et al. Germline FAS gene mutation in a case of ALPS and NLP Hodgkin lymphoma. Blood. 2002 Feb 15;99(4):1492–4. PMID:11830507
4144. van den Berg A, Tamminga R, de Jong D, et al. FAS gene mutation in a case of autoimmune lymphoproliferative syndrome type IA with accumulation of gammadelta+ T cells. Am J Surg Pathol. 2003 Apr;27(4):546–53. PMID:12657942
4145. van den Brand M, Rijntjes J, Hebeda KM, et al. Recurrent mutations in genes involved in nuclear factor-κB signalling in nodal marginal zone lymphoma-diagnostic and therapeutic implications. Histopathology. 2017 Jan;70(2):174–84. PMID:27297871
4146. van den Brand M, van der Velden WJ, Diets IJ, et al. Clinical features of patients with nodal marginal zone lymphoma compared to follicular lymphoma: similar presentation, but differences in prognostic factors and rate of transformation. Leuk Lymphoma. 2016 Jul;57(7):1649–56. PMID:26694256
4147. van den Elshout-den Uyl D, Spoto CPE, de Boer M, et al. First report of IgG4 related disease primary presenting as vertebral bone marrow lesions. Front Immunol. 2019 Aug 13;10:1910. PMID:31456806
4148. van der Krogt JA, Bempt MV, Ferreiro JF, et al. Anaplastic lymphoma kinase-positive anaplastic large cell lymphoma with the variant RNF213-, ATIC- and TPM3-ALK fusions is characterized by copy number gain of the rearranged ALK gene. Haematologica. 2017 Sep;102(9):1605–16. PMID:28659337
4149. Van Der Nest BM, Leslie C, Joske D, et al. Peripheral T-cell lymphoma arising in patients with chronic lymphocytic leukemia. Am J Clin Pathol. 2019 Nov 4;152(6):818–27. PMID:31433844
4150. van der Veer A, Waanders E, Pieters R, et al. Independent prognostic value of BCR-ABL1-like signature and IKZF1 deletion, but not high CRLF2 expression, in children with B-cell precursor ALL. Blood. 2013 Oct 10;122(15):2622–9. PMID:23974192
4151. van der Veer A, Zaliova M, Mottadelli F, et al. IKZF1 status as a prognostic feature in BCR-ABL1-positive childhood ALL. Blood. 2014 Mar 13;123(11):1691–8. PMID:24366361
4152. van der Weyden L, Giotopoulos G, Rust AG, et al. Modeling the evolution of ETV6-RUNX1-induced B-cell precursor acute lymphoblastic leukemia in mice. Blood. 2011 Jul 28;118(4):1041–51. PMID:21628403
4153. van der Weyden L, Giotopoulos G, Wong K, et al. Somatic drivers of B-ALL in a model of ETV6-RUNX1; Pax5(+/-) leukemia. BMC Cancer. 2015 Aug 13;15:585. PMID:26269126
4154. van Dongen JJ, Lhermitte L, Böttcher S, et al. EuroFlow antibody panels for standardized n-dimensional flow cytometric immunophenotyping of normal, reactive and malignant leukocytes. Leukemia. 2012 Sep;26(9):1908–75. PMID:22552007
4155. van Dongen JJ, Seriu T, Panzer-Grümayer ER, et al. Prognostic value of minimal residual disease in acute lymphoblastic leukaemia in childhood. Lancet. 1998 Nov 28;352(9142):1731–8. PMID:9848348
4156. van Galen JC, Dukers DF, Giroth C, et al. Distinct expression patterns of polycomb oncoproteins and their binding partners during the germinal center reaction. Eur J Immunol. 2004 Jul;34(7):1870–81. PMID:15214035
4157. van Gorp J, Weiping L, Jacobse K, et al. Epstein-Barr virus in nasal T-cell lymphomas (polymorphic reticulosis/midline malignant reticulosis) in western China. J Pathol. 1994 Jun;173(2):81–7. PMID:7522272
4158. Van Heerden JA, Longo MF, Cardoza F, et al. The abdominal mass in the patient with tuberous sclerosis. Surgical implications and report of a case. Arch Surg. 1967 Aug;95(2):317–9. PMID:16097309
4159. van Keimpema M, Grüneberg LJ, Mokry M, et al. FOXP1 directly represses transcription of proapoptotic genes and cooperates with NF-κB to promote survival of human B cells. Blood. 2014 Nov 27;124(23):3431–40. PMID:25267198
4160. van Kester MS, Tensen CP, Vermeer MH, et al. Cutaneous anaplastic large cell lymphoma and peripheral T-cell lymphoma NOS show distinct chromosomal alterations and differential expression of chemokine receptors and apoptosis regulators. J Invest Dermatol. 2010 Feb;130(2):563–75. PMID:19710685
4161. Van Loo P, Tousseyn T, Vanhentenrijk V, et al. T-cell/histiocyte-rich large B-cell lymphoma shows transcriptional features suggestive of a tolerogenic host immune response. Haematologica. 2010 Mar;95(3):440–8. PMID:19797726
4162. van Maldegem F, van Dijk R, Wormhoudt TA, et al. The majority of cutaneous marginal zone B-cell lymphomas expresses class-switched immunoglobulins and develops in a T-helper type 2 inflammatory environment. Blood. 2008 Oct 15;112(8):3355–61. PMID:18687986
4163. van Maldegem F, Wormhoudt TA, Mulder MM, et al. Chlamydia psittaci-negative ocular adnexal marginal zone B-cell lymphomas have biased VH4-34 immunoglobulin gene expression and proliferate in a distinct inflammatory environment. Leukemia. 2012 Jul;26(7):1647–53. PMID:22382892
4164. Van Neer FJ, Toonstra J, Van Voorst Vader PC, et al. Lymphomatoid papulosis in children: a study of 10 children registered by the Dutch Cutaneous Lymphoma Working Group. Br J Dermatol. 2001 Feb;144(2):351–4. PMID:11251571
4165. van Rhee F, Oksenhendler E, Srkalovic G, et al. International evidence-based consensus diagnostic and treatment guidelines for unicentric Castleman disease. Blood Adv. 2020 Dec 8;4(23):6039–50. PMID:33284946
4166. van Rhee F, Voorhees P, Dispenzieri A, et al. International, evidence-based consensus treatment guidelines for idiopathic multicentric Castleman disease. Blood. 2018 Nov 15;132(20):2115–24. PMID:30181172
4167. van Rhee F, Wong RS, Munshi N, et al. Siltuximab for multicentric Castleman's disease: a randomised, double-blind, placebo-controlled trial. Lancet Oncol. 2014 Aug;15(9):966–74. PMID:25042199
4168. van Santen S, Jansen PM, Quint KD, et al. Plaque stage folliculotropic mycosis fungoides: histopathologic features and prognostic factors in a series of 40 patients. J Cutan Pathol. 2020 Mar;47(3):241–50. PMID:31755567
4169. van Santen S, Roach RE, van Doorn R, et al. Clinical staging and prognostic factors in folliculotropic mycosis fungoides. JAMA Dermatol. 2016 Sep 1;152(9):992–1000. PMID:27276223
4170. van Santen S, van Doorn R, Neelis KJ, et al. Recommendations for treatment in folliculotropic mycosis fungoides: report of the Dutch Cutaneous Lymphoma Group. Br J Dermatol. 2017 Jul;177(1):223–8. PMID:28132406
4171. Van Slambrouck C, Huh J, Suh C, et al. Diagnostic utility of STAT6YE361 expression in classical Hodgkin lymphoma and related entities. Mod Pathol. 2020 May;33(5):834–45. PMID:31822802
4172. van Stigt AC, Dik WA, Kamphuis LSJ, et al. What works when treating granulomatous disease in genetically undefined CVID? A systematic review. Front Immunol. 2020 Dec 17;11:606389. PMID:33391274
4173. Van Vlierberghe P, Pieters R, Beverloo HB, et al. Molecular-genetic insights in paediatric T-cell acute lymphoblastic leukaemia. Br J Haematol. 2008 Oct;143(2):153–68. PMID:18691165
4174. van Wanrooij RL, de Jong D, Langerak AW, et al. Novel variant of EATL evolving from mucosal γδ-T-cells in a patient with type I RCD. BMJ Open Gastroenterol. 2015 Jun 9;2(1):e000026. PMID:26462278
4175. van Wanrooij RL, Müller DM, Neefjes-Borst EA, et al. Optimal strategies to identify aberrant intra-epithelial lymphocytes in refractory coeliac disease. J Clin Immunol. 2014 Oct;34(7):828–35. PMID:25062848
4176. Van Arnam JS, Lim MS, Elenitoba-Johnson KSJ. Novel insights into the pathogenesis of T-cell lymphomas. Blood. 2018 May 24;131(21):2320–30. PMID:29666117
4177. Van Baeten C, Van Dorpe J. Splenic Epstein-Barr virus-associated inflammatory pseudotumor. Arch Pathol Lab Med. 2017 May;141(5):722–7. PMID:28447898
4178. Vandenberghe E, De Wolf-Peeters C, van den Oord J, et al. Translocation (11;14): a cytogenetic anomaly associated with B-cell lymphomas of non-follicle centre cell lineage. J Pathol. 1991 Jan;163(1):13–8. PMID:2002419
4179. van den Brand M, van Krieken JH. Recognizing nodal marginal zone lymphoma: recent advances and pitfalls. A systematic review. Haematologica. 2013 Jul;98(7):1003–13. PMID:23813646
4180. Vandermolen L, Rice L, Lynch EC. Plasma cell dyscrasia with marrow fibrosis. Clinicopathologic syndrome. Am J Med. 1985 Sep;79(3):297–302. PMID:4036981
4181. van Nierop K, de Groot C. Human follicular dendritic cells: function, origin and development. Semin Immunol. 2002 Aug;14(4):251–7. PMID:12163300
4182. van Rhee F, Greenway A, Stone K. Treatment of idiopathic Castleman disease. Hematol Oncol Clin North Am. 2018 Feb;32(1):89–106. PMID:29157622
4183. van Zelm MC, Condino-Neto A, Barbouche MR. Editorial: Primary immunodeficiencies worldwide. Front Immunol. 2020 Jan 22;10:3148. PMID:32038648
4184. Vaqué JP, Gómez-López G, Monsálvez V, et al. PLCG1 mutations in cutaneous T-cell lymphomas. Blood. 2014 Mar 27;123(13):2034–43. PMID:24497536
4185. Vardi A, Dagklis A, Scarfò L, et al. Immunogenetics shows that not all MBL are equal: the larger the clone, the more similar to CLL. Blood. 2013 May 30;121(22):4521–8. PMID:23596047
4186. Varettoni M, Boveri E, Zibellini S, et al. Clinical and molecular characteristics of lymphoplasmacytic lymphoma not associated with an IgM monoclonal protein: a multicentric study of the Rete Ematologica Lombarda (REL) network. Am J Hematol. 2019 Nov;94(11):1193–9. PMID:31378966
4187. Varettoni M, Zibellini S, Arcaini L, et al. MYD88 (L265P) mutation is an independent risk factor for progression in patients with IgM monoclonal gammopathy of undetermined significance. Blood. 2013 Sep 26;122(13):2284–5. PMID:24072850
4188. Vaskova M, Mejstrikova E, Kalina T, et al. Transfer of genomics information to flow cytometry: expression of CD27 and CD44 discriminates subtypes of acute lymphoblastic leukemia. Leukemia. 2005 May;19(5):876–8. PMID:15759032
4189. Vasmatzis G, Johnson SH, Knudson RA, et al. Genome-wide analysis reveals recurrent structural abnormalities of TP63 and other p53-related genes in peripheral T-cell lymphomas. Blood. 2012 Sep 13;120(11):2280–9. PMID:22855598
4190. Vater I, Montesinos-Rongen M, Schlesner M, et al. The mutational pattern of primary lymphoma of the central nervous system determined by whole-exome sequencing. Leukemia.

2015 Mar;29(3):677–85. PMID:25189415
4191. Vavassori S, Galson JD, Trück J, et al. Lymphadenopathy driven by TCR-Vγ8Vδ1 T-cell expansion in FAS-related autoimmune lymphoproliferative syndrome. Blood Adv. 2017 Jun 22;1(15):1101–6. PMID:29296752
4192. Vega F, Amador C, Chadburn A, et al. American Registry of Pathology Expert Opinions: Recommendations for the diagnostic workup of mature T cell neoplasms. Ann Diagn Pathol. 2020 Dec;49:151623. PMID:32947231
4193. Vega F, Amador C, Chadburn A, et al. Genetic profiling and biomarkers in peripheral T-cell lymphomas: current role in the diagnostic work-up. Mod Pathol. 2022 Mar;35(3):306–18. PMID:34584212
4194. Vega F, Chang CC, Medeiros LJ, et al. Plasmablastic lymphomas and plasmablastic plasma cell myelomas have nearly identical immunophenotypic profiles. Mod Pathol. 2005 Jun;18(6):806–15. PMID:15578069
4195. Vega F, Chang CC, Schwartz MR, et al. Atypical NK-cell proliferation of the gastrointestinal tract in a patient with antigliadin antibodies but not celiac disease. Am J Surg Pathol. 2006 Apr;30(4):539–44. PMID:16625103
4196. Vega F, Cho-Vega JH, Lennon PA, et al. Splenic marginal zone lymphomas are characterized by loss of interstitial regions of chromosome 7q, 7q31.32 and 7q36.2 that include the protection of telomere 1 (POT1) and sonic hedgehog (SHH) genes. Br J Haematol. 2008 Jun;142(2):216–26. PMID:18492102
4197. Vega F, Medeiros LJ, Bueso-Ramos C, et al. Hepatosplenic gamma/delta T-cell lymphoma in bone marrow. A sinusoidal neoplasm with blastic cytologic features. Am J Clin Pathol. 2001 Sep;116(3):410–9. PMID:11554170
4198. Vega F, Medeiros LJ, Gaulard P. Hepatosplenic and other gammadelta T-cell lymphomas. Am J Clin Pathol. 2007 Jun;127(6):869–80. PMID:17509984
4199. Vegliante MC, Palomero J, Pérez-Galán P, et al. SOX11 regulates PAX5 expression and blocks terminal B-cell differentiation in aggressive mantle cell lymphoma. Blood. 2013 Mar 21;121(12):2175–85. PMID:23321250
4200. Vela V, Juskevicius D, Dirnhofer S, et al. Mutational landscape of marginal zone B-cell lymphomas of various origin: organotypic alterations and diagnostic potential for assignment of organ origin. Virchows Arch. 2022 Feb;480(2):403–13. PMID:34494161
4201. Vela-Chávez T, Adam P, Kremer M, et al. Cyclin D1 positive diffuse large B-cell lymphoma is a post-germinal center-type lymphoma without alterations in the CCND1 gene locus. Leuk Lymphoma. 2011 Mar;52(3):458–66. PMID:21281227
4202. Velankar MM, Nathwani BN, Schlutz MJ, et al. Indolent T-lymphoblastic proliferation: report of a case with a 16-year course without cytotoxic therapy. Am J Surg Pathol. 1999 Aug;23(8):977–81. PMID:10435569
4203. Veloza L, Cavalieri D, Missiaglia E, et al. Monomorphic epitheliotropic intestinal T-cell lymphoma comprises morphologic and genomic heterogeneity impacting outcome. Haematologica. 2023 Jan 1;108(1):181–95. PMID:35708139
4204. Veloza L, Tsai CY, Bisig B, et al. EBV-positive large B-cell lymphoma with an unusual intravascular presentation and associated haemophagocytic syndrome in an HIV-positive patient: report of a case expanding the spectrum of EBV-positive immunodeficiency-associated lymphoproliferative disorders. Virchows Arch. 2022 Mar;480(3):699–705. PMID:34148126
4205. Velusamy T, Kiel MJ, Sahasrabuddhe AA, et al. A novel recurrent NPM1-TYK2 gene fusion in cutaneous CD30-positive lymphoproliferative disorders. Blood. 2014 Dec 11;124(25):3768–71. PMID:25349176
4206. Vempati P, Knoll MA, Alqatari M, et al. MALT lymphoma of the bladder: a case report and review of the literature. Case Rep Hematol. 2015;2015:934374. PMID:26417464
4207. Venkataraman G, Aguhar C, Kreitman RJ, et al. Characteristic CD103 and CD123 expression pattern defines hairy cell leukemia: usefulness of CD123 and CD103 in the diagnosis of mature B-cell lymphoproliferative disorders. Am J Clin Pathol. 2011 Oct;136(4):625–30. PMID:21917686
4208. Venkataraman G, McClain KL, Pittaluga S, et al. Development of disseminated histiocytic sarcoma in a patient with autoimmune lymphoproliferative syndrome and associated Rosai-Dorfman disease. Am J Surg Pathol. 2010 Apr;34(4):589–94. PMID:20216376
4209. Venkataraman G, Raffeld M, Pittaluga S, et al. CD15-expressing nodular lymphocyte-predominant Hodgkin lymphoma. Histopathology. 2011 Apr;58(5):803–5. PMID:21457163
4210. Venkataraman G, Rizzo KA, Chavez JJ, et al. Marginal zone lymphomas involving meningeal dura: possible link to IgG4-related diseases. Mod Pathol. 2011 Mar;24(3):355–66. PMID:21102421
4211. Venkataraman G, Song JY, Tzankov A, et al. Aberrant T-cell antigen expression in classical Hodgkin lymphoma is associated with decreased event-free survival and overall survival. Blood. 2013 Mar 7;121(10):1795–804. PMID:23305738
4212. Venturutti L, Melnick AM. The dangers of déjà vu: memory B cells as the cells of origin of ABC-DLBCLs. Blood. 2020 Nov 12;136(20):2263–74. PMID:32932517
4213. Venturutti L, Teater M, Zhai A, et al. TBL1XR1 mutations drive extranodal lymphoma by inducing a pro-tumorigenic memory fate. Cell. 2020 Jul 23;182(2):297–316.e27. PMID:32619424
4214. Verbeek WH, Goerres MS, von Blomberg BM, et al. Flow cytometric determination of aberrant intra-epithelial lymphocytes predicts T-cell lymphoma development more accurately than T-cell clonality analysis in refractory celiac disease. Clin Immunol. 2008 Jan;126(1):48–56. PMID:18024205
4215. Verbeek WH, Van De Water JM, Al-Toma A, et al. Incidence of enteropathy–associated T-cell lymphoma: a nation-wide study of a population-based registry in the Netherlands. Scand J Gastroenterol. 2008;43(11):1322–8. PMID:18618372
4216. Verbeek WH, von Blomberg BM, Coupe VM, et al. Aberrant T-lymphocytes in refractory coeliac disease are not strictly confined to a small intestinal intraepithelial localization. Cytometry B Clin Cytom. 2009 Nov;76(6):367–74. PMID:19444812
4217. Vergier B, Belaud-Rotureau MA, Benassy MN, et al. Neoplastic cells do not carry bcl2-JH rearrangements detected in a subset of primary cutaneous follicle center B-cell lymphomas. Am J Surg Pathol. 2004 Jun;28(6):748–55. PMID:15166666
4218. Vergneault H, Bengoufa D, Frazier-Mironer A, et al. Light chain proteinuria revealing mu-heavy chain disease: an atypical presentation of Waldenström macroglobulinemia in two cases. Haematologica. 2021 Jul 1;106(7):2034–6. PMID:33596645
4219. Verkarre V, Asnafi V, Lecomte T, et al. Refractory coeliac sprue is a diffuse gastrointestinal disease. Gut. 2003 Feb;52(2):205–11. PMID:12524401
4220. Verkarre V, Romana SP, Cellier C, et al. Recurrent partial trisomy 1q22-q44 in clonal intraepithelial lymphocytes in refractory celiac sprue. Gastroenterology. 2003 Jul;125(1):40–6. PMID:12851869
4221. Verma NK, Davies AM, Long A, et al. STAT3 knockdown by siRNA induces apoptosis in human cutaneous T-cell lymphoma line Hut78 via downregulation of Bcl-xL. Cell Mol Biol Lett. 2010 Jun;15(2):342–55. PMID:20213502
4222. Verma S, Frambach GE, Seilstad KH, et al. Epstein–Barr virus-associated B-cell lymphoma in the setting of iatrogenic immune dysregulation presenting initially in the skin. J Cutan Pathol. 2005 Aug;32(7):474–83. PMID:16008691
4223. Vermaat JS, Somers SF, de Wreede LC, et al. MYD88 mutations identify a molecular subgroup of diffuse large B-cell lymphoma with an unfavorable prognosis. Haematologica. 2020 Jan 31;105(2):424–34. PMID:31123031
4224. Vermeer MH, Geelen FA, van Haselen CW, et al. Primary cutaneous large B-cell lymphomas of the legs. A distinct type of cutaneous B-cell lymphoma with an intermediate prognosis. Arch Dermatol. 1996 Nov;132(11):1304–8. PMID:8915307
4225. Vermeer MH, van Doorn R, Dijkman R, et al. Novel and highly recurrent chromosomal alterations in Sézary syndrome. Cancer Res. 2008 Apr 15;68(8):2689–98. PMID:18413736
4226. Vermi W, Giurisato E, Lonardi S, et al. Ligand-dependent activation of EGFR in follicular dendritic cells sarcoma is sustained by local production of cognate ligands. Clin Cancer Res. 2013 Sep 15;19(18):5027–38. PMID:23888072
4227. Vermi W, Lonardi S, Bosisio D, et al. Identification of CXCL13 as a new marker for follicular dendritic cell sarcoma. J Pathol. 2008 Nov;216(3):356–64. PMID:18792075
4228. Vesely C, Frech C, Eckert C, et al. Genomic and transcriptional landscape of P2RY8-CRLF2-positive childhood acute lymphoblastic leukemia. Leukemia. 2017 Jul;31(7):1491–501. PMID:27899802
4229. Vidal R, Goñi F, Stevens F, et al. Somatic mutations of the L12a gene in V-kappa(1) light chain deposition disease: potential effects on aberrant protein conformation and deposition. Am J Pathol. 1999 Dec;155(6):2009–17. PMID:10595931
4230. Vigliar E, Cozzolino I, Picardi M, et al. Lymph node fine needle cytology in the staging and follow-up of cutaneous lymphomas. BMC Cancer. 2014 Jan 6;14:8. PMID:24393425
4231. Viglietti D, Sverzut JM, Peraldi MN. Perirenal fluid collections and monoclonal gammopathy. Nephrol Dial Transplant. 2012 Jan;27(1):448–9. PMID:21810768
4232. Vijai J, Wang Z, Berndt SI, et al. A genome-wide association study of marginal zone lymphoma shows association to the HLA region. Nat Commun. 2015 Jan 8;6:5751. PMID:25569183
4233. Villano JL, Koshy M, Shaikh H, et al. Age, gender, and racial differences in incidence and survival in primary CNS lymphoma. Br J Cancer. 2011 Oct 25;105(9):1414–8. PMID:21915121
4234. Villemagne B, Bay JO, Tournilhac O, et al. Two new cases of familial hairy cell leukemia associated with HLA haplotypes A2, B7, Bw4, Bw6. Leuk Lymphoma. 2005 Feb;46(2):243–5. PMID:15621808
4235. Viny AD, Lichtin A, Pohlman B, et al. Chronic B-cell dyscrasias are an important clinical feature of T-LGL leukemia. Leuk Lymphoma. 2008 May;49(5):932–8. PMID:18452068
4236. Viola P, Vroobel KM, Devaraj A, et al. Follicular dendritic cell tumour/sarcoma: a commonly misdiagnosed tumour in the thorax. Histopathology. 2016 Nov;69(5):752–61. PMID:27206572
4237. Virgilio L, Lazzeri C, Bichi R, et al. Deregulated expression of TCL1 causes T cell leukemia in mice. Proc Natl Acad Sci U S A. 1998 Mar 31;95(7):3885–9. PMID:9520462
4238. Virmani P, Jawed S, Myskowski PL, et al. Long-term follow-up and management of small and medium-sized CD4+ T cell lymphoma and CD8+ lymphoid proliferations of acral sites: a multicenter experience. Int J Dermatol. 2016 Nov;55(11):1248–54. PMID:27369070
4239. Visco C, Hoeller S, Malik JT, et al. Molecular characteristics of mantle cell lymphoma presenting with clonal plasma cell component. Am J Surg Pathol. 2011 Feb;35(2):177–89. PMID:21263238
4240. Visco C, Ruggeri M, Laura Evangelista M, et al. Impact of immune thrombocytopenia on the clinical course of chronic lymphocytic leukemia. Blood. 2008 Feb 1;111(3):1110–6. PMID:17986663
4241. Visser L, Rutgers B, Diepstra A, et al. Characterization of the microenvironment of nodular lymphocyte predominant Hodgkin lymphoma. Int J Mol Sci. 2016 Dec 16;17(12):2127. PMID:27999289
4242. Vitolo U, Chiappella A, Ferreri AJ, et al. First-line treatment for primary testicular diffuse large B-cell lymphoma with rituximab-CHOP, CNS prophylaxis, and contralateral testis irradiation: final results of an international phase II trial. J Clin Oncol. 2011 Jul 10;29(20):2766–72. PMID:21646602
4243. Vivian LF, Magnoli F, Campiotti L, et al. Composite follicular lymphoma and "early" (in situ and mantle zone growth pattern) mantle cell neoplasia: a rare entity with peculiar cytogenetic and clinical features. Pathol Res Pract. 2020 Sep;216(9):153067. PMID:32825940
4244. Vizcarra E, Martínez-Climent JA, Benet I, et al. Identification of two subgroups of mantle cell leukemia with distinct clinical and biological features. Hematol J. 2001;2(4):234–41. PMID:11920255
4245. Vogelsberg A, Steinhilber J, Mankel B, et al. Genetic evolution of in situ follicular neoplasia to aggressive B-cell lymphoma of germinal center subtype. Haematologica. 2021 Oct 1;106(10):2673–81. PMID:32855278
4246. Vogelstein B, Lane D, Levine AJ. Surfing the p53 network. Nature. 2000 Nov 16;408(6810):307–10. PMID:11099028
4247. Vogt J, Wagener R, Montesinos-Rongen M, et al. Array-based profiling of the lymphoma cell DNA methylome does not unequivocally distinguish primary lymphomas of the central nervous system from non-CNS diffuse large B-cell lymphomas. Genes Chromosomes Cancer. 2019 Jan;58(1):66–9. PMID:30284345
4248. Vogt N, Klapper W. Variability in morphology and cell proliferation in sequential biopsies of mantle cell lymphoma at diagnosis and relapse: clinical correlation and insights into disease progression. Histopathology. 2013 Jan;62(2):334–42. PMID:23240716
4249. Volaric A, Bacchi CE, Gru AA. PD-1 and PD-L1 immunohistochemistry as a diagnostic tool for classic Hodgkin lymphoma in small-volume biopsies. Am J Surg Pathol. 2020 Oct;44(10):1353–66. PMID:32649320
4250. Volk T, Pannicke U, Reisli I, et al. DCLRE1C (ARTEMIS) mutations causing phenotypes ranging from atypical severe combined immunodeficiency to mere antibody deficiency. Hum Mol Genet. 2015 Dec 20;24(25):7361–72. PMID:26476407
4251. Völkl S, Rensing-Ehl A, Allgäuer A, et al. Hyperactive mTOR pathway promotes lymphoproliferation and abnormal differentiation in autoimmune lymphoproliferative syndrome. Blood. 2016 Jul 14;128(2):227–38. PMID:27099149
4252. Voltin CA, Goergen H, Baues C, et al. Value of bone marrow biopsy in Hodgkin lymphoma patients staged by FDG PET: results from the German Hodgkin Study Group trials HD16, HD17, and HD18. Ann Oncol. 2018 Sep

1;29(9):1926–31. PMID:30010775
4253. Vonderheid EC, Pena J, Nowell P. Sézary cell counts in erythrodermic cutaneous T-cell lymphoma: implications for prognosis and staging. Leuk Lymphoma. 2006 Sep;47(9):1841–56. PMID:17064997
4254. von Holstein SL, Rasmussen PK, Heegaard S. Tumors of the lacrimal gland. Semin Diagn Pathol. 2016 May;33(3):156–63. PMID:26849904
4255. Voorhees TJ, Ghosh N, Grover N, et al. Long-term remission in multiply relapsed enteropathy-associated T-cell lymphoma following CD30 CAR T-cell therapy. Blood Adv. 2020 Dec 8;4(23):5925–8. PMID:33259598
4256. Vos JM, Gustine J, Rennke HG, et al. Renal disease related to Waldenström macroglobulinaemia: incidence, pathology and clinical outcomes. Br J Haematol. 2016 Nov;175(4):623–30. PMID:27468978
4257. Vose J, Armitage J, Weisenburger D. International peripheral T-cell and natural killer/T-cell lymphoma study: pathology findings and clinical outcomes. J Clin Oncol. 2008 Sep 1;26(25):4124–30. PMID:18626005
4258. Vrana JA, Gamez JD, Madden BJ, et al. Classification of amyloidosis by laser microdissection and mass spectrometry-based proteomic analysis in clinical biopsy specimens. Blood. 2009 Dec 3;114(24):4957–9. PMID:19797517
4259. Vremec D, O'Keeffe M, Hochrein H, et al. Production of interferons by dendritic cells, plasmacytoid cells, natural killer cells, and interferon-producing killer dendritic cells. Blood. 2007 Feb 1;109(3):1165–73. PMID:17038535
4260. Wada DA, Law ME, Hsi ED, et al. Specificity of IRF4 translocations for primary cutaneous anaplastic large cell lymphoma: a multicenter study of 204 skin biopsies. Mod Pathol. 2011 Apr;24(4):596–605. PMID:21169992
4261. Wada H, Masuda K, Satoh R, et al. Adult T-cell progenitors retain myeloid potential. Nature. 2008 Apr 10;452(7188):768–72. PMID:18401412
4262. Wada T, Toga A, Sakakibara Y, et al. Clonal expansion of Epstein-Barr virus (EBV)-infected γδ T cells in patients with chronic active EBV disease and hydroa vacciniforme-like eruptions. Int J Hematol. 2012 Oct;96(4):443–9. PMID:22886572
4263. Wada T, Toma T, Miyazawa H, et al. Characterization of skin blister fluids from children with Epstein-Barr virus-associated lymphoproliferative disease. J Dermatol. 2018 Apr;45(4):444–9. PMID:29352500
4264. Wagener R, Bens S, Toprak UH, et al. Cryptic insertion of MYC exons 2 and 3 into the immunoglobulin heavy chain locus detected by whole genome sequencing in a case of "MYC-negative" Burkitt lymphoma. Haematologica. 2020 Apr;105(4):e202–5. PMID:31073073
4265. Wagener R, López C, Kleinheinz K, et al. IG-MYC + neoplasms with precursor B-cell phenotype are molecularly distinct from Burkitt lymphomas. Blood. 2018 Nov 22;132(21):2280–5. PMID:30282799
4266. Wagener R, Seufert J, Raimondi F, et al. The mutational landscape of Burkitt-like lymphoma with 11q aberration is distinct from that of Burkitt lymphoma. Blood. 2019 Feb 28;133(9):962–6. PMID:30567752
4267. Wagner-Johnston ND, Link BK, Byrtek M, et al. Outcomes of transformed follicular lymphoma in the modern era: a report from the National LymphoCare Study (NLCS). Blood. 2015 Aug 13;126(7):851–7. PMID:26105149
4268. Wahlin BE, Yri OE, Kimby E, et al. Clinical significance of the WHO grades of follicular lymphoma in a population-based cohort of 505 patients with long follow-up times. Br J Haematol. 2012 Jan;156(2):225–33. PMID:22126847
4269. Wahner-Roedler DL, Kyle RA. Heavy chain diseases. Best Pract Res Clin Haematol. 2005;18(4):729–46. PMID:16026747
4270. Wahner-Roedler DL, Kyle RA. Mu-heavy chain disease: presentation as a benign monoclonal gammopathy. Am J Hematol. 1992 May;40(1):56–60. PMID:1566748
4271. Wahner-Roedler DL, Witzig TE, Loehrer LL, et al. Gamma-heavy chain disease: review of 23 cases. Medicine (Baltimore). 2003 Jul;82(4):236–50. PMID:12861101
4272. Wahnschaffe L, Braun T, Timonen S, et al. JAK/STAT-activating genomic alterations are a hallmark of T-PLL. Cancers (Basel). 2019 Nov 21;11(12):1833. PMID:31766351
4273. Wai CMM, Chen S, Phyu T, et al. Immune pathway upregulation and lower genomic instability distinguish EBV-positive nodal T/NK-cell lymphoma from ENKTL and PTCL-NOS. Haematologica. 2022 Aug 1;107(8):1864–79. PMID:35021606
4274. Wakely PE Jr, Kornstein MJ. Aspiration cytopathology of lymphoblastic lymphoma and leukemia: the MCV experience. Pediatr Pathol Lab Med. 1996 Mar-Apr;16(2):243–52. PMID:9025830
4275. Waldmann TA, Chen J. Disorders of the JAK/STAT pathway in T cell lymphoma pathogenesis: implications for immunotherapy. Annu Rev Immunol. 2017 Apr 26;35:533–50. PMID:28182501
4276. Walker BA, Leone PE, Chiecchio L, et al. A compendium of myeloma-associated chromosomal copy number abnormalities and their prognostic value. Blood. 2010 Oct 14;116(15):e56–65. PMID:20616218
4277. Walker BA, Mavrommatis K, Wardell CP, et al. A high-risk, double-hit, group of newly diagnosed myeloma identified by genomic analysis. Leukemia. 2019 Jan;33(1):159–70. PMID:29967379
4278. Walker BA, Mavrommatis K, Wardell CP, et al. Identification of novel mutational drivers reveals oncogene dependencies in multiple myeloma. Blood. 2018 Aug 9;132(6):587–97. PMID:29884741
4279. Walker BA, Wardell CP, Melchor L, et al. Intraclonal heterogeneity is a critical early event in the development of myeloma and precedes the development of clinical symptoms. Leukemia. 2014 Feb;28(2):384–90. PMID:23817176
4280. Walker CJ, Martinez-Escala ME, Tan TL, et al. High incidence of adnexotropism in cytotoxic cutaneous lymphomas. J Cutan Pathol. 2021 Oct;48(10):1231–8. PMID:33759218
4281. Walker JN, Hanson BM, Pinkner CL, et al. Insights into the microbiome of breast implants and periprosthetic tissue in breast implant-associated anaplastic large cell lymphoma. Sci Rep. 2019 Jul 17;9(1):10393. PMID:31316085
4282. Wallace ZS, Deshpande V, Mattoo H, et al. IgG4-related disease: clinical and laboratory features in one hundred twenty-five patients. Arthritis Rheumatol. 2015 Sep;67(9):2466–75. PMID:25988916
4283. Wallace ZS, Zhang Y, Perugino CA, et al. Clinical phenotypes of IgG4-related disease: an analysis of two international cross-sectional cohorts. Ann Rheum Dis. 2019 Mar;78(3):406–12. PMID:30612117
4284. Walters M, Pittelkow MR, Hasserjian RP, et al. Follicular dendritic cell sarcoma with indolent T-lymphoblastic proliferation is associated with paraneoplastic autoimmune multiorgan syndrome. Am J Surg Pathol. 2018 Dec;42(12):1647–52. PMID:30222603
4285. Wang C, McKeithan TW, Gong Q, et al. IDH2R172 mutations define a unique subgroup of patients with angioimmunoblastic T-cell lymphoma. Blood. 2015 Oct 8;126(15):1741–52. PMID:26268241
4286. Wang C, Zhou YL, Cai H, et al. Markedly elevated serum total N-terminal propeptide of type I collagen is a novel marker for the diagnosis and follow up of patients with POEMS syndrome. Haematologica. 2014 Jun;99(6):e78–80. PMID:24658817
4287. Wang CC, Tien HF, Lin MT, et al. Consistent presence of isochromosome 7q in hepatosplenic T gamma/delta lymphoma: a new cytogenetic-clinicopathologic entity. Genes Chromosomes Cancer. 1995 Mar;12(3):161–4. PMID:7536454
4288. Wang GN, Cui Y, Zhao WG, et al. Clinicopathological analysis of the hydroa vacciniforme-like lymphoproliferative disorder with natural killer cell phenotype compared with cutaneous natural killer T-cell lymphoma. Exp Ther Med. 2018 Dec;16(6):4772–8. PMID:30542432
4289. Wang HH, Myers T, Lach LJ, et al. Increased risk of lymphoid and nonlymphoid malignancies in patients with lymphomatoid papulosis. Cancer. 1999 Oct 1;86(7):1240–5. PMID:10506709
4290. Wang HP, Zhou YL, Huang X, et al. CDKN2A deletions are associated with poor outcomes in 101 adults with T-cell acute lymphoblastic leukemia. Am J Hematol. 2021 Mar 1;96(3):312–9. PMID:33306218
4291. Wang HW, Balakrishna JP, Pittaluga S, et al. Diagnosis of Hodgkin lymphoma in the modern era. Br J Haematol. 2019 Jan;184(1):45–59. PMID:30407610
4292. Wang HW, Lin P. Flow cytometric immunophenotypic analysis in the diagnosis and prognostication of plasma cell neoplasms. Cytometry B Clin Cytom. 2019 Sep;96(5):338–50. PMID:31566910
4293. Wang HW, Raffeld M. Molecular assessment of clonality in lymphoid neoplasms. Semin Hematol. 2019 Jan;56(1):37–45. PMID:30573043
4294. Wang J, Bu DF, Li T, et al. Autoantibody production from a thymoma and a follicular dendritic cell sarcoma associated with paraneoplastic pemphigus. Br J Dermatol. 2005 Sep;153(3):558–64. PMID:16120143
4295. Wang JH, Wang L, Liu CC, et al. Efficacy of combined gemcitabine, oxaliplatin and pegaspargase (P-gemox regimen) in patients with newly diagnosed advanced-stage or relapsed/refractory extranodal NK/T-cell lymphoma. Oncotarget. 2016 May 17;7(20):29092–101. PMID:27093153
4296. Wang JJ, Dong M, He XH, et al. GDP (gemcitabine, dexamethasone, and cisplatin) is highly effective and well-tolerated for newly diagnosed stage IV and relapsed/refractory extranodal natural killer/T-cell lymphoma, nasal type. Medicine (Baltimore). 2016 Feb;95(6):e2787. PMID:26871836
4297. Wang L, Li C, Gao T. Cutaneous intravascular anaplastic large cell lymphoma. J Cutan Pathol. 2011 Feb;38(2):221–6. PMID:20337769
4298. Wang L, Ni X, Covington KR, et al. Genomic profiling of Sézary syndrome identifies alterations of key T cell signaling and differentiation genes. Nat Genet. 2015 Dec;47(12):1426–34. PMID:26551670
4299. Wang L, Tang G, Medeiros LJ, et al. MYC rearrangement but not extra MYC copies is an independent prognostic factor in patients with mantle cell lymphoma. Haematologica. 2021 May 1;106(5):1381–9. PMID:32273477
4300. Wang L, Wang H, Li PF, et al. CD38 expression predicts poor prognosis and might be a potential therapy target in extranodal NK/T cell lymphoma, nasal type. Ann Hematol. 2015 Aug;94(8):1381–8. PMID:25865943
4301. Wang S, Medeiros LJ, Xu-Monette ZY, et al. Epstein-Barr virus-positive nodular lymphocyte predominant Hodgkin lymphoma. Ann Diagn Pathol. 2014 Aug;18(4):203–9. PMID:24852241
4302. Wang SA, Wang L, Hochberg EP, et al. Low histologic grade follicular lymphoma with high proliferation index: morphologic and clinical features. Am J Surg Pathol. 2005 Nov;29(11):1490–6. PMID:16224216
4303. Wang SS, Deapen D, Voutsinas J, et al. Breast implants and anaplastic large cell lymphomas among females in the California Teachers Study cohort. Br J Haematol. 2016 Aug;174(3):480–3. PMID:26456010
4304. Wang T, Chen X, Chen W, et al. A retrospective study of 44 patients with head and neck Castleman's disease. Eur Arch Otorhinolaryngol. 2022 May;279(5):2625–30. PMID:34480599
4305. Wang T, Feldman AL, Wada DA, et al. GATA-3 expression identifies a high-risk subset of PTCL, NOS with distinct molecular and clinical features. Blood. 2014 May 8;123(19):3007–15. PMID:24497534
4306. Wang V, Davis DA, Deleage C, et al. Induction of Kaposi's sarcoma-associated herpesvirus-encoded thymidine kinase (ORF21) by X-box binding protein 1. J Virol. 2020 Feb 14;94(5):e01555-19. PMID:31801863
4307. Wang W, Kanagal-Shamanna R, Medeiros LJ. Lymphoproliferative disorders with concurrent HHV8 and EBV infection: beyond primary effusion lymphoma and germinotropic lymphoproliferative disorder. Histopathology. 2018 Apr;72(5):855–61. PMID:29105119
4308. Wang W, Medeiros LJ. Castleman disease. Surg Pathol Clin. 2019 Sep;12(3):849–63. PMID:31352991
4309. Wang X, Asplund AC, Porwit A, et al. The subcellular Sox11 distribution pattern identifies subsets of mantle cell lymphoma: correlation to overall survival. Br J Haematol. 2008 Oct;143(2):248–52. PMID:18729857
4310. Wang X, Miao Y, Cao Z, et al. Characterization of molecular genetics and clinicopathology in thymic MALT lymphoma. Ann Hematol. 2022 Jan;101(1):91–7. PMID:34605949
4311. Wang XJ, Medeiros LJ, Lin P, et al. MYC cytogenetic status correlates with expression and has prognostic significance in patients with MYC/BCL2 protein double-positive diffuse large B-cell lymphoma. Am J Surg Pathol. 2015 Sep;39(9):1250–8. PMID:25828389
4312. Wang Y, Li T, Tu P, et al. Primary cutaneous aggressive epidermotropic CD8+ cytotoxic T-cell lymphoma clinically simulating pyoderma gangrenosum. Clin Exp Dermatol. 2009 Oct;34(7):e261–2. PMID:19438529
4313. Wang Y, Sinha S, Wellik LE, et al. Distinct immune signatures in chronic lymphocytic leukemia and Richter syndrome. Blood Cancer J. 2021 May 10;11(5):86. PMID:33972504
4314. Wang Y, Wenzl K, Manske MK, et al. Amplification of 9p24.1 in diffuse large B-cell lymphoma identifies a unique subset of cases that resemble primary mediastinal large B-cell lymphoma. Blood Cancer J. 2019 Aug 30;9(9):73. PMID:31471540
4315. Wang Y, Xue YJ, Lu AD, et al. Long-term results of the risk-stratified treatment of TCF3-PBX1-positive pediatric acute lymphoblastic leukemia in China. Clin Lymphoma Myeloma Leuk. 2021 Feb;21(2):e137–44. PMID:33221150
4316. Wang Z, Cook JR. IRTA1 and MNDA expression in marginal zone lymphoma: utility in differential diagnosis and implications for classification. Am J Clin Pathol. 2019 Feb 4;151(3):337–43. PMID:30346478
4317. Wang Z, Kimura S, Iwasaki H, et al. Clinicopathological findings of systemic Epstein-Barr virus-positive T-lymphoproliferative

diseases in younger and older adults. Diagn Pathol. 2021 Jun 4;16(1):48. PMID:34088321
4318. Wang Z, Zhang L, Zhang B, et al. Hemangioendothelioma arising from the spleen: a case report and literature review. Oncol Lett. 2015 Jan;9(1):209–12. PMID:25435960
4319. Wang ZM, Xiao WB, Zheng SS, et al. Hepatocellular carcinoma with indolent T-lymphoblastic proliferation. Leuk Lymphoma. 2006 Nov;47(11):2424–6. PMID:17107923
4320. Ward ZJ, Yeh JM, Bhakta N, et al. Estimating the total incidence of global childhood cancer: a simulation-based analysis. Lancet Oncol. 2019 Apr;20(4):483–93. PMID:30824204
4321. Warsame R, Gertz MA, Lacy MQ, et al. Trends and outcomes of modern staging of solitary plasmacytoma of bone. Am J Hematol. 2012 Jul;87(7):647–51. PMID:22549792
4322. Wasco MJ, Fullen D, Su L, et al. The expression of MUM1 in cutaneous T-cell lymphoproliferative disorders. Hum Pathol. 2008 Apr;39(4):557–63. PMID:18234282
4323. Washington K, Stenzel TT, Buckley RH, et al. Gastrointestinal pathology in patients with common variable immunodeficiency and X-linked agammaglobulinemia. Am J Surg Pathol. 1996 Oct;20(10):1240–52. PMID:8827031
4324. Wasman J, Rosenthal NS, Farhi DC. Mantle cell lymphoma. Morphologic findings in bone marrow involvement. Am J Clin Pathol. 1996 Aug;106(2):196–200. PMID:8712173
4325. Wass M, Behlendorf T, Schädlich B, et al. Crizotinib in refractory ALK-positive diffuse large B-cell lymphoma: a case report with a short-term response. Eur J Haematol. 2014 Mar;92(3):268–70. PMID:24330038
4326. Watanabe N, Noh JY, Narimatsu H, et al. Clinicopathological features of 171 cases of primary thyroid lymphoma: a long-term study involving 24553 patients with Hashimoto's disease. Br J Haematol. 2011 Apr;153(2):236–43. PMID:21371004
4327. Watatani Y, Sato Y, Miyoshi H, et al. Molecular heterogeneity in peripheral T-cell lymphoma, not otherwise specified revealed by comprehensive genetic profiling. Leukemia. 2019 Dec;33(12):2867–83. PMID:31092896
4328. Waterfall JJ, Arons E, Walker RL, et al. High prevalence of MAP2K1 mutations in variant and IGHV4-34-expressing hairy-cell leukemias. Nat Genet. 2014 Jan;46(1):8–10. PMID:24241536
4329. Watkins AJ, Hamoudi RA, Zeng N, et al. An integrated genomic and expression analysis of 7q deletion in splenic marginal zone lymphoma. PLoS One. 2012;7(9):e44997. PMID:23028731
4330. Watkins AJ, Huang Y, Ye H, et al. Splenic marginal zone lymphoma: characterization of 7q deletion and its value in diagnosis. J Pathol. 2010 Mar;220(4):461–74. PMID:20077527
4331. Webber SA, Naftel DC, Fricker FJ, et al. Lymphoproliferative disorders after paediatric heart transplantation: a multi-institutional study. Lancet. 2006 Jan 21;367(9506):233–9. PMID:16427492
4332. Weber DM. Solitary bone and extramedullary plasmacytoma. Hematology Am Soc Hematol Educ Program. 2005:373–6. PMID:16304406
4333. Weber-Matthiesen K, Deerberg J, Poetsch M, et al. Numerical chromosome aberrations are present within the CD30+ Hodgkin and Reed-Sternberg cells in 100% of analyzed cases of Hodgkin's disease. Blood. 1995 Aug 15;86(4):1464–8. PMID:7632954
4334. Wechalekar AD, Gillmore JD, Hawkins PN. Systemic amyloidosis. Lancet. 2016 Jun 25;387(10038):2641–54. PMID:26719234
4335. Wechalekar AD, Schonland SO, Kastritis E, et al. A European collaborative study of treatment outcomes in 346 patients with cardiac stage III AL amyloidosis. Blood. 2013 Apr 25;121(17):3420–7. PMID:23479568
4336. Wegehaupt O, Groß M, Wehr C, et al. TIM-3 deficiency presenting with two clonally unrelated episodes of mesenteric and subcutaneous panniculitis-like T-cell lymphoma and hemophagocytic lymphohistiocytosis. Pediatr Blood Cancer. 2020 Jun;67(6):e28302. PMID:32285995
4337. Wehkamp U, Pott C, Unterhalt M, et al. Skin involvement of mantle cell lymphoma may mimic primary cutaneous diffuse large B-cell lymphoma, leg type. Am J Surg Pathol. 2015 Aug;39(8):1093–101. PMID:26034867
4338. Wehr C, Houet L, Unger S, et al. Altered spectrum of lymphoid neoplasms in a single-center cohort of common variable immunodeficiency with immune dysregulation. J Clin Immunol. 2021 Aug;41(6):1250–65. PMID:33876323
4339. Wehr C, Kivioja T, Schmitt C, et al. The EUROclass trial: defining subgroups in common variable immunodeficiency. Blood. 2008 Jan 1;111(1):77–85. PMID:17898316
4340. Wei XJ, Zhou XG, Xie JL, et al. Aberrant phenotypes in Kikuchi's disease. Int J Clin Exp Pathol. 2014 Aug 15;7(9):5557–63. PMID:25337197
4341. Weidmann E. Hepatosplenic T cell lymphoma. A review on 45 cases since the first report describing the disease as a distinct lymphoma entity in 1990. Leukemia. 2000 Jun;14(6):991–7. PMID:10865963
4342. Weigert O, Kopp N, Lane AA, et al. Molecular ontogeny of donor-derived follicular lymphomas occurring after hematopoietic cell transplantation. Cancer Discov. 2012 Jan;2(1):47–55. PMID:22585168
4343. Weigert O, Weinstock DM. The promises and challenges of using gene mutations for patient stratification in follicular lymphoma. Blood. 2017 Sep 28;130(13):1491–8. PMID:28784599
4344. Weilemann A, Grau M, Erdmann T, et al. Essential role of IRF4 and MYC signaling for survival of anaplastic large cell lymphoma. Blood. 2015 Jan 1;125(1):124–32. PMID:25359993
4345. Weinberg OK, Ma L, Seo K, et al. Low stage follicular lymphoma: biologic and clinical characterization according to nodal or extranodal primary origin. Am J Surg Pathol. 2009 Apr;33(4):591–8. PMID:19065102
4346. Weisenburger DD, Savage KJ, Harris NL, et al. Peripheral T-cell lymphoma, not otherwise specified: a report of 340 cases from the International Peripheral T-cell Lymphoma Project. Blood. 2011 Mar 24;117(12):3402–8. PMID:21270441
4347. Weiss BM, Abadie J, Verma P, et al. A monoclonal gammopathy precedes multiple myeloma in most patients. Blood. 2009 May 28;113(22):5418–22. PMID:19234139
4348. Weiss LM, Berry GJ, Dorfman RF, et al. Spindle cell neoplasms of lymph nodes of probable reticulum cell lineage. True reticulum cell sarcoma? Am J Surg Pathol. 1990 May;14(5):405–14. PMID:2158241
4349. Weiss LM, Movahed LA, Warnke RA, et al. Detection of Epstein-Barr viral genomes in Reed-Sternberg cells of Hodgkin's disease. N Engl J Med. 1989 Feb 23;320(8):502–6. PMID:2536894
4350. Weiss SW, Gnepp DR, Bratthauer GL. Palisaded myofibroblastoma. A benign mesenchymal tumor of lymph node. Am J Surg Pathol. 1989 May;13(5):341–6. PMID:2712186
4351. Wellmann A, Thieblemont C, Pittaluga S, et al. Detection of differentially expressed genes in lymphomas using cDNA arrays: identification of clusterin as a new diagnostic marker for anaplastic large-cell lymphomas. Blood. 2000 Jul 15;96(2):398–404. PMID:10887098
4352. Wells J, Jain N, Konopleva M. Philadelphia chromosome-like acute lymphoblastic leukemia: progress in a new cancer subtype. Clin Adv Hematol Oncol. 2017 Jul;15(7):554–61. PMID:28749919
4353. Weng AP, Ferrando AA, Lee W, et al. Activating mutations of NOTCH1 in human T cell acute lymphoblastic leukemia. Science. 2004 Oct 8;306(5694):269–71. PMID:15472075
4354. Weng AP, Millholland JM, Yashiro-Ohtani Y, et al. c-Myc is an important direct target of Notch1 in T-cell acute lymphoblastic leukemia/lymphoma. Genes Dev. 2006 Aug 1;20(15):2096–109. PMID:16847353
4355. Weniger MA, Gesk S, Ehrlich S, et al. Gains of REL in primary mediastinal B-cell lymphoma coincide with nuclear accumulation of REL protein. Genes Chromosomes Cancer. 2007 Apr;46(4):406–15. PMID:17243160
4356. Weniger MA, Küppers R. Molecular biology of Hodgkin lymphoma. Leukemia. 2021 Apr;35(4):968–81. PMID:33686198
4357. Weniger MA, Melzner I, Menz CK, et al. Mutations of the tumor suppressor gene SOCS-1 in classical Hodgkin lymphoma are frequent and associated with nuclear phospho-STAT5 accumulation. Oncogene. 2006 Apr 27;25(18):2679–84. PMID:16532038
4358. Went M, Sud A, Försti A, et al. Identification of multiple risk loci and regulatory mechanisms influencing susceptibility to multiple myeloma. Nat Commun. 2018 Sep 13;9(1):3707. PMID:30213928
4359. Went P, Agostinelli C, Gallamini A, et al. Marker expression in peripheral T-cell lymphoma: a proposed clinical-pathologic prognostic score. J Clin Oncol. 2006 Jun 1;24(16):2472–9. PMID:16636342
4360. Wenzel C, Dieckmann K, Fiebiger W, et al. CD5 expression in a lymphoma of the mucosa-associated lymphoid tissue (MALT)-type as a marker for early dissemination and aggressive clinical behaviour. Leuk Lymphoma. 2001 Aug;42(4):823–9. PMID:11697516
4361. Werner B, Massone C, Kerl H, et al. Large CD30-positive cells in benign, atypical lymphoid infiltrates of the skin. J Cutan Pathol. 2008 Dec;35(12):1100–7. PMID:18616762
4362. Wetzler M, Dodge RK, Mrózek K, et al. Additional cytogenetic abnormalities in adults with Philadelphia chromosome-positive acute lymphoblastic leukaemia: a study of the Cancer and Leukaemia Group B. Br J Haematol. 2004 Feb;124(3):275–88. PMID:14717774
4363. Whitaker JA, Parikh SA, Shanafelt TD, et al. The humoral immune response to high-dose influenza vaccine in persons with monoclonal B-cell lymphocytosis (MBL) and chronic lymphocytic leukemia (CLL). Vaccine. 2021 Feb 12;39(7):1122–30. PMID:33461835
4364. White RE, Rämer PC, Naresh KN, et al. EBNA3B-deficient EBV promotes B cell lymphomagenesis in humanized mice and is found in human tumors. J Clin Invest. 2012 Apr;122(4):1487–502. PMID:22406538
4365. Whittaker SJ, Smith NP. Diagnostic value of T-cell receptor beta gene rearrangement analysis on peripheral blood lymphocytes of patients with erythroderma. J Invest Dermatol. 1992 Sep;99(3):361–2. PMID:1324964
4366. Whittaker SJ, Smith NP, Jones RR, et al. Analysis of beta, gamma, and delta T-cell receptor genes in mycosis fungoides and Sezary syndrome. Cancer. 1991 Oct 1;68(7):1572–82. PMID:1654197
4367. WHO. Technical Report: Human T-lymphotropic virus type 1. Geneva (Switzerland): WHO; 2021. Available from: https://apps.who.int/iris/handle/10665/339773.
4368. Wick MR, Scheithauer BW, Smith SL, et al. Primary nonlymphoreticular malignant neoplasms of the spleen. Am J Surg Pathol. 1982 Apr;6(3):229–42. PMID:6285748
4369. Wiemels JL, Cazzaniga G, Daniotti M, et al. Prenatal origin of acute lymphoblastic leukaemia in children. Lancet. 1999 Oct 30;354(9189):1499–503. PMID:10551495
4370. Wieser I, Oh CW, Talpur R, et al. Lymphomatoid papulosis: treatment response and associated lymphomas in a study of 180 patients. J Am Acad Dermatol. 2016 Jan;74(1):59–67. PMID:26518172
4371. Wieser I, Wohlmuth C, Nunez CA, et al. Lymphomatoid papulosis in children and adolescents: a systematic review. Am J Clin Dermatol. 2016 Aug;17(4):319–27. PMID:27138554
4372. Wiestner A, Tehrani M, Chiorazzi M, et al. Point mutations and genomic deletions in CCND1 create stable truncated cyclin D1 mRNAs that are associated with increased proliferation rate and shorter survival. Blood. 2007 Jun 1;109(11):4599–606. PMID:17299095
4373. Wilcox RA. Cutaneous B-cell lymphomas: 2019 update on diagnosis, risk stratification, and management. Am J Hematol. 2018 Nov;93(11):1427–30. PMID:30039522
4374. Wilks R, Hanchard B, Morgan O, et al. Patterns of HTLV-I infection among family members of patients with adult T-cell leukemia/lymphoma and HTLV-I associated myelopathy/tropical spastic paraparesis. Int J Cancer. 1996 Jan 17;65(2):272–3. PMID:8567128
4375. Willemse MJ, Seriu T, Hettinger K, et al. Detection of minimal residual disease identifies differences in treatment response between T-ALL and precursor B-ALL. Blood. 2002 Jun 15;99(12):4386–93. PMID:12036866
4376. Willemze R. Mycosis fungoides variants-clinicopathologic features, differential diagnosis, and treatment. Semin Cutan Med Surg. 2018 Mar;37(1):11–7. PMID:29719015
4377. Willemze R, Cerroni L, Kempf W, et al. The 2018 update of the WHO-EORTC classification for primary cutaneous lymphomas. Blood. 2019 Apr 18;133(16):1703–14. PMID:30635287
4378. Willemze R, Cerroni L, Kempf W, et al. The 2018 update of the WHO-EORTC classification for primary cutaneous lymphomas. Blood. 2019 Sep 26;134(13):1112. Erratum for: Blood. 2019 Apr 18;133(16):1703–14. PMID:31558559
4379. Willemze R, Jaffe ES, Burg G, et al. WHO-EORTC classification for cutaneous lymphomas. Blood. 2005 May 15;105(10):3768–85. PMID:15692063
4380. Willemze R, Jansen PM, Cerroni L, et al. Subcutaneous panniculitis-like T-cell lymphoma: definition, classification, and prognostic factors: an EORTC Cutaneous Lymphoma Group study of 83 cases. Blood. 2008 Jan 15;111(2):838–45. PMID:17934071
4381. Willemze R, Kerl H, Sterry W, et al. EORTC classification for primary cutaneous lymphomas: a proposal from the Cutaneous Lymphoma Study Group of the European Organization for Research and Treatment of Cancer. Blood. 1997 Jul 1;90(1):354–71. PMID:9207472
4382. Willemze R, Meijer CJ. Primary cutaneous CD30-positive lymphoproliferative disorders. Hematol Oncol Clin North Am. 2003 Dec;17(6):1319–32, vii–viii. PMID:14710887
4383. Willemze R, Meyer CJ, Van Vloten WA, et al. The clinical and histological spectrum of lymphomatoid papulosis. Br J Dermatol. 1982 Aug;107(2):131–44. PMID:7104214
4384. Williams D, Mori T, Reiter A, et al. Central nervous system involvement in anaplastic large cell lymphoma in childhood: results from a multicentre European and

Japanese study. Pediatr Blood Cancer. 2013 Oct;60(10):E118–21. PMID:23720354
4385. Wilson KS, McKenna RW, Kroft SH, et al. Primary effusion lymphomas exhibit complex and recurrent cytogenetic abnormalities. Br J Haematol. 2002 Jan;116(1):113–21. PMID:11841403
4386. Wilson WH, Kingma DW, Raffeld M, et al. Association of lymphomatoid granulomatosis with Epstein-Barr viral infection of B lymphocytes and response to interferon-alpha 2b. Blood. 1996 Jun 1;87(11):4531–7. PMID:8639820
4387. Wilson WH, Pittaluga S, Nicolae A, et al. A prospective study of mediastinal gray-zone lymphoma. Blood. 2014 Sep 4;124(10):1563–9. PMID:25024303
4388. Winters AC, Bernt KM. MLL-rearranged leukemias-an update on science and clinical approaches. Front Pediatr. 2017 Feb 9;5:4. PMID:28232907
4389. Wirth A, Foo M, Seymour JF, et al. Impact of [18f] fluorodeoxyglucose positron emission tomography on staging and management of early-stage follicular non-Hodgkin lymphoma. Int J Radiat Oncol Biol Phys. 2008 May 1;71(1):213–9. PMID:18295982
4390. Witte HM, Merz H, Biersack H, et al. Impact of treatment variability and clinicopathological characteristics on survival in patients with Epstein-Barr-virus positive diffuse large B cell lymphoma. Br J Haematol. 2020 Apr;189(2):257–68. PMID:31958882
4391. Witzens M, Egerer G, Stahl D, et al. A case of mu heavy-chain disease associated with hyperglobulinemia, anemia, and a positive Coombs test. Ann Hematol. 1998 Nov;77(5):231–4. PMID:9858149
4392. Wlodarska I, Nooyen P, Maes B, et al. Frequent occurrence of BCL6 rearrangements in nodular lymphocyte predominance Hodgkin lymphoma but not in classical Hodgkin lymphoma. Blood. 2003 Jan 15;101(2):706–10. PMID:12393409
4393. Wobser M, Petrella T, Kneitz H, et al. Extrafacial indolent CD8-positive cutaneous lymphoid proliferation with unusual symmetrical presentation involving both feet. J Cutan Pathol. 2013 Nov;40(11):955–61. PMID:24102688
4394. Wobser M, Roth S, Reinartz T, et al. CD68 expression is a discriminative feature of indolent cutaneous CD8-positive lymphoid proliferation and distinguishes this lymphoma subtype from other CD8-positive cutaneous lymphomas. Br J Dermatol. 2015 Jun;172(6):1573–80. PMID:25524664
4395. Woellner C, Gertz EM, Schäffer AA, et al. Mutations in STAT3 and diagnostic guidelines for hyper-IgE syndrome. J Allergy Clin Immunol. 2010 Feb;125(2):424–432.e8. PMID:20159255
4396. Woessmann W, Quintanilla-Martinez L. Rare mature B-cell lymphomas in children and adolescents. Hematol Oncol. 2019 Jun;37 Suppl 1:53–61. PMID:31187530
4398. Wöhrer S, Streubel B, Bartsch R, et al. Monoclonal immunoglobulin production is a frequent event in patients with mucosa-associated lymphoid tissue lymphoma. Clin Cancer Res. 2004 Nov 1;10(21):7179–81. PMID:15534090
4399. Wolf BC, Kumar A, Vera JC, et al. Bone marrow morphology and immunology in systemic amyloidosis. Am J Clin Pathol. 1986 Jul;86(1):84–8. PMID:3524195
4400. Wolfe F, Michaud K. The effect of methotrexate and anti-tumor necrosis factor therapy on the risk of lymphoma in rheumatoid arthritis in 19,562 patients during 89,710 person-years of observation. Arthritis Rheum. 2007 May;56(5):1433–9. PMID:17469100
4400A. Wolfram D, Rabensteiner E, Grundtman C, et al. T regulatory cells and TH17 cells in peri-silicone implant capsular fibrosis. Plast Reconstr Surg. 2012 Feb;129(2):327e–37e. PMID:22286447
4401. Wong AK, Kerkoutian S, Said J, et al. Risk of lymphoma in patients receiving antitumor necrosis factor therapy: a meta-analysis of published randomized controlled studies. Clin Rheumatol. 2012 Apr;31(4):631–6. PMID:22147207
4402. Wong CY, Law GT, Shum TT, et al. Pulmonary haemorrhage in a patient with Kikuchi disease. Monaldi Arch Chest Dis. 2001 Apr;56(2):118–20. PMID:11499298
4403. Wong NC, Ashley D, Chatterton Z, et al. A distinct DNA methylation signature defines pediatric pre-B cell acute lymphoblastic leukemia. Epigenetics. 2012 Jun 1;7(6):535–41. PMID:22531296
4404. Woo CG, Huh J. TdT+ T-lymphoblastic proliferation in Castleman disease. J Pathol Transl Med. 2015 Jan;49(1):1–4. PMID:25812651
4405. Woo DK, Jones CR, Vanoli-Storz MN, et al. Prognostic factors in primary cutaneous anaplastic large cell lymphoma: characterization of clinical subset with worse outcome. Arch Dermatol. 2009 Jun;145(6):667–74. PMID:19528422
4406. Wood GS, Kamath NV, Guitart J, et al. Absence of Borrelia burgdorferi DNA in cutaneous B-cell lymphomas from the United States. J Cutan Pathol. 2001 Nov;28(10):502–7. PMID:11737518
4407. Woods CG, Bundey SE, Taylor AM. Unusual features in the inheritance of ataxia telangiectasia. Hum Genet. 1990 May;84(6):555–62. PMID:2338342
4408. Woollard WJ, Pullabhatla V, Lorenc A, et al. Candidate driver genes involved in genome maintenance and DNA repair in Sézary syndrome. Blood. 2016 Jun 30;127(26):3387–97. PMID:27121473
4409. Wotherspoon A, Attygalle A, Mendes LS. Bone marrow and splenic histology in hairy cell leukaemia. Best Pract Res Clin Haematol. 2015 Dec;28(4):200–7. PMID:26614898
4410. Wotherspoon AC, Doglioni C, Diss TC, et al. Regression of primary low-grade B-cell gastric lymphoma of mucosa-associated lymphoid tissue type after eradication of Helicobacter pylori. Lancet. 1993 Sep 4;342(8871):575–7. PMID:8102719
4411. Wotherspoon AC, Ortiz-Hidalgo C, Falzon MR, et al. Helicobacter pylori-associated gastritis and primary B-cell gastric lymphoma. Lancet. 1991 Nov 9;338(8776):1175–6. PMID:1682595
4412. Woyach JA, Furman RR, Liu TM, et al. Resistance mechanisms for the Bruton's tyrosine kinase inhibitor ibrutinib. N Engl J Med. 2014 Jun 12;370(24):2286–94. PMID:24869598
4413. Woyach JA, Ruppert AS, Guinn D, et al. BTKC481S-mediated resistance to ibrutinib in chronic lymphocytic leukemia. J Clin Oncol. 2017 May 1;35(13):1437–43. PMID:28418267
4414. Woyach JA, Ruppert AS, Heerema NA, et al. Ibrutinib regimens versus chemoimmunotherapy in older patients with untreated CLL. N Engl J Med. 2018 Dec 27;379(26):2517–28. PMID:30501481
4415. Wren WS, McShane AJ. Induction of anesthesia with isoflurane in children. Anesth Analg. 1986 Dec;65(12):1365–6. PMID:3777471
4416. Wright DH. What is Burkitt's lymphoma and when is it endemic? Blood. 1999 Jan 15;93(2):758. PMID:10215347
4417. Wright GW, Huang DW, Phelan JD, et al. A probabilistic classification tool for genetic subtypes of diffuse large B cell lymphoma with therapeutic implications. Cancer Cell. 2020 Apr 13;37(4):551–568.e14. PMID:32289277
4418. Wu A, Pullarkat S. Follicular dendritic cell sarcoma. Arch Pathol Lab Med. 2016 Feb;140(2):186–90. PMID:26910224
4419. Wu B, Vallangeon B, Galeotti J, et al. Epstein-Barr virus-negative diffuse large B cell lymphoma with aberrant expression of CD3 and other T cell-associated antigens: report of three cases with a review of the literature. Ann Hematol. 2016 Oct;95(10):1671–83. PMID:27431583
4420. Wu D, Lim MS, Jaffe ES. Pathology of Castleman disease. Hematol Oncol Clin North Am. 2018 Feb;32(1):37–52. PMID:29157618
4421. Wu D, Sherwood A, Fromm JR, et al. High-throughput sequencing detects minimal residual disease in acute T lymphoblastic leukemia. Sci Transl Med. 2012 May 16;4(134):134ra63. PMID:22593176
4422. Wu D, Thomas A, Fromm JR. Reactive T cells by flow cytometry distinguish Hodgkin lymphomas from T cell/histiocyte-rich large B cell lymphoma. Cytometry B Clin Cytom. 2016 Sep;90(5):424–32. PMID:26084540
4423. Wu F, Watanabe N, Tzioni MM, et al. Thyroid MALT lymphoma: self-harm to gain potential T-cell help. Leukemia. 2021 Dec;35(12):3497–508. PMID:34021249
4424. Wu JH, Cohen BA, Sweren RJ. Mycosis fungoides in pediatric patients: clinical features, diagnostic challenges, and advances in therapeutic management. Pediatr Dermatol. 2020 Jan;37(1):18–28. PMID:31630432
4425. Wu SS, Brady K, Anderson JJ, et al. The predictive value of bone marrow morphologic characteristics and immunostaining in primary (AL) amyloidosis. Am J Clin Pathol. 1991 Jul;96(1):95–9. PMID:1712547
4426. Wu W, Youm W, Rezk SA, et al. Human herpesvirus 8-unrelated primary effusion lymphoma-like lymphoma: report of a rare case and review of 54 cases in the literature. Am J Clin Pathol. 2013 Aug;140(2):258–73. PMID:23897264
4427. Wulf GG, Altmann B, Ziepert M, et al. Alemtuzumab plus CHOP versus CHOP in elderly patients with peripheral T-cell lymphoma: the DSHNHL2006-1B/ACT-2 trial. Leukemia. 2021 Jan;35(1):143–55. PMID:32382083
4428. Wündisch T, Thiede C, Morgner A, et al. Long-term follow-up of gastric MALT lymphoma after Helicobacter pylori eradication. J Clin Oncol. 2005 Nov 1;23(31):8018–24. PMID:16204012
4429. Wylin RF, Greene MH, Palutke M, et al. Hairy cell leukemia in three siblings: an apparent HLA-linked disease. Cancer. 1982 Feb 1;49(3):538–42. PMID:6977406
4430. Xerri L, Bachy E, Fabiani B, et al. Identification of MUM1 as a prognostic immunohistochemical marker in follicular lymphoma using computerized image analysis. Hum Pathol. 2014 Oct;45(10):2085–93. PMID:25149549
4431. Xerri L, Chetaille B, Serriari N, et al. Programmed death 1 is a marker of angioimmunoblastic T-cell lymphoma and B-cell small lymphocytic lymphoma/chronic lymphocytic leukemia. Hum Pathol. 2008 Jul;39(7):1050–8. PMID:18479731
4432. Xerri L, Dirnhofer S, Quintanilla-Martinez L, et al. The heterogeneity of follicular lymphomas: from early development to transformation. Virchows Arch. 2016 Feb;468(2):127–39. PMID:26481245
4433. Xerri L, Huet S, Venstrom JM, et al. Rituximab treatment circumvents the prognostic impact of tumor-infiltrating T-cells in follicular lymphoma patients. Hum Pathol. 2017 Jun;64:128–36. PMID:28414090
4434. Xi L, Arons E, Navarro W, et al. Both variant and IGHV4-34-expressing hairy cell leukemia lack the BRAF V600E mutation. Blood. 2012 Apr 5;119(14):3330–2. PMID:22210875
4435. Xia D, Morgan EA, Berger D, et al. NK-cell enteropathy and similar indolent lymphoproliferative disorders: a case series with literature review. Am J Clin Pathol. 2019 Jan 1;151(1):75–85. PMID:30212873
4436. Xia D, Sayed S, Moloo Z, et al. Geographic variability of nodular lymphocyte-predominant Hodgkin lymphoma. Am J Clin Pathol. 2022 Feb 3;157(2):231–43. PMID:34542569
4437. Xian RR, Xie Y, Haley LM, et al. CREBBP and STAT6 co-mutation and 16p13 and 1p36 loss define the t(14;18)-negative diffuse variant of follicular lymphoma. Blood Cancer J. 2020 Jun 17;10(6):69. PMID:32555149
4438. Xiang CX, Chen ZH, Zhao S, et al. Laryngeal extranodal nasal-type natural killer/T-cell lymphoma: a clinicopathologic study of 31 cases in China. Am J Surg Pathol. 2019 Jul;43(7):995–1004. PMID:31045893
4439. Xiao W, Gupta GK, Yao J, et al. Recurrent somatic JAK3 mutations in NK-cell enteropathy. Blood. 2019 Sep 19;134(12):986–91. PMID:31383643
4440. Xie J, Pu C, Silverman JF. Fine-needle aspiration cytology of intranodal palisaded myofibroblastoma of the inguinal lymph node. Acta Cytol. 2016;60(1):89–92. PMID:27027816
4441. Xie L, Wang H, Jiang J. Does radiotherapy with surgery improve survival and decrease progression to multiple myeloma in patients with solitary plasmacytoma of bone of the spine? World Neurosurg. 2020 Feb;134:e790–8. PMID:31715413
4442. Xie Y, Pittaluga S, Jaffe ES. The histological classification of diffuse large B-cell lymphomas. Semin Hematol. 2015 Apr;52(2):57–66. PMID:25805585
4443. Xie Y, Pittaluga S, Price S, et al. Bone marrow findings in autoimmune lymphoproliferative syndrome with germline FAS mutation. Haematologica. 2017 Feb;102(2):364–72. PMID:27846610
4444. Xing KH, Connors JM, Lai A, et al. Advanced-stage nodular lymphocyte predominant Hodgkin lymphoma compared with classical Hodgkin lymphoma: a matched pair outcome analysis. Blood. 2014 Jun 5;123(23):3567–73. PMID:24713929
4445. Xiong J, Cui BW, Wang N, et al. Genomic and transcriptomic characterization of natural killer T cell lymphoma. Cancer Cell. 2020 Mar 16;37(3):403–419.e6. PMID:32183952
4446. Xochelli A, Bikos V, Polychronidou E, et al. Disease-biased and shared characteristics of the immunoglobulin gene repertoires in marginal zone B cell lymphoproliferations. J Pathol. 2019 Apr;247(4):416–21. PMID:30484876
4447. Xochelli A, Kalpadakis C, Gardiner A, et al. Clonal B-cell lymphocytosis exhibiting immunophenotypic features consistent with a marginal-zone origin: Is this a distinct entity? Blood. 2014 Feb 20;123(8):1199–206. PMID:24300853
4448. Xochelli A, Oscier D, Stamatopoulos K. Clonal B-cell lymphocytosis of marginal zone origin. Best Pract Res Clin Haematol. 2017 Mar-Jun;30(1-2):77–83. PMID:28288720
4449. Xochelli A, Sutton LA, Agathangelidis A, et al. Molecular evidence for antigen drive in the natural history of mantle cell lymphoma. Am J Pathol. 2015 Jun;185(6):1740–8. PMID:25843681
4450. Xu H, Chaudhri VK, Wu Z, et al. Regulation of bifurcating B cell trajectories by mutual antagonism between transcription factors IRF4 and IRF8. Nat Immunol. 2015 Dec;16(12):1274–81. PMID:26437243
4451. Xu J, Li J, Wei Z, et al. Screening for monoclonal B-lymphocyte expansion in a hospital-based Chinese population with lymphocytosis: an observational cohort study. BMJ Open. 2020 Sep 15;10(9):e036006. PMID:32933958
4452. Xu J, Li P, Chai J, et al. The

clinicopathological and molecular features of sinusoidal large B-cell lymphoma. Mod Pathol. 2021 May;34(5):922–33. PMID:32973328
4453. Xu JX, Hoshida Y, Yang WI, et al. Life-style and environmental factors in the development of nasal NK/T-cell lymphoma: a case-control study in East Asia. Int J Cancer. 2007 Jan 15;120(2):406–10. PMID:17066445
4454. Xu X, Paxton CN, Hayashi RJ, et al. Genomic and clinical characterization of early T-cell precursor lymphoblastic lymphoma. Blood Adv. 2021 Jul 27;5(14):2890–900. PMID:34297047
4455. Xu Z, Lian S. Epstein-Barr virus-associated hydroa vacciniforme-like cutaneous lymphoma in seven Chinese children. Pediatr Dermatol. 2010 Sep-Oct;27(5):463–9. PMID:20497358
4456. Xu-Monette ZY, Tu M, Jabbar KJ, et al. Clinical and biological significance of de novo CD5+ diffuse large B-cell lymphoma in western countries. Oncotarget. 2015 Mar 20;6(8):5615–33. PMID:25760242
4457. Xu-Monette ZY, Wu L, Visco C, et al. Mutational profile and prognostic significance of TP53 in diffuse large B-cell lymphoma patients treated with R-CHOP: report from an International DLBCL Rituximab-CHOP Consortium Program study. Blood. 2012 Nov 8;120(19):3986–96. PMID:22955915
4458. Yabe M, Gao Q, Ozkaya N, et al. Bright PD-1 expression by flow cytometry is a powerful tool for diagnosis and monitoring of angioimmunoblastic T-cell lymphoma. Blood Cancer J. 2020 Mar 6;10(3):32. PMID:32144240
4459. Yabe M, Medeiros LJ, Daneshbod Y, et al. Hepatosplenic T-cell lymphoma arising in patients with immunodysregulatory disorders: a study of 7 patients who did not receive tumor necrosis factor-α inhibitor therapy and literature review. Ann Diagn Pathol. 2017 Feb;26:16–22. PMID:28038706
4460. Yabe M, Medeiros LJ, Tang G, et al. Dyspoietic changes associated with hepatosplenic T-cell lymphoma are not a manifestation of a myelodysplastic syndrome: analysis of 25 patients. Hum Pathol. 2016 Apr;50:109–17. PMID:26997444
4461. Yabe M, Medeiros LJ, Tang G, et al. Prognostic factors of hepatosplenic T-cell lymphoma: clinicopathologic study of 28 cases. Am J Surg Pathol. 2016 May;40(5):676–88. PMID:26872013
4462. Yabe M, Medeiros LJ, Wang SA, et al. Distinguishing between hepatosplenic T-cell lymphoma and γδ T-cell large granular lymphocytic leukemia: a clinicopathologic, immunophenotypic, and molecular analysis. Am J Surg Pathol. 2017 Jan;41(1):82–93. PMID:27755009
4463. Yabe M, Miranda RN, Medeiros LJ. Hepatosplenic T-cell lymphoma: a review of clinicopathologic features, pathogenesis, and prognostic factors. Hum Pathol. 2018 Apr;74:5–16. PMID:29337025
4464. Yabe M, Ozkaya N, de Jong D, et al. Localized peritumoral AL amyloidosis associated with mantle cell lymphoma with plasmacytic differentiation. Am J Surg Pathol. 2021 Jul 1;45(7):939–44. PMID:33739787
4465. Yakaboski E, Fuleihan RL, Sullivan KE, et al. Lymphoproliferative disease in CVID: a report of types and frequencies from a US patient registry. J Clin Immunol. 2020 Apr;40(3):524–30. PMID:32185577
4466. Yamada K, Miyoshi H, Yoshida N, et al. Human T-cell lymphotropic virus HBZ and tax mRNA expression are associated with specific clinicopathological features in adult T-cell leukemia/lymphoma. Mod Pathol. 2021 Feb;34(2):314–26. PMID:32973330
4467. Yamada K, Yamamoto M, Saeki T, et al. New clues to the nature of immunoglobulin G4-related disease: a retrospective Japanese multicenter study of baseline clinical features of 334 cases. Arthritis Res Ther. 2017 Dec 1;19(1):262. PMID:29191210
4468. Yamada M, Ishikawa Y, Imadome KI. Hypersensitivity to mosquito bites: a versatile Epstein-Barr virus disease with allergy, inflammation, and malignancy. Allergol Int. 2021 Oct;70(4):430–8. PMID:34334322
4469. Yamagishi M, Nakano K, Miyake A, et al. Polycomb-mediated loss of miR-31 activates NIK-dependent NF-κB pathway in adult T cell leukemia and other cancers. Cancer Cell. 2012 Jan 17;21(1):121–35. PMID:22264793
4470. Yamaguchi M, Kwong YL, Kim WS, et al. Phase II study of SMILE chemotherapy for newly diagnosed stage IV, relapsed, or refractory extranodal natural killer (NK)/T-cell lymphoma, nasal type: the NK-Cell Tumor Study Group study. J Clin Oncol. 2011 Nov 20;29(33):4410–6. PMID:21990393
4471. Yamaguchi M, Seto M, Okamoto M, et al. De novo CD5+ diffuse large B-cell lymphoma: a clinicopathologic study of 109 patients. Blood. 2002 Feb 1;99(3):815–21. PMID:11806981
4472. Yamaguchi M, Suzuki R, Oguchi M, et al. Treatments and outcomes of patients with extranodal natural killer/T-cell lymphoma diagnosed between 2000 and 2013: a cooperative study in Japan. J Clin Oncol. 2017 Jan;35(1):32–9. PMID:28034070
4473. Yamaguchi M, Tobinai K, Oguchi M, et al. Concurrent chemoradiotherapy for localized nasal natural killer/T-cell lymphoma: an updated analysis of the Japan clinical oncology group study JCOG0211. J Clin Oncol. 2012 Nov 10;30(32):4044–6. PMID:23045573
4474. Yamakawa N, Fujimoto M, Kawabata D, et al. A clinical, pathological, and genetic characterization of methotrexate-associated lymphoproliferative disorders. J Rheumatol. 2014 Feb;41(2):293–9. PMID:24334644
4475. Yamanaka Y, Tagawa H, Takahashi N, et al. Aberrant overexpression of microRNAs activate AKT signaling via down-regulation of tumor suppressors in natural killer-cell lymphoma/leukemia. Blood. 2009 Oct 8;114(15):3265–75. PMID:19641183
4476. Yamane T, Kawakami T, Sekiguchi N, et al. High frequency of STAT3 gene mutations in T-cell receptor (TCR)γδ-type T-cell large granular lymphocytic leukaemia: implications for molecular diagnostics. Br J Haematol. 2020 Sep;190(5):e301–4. PMID:32478405
4477. Yamashita D, Shimada K, Takata K, et al. Reappraisal of nodal Epstein-Barr virus-negative cytotoxic T-cell lymphoma: identification of indolent CD5+ diseases. Cancer Sci. 2018 Aug;109(8):2599–610. PMID:29845715
4478. Yan B, Tan SY, Yau EX, et al. EBV-positive plasmacytoma of the submandibular gland–report of a rare case with molecular genetic characterization. Head Neck Pathol. 2011 Dec;5(4):389–94. PMID:21442194
4479. Yan J, Li B, Lin B, et al. EZH2 phosphorylation by JAK3 mediates a switch to noncanonical function in natural killer/T-cell lymphoma. Blood. 2016 Aug 18;128(7):948–58. PMID:27297789
4480. Yan J, Luo D, Zhang F, et al. Diffuse large B cell lymphoma associated with chronic inflammation arising within atrial myxoma: aggressive histological features but indolent clinical behaviour. Histopathology. 2017 Dec;71(6):951–9. PMID:28782131
4481. Yan J, Ng SB, Tay JL, et al. EZH2 overexpression in natural killer/T-cell lymphoma confers growth advantage independently of histone methyltransferase activity. Blood. 2013 May 30;121(22):4512–20. PMID:23529930
4482. Yang F, Liu T, Zhao H, et al. Indolent T-lymphblastic proliferation: report of a case involving the upper aerodigestive tract. Int J Clin Exp Pathol. 2014 Aug 15;7(9):6350–6. PMID:25337290
4483. Yang J, Liu X, Nyland SB, et al. Platelet-derived growth factor mediates survival of leukemic large granular lymphocytes via an autocrine regulatory pathway. Blood. 2010 Jan 7;115(1):51–60. PMID:19880494
4484. Yang L, Zhao H, He Y, et al. Contrast-enhanced ultrasound in the differential diagnosis of primary thyroid lymphoma and nodular Hashimoto's thyroiditis in a background of heterogeneous parenchyma. Front Oncol. 2021 Jan 7;10:597975. PMID:33489895
4485. Yang QP, Zhang WY, Yu JB, et al. Subtype distribution of lymphomas in Southwest China: analysis of 6,382 cases using WHO classification in a single institution. Diagn Pathol. 2011 Aug 22;6:77. PMID:21854649
4486. Yang S, Varghese AM, Sood N, et al. Ethnic and geographic diversity of chronic lymphocytic leukaemia. Leukemia. 2021 Feb;35(2):433–9. PMID:33077870
4487. Yao WQ, Wu F, Zhang W, et al. Angioimmunoblastic T-cell lymphoma contains multiple clonal T-cell populations derived from a common TET2 mutant progenitor cell. J Pathol. 2020 Mar;250(3):346–57. PMID:31859368
4488. Yasuda H, Tsutsui M, Ota Y, et al. Indolent T-lymphoblastic proliferation concomitant with acinic cell carcinoma mimicking T-lymphoblastic lymphoma: case report and literature review. Histopathology. 2018 Apr;72(5):862–6. PMID:29143359
4489. Yasuda T, Tsuzuki S, Kawazu M, et al. Recurrent DUX4 fusions in B cell acute lymphoblastic leukemia of adolescents and young adults. Nat Genet. 2016 May;48(5):569–74. PMID:27019113
4490. Ye H, Dogan A, Karran L, et al. BCL10 expression in normal and neoplastic lymphoid tissue. Nuclear localization in MALT lymphoma. Am J Pathol. 2000 Oct;157(4):1147–54. PMID:11021819
4491. Ye H, Gong L, Liu H, et al. MALT lymphoma with t(14;18)(q32;q21)/IGH-MALT1 is characterized by strong cytoplasmic MALT1 and BCL10 expression. J Pathol. 2005 Feb;205(3):293–301. PMID:15682443
4492. Ye H, Liu H, Attygalle A, et al. Variable frequencies of t(11;18)(q21;q21) in MALT lymphomas of different sites: significant association with CagA strains of H pylori in gastric MALT lymphoma. Blood. 2003 Aug 1;102(3):1012–8. PMID:12676782
4493. Ye P, Miao H, Chen Y. An unusual case of symptomatic portal hypertension. Gastroenterology. 2022 Mar;162(3):e11–3. PMID:34280388
4494. Ye Q, Xu-Monette ZY, Tzankov A, et al. Prognostic impact of concurrent MYC and BCL6 rearrangements and expression in de novo diffuse large B-cell lymphoma. Oncotarget. 2016 Jan 19;7(3):2401–16. PMID:26573234
4495. Yeoh EJ, Ross ME, Shurtleff SA, et al. Classification, subtype discovery, and prediction of outcome in pediatric acute lymphoblastic leukemia by gene expression profiling. Cancer Cell. 2002 Mar;1(2):133–43. PMID:12086872
4496. Yewdell WT, Kim Y, Chowdhury P, et al. A hyper-IgM syndrome mutation in activation-induced cytidine deaminase disrupts G-quadruplex binding and genome-wide chromatin localization. Immunity. 2020 Nov 17;53(5):952–970.e11. PMID:33098766
4497. Yi JH, Lee GW, Do YR, et al. Multicenter retrospective analysis of the clinicopathologic features of monomorphic epitheliotropic intestinal T-cell lymphoma. Ann Hematol. 2019 Nov;98(11):2541–50. PMID:31493002
4498. Yigit N, Covey S, Tam W. Massive splenic hamartoma with bizarre stromal cells. Int J Hematol. 2015 Apr;101(4):315–6. PMID:25637257
4499. Yilmaz M, Kantarjian HM, Toruner G, et al. Translocation t(1;19)(q23;p13) in adult acute lymphoblastic leukemia - a distinct subtype with favorable prognosis. Leuk Lymphoma. 2021 Jan;62(1):224–8. PMID:32955970
4500. Yoda A, Yoda Y, Chiaretti S, et al. Functional screening identifies CRLF2 in precursor B-cell acute lymphoblastic leukemia. Proc Natl Acad Sci U S A. 2010 Jan 5;107(1):252–7. PMID:20018760
4501. Yonal-Hindilerden I, Hindilerden F, Bulut-Dereli S, et al. Hairy cell leukemia presenting with isolated skeletal involvement successfully treated by radiation therapy and cladribine: a case report and review of the literature. Case Rep Hematol. 2015;2015:803921. PMID:26788382
4502. Yonese I, Sakashita C, Imadome KI, et al. Nationwide survey of systemic chronic active EBV infection in Japan in accordance with the new WHO classification. Blood Adv. 2020 Jul 14;4(13):2918–26. PMID:32598475
4503. Yoo HY, Kim P, Kim WS, et al. Frequent CTLA4-CD28 gene fusion in diverse types of T-cell lymphoma. Haematologica. 2016 Jun;101(6):757–63. PMID:26819049
4504. Yoo HY, Sung MK, Lee SH, et al. A recurrent inactivating mutation in RHOA GTPase in angioimmunoblastic T cell lymphoma. Nat Genet. 2014 Apr;46(4):371–5. PMID:24584070
4505. Yoo KH, Lee H, Suh C. Lymphoma epidemiology in Korea and the real clinical field including the Consortium for Improving Survival of Lymphoma (CISL) trial. Int J Hematol. 2018 Apr;107(4):395–404. PMID:29357080
4506. Yoon DH, Choi DR, Ahn HJ, et al. Ki-67 expression as a prognostic factor in diffuse large B-cell lymphoma patients treated with rituximab plus CHOP. Eur J Haematol. 2010 Aug;85(2):149–57. PMID:20477862
4507. Yoon SE, Cho J, Kim YJ, et al. Comprehensive analysis of clinical, pathological, and genomic characteristics of follicular helper T-cell derived lymphomas. Exp Hematol Oncol. 2021 May 14;10(1):33. PMID:33990228
4508. Yoon SE, Song Y, Kim SJ, et al. Comprehensive analysis of peripheral T-cell and natural killer/T-cell lymphoma in Asian patients: a multinational, multicenter, prospective registry study in Asia. Lancet Reg Health West Pac. 2021 Mar 22;10:100126. PMID:34327343
4509. Yoon SO, Suh C, Lee DH, et al. Distribution of lymphoid neoplasms in the Republic of Korea: analysis of 5318 cases according to the World Health Organization classification. Am J Hematol. 2010 Oct;85(10):760–4. PMID:20806229
4510. Yoshida M, Osumi T, Imadome KI, et al. Successful treatment of systemic EBV positive T-cell lymphoma of childhood using the SMILE regimen. Pediatr Hematol Oncol. 2018 Mar;35(2):121–4. PMID:29648917
4511. You MJ, Medeiros LJ, Hsi ED. T-lymphoblastic leukemia/lymphoma. Am J Clin Pathol. 2015 Sep;144(3):411–22. PMID:26276771
4512. Younes A, Sehn LH, Johnson P, et al. Randomized phase III trial of ibrutinib and rituximab plus cyclophosphamide, doxorubicin, vincristine, and prednisone in non-germinal center B-cell diffuse large B-cell lymphoma. J Clin Oncol. 2019 May 20;37(15):1285–95. PMID:30901302
4513. Younes SF, Beck AH, Lossos IS, et al. Immunoarchitectural patterns in follicular lymphoma: efficacy of HGAL and LMO2 in the detection of the interfollicular and diffuse components. Am J Surg Pathol. 2010 Sep;34(9):1266–76. PMID:20697248
4514. Younes SF, Beck AH, Ohgami RS, et al. The efficacy of HGAL and LMO2 in the separation of lymphomas derived from small

B cells in nodal and extranodal sites, including the bone marrow. Am J Clin Pathol. 2011 May;135(5):697–708. PMID:21502424
4515. Young KH, Chan WC, Fu K, et al. Mantle cell lymphoma with plasma cell differentiation. Am J Surg Pathol. 2006 Aug;30(8):954–61. PMID:16861965
4516. Young KH, Leroy K, Møller MB, et al. Structural profiles of TP53 gene mutations predict clinical outcome in diffuse large B-cell lymphoma: an international collaborative study. Blood. 2008 Oct 15;112(8):3088–98. PMID:18559976
4517. Young RH, Harris NL, Scully RE. Lymphoma-like lesions of the lower female genital tract: a report of 16 cases. Int J Gynecol Pathol. 1985;4(4):289–99. PMID:4086158
4518. Yousem SA, Weiss LM, Warnke RA. Primary mediastinal non-Hodgkin's lymphomas: a morphologic and immunologic study of 19 cases. Am J Clin Pathol. 1985 Jun;83(6):676–80. PMID:3923821
4519. Yu CH, Lin TK, Jou ST, et al. MLPA and DNA index improve the molecular diagnosis of childhood B-cell acute lymphoblastic leukemia. Sci Rep. 2020 Jul 13;10(1):11501. PMID:32661308
4520. Yu H, Gibson JA, Pinkus GS, et al. Podoplanin (D2-40) is a novel marker for follicular dendritic cell tumors. Am J Clin Pathol. 2007 Nov;128(5):776–82. PMID:17951199
4521. Yu H, Wertheim G, Shankar S, et al. Marked eosinophilia masking B lymphoblastic leukemia. Am J Hematol. 2016 May;91(5):543–4. PMID:26662494
4522. Yu HL, Lee SS, Tsai HC, et al. Clinical manifestations of Kikuchi's disease in southern Taiwan. J Microbiol Immunol Infect. 2005 Feb;38(1):35–40. PMID:15692625
4523. Yu L, Shi M, Cai Q, et al. A novel predictive model for idiopathic multicentric Castleman disease: the International Castleman Disease Consortium study. Oncologist. 2020 Nov;25(11):963–73. PMID:32852137
4524. Yu L, Tu M, Cortes J, et al. Clinical and pathological characteristics of HIV- and HHV-8-negative Castleman disease. Blood. 2017 Mar 23;129(12):1658–68. PMID:28100459
4525. Yu M, Hazelton WD, Luebeck GE, et al. Epigenetic aging: more than just a clock when it comes to cancer. Cancer Res. 2020 Feb 1;80(3):367–74. PMID:31694907
4526. Yu WW, Hsieh PP, Chuang SS. Cutaneous EBV-positive γδ T-cell lymphoma vs. extranodal NK/T-cell lymphoma: a case report and literature review. J Cutan Pathol. 2013 Mar;40(3):310–6. PMID:23240992
4527. Yu YT, Sakata S, Takeuchi K, et al. Tonsillar follicular large B-cell lymphoma with IRF4 rearrangement causing sleep apnoea. J Clin Pathol. 2020 Feb;73(2):120. PMID:31324665
4528. Yuan J, Li S, Liu X, et al. Mantle cell lymphoma with mantle zone growth pattern. Am J Clin Pathol. 2019 Jul 5;152(2):132–45. PMID:31140550
4529. Yui MA, Rothenberg EV. Developmental gene networks: a triathlon on the course to T cell identity. Nat Rev Immunol. 2014 Aug;14(8):529–45. PMID:25060579
4530. Zaliova M, Kotrova M, Bresolin S, et al. ETV6/RUNX1-like acute lymphoblastic leukemia: a novel B-cell precursor leukemia subtype associated with the CD27/CD44 immunophenotype. Genes Chromosomes Cancer. 2017 Aug;56(8):608–16. PMID:28395118
4531. Zaliova M, Potuckova E, Hovorkova L, et al. ERG deletions in childhood acute lymphoblastic leukemia with DUX4 rearrangements are mostly polyclonal, prognostically relevant and their detection rate strongly depends on screening method sensitivity. Haematologica. 2019 Jul;104(7):1407–16. PMID:30630977
4532. Zaliova M, Stuchly J, Winkowska L, et al. Genomic landscape of pediatric B-other acute lymphoblastic leukemia in a consecutive European cohort. Haematologica. 2019 Jul;104(7):1396–406. PMID:30630978
4533. Zaliova M, Winkowska L, Stuchly J, et al. A novel class of ZNF384 aberrations in acute leukemia. Blood Adv. 2021 Nov 9;5(21):4393–7. PMID:34529760
4534. Zamagni E, Nanni C, Dozza L, et al. Standardization of 18F-FDG-PET/CT according to Deauville criteria for metabolic complete response definition in newly diagnosed multiple myeloma. J Clin Oncol. 2021 Jan 10;39(2):116–25. PMID:33151787
4535. Zamagni E, Patriarca F, Nanni C, et al. Prognostic relevance of 18-F FDG PET/CT in newly diagnosed multiple myeloma patients treated with up-front autologous transplantation. Blood. 2011 Dec 1;118(23):5989–95. PMID:21900189
4536. Zambello R, Falco M, Della Chiesa M, et al. Expression and function of KIR and natural cytotoxicity receptors in NK-type lymphoproliferative diseases of granular lymphocytes. Blood. 2003 Sep 1;102(5):1797–805. PMID:12750175
4537. Zambello R, Teramo A, Barilà G, et al. Activating KIRs in chronic lymphoproliferative disorder of NK cells: protection from viruses and disease induction? Front Immunol. 2014 Feb 26;5:72. PMID:24616720
4538. Zamò A, Pischimarov J, Horn H, et al. The exomic landscape of t(14;18)-negative diffuse follicular lymphoma with 1p36 deletion. Br J Haematol. 2018 Feb;180(3):391–4. PMID:29193015
4539. Zamò A, Pischimarov J, Schlesner M, et al. Differences between BCL2-break positive and negative follicular lymphoma unraveled by whole-exome sequencing. Leukemia. 2018 Mar;32(3):685–93. PMID:28824170
4540. Zand L, Nasr SH, Gertz MA, et al. Clinical and prognostic differences among patients with light chain deposition disease, myeloma cast nephropathy and both. Leuk Lymphoma. 2015;56(12):3357–64. PMID:25860232
4541. Zanelli M, Mengoli MC, Del Sordo R, et al. Intravascular NK/T-cell lymphoma, Epstein-Barr virus positive with multiorgan involvement: a clinical dilemma. BMC Cancer. 2018 Nov 15;18(1):1115. PMID:30442097
4542. Zanelli M, Sanguedolce F, Zizzo M, et al. Primary effusion lymphoma occurring in the setting of transplanted patients: a systematic review of a rare, life-threatening post-transplantation occurrence. BMC Cancer. 2021 Apr 27;21(1):468. PMID:33906629
4543. Zanelli M, Zizzo M, Bisagni A, et al. Germinotropic lymphoproliferative disorder: a systematic review. Ann Hematol. 2020 Oct;99(10):2243–53. PMID:32307569
4544. Zanelli M, Zizzo M, Montanaro M, et al. Fibrin-associated large B-cell lymphoma: first case report within a cerebral artery aneurysm and literature review. BMC Cancer. 2019 Sep 13;19(1):916. PMID:31519155
4545. Zangrando A, Intini F, te Kronnie G, et al. Validation of NG2 antigen in identifying BP-ALL patients with MLL rearrangements using qualitative and quantitative flow cytometry: a prospective study. Leukemia. 2008 Apr;22(4):858–61. PMID:17851550
4546. Zavidij O, Haradhvala NJ, Mouhieddine TH, et al. Single-cell RNA sequencing reveals compromised immune microenvironment in precursor stages of multiple myeloma. Nat Cancer. 2020 May;1(5):493–506. PMID:33409501
4547. Zelent A, Greaves M, Enver T. Role of the TEL-AML1 fusion gene in the molecular pathogenesis of childhood acute lymphoblastic leukaemia. Oncogene. 2004 May 24;23(24):4275–83. PMID:15156184
4548. Zen Y, Nakanuma Y. IgG4-related disease: a cross-sectional study of 114 cases. Am J Surg Pathol. 2010 Dec;34(12):1812–9. PMID:21107087
4549. Zenz T, Eichhorst B, Busch R, et al. TP53 mutation and survival in chronic lymphocytic leukemia. J Clin Oncol. 2010 Oct 10;28(29):4473–9. PMID:20697090
4550. Zettl A, Lee SS, Rüdiger T, et al. Epstein-Barr virus-associated B-cell lymphoproliferative disorders in angloimmunoblastic T-cell lymphoma and peripheral T-cell lymphoma, unspecified. Am J Clin Pathol. 2002 Mar;117(3):368–79. PMID:11888076
4551. Zettl A, Rüdiger T, Konrad MA, et al. Genomic profiling of peripheral T-cell lymphoma, unspecified, and anaplastic large T-cell lymphoma delineates novel recurrent chromosomal alterations. Am J Pathol. 2004 May;164(5):1837–48. PMID:15111330
4552. Zettl A, Rüdiger T, Marx A, et al. Composite marginal zone B-cell lymphoma and classical Hodgkin's lymphoma: a clinicopathological study of 12 cases. Histopathology. 2005 Feb;46(2):217–28. PMID:15693895
4553. Zhan FH, Barlogie B, John D S Jr. Gene expression profiling defines a high-risk entity of multiple myeloma. Zhong Nan Da Xue Xue Bao Yi Xue Ban. 2007 Apr;32(2):191–203. PMID:17478923
4554. Zhang C, Amos Burke GA. Pediatric precursor B-cell acute lymphoblastic leukemia with MYC 8q24 translocation - How to treat? Leuk Lymphoma. 2018 Aug;59(8):1807–13. PMID:29022749
4555. Zhang C, Stelloo E, Barrans S, et al. Non-IG:MYC in diffuse large B-cell lymphoma confers variable genomic configurations and MYC transactivation potential. Leukemia. 2024 Mar;38(3):621–9. PMID:38184753
4556. Zhang C, Xia R, Gu T, et al. Clinicopathological aspects of primary mucosa-associated lymphoid tissue lymphoma of the salivary gland: a retrospective single-center analysis of 72 cases. J Oral Pathol Med. 2021 Aug;50(7):723–30. PMID:33730431
4557. Zhang J, Ding L, Holmfeldt L, et al. The genetic basis of early T-cell precursor acute lymphoblastic leukaemia. Nature. 2012 Jan 11;481(7380):157–63. PMID:22237106
4558. Zhang J, Dominguez-Sola D, Hussein S, et al. Disruption of KMT2D perturbs germinal center B cell development and promotes lymphomagenesis. Nat Med. 2015 Oct;21(10):1190–8. PMID:26366712
4559. Zhang J, McCastlain K, Yoshihara H, et al. Deregulation of DUX4 and ERG in acute lymphoblastic leukemia. Nat Genet. 2016 Dec;48(12):1481–9. PMID:27776115
4560. Zhang J, Weng Z, Huang Y, et al. High-grade B-cell lymphoma with MYC, BCL2, and/or BCL6 translocations/rearrangements: clinicopathologic features of 51 cases in a single institution of South China. Am J Surg Pathol. 2020 Dec;44(12):1602–11. PMID:32991338
4561. Zhang J, Xu X, Shi M, et al. CD13hi Neutrophil-like myeloid-derived suppressor cells exert immune suppression through arginase 1 expression in pancreatic ductal adenocarcinoma. Oncoimmunology. 2017 Jan 9;6(2):e1258504. PMID:28344866
4562. Zhang M, Jin L, Duan YL, et al. Diagnosis and treatment of pediatric anaplastic lymphoma kinase-positive large B-cell lymphoma: a case report. World J Clin Cases. 2021 Jun 16;9(17):4268–78. PMID:34141790
4563. Zhang M, Zhang H, Li Z, et al. Functional, structural, and molecular characterizations of the leukemogenic driver MEF2D-HNRNPUL1 fusion. Blood. 2022 Sep 22;140(12):1390–407. PMID:35544603
4564. Zhang MY, Jia MN, Chen J, et al. UCD with MCD-like inflammatory state: surgical excision is highly effective. Blood Adv. 2021 Jan 12;5(1):122–8. PMID:33570636
4565. Zhang Q, Raghunath PN, Xue L, et al. Multilevel dysregulation of STAT3 activation in anaplastic lymphoma kinase-positive T/null-cell lymphoma. J Immunol. 2002 Jan 1;168(1):466–74. PMID:11751994
4566. Zhang S, Sun J, Fang Y, et al. Signet-ring cell lymphoma: clinicopathologic, immunohistochemical, and fluorescence in situ hybridization studies of 7 cases. Ann Diagn Pathol. 2017 Feb;26:38–42. PMID:28038709
4567. Zhang W, Jang E. Association of minimal residual disease with clinical outcomes in Philadelphia chromosome positive acute lymphoblastic leukemia in the tyrosine kinase inhibitor era: a systemic literature review and meta-analysis. PLoS One. 2021 Aug 26;16(8):e0256801. PMID:34437635
4568. Zhang WP, Wang JH, Wang WQ, et al. An association between parvovirus B19 and Kikuchi-Fujimoto disease. Viral Immunol. 2007 Sep;20(3):421–8. PMID:17931112
4569. Zhang X, Rao H, Xu X, et al. Clinical characteristics and outcomes of Castleman disease: a multicenter study of 185 Chinese patients. Cancer Sci. 2018 Jan;109(1):199–206. PMID:29124835
4570. Zhang Y, Li X, Liang D, et al. Heavy chain deposition disease: clinicopathologic characteristics of a Chinese case series. Am J Kidney Dis. 2020 May;75(5):736–43. PMID:31699519
4571. Zhang Y, Qian JJ, Zhou YL, et al. Comparison of early T-cell precursor and non-ETP subtypes among 122 Chinese adults with acute lymphoblastic leukemia. Front Oncol. 2020 Aug 21;10:1423. PMID:32974153
4572. Zhang Y, Sanjose SD, Bracci PM, et al. Personal use of hair dye and the risk of certain subtypes of non-Hodgkin lymphoma. Am J Epidemiol. 2008 Jun 1;167(11):1321–31. PMID:18408225
4573. Zhang Y, Wang Y, Yu R, et al. Molecular markers of early-stage mycosis fungoides. J Invest Dermatol. 2012 Jun;132(6):1698–706. PMID:22377759
4574. Zhang Z, Shi Q, An X, et al. NK/T-cell lymphoma in a child with hypersensitivity to mosquito bites. J Pediatr Hematol Oncol. 2009 Nov;31(11):855–7. PMID:19636274
4575. Zhang Z, Wang W, Li Y, et al. A nodal EBV-positive T cell lymphoma with a T follicular helper cell phenotype. Histopathology. 2023 Jul;83(1):137–42. PMID:37071061
4576. Zhao R, Chen Z, Zhao S, et al. Prognosis of solitary bone plasmacytoma of the extremities: a SEER-based study. Medicine (Baltimore). 2021 Jul 2;100(26):e26568. PMID:34190199
4577. Zhao S, Kanagal-Shamanna R, Navsaria L, et al. Efficacy of venetoclax in high risk relapsed mantle cell lymphoma (MCL) - outcomes and mutation profile from venetoclax resistant MCL patients. Am J Hematol. 2020 Jun;95(6):623–9. PMID:32239765
4578. Zheng G, Wang Y, Zhao Y, et al. Clinicopathological features, treatment strategy, and prognosis of primary non-Hodgkin's lymphoma of the duodenum: a SEER database analysis. Can J Gastroenterol Hepatol. 2020 Jan 13;2020:9327868. PMID:32399459
4579. Zhou B, Chu X, Tian H, et al. The clinical outcomes and genomic landscapes of acute lymphoblastic leukemia patients with E2A-PBX1: a 10-year retrospective study. Am J Hematol. 2021 Nov 1;96(11):1461–71. PMID:34406703
4580. Zhou L, Gu B, Shen X, et al. B cell lymphoma with IRF4 rearrangement: a

clinicopathological study of 13 cases. Pathol Int. 2021 Mar;71(3):183–90. PMID:33503299
4581. Zhou L, Yu Q, Wei G, et al. Measuring the global, regional, and national burden of multiple myeloma from 1990 to 2019. BMC Cancer. 2021 May 25;21(1):606. PMID:34034700
4582. Zhou XA, Louissaint A Jr, Wenzel A, et al. Genomic analyses identify recurrent alterations in immune evasion genes in diffuse large B-cell lymphoma, leg type. J Invest Dermatol. 2018 Nov;138(11):2365–76. PMID:29857068
4583. Zhou XA, Yang J, Ringbloom KG, et al. Genomic landscape of cutaneous follicular lymphomas reveals 2 subgroups with clinically predictive molecular features. Blood Adv. 2021 Feb 9;5(3):649–61. PMID:33560380
4584. Zhou Y, Xu Z, Lin W, et al. Comprehensive genomic profiling of EBV-positive diffuse large B-cell lymphoma and the expression and clinicopathological correlations of some related genes. Front Oncol. 2019 Jul 25;9:683. PMID:31403034
4585. Zhu D, Lossos C, Chapman-Fredricks JR, et al. Biased use of the IGHV4 family and evidence for antigen selection in Chlamydophila psittaci-negative ocular adnexal extranodal marginal zone lymphomas. PLoS One. 2011;6(12):e29114. PMID:22216179
4586. Zhu Y, Gao Q, Hu J, et al. Clinical features and treatment outcomes in patients with T-cell large granular lymphocytic leukemia: a single-institution experience. Leuk Res. 2020 Mar;90:106299. PMID:32035354
4587. Ziepert M, Lazzi S, Santi R, et al. A 70% cut-off for MYC protein expression in diffuse large B cell lymphoma identifies a high-risk group of patients. Haematologica. 2020 Nov 1;105(11):2667–70. PMID:33131258
4588. Ziino O, Rondelli R, Micalizzi C, et al. Acute lymphoblastic leukemia in children with associated genetic conditions other than Down's syndrome. The AIEOP experience. Haematologica. 2006 Jan;91(1):139–40. PMID:16434385
4589. Zinzani PL, Quaglino P, Pimpinelli N, et al. Prognostic factors in primary cutaneous B-cell lymphoma: the Italian Study Group for Cutaneous Lymphomas. J Clin Oncol. 2006 Mar 20;24(9):1376–82. PMID:16492713
4590. Zinzani PL, Santoro A, Gritti G, et al. Nivolumab combined with brentuximab vedotin for relapsed/refractory primary mediastinal large B-cell lymphoma: efficacy and safety from the phase II CheckMate 436 study. J Clin Oncol. 2019 Nov 20;37(33):3081–9. PMID:31398081
4591. Ziogas DC, Kastritis E, Terpos E, et al. Hematologic and renal improvement of monoclonal immunoglobulin deposition disease after treatment with bortezomib-based regimens. Leuk Lymphoma. 2017 Aug;58(8):1832–9. PMID:27967286
4592. Ziol M, Poirel H, Kountchou GN, et al. Intrasinusoidal cytotoxic CD8+ T cells in nodular regenerative hyperplasia of the liver. Hum Pathol. 2004 Oct;35(10):1241–51. PMID:15492992
4593. Zubair M, Din NU, Arshad S, et al. Intra-abdominal follicular dendritic cell sarcoma (FDCS): series of 18 cases of a rare entity from Pakistan. Ann Diagn Pathol. 2020 Dec;49:151595. PMID:32905993
4594. Zucca E, Arcaini L, Buske C, et al. Marginal zone lymphomas: ESMO Clinical Practice Guidelines for diagnosis, treatment and follow-up. Ann Oncol. 2020 Jan;31(1):17–29. PMID:31912792
4595. Zuckerman T, Rowe JM. Pathogenesis and prognostication in acute lymphoblastic leukemia. F1000Prime Rep. 2014 Jul 8;6:59. PMID:25184049
4596. Zukerberg LR, Collins AB, Ferry JA, et al. Coexpression of CD15 and CD20 by Reed-Sternberg cells in Hodgkin's disease. Am J Pathol. 1991 Sep;139(3):475–83. PMID:1716042
4597. Zukerberg LR, Kaynor BL, Silverman ML, et al. Splenic hamartoma and capillary hemangioma are distinct entities: immunohistochemical analysis of CD8 expression by endothelial cells. Hum Pathol. 1991 Dec;22(12):1258–61. PMID:1748432
4598. Zullo A, Hassan C, Andriani A, et al. Primary low-grade and high-grade gastric MALT-lymphoma presentation. J Clin Gastroenterol. 2010 May-Jun;44(5):340–4. PMID:19745757
4599. Zuurbier L, Gutierrez A, Mullighan CG, et al. Immature MEF2C-dysregulated T-cell leukemia patients have an early T-cell precursor acute lymphoblastic leukemia gene signature and typically have non-rearranged T-cell receptors. Haematologica. 2014 Jan;99(1):94–102. PMID:23975177

Subject index

Bold page numbers indicate the main discussion(s) of the topic.

C

D

E

N

The World Health Organization Classification of Tumours

Skin

Elder DE, Massi D, Scolyer RA, et al., editors. WHO classification of skin tumours. Lyon (France): International Agency for Research on Cancer; 2018. (WHO classification of tumours series, 4th ed.; vol. 11). https://publications.iarc.who.int/560.

Eye

Grossniklaus HE, Eberhart CG, Kivelä TT, editors. WHO classification of tumours of the eye. Lyon (France): International Agency for Research on Cancer; 2018. (WHO classification of tumours series, 4th ed.; vol. 12). https://publications.iarc.who.int/561.

Digestive system

WHO Classification of Tumours Editorial Board. Digestive system tumours. Lyon (France): International Agency for Research on Cancer; 2019. (WHO classification of tumours series, 5th ed.; vol. 1). https://publications.iarc.who.int/579.

Breast

WHO Classification of Tumours Editorial Board. Breast tumours. Lyon (France): International Agency for Research on Cancer; 2019. (WHO classification of tumours series, 5th ed.; vol. 2). https://publications.iarc.who.int/581.

Soft tissue and bone

WHO Classification of Tumours Editorial Board. Soft tissue and bone tumours. Lyon (France): International Agency for Research on Cancer; 2020. (WHO classification of tumours series, 5th ed.; vol. 3). https://publications.iarc.who.int/588.

Female genital tract

WHO Classification of Tumours Editorial Board. Female genital tumours. Lyon (France): International Agency for Research on Cancer; 2020. (WHO classification of tumours series, 5th ed.; vol. 4). https://publications.iarc.who.int/592.

Thorax

WHO Classification of Tumours Editorial Board. Thoracic tumours. Lyon (France): International Agency for Research on Cancer; 2021. (WHO classification of tumours series, 5th ed.; vol. 5). https://publications.iarc.who.int/595.

Central nervous system

WHO Classification of Tumours Editorial Board. Central nervous system tumours. Lyon (France): International Agency for Research on Cancer; 2021. (WHO classification of tumours series, 5th ed.; vol. 6). https://publications.iarc.who.int/601.

Paediatric tumours

WHO Classification of Tumours Editorial Board. Paediatric tumours. Lyon (France): International Agency for Research on Cancer; 2022. (WHO classification of tumours series, 5th ed.; vol. 7). https://publications.iarc.who.int/608.

Urinary and male genital tracts

WHO Classification of Tumours Editorial Board. Urinary and male genital tumours. Lyon (France): International Agency for Research on Cancer; 2022. (WHO classification of tumours series, 5th ed.; vol. 8). https://publications.iarc.who.int/610.

Head and neck

WHO Classification of Tumours Editorial Board. Head and neck tumours. Lyon (France): International Agency for Research on Cancer; 2024. (WHO classification of tumours series, 5th ed.; vol. 9). https://publications.iarc.who.int/629.

Endocrine and neuroendocrine tumours

WHO Classification of Tumours Editorial Board. Endocrine and neuroendocrine tumours. Lyon (France): International Agency for Research on Cancer; forthcoming. (WHO classification of tumours series, 5th ed.; vol. 10). https://publications.iarc.who.int.

Haematopoietic and lymphoid tissues

WHO Classification of Tumours Editorial Board. Haematolymphoid tumours. Lyon (France): International Agency for Research on Cancer; 2024. (WHO classification of tumours series, 5th ed.; vol. 11). https://publications.iarc.who.int/637.

WHO Classification of Tumours Online

The content of this renowned classification series is now also available in a convenient digital format: https://tumourclassification.iarc.who.int